MEDICAL-SURGICAL
NURSING CARE
PLANNING GUIDES

MEDICAL-SURGICAL
NURSING CARE
PLANNING GUIDES

4th Edition

Susan Puderbaugh Ulrich, RN, MSN
Nurse Educator and Consultant
Lane Community College
Eugene, Oregon

Suzanne Weyland Canale, RN, MSN
Nurse Educator and Consultant
Lane Community College
Eugene, Oregon

Sharon Andrea Wendell, RN, MSN
Nurse Educator, Consultant, and
Oncology Nurse Clinician
Lane Community College
Eugene, Oregon

W.B. SAUNDERS COMPANY
A Division of Harcourt Brace & Company
Philadelphia London Toronto Montreal Sydney Tokyo

W.B. SAUNDERS COMPANY
A Division of Harcourt Brace & Company

The Curtis Center
Independence Square West
Philadelphia, Pennsylvania 19106

Library of Congress Cataloging-in-Publication Data

Ulrich, Susan Puderbaugh.

Medical-surgical nursing care planning guides / Susan Puderbaugh Ulrich, Suzanne Weyland Canale, Sharon Andrea Wendell.—4th ed.

p.   cm.

Includes bibliographical references and index.

ISBN 0–7216–6031–2

1. Nursing care plans—Handbooks, manuals, etc.   2. Nursing diagnosis—Handbooks, manuals, etc.   I. Canale, Suzanne Weyland.   II. Wendell, Sharon Andrea.   III. Title.   [DNLM: 1. Nursing Care—handbooks. 2. Nursing Diagnosis—handbooks.   WY 49 U45m 1998]

RT49.U47 1998

610.73—dc21

DNLM/DLC   97-7514

MEDICAL-SURGICAL NURSING CARE PLANNING GUIDES   ISBN 0–7216–6031–2

Printed in the United States of America.

Last digit is the print number: 9   8   7   6   5   4   3   2   1

Preface

Medical-Surgical Nursing Care Planning Guides is a comprehensive reference to guide the planning of nursing care for hospitalized adults with commonly recurring medical-surgical conditions. The book has been updated to include recent changes in nursing diagnoses and advances in nursing, medicine, and other areas of health care. The care plans provide standards of care that the nursing student and practitioner should modify as needed when planning and implementing care for individual clients.

There are a total of 60 nursing care plans included in this book. Unit One provides guidelines for individualizing the care plans. It uses a case study format to demonstrate the selection of pertinent diagnostic labels and the individualization of etiology statements, desired outcomes, and nursing actions.

Unit Two addresses 24 of the most commonly used nursing diagnoses in the acute care setting. The primary purposes of this unit are twofold: to provide the reader with a rationale for each action and to provide documentation guidelines that meet professional, accreditation, and legal standards. The definition of the label and a desired client outcome are also included for each diagnosis. This unit also facilitates the planning of individualized care for the client with a medical-surgical condition that is not addressed in this text.

Unit Three focuses on care of the elderly client and the biopsychosocial changes that occur with aging. The care plan is directed toward the client who is hospitalized for management of a medical-surgical condition but it can easily be used to plan care for the elderly client in a variety of health care settings. Units Four to Seven include care plans that provide standardized information regarding conditions or treatment modalities. The standardized care plans in Unit Four on Preoperative and Postoperative Care should be used in conjunction with each surgical care plan in the text. The care plans on Immobility and Terminal Care (Units Five and Six) are applicable to a wide range of conditions and should be utilized whenever appropriate. The care plans in Unit Seven cover treatment modalities for neoplastic disorders and are referred to when appropriate in subsequent care plans involving neoplastic disease. Each of the standardized care plans in these units can be used in planning care for a client with a condition not covered in this text. When care plans in Units Four to Seven are to be used with a care plan in Units Eight to Nineteen, the authors indicate this at the beginning of the plan by the phrase **Use in conjunction with** or **Refer to**.

Units Eight to Nineteen are divided according to body systems. Care plans within each unit deal with conditions that are frequently seen in an acute care setting. Each care plan is organized as follows:

INTRODUCTION

The introduction provides the reader with an overview of the condition including a basic definition and discussion of the pathophysiological mechanisms involved and/or a description of the surgical procedure or selected treatment modality. This overview is not intended to be a substitute for the information provided in medical-surgical nursing texts or other references but rather a quick refresher or a starting point for additional research. Within this section, the reader will also find the focus of the care plan (highlighted in bold print) and the overall goals of care.

DIAGNOSTIC TESTS

Diagnostic tests included in this section are those commonly performed either prior to or during hospitalization to confirm the presence of a disease process or the need for the surgical procedure or treatment modality.

DISCHARGE CRITERIA

This section includes criteria that serve as a guide for determining the client's readiness for discharge from the acute care setting. Recognizing that client education is a vital aspect of health care, the authors use these criteria as the basis for the detailed discharge teaching that is included at the end of each care plan.

NURSING AND COLLABORATIVE DIAGNOSES

The nursing and collaborative diagnoses describe the actual or potential health problems that a client with a particular condition may experience. The nursing diagnoses were selected from those approved by the North American Nursing Diagnosis Association (NANDA) through 1996. In a few instances the authors have included nursing diagnoses that have been modified or are not currently on the NANDA list. These diagnostic labels are usually noted in the text by an asterisk (*) and an explanatory footnote. Nursing diagnoses that are not unique to a particular condition but that may be relevant for a client (e.g. spiritual distress) have not consistently been included but should be considered when individualizing each care plan. Collaborative diagnoses have been included to incorporate potential complications and electrolyte imbalances for which there are no established nursing diagnostic labels. Specific etiology statements that incorporate possible causal pathophysiological and psychosocial factors are identified for the majority of the nursing and collaborative diagnosis labels. As with other portions of the standardized care plans, these etiologies need to be individualized for each client. The authors did not include etiologies for those nursing diagnosis labels that deal most directly with client teaching (i.e. knowledge deficit, altered health maintenance, ineffective management of therapeutic regimen) because of the numerous individual variables that affect the teaching-learning process.

In order to provide consistency in the care plans, the nursing and collaborative diagnoses statements have usually been listed in the same order in all the care plans. No attempt has been made to prioritize the diagnoses. Priorities will need to be established by the student and practitioner based on the individual client's current needs.

DESIRED OUTCOMES

The desired outcomes for the nursing and collaborative diagnoses provide specific, measurable criteria for evaluating client progress and identifying when goals of care have been met. The outcome criteria for the nursing diagnoses are based on the defining characteristics approved by NANDA. The student and practitioner should modify the goal and specific outcome criteria as needed to reflect what is achievable for each individual client. Target dates for the desired outcomes have not been included since these are determined by the client's current status.

NURSING ACTIONS AND SELECTED PURPOSES/RATIONALES

Included in this section are nursing actions that can assist the client to achieve the desired outcomes. The actions include detailed assessments that are based on the defining characteristics for the label as defined by NANDA. These assessments assist the user to determine if the nursing or collaborative diagnosis is an actual problem or if the client is at risk for developing it. The nursing interventions are specific and realistic yet global enough to allow for regional and multidisciplinary variations in standards of care. The selected purposes or rationales, which appear in italics, have been included to clarify actions that may not be fundamental nursing knowledge.

CLIENT TEACHING

Although client teaching is included throughout the care plans, the majority of the teaching is found in the actions for the nursing diagnoses of knowledge deficit, altered health maintenance, and ineffective management of therapeutic regimen. The client teaching included uses terminology that most clients can understand.

*   *   *

An appendix of alphabetically arranged, NANDA-approved nursing diagnoses with definitions, defining characteristics, related factors, and risk factors has been included in this edition to facilitate the use and individualization of the standardized care plans in this book. A comprehensive index assists the reader to easily locate specific care plans and nursing and collaborative diagnoses.

Ultimately, the value of a systematic approach to individualized client care is measured by its effect on the quality of care provided to the client. The authors hope that the fourth edition of this book will assist with the integration of the numerous aspects of client care, facilitate critical thinking and implementation of the nursing process, and provide both the student and the practitioner with a guide for planning and implementing high-quality client care.

≣ Acknowledgments

To our numerous readers who shared their expertise.
To our students who are a continual source of inspiration.
To our friends for their support and encouragement.
To Sharon Wendell for her participation in the previous editions of this book.
Most importantly, to our families for their love, patience, and encouragement:

Curt, Shannon, and Chad Ulrich
Joe and Christopher Canale

Sue Ulrich
Suzanne Canale

Contributors

Revision of Care Plans on Pneumonia and Amputation
Glenna Sandgathe Clemens, RN, MN
Lane Community College
Eugene, Oregon

Revision of Care Plans on Brachytherapy, Chemotherapy, and External Radiation Therapy
Janice L. Kinman, RN, MS
Lane Community College
Eugene, Oregon

Revision of Care Plans on Thoracic Surgery and Pneumothorax
Julia P. Munkvold, BSN, MS
Lane Community College
Eugene, Oregon

FOURTH EDITION REVIEWERS

Suzanne C. Beyea, PhD, RN, CS
Saint Anselm College
Manchester, New Hampshire, and
University of New Hampshire
Durham, New Hampshire

Mary Gardner Cantley, RN, MSN
School of Nursing
Anderson University
Anderson, Indiana

Susan M. Chappell, RN, MSN, CDE
The University of Texas at Arlington
School of Nursing
Arlington, Texas

Kimberly K. Cribb, RN, MSN, CEN
Darton College
Albany, Georgia

Sherill Nones Cronin, PhD, RNC
Bellarmine College/Jewish Hospital
Louisville, Kentucky

Linda Ann Ellsworth, RN, BSN
Ohio Organization of Practical Nurse Educators
(O.O.P.N.E.)
Columbus, Ohio

Sue A. Hughes, MS, RN, OCN
Jewish Hospital
Louisville, Kentucky

Nancy Jo Kastor, RN, BSN
Portage Lakes Career Center
W. Howard Nicol School of Practical Nursing
Green, Ohio

Anne M. Larson, RN, BA, MS, PhD
Midland Lutheran College
Fremont, Nebraska

Karen M. T. Lavallee, RNC, BSN
New Hampshire Technical Institute
Concord, New Hampshire

Teresita F. Proctor, MS, RN, CS
School of Nursing
Elizabeth General Medical Center
Elizabeth, New Jersey

Donna Norwood Roddy, RN, MSN
Chattanooga State Community College
Chattanooga, Tennessee

Ann H. White, RN, MSN, MBA, CNA
University of Southern Indiana
Evansville, Indiana

Contents

INDIVIDUALIZING A STANDARDIZED CARE PLAN

▶ Steps in Individualizing a Standardized Care Plan

Planning nursing care is an exciting challenge and a rewarding experience when one sees high quality client care provided as a result of the efforts. However, planning care that is individualized and comprehensive can be a tedious process because of lack of time and adequate resources. This book is intended to facilitate the care planning process of adult clients with common recurring medical-surgical conditions. Within each care plan are nursing and collaborative diagnoses with etiological factors, desired outcomes with measurable behavioral criteria, and appropriate nursing actions with selected purposes or rationales. Safe, comprehensive client care can be planned in a minimal amount of time using this book.

To be most effective, the standardized nursing care plan must be adapted to the client's individual needs. A process for planning individualized client care follows:

1. read the admission sheet and the medication administration record of the assigned client

2. review the history, current diagnostic test results, nurses' notes for the last 48 hours, physician's progress notes, and current consultations

3. interview the client and complete an assessment using the tool provided by your nursing school or clinical facility

4. highlight pertinent data obtained

5. read about the client's diagnosis in a current medical-surgical nursing text

6. select the appropriate standardized care plan(s) from this text and read the introductory information at the beginning of the care plan(s)

7. select the nursing and collaborative diagnoses that are appropriate for your client; choose the etiological factors that are relevant and modify them as appropriate

8. set priorities for the nursing/collaborative diagnoses

9. modify the desired outcomes so that they are measurable and realistic for your client; establish appropriate target dates

10. select the nursing actions that are relevant to the client's care; add to or modify the actions to meet the needs of your particular client; include medications, treatments, client preferences, and actions that will facilitate the achievement of the desired client outcomes.

The following situation is used to illustrate how these standardized nursing care plans can be used by the student and the practitioner in planning individualized client care:

Mary G. is a 50-year-old woman who has been hospitalized in the terminal stages of cancer of the lung. She has been bedridden for the past 3 weeks because of severe bone pain due to metastatic lesions. She has four children ranging in age from 13 to 19 years. Both Mary and her husband have been trying to prepare the children for her death. They have no other family members living nearby.

1. **Read the admission sheet and the medication administration record of the assigned client.**
   It is determined that Mary is a 50-year-old *married* woman. Her religious preference is Protestant. Her diagnosis is *stage IV cancer of the lung.* She is *receiving morphine sulfate, 15 mg q2h, for pain relief.* She is also receiving *Dialose, 1 capsule/day; Phenergan, 25 mg IM q6h prn; and milk of magnesia, 30 ml p.o. every evening.*

2. **Review the history, current diagnostic test results, nurses' notes for the last 48 hours, physician's progress notes, and current consultations.**
   From the history it is determined that Mary had a *lobectomy 3 years ago* and experienced *disease recurrence 1 year ago.* She was treated with chemotherapeutic drugs until 3 months ago when she *elected to stop treatment.* She has *metastasis to the spine, ribs, and pelvis* and has been *bedridden for the last 3 weeks.* The progress notes indicate that Mary's *condition is steadily deteriorating* and the goal of care is to keep her comfortable.
   Diagnostic test results reveal that Mary's *RBC, Hb, Hct, and serum protein levels are decreased.*

The nurses' notes reveal that Mary *needs assistance with all activities.* She is able to feed herself but is only *consuming 10% of her meals.* She *has not had a bowel movement for 6 days.* Mary is voiding adequate amounts and her intake and output are balanced. She has been *crying frequently* and *states that neither she nor her husband is ready for her death.*

3. **Interview the client and complete an assessment using the tool provided by your nursing school or clinical facility.**
   The interview and physical assessment reveal that Mary has *persistent red-dened areas on her left hip and coccyx; diminished breath sounds in the bases; shallow respirations of 24/minute; crackles [rales] in both lungs; and a cough that is productive of yellow, foul-smelling sputum.* She has *hypoactive bowel sounds and a firm, distended abdomen* and states that she usually has a bowel movement every other day after breakfast. Mary is alert and oriented and able to move all extremities. She *complains of pain in her back, rib, and pelvic area.*

4. **Highlight pertinent data obtained.**
   Pertinent data for the nursing diagnoses included in step 7 are designated in italics in steps 1 through 3.

5. **Read about the client's diagnosis in a current medical-surgical nursing text.**
   Review cancer of the lung and care of the terminally ill client and the immobile client.

6. **Select the appropriate standardized care plan(s) from this text and read the introductory information at the beginning of the care plan(s).**
   Based on the physician's statement that Mary has been admitted for pain control and terminal care and will have no further palliative treatment, it is determined that the appropriate care plans for Mary are Cancer of the Lung, Terminal Care, and Immobility.

7. **Select the nursing and collaborative diagnoses that are appropriate for your client. Choose the etiological factors that are relevant and modify them as appropriate.**
   It is determined that there are numerous diagnoses and etiological factors from the care plans on Cancer of the Lung, Terminal Care, and Immobility that are appropriate. Examples of some of these nursing diagnoses follow. The etiological factors have been modified to reflect Mary's situation.
   a. **Ineffective breathing pattern** related to:
      1. increased rate and decreased depth of respirations associated with fear, anxiety, and pain;
      2. decreased rate and depth of respirations associated with depressant effect of morphine sulfate;
      3. diminished lung/chest wall expansion associated with compression of lung tissue by the tumor, recumbent positioning, weakness, fatigue, abdominal distention, and reluctance to breathe deeply because of pain.
   b. **Ineffective airway clearance** related to:
      1. excessive mucus production associated with inflammation of lung tissue resulting from the disease process;
      2. stasis of secretions associated with decreased mobility, difficulty coughing up secretions, and impaired ciliary function;
      3. invasion of and/or pressure on airways by tumor.
   c. **Pain: back, rib, and pelvic** related to bone metastasis.
   d. **Constipation** related to:
      1. diminished defecation reflex associated with decreased nervous system responses in terminal state, suppression of urge to defecate because of increased back and pelvic pain when attempting to use bedpan, and decreased gravity filling of lower rectum resulting from horizontal positioning;
      2. decreased ability to respond to urge to defecate associated with weakened abdominal muscles and impaired physical mobility;
      3. decreased gastrointestinal motility associated with decreased activity, use of morphine sulfate, and increased sympathetic nervous system activity that occurs with anxiety and pain;
      4. decreased intake of fluids and foods high in fiber associated with anorexia.
   e. **Grieving** related to loss of control over life and body functioning, changes in body image, loss of significant others, and imminent death.

The process for individualization of etiologies is demonstrated below using the nursing diagnosis of **Constipation** as a prototype.

STANDARDIZED	**INDIVIDUALIZED**

(etiologies from Care Plan on Immobility)

Constipation related to:
a. diminished defecation reflex associated with:
  1. suppression of urge to defecate because of reluctance to use bedpan

  2. decreased gravity filling of lower rectum resulting from horizontal positioning
b. weakened abdominal muscles associated with generalized loss of muscle tone resulting from prolonged immobility
c. decreased gastrointestinal motility associated with decreased activity and the increased sympathetic nervous system activity that occurs with anxiety.

Constipation related to:
a. diminished defecation reflex associated with:
  1. suppression of urge to defecate because of increased back and pelvic pain when attempting to use bedpan
  2. decreased gravity filling of lower rectum resulting from horizontal positioning
b. weakened abdominal muscles associated with generalized loss of muscle tone resulting from prolonged immobility
c. decreased gastrointestinal motility associated with decreased activity and increased sympathetic nervous system activity that occurs with anxiety and pain.

(etiologies from Care Plan on Terminal Care)

a. diminished defecation reflex associated with decreased nervous system responses in terminal state, suppression of the urge to defecate because of reluctance to use bedpan, and decreased gravity filling of lower rectum resulting from horizontal positioning

b. decreased ability to respond to the urge to defecate associated with weakened abdominal muscles, impaired physical mobility, and decreased level of consciousness
c. decreased gastrointestinal motility associated with decreased activity, increased sympathetic nervous system activity that occurs with anxiety, and use of some medications (e.g. narcotic [opioid] analgesics, antacids containing aluminum or calcium)
d. decreased intake of fluid and foods high in fiber.

a. diminished defecation reflex associated with decreased nervous system responses in terminal state, suppression of the urge to defecate because of increased back and pelvic pain when attempting to use bedpan, and decreased gravity filling of lower rectum resulting from horizontal positioning
b. decreased ability to respond to the urge to defecate associated with weakened abdominal muscles and impaired physical mobility

c. decreased gastrointestinal motility associated with decreased activity, use of morphine sulfate, and increased sympathetic nervous system activity that occurs with anxiety and pain

d. decreased intake of fluid and foods high in fiber associated with anorexia.

8. **Set priorities for the nursing/collaborative diagnoses.**
   Because Mary is terminally ill, the top four priorities are:
   a. Pain: back, rib, and pelvic
   b. Grieving
   c. Ineffective airway clearance
   d. Constipation

9. **Modify the desired outcomes so that they are measurable and realistic for your client. Establish appropriate target dates.**
   The process for individualization of a desired outcome is demonstrated next using the nursing diagnosis of **Constipation** as a prototype.

STANDARDIZED

(outcome from Care Plan on Immobility)

The client will not experience constipation as evidenced by:
a. usual frequency of bowel
movements
b. passage of soft, formed stool
c. absence of abdominal distention
and pain, feeling of rectal fullness
or pressure, and straining during
defecation.

(outcome from Care Plan on Terminal Care)

The client will maintain a bowel routine that provides optimal comfort.

INDIVIDUALIZED

Mary will have resolution of
constipation as evidenced by:
a. passing a soft, formed stool at least
every other day
b. absence of increased abdominal
distention, abdominal pain, feeling
of rectal fullness or pressure, and
straining during defecation.

Same as above.

10. Select the nursing actions that are relevant to the client's care. Add to or modify the actions to meet the needs of your particular client. Include medications, treatments, client preferences, and actions that will facilitate the achievement of the desired client outcomes.

The process for individualization of nursing actions is demonstrated below using the nursing diagnosis of **Constipation** as a prototype.

STANDARDIZED

(actions from Care Plan on Immobility)

a. Ascertain client's usual bowel
elimination habits.
b. Assess for signs and symptoms of
constipation (e.g. decrease in
frequency of bowel movements;
passage of hard, formed stools;
anorexia; abdominal distention and
pain; feeling of fullness or pressure
in rectum; straining during
defecation).
c. Assess bowel sounds. Report a
pattern of decreasing bowel
sounds.
d. Implement measures to prevent
constipation:
1. encourage client to defecate
whenever the urge is felt
2. place client in high Fowler's
position for bowel movements
unless contraindicated
3. encourage client to relax,
provide privacy, and have call
signal within reach during
attempts to defecate (*measures
to promote relaxation enable
client to relax the levator ani
muscle and external anal
sphincter, which facilitates
evacuation of stool*)
4. encourage client to establish a
regular time for defecation,
preferably an hour after a meal
5. instruct client to increase
intake of foods high in fiber
(e.g. bran, whole-grain breads
and cereals, fresh fruits

INDIVIDUALIZED*

a. Omit—bowel habits already
known.
b. Assess Mary every shift for signs
and symptoms of continuing
constipation (e.g. absence of bowel
movement; passage of hard, formed
stool; increased anorexia and
abdominal distention; abdominal
pain; feeling of fullness or pressure
in rectum; straining during
defecation).
c. Assess bowel sounds. Report a
pattern of decreasing bowel
sounds.
d. Implement measures to relieve
Mary's constipation:
1. encourage Mary to defecate
whenever the urge is felt
2. place Mary on bedpan in high
Fowler's position for bowel
movements
3. turn on soft music, provide
privacy, and have call signal
within reach during attempts
to defecate

4. encourage Mary to attempt to
defecate about an hour after
breakfast
5. offer bran cereal and fresh fruit
for breakfast; encourage Mary
to select foods high in fiber for
lunch and dinner

*The italicized information from the standardized action is a purpose or rationale and is omitted here. It should be placed in the rationale column of an individualized care plan.

STANDARDIZED	**INDIVIDUALIZED**
(actions from Care Plan on Immobility)—cont'd	
and vegetables) unless contraindicated	
6. instruct client to maintain a minimum fluid intake of 2500 ml/day unless contraindicated	6. encourage Mary to increase her fluid intake; offer 200 ml of apple juice, orange juice, or water every hour while she is awake
7. encourage client to drink hot liquids upon arising in the morning *in order to stimulate peristalsis*	7. offer hot tea with breakfast
8. encourage client to perform isometric abdominal strengthening exercises unless contraindicated	8. omit—not applicable for terminally ill client
9. increase activity as allowed	9. omit—not applicable
10. administer laxatives or cathartics and/or enemas if ordered.	10. administer milk of magnesia, 30 ml p.o. each evening and Dialose, 1 capsule p.o. each morning; consult physician about increasing dose of Dialose if constipation persists.
e. Consult physician about checking for an impaction and digitally removing stool if client has not had a bowel movement in 3 days, if he/she is passing liquid stool, or if other signs and symptoms of constipation are present.	e. Consult physician about checking for an impaction and digitally removing stool since Mary has not had a bowel movement for 6 days and other signs and symptoms of constipation are present.

STANDARDIZED	**INDIVIDUALIZED**
(actions from Care Plan on Terminal Care)	
a. Refer to Care Plan on Immobility, Nursing Diagnosis 9 (pp. 133–134), for measures related to assessment, prevention, and management of constipation.	a. Omit—individualization of these actions from the Care Plan on Immobility has already been completed above.
b. Assist client to toilet or bedside commode or place in high Fowler's position on bedpan for bowel movements unless contraindicated.	b. Omit—action already covered by referral to Care Plan on Immobility since Mary is not able to get to the bathroom or sit on bedside commode.
c. If client is taking antacids containing aluminum or calcium, consult physician about alternating them with antacids containing magnesium.	c. Omit—not applicable.

Individualized care plan for Mary for the nursing diagnosis of Constipation:

DATA	NURSING DIAGNOSIS	DESIRED OUTCOME	NURSING ACTIONS
States has not had bowel movement for 6 days Bowel sounds hypoactive Physician's order: milk of magnesia, 30 ml each evening prn—taking every evening; Dialose, 1 capsule p.o. every morning Abdomen firm and distended Bedridden for 3 weeks Consuming only 10% of meals States usually has bowel movement q.o.d. after breakfast Activity—bed rest; requires assistance with all activities Receiving morphine sulfate every 2 hours	Constipation related to: a. diminished defecation reflex associated with decreased nervous system responses in terminal state, suppression of urge to defecate because of increased back and pelvic pain when attempting to use bedpan, and decreased gravity filling of lower rectum resulting from horizontal positioning; b. decreased ability to respond to urge to defecate associated with weakened abdominal muscles and impaired physical mobility; c. decreased gastrointestinal motility associated with decreased activity, use of morphine sulfate, and increased sympathetic nervous system activity that occurs with anxiety and pain; d. decreased intake of fluids and foods high in fiber associated with anorexia.	Mary will have resolution of constipation as evidenced by: a. passing a soft, formed stool at least every other day b. absence of increased abdominal distention, abdominal pain, feeling of rectal fullness or pressure, and straining during defecation.	1. Assess Mary every shift for signs and symptoms of continuing constipation (e.g. absence of a bowel movement; passage of hard, formed stool; increased anorexia and abdominal distention; abdominal pain; feeling of fullness or pressure in rectum; straining during defecation). 2. Assess bowel sounds. Report a pattern of decreasing bowel sounds. 3. Implement measures to relieve Mary's constipation: a. encourage Mary to defecate whenever the urge is felt b. place Mary on bedpan in high Fowler's position for bowel movements c. turn on soft music, provide privacy, and have call signal within reach during attempts to defecate d. encourage Mary to attempt to defecate about an hour after breakfast e. offer bran cereal and fresh fruit for breakfast; encourage Mary to select foods high in fiber for lunch and dinner f. encourage Mary to increase her fluid intake; offer 200 ml of apple juice, orange juice, or water every hour while she is awake g. offer hot tea with breakfast h. administer milk of magnesia, 30 ml p.o. each evening and Dialose, 1 capsule p.o. each morning; consult physician about increasing dose of Dialose if constipation persists. 4. Consult physician about checking for an impaction and digitally removing stool since Mary has not had a bowel movement for 6 days and other signs and symptoms of constipation are present.

UNIT TWO

ACTIONS, RATIONALES, AND DOCUMENTATION FOR SELECTED NURSING DIAGNOSES

▶ Nursing Diagnosis: *Activity Intolerance*

Definition

A state in which an individual has insufficient physiological or psychological energy to endure or complete required or desired daily activities.

Defining Characteristics

Refer to Appendix.

Desired Outcome

The client will demonstrate an increased tolerance for activity as evidenced by:
a. verbalization of feeling less fatigued and weak
b. ability to perform activities of daily living without exertional dyspnea, chest pain, diaphoresis, dizziness, and significant change in vital signs.

Documentation

a. Activity level
b. Statements of weakness and fatigue
c. Exertional dyspnea, chest pain, diaphoresis, or dizziness
d. Vital signs before and after activity
e. Therapeutic interventions
f. Client teaching

NURSING ACTIONS

Assessments

1. Assess for signs and symptoms of activity intolerance:
   a. statements of fatigue or weakness
   b. exertional dyspnea, chest pain, diaphoresis, or dizziness
   c. abnormal heart rate response to activity (e.g. increase in rate of 20 beats/minute above resting rate, rate not returning to preactivity level within 3 minutes after stopping activity, change from regular to irregular rate)
   d. decreased systolic B/P or a significant increase (10–15 mm Hg) in diastolic pressure with activity.

Prevention/Treatment

2. Implement measures to promote rest and/or conserve energy (e.g. maintain prescribed activity restrictions, minimize environmental activity and noise, provide uninterrupted rest periods, assist with care, limit the number of visitors).
3. Implement measures to increase cardiac output (e.g. administer positive inotropic agents, vasodilators, or antiarrhythmics as ordered; elevate head of bed) if decreased cardiac output is contributing to client's activity intolerance.
4. Implement measures to reduce fever if present (e.g. administer tepid sponge bath, administer antipyretics as ordered).

5. Discourage smoking and excessive

RATIONALES

1. Early recognition of signs and symptoms of activity intolerance allows for prompt intervention.

2. Cells utilize oxygen and fat, protein, and carbohydrate to produce the energy needed for all body activities. Rest and activities that conserve energy result in a lower metabolic rate, which preserves nutrients and oxygen for necessary activities.
3. Sufficient cardiac output is necessary to maintain an adequate blood flow and oxygen supply to the tissues. Adequate tissue oxygenation promotes more efficient energy production, which subsequently improves the client's activity tolerance.
4. An elevated temperature increases the metabolic rate with subsequent depletion of available energy and a decrease in ability to tolerate activity.

5. Both nicotine and excessive

intake of beverages high in caffeine such as coffee, tea, and colas.

6. Maintain oxygen therapy as ordered.

7. Implement measures to improve respiratory status (e.g. encourage use of incentive spirometer; elevate head of bed; assist with turning, coughing, and deep breathing) if ineffective breathing pattern, ineffective airway clearance, or impaired gas exchange is contributing to client's activity intolerance.

8. Implement measures to maintain an adequate nutritional status (e.g. provide a diet high in essential nutrients, provide dietary supplements as indicated, administer vitamins and minerals as ordered).

9. Implement measures to treat anemia if present (e.g. administer prescribed iron, folic acid, and/or vitamin B_{12}; administer whole blood or packed red cells as ordered).

10. Increase client's activity gradually as allowed and tolerated.

11. Instruct client to report a decreased tolerance for activity and to stop any activity that causes chest pain, shortness of breath, dizziness, or extreme fatigue or weakness.

12. Consult physician if signs and symptoms of activity intolerance persist or worsen.

caffeine intake can increase cardiac workload and myocardial oxygen utilization, thereby decreasing the amount of oxygen available for energy production.

6. An oxygen deficiency results in anaerobic metabolism, which is less efficient than the aerobic mechanism of energy supply. Supplemental oxygen helps restore the more efficient aerobic metabolism, thereby improving energy levels and activity tolerance.

7. Altered respiratory function can lead to inadequate tissue oxygenation, which results in less efficient energy production and a reduced ability to tolerate activity. Improving respiratory status increases the amount of oxygen available for energy production. It also eases the work of breathing, which reduces energy expenditure.

8. Metabolism is the process by which nutrients are transformed into energy. If nutrition is inadequate, energy production is decreased, which subsequently reduces one's ability to tolerate activity.

9. Anemia reduces the oxygen-carrying capacity of the blood. Resolution of anemia increases oxygen availability to the cells, which increases the efficiency of energy production and subsequently improves activity tolerance.

10. A gradual increase in activity helps prevent a sudden increase in cardiac workload and myocardial oxygen consumption and the subsequent imbalance between oxygen supply and demand. Progressive activity also helps strengthen the myocardium, which enhances cardiac output and subsequently improves activity tolerance.

11. These symptoms indicate that insufficient oxygen is reaching the tissues and that activity has been increased beyond a therapeutic level.

12. Notifying the physician allows for modification of treatment plan.

▶ Nursing Diagnosis: *Airway Clearance, Ineffective*

Definition

A state in which an individual is unable to clear secretions or obstructions from the respiratory tract.

Defining Characteristics

Refer to Appendix.

Desired Outcome

The client will maintain clear, open airways as evidenced by:
a. normal breath sounds
b. normal rate and depth of respirations
c. absence of dyspnea.

Documentation

a. Breath sounds
b. Rate, depth, and ease of respirations
c. Characteristics of cough
d. Description of sputum
e. Therapeutic interventions
f. Client teaching

NURSING ACTIONS

Assessments

1. Assess for and report signs and symptoms of ineffective airway clearance (e.g. abnormal breath sounds; rapid, shallow respirations; dyspnea; cough).

Prevention/Treatment

2. Implement measures to decrease pain if present (e.g. splint chest or abdominal incision with pillow when coughing and deep breathing, administer prescribed analgesics before planned activity).

3. Instruct and assist client to turn, deep breathe, and cough or "huff" every 1–2 hours.

4. Increase activity as allowed and tolerated.

5. Implement measures to thin secretions and maintain adequate moisture of the respiratory mucous membranes (e.g. maintain a fluid intake of 2500 ml/day, humidify inspired air).

6. Assist with administration of mucolytics and diluent or hydrating agents via nebulizer as ordered.

7. Assist with or perform postural drainage therapy (PDT) if ordered.

RATIONALES

1. Early recognition and reporting of signs and symptoms of ineffective airway clearance allow for prompt intervention.

2. Pain often interferes with a client's willingness to move, cough, and deep breathe. Pain reduction enables the client to increase activity and cough and deep breathe more effectively, which all help promote effective airway clearance.

3. Turning mobilizes secretions. Deep breathing loosens secretions and enhances the effectiveness of coughing. Coughing or "huffing" (a forced expiration technique) accelerates airflow through the airways, which rids the larger airways of mucus and foreign matter.

4. Activity helps mobilize secretions and promotes deeper breathing. Deep breathing loosens secretions and also enhances the effectiveness of coughing.

5. Adequate hydration and humidified inspired air help thin secretions, which facilitates their mobilization and expectoration. These actions also reduce drying of the respiratory mucous membrane, which helps enhance mucociliary clearance.

6. Mucolytics and diluent or hydrating agents (e.g. water, saline) are mucokinetic substances that reduce the viscosity of mucus and subsequently make it easier for the client to mobilize and clear secretions from the respiratory tract.

7. Postural drainage therapy techniques (e.g. vibration, percussion, postural drainage) utilize the forces of motion and gravity to mobilize secretions

8. Perform suctioning if needed.

8. Suctioning removes secretions from the large airways. It also stimulates coughing, which helps clear airways of mucus and foreign matter.

from the periphery of the lungs to the central airways where they can be removed by coughing or suctioning.

9. Administer expectorants if ordered.

9. Expectorants indirectly stimulate the bronchial glands to secrete more serous fluid, which dilutes respiratory secretions, making them less viscous and easier to expectorate.

10. Discourage smoking.

10. Irritants present in smoke increase mucus production, impair ciliary function, and can cause inflammation and damage to the bronchial walls. This results in narrowed airways and stasis of pulmonary secretions.

11. Administer the following medications if ordered:
    a. methylxanthines (e.g. theophylline)
    b. adrenergic (sympathomimetic) bronchodilators (e.g. albuterol, terbutaline)
    c. antimuscarinic agents (e.g. ipratropium bromide [Atrovent])
    d. corticosteroids (e.g. methylprednisolone, prednisone).

11. These medications increase the patency of the airways and enhance bronchial airflow. Methylxanthines and sympathomimetics are thought to increase the intracellular concentration of cAMP, which results in bronchial smooth muscle relaxation. Antimuscarinic agents inhibit the cholinergic component of airway constriction and corticosteroids reduce inflammation in the airways.

12. Administer central nervous system depressants judiciously.

12. Central nervous system depressants depress the cough reflex, which can result in stasis of secretions.

13. Consult physician if signs and symptoms of ineffective airway clearance persist.

13. Notifying the physician allows for modification of the treatment plan.

▶ Nursing Diagnosis: *Anxiety*

Definition

A vague, uneasy feeling whose source is often nonspecific or unknown to the individual.

Defining Characteristics

Refer to Appendix.

Desired Outcome

The client will experience a reduction in anxiety as evidenced by:
a. verbalization of feeling less anxious
b. usual sleep pattern
c. relaxed facial expression and body movements
d. stable vital signs
e. usual perceptual ability and interactions with others.

Documentation

a. Verbalization of feeling anxious
b. Sleep pattern
c. Facial expression and body movement
d. Vital signs
e. Focus on self
f. Client's perception of precipitating factors
g. Therapeutic interventions
h. Client/family teaching

NURSING ACTIONS	RATIONALES

Assessments

1. Assess client for signs and symptoms of anxiety (e.g. verbalization of feeling anxious, insomnia, tenseness, shakiness, restlessness, diaphoresis, tachycardia, elevated B/P, facial pallor, self-focused behaviors).

1. Early recognition of signs and symptoms of anxiety allows for prompt intervention.

Prevention/Treatment

2. Encourage verbalization of feelings and concerns and assist client to identify specific stressors that may be causing anxiety. Provide feedback.

2. Verbalization of feelings and concerns helps the client focus on factors that may be causing anxiety. Providing feedback helps the client clarify and validate his/her feelings and concerns and identify techniques that can reduce anxiety.

3. Orient client to hospital environment, equipment, and routines.

3. Familiarity with the environment and usual routines reduces the client's anxiety about the unknown, provides a sense of security, and increases his/her sense of control, which all help to decrease anxiety.

4. Introduce staff who will be participating in the client's care. If possible, maintain consistency in staff assigned to his/her care.

4. Introduction of the staff familiarizes the client with those people who will be working with him/her, which provides a sense of comfort with the environment. Consistency in staff assignment provides the client with a feeling of stability, which reduces the anxiety that typically occurs with change.

5. Assure client that staff members are nearby. Respond to call signal as soon as possible.

5. Close contact and a prompt response to requests provide a sense of security and facilitate the development of trust, which help to reduce feelings of anxiety.

6. Maintain a calm, supportive, confident manner when interacting with client.

6. A sense of calmness and confidence conveys to the client that someone is in control of the situation, which helps to reduce feelings of anxiety.

7. Reinforce physician's explanations and clarify misconceptions the client has about the diagnostic tests, disease condition, treatment plan, surgical procedure, and/or prognosis.

7. Factual information and an awareness of what to expect help to decrease the anxiety that arises from uncertainty.

8. Implement measures to reduce respiratory distress if present (e.g. elevate head of bed, encourage client to breathe deeply and more slowly, administer oxygen as ordered).

8. Improvement of respiratory status helps relieve the anxiety associated with the feeling of not being able to breathe.

9. Implement measures to reduce pain if present (e.g. administer prescribed analgesics, instruct and assist with relaxation techniques).

9. Pain can create anxiety because it is often perceived as a threat to well-being. Pain also causes sympathetic nervous system stimulation with subsequent feelings of tenseness and increased anxiety.

10. Provide a calm, restful environment.

10. A calm, restful environment allows the client to relax and

11. Instruct client in relaxation techniques and encourage participation in diversional activities.

11. Relaxation techniques reduce muscle tension and other physiological effects of anxiety. Activities that the client enjoys provide a means of distraction, which may minimize feelings of anxiety.

12. When appropriate, assist client to meet spiritual needs (e.g. arrange for a visit from clergy).

12. Spiritual support is a source of comfort and security for many people and can help reduce client's feeling of anxiety.

13. Initiate a financial and/or social service referral if indicated.

13. Concerns about financial matters can be a source of great anxiety. Assistance with resolution of these concerns helps to allay anxiety.

14. Encourage significant others to project a caring, concerned attitude without obvious anxiousness.

14. Anxiety is easily transferable from one person to another. If significant others convey empathy, provide reassurance, and do not appear anxious, they can help reduce the client's anxiety.

15. Administer prescribed antianxiety agents if indicated.

15. Benzodiazepines, the drugs of choice to treat anxiety, augment the inhibitory effect of gamma-aminobutyric acid (GABA) on cell membrane responses to excitatory neurotransmitters.

16. Include significant others in orientation and teaching sessions and encourage their continued support of the client.

16. The presence of significant others provides the client with a sense of support, which helps reduce anxiety. In addition, significant others can reinforce information given if anxiety has reduced the client's ability to concentrate on, recall, and learn information.

17. Provide information based on current needs of client and significant others at a level they can understand. Encourage questions and clarification of information provided.

17. Providing the client and significant others with information they are not ready to process or are unable to understand tends to increase anxiety. Being able to ask questions and clarify information helps reduce anxiety.

18. Consult physician if above actions fail to control anxiety.

18. Notifying the physician allows for modification of the treatment plan.

▶ Nursing Diagnosis: *Aspiration, Risk for*

Definition

The state in which an individual is at risk for entry of gastrointestinal secretions, oropharyngeal secretions, or solids or fluids into tracheobronchial passages.

Defining Characteristics

Refer to Appendix.

Desired Outcome

The client will not aspirate secretions or foods/fluids as evidenced by:

Documentation

a. Breath sounds
b. Percussion note over lungs

Desired Outcome

a. clear breath sounds
b. resonant percussion note over lungs
c. absence of cough, tachypnea, and dyspnea.

Documentation

c. Respiratory rate and effort
d. Presence of cough
e. Pulse rate
f. Color of tracheal aspirate
g. Therapeutic interventions
h. Client/family teaching

NURSING ACTIONS

Assessments

1. Assess for and report signs and symptoms of aspiration of secretions or foods/fluids (e.g. rhonchi, dull percussion note over affected lung area, cough, tachypnea, dyspnea, tachycardia, presence of tube feeding in tracheal aspirate).

2. If client is receiving tube feedings, add food coloring to the solution according to hospital policy.

3. Assist with diagnostic studies that show whether aspiration is occurring during swallowing (e.g. videofluoroscopy) if ordered.

4. Monitor chest x-ray results. Report findings of pulmonary infiltrate.

Prevention

5. Implement the following measures to prevent aspiration if client has a depressed or absent gag reflex, severe dysphagia, and/ or decreased level of consciousness:
   a. withhold oral foods/fluids

   b. place client in a side-lying position

   c. perform oral hygiene and/or oropharyngeal suctioning as often as needed to remove excess secretions.
6. Implement measures to prevent vomiting (e.g. eliminate noxious sights and odors, administer antiemetics as ordered).

7. If client is receiving tube feedings,

RATIONALES

1. Early recognition and reporting of signs and symptoms of aspiration allow for prompt intervention.

2. The addition of food coloring helps differentiate the tube feeding solution from respiratory secretions, which allows for early recognition of aspiration and prompt intervention.

3. Aspiration of foods/fluids during the swallowing process is evident on studies such as videofluoroscopy. Knowing when aspiration occurs during the swallowing process aids in the development of an individualized plan of care to prevent further aspiration.

4. Evidence of pulmonary infiltrate on chest x-ray results can indicate that aspiration has occurred.

5. The risk for aspiration is high when mechanisms to protect the client's airway (e.g. gag reflex, swallowing reflex) are impaired or he/she has a decreased level of consciousness.
   a. Withholding oral foods/fluids eliminates the possibility of aspiration of same.
   b. Placing the client in a side-lying position allows oral secretions to accumulate in the mouth where they can be expectorated or removed by suctioning rather than flow into the pharynx, where they can be aspirated.
   c. Removing excess secretions from the mouth and pharynx prevents them from entering the larynx and being aspirated.
6. When the client vomits, gastric contents travel up the esophagus, through the pharynx, and into the mouth. While vomitus is in the pharynx, it can spill into the larynx resulting in aspiration.
7. Verification of feeding tube

check tube placement before each feeding or on a routine basis if tube feeding is continuous.

8. Implement measures to reduce the risk of regurgitation (e.g. maintain gastric decompression as ordered, provide small meals rather than large ones, do not administer gastric tube feedings if the residual exceeds specified amount [usually 75–100 ml], maintain client in high Fowler's position for at least 30 minutes after meals and tube feedings, administer upper gastrointestinal stimulants as ordered).

9. Implement measures to prevent aspiration when client is eating and drinking:

   a. perform actions to improve swallowing if indicated (e.g. select foods/fluids appropriate to client's swallowing ability, reinforce exercises to strengthen and develop muscles used in swallowing)

   b. place client in high Fowler's position

   c. instruct client to avoid laughing or talking when swallowing

   d. encourage client to concentrate on eating and drinking and allow ample time for meals and snacks

   e. instruct client to dry swallow, cough twice, or clear his/her

placement ensures that the tube feeding solution goes into the alimentary tract rather than the lungs.

8. As gastric secretions or foods/fluids accumulate in the stomach, upward pressure is placed on the lower esophageal sphincter (LES). If the pressure increases significantly and/or the client has an incompetent LES, regurgitation can occur. Contents that move up through the esophagus into the pharynx can spill into the larynx, resulting in aspiration.

9. When the client is eating and drinking, he/she is at high risk for aspiration before the swallowing reflex is triggered (the larynx and pharynx are at rest and the airway is open at this time), during swallowing if the larynx does not close completely, and after swallowing when the larynx opens again.

   a. Improving the client's ability to swallow helps ensure that foods/fluids do not enter the larynx when he/she is eating and drinking.

   b. This position uses gravity to facilitate movement of foods/fluids through the pharynx into the esophagus where the risk for aspiration is greatly reduced.

   c. Normally, when the swallowing reflex is triggered, the folds of the larynx that form its three valves contract so that aspiration does not occur as foods/fluids pass from the back of the mouth through the pharynx. When the client talks and laughs, air is forced through the trachea and the larynx opens. Instructing the client to avoid talking and laughing when swallowing reduces the risk of having his/her airway open when food/fluid is in the pharynx.

   d. If the client becomes distracted and/or is rushed during meals or snacks, swallowing and breathing attempts can become uncoordinated. This results in the larynx being open when the food/fluid is in the pharynx, which greatly increases the risk for aspiration.

   e. If the client has a swallowing impairment such as decreased

NURSING ACTIONS
Prevention—*cont'd*

throat after swallowing if
indicated.

10. Instruct and assist client to
perform oral hygiene after meals.

RATIONALES

pharyngeal peristalsis, residual
food/fluid can remain in the
pharyngeal recesses after the
swallowing reflex has occurred.
Dry swallowing, coughing, or
clearing the throat helps
ensure that the pharynx is
clear after swallowing, which
reduces the risk for aspiration.

10. Good oral hygiene after meals
removes remaining food particles
that could enter the larynx and be
aspirated into the lungs.

▶ Nursing Diagnosis: *Breathing Pattern, Ineffective*

Definition

A state in which the rate, depth, timing, rhythm, or chest/abdominal wall
excursion during inspiration, expiration, or both does not maintain optimum
ventilation for the individual.

Defining Characteristics

Refer to Appendix.

Desired Outcome

The client will maintain an effective
breathing pattern as evidenced by:
a. normal rate and depth of
respirations
b. absence of dyspnea
c. blood gases within normal range.

Documentation

a. Rate, depth, and ease of
respirations
b. Oximetry results
c. Therapeutic interventions
d. Client teaching

NURSING ACTIONS

Assessments

1. Assess for signs and symptoms of
an ineffective breathing pattern
(e.g. shallow respirations,
tachypnea, dyspnea, use of
accessory muscles when
breathing).
2. Monitor for and report abnormal
blood gases.

3. Monitor for and report a
significant decrease in oximetry
results.

Prevention/Treatment

4. Implement measures to reduce
chest or upper abdominal pain if
present (e.g. splint incision with
pillow during coughing and deep
breathing, administer prescribed
analgesics before planned
activity).
5. Implement measures to decrease
fear and anxiety (e.g. assure client

RATIONALES

1. Early recognition of signs and
symptoms of an ineffective
breathing pattern allows for
prompt intervention.

2. Typical components of an arterial
blood gas analysis include Pa_{O_2},
Pa_{CO_2}, pH, HCO_3^-, and Sa_{O_2}.
These values provide information
about actual blood gases as well
as acid-base balance and are
useful tools in assessing a client's
respiratory status.
3. Oximetry is a noninvasive method
of measuring arterial oxygen
saturation. The results assist in
evaluating respiratory status.

4. A client with chest or upper
abdominal pain often guards
respiratory efforts and breathes
shallowly in an attempt to
prevent additional discomfort.
Pain reduction enables the client
to breathe more deeply.
5. Fear and anxiety may cause a
client to breathe shallowly or to

that breathing deeply will not dislodge tubes or cause incision to break open, interact with client in a confident manner).

6. Implement measures to increase strength and activity tolerance if client is weak and fatigued (e.g. provide uninterrupted rest periods, maintain optimal nutrition).

7. Place client in a semi- to high Fowler's position unless contraindicated. Position with pillows to prevent slumping.

8. Assist client to turn from side to side at least every 2 hours while in bed.

9. Instruct client to deep breathe or use incentive spirometer every 1–2 hours.

10. Assist with positive airway pressure techniques (e.g. IPPB, continuous positive airway pressure [CPAP], biphasic positive airway pressure [BiPAP], expiratory positive airway pressure [EPAP]) if ordered.

11. Instruct client in and assist with diaphragmatic and pursed-lip breathing techniques if appropriate. NOTE: Diaphragmatic breathing is most often indicated for clients who have had thoracic surgery or clients who have chronic airflow limitation (e.g. emphysema) or certain neuromuscular conditions that may cause fixation or weakening of the diaphragm.

12. Instruct client to breathe slowly if hyperventilating.

13. Instruct client in and assist with segmental or localized breathing exercises if appropriate (may be indicated for clients with painful respiratory conditions or clients who have had thoracic or abdominal surgery).

hyperventilate. Decreasing fear and anxiety allows the client to focus on breathing more slowly and taking deeper breaths.

6. An increase in strength and activity tolerance enables the client to breathe more deeply and participate in activities to improve breathing pattern.

7. A semi- to high Fowler's position allows for maximum diaphragmatic excursion and lung expansion. Prevention of slumping is essential because slumping causes the abdominal contents to be pushed up against the diaphragm and restrict lung expansion.

8. Compression of the thorax and subsequent limited chest wall and lung expansion occur when the client lies in one position. Turning from side to side allows for increased expansion of the lung in the nondependent ("up") position.

9. Deep breathing and use of an incentive spirometer promote maximum inhalation and lung expansion. Deep inhalation also stimulates surfactant production, which lowers alveolar surface tension and subsequently helps prevent collapse of the alveoli.

10. Positive airway pressure techniques increase the transpulmonary pressure gradient by raising pressure inside the alveoli. These techniques are used to re-expand collapsed alveoli and prevent further alveolar collapse.

11. Diaphragmatic breathing promotes greater use of the diaphragm and decreases the use of accessory muscles for inspiration. Use of this technique eases the work of breathing and ultimately promotes an increased efficiency of alveolar ventilation. Pursed-lip breathing causes a mild resistance to exhalation, which creates positive pressure in the airways. This pressure helps prevent airway collapse and subsequently promotes more complete alveolar emptying.

12. Hyperventilation is an ineffective breathing pattern that can eventually lead to respiratory alkalosis. The client can often slow breathing rate if he/she concentrates on doing so.

13. Segmental or localized breathing exercises improve expansion of apical and/or basal areas of the lung by having the client focus on selectively expanding these areas of the chest.

NURSING ACTIONS
Prevention/Treatment—*cont'd*

RATIONALES

14. Increase activity as allowed and tolerated.

14. During activity, especially ambulation, the client usually takes deeper breaths, thus increasing lung expansion.

15. Administer central nervous system depressants judiciously. Hold medication and consult physician if respiratory rate is less than 12/minute.

15. Central nervous system depressants cause depression of the respiratory center in the brainstem, which can result in a decreased rate and depth of respiration.

16. Consult physician if ineffective breathing pattern continues.

16. Notifying the physician allows for modification of treatment plan.

▶ Nursing Diagnosis: *Cardiac Output, Decreased*

Definition

A state in which the blood pumped by the heart is inadequate to meet the metabolic demands of the body.

Defining Characteristics

Refer to Appendix.

Desired Outcome

The client will maintain adequate cardiac output as evidenced by:
a. B/P within normal range for client
b. apical pulse regular and between 60–100 beats/minute
c. absence of gallop rhythms
d. absence of fatigue and weakness
e. unlabored respirations at 14–20/minute
f. clear, audible breath sounds
g. usual mental status
h. absence of vertigo and syncope
i. palpable peripheral pulses
j. skin warm, dry, and usual color
k. capillary refill time less than 3 seconds
l. urine output at least 30 ml/hour
m. absence of edema and jugular vein distention
n. central venous pressure (CVP) within normal range.

Documentation

a. Vital signs
b. Heart sounds
c. Activity tolerance
d. Breath sounds
e. Ease of respirations
f. Mental status
g. Peripheral pulses
h. Capillary refill time
i. Skin color and temperature
j. Urine output
k. Presence of edema
l. Presence of jugular vein distention
m. Central venous pressure (CVP)
n. Therapeutic interventions
o. Client teaching

NURSING ACTIONS
Assessments

RATIONALES

1. Assess for and report signs and symptoms of decreased cardiac output:
   a. variations in B/P (may be increased because of compensatory vasoconstriction; may be decreased when compensatory mechanisms and pump fail)
   b. tachycardia
   c. presence of gallop rhythm
   d. fatigue and weakness
   e. dyspnea, tachypnea
   f. crackles (rales)

1. Early recognition and reporting of signs and symptoms of decreased cardiac output allow for prompt intervention.

g. restlessness, change in mental status
h. vertigo, syncope
i. diminished or absent peripheral pulses
j. cool, moist skin
k. pallor or cyanosis of skin
l. capillary refill time greater than 3 seconds
m. oliguria
n. edema
o. jugular vein distention (JVD)
p. increased CVP (use internal jugular vein pulsation method to estimate CVP if monitoring device not present).

2. Monitor ECG readings and report significant abnormalities.

2. ECG readings provide data regarding functioning of the heart's electrical conduction system. Altered generation or transmission of electrical impulses often causes an abnormal heart rate or rhythm that can lead to decreased cardiac output.

3. Monitor chest x-ray results. Report findings of cardiomegaly, pleural effusion, or pulmonary edema.

3. Chest x-ray films provide data regarding size of the heart and fluid accumulation in the pleural space, pulmonary interstitium, and alveoli. The presence of cardiomegaly, pleural effusion, and/or pulmonary edema can contribute to or be caused by decreased cardiac output.

Prevention/Treatment

4. Implement measures to reduce cardiac workload:

4. Cardiac workload is the effort the heart expends to pump blood. The work of the heart is determined largely by the volume of blood distending the ventricles at the end of diastole (preload) and the amount of tension the ventricle must pump against to eject blood (afterload). Decreasing cardiac workload reduces the work that the compromised heart must perform in order to pump an adequate amount of blood. This results in increased cardiac output.

a. place client in a semi- to high Fowler's position

a. Elevation of client's upper body reduces cardiac workload by:
1. decreasing venous return from the periphery and subsequently reducing preload
2. reducing venous pooling in the lungs and subsequently lowering pulmonary vascular congestion and resistance
3. lowering the diaphragm, which enhances ventilation, thereby increasing oxygen availability.

b. instruct client to avoid activities that create a Valsalva response (e.g. straining to have

b. When a client exhales following the Valsalva maneuver, the intrathoracic

NURSING ACTIONS
Prevention/Treatment—*cont'd*

a bowel movement, holding breath while moving up in bed)

c. perform actions to promote physical and emotional rest (e.g. maintain a calm, quiet environment; limit the number of visitors; maintain activity restrictions)

d. perform actions to promote adequate tissue oxygenation (e.g. maintain oxygen therapy as ordered, encourage deep breathing exercises and use of incentive spirometer)
e. discourage smoking

f. discourage excessive intake of beverages high in caffeine such as coffee, tea, and colas

g. perform actions to prevent or treat fluid volume excess (e.g. maintain prescribed fluid and dietary sodium restrictions, administer diuretics as ordered)

h. increase activity gradually as allowed and tolerated.

5. Administer the following medications if ordered:
   a. positive inotropic agents (e.g. digitalis preparations, dobutamine, dopamine, amrinone)
   b. nitrates (e.g. nitroglycerin, isosorbide dinitrate)

RATIONALES

pressure falls, causing a sudden increase in venous return and a subsequent increase in preload and cardiac workload.

c. Physical rest reduces cardiac workload by lowering the body's energy requirements and subsequent need for oxygen. Promoting emotional rest reduces cardiac workload by preventing the increase in heart rate and blood pressure that accompany stress-induced sympathetic nervous system stimulation.

d. When tissue oxygenation is adequate, the heart does not need to work as hard to supply oxygen to the tissues and more oxygen is available for myocardial use.
e. Nicotine stimulates catecholamine output, which increases heart rate and causes vasoconstriction and subsequently increases cardiac workload. Smoking also reduces oxygen availability because hemoglobin has a greater affinity for the carbon monoxide in smoke than for oxygen. This increases cardiac workload as the heart tries to compensate for the reduced oxygen levels.

f. Excessive caffeine can increase cardiac workload because caffeine is a myocardial stimulant and can increase the rate and force of myocardial contractions.

g. Preventing or treating fluid volume excess reduces vascular volume, which decreases preload and afterload and subsequently lessens cardiac workload.

h. A gradual increase in activity prevents a sudden increase in cardiac workload. A graded activity program also helps strengthen and tone the myocardium, which ultimately increases cardiac output.

5. a. Positive inotropic agents increase cardiac output by improving myocardial contractility.
   b. The primary effect of nitrates is to decrease cardiac workload and myocardial oxygen demands by relaxing peripheral veins and, to a lesser extent, arterioles. This reduces venous return (preload) and peripheral

c. direct-acting vasodilators (e.g. sodium nitroprusside, hydralazine) or central- or alpha-adrenergic inhibitors (e.g. clonidine, prazosin)

d. angiotensin-converting enzyme (ACE) inhibitors (e.g. captopril, enalapril, lisinopril)

e. beta-adrenergic blocking agents (e.g. propranolol, acebutolol, metoprolol, atenolol, nadolol)

f. anticholinergic agents (e.g. atropine) and sympathomimetics (e.g. isoproterenol)

g. antidysrhythmics (e.g. quinidine, flecainide, lidocaine, disopyramide, procainamide, amiodarone, sotalol, adenosine)

h. calcium channel blocking agents (e.g. nifedepine, verapamil, diltiazem, nicardipine, amlodipine).

vascular resistance (afterload). Nitrates also dilate nonsclerosed coronary arteries, which improves blood flow to underperfused portions of the heart.

c. Vasodilators reduce cardiac workload by dilating the arterioles and subsequently decreasing peripheral vascular resistance (afterload). Certain vasodilators also dilate the veins which decreases venous return and lowers diastolic ventricular filling pressure (preload).

d. ACE inhibitors block the formation of angiotensin II (a potent vasoconstrictor), which subsequently also causes a decrease in aldosterone output. The reduction in angiotensin II and aldosterone results in a decrease in total peripheral vascular resistance and reduced sodium and water retention, which leads to decreased cardiac workload.

e. Beta-adrenergic blockers reduce cardiac workload by blocking sympathetic nervous system stimulation of beta receptors in the heart.

f. Cardiac output is dependent on stroke volume and heart rate. Drugs such as anticholinergics and sympathomimetics that increase the heart rate (have a positive chronotropic effect) may be used to increase cardiac output in clients with bradyarrhythmias.

g. Antidysrhythmics improve cardiac output by correcting automaticity and/or conduction abnormalities in the heart. By slowing the heart rate and/or decreasing irregularity of the heart rate, the diastolic filling time is prolonged, resulting in an increased preload and stroke volume.

h. Calcium channel blockers dilate the coronary arteries, thus improving coronary blood flow and myocardial oxygen supply. They also reduce cardiac workload by dilating peripheral arteries and subsequently reducing afterload. Certain calcium channel blockers (e.g. verapamil) also have an antidysrhythmic effect, which subsequently increases cardiac output by helping restore normal heart rate and rhythm.

NURSING ACTIONS

Prevention/Treatment—*cont'd*

6. Consult physician if signs and symptoms of decreased cardiac output persist or worsen.

RATIONALES

6. Notifying the physician allows for modification of treatment plan.

▶ Nursing Diagnosis: *Constipation*

Definition

A state in which an individual experiences a change in normal bowel habits characterized by a decrease in frequency and/or passage of hard, dry stools.

Defining Characteristics

Refer to Appendix.

Desired Outcome

The client will maintain usual bowel elimination pattern as evidenced by:
  a. usual frequency of bowel movements
  b. passage of soft, formed stool
  c. absence of abdominal distention and pain, feeling of rectal fullness or pressure, and straining during defecation.

Documentation

  a. Occurrence of last bowel movement
  b. Characteristics of stool
  c. Abdominal distention or pain
  d. Reports of fullness or pressure in rectum
  e. Reports of straining at stool
  f. Bowel sounds
  g. Therapeutic interventions
  h. Client teaching

NURSING ACTIONS

Assessments

1. Ascertain client's usual bowel elimination habits.

2. Assess for signs and symptoms of constipation (e.g. decrease in frequency of bowel movements; passage of hard, formed stools; anorexia; abdominal distention and pain; feeling of fullness or pressure in rectum; straining during defecation).

3. Assess bowel sounds. Report a pattern of decreasing bowel sounds.

Prevention/Treatment

4. Encourage client to defecate whenever the urge is felt.

RATIONALES

1. Knowledge of the client's usual bowel elimination habits is essential in determining if constipation is present because the frequency of defecation varies among individuals.

2. Early recognition of signs and symptoms of constipation allows for prompt intervention.

3. Bowel sounds are produced by peristaltic activity. A pattern of decreasing bowel sounds indicates a decrease in bowel motility, which can lead to and be present with constipation.

4. If the client feels the urge to defecate but suppresses it by contracting the external anal sphincter, the defecation reflex will subside after a few minutes and will not recur again for several hours or until additional feces enters the rectum. Repeated inhibition of the defecation reflex results in progressive weakening of the reflex. In addition, when the defecation reflex is inhibited, feces remains in the colon longer and water continues to be absorbed from the feces, making

5. Assist client to toilet or bedside commode or place in high Fowler's position on bedpan for bowel movements unless contraindicated.

6. Encourage client to relax, provide privacy, and have call light within reach during attempts to defecate.

7. Encourage client to establish a regular time for defecation, preferably within an hour after a meal.

8. Instruct client to increase intake of foods high in fiber (e.g. bran, whole-grain breads and cereals, fresh fruits and vegetables) unless contraindicated.

9. Instruct client to maintain a minimum fluid intake of 2500 ml/day unless contraindicated.

10. Encourage client to drink hot liquids (e.g. coffee, tea) upon arising in the morning.

11. Increase activity as allowed and tolerated.

12. When appropriate, encourage the use of nonnarcotic rather than narcotic (opioid) analgesics for pain management.

13. Administer laxatives or cathartics (e.g. stool softeners, bulk-forming agents, irritants/stimulants, saline/osmotic agents) as ordered.

14. Administer cleansing and/or oil retention enemas if ordered.

the stool drier, harder, and subsequently more difficult to evacuate.

5. A sitting or high Fowler's position aids in the expulsion of stool by enhancing the client's ability to contract the abdominal muscles, which subsequently increases intra-abdominal pressure and forces the fecal contents downward and into the rectum where the defecation reflex is then elicited.

6. If the client is able to relax during attempts to defecate, he/she will be able to relax the levator ani muscle and external anal sphincter, which subsequently facilitates the evacuation of stool.

7. Attempting to have a bowel movement within an hour after a meal, particularly breakfast, takes advantage of mass peristalsis, which occurs only a few times a day and is strongest after meals. Mass peristalsis is stimulated by the gastrocolic reflex, which is initiated by the presence of foods/fluids in the stomach.

8. Foods high in fiber provide bulk to the fecal mass and keep the stool soft because of the ability of fiber to absorb water. The increased bulkiness (mass) of the stools stimulates peristalsis, which promotes more rapid movement of stool through the colon. Also, the shorter the time that feces remains in the intestine, the less water is absorbed from it, which helps prevent the formation of hard, dry stools that are difficult to expel.

9. Inadequate fluid intake reduces the water content of feces, which results in hard, dry stool that is difficult to evacuate.

10. Ingestion of hot fluids can stimulate peristalsis.

11. Ambulation stimulates peristalsis, which promotes the passage of stool through the intestines.

12. Narcotic analgesics inhibit peristalsis, which delays transit of intestinal contents. This delay also results in increased absorption of fluid from the fecal mass with the subsequent formation of hard, dry stool.

13. Laxatives/cathartics act in a variety of ways to soften the stool, increase stool bulk, stimulate bowel motility, and/or lubricate the fecal mass and thereby promote the evacuation of stool.

14. A cleansing enema is the instillation of a large volume of

NURSING ACTIONS **Prevention/Treatment**—*cont'd*	**RATIONALES**
	solution into the lower bowel. The resultant irritation and distention of the lower bowel stimulates peristalsis and promotes evacuation of stool. An oil retention enema facilitates the passage of stool by softening the fecal mass and lubricating the rectum and anal canal.
15. Consult physician about checking for an impaction and digitally removing stool if the client has not had a bowel movement in 3 days, if he/she is passing liquid stool, or if other signs and symptoms of constipation are present.	15. An impaction prohibits the normal passage of feces. Digital removal of an impacted fecal mass may be necessary before normal passage of stool can occur.
16. Consult physician if signs and symptoms of constipation persist.	16. Notifying the physician allows for modification of treatment plan.

▶ Nursing Diagnosis: *Coping, Ineffective Individual*

Definition

Impairment of adaptive behaviors and abilities of a person in meeting life's demands and roles.

Defining Characteristics

Refer to Appendix.

Desired Outcome	**Documentation**
The client will demonstrate effective coping as evidenced by: a. verbalization of ability to cope b. use of appropriate problem-solving techniques c. willingness to participate in treatment plan and meet basic needs d. absence of destructive behavior toward self and others e. appropriate use of defense mechanisms f. use of available support systems.	a. Client statements related to coping ability b. Ability to meet basic needs and problem solve c. Factors inhibiting successful coping d. Current coping strategies used e. Sleep pattern f. Interactions with others g. Support systems used h. Therapeutic interventions i. Client/family teaching

NURSING ACTIONS **Assessments**	**RATIONALES**
1. Assess for and report signs and symptoms of ineffective individual coping (e.g. verbalization of inability to cope; inability to ask for help, problem solve, or meet basic needs; insomnia; withdrawal; destructive behavior toward self or others; inappropriate use of defense mechanisms).	1. Early recognition and reporting of signs and symptoms of ineffective individual coping allow for prompt intervention.
2. Assess client's perception of current situation.	2. The client's perception of the situation is the major determinant of his/her response. An awareness of the situation from the client's point of view helps the nurse develop interventions that will facilitate coping.

Prevention/Treatment

3. Allow time for client to begin to adjust to his/her situation. Recognize that the amount of time needed will vary from client to client.

3. Time is necessary for cognitive appraisal of the situation and development of effective coping strategies.

4. Assist client to recognize and manage inappropriate denial if it is present.

4. Denial is a major defense mechanism used to deal with illness, particularly when the client is unable to deal with the realities of his/her situation or is grieving. If denial persists or is inappropriate, it inhibits the client's ability to cope.

5. Implement measures to reduce fear and anxiety (e.g. encourage verbalization about the situation, instruct in relaxation techniques, administer antianxiety agents as ordered).

5. Fear and anxiety inhibit clarity of thought and problem solving and the subsequent development of effective coping techniques.

6. Implement measures to reduce discomfort (e.g. administer prescribed analgesics, encourage use of relaxation techniques).

6. The presence of discomfort, particularly if it continues, can reduce the client's ability to effectively identify and use coping strategies.

7. Encourage verbalization about current situation and ways comparable situations have been handled in the past.

7. Verbalization assists the client to reflect on the situation he/she is dealing with and to develop coping strategies based on previous successful experiences.

8. Assist client to identify personal strengths and resources that can be used to facilitate coping with the current situation.

8. The development of effective coping strategies is dependent on the client's ability to recognize and use personal strengths and resources.

9. Demonstrate acceptance of client and create an atmosphere of trust and support.

9. An environment where acceptance, trust, and support exist is essential for the client to feel free to express his/her feelings and concerns and subsequently begin to cope with his/her situation.

10. If acceptable to client, arrange for a visit with another individual who has successfully adjusted to a similar situation.

10. Contact with another individual who has experienced and successfully adjusted to a similar situation provides the client with support and insight into ways to effectively cope with his/her situation.

11. Include client in planning of care, encourage maximum participation in treatment plan, and allow choices when possible.

11. Active participation in the planning of care allows the client to maintain a sense of control. This enhances his/her self-esteem and subsequent ability to cope.

12. Instruct client in effective problem-solving techniques (e.g. accurate identification of stressors, determination of various options to solve problem).

12. Effective problem-solving skills are essential to the development of useful coping strategies because they enable the client to identify the problem clearly and select and implement viable options for solving it.

13. Assist client to identify priorities and attainable goals as he/she starts to plan for necessary life-style and role changes.

13. The setting of appropriate priorities and realistic goals is necessary if the client is to cope effectively with the changes being experienced.

14. Assist client and significant others

14. Adjustment rather than

NURSING ACTIONS Prevention/Treatment—*cont'd*	RATIONALES
to identify ways that personal and family goals can be adjusted rather than abandoned.	abandonment of personal and family goals reduces the feeling of loss and increases the probability of positive adaptation to the situation being experienced.
15. Assist client, through methods such as role playing, to practice coping strategies.	15. Practicing coping strategies in a safe environment helps the client to integrate these skills so that they are more easily implemented when the need arises.
16. Assist client to identify and use available support systems. Provide information about available community resources that can assist client and significant others in coping with the situation at hand.	16. Social support provides a sense of acceptance and reduces the feelings of aloneness, which are often experienced in a crisis situation. Community resources are usually able to provide both information and psychological support for the client and significant others and subsequently facilitate the development and success of coping strategies.
17. Encourage client to share with significant others the kind of support that would be most beneficial (e.g. listening, inspiring hope, providing reassurance and accurate information).	17. Techniques or behaviors that facilitate one's coping ability vary from person to person and need to be clearly communicated to significant others in order to maximize their support.
18. Support behaviors indicative of effective coping (e.g. participation in treatment plan and self-care activities, communication of the ability to cope, use of effective problem-solving strategies).	18. Positive reinforcement of effective coping strategies increases the likelihood of continued use and enhancement of these strategies.
19. Consult physician about psychological and vocational counseling if appropriate. Initiate a referral if necessary.	19. If client is unable to cope effectively and/or is unable to pursue his/her vocation, additional counseling may be necessary. Consulting with physician and making referrals can help the client to meet his/her needs and cope effectively.

▶ Nursing Diagnosis: *Diarrhea*

Definition

A state in which an individual experiences a change in normal bowel habits characterized by the frequent passage of loose, fluid, unformed stools.

Defining Characteristics

Refer to Appendix.

Desired Outcome

The client will have fewer bowel movements and more formed stool.

Documentation

a. Frequency of defecation
b. Characteristics of stool
c. Complaints of abdominal cramping
d. Bowel sounds
e. Therapeutic interventions
f. Client teaching

NURSING ACTIONS Assessments	RATIONALES
1. Ascertain client's usual bowel elimination habits.	1. Knowledge of the client's usual bowel elimination habits helps

2. Assess for and report signs and symptoms of diarrhea (e.g. frequent, loose stools; urgency; abdominal cramping; hyperactive bowel sounds).

determine the severity of the diarrhea.

2. Early recognition and reporting of signs and symptoms of diarrhea allow for prompt intervention.

Prevention/Treatment

3. Restrict oral intake if ordered.

3. Peristalsis is stimulated by the presence of foods/fluids in the stomach and duodenum. Restricting oral intake helps decrease peristalsis and subsequently lessens the episodes of diarrhea.

4. When oral intake is allowed, gradually progress from fluids to small meals.

4. Gradual introduction of small amounts of fluid and then food helps prevent a sudden increase in peristalsis and subsequent diarrhea.

5. Instruct client to avoid the following foods/fluids:
   a. those that are spicy or extremely hot or cold

5. a. Spicy foods can irritate the bowel, which results in increased peristalsis and excessive mucus secretion with subsequent increased liquidity of intestinal contents. Extremes in temperature of ingested foods/fluids can also stimulate peristalsis.

   b. those high in lactose (e.g. milk, milk products)

   b. Diarrhea may temporarily deplete the gastrointestinal enzyme lactase, which is essential for the hydrolysis and subsequent absorption of lactose. The nonabsorbed lactose has an osmotic effect and draws water into the colon, which results in more liquid stool. The lactose also serves as a base for bacterial fermentation in the colon. The lactic and fatty acids produced by this fermentation process irritate the colon with a subsequent increase in bowel motility and diarrhea.

   c. those high in fiber (e.g. whole-grain cereals, raw fruits and vegetables).

   c. Fiber increases bulk of the stool because of its ability to absorb water. The increased mass (bulk) of the stools stimulates peristalsis. Limiting fiber intake decreases the water content of the stool, which results in the stools being drier, firmer, and less bulky. The decrease in bulk (mass) results in less stimulation of peristalsis and the dryness of the stools slows intestinal transit time.

6. Implement measures to reduce fear and anxiety (e.g. provide client teaching, interact with

6. Parasympathetic activity may dominate in some stressful situations and cause increased

NURSING ACTIONS	**RATIONALES**
Prevention/Treatment—*cont'd*	
client in a calm manner, administer prescribed antianxiety agents).	gastrointestinal motility and diarrhea.
7. Encourage client to rest.	7. Physical activity stimulates peristalsis.
8. Discourage smoking.	8. Nicotine excites the sympathetic and the parasympathetic postganglionic neurons simultaneously. If the parasympathetic effect is dominant, peristalsis increases, which results in increased propulsion of feces through the gastrointestinal tract.
9. If the client is receiving tube feeding, administer the solution at room temperature. Consult physician about reducing the concentration and/or rate of administration of the tube-feeding solution if diarrhea occurs.	9. Tube feedings can increase peristalsis if the solution is given while cold or if large amounts are given too quickly. Full-strength tube-feeding solution can sometimes produce an osmotic diarrhea.
10. Consult physician regarding measures to remove fecal impaction if present (e.g. digital removal of stool, oil retention enema).	10. When a fecal impaction is present, the secretory activity of the bowel increases in an attempt to lubricate and promote evacuation of the impacted feces. The liquid portion of the feces above the mass then leaks around the impaction, resulting in a continuous oozing of diarrheal stool.
11. Administer the following antidiarrheal agents if ordered: a. opiate or opiate derivatives (e.g. paregoric, loperamide, diphenoxylate hydrochloride)	11. a. Opiates and their derivatives decrease gastrointestinal motility, which delays the passage of intestinal contents and subsequently allows more time for water to be absorbed from the feces. This results in fewer bowel movements and more formed stool.
b. bulk-forming agents (e.g. methylcellulose, psyllium hydrophilic mucilloid, calcium polycarbophil)	b. Bulk-forming agents absorb water in the bowel, which results in a more formed stool.
c. adsorbents (e.g. kaolin, pectin, attapulgite [Kaopectate], bismuth subsalicylate [Pepto-Bismol]).	c. Adsorbents act locally in the gastrointestinal tract to absorb toxins that are stimulating gut motility and/or secretions.
12. Consult physician if diarrhea persists.	12. Notifying physician allows for modification of the treatment plan.

▶ Nursing Diagnosis: *Fluid Volume Deficit*

NANDA's definition of this diagnostic label has been altered slightly to reflect information in current resources.

Definition

The state in which an individual experiences decreased intravascular, interstitial and/or intracellular fluid.

Defining Characteristics

Refer to Appendix.

Desired Outcome

The client will not experience a fluid volume deficit as evidenced by:

a. normal skin turgor
b. moist mucous membranes
c. stable weight
d. B/P and pulse within normal range for client and stable with position change
e. hand vein filling time less than 3–5 seconds
f. usual mental status
g. BUN and Hct within normal range
h. balanced intake and output
i. urine specific gravity within normal range.

Documentation

a. Vital signs
b. Condition of skin and mucous membranes
c. Weight
d. Hand vein filling time
e. Mental status
f. Intake and output
g. Presence of nausea, vomiting, or other contributing factors
h. Intravenous fluid therapy
i. Client teaching

NURSING ACTIONS

Assessments

1. Assess for and report signs and symptoms of fluid volume deficit:
   a. decreased skin turgor
   b. dry mucous membranes, thirst
   c. sudden weight loss of 2% or greater
   d. postural hypotension and/or low B/P
   e. weak, rapid pulse
   f. delayed hand vein filling time (longer than 3–5 seconds)
   g. change in mental status
   h. elevated BUN and Hct
   i. decreased urine output with a change in specific gravity (the specific gravity will usually be increased with an actual fluid volume deficit but may be decreased depending on the cause of the deficit).

Prevention/Treatment

2. Implement measures to reduce nausea and vomiting if present (e.g. administer antiemetics as ordered, instruct client to ingest foods/fluids slowly, eliminate noxious sights and odors).
3. Implement measures to control diarrhea if present (e.g. administer antidiarrheal agents as ordered, discourage intake of spicy foods and foods high in fiber, discourage smoking).
4. Implement measures to reduce fever if present (e.g. administer antipyretics as ordered, sponge client with tepid water, remove excessive clothing or bedcovers).
5. Maintain a fluid intake of at least 2500 ml/day unless contraindicated. If oral intake is inadequate, maintain intravenous fluid therapy as ordered.
6. Consult physician if signs and symptoms of fluid volume deficit persist or worsen.

RATIONALES

1. Early recognition and reporting of signs and symptoms of fluid volume deficit allow for prompt intervention.

2. Nausea often causes the client to have decreased fluid intake. Persistent vomiting results in excessive loss of fluid.

3. Persistent or severe diarrhea results in excessive loss of gastrointestinal fluid.

4. Fever may be accompanied by diaphoresis, which can result in excessive loss of fluid.

5. Adequate fluid intake needs to be provided in order to replace losses and/or ensure adequate hydration.

6. Notifying the physician allows for modification of treatment plan.

▶ Nursing Diagnosis: *Fluid Volume Excess*

Definition

The state in which an individual experiences increased isotonic fluid retention.

Defining Characteristics

Refer to Appendix.

Desired Outcome

The client will not experience fluid volume excess as evidenced by:
a. stable weight
b. B/P within normal range for client
c. absence of S_3 heart sound
d. normal pulse volume
e. balanced intake and output
f. usual mental status
g. normal breath sounds
h. BUN and Hct within normal range
i. absence of dyspnea, orthopnea, peripheral edema, and distended neck veins
j. hand vein emptying time less than 3–5 seconds
k. CVP within normal range.

Documentation

a. Blood pressure
b. Weight
c. Heart sounds
d. Pulse volume
e. Intake and output
f. Mental status
g. Breath sounds, ease of respirations
h. Presence of edema and neck vein distention
i. Hand vein emptying time
j. CVP readings
k. Therapeutic interventions
l. Client teaching

NURSING ACTIONS

Assessments

1. Assess for and report signs and symptoms of fluid volume excess:
   a. weight gain of 2% or greater in a short period
   b. elevated B/P (B/P may not be elevated if fluid has shifted out of vascular space)
   c. presence of an S_3 heart sound
   d. full, bounding pulse
   e. intake greater than output
   f. change in mental status
   g. crackles (rales), diminished or absent breath sounds
   h. decreased BUN and Hct
   i. dyspnea, orthopnea
   j. peripheral edema
   k. distended neck veins
   l. delayed hand vein emptying time (longer than 3–5 seconds)
   m. elevated CVP.
2. Monitor chest x-ray results. Report findings of pulmonary vascular congestion, pleural effusion, or pulmonary edema.

Prevention/Treatment

3. Maintain fluid restrictions as ordered.

4. Restrict sodium intake as ordered.

RATIONALES

1. Early recognition and reporting of signs and symptoms of fluid volume excess allow for prompt intervention.

2. Chest x-ray films provide data about pulmonary vascular status and fluid accumulation in the pleural space, pulmonary interstitium, and alveoli.

3. Fluid restriction helps to reduce total body water and prevent the accumulation of excess fluid.
4. When blood filters through the kidneys, the majority of sodium ions are reabsorbed by the renal tubules. Water is attracted to sodium and is also reabsorbed. Restriction of sodium intake

5. Administer diuretics if ordered.

6. Consult physician if signs and symptoms of fluid volume excess persist or worsen.

reduces the amount of sodium that passes through and is reabsorbed by the kidney. This results in decreased retention of water.

5. Most diuretics inhibit sodium reabsorption in the renal tubules. This results in decreased water reabsorption and subsequent excretion of excess fluid.

6. Notifying the physician allows for modification of treatment plan.

▶ Nursing Diagnosis: *Gas Exchange, Impaired*

NANDA's definition of this diagnostic label has been altered slightly to reflect information in current resources.

Definition

A state in which an individual experiences an imbalance in oxygenation and/or carbon dioxide elimination at the alveolar-capillary membrane.

Defining Characteristics

Refer to Appendix.

Desired Outcome

The client will experience adequate gas (O_2/CO_2) exchange as evidenced by:
a. usual mental status
b. unlabored respirations at 14–20/ minute
c. blood gases within normal range.

Documentation

a. Respiratory rate
b. Difficulty breathing
c. Mental status
d. Oximetry results
e. Route and rate of oxygen administration
f. Therapeutic interventions
g. Client teaching

NURSING ACTIONS

Assessments

1. Assess for and report signs and symptoms of impaired gas (O_2/CO_2) exchange:
   a. restlessness, irritability
   b. confusion, somnolence
   c. tachypnea, dyspnea
   d. decreased PaO_2 and/or increased $PaCO_2$.
2. Monitor for and report a significant decrease in oximetry results.

Prevention/Treatment

3. Place client in a semi- to high Fowler's position unless contraindicated. Position with pillows to prevent slumping. If client is experiencing dyspnea or orthopnea, position overbed table

RATIONALES

1. Early recognition and reporting of signs and symptoms of impaired gas exchange allow for prompt intervention.

2. Oximetry is a noninvasive method of measuring arterial oxygen saturation. The results assist in evaluating respiratory status.

3. These positions allow for increased diaphragmatic excursion and maximum lung expansion, which promotes optimal alveolar ventilation and O_2/CO_2 exchange.

NURSING ACTIONS	RATIONALES
Prevention/Treatment—*cont'd*	

so he/she can lean on it if desired.

4. Instruct and assist client to turn, deep breathe, and cough or "huff" every 1–2 hours.

4. Turning from side to side mobilizes secretions and allows for increased expansion of the lung in the nondependent ("up") position. Deep breathing loosens secretions, increases the forcefulness of a cough, promotes maximum lung expansion, and stimulates surfactant production, which helps prevent alveolar collapse. Coughing or "huffing" (a forced expiration technique) mobilizes secretions and facilitates removal of these secretions from the respiratory tract. These actions promote optimal alveolar ventilation and O_2/CO_2 exchange.

5. Reinforce correct use of incentive spirometer every 1–2 hours.

5. Incentive spirometer use promotes slow, deep inhalation, which improves lung expansion and helps clear airways by loosening secretions and promoting a more effective cough. These actions enhance alveolar ventilation and the exchange of O_2/CO_2.

6. Implement measures to facilitate removal of pulmonary secretions (e.g. suction, postural drainage, percussion, vibration) if ordered.

6. Excessive secretions and/or client's inability to clear secretions from the respiratory tract lead to stasis of secretions, which can impair O_2/CO_2 exchange. Suction and chest physical therapy may be necessary to facilitate removal of pulmonary secretions and thereby promote adequate gas exchange.

7. Assist with positive airway pressure techniques (e.g. IPPB, continuous positive airway pressure [CPAP], biphasic positive airway pressure [BiPAP], expiratory positive airway pressure [EPAP]) if ordered.

7. Positive airway pressure techniques increase the transpulmonary pressure gradient by raising pressure inside the alveoli. These techniques are used to re-expand collapsed alveoli and prevent further alveolar collapse so that gas exchange can take place.

8. Maintain oxygen therapy as ordered.

8. Supplemental oxygen increases the amount of oxygen available for gas exchange.

9. Maintain activity restrictions as ordered. Increase activity gradually as allowed and tolerated.

9. Restricting activity lowers the body's oxygen requirements and thus increases the amount of oxygen available for gas exchange. A gradual increase in activity conserves energy and thereby lessens oxygen utilization, yet promotes mobilization of secretions and deeper breathing.

10. Discourage smoking.

10. Smoking impairs gas exchange because it:
    a. reduces effective airway clearance by increasing mucus production and impairing ciliary function
    b. decreases oxygen availability (hemoglobin binds with the

carbon monoxide in smoke
rather than with oxygen)
c. causes damage to the bronchial
and alveolar walls
d. causes vasoconstriction and
subsequently reduces
pulmonary blood flow.

11. Administer central nervous
system depressants judiciously.
Hold medication and consult
physician if respiratory rate is less
than 12/minute.

11. Central nervous system
depressants cause depression of
the respiratory center and cough
reflex. This can result in
hypoventilation and stasis of
secretions with subsequent
impaired gas exchange.

12. Consult physician if signs and
symptoms of impaired gas
exchange persist or worsen.

12. Notifying the physician allows for
modification of treatment plan.

▶ Nursing Diagnosis: *Grieving*

This diagnostic label includes anticipatory grieving and grieving following the actual loss.

Definition

Intellectual and emotional responses and behaviors by which individuals (families, communities) work through or attempt to work through the process of modifying self-concept based on the perception of potential or actual loss.

Defining Characteristics

Refer to Appendix.

Desired Outcome

The client will demonstrate beginning progression through the grieving process as evidenced by:
a. verbalization of feelings about the loss
b. usual sleep pattern
c. participation in treatment plan and self-care activities
d. use of available support systems.

Documentation

a. Verbalization of feelings of loss
b. Participation in activities
c. Eating pattern
d. Sleep pattern
e. Interaction with others
f. Measures used to adapt to loss
g. Client/family teaching

NURSING ACTIONS

Assessments

1. Assess for signs and symptoms of grieving (e.g. change in eating habits, inability to concentrate, insomnia, anger, sadness, withdrawal from significant others, denial of loss).

2. Assess for factors that may hinder and facilitate client's acknowledgment of the loss.

RATIONALES

1. Assessment of signs and symptoms of grieving helps the nurse determine the phase of grieving the client is experiencing. This knowledge aids in the development of effective strategies that can assist the client to progress through the phases of grieving.

2. In order for grief work to begin, the client needs to acknowledge the loss. An awareness of factors that may hinder and facilitate this acknowledgment assists the nurse to develop effective strategies to accomplish this goal.

NURSING ACTIONS	RATIONALES
Prevention/Treatment—*cont'd*	
3. Assist client to acknowledge the loss (e.g. encourage conversation about the loss including how or why it occurred and its impact on his/her future).	3. The client needs to acknowledge the loss in order for grief work to begin.
4. Discuss the grieving process and assist client to accept the phases of grieving as an expected response to an actual and/or anticipated loss.	4. An awareness of the feelings and behaviors commonly associated with each phase of the grieving process assists the client to accept his/her responses to the loss.
5. Allow time for client to progress through the phases of grieving (phases vary among theorists but progress from shock and alarm to acceptance).	5. Grieving is a process that occurs in a sequence of phases or stages that progress over time. Some phases may not be experienced by the client and some may overlap or recur. The amount of time necessary to reach resolution of grief is very individual, may take months to years, and must be allowed to occur in order to reduce the risk for dysfunctional grieving.
6. Provide an atmosphere of care and concern (e.g. provide privacy, be available and nonjudgmental, display empathy and respect).	6. A supportive, nonthreatening environment provides the basis for a constructive, therapeutic relationship between the client and nurse. This allows the client to express his/her feelings of grief and work toward its resolution.
7. Implement measures to promote trust (e.g. answer questions honestly, provide requested information).	7. A feeling of trust in the caregiver promotes the development of a therapeutic nurse/client relationship in which the client can feel free to verbalize his/her feelings. This facilitates the progression of grief work.
8. Encourage the verbal expression of anger and sadness about the loss experienced. Recognize displacement of anger and assist client to see the actual cause of angry feelings and resentment. Establish limits on abusive behavior if demonstrated.	8. The verbal expression of feelings of anger and sadness facilitates movement toward resolution of grief. Displacement of angry feelings needs to be acknowledged so that grieving can progress but should not be allowed to interfere with the therapeutic process.
9. Encourage client to express his/her feelings in whatever ways are comfortable (e.g. writing, drawing, conversation).	9. Expression of feelings helps the client integrate both positive and negative aspects of the loss and move toward its acceptance.
10. Assist client to identify and utilize techniques that have helped him/her cope in previous situations of loss.	10. The identification and utilization of coping techniques that help deal with the current loss can facilitate progression through the grieving process.
11. Support behaviors suggesting successful grief work (e.g. verbalizing feelings about loss, focusing on ways to adapt to loss, learning needed skills, developing or renewing relationships).	11. Positive feedback about behaviors that suggest successful grief work reinforces those behaviors and promotes positive adaptation to loss.
12. Explain the phases of the grieving process to significant others. Encourage their support and understanding.	12. When significant others are knowledgeable about the phases of the grieving process, they are more likely to understand and accept the client's behavior and assist him/her to move toward resolution of grief.

13. Facilitate communication between the client and significant others.

13. Effective communication between the client and significant others enhances the client's ability to express feelings and successfully move through the phases of grieving.

14. Provide information about counseling services and support groups that might assist client in working through grief.

14. Counseling and support groups can assist the client in working through grief by:
    a. providing insight into his/her responses to the loss
    b. decreasing the feelings of aloneness and isolation that frequently accompany a loss
    c. helping to identify methods or skills he/she can use to cope with the loss.

15. When appropriate, assist client to meet spiritual needs (e.g. arrange for a visit from clergy).

15. Spiritual support can be a source of strength and solace to the client and can facilitate resolution of grief.

16. Consult physician if signs of dysfunctional grieving (e.g. persistent denial of losses, excessive anger or sadness, emotional lability) occur.

16. Notifying the physician allows for modification of the treatment plan.

▶ Nursing Diagnosis: *Infection, Risk for*

Definition

The state in which an individual is at increased risk for being invaded by pathogenic organisms.

Defining Characteristics

Refer to Appendix.

Desired Outcome

The client will remain free of infection as evidenced by:
a. absence of fever and chills
b. pulse within normal limits
c. usual mental status
d. normal breath sounds
e. cough productive of clear mucus only
f. voiding clear urine without reports of frequency, urgency, and burning
g. absence of heat, pain, redness, swelling, and unusual drainage in any area
h. WBC and differential counts within normal range for client
i. negative results of cultured specimens.

Documentation

a. Temperature
b. Pulse rate
c. Presence of chills
d. Mental status
e. Breath sounds
f. Characteristics of urine, sputum, and wound drainage
g. Evidence of inflammation in any area
h. Evidence of unusual drainage from any area
i. Therapeutic interventions
j. Client/family teaching

NURSING ACTIONS

Assessments

1. Assess for and report signs and symptoms of infection (be aware that some signs and symptoms vary depending on the site of infection, the causative agent, and the age and immune status of the client):
   a. elevated temperature

RATIONALES

1. Early recognition and reporting of signs and symptoms of infection allow for prompt intervention.

NURSING ACTIONS	**RATIONALES**

Assessment—*cont'd*

b. chills
c. increased pulse
d. malaise, lethargy, acute confusion
e. loss of appetite
f. abnormal breath sounds
g. productive cough of purulent, green, or rust-colored sputum
h. cloudy, foul-smelling urine
i. reports of frequency, urgency, or burning when urinating
j. presence of WBCs, bacteria, and/or nitrites in urine
k. heat, pain, redness, swelling, or unusual drainage in any area
l. elevated WBC count and/or significant change in differential.

2. Obtain specimens (e.g. urine, vaginal drainage, sputum, blood) for culture as ordered. Report positive results.

2. Cultures are done to identify the specific organism(s) causing the infection. Culture results provide the physician with information necessary to determine the most effective treatment.

Prevention

3. Maintain a fluid intake of at least 2500 ml/day unless contraindicated.

3. Adequate hydration helps prevent infection by:
   a. helping maintain adequate blood flow and nutrient supply to the tissues
   b. promoting urine formation and subsequent voiding, which flushes pathogens from the bladder and urethra
   c. thinning respiratory secretions, which facilitates removal of secretions.

4. Use good handwashing technique and encourage client to do the same.

4. Good handwashing removes transient flora, which reduces the risk of transmission of pathogens.

5. Use sterile technique (surgical asepsis) during invasive procedures (e.g. urinary catheterizations, venous and arterial punctures, injections, tracheal suctioning, wound care).

5. Use of sterile technique during invasive procedures reduces the possibility of introducing pathogens into the body.

6. Anchor catheters/tubings (e.g. urinary, intravenous, wound drainage) securely.

6. Catheters/tubings that are not securely anchored have some degree of in-and-out movement. This movement increases the risk of infection because it allows for the introduction of pathogens into the body. It can also cause tissue trauma, which can result in colonization of microorganisms.

7. Change equipment, tubings, and solutions used for treatments such as intravenous infusions, respiratory care, irrigations, and enteral feedings according to hospital policy.

7. The longer that equipment, tubings, and solutions are in use, the greater the chance of colonization of microorganisms, which can then be introduced into the body.

8. Maintain a closed system for drains (e.g. wound, chest tubes, urinary catheters) and intravenous infusions whenever possible.

8. Each time a drainage or infusion system is opened, pathogens from the external environment have an opportunity to enter the body.

9. Rotate intravenous insertion sites according to hospital policy.

10. Implement measures to promote wound healing (e.g. use dressing materials that maintain a moist wound surface, assist with debridement of necrotic tissue, use dressing materials that absorb excess exudate, protect granulating tissue from trauma and contamination, maintain patency of wound drains).

11. Protect client from others with infections.

12. Implement measures to maintain healthy, intact skin (e.g. keep skin lubricated, clean, and dry; instruct or assist client to turn every 2 hours; keep bed linens dry and wrinkle-free).

13. Implement measures to reduce stress (e.g. reduce fear, anxiety, and pain; help client identify and use effective coping mechanisms).

14. Maintain an optimal nutritional status. Administer vitamins and minerals as ordered.

15. Instruct and assist client to perform good perineal care routinely and after each bowel movement.

16. Instruct and assist client to perform good oral hygiene as often as needed.

Maintaining a closed system decreases this risk, which reduces the possibility of infection.

9. Intravenous insertion sites need to be changed routinely in order to reduce persistent irritation of one area of a vein wall and the resultant colonization of microorganisms at that site.

10. Proper wound care facilitates healing of the wound and also reduces the number of pathogens present, which reduces the risk of the wound becoming infected.

11. Protecting the client from others with infections reduces his/her risk of exposure to pathogens.

12. Healthy, intact skin reduces the risk for infection by:
    a. providing a physical barrier against the introduction of pathogens into the body
    b. removing many of the microorganisms on the surface of the skin during the constant shedding of the epidermis
    c. inhibiting the growth of some bacteria (sebum contains fatty acids, which create a slightly acidic environment that inhibits the growth of some bacteria)
    d. destroying some bacteria and fungi on the skin (sweat and sebaceous glands secrete substances such as lysozyme that act as chemical barriers against infection).

13. Stress causes an increased secretion of cortisol. Cortisol interferes with the immune response, which subsequently increases the client's susceptibility to infection.

14. Adequate nutrition is needed to maintain normal function of the immune system.

15. The perineal area contains a large number of organisms. Routine cleansing of the area reduces the risk of colonization of the organisms and subsequent perineal, urinary tract, and/or vaginal infection.

16. Frequent oral hygiene helps prevent infection by removing most of the food, debris, and many of the microorganisms that are present in the mouth. It also helps maintain the integrity of the oral mucosa, which provides a physical and chemical barrier to pathogens.

NURSING ACTIONS
Prevention—*cont'd*.

RATIONALES

17. Implement measures to prevent urinary retention (e.g. instruct client to urinate when the urge is felt, promote relaxation during voiding attempts, administer bethanechol as ordered).

17. A client experiencing urinary retention is at increased risk for urinary tract infection because:
    a. blood flow to the bladder wall is decreased as the bladder becomes distended; the resultant ischemic tissue is vulnerable to infection
    b. the urine that accumulates in the bladder creates an environment conducive to the growth and colonization of microorganisms
    c. voiding does not occur so microorganisms are not flushed from the mucous lining of the urethra; these microorganisms can colonize and ascend into the bladder.

18. Implement measures to prevent stasis of respiratory secretions (e.g. assist client to turn, cough, and deep breathe; increase activity as allowed and tolerated).

18. Respiratory secretions provide a good medium for growth of microorganisms. By preventing stasis, there is less chance of colonization of the microorganisms and a decreased risk for development of respiratory tract infection.

19. Instruct client to receive immunizations (e.g. influenza vaccine, pneumococcal vaccine) if appropriate.

19. Immunizations are often recommended to reduce the possibility of some infections in high-risk clients (e.g. those clients who are immunosuppressed, elderly, or have a chronic disease).

20. Administer antimicrobials as ordered.

20. Most antimicrobials disrupt cell wall synthesis, which halts the growth of or kills microorganisms.

▶ Nursing Diagnosis: *Nutrition, Altered: Less Than Body Requirements*

Definition

The state in which an individual experiences an intake of nutrients insufficient to meet metabolic needs.

Defining Characteristics

Refer to Appendix.

Desired Outcome

The client will maintain an adequate nutritional status as evidenced by:
a. weight within normal range for client's age, height, and body frame
b. normal BUN and serum albumin, Hct, Hb, transferrin, and lymphocyte levels
c. usual strength and activity tolerance
d. healthy oral mucous membrane.

Documentation

a. Weight
b. Activity tolerance
c. Condition of oral mucous membrane
d. Type of diet and amount consumed
e. Therapeutic interventions
f. Client/family teaching

NURSING ACTIONS
Assessments

1. Assess for and report signs and symptoms of malnutrition:

RATIONALES

1. Early recognition and reporting of signs and symptoms of

a. weight below normal for client's age, height, and body frame
b. abnormal BUN and low serum albumin, Hct, Hb, transferrin, and lymphocyte levels
c. weakness and fatigue
d. sore, inflamed oral mucous membrane
e. pale conjunctiva.
2. Monitor percentage of meals and snacks client consumes. Report a pattern of inadequate intake.

3. Measure client's skinfold thickness and mid arm circumference (MAC) if indicated. Report measurements lower than normal.

Prevention/Treatment

4. Implement measures to prevent vomiting if indicated (e.g. administer antiemetics as ordered, eliminate noxious sights and odors).
5. Implement measures to control diarrhea if present (e.g. administer antidiarrheal agents as ordered, discourage intake of spicy foods and foods high in fiber).

6. Implement measures to improve oral intake:

a. perform actions to reduce nausea, pain, fear, and anxiety if present

b. perform actions to relieve gastrointestinal distention if present (e.g. encourage and assist client with frequent ambulation unless contraindicated, administer gastrointestinal stimulants as ordered)

c. increase activity as allowed and tolerated

d. maintain a clean environment and a relaxed, pleasant atmosphere

malnutrition allow for prompt intervention.

2. An awareness of the amount of foods/fluids the client consumes alerts the nurse to deficits in nutritional intake. Reporting an inadequate intake allows for prompt intervention.
3. Anthropometric measurements such as skinfold thickness and mid arm circumference provide information about the amount of muscle mass, body fat, and protein reserves the client has. These assessments assist in evaluating the client's nutritional status.

4. Vomiting results in an actual loss of nutrients.

5. The increased intestinal motility that occurs with or causes diarrhea results in a decreased absorption of nutrients in the bowel. In addition, diarrhea causes an actual loss of nutrients.
6. The client is more likely to achieve or maintain a good nutritional status if he/she has a good oral intake.
a. Nausea, pain, fear, and/or anxiety can decrease the client's appetite and result in a decreased oral intake.
b. Distention of the gastrointestinal tract (especially the stomach and duodenum) can result in stimulation of the satiety center and subsequent inhibition of the feeding center in the hypothalamus. This effect, along with the discomfort that occurs with distention, decreases appetite.
c. Activity usually promotes a general feeling of well-being, which can result in improved appetite.
d. Noxious sights and odors can inhibit the feeding center in the hypothalamus. Maintaining a clean environment helps prevent this from occurring. In addition, maintaining a

relaxed, pleasant atmosphere reduces the client's stress and promotes a feeling of well-being, which tends to improve appetite and oral intake.

e. encourage a rest period before meals if indicated

e. The physical activity of eating requires some expenditure of energy. If the client is fatigued, he/she is less likely to continue eating.

f. provide oral hygiene before meals

f. Oral hygiene freshens the mouth by moistening the oral mucous membrane and removing unpleasant tastes. This can improve the taste of foods/fluids, which helps stimulate appetite and increase oral intake.

g. serve foods/fluids that are appealing to the client and adhere to personal and cultural (e.g. religious, ethnic) preferences whenever possible

g. Foods/fluids that appeal to the client's senses (especially sight and smell) and are in accordance with his/her personal and cultural preferences are most likely to stimulate appetite and promote interest in eating.

h. serve frequent, small meals rather than large ones if client is weak, fatigues easily, and/or has a poor appetite

h. Providing small rather than large meals can enable a client who is weak or fatigues easily to finish a meal. Also, a client who has a poor appetite is often more willing to attempt to eat smaller meals because they seem less overwhelming than larger ones. If smaller meals are served, the number of meals per day should be increased to help ensure adequate nutrition.

i. encourage significant others to bring in client's favorite foods unless contraindicated and eat with him/her if client desires

i. A client's favorite foods/fluids tend to stimulate his/her appetite more than institutional foods/fluids. The presence of significant others during meals helps create a familiar social environment that can stimulate appetite and improve oral intake.

j. if client is experiencing dyspnea, place him/her in a high Fowler's position and provide supplemental oxygen therapy during meals if indicated

j. Because a person cannot swallow and breathe at the same time, relief of the client's dyspnea increases the likelihood of his/her maintaining a good oral intake. In addition, relieving dyspnea decreases the client's anxiety about and preoccupation with breathing efforts and increases the ability to focus on eating and drinking.

k. perform actions to compensate for taste alterations if present (e.g. add extra sweeteners to foods unless contraindicated, encourage client to experiment with different flavorings and seasonings,

k. Enhancing the taste of foods/fluids and providing nutritious alternatives to those that taste unusual to the client help to stimulate his/her appetite and improve oral intake.

provide alternative sources of protein if meats such as beef or pork taste bitter or rancid)

l. allow adequate time for meals; reheat foods/fluids if necessary

m. limit fluid intake with meals unless the fluid has a high nutritional value.

l. If the client feels rushed during meals, he/she tends to become anxious, lose his/her appetite, and stop eating. Appetite is also suppressed if foods/fluids normally served hot or warm become cold and do not appeal to the client.

m. When the stomach becomes distended, its volume receptors stimulate the satiety center in the hypothalamus and the client reduces his/her oral intake. Drinking liquids with meals distends the stomach and may cause satiety before an adequate amount of food is consumed.

7. Ensure that meals are well balanced and high in essential nutrients. Offer dietary supplements if indicated.

7. The client must consume a diet that is well balanced and high in essential nutrients in order to meet his/her nutritional needs. Dietary supplements are often needed to help the client accomplish this.

8. Administer vitamins and minerals if ordered.

8. Vitamins and minerals are nutritional substances that are needed to maintain metabolic functioning. If the client's dietary intake does not provide adequate amounts of them, oral and/or parenteral supplements may be necessary.

9. Allow the client to assist in the selection of foods/fluids that meet nutritional needs. Obtain a dietary consult if necessary.

9. The client who is actively involved in menu planning is more likely to comply with the diet plan. In addition, the involvement increases his/her sense of control, which promotes a feeling of well-being and can lead to an increased oral intake. A dietitian is best able to evaluate whether the foods/fluids selected will meet the client's nutritional needs.

10. Perform a calorie count if ordered. Report information to dietitian and physician.

10. A calorie count provides information about the caloric and nutritional value of the foods/fluids the client consumes. The information obtained helps the dietitian and physician determine if an alternative method of nutritional support is needed.

11. Consult physician about an alternative method of providing nutrition (e.g. parenteral nutrition, tube feedings) if client does not consume enough food or fluids to meet nutritional needs.

11. If the client's oral intake is inadequate, an alternative method of providing nutrients needs to be implemented.

▶ Nursing Diagnosis: *Oral Mucous Membrane, Altered*

Definition

The state in which an individual experiences disruptions in the tissue layers of the oral cavity.

Defining Characteristics

Refer to Appendix.

Desired Outcome

The client will maintain a healthy oral cavity as evidenced by:
a. absence of inflammation and discomfort
b. pink, moist, intact mucosa.

Documentation

a. Client reports oral dryness and/or discomfort
b. Condition of oral mucous membrane
c. Therapeutic interventions
d. Client teaching

NURSING ACTIONS

Assessments

1. Assess client for signs and symptoms of altered oral mucous membrane (e.g. reports of oral dryness and discomfort, coated tongue, inflamed and/or ulcerated oral mucosa).
2. Culture oral lesions as ordered. Report positive results.

Prevention/Treatment

3. Instruct and assist client to perform oral hygiene as often as needed (e.g. after meals and at bedtime, at least every 2 hours if NPO).

4. Use a soft bristle brush, sponge-tipped applicator, or low-pressure power spray for oral hygiene if indicated.

5. Avoid use of mouthwashes containing alcohol and oral care products that contain lemon and glycerin.

6. Encourage client to rinse mouth frequently with water.

7. Lubricate client's lips frequently.

8. Encourage client to breathe through nose rather than mouth.

RATIONALES

1. Early recognition of signs and symptoms of altered oral mucous membrane allows for prompt intervention.

2. A positive culture reveals the organisms present in a lesion, which provides direction for the treatment plan.

3. Good oral hygiene helps maintain health of the oral mucous membrane by removing food particles and debris that harbor or promote the growth of bacteria that can cause inflammation and infection. Brushing the teeth also stimulates circulation to the gums, which helps maintain the integrity of the oral mucosa.

4. These devices are useful for removing food particles and debris from client's mouth without causing trauma to the oral mucous membrane.

5. Mouthwashes containing alcohol and oral care products containing lemon and glycerin have a drying and irritating effect on the oral mucous membrane. Excessive use of the lemon-glycerin products also increases acidity in the mouth, which results in further irritation of the oral mucosa.

6. Frequent rinsing of the mouth helps alleviate dryness, which reduces the risk for cracking and breakdown of the oral mucosa. Rinsing also helps prevent inflammation and infection in the mouth by removing food particles and debris that can harbor or promote the growth of organisms.

7. Lubricating the client's lips helps keep them moist, which helps maintain integrity of the lips.

8. Air inspired through the nose is humidified by the layer of mucus that coats the lining of the nasal cavity. Air inspired through the mouth lacks this moisture and is

9. Encourage client not to smoke.

9. Smoking dries and irritates the oral mucous membrane.

10. Encourage a fluid intake of at least 2500 ml/day unless contraindicated.

10. Adequate hydration helps keep the oral mucosa moist, which reduces the risk of cracking and breakdown.

11. Encourage client to suck on hard candy if allowed.

11. Sucking on hard candy stimulates salivation, which helps alleviate dryness of the oral mucosa and the subsequent risk of cracking and breakdown.

12. Encourage client to use artificial saliva if indicated.

12. Artificial saliva lubricates the oral mucous membrane in the absence of normal salivary flow. This helps reduce dryness and the subsequent risk of cracking and breakdown.

13. Assist client to select foods of moderate temperature and those that are soft and bland.

13. Foods that are extremely hot or cold; hard, crusty, or rough; spicy; and/or acidic may cause thermal, mechanical, or chemical trauma to the oral mucosa.

14. Encourage client to maintain an optimal nutritional status.

14. Adequate nutrition is needed to maintain the high cellular turnover of the oral mucous membrane. Good nutrition also promotes optimal function of the immune system, which reduces the client's risk of oral cavity infection.

15. Inspect client's dentures. Obtain a dental consult if dentures are rough, cracked, or ill-fitting.

15. Rough, cracked, or ill-fitting dentures can cause mechanical trauma to the oral mucosa. This can result in a decreased oral intake, which compromises the health of the oral mucosa.

16. Administer topical anesthetics, oral protective agents, analgesics, and antimicrobials if ordered.

16. Topical anesthetics, oral protective agents, and analgesics promote comfort if the oral mucous membrane is inflamed or if breakdown is present. The increased comfort can result in an improved oral intake, which helps maintain health of the oral mucosa. Antimicrobials prevent or treat infection of the oral mucosa.

17. Consult physician if dryness, irritation, discomfort, and/or breakdown of the oral cavity persist or worsen.

17. Notifying the physician allows for modification of the treatment plan.

▶ Nursing Diagnosis: *Pain*

Definition

An unpleasant sensory and emotional experience arising from actual or potential tissue damage or described in terms of such damage (International Association for the Study of Pain); sudden or slow onset of any intensity from mild to severe with an anticipated or predictable end and a duration of less than 6 months.

Defining Characteristics

Refer to Appendix.

Desired Outcome

The client will experience diminished pain as evidenced by:
a. verbalization of decrease in or absence of pain
b. relaxed facial expression and body positioning
c. increased participation in activities
d. stable vital signs.

Documentation

a. Verbal description of pain
b. Rating of pain intensity
c. Facial expression
d. Body movement and position
e. Vital signs
f. Participation in activities
g. Factors that precipitate, aggravate, and alleviate pain
h. Therapeutic interventions
i. Client/family teaching

NURSING ACTIONS

Assessments

1. Assess for signs and symptoms of pain (e.g. verbalization of pain, grimacing, reluctance to move, restlessness, diaphoresis, facial pallor, increased B/P, tachycardia).
2. Assess client's perception of the severity of pain using a pain intensity rating scale.

3. Assess the client's pain pattern (e.g. location, quality, onset, duration, precipitating factors, aggravating factors, alleviating factors).
4. Ask the client to describe previous pain experiences and methods used to manage pain effectively.

Prevention/Treatment

5. Implement measures to reduce fear and anxiety (e.g. assure client that his/her need for pain relief is understood, plan methods for achieving pain control with client, provide a calm environment).
6. Implement measures to promote rest (e.g. minimize environmental activity and noise).

RATIONALES

1. Early recognition of signs and symptoms of pain allows for prompt intervention and improved pain control.

2. An awareness of the severity of pain being experienced helps determine the most appropriate intervention(s) for pain management. Use of a pain intensity rating scale provides as objective a description as possible for a subjective experience. This gives the nurse a clearer understanding of the pain being experienced and promotes consistency when communicating with others about the client's pain experience.
3. Knowledge of the client's pain pattern assists in the identification of effective pain management interventions.

4. Many variables affect a client's response to pain (e.g. age, sex, coping style, previous experience with pain, culture, cause of pain). An understanding of the client's usual response to pain enables the nurse to evaluate the client's pain more accurately and facilitates the identification of effective strategies for pain management.

5. Fear and anxiety can decrease the client's threshold and tolerance for pain and thereby heighten the perception of pain. In addition, pain management methods are not as effective if the client is tense and unable to relax.
6. Fatigue can decrease the client's threshold and tolerance for pain and thereby heighten the perception of pain. If the client is well rested, he/she often experiences decreased pain and increased effectiveness of pain management measures.

7. Administer analgesics before activities and procedures that can cause pain and before pain becomes severe.

7. The administration of analgesics before a pain-producing event helps minimize the pain that will be experienced. Analgesics are also more effective if given before pain becomes severe because mild to moderate pain is controlled more quickly and effectively than severe pain.

8. Provide or assist with nonpharmacologic methods for pain relief. Examples include:
   a. cutaneous stimulation measures (e.g. pressure, massage, heat and cold applications, transcutaneous electrical nerve stimulation [TENS], acupuncture)
   b. relaxation techniques (e.g. progressive relaxation exercises, meditation, guided imagery)
   c. distraction measures (e.g. listening to music, conversing, watching television, playing cards, reading)
   d. position change.

8. Nonpharmacologic pain management includes a variety of interventions. It is believed that most of these are effective because they stimulate closure of the gating mechanism in the spinal cord and subsequently block the transmission of pain impulses. In addition, some interventions are thought to stimulate the release of endogenous analgesics (e.g. endorphins) that inhibit the transmission of pain impulses and/or alter the client's perception of pain. Many of the nonpharmacologic interventions also help decrease pain by promoting relaxation.

9. Administer the following analgesics as ordered:

   a. opioid (narcotic) analgesics

   b. nonopioid (nonnarcotic) analgesics such as salicylates, acetaminophen, and nonsteroidal anti-inflammatory agents.

9. Pharmacologic therapy is an effective method of reducing or relieving pain.
   a. Opioid analgesics act mainly by altering the client's perception of pain and his/her emotional response to the pain experience.
   b. Nonopioid analgesics are thought to interfere with the transmission of pain impulses by inhibiting prostaglandin synthesis.

10. Consult physician about an order for patient-controlled analgesia (PCA) if indicated.

10. The use of PCA allows the client to self-administer analgesics within parameters established by the physician. This method facilitates pain management by ensuring prompt administration of drug when needed, providing more continuous pain relief, and increasing the client's control over the pain.

11. Consult physician if above measures fail to provide adequate pain relief.

11. Notifying the physician allows for modification of the treatment plan.

▶ Nursing Diagnosis: *Self-Concept Disturbance*

This diagnostic label includes the nursing diagnoses of body image disturbance, self-esteem disturbance, and altered role performance.

Definitions

Body Image Disturbance: Disruption in the way one perceives one's body image.

Self-Esteem Disturbance: Negative self-evaluation/feelings about self or self-capabilities, which may be directly or indirectly expressed.

Altered Role Performance: Disruption in the way one perceives one's role performance.

Defining Characteristics

Refer to Appendix.

Desired Outcome

The client will demonstrate beginning adaptation to changes in appearance, level of independence, body functioning, life style, and roles as evidenced by:
a. verbalization of feelings of self-worth
b. maintenance of relationships with significant others
c. active participation in activities of daily living
d. verbalization of a beginning plan for adapting life style to changes resulting from the injury or disease and/or its treatment.

Documentation

a. Verbalization about changes that have occurred
b. Interactions with significant others
c. Reaction of significant others to changes in client's body functioning and/or appearance
d. Participation in activities of daily living
e. Client/family teaching
f. Referrals to community agencies

NURSING ACTIONS

Assessments

1. Assess for signs and symptoms of a self-concept disturbance (e.g. verbalization of negative feelings about self, refusal to look at or touch a body part, withdrawal from significant others, lack of participation in activities of daily living, lack of plan for adapting to necessary changes in life style).
2. Determine the meaning of the change in body image and/or functioning to the client by encouraging the verbalization of feelings and by noting nonverbal responses to changes experienced.

Prevention/Treatment

3. Implement measures to assist client through the beginning phases of grieving (e.g. shock, disbelief, denial, anger, sadness, depression).

4. Discuss with client improvements in appearance and/or body functioning that can realistically be expected.

5. Implement measures to assist client to increase self-esteem (e.g. limit negative self-assessment, encourage positive comments about self, assist to identify strengths, give positive feedback

RATIONALES

1. Early recognition of signs and symptoms of self-concept disturbance allows for prompt intervention.

2. An understanding of what the change means to the client provides a basis for planning care.

3. A change in appearance, body functioning, and/or role can initiate a grieving response. Successful resolution of grief assists the client to accept changes experienced and integrate the changes into self-concept.
4. Realistic expectations about appearance and/or body functioning facilitate goal setting and are essential for positive adaptation to the changes experienced and integration of these changes into self-concept.
5. Self-esteem is a major component of one's view of self. It is a product of self-evaluation, reflected appraisals, social expectations, and perceptions of personal competence. An increase

about accomplishments and behaviors that are indicative of high self-esteem).

6. Assist client to identify and use coping techniques that have been helpful in the past.

7. Implement measures to assist client to adjust to alteration(s) in sexual functioning if appropriate (e.g. encourage questions and discussion about changes experienced, facilitate communication between client and his/her partner, discuss ways to be creative in expressing sexuality).

8. Implement measures to assist client to adapt to changes in body functioning and/or appearance (e.g. instruct in use of assistive devices, assist with clothing selection that minimizes changes in body contour).

9. Assist client with usual grooming and makeup habits if necessary.

10. Promote activities that require client to confront the body changes that have occurred (e.g. exercise, grooming, bathing). Be aware that the integration of changes in body image do not usually occur until 2–6 months after the actual physical change has occurred.

11. Demonstrate acceptance of client with techniques such as touch and frequent visits. Encourage significant others to do the same.

12. Support behaviors suggesting positive adaptation to changes that have occurred (e.g. willingness to care for wounds, compliance with treatment plan, verbalization of feelings of self-worth, maintenance of relationships with significant others).

13. Encourage significant others to allow client to do what he/she is able.

14. Encourage client contact with others if a change in appearance

---

in self-esteem has a positive effect on the client's self-concept.

6. Coping techniques help the client to manage or reduce the anxiety and stress that result when changes in appearance and/or body functioning occur. This reduction in anxiety and stress facilitates adaptation to these changes and development of a positive self-concept.

7. Sexual functioning is an important component of one's sense of self. Assistance may be necessary to help the client adjust to changes experienced and/or identify alternative ways of sexual expression.

8. Measures that help minimize changes in appearance and/or body functioning reduce the impact of these changes on self-concept.

9. Appearance is an essential component of self-esteem and one's concept of self. Maintaining an appearance he/she is comfortable with has a positive effect on the client's self-concept.

10. Activities that require the client to acknowledge and deal with the changes that have occurred in his/her body facilitate the incorporation of the changes into the brain's schemata of the body.

11. Frequent visits and the use of touch convey a feeling of acceptance to the client. This enhances his/her feelings of self-worth and assists in the development of a positive self-concept.

12. Supporting behaviors indicative of positive adaptation to changes encourages the client to repeat these behaviors. Repetition of positive adaptive behaviors facilitates the development of a positive self-concept.

13. Allowing the client to do as much as he/she is able facilitates the re-establishment of independence, which enhances feelings of self-esteem.

14. Feedback from others is often a critical factor in the development

NURSING ACTIONS
Prevention/Treatment—*cont'd*

RATIONALES

and body functioning has occurred.

of one's self-image. When a change in appearance and/or body functioning has occurred, contact with others provides the client with the opportunity to obtain feedback, test and establish a new self-image, and begin to adapt to the changes that have occurred.

15. Assist client's and significant others' adjustment by listening, facilitating communication, and providing information.

15. Listening, facilitating communication, and providing information assist the client and significant others to cope with the present situation. Effective coping facilitates their integration of the changes that have occurred.

16. Assist client and significant others to have similar expectations and understanding of future life style and to identify ways that personal and family goals can be adjusted rather than abandoned.

16. Congruent expectations of client and significant others facilitates their working together to meet common goals. Adjustment, rather than abandonment, of personal and family goals reduces the feeling of loss and increases the probability of positive adaptation to the changes that have occurred.

17. Teach client the rationale for treatments, encourage maximum participation in treatment regimen, and allow choices whenever possible.

17. An understanding of the reasons for treatments, active participation in treatment regimen, and the opportunity to make choices on one's behalf enable the client to maintain a sense of control, which enhances his/her self-esteem.

18. Encourage client to pursue usual roles and interests and to continue involvement in social activities. If previous roles, interests, and hobbies cannot be pursued, encourage development of new ones.

18. The ability to pursue usual roles and activities has a positive effect on the client's self-esteem. The same effect can be achieved if the client is successful in new roles and activities that he/she chooses.

19. Provide information about and encourage use of community agencies and support groups (e.g. vocational rehabilitation; sexual, family, individual, and/or financial counseling).

19. Community agencies and support groups provide the opportunity for the client to see that he/she is not experiencing a unique problem, to share feelings and concerns, to profit from the experience of others with similar difficulties, and to learn new skills necessary to rebuild self-esteem. All of these factors help the client to establish a positive self-concept.

20. Consult physician about psychological counseling if client desires or if he/she seems unwilling or unable to adapt to changes resulting from the disease process and/or its treatment.

20. Psychological counseling may be necessary to facilitate positive adaptation to the changes in appearance and/or body functioning that have occurred.

▶ Nursing Diagnosis: *Skin Integrity, Impaired, Risk for*

Definition

A state in which the individual's skin is at risk of being adversely altered.

Defining Characteristics

Refer to Appendix.

Desired Outcome

The client will maintain skin integrity as evidenced by:

a. absence of redness and irritation

b. no skin breakdown.

NURSING ACTIONS

Assessments

1. Inspect the skin (especially bony prominences, dependent areas, pruritic areas, perineum, and areas of decreased sensation and/or edema) for pallor, redness, and breakdown.

Prevention

2. Implement measures to prevent prolonged and/or excessive pressure on any area of the skin:
   a. assist client to turn at least every 2 hours unless contraindicated
   b. instruct or assist client to shift weight at least every 30 minutes
   c. position client properly using supportive devices such as pillows and pads as needed
   d. keep bed linens wrinkle-free
   e. ensure that external devices such as braces, casts, and restraints are applied properly
   f. use pressure-reducing or pressure-relieving devices (e.g. gel or foam cushions, alternating pressure mattress, air-fluidized bed) if indicated.

3. Gently massage around reddened areas at least every 2 hours.

4. Implement measures to prevent shearing:

   a. perform actions to keep skin from adhering to the bottom sheet when client moves (e.g. apply thin layer of cornstarch to bottom sheet or skin, lift and move client carefully using turn sheet and adequate assistance)
   b. limit length of time client is in semi-Fowler's position to 30-minute intervals.

Documentation

a. Appearance of skin

b. Therapeutic interventions

c. Client/family teaching

RATIONALES

1. Early recognition of signs of impaired skin integrity allows for prompt intervention.

2. Prolonged and/or excessive pressure on the skin obstructs capillary blood flow to that area. The resultant hypoxia, impaired flow of nutrients, and accumulation of waste products in the area of obstructed blood flow make that tissue more susceptible to breakdown. Measures that prevent the excessive pressure or ensure that pressure is relieved often enough to avoid obstruction of capillary flow help maintain skin integrity.

3. Massage stimulates circulation to the skin and underlying tissues. The improved blood flow helps maintain skin integrity by increasing the supply of oxygen and nutrients available to the cells and by removing waste products of metabolism. To avoid damaging the capillaries, massage should be gentle rather than deep and massage over reddened areas should be avoided.

4. When shearing (one tissue layer sliding past another in an opposite direction) occurs, the capillaries in the affected area are kinked, stretched, or severed. This compromises the area's blood supply and increases the risk of tissue breakdown.
   a. Keeping the skin from adhering to the sheet when the client changes position ensures that the skin and underlying tissue move in the same direction as the client moves.

   b. A client in a semi-Fowler's position often slides down in the bed. When this occurs, his/

NURSING ACTIONS
Prevention—*cont'd*

RATIONALES

her skin tends to remain stationary while the underlying tissues and skeletal structures shift position.

5. Implement measures to reduce friction between the skin and another surface (e.g. place sheepskin under client, apply thin layer of cornstarch to bottom sheet or client's skin, lift and move client carefully using turn sheet and adequate assistance, adequately secure restraints and tubings, pat skin dry rather than rub).

5. The outermost layers of skin can be damaged when dragged along or rubbed against another surface. Reducing friction helps prevent skin surface irritation and abrasion.

6. Keep client's skin clean.

6. Microorganisms are present in sebum and dead skin cells. Keeping the skin clean removes many of these microorganisms, which, if allowed to accumulate, increase the risk of irritation or infection and subsequent skin breakdown.

7. Implement measures to keep skin free of excessive moisture:
   a. apply a thin layer of cornstarch to bottom sheet or skin and to opposing skin surfaces
   b. keep bed linens dry
   c. protect skin surrounding wound from drainage (e.g. change dressing when damp, apply a drainage collection device if needed).

7. Excessive moisture on the skin or prolonged exposure of the skin to moisture softens the epidermal cells and makes them less resistant to damage. Moisture also harbors microorganisms that can cause irritation or infection, and it increases the possibility of friction between the skin and the surface it is against. Removing excessive moisture and protecting the skin from prolonged contact with moisture reduces the risk of skin irritation and subsequent breakdown.

8. Increase activity as allowed and tolerated.

8. Activity stimulates circulation, which helps maintain skin integrity by increasing the flow of oxygen and nutrients to the skin and underlying tissues. In addition, increasing activity reduces the possibility of prolonged pressure on any area as a result of decreased mobility.

9. Maintain an optimal nutritional status.

9. An inadequate nutritional status results in muscle atrophy, a decrease in the amount of subcutaneous tissue, and skin that is thin and less elastic. Subsequently, the skin and tissue are more vulnerable to injury because they are less able to withstand minor trauma. In addition, a malnourished client is more susceptible to the effects of pressure because there is less padding between the skin and underlying bone.

10. Implement measures to prevent drying of the skin:

    a. encourage a fluid intake of 2500 ml/day unless contraindicated

10. Dry skin is more prone to cracking and has decreased elasticity, which make it susceptible to damage.

    a. An adequate fluid intake helps ensure that the skin remains well hydrated.

b. provide a mild soap for bathing

b. Sebum has a lubricating effect on the skin. Using a mild rather than a harsh soap allows some sebum to remain on the skin, which helps prevent dryness.

c. apply a moisturizing lotion and/or emollient to skin at least once a day.

c. Moisturizing lotion and some emollients provide a source of moisture to the skin. Emollients also form a protective barrier on the epidermis, which reduces the evaporation of moisture.

11. Protect skin from contact with urine and feces (e.g. perform actions to prevent incontinence and/or diarrhea, keep perineal area clean and dry, apply a protective ointment or cream to perineal area).

11. The moisture in urine and feces softens epidermal cells and increases friction between opposing skin surfaces and between the skin and bed linen. In addition, the normal acidity of urine and the digestive enzymes present in feces irritate the skin.

12. If edema is present, handle edematous areas carefully and implement measures to reduce fluid accumulation in dependent areas (e.g. instruct client in and assist with range of motion exercises, elevate affected extremities whenever possible).

12. Edematous areas have an increased risk for skin breakdown because the oxygen and nutrient supply to the skin is compromised by the increased distance that exists between the capillaries and the cells. Handling edematous areas carefully and implementing measures to reduce edema decrease the risk for skin breakdown.

13. If the client is experiencing pruritus, implement measures to reduce the itching sensation (e.g. apply cool compress to pruritic area, administer prescribed antihistamines), keep his/her nails trimmed, and apply mittens if necessary.

13. The client experiencing pruritus is likely to scratch the affected areas, which irritates the skin and can cause excoriation. Implementing measures to reduce the itching sensation helps prevent scratching. Trimming the client's nails and applying mittens if necessary reduces the risk of trauma to the skin if he/she does scratch the pruritic areas.

14. Notify physician if skin breakdown occurs.

14. Notifying the physician allows for modification of treatment plan.

▶ Nursing Diagnosis: *Sleep Pattern Disturbance*

Definition

Disruption of sleep time causes discomfort or interferes with desired life style.

Defining Characteristics

Refer to Appendix.

Desired Outcome

The client will attain optimal amounts of sleep as evidenced by:
a. statements of feeling well rested
b. usual mental status
c. absence of frequent yawning, dark circles under eyes, and hand tremors.

Documentation

a. Statements of difficulty falling asleep, interruptions in sleep, and/ or not feeling well rested
b. Mental status
c. Frequent yawning
d. Presence of dark circles under eyes or hand tremors
e. Therapeutic interventions
f. Client teaching

NURSING ACTIONS
Assessments

1. Assess for signs and symptoms of a sleep pattern disturbance (e.g. statements of difficulty falling asleep, sleep interruptions, or not feeling well rested; irritability; lethargy; disorientation; frequent yawning; dark circles under eyes; slight hand tremors).
2. Determine client's usual sleep habits.

Prevention/Treatment

3. Discourage long periods of sleep during the day unless signs and symptoms of sleep deprivation exist or daytime sleep is usual for client.

4. Implement measures to reduce fear and anxiety (e.g. maintain a calm, confident manner when working with client; assist client to identify specific stressors and ways to cope with them).

5. Encourage participation in relaxing diversional activities during the evening.
6. Discourage intake of fluids high in caffeine (e.g. coffee, tea, colas), especially in the evening.

7. Offer client an evening snack that includes milk or cheese unless contraindicated.

8. Allow client to continue usual sleep practices (e.g. position; time; presleep routines such as reading, watching television, listening to music, and meditating) unless contraindicated.
9. Satisfy basic needs such as comfort and warmth before sleep.

10. Encourage client to urinate just before bedtime.

RATIONALES

1. Early recognition of signs and symptoms of a sleep pattern disturbance allows for prompt intervention.

2. Knowledge of the client's usual sleep-wake cycle and the routines that help induce and maintain his/her sleep helps the nurse plan interventions aimed at preventing a sleep pattern disturbance.

3. Long periods of sleep during the day are often a change in the client's usual sleep-wake cycle and cause desynchronization of his/her circadian rhythm. This can result in a poorer quality of sleep.
4. Fear and anxiety stimulate the sympathetic nervous system, which increases alertness and makes it difficult for the client to fall asleep. Sympathetic nervous system stimulation is also believed to shorten the duration of nonrapid eye movement (NREM) and rapid eye movement (REM) sleep, which results in a poorer quality of sleep.
5. Involvement in relaxing activities in the evening helps the client fall asleep more easily.
6. Caffeine acts as a central nervous system stimulant and can interfere with relaxation and subsequent sleep induction. Caffeine also acts as a diuretic, which can cause an interruption in sleep if the client awakens in response to the urge to urinate.
7. Foods/fluids such as milk and cheese contain the amino acid L-tryptophan, which is believed to help induce and maintain sleep.
8. Adherence to usual sleep practices promotes mental and physical relaxation that assists the client to maintain his/her usual sleep-wake cycle.

9. When basic needs are met, the client is usually more comfortable and better able to relax. This facilitates sleep induction and reduces the probability of frequent awakenings.
10. A full bladder stimulates an urge to urinate, which can interrupt

11. Reduce environmental distractions (e.g. close door to client's room; use night light rather than overhead light whenever possible; lower volume of paging system; keep staff conversations at a low level and away from client's room; close curtains between clients in a semi-private room or ward; keep beepers and alarms on low volume; provide client with "white noise" such as a fan, soft music, or tape-recorded sounds of the ocean or rain; have sleep mask and earplugs available for client if needed).

12. If client has orthopnea, assist him/her to assume a position that facilitates breathing (e.g. head of bed elevated with arms supported on pillows, resting forward on overbed table with good pillow support, sitting in a chair) and maintain oxygen therapy during sleep.

13. Administer prescribed sedative-hypnotics if indicated.

14. Implement measures to reduce interruptions during sleep (e.g. restrict visitors, group care whenever possible) so that client is able to sleep undisturbed for 80- to 100-minute intervals.

15. Consult physician if signs and symptoms of sleep deprivation persist or worsen.

---

the client's sleep. Emptying the bladder just before bedtime reduces the risk of the client awakening more frequently and/or earlier than desired.

11. Environmental activity, noise, and light can interfere with the client's ability to fall asleep and stay asleep. Reducing stimuli helps prevent a sleep pattern disturbance.

12. Hypoxemia stimulates the client's arousal system and can make it difficult for him/her to fall asleep and stay asleep. Proper positioning and administration of supplemental oxygen help ease breathing efforts and reduce hypoxemia, which makes it easier for the client to fall asleep and reduces the number of awakenings.

13. Sedative-hypnotics are central nervous system depressants that promote sleep by reducing anxiety, shortening sleep induction, and/or reducing arousal level (wakefulness). These medications should be used for only a short time because they interfere with the length of REM sleep and can actually create a disturbance in the client's sleep-wake cycle.

14. One sleep cycle takes about 80–100 minutes to complete. Each time the cycle is interrupted, it begins again with NREM stage 1 sleep so the client loses portions of NREM and/or REM sleep. When the client is deprived of NREM sleep, lethargy and depression occur. Loss of REM sleep results in irritability and anxiety. Reducing the frequency of sleep interruptions helps ensure that the client progresses through all of the sleep stages and does not experience a sleep pattern disturbance.

15. Notifying the physician allows for modification of treatment plan.

▶ Nursing Diagnosis: *Swallowing, Impaired*

Definition

The state in which an individual has decreased ability to voluntarily pass fluids and/or solids from the mouth to the stomach.

Defining Characteristics

Refer to Appendix.

Desired Outcome

The client will experience an improvement in swallowing as evidenced by:
a. verbalization of same
b. absence of food in oral cavity after swallowing
c. absence of coughing and choking when eating and drinking.

Documentation

a. Verbalization of difficulty swallowing
b. Stasis of food in oral cavity
c. Coughing or choking when eating or drinking
d. Consistency of foods/fluids client is able to swallow without difficulty
e. Therapeutic interventions
f. Client/family teaching

NURSING ACTIONS

Assessments

1. Assess for signs and symptoms of impaired swallowing (e.g. statements of difficulty swallowing, stasis of food in oral cavity, coughing or choking when eating or drinking).
2. Assist with tests to evaluate client's swallowing (e.g. videofluoroscopy, manometry) if ordered.

Prevention/Treatment

3. Implement measures to reduce oral and pharyngeal discomfort if indicated (e.g. instruct client to gargle with a saline solution, administer topical and/or systemic analgesics as ordered).
4. If client has viscous oral secretions, implement measures to liquefy these secretions (e.g. encourage a fluid intake of 2500 ml/day unless contraindicated, administer a papain product before meals as ordered).

5. If client's mouth is dry, implement measures to stimulate salivation (e.g. provide oral care before meals, give client a piece of hard candy to suck on just before meals).

RATIONALES

1. Early recognition of signs and symptoms of impaired swallowing allows for prompt intervention.

2. Swallowing is a complex act that consists of voluntary and involuntary neuromotor components. Studies that evaluate the client's ability to swallow help identify the specific physiological dysfunction, which aids in planning effective interventions.

3. Oral and pharyngeal discomfort can interfere with the client's ability to chew and move the foods/fluids to the back of the mouth.

4. Thick, ropy oral secretions interfere with movement of food in the mouth. Liquefying these secretions makes it easier for a bolus of food to be formed and moved to the back of the mouth. Liquefying the secretions also helps ensure that the bolus that is formed is moist so that it stays intact and triggers an effective swallowing reflex.

5. Saliva lubricates food, which makes it easier to chew, form into a bolus, and manipulate toward the back of the mouth. A formed, moist bolus more effectively triggers the swallowing reflex and moves more easily through the esophagus.

6. Consult speech pathologist about methods for dealing with client's specific swallowing impairment.

7. Instruct and assist client to select foods/fluids that are appropriate for his/her swallowing ability. Some general guidelines include:

    a. avoiding foods that tend to fall apart in mouth (e.g. applesauce, cake, muffins) and those that consist of small food particles (e.g. rice, peas, nuts) if client has impaired tongue control

    b. avoiding foods that are sticky (e.g. peanut butter, soft bread, honey)

    c. moistening dry foods with gravy or sauces (e.g. catsup, sour cream, salad dressing)

    d. selecting thick rather than thin fluids or adding a thickening agent (e.g. "Thick-it," gelatin, baby cereal) if client has a delayed swallowing reflex and/or poor tongue control.

8. Place client in a high Fowler's position for meals and snacks unless contraindicated.

9. If client has difficulty chewing and maneuvering a bolus of food to the back of the mouth, instruct him/her to tilt head down when chewing and forming a bolus, then tilt head back when ready to swallow.

10. Serve foods/fluids that are hot or cold instead of room temperature.

6. Consulting with persons who are knowledgeable about the management of swallowing difficulties aids in the development of an individualized plan of care to improve the client's swallowing.

7. Impaired swallowing can result from structural or neurological problems. The types of foods/fluids a client can swallow effectively varies depending on his/her particular swallowing difficulty.

    a. Clients with impaired tongue movement have difficulty keeping foods that tend to fall apart in the mouth or consist of small pieces in a bolus that can be transferred to the back of the mouth. Some small pieces of food may fall to the back of the mouth, but because the food is not in a bolus, it will not trigger a strong swallowing reflex.

    b. Sticky foods are difficult to propel through the mouth because they tend to adhere to various structures, especially the hard palate. It is also difficult to form these foods into the distinct bolus needed to trigger the swallowing reflex.

    c. Moist foods are more easily formed into a bolus and moved through the mouth and esophagus.

    d. Thin fluids pass rapidly through the mouth and can pour over the back of the tongue without triggering an effective swallow. Thick fluids remain more cohesive and are able to stimulate the swallowing reflex more effectively.

8. A high Fowler's position uses gravity to aid in the flow of foods/fluids through the esophagus.

9. Tilting the head down allows client more time to chew and form a bolus because the food is in the front of the mouth where it does not trigger the swallowing reflex. Tilting the head back facilitates movement of the bolus to the back of the mouth so that the swallowing reflex can be triggered. NOTE: Tilting head back is safe only if the client is unlikely to aspirate.

10. Foods/fluids that are hot or cold trigger a more effective swallowing reflex because they have a greater stimulatory effect

NURSING ACTIONS
Prevention/Treatment—*cont'd*

RATIONALES

on the sensory receptors in the mouth.

11. Instruct and assist client to use assistive devices such as a long-handled spoon to place food that does not need to be chewed (e.g. gelatin, mashed potatoes, custard) in the back of his/her mouth if tongue movement is impaired.

11. The swallowing reflex is triggered when a bolus of food is pressed against the posterior wall of the mouth. Placing food that can be swallowed safely without chewing in the back of the mouth facilitates swallowing if the client is unable to effectively move food posteriorly with his/her tongue.

12. If client has motor and sensory dysfunction of one side of the mouth or face, instruct and assist him/her to tilt head toward the unaffected side when eating and drinking and to place food in the unaffected side of the mouth.

12. When foods/fluids are directed toward the unaffected side of the mouth, the client is able to more effectively chew and use his/her tongue to form a bolus and move it to the back of the mouth. The unaffected side of the mouth also has more tension in the buccal musculature so foods/fluids are more likely to get to the back of the mouth rather than collect between the cheek and the mandible. Sensory receptors on the unaffected side also trigger a stronger swallowing reflex than those on the affected side.

13. Encourage client to concentrate on the act of swallowing.

13. The client can achieve a more effective swallow by focusing on chewing and moving foods/fluids to the back of the mouth where the swallowing reflex is triggered.

14. Instruct client to avoid putting too much food/fluid in mouth at one time.

14. Overfilling the mouth makes it difficult for the client to form a distinct bolus and effectively move it along to the back of the mouth where it triggers the swallowing reflex.

15. Encourage client to perform exercises to strengthen tongue and facial muscles if indicated (e.g. drinking through a straw; opening mouth and moving tongue anteriorly, posteriorly, and laterally; pushing tongue upward against resistance using an object such as a tongue blade, popsicle, or sucker).

15. Strong tongue and facial muscles increase the client's ability to chew food, form a bolus, and direct the bolus to the back of the mouth, where it triggers the swallowing reflex.

16. Consult physician if swallowing difficulties persist or worsen.

16. Notifying the physician allows for modification of treatment plan.

▶ Nursing Diagnosis: *Tissue Perfusion, Altered*

NANDA identifies five types of altered tissue perfusion (renal, cerebral, cardiopulmonary, gastrointestinal, peripheral). A client can experience more than one type of altered tissue perfusion and the actions for the various types are often similar. The information presented here focuses on altered tissue perfusion in general rather than a specific type.

Definition

The state in which an individual experiences a decrease in nutrition and oxygenation at the cellular level due to a deficit in capillary blood supply.

Defining Characteristics

Refer to Appendix.

Desired Outcome

The client will maintain adequate systemic tissue perfusion as evidenced by:
a. B/P within normal range
b. usual mental status
c. extremities warm with absence of pallor and cyanosis
d. palpable peripheral pulses
e. capillary refill time less than 3 seconds
f. absence of edema
g. absence of exercise-induced pain
h. urine output at least 30 ml/hour.

Documentation

a. Blood pressure
b. Mental status
c. Skin color and temperature
d. Peripheral pulses
e. Capillary refill time
f. Presence of edema
g. Exercise-induced pain
h. Urine output
i. Therapeutic interventions
j. Client teaching

NURSING ACTIONS

Assessments

1. Assess for and report signs and symptoms of diminished tissue perfusion (e.g. hypotension, restlessness, confusion, cool extremities, pallor or cyanosis of extremities, diminished or absent peripheral pulses, slow capillary refill, edema, claudication, angina, oliguria).

Prevention/Treatment

2. Administer intravenous fluids and/or blood if ordered.

3. Maintain a minimum fluid intake of 2500 ml/day unless contraindicated.

4. Instruct client to change from a supine to an upright position slowly if he/she has postural hypotension.

5. Discourage positions such as crossing legs, pillows under knees, and use of knee gatch.
6. Encourage client to avoid sitting or standing for prolonged periods.
7. If client is on bed rest, instruct and assist with range of motion exercises at least 3 times/day and active foot and leg exercises every 1–2 hours. Elevate foot of bed for 20-minute intervals several times/shift unless contraindicated.

8. If client's activity is limited and/or venous insufficiency is a

RATIONALES

1. Early recognition and reporting of signs and symptoms of diminished tissue perfusion allow for prompt intervention.

2. Intravenous fluids and/or blood help maintain vascular volume, which is essential for adequate tissue perfusion.
3. Adequate hydration is essential for maintenance of a vascular volume sufficient to maintain adequate tissue perfusion.
4. Changing from a supine to a sitting or standing position slowly allows time for the baroreceptors to adjust to an upright position and thereby helps keep the blood pressure at a level sufficient to maintain adequate tissue perfusion.
5. These positions exert pressure on vessels in the lower extremities, which compromises blood flow.
6. Prolonged sitting or standing causes venous stasis.
7. When a client is on bed rest, blood pools in the extremities as a result of decreased muscle activity. Range of motion exercises help reduce venous stasis. The rhythmic muscle contractions that occur during active foot and leg exercises cause intermittent compression of the veins, which improves venous return. Elevation of the lower extremities promotes venous return by gravity flow.
8. Elastic stockings and sequential compression devices promote

NURSING ACTIONS
Prevention/Treatment—*cont'd*

problem, consult physician about an order for elastic stockings or a sequential compression device.

9. Encourage and assist client with ambulation as soon as allowed and tolerated.

10. Implement measures to improve cardiac output (e.g. administer positive inotropic agents, vasodilators, and/or antiarrhythmics if ordered; promote rest) if decreased cardiac output is contributing to inadequate tissue perfusion.

11. Implement measures to prevent vasoconstriction:

    a. perform actions to reduce stress

    b. discourage smoking

    c. perform actions to keep client from getting cold (e.g. maintain a comfortable room temperature, provide adequate clothing and blankets).

12. Consult physician if signs and symptoms of diminished tissue perfusion persist or worsen.

RATIONALES

venous return by exerting either a constant pressure or an intermittent pumping effect on the vessels in the lower extremities.

9. Ambulation causes rhythmic contractions of the leg muscles. This creates a pumping effect on the leg veins, which subsequently increases venous return.

10. Improved cardiac output enhances tissue perfusion by increasing arterial and venous blood flow.

11. Vasoconstriction narrows vessel lumens, which results in diminished blood flow through the affected vessels. Vasoconstriction may also increase afterload, which can decrease cardiac output and systemic tissue perfusion.

    a. Stress stimulates the sympathetic nervous system, which results in vasoconstriction.

    b. Nicotine increases catecholamine output, which subsequently causes vasoconstriction.

    c. When the body is cold, peripheral vasoconstriction occurs in an attempt to contain body heat.

12. Notifying the physician allows for modification of treatment plan.

▶ Nursing Diagnosis: *Urinary Elimination, Altered: Incontinence*

NANDA identifies five types of urinary incontinence (stress, reflex, urge, functional, and total). A client can experience a combination of types of incontinence and the actions for various types often are similar. The information presented here focuses on incontinence in general rather than a specific type.

Definition

The state in which the individual experiences an involuntary loss or passage of urine.

Defining Characteristics

Refer to Appendix.

Desired Outcome

The client will experience urinary continence.

NURSING ACTIONS

Assessments

1. Assess for and report urinary incontinence.

2. Monitor client's patterns of fluid intake and urination (e.g. times and amounts of fluid intake, types of fluids consumed, times and amounts of voluntary and involuntary voiding, reports of sensation of need to void, activities preceding incontinence).

3. Assist with urodynamic studies (e.g. cystometrogram) if ordered.

Prevention/Treatment

4. Offer bedpan or urinal or assist client to bedside commode or bathroom every 2–4 hours if indicated.

5. Allow client to assume a normal position for voiding (usually sitting for females and standing for males) unless contraindicated.

6. Implement measures to reduce delays in toileting (e.g. have call signal within client's reach and respond promptly to requests for assistance; have bedpan, urinal, or bedside commode readily available to client; provide easy access to bathroom; provide client with easy-to-remove clothing such as pajamas with Velcro closures or an elastic waistband).

7. Instruct client to perform pelvic muscle exercises (e.g. stopping and starting stream during voiding; squeezing buttocks together, then relaxing the muscles) if appropriate.

8. Instruct client to space fluids evenly throughout the day rather than drinking a large quantity at one time.

9. Limit oral fluid intake in the evening.

Documentation

a. Episodes of urinary incontinence
b. Statements of being unable to control urinary elimination
c. Therapeutic interventions
d. Client teaching

RATIONALES

1. Early recognition and reporting of urinary incontinence allow for prompt intervention.

2. Knowledge of the client's fluid intake and urination patterns assists in the identification of factors that may be causing or contributing to urinary incontinence. This information helps the nurse plan individualized interventions that promote urinary continence.

3. Urodynamic studies may be done to determine the cause(s) of urinary incontinence. The studies provide information about bladder filling, capacity, and emptying.

4. Urinary incontinence occurs when the pressure within the bladder becomes greater than the pressure exerted by the urinary sphincters. Emptying the bladder before the pressure becomes too great reduces the risk of incontinence.

5. A sitting or standing position uses gravity to facilitate bladder emptying. The more completely the bladder is emptied, the less risk there is of incontinence.

6. If client is having difficulty controlling urination, any delay in toileting increases the risk of incontinence. Measures that assist the client to use a bedpan, urinal, bedside commode, or toilet in a timely manner help reduce the risk of incontinence.

7. Pelvic muscle exercises help strengthen the pelvic floor muscles and improve the tone of the external urinary sphincter. As this is achieved, the risk for incontinence decreases.

8. Drinking a large amount of fluid at one time results in rapid filling of the bladder, which increases bladder pressure and the subsequent risk of incontinence.

9. As the client's bladder fills and bladder pressure increases during sleep, he/she is less likely to be

NURSING ACTIONS
Prevention/Treatment—*cont'd*

RATIONALES

aware of and/or able to respond to the urge to urinate. By limiting fluid intake in the evening, bladder filling during the night is decreased, which reduces the risk of incontinence.

10. Instruct client to avoid drinking beverages containing caffeine such as colas, coffee, and tea.

10. Caffeinated beverages increase urine formation because of their mild diuretic effect. With increased urine formation, bladder filling increases, causing a rise in pressure in the bladder, which subsequently increases the risk of incontinence. Caffeine also acts as a chemical irritant to the bladder and contributes to urge incontinence.

11. Administer the following medications if ordered:
   a. cholinergics (e.g. bethanechol)

11. a. If incontinence results from incomplete bladder emptying, cholinergic drugs may be prescribed to stimulate contraction of the detrusor muscle (smooth muscle of the bladder). This enhances bladder emptying and reduces the risk of incontinence.

   b. muscle relaxants (e.g. oxybutynin, flavoxate hydrochloride, dicyclomine) and/or sympathomimetic agents (e.g. ephedrine).

   b. Hyperactivity of the detrusor muscle can cause a sudden increase in pressure in the bladder and result in incontinence, especially if there is decreased bladder outlet resistance. Muscle relaxants may be prescribed to reduce detrusor muscle activity and thereby reduce the risk of incontinence. If decreased bladder outlet resistance is contributing to the incontinence, sympathomimetic agents may be given to increase the tone of the urinary sphincters.

12. Consult physician if urinary incontinence persists.

12. Notifying the physician allows for modification of treatment plan.

▶ Nursing Diagnosis: *Urinary Retention*

Definition

The state in which the individual experiences incomplete emptying of the bladder.

Defining Characteristics

Refer to Appendix.

Desired Outcome

The client will not experience urinary retention as evidenced by:
a. voiding at normal intervals
b. no reports of bladder fullness and suprapubic discomfort
c. absence of bladder distention and dribbling of urine

Documentation

a. Frequency of urination and amount voided each time
b. Reports of bladder fullness and/or suprapubic discomfort
c. Bladder distention
d. Evidence or statements of dribbling of urine

d. balanced intake and output.

e. Patency of urinary catheter if present
f. Intake and output
g. Therapeutic interventions
h. Client teaching

NURSING ACTIONS

Assessments

1. Assess for signs and symptoms of urinary retention:
   a. frequent voiding of small amounts (25–60 ml) of urine
   b. reports of bladder fullness or suprapubic discomfort
   c. bladder distention
   d. dribbling of urine
   e. output less than intake.
2. Assist with urodynamic studies (e.g. cystometrogram) if ordered.

Prevention/Treatment

3. Instruct client to urinate when the urge is first felt.

4. Implement measures to promote relaxation during voiding attempts (e.g. provide privacy, hold a warm blanket against abdomen, administer prescribed analgesic if client is painful, encourage client to read).
5. If client is having difficulty voiding, run water, place his/her hands in warm water, and/or pour warm water over his/her perineum unless contraindicated.

6. Allow client to assume a normal position for voiding (usually sitting for females and standing for males) unless contraindicated.

7. Instruct client to lean his/her upper body forward and/or gently press downward on the lower abdomen when attempting to void unless contraindicated.

8. Administer cholinergic drugs (e.g. bethanechol) if ordered.

RATIONALES

1. Early recognition of signs and symptoms of urinary retention allows for prompt intervention.

2. Urodynamic studies may be indicated when neurogenic dysfunction is the suspected cause of urinary retention. The studies provide information about bladder filling, capacity, and emptying.

3. If the client feels the urge to urinate but suppresses it by contracting the external urinary sphincter, the urge will subside and not recur until the bladder fills more. If the client repeatedly suppresses the urge to urinate and the bladder fills too much or is chronically distended, the micturition reflex becomes less sensitive and does not effectively stimulate urination when the bladder fills.
4. When the client is relaxed, he/she is better able to relax the perineal muscles and external urinary sphincter and allow voiding to occur.

5. These measures have been found to trigger the micturition reflex and thereby promote voiding. They also promote a sense of relaxation, which facilitates voiding.

6. A sitting or standing position uses gravity to facilitate bladder emptying. Allowing the client to assume a normal voiding position also promotes relaxation, which facilitates voiding.

7. Leaning forward or gently pressing downward on the lower abdomen increases pressure on the bladder. This pressure helps create a sensation of bladder fullness, which stimulates the micturition reflex.

8. Cholinergic drugs promote urination by stimulating

NURSING ACTIONS
Prevention/Treatment—*cont'd*

RATIONALES

                    contraction of the detrusor muscle.

9. If an indwelling urinary catheter is present, implement measures to ensure its patency (e.g. keep tubing free of kinks, keep collection bag below bladder level, irrigate catheter if indicated).

9. Maintaining patency of the indwelling catheter prevents urinary retention.

10. Consult physician if signs and symptoms of urinary retention persist.

10. Notifying the physician allows for modification of treatment plan.

UNIT THREE

NURSING CARE OF
THE ELDERLY CLIENT

▨ THE ELDERLY CLIENT

The elderly client is a common recipient of health care in the United States today because of the marked shift in the age distribution of the population. Older persons are in the final stage of development, the stage during which many adaptations need to be made by the client because of the inevitable physiological changes that occur with aging. The extent or degree of the changes that take place depends on genetic and environmental factors as well as on the client's previous attention to health maintenance. As a client reaches old age, there may also be many changes in roles, relationships, and ability to maintain his/her usual life style. These

factors create psychosocial concerns that need to be addressed.

This care plan focuses on the elderly client hospitalized for management of a medical-surgical condition. It includes the nursing diagnoses that reflect the biopsychosocial changes that commonly occur with old age and are intensified with the stressors of an acute illness and hospitalization. **This care plan should be used in conjunction with the medical and/or surgical care plans in this text that are appropriate to the client's specific diagnosis.**

1. NURSING DIAGNOSIS: **Altered tissue perfusion**

related to:
a. decreased cardiac output associated with:
   1. decrease in contractile strength and reduced compliance of the myocardium
   2. increased cardiac workload resulting from an increase in vascular resistance, thickened and rigid cardiac valves, and stress of current illness;
b. decreased elasticity and narrowing of arterial vessels associated with degeneration of elastin, changes in collagen deposition, and/or accumulation of substances such as calcium and lipids;
c. decrease in baroreceptor sensitivity;
d. peripheral pooling of blood associated with loss of muscle tone in extremities, decreased competency of venous valves, decreased baroreceptor sensitivity, and venous dilation (results from loss of vascular elasticity).

Desired Outcome	Nursing Actions and *Selected Purposes/Rationales*

1. The client will maintain adequate tissue perfusion as evidenced by:
   a. B/P within normal range for client
   b. usual mental status
   c. absence of vertigo and syncope
   d. extremities warm with absence of pallor and cyanosis
   e. palpable peripheral pulses
   f. capillary refill time less than 3 seconds
   g. absence of edema
   h. BUN and serum creatinine within normal limits for an elderly client
   i. urine output at least 30 ml/hour
   j. absence of exercise-induced pain.

1.a. Assess for and report signs and symptoms of:
   1. decreased cardiac output (can lead to diminished tissue perfusion):
      a. variations in B/P (may be increased because of compensatory vasoconstriction; may be decreased when compensatory mechanisms and pump fail)
      b. irregular, rapid, or slow pulse (the incidence of dysrhythmias increases with age and is of concern *because of the coexisting decrease in cardiac reserve*)
      c. increase in loudness of existing systolic murmurs or presence of diastolic murmur (soft systolic murmurs are often present in elderly clients *because of sclerosed valves*)
      d. development of or an increase in loudness of S_3 and/or S_4 gallop rhythm (an S_4 can be present in a healthy elderly client)
      e. development of or increase in fatigue and weakness
      f. development of or increase in dyspnea
      g. increased crackles (crackles in the morning are a common finding in an elderly client)
      h. edema
      i. jugular vein distention (JVD)
      j. abnormal ECG readings (expected age-related changes include left axis deviation, some prolongation of all conduction intervals, and lower voltage of waves)
      k. chest x-ray results showing cardiomegaly, pleural effusion, or pulmonary edema
   2. diminished tissue perfusion:
      a. significant decrease in B/P (elevated systolic and diastolic pressures are often present in elderly clients *because of the age-related thickening and stiffening of the arteries*)
      b. decline in systolic B/P of greater than 20 mm Hg when client changes from a lying to sitting or standing position (in an elderly client, there is often a decline in systolic B/P of 15–20 mm Hg with this position change *because of a decrease in baroreceptor sensitivity and vasomotor tone*)
      c. restlessness, confusion, or other change in mental status
      d. vertigo, syncope
      e. cool, pale, or cyanotic skin
      f. diminished or absent peripheral pulses
      g. capillary refill time greater than 3 seconds
      h. edema
      i. elevated BUN and serum creatinine (BUN and serum creatinine tend

Desired Outcome	Nursing Actions and *Selected Purposes/Rationales*

to be slightly elevated *because of the age-related decline in renal function*)
    j. oliguria
    k. claudication
    l. angina.
  b. Implement measures *to maintain adequate tissue perfusion*:
    1. perform actions *to reduce cardiac workload and help maintain an adequate cardiac output*:
      a. maintain client in a semi- to high Fowler's position unless contraindicated
      b. instruct client to avoid activities that create a Valsalva response (e.g. straining to have a bowel movement, holding breath while moving up in bed) *in order to prevent the marked increase in venous return and preload that occurs with exhalation*
      c. implement measures to promote rest and conserve energy (see Nursing Diagnosis 9, action b.1)
      d. implement measures to maintain an adequate respiratory status (see Nursing Diagnosis 2, action c) *in order to promote adequate tissue oxygenation*
      e. discourage smoking (*smoke has a cardiostimulatory effect, causes vasoconstriction, and reduces oxygen availability*)
      f. discourage excessive intake of beverages high in caffeine such as coffee, tea, and colas (*caffeine is a myocardial stimulant and can increase myocardial oxygen consumption*)
      g. increase activity gradually as allowed and tolerated
    2. maintain a fluid intake of 1500–2000 ml/day unless contraindicated; if oral intake is inadequate or contraindicated, maintain intravenous fluid therapy as ordered (be alert to the greater risk for fluid overload in the elderly client *because of the age-related decline in the kidney's ability to excrete large volumes of water in response to sudden volume excess*)
    3. perform actions *to reduce peripheral pooling of blood and increase venous return*:
      a. instruct client in and assist with active foot and leg exercises every 1–2 hours during periods of decreased activity
      b. consult physician about order for elastic stockings
      c. if client is on bed rest, elevate foot of bed for 20-minute intervals several times a shift unless contraindicated
      d. encourage ambulation as allowed and tolerated
    4. instruct and assist client to change from a supine to an upright position slowly *in order to allow time for autoregulatory mechanisms to adjust to upright position*
    5. discourage positions that compromise blood flow in lower extremities (e.g. crossing legs, pillow under knees, use of knee gatch, sitting for long periods, prolonged standing)
    6. maintain a comfortable room temperature and provide client with adequate clothing and blankets (*exposure to cold causes generalized vasoconstriction*).
  c. Consult physician if signs and symptoms of diminished tissue perfusion persist or worsen.

---

2. NURSING DIAGNOSIS:

Impaired respiratory function:*

  a. **ineffective breathing pattern** related to:
    1. loss of alveolar elasticity (results in reduced efficiency of air expulsion)
    2. decreased chest expansion associated with calcification of costal cartilage and weakened respiratory muscles

---

*This diagnostic label includes the following nursing diagnoses: ineffective breathing pattern, ineffective airway clearance, and impaired gas exchange.

   3. decreased responsiveness of chemoreceptors to hypoxia and hypercapnea;
b. **ineffective airway clearance** related to stasis of secretions associated with decreased activity and an age-related decrease in ciliary activity and cough effectiveness;
c. **impaired gas exchange** related to:
   1. loss of effective lung surface associated with a reduced number of alveoli, changes in the alveolar walls, and accumulation of secretions in the bronchioles and alveoli
   2. reduced airflow associated with loss of alveolar elasticity, restricted chest expansion, and premature closure of small airways
   3. decreased pulmonary blood flow (especially in bases) associated with a decrease in the number of capillaries surrounding the alveoli and a generalized decrease in tissue perfusion.

Desired Outcome	Nursing Actions and *Selected Purposes/Rationales*

2. The client will experience adequate respiratory function as evidenced by:
a. normal rate and depth of respirations
b. absence of dyspnea
c. usual or improved breath sounds
d. usual mental status
e. usual skin color
f. blood gases within normal range for an elderly client.
	2.a. Assess for and report signs and symptoms of impaired respiratory function:
	  1. rapid, shallow, or slow respirations
	  2. dyspnea, orthopnea
	  3. use of accessory muscles when breathing
	  4. adventitious breath sounds (e.g. crackles [rales], rhonchi); crackles may be heard, especially on initial morning assessment, *as a result of some alveolar collapse associated with age-related hypoventilation and decreased activity*
	  5. diminished or absent breath sounds (diminished sounds are often present in the elderly client *because of reduced airflow*)
	  6. cough
	  7. restlessness, irritability
	  8. confusion, somnolence
	  9. central cyanosis (a late sign).
	b. Monitor for and report the following:
	  1. abnormal blood gases (PaO$_2$ is normally lower in the elderly client)
	  2. significant decrease in oximetry results (oxygen saturation is normally lower in the elderly client)
	  3. abnormal chest x-ray results.
	c. Implement measures *to maintain an adequate respiratory status*:
	  1. place client in a semi- to high Fowler's position unless contraindicated; position with pillows *to prevent slumping*
	  2. assist client to turn from side to side at least every 2 hours while in bed
	  3. instruct client to deep breathe or use incentive spirometer every 1–2 hours
	  4. instruct client in and assist with diaphragmatic and pursed-lip breathing techniques if indicated
	  5. perform actions *to facilitate removal of pulmonary secretions*:
	    a. instruct and assist client to cough or "huff" every 1–2 hours
	    b. implement measures *to thin tenacious secretions and reduce dryness of the respiratory mucous membrane*:
	      1. maintain a fluid intake of 1500–2000 ml/day unless contraindicated
	      2. humidify inspired air if ordered
	    c. if client has difficulty mobilizing secretions:
	      1. assist with or perform postural drainage therapy (PDT) if ordered
	      2. consult physician about use of a mucolytic or diluent or hydrating agent via nebulizer
	      3. suction as needed
	  6. assist with positive airway pressure techniques (e.g. IPPB, continuous positive airway pressure [CPAP], biphasic positive airway pressure [BiPAP], expiratory positive airway pressure [EPAP]) if ordered

Desired Outcome	Nursing Actions and **Selected Purposes/Rationales**

7. discourage smoking (*smoke increases mucus production, further impairs ciliary function, decreases oxygen availability, and can cause inflammation and damage to the bronchial walls*)
8. maintain oxygen therapy if ordered
9. instruct client to avoid intake of gas-forming foods (e.g. beans, cabbage, cauliflower, onions), carbonated beverages, and large meals *in order to prevent gastric distention and pressure on the diaphragm*
10. maintain activity restrictions as ordered; increase activity gradually as allowed and tolerated
11. administer central nervous system depressants judiciously *because of their respiratory depressant effect* (the possibility of respiratory depression is increased in elderly clients *because of their altered metabolism, distribution, and excretion of drugs and decreased responsiveness of chemoreceptors to hypoxia and hypercapnea*); hold medication and consult physician if respiratory rate is less than 12/minute.

d. Consult physician if signs and symptoms of impaired respiratory function persist or worsen.

---

3. NURSING DIAGNOSIS:

Risk for fluid volume deficit

related to:
a. age-related decrease in total body water;
b. decreased fluid intake associated with:
   1. restrictions imposed by current illness and/or treatment plan
   2. diminished thirst sensation
   3. desire to avoid nocturia and/or urinary incontinence;
c. age-related decline in kidney's ability to conserve water when a deficit is caused by disease or environmental factors.

Desired Outcome	Nursing Actions and **Selected Purposes/Rationales**

3. The client will not experience a fluid volume deficit as evidenced by:
   a. normal skin and tongue turgor for client
   b. moist mucous membranes
   c. stable weight
   d. B/P and pulse within normal range for client with no further increase in postural hypotension
   e. hand vein filling time less than 3–5 seconds
   f. BUN and Hct within normal range for age
   g. usual mental status
   h. balanced intake and output.

3.a. Assess for and report signs and symptoms of fluid volume deficit:
   1. decreased skin turgor (not always a reliable indicator *because decreased skin turgor is a normal age-related change*; turgor is best assessed over the forehead or sternum in an elderly client)
   2. decreased tongue turgor (the tongue will be smaller than usual and have more than one longitudinal furrow)
   3. dry mucous membranes, thirst (may not be reliable indicators *because saliva production and sensation of thirst are diminished in elderly clients*)
   4. sudden weight loss of 2% or greater
   5. low B/P and/or decline in systolic B/P of greater than 20 mm Hg when client sits up (not a reliable indicator of fluid volume unless compared with client's baseline B/P *because postural hypotension often occurs in elderly clients*)
   6. weak, rapid pulse
   7. delayed hand vein filling time (longer than 3–5 seconds)
   8. elevated BUN and Hct
   9. change in mental status (e.g. confusion)
   10. decreased urine output (reflects an actual rather than potential fluid volume deficit).
b. Implement measures *to prevent fluid volume deficit*:
   1. maintain a fluid intake of 1500–2000 ml/day and instruct client to adhere to this regimen following discharge unless contraindicated
   2. maintain intravenous fluid therapy if ordered (administer intravenous

fluids cautiously *because the elderly client is also at risk for fluid overload*).

---

4. NURSING DIAGNOSIS: **Altered nutrition: less than body requirements**

related to:
a. decreased oral intake associated with:
 1. anorexia resulting from factors such as depression, loneliness, diminished sense of smell and/or taste, early satiety, and dyspepsia
 2. difficulty chewing and swallowing food resulting from poor dentition, a decreased amount of saliva, and weakened chewing and swallowing muscles
 3. decreased ability to purchase and/or prepare healthy foods;
b. decreased utilization of nutrients associated with impaired digestion resulting from:
 1. decreased ability to chew foods thoroughly
 2. reduced secretion of digestive enzymes (e.g. salivary ptyalin, hydrochloric acid, pepsin, lipase);
c. reduced absorption of nutrients associated with hypochlorhydria and atrophy of the absorptive surface of the intestine.

Desired Outcome	Nursing Actions and *Selected Purposes/Rationales*

4. The client will maintain an adequate nutritional status as evidenced by:
 a. weight within normal range for client's age, height, and body frame
 b. normal serum albumin, Hct, Hb, and lymphocyte levels for client's age
 c. usual strength and activity tolerance
 d. healthy oral mucous membrane.

4.a. Assess for and report signs and symptoms of malnutrition:
 1. weight below normal for client's age, height, and body frame; when using height and weight charts, be aware that weight is expected to decline gradually with age
 2. low serum albumin, Hct, Hb, and lymphocyte levels
 3. weakness and fatigue
 4. sore, inflamed oral mucous membrane
 5. pale conjunctiva.
 b. Monitor percentage of meals and snacks client consumes. Report a pattern of inadequate intake.
 c. Implement measures *to maintain an adequate nutritional status*:
 1. perform actions *to improve oral intake*:
 a. implement measures to relieve dyspepsia, gastric fullness, and gas pain (see Nursing Diagnosis 5, action c)
 b. increase activity as allowed and tolerated (*activity usually promotes a sense of well-being and stimulates appetite; it also promotes gastric emptying, which reduces feeling of gastric fullness*)
 c. obtain a dietary consult if necessary to assist client in selecting foods/fluids that meet nutritional needs as well as personal and cultural preferences whenever possible
 d. maintain a clean environment and a relaxed, pleasant atmosphere
 e. implement measures to reduce fear and anxiety (see Nursing Diagnosis 18, action b) and decrease social isolation and sense of aloneness (see Nursing Diagnosis 21, action c) *in order to promote a sense of well-being and stimulate appetite*
 f. provide oral hygiene before meals
 g. serve foods/fluids that are appealing to client (visual appeal is especially important if sense of smell is diminished)
 h. encourage significant others to bring in client's favorite foods unless contraindicated and eat with him/her *to make eating more of a familiar social experience*
 i. if client has dentures, assist him/her to put them in before meals; if dentures do not fit properly, consult physician about referral to a dentist

Desired Outcome	Nursing Actions and *Selected Purposes/Rationales*

	j. provide a soft, ground, or pureed diet if client has difficulty chewing
	k. implement measures *to compensate for taste alterations and/or dislike of prescribed diet*:
	   1. serve foods warm *to stimulate sense of smell*
	   2. encourage client to experiment with different flavorings and seasonings
	   3. instruct client to use salt substitutes and salt-free herbs and spices if he/she is on low-sodium diet
	   4. encourage client to add extra sweeteners to foods unless contraindicated
	  l. limit fluid intake with meals (unless the fluid has high nutritional value) *to reduce early satiety and subsequent decreased food intake*
	  m. allow adequate time for meals; reheat food/fluids if necessary
	2. ensure that meals are well balanced and high in essential nutrients; offer high-protein supplements if client is having difficulty maintaining an adequate caloric intake
	3. administer vitamins and minerals if ordered.
	d. Perform a calorie count if ordered. Report information to dietitian and physician.
	e. Consult physician regarding an alternative method of providing nutrition (e.g. parenteral nutrition, tube feedings) if client does not consume enough food or fluids to meet nutritional needs.

---

5. NURSING DIAGNOSIS:

Altered comfort: dyspepsia, gastric fullness, and/or gas pain

related to:
a. increased gastroesophageal sensitivity to irritants associated with thinning of the esophageal and gastric mucosa;
b. gastroesophageal reflux associated with decreased tone of the cardiac sphincter;
c. impaired digestion of many foods associated with reduced secretion of digestive enzymes (e.g. hydrochloric acid, pepsin, lipase);
d. delayed esophageal and gastric emptying associated with altered lower esophageal sphincter pressure and decreased gastroesophageal motility;
e. accumulation of intestinal gas associated with decreased peristalsis.

Desired Outcome	Nursing Actions and *Selected Purposes/Rationales*

5. The client will experience diminished dyspepsia, gastric fullness, and gas pain as evidenced by:
  a. verbalization of same
  b. relaxed facial expression and body positioning
  c. diminished eructation.
	5.a. Assess for verbal reports of indigestion, fullness, or gas pain.
	  b. Assess for nonverbal signs of dyspepsia, gastric fullness, or gas pain (e.g. grimacing, clutching and guarding of abdomen, rubbing epigastric area, restlessness, reluctance to move, frequent eructation, reluctance to eat).
	  c. Implement measures *to reduce dyspepsia, gastric fullness, and gas pain*:
	   1. perform actions *to reduce gastroesophageal reflux*:
	    a. provide small, frequent meals rather than 3 large ones
	    b. instruct client to ingest foods and fluids slowly
	    c. maintain client in high Fowler's position during and for at least 30 minutes after meals and snacks
	   2. instruct client to avoid the following foods/fluids:
	    a. those that may irritate the gastroesophageal mucosa (e.g. spicy foods; caffeine-containing beverages such as coffee, tea, and colas)
	    b. those that are hard to digest (e.g. fried foods)
	   3. perform actions *to reduce accumulation of gas and fluid in gastrointestinal tract*:
	    a. encourage and assist client with frequent position changes and

ambulation as allowed and tolerated (*activity stimulates peristalsis and expulsion of flatus*)

b. instruct client to avoid activities such as gum-chewing and smoking *in order to reduce air swallowing*

c. instruct client to avoid intake of carbonated beverages and gas-producing foods (e.g. cabbage, onions, beans)

d. encourage client to eructate and expel flatus whenever the urge is felt

4. administer the following medications if ordered:

a. antacids and cytoprotective agents (e.g. sucralfate, misoprostol) *to protect the gastroesophageal mucosa*

b. antiflatulents (e.g. simethicone) *to reduce gas accumulation*

c. gastrointestinal stimulants (e.g. metoclopramide, cisapride) *to promote gastric emptying.*

d. Consult physician if signs and symptoms of dyspepsia, gastric fullness, or gas pain persist or worsen.

---

6. NURSING DIAGNOSIS:

Sensory/perceptual alterations:

a. **visual** related to the lens becoming more opaque, losing elasticity, and yellowing; loss of ciliary muscle tone; decreased pupil size; and changes in the cornea, retina, macula, and vitreous humor;

b. **auditory** related to degenerative changes in sensorineural and conduction pathways in the ear and cerumen accumulation;

c. **gustatory** related to a diminished sense of smell and atrophy of the taste buds (there is usually only a modest, quality-specific loss of taste in healthy elderly clients);

d. **olfactory** related to a decline in olfactory nerve function and a decreased number of sensory cells in the nasal lining;

e. **kinesthetic** related to a decreased central nervous system response to vestibular and kinesthetic stimuli;

f. **tactile** related to a decreased number of nerve endings in the fingertips, palms, and lower extremities.

Desired Outcome	Nursing Actions and *Selected Purposes/Rationales*

6. The client will demonstrate adaptation to altered sensory/perceptual function as evidenced by:

a. appropriate verbal and nonverbal responses

b. expected level of participation in self-care activities and treatment plan

c. safe responses to environmental stimuli.

6.a. Assess client for the following:

1. vision changes (e.g. statements of decreased visual acuity, altered depth perception, inability to adjust to changes in lighting, increased sensitivity to glare, or altered color perception; overreaching or underreaching for objects)

2. decreased auditory ability (e.g. statements of not being able to hear or understand what others are saying, inappropriate responses to auditory stimuli, irritability, increased volume of speech, staring at other person's lips during conversation, moving closer to others when they speak)

3. altered taste and smell (e.g. statements of same, decreased food intake, heavy use of sugar or seasonings)

4. diminished kinesthetic sense (e.g. unsteadiness on feet, swaying, lack of coordination)

5. diminished tactile sensation (e.g. statements of diminished feeling in extremities, holding or touching very hot objects, use of heating pad at higher than expected temperatures).

b. If client's vision is impaired:

1. ensure that lighting is adequate but not too bright (*elderly persons have increased sensitivity to glare*)

Desired Outcome	Nursing Actions and *Selected Purposes/Rationales*

2. avoid sudden changes in light intensity (*elderly clients often adjust more slowly to changes in lighting*)
3. reduce the glare from windows by partially closing blinds or curtains
4. provide a night light *to facilitate adaptation to a darkened environment and improve night vision*
5. provide large-print reading material if available
6. keep frequently used items within the visual field (*the visual field narrows with aging*)
7. encourage client to wear his/her glasses; make sure glasses are clean
8. provide auditory rather than visual diversionary activities if indicated
9. inform client of resources available if he/she desires additional information about visual aids (e.g. American Foundation for the Blind)
10. assist with activities such as filling out menus and reading mail and legal documents as needed.

c. If client's hearing is impaired:
1. assess auditory canal for excessive cerumen accumulation; if present, consult physician regarding removal of ear wax
2. implement measures *to facilitate communication*:
   a. provide adequate lighting in room *so client can read lips and see facial expressions and gestures*
   b. reduce environmental noise
   c. get client's attention (e.g. touch his/her shoulder, stand within visual field) before beginning conversation
   d. remind client to use his/her hearing aid; ensure that it is functioning well, positioned correctly, and free of cerumen
   e. face client and stay within 3–6 feet of him/her while speaking
   f. avoid chewing gum, eating, and covering mouth while talking to client
   g. lower tone of voice, speak slightly louder than usual, and avoid talking rapidly
   h. avoid lowering voice at end of sentences
   i. use simple sentences
   j. articulate clearly but avoid overenunciation of words
   k. rephrase sentences if client does not understand what is being said
   l. employ related nonverbal cues such as gestures when appropriate
   m. use alternative forms of communication (e.g. word cards, paper and pencil, magic slate) if indicated
   n. respond to client's call signal in person rather than over intercommunication system
3. encourage client to have an audiometric examination if indicated; provide client and significant others with information about available resources (e.g. audiologists, local chapter of hearing association).

d. Implement measures to compensate for taste alterations if present (see Nursing Diagnosis 4, action c.1.k).
e. Implement measures to prevent burns (see Nursing Diagnosis 16, action a.1.b) if client has diminished tactile sensation.
f. Implement measures to reduce the risk for falls (see Nursing Diagnosis 16, action a.1.a) if client's vision and/or sense of position or balance seems impaired.
g. Instruct client and significant others in above methods of adapting to sensory/perceptual alterations.
h. Consult physician if sensory/perceptual alterations worsen.

■

7. NURSING DIAGNOSIS: **Risk for impaired skin integrity**

related to:
a. increased fragility of the skin associated with decreased nutritional status and age-related dryness, loss of elasticity, and thinning of skin;

b. frequent contact with irritants if urinary incontinence is present;
c. accumulation of waste products and decreased oxygen and nutrient supply to the skin and subcutaneous tissue associated with decreased tissue perfusion and prolonged pressure on tissues if mobility is decreased.

Desired Outcome	Nursing Actions and *Selected Purposes/Rationales*

7. The client will maintain skin integrity as evidenced by:
  a. absence of redness and irritation
  b. no skin breakdown.
	7.a. Inspect the skin (especially bony prominences, dependent areas, edematous areas, and perineum) for pallor, redness, and breakdown.
	  b. Implement measures *to prevent skin breakdown*:

1. assist client to turn at least every 2 hours (elderly clients may require more frequent position change *because of decreased tissue perfusion and reduced amounts of protective subcutaneous fat*)
2. position client properly; use pressure-reducing or pressure-relieving devices (e.g. pillows, gel or foam cushions, alternating pressure mattress, air-fluidized bed) if indicated
3. gently massage around reddened areas at least every 2 hours
4. apply a thin layer of powder or cornstarch to bottom sheet or skin and to opposing skin surfaces (e.g. axillae, beneath breasts) if indicated *to absorb moisture and/or reduce friction*
5. lift and move client carefully using a turn sheet and adequate assistance
6. limit length of time client is in semi-Fowler's position to 30 minutes (*in this position, client tends to slide down in bed, which can cause skin surface abrasion and shearing*)
7. instruct or assist client to shift weight at least every 30 minutes
8. keep skin clean and dry; pat skin dry rather than rub
9. keep bed linens dry and wrinkle-free
10. ensure that external devices such as braces, casts, and restraints are applied properly
11. provide elbow and heel protectors if indicated
12. encourage client to wear socks while in bed (*helps reduce friction on heels*)
13. increase activity as allowed and tolerated
14. perform actions *to reduce dryness of the skin*:
  a. avoid use of harsh soaps and hot water; use superfatted soap and tepid water for bathing
  b. apply moisturizing lotion and/or emollient to skin at least once a day
  c. assist client with total bath or shower every other day rather than daily
  d. encourage a fluid intake of 1500–2000 ml/day unless contraindicated
15. perform actions *to prevent skin irritation resulting from urinary incontinence if present*:
  a. implement measures to reduce episodes of urinary incontinence (see Nursing Diagnosis 12, action f.2)
  b. assist client to thoroughly cleanse and dry perineal area with soft tissue or cloth after each episode of incontinence; apply a protective ointment or cream
  c. provide incontinence pads if needed to absorb moisture; do not allow skin to come in contact with plastic portion of the pads
16. use caution with application of heat or cold to areas of decreased sensation or circulatory impairment
17. perform actions to maintain an adequate nutritional status (see Nursing Diagnosis 4, action c)
18. perform actions to maintain adequate tissue perfusion (see Nursing Diagnosis 1, action b).

Desired Outcome	Nursing Actions and *Selected Purposes/Rationales*

    c. If skin breakdown occurs:
      1. notify physician
      2. continue with above measures to prevent further irritation and breakdown
      3. perform care of involved area(s) as ordered or per standard hospital procedure
      4. assess client closely and report signs and symptoms of infection (e.g. elevated temperature; redness, heat, pain, and swelling around area of breakdown; unusual drainage from site).

---

8. NURSING DIAGNOSIS: **Altered oral mucous membrane: dryness, irritation, and breakdown**

related to:
a. thinning of the oral mucosa associated with epithelial atrophy;
b. decreased saliva production associated with a gradual decline in salivary gland activity.

Desired Outcome	Nursing Actions and *Selected Purposes/Rationales*

8. The client will maintain a moist, intact oral mucous membrane.

8.a. Assess client for dryness, irritation, and breakdown of the oral mucosa.
   b. Implement measures *to decrease dryness and irritation of the oral mucous membrane*:
     1. instruct and assist client to perform oral hygiene as often as needed; avoid products that contain lemon and glycerin and mouthwashes containing alcohol (*these products have a drying and irritating effect on the oral mucous membrane*)
     2. encourage client to rinse mouth frequently with water
     3. lubricate client's lips frequently
     4. encourage client to breathe through nose rather than mouth
     5. encourage client not to smoke (*smoking irritates and dries the mucosa*)
     6. encourage a fluid intake of 1500–2000 ml/day unless contraindicated
     7. encourage client to chew sugarless gum or suck on sugarless hard candy *in order to stimulate salivation*
     8. encourage client to use artificial saliva *to lubricate the mucous membrane*
     9. inspect client's dentures; obtain a dental consult if dentures are rough, cracked, or ill-fitting.
   c. If oral mucosa is irritated or cracked, implement measures *to relieve discomfort and promote healing*:
     1. assist client to select soft, bland foods
     2. instruct client to avoid foods/fluids that are extremely hot
     3. use a soft bristle brush, sponge-tipped applicator, or low-pressure power spray for oral hygiene
     4. if client has dentures that fit poorly, remove and replace only for meals
     5. administer topical anesthetics, oral protective agents, and analgesics if ordered.
   d. Consult physician if dryness, irritation, breakdown, or discomfort persists.

---

9. NURSING DIAGNOSIS: **Risk for activity intolerance**

related to:
a. decreased tissue oxygenation associated with diminished functional reserve capacity of the respiratory and cardiac systems during stress/illness;

b. decrease in strength and endurance associated with the loss of muscle mass that occurs with aging;

c. inadequate nutritional status;

d. inadequate rest and sleep associated with age-related changes in sleep pattern and effects of current illness and hospitalization on sleep pattern.

Desired Outcome	Nursing Actions and *Selected Purposes/Rationales*

9. The client will not experience activity intolerance as evidenced by:
a. no reports of fatigue and weakness
b. ability to perform activities of daily living without exertional dyspnea, chest pain, diaphoresis, dizziness, and a significant change in vital signs.
	9.a. Assess for signs and symptoms of activity intolerance:
	  1. statements of fatigue or weakness
	  2. exertional dyspnea, chest pain, diaphoresis, or dizziness
	  3. abnormal heart rate response to activity (e.g. increase in rate of 20 beats/minute above resting rate, rate not returning to preactivity level within 10 minutes after stopping activity, change from regular to irregular rate); be aware that the pulse rate increases only slightly with activity and returns to preactivity level slowly in an elderly client
	  4. decreased systolic B/P or a significant increase (10–15 mm Hg) in diastolic pressure with activity.
	  b. Implement measures *to maintain adequate activity tolerance*:
	    1. perform actions *to promote rest and/or conserve energy*:
	      a. maintain activity restrictions as ordered
	      b. minimize environmental activity and noise
	      c. organize nursing care to allow for periods of uninterrupted rest
	      d. limit the number of visitors and their length of stay
	      e. assist client with self-care activities as needed
	      f. keep supplies and personal articles within easy reach
	      g. instruct client in energy-saving techniques (e.g. using shower chair when showering, sitting to brush teeth or comb hair)
	      h. implement measures to reduce fear and anxiety (see Nursing Diagnosis 18, action b)
	      i. implement measures to promote sleep (see Nursing Diagnosis 14, action c)
	    2. perform actions to maintain adequate cardiac output and tissue perfusion (see Nursing Diagnosis 1, action b)
	    3. perform actions to maintain an adequate respiratory status (see Nursing Diagnosis 2, action c)
	    4. perform actions to maintain an adequate nutritional status (see Nursing Diagnosis 4, action c)
	    5. increase client's activity gradually as allowed and tolerated; periods of activity should be short, frequent, and interspersed with rest periods.
	  c. Instruct client to:
	    1. report a decreased tolerance for activity; caution client that tolerance for vigorous activity may be diminished *because of age-related changes in thermoregulatory mechanisms and sympathetic nervous system responses*
	    2. stop any activity that causes chest pain, shortness of breath, dizziness, or extreme fatigue or weakness
	    3. continue with a regular exercise program following discharge to improve activity tolerance.
	  d. Consult physician if signs and symptoms of activity intolerance persist or worsen.

---

10. NURSING DIAGNOSIS: **Impaired physical mobility**

related to:

a. decreased muscle strength associated with the loss of muscle mass that occurs with aging;

b. activity intolerance associated with decreased functional reserve capacity of the respiratory and cardiac systems during stress and illness, inadequate nutritional status, and difficulty resting and sleeping;
c. joint aching and stiffness that may be present as a result of degenerative changes in the joints;
d. fear of falling;
e. activity limitations imposed by current diagnosis and/or treatment plan.

Desired Outcome	Nursing Actions and *Selected Purposes/Rationales*

10. The client will maintain an optimal level of physical mobility within prescribed activity restrictions.	10.a. Implement measures *to maintain an optimal level of physical mobility*:
	1. perform actions to maintain adequate strength and activity tolerance (see Nursing Diagnosis 9, action b)
	2. perform actions to prevent falls (see Nursing Diagnosis 16, action a.1.a) *in order to reduce client's fear of injury*
	3. instruct client in and assist with use of mobility aids (e.g. cane, walker) if indicated
	4. instruct client in and assist with range of motion exercises at least 3 times/day unless contraindicated
	5. if client complains of joint aching or stiffness:
	  a. encourage him/her to perform mild exercise of affected joint(s) upon awakening in the morning *in order to reduce stiffness*
	  b. consult physician regarding application of heat to affected joint(s)
	  c. administer analgesics (e.g. nonsteroidal anti-inflammatories) if ordered
	6. encourage activity and participation in self-care as allowed and tolerated
	7. encourage client to continue a regular exercise program following discharge.
	b. Provide praise and encouragement for all efforts to increase physical mobility.
	c. Encourage the support of significant others. Allow them to assist with range of motion exercises, positioning, and activity if desired.
	d. Consult physician if client is unable to achieve expected level of mobility or if range of motion becomes more restricted.

11. NURSING DIAGNOSIS: **Self-care deficit**

related to:
a. impaired physical mobility;
b. decreased activity tolerance;
c. lack of motivation and/or presence of cognitive impairments that result in the elderly client attaching less importance to or forgetting usual grooming and hygiene practices.

Desired Outcome	Nursing Actions and *Selected Purposes/Rationales*
11. The client will perform self-care activities within physical limitations and activity restrictions imposed by the treatment plan.	11.a. With client, develop a realistic plan for meeting daily physical needs. b. Implement measures *to facilitate client's ability to perform self-care activities*: 1. schedule care at a time when client is most likely to be able to participate (e.g. after rest periods, not immediately after meals or treatments) 2. keep needed objects within easy reach

3. consult occupational therapist about assistive devices available (e.g. long-handled hairbrush and shoehorn) if indicated
4. allow adequate time for the accomplishment of self-care activities, remembering that elderly clients tend to be slower in reacting to stimuli and in moving
5. perform actions to maintain an optimal level of mobility (see Nursing Diagnosis 10, action a)
6. perform actions to maintain adequate activity tolerance (see Nursing Diagnosis 9, action b).

c. Encourage maximum independence within physical limitations and prescribed activity restrictions. Provide positive feedback for all efforts and accomplishments of self-care.

d. Assist the client with activities he/she is unable to perform independently.

e. Inform significant others of client's abilities to perform own care. Explain the importance of encouraging and allowing client to maintain an optimal level of independence and allowing client to complete activities at his/her own pace.

---

12. NURSING DIAGNOSIS: **Altered urinary elimination:**

a. **frequency and urgency** related to an age-related decrease in bladder capacity and presence of an enlarged prostate in men;

b. **retention** related to age-related loss of bladder muscle tone, obstruction of the bladder outlet by an enlarged prostate in men, and difficulty urinating associated with anxiety about having to use a bedpan or urinal;

c. **incontinence (stress, urge, functional)** related to:
   1. decreased tone of the external urinary sphincter and an incompetent bladder outlet (a result of lessening of the urethrovesical junction angle in women) associated with degenerative changes in the pelvic floor muscles and structural supports of the bladder (occurs more in women as a result of childbearing and estrogen deficiency)
   2. decreased bladder capacity and diminished sensation of the urge to void until bladder is full
   3. overflow of urine associated with overdistention of the bladder if urinary retention is present
   4. delays in toileting associated with:
      a. inability to get to the toilet in time to urinate associated with unfamiliar environment and impaired physical mobility
      b. difficulty removing clothing in a timely manner when needing to urinate resulting from reduced manual dexterity.

Desired Outcome	Nursing Actions and *Selected Purposes/Rationales*
12. The client will maintain or regain optimal urinary elimination as evidenced by: a. voiding at normal intervals b. no reports of urgency, frequency, bladder fullness, and suprapubic discomfort c. absence of bladder distention	12.a. Determine client's usual urinary elimination pattern. b. Assess for signs and symptoms of altered urinary elimination: 1. frequent voiding of small amounts (25–60 ml) of urine 2. nocturia 3. reports of urgency, frequency, bladder fullness, or suprapubic discomfort 4. bladder distention 5. incontinence 6. output less than intake. c. Monitor client's patterns of fluid intake and urination (e.g. times and amounts of fluid intake, types of fluids consumed, times and amounts of

Desired Outcome	Nursing Actions and *Selected Purposes/Rationales*

d. absence of incontinence
e. balanced intake and output.

voluntary and involuntary voiding, reports of sensation of need to void, activities preceding incontinence).

d. Catheterize client if ordered *to determine the amount of residual urine.*

e. Assist with urodynamic studies (e.g. cystometrogram) if performed *to determine cause for altered urinary elimination.*

f. Implement measures *to promote optimal urinary elimination*:

1. perform actions *to prevent or treat urinary retention*:
   a. offer bedpan or urinal or assist client to bedside commode or bathroom every 2–3 hours if indicated
   b. instruct client to urinate when urge is first felt
   c. perform actions *to promote relaxation during voiding attempts* (e.g. provide privacy, encourage client to read)
   d. perform actions *that may help trigger the micturition reflex and promote a sense of relaxation during voiding attempts* (e.g. run water, place client's hands in warm water, pour warm water over perineum)
   e. allow client to assume a normal position for voiding unless contraindicated
   f. instruct client to lean his/her upper body forward and/or gently press downward on lower abdomen during voiding attempts unless contraindicated *in order to put pressure on the bladder (pressure helps create a sensation of bladder fullness, which stimulates the micturition reflex)*
   g. perform actions to prevent or treat constipation (see Nursing Diagnosis 13, actions d and e) *in order to prevent increased pressure on bladder outlet*
   h. administer cholinergic drugs (e.g. bethanechol) if ordered *to stimulate bladder contraction*
   i. consult physician about intermittent catheterization or insertion of an indwelling catheter if signs and symptoms of urinary retention persist

2. perform actions *to prevent or treat urinary incontinence*:
   a. offer bedpan or urinal or assist client to bedside commode or bathroom every 2–3 hours or more frequently depending on the client's usual urinary elimination pattern
   b. allow client to assume a normal position for voiding unless contraindicated *in order to promote complete bladder emptying*
   c. implement measures *to reduce delays in toileting* (e.g. have call signal within client's reach and respond promptly to requests for assistance; have bedpan, urinal, or bedside commode readily available to client; provide easy access to bathroom; provide client with easy-to-remove clothing such as pajamas with Velcro closures or an elastic waistband)
   d. instruct client to perform pelvic muscle exercises (e.g. stopping and starting stream during voiding; squeezing buttocks together, then relaxing the muscles) several times a day if appropriate *in order to strengthen pelvic floor muscles and improve tone of the external urinary sphincter*; instruct client to continue these exercises following discharge, emphasizing that it will take several weeks of exercise before improvement may be noted
   e. instruct client to space fluids evenly throughout the day rather than drinking a large quantity at one time (*rapid filling of bladder can result in incontinence if client has decreased urinary sphincter control*)
   f. limit oral fluid intake in the evening *to decrease the possibility of nighttime incontinence*
   g. instruct client to avoid drinking beverages containing caffeine (*caffeine is a mild diuretic and an irritant to the bladder; both effects may make urinary control more difficult*)
   h. administer the following medications if ordered:
      1. cholinergic agents (e.g. bethanechol) *to stimulate bladder*

contractions and promote complete bladder emptying if incontinence is associated with urinary retention
   2. estrogen preparations (*may be used to treat urge incontinence in postmenopausal women*)
  i. if urinary incontinence persists:
    1. utilize biofeedback techniques if appropriate *to assist client to regain control over the pelvic floor musculature and external urinary sphincter*
    2. instruct and assist client with bladder retraining program if appropriate
    3. consult physician regarding intermittent catheterization, insertion of an indwelling catheter, or use of an external catheter or penile clamp.

---

13. NURSING DIAGNOSIS: **Constipation**

related to:
a. decreased gastrointestinal motility associated with age and exacerbated by decreased activity and anxiety during hospitalization;
b. failure to respond to the urge to defecate associated with dulling of the impulses that sense the signal to defecate, inability to get to the toilet independently, and/or reluctance to use the bedpan or bedside commode;
c. difficulty evacuating stool associated with weakened abdominal and pelvic floor muscles and decreased lubrication of stools (a result of diminished intestinal mucus production);
d. decreased intake of fiber and fluids;
e. chronic laxative use.

Desired Outcome	Nursing Actions and *Selected Purposes/Rationales*

13. The client will not experience constipation as evidenced by:
a. usual frequency of bowel movements
b. passage of soft, formed stool
c. absence of abdominal distention and pain, feeling of rectal fullness or pressure, and straining during defecation.
	13.a. Ascertain client's usual bowel elimination habits.
	  b. Assess for signs and symptoms of constipation (e.g. decrease in frequency of bowel movements; passage of hard, formed stools; anorexia; abdominal distention and pain; feeling of fullness or pressure in rectum; straining during defecation).
	  c. Assess bowel sounds. Report a pattern of decreasing bowel sounds.
	  d. Implement measures *to prevent constipation*:
	    1. encourage client to defecate whenever the urge is felt
	    2. assist client to toilet or bedside commode or place in high Fowler's position on bedpan for bowel movements unless contraindicated
	    3. encourage client to relax, provide privacy, and have call signal within reach during attempts to defecate (*measures to promote relaxation enable client to relax the levator ani muscle and external anal sphincter, which facilitates evacuation of stool*)
	    4. encourage client to establish a regular time for defecation, preferably an hour after a meal
	    5. instruct client to increase intake of foods high in fiber (e.g. bran, whole grains, fresh fruits and vegetables) unless contraindicated
	    6. instruct client to maintain a minimum fluid intake of 1500–2000 ml/day unless contraindicated
	    7. increase activity as allowed and tolerated
	    8. encourage client to perform isometric abdominal strengthening exercises unless contraindicated
	    9. perform actions to reduce fear and anxiety (see Nursing Diagnosis 18, action b)
	   10. administer laxatives or cathartics and/or enemas if ordered

Desired Outcome	Nursing Actions and *Selected Purposes/Rationales*

11. instruct client to continue with actions to promote regular bowel function following discharge (e.g. maintain a fluid intake of at least 6–8 glasses/day, increase intake of foods high in fiber, participate in regular exercise program).
   e. Consult physician about checking for an impaction and digitally removing stool if client has not had a bowel movement in 3 days, if he/she is passing liquid stool, or if other signs and symptoms of constipation are present.

---

14. NURSING DIAGNOSIS: **Sleep pattern disturbance**

related to:
a. fear, anxiety, decreased activity, unfamiliar environment, and discomfort associated with present illness;
b. age-related nocturia;
c. age-related changes in the stages of sleep resulting in frequent awakenings and less deep restorative sleep.

Desired Outcome	Nursing Actions and *Selected Purposes/Rationales*

14. The client will attain optimal amounts of sleep as evidenced by:
   a. statements of feeling well rested
   b. usual mental status
   c. absence of frequent yawning, dark circles under eyes, and hand tremors.

14.a. Assess for signs and symptoms of a sleep pattern disturbance (e.g. statements of difficulty falling asleep, sleep interruptions, or not feeling well rested; irritability; lethargy; disorientation; frequent yawning; dark circles under eyes; slight hand tremors).
   b. Determine the client's usual sleep habits.
   c. Implement measures *to promote sleep*:
      1. assist client to determine the part of the night that he/she sleeps the best; arrange time of sleep to coincide with his/her particular body rhythms whenever possible
      2. discourage excessive napping during the day unless signs and symptoms of sleep deprivation exist
      3. perform actions to reduce fear and anxiety (see Nursing Diagnosis 18, action b)
      4. perform actions to reduce dyspepsia, gastric fullness, and gas pain if present (see Nursing Diagnosis 5, action c) and discomfort associated with client's diagnosis and treatment
      5. inform client of normal changes in sleep pattern that occur with aging *in order to reduce concerns about quantity of sleep necessary to maintain health*
      6. encourage participation in relaxing diversional activities during the evening
      7. discourage intake of fluids high in caffeine (e.g. coffee, tea, colas), especially in the evening
      8. offer client an evening snack that includes milk or cheese unless contraindicated (*the L-tryptophan in milk and cheese helps induce and maintain sleep*)
      9. allow client to continue usual sleep practices (e.g. position; time; presleep routines such as reading, watching television, and listening to music) unless contraindicated
      10. satisfy basic needs such as comfort and warmth before sleep
      11. instruct client to limit intake of fluids in the evening and urinate just before bedtime *in order to reduce nocturia*
      12. reduce environmental distractions (e.g. close door to client's room; use night light rather than overhead light whenever possible; lower volume of paging system; keep staff conversations at a low level and

away from client's room; close curtains between clients in a semi-private room or ward; keep beepers and alarms on low volume; have earplugs available for client if needed)

13. administer prescribed sedative-hypnotics if indicated; administer these agents cautiously *because the metabolism, distribution, and excretion of drugs are often altered in the elderly client*

14. perform actions *to reduce interruptions during sleep (80–100 minutes of uninterrupted sleep is usually needed to complete one sleep cycle)*:
    a. restrict visitors
    b. group care (e.g. medications, treatments, physical care, assessments) whenever possible.

d. Consult physician if signs and symptoms of sleep deprivation persist or worsen.

---

15. NURSING DIAGNOSIS:	**Risk for infection**

related to:

a. stasis of respiratory secretions associated with decreased activity and age-related decrease in ciliary activity and cough effectiveness;
b. decrease in cell-mediated immunity associated with changes in T-cell activity;
c. inadequate nutritional status;
d. urinary stasis associated with incomplete bladder emptying and decreased activity;
e. favorable environment for growth of pathogens in vagina associated with an increase in the pH of vaginal secretions (results from age-related estrogen depletion).

Desired Outcome	Nursing Actions and *Selected Purposes/Rationales*

15. The client will remain free of infection as evidenced by:
    a. absence of fever and chills
    b. pulse within normal limits
    c. normal breath sounds
    d. cough productive of clear mucus only
    e. voiding clear urine without reports of burning and increased frequency and urgency
    f. absence of heat, pain, redness, swelling, and unusual drainage in any area
    g. usual mental status
    h. WBC and differential counts within normal range for elderly client
    i. negative results of cultured specimens.

15.a. Assess for and report signs and symptoms of infection (be aware that some signs and symptoms vary *because of an age-related decline in thermoregulatory, immune, and sympathetic nervous system responses*; some signs and symptoms also vary depending on the site of infection and causative organism):
   1. increase in temperature above client's usual level (be aware that normal temperature in the elderly client may be less than 37° C)
   2. chills (may not be present in the elderly *because they may have a diminished shivering reflex*)
   3. increased pulse (the elderly client may not demonstrate the classic elevation in pulse rate that occurs with infection *because of his/her decreased sympathetic nervous system responses*)
   4. abnormal breath sounds
   5. cough productive of purulent, green, or rust-colored sputum
   6. loss of appetite
   7. cloudy, foul-smelling urine
   8. reports of burning when urinating
   9. reports of increased urinary frequency or urgency
   10. presence of WBCs, bacteria, and/or nitrites in urine
   11. heat, pain, redness, swelling, or unusual drainage in any area
   12. malaise, lethargy, acute confusion
   13. elevated WBC count and/or significant change in differential.

b. Obtain specimens (e.g. urine, vaginal drainage, sputum, blood) for culture as ordered. Report positive results.

c. Implement measures *to prevent infection*:
   1. maintain a fluid intake of at least 1500–2000 ml/day unless contraindicated

Desired Outcome	Nursing Actions and *Selected Purposes/Rationales*

2. use good handwashing technique and encourage client to do the same
3. use sterile technique during all invasive procedures (e.g. urinary catheterizations, venous and arterial punctures, injections, wound care)
4. anchor catheters/tubings (e.g. urinary, intravenous, wound drainage) securely *in order to reduce the risk for trauma to the tissues and the risk for introduction of pathogens associated with in-and-out movement of the tubing*
5. change equipment, tubings, and solutions used for treatments such as intravenous infusions, respiratory care, irrigations, and enteral feedings according to hospital policy
6. rotate intravenous insertion sites according to hospital policy
7. maintain a closed system for drains (e.g. wound, chest tube, urinary catheter) and intravenous infusions whenever possible
8. protect client from others with infections and instruct him/her to continue this after discharge
9. perform actions to maintain an adequate nutritional status (see Nursing Diagnosis 4, action c)
10. perform actions to prevent and treat irritation and breakdown of the oral mucous membrane (see Nursing Diagnosis 8, actions b and c)
11. instruct and assist client to perform good perineal care routinely and after each bowel movement
12. perform actions to maintain an adequate respiratory status (see Nursing Diagnosis 2, action c) *in order to reduce the risk of respiratory tract infection*
13. perform actions to prevent or treat urinary retention (see Nursing Diagnosis 12, action f.1) *in order to prevent urinary stasis*
14. perform actions to prevent skin breakdown (see Nursing Diagnosis 7, action b)
15. instruct client to receive vaccinations (e.g. pneumococcal pneumonia, tetanus, influenza) at recommended intervals if appropriate.

---

16. NURSING DIAGNOSIS: **Risk for injury:**

a. **falls** related to:
1. dizziness, syncope, or drop attacks (sudden, unexplained fall without loss of consciousness) associated with decreased cerebral tissue perfusion (can occur because of age-related decrease in cardiac output, vascular changes, and postural hypotension)
2. impaired vision (e.g. decreased visual acuity, peripheral and night vision, and depth perception; glare intolerance)
3. loss of balance and tripping associated with gait abnormalities (e.g. decreased step height and length), delayed reaction time, reduced coordination, and impaired proprioception
4. weakness associated with decreased muscle strength and the general deconditioning that occurs with reduced physical activity;
b. **burns** related to age-related decrease in tactile sensation;
c. **aspiration** related to a diminished gag reflex and gastroesophageal reflux (can occur as a result of delayed esophageal and gastric emptying);
d. **pathologic fractures** related to osteoporosis associated with an imbalance between bone resorption and bone formation resulting from decreased estrogen levels in women, calcium deficiency (results from decreased dietary intake and decreased absorption due to vitamin D deficiency), and decreased activity;
e. **drug toxicity** related to:
1. increase in cell receptor sensitivity to many drugs and change in usual distribution of drugs

2. impaired metabolism and excretion of drugs associated with diminished liver and kidney function
3. synergistic effect that occurs with some combinations of medications (elderly clients are often taking a number of medications).

Desired Outcomes	Nursing Actions and *Selected Purposes/Rationales*

16.a. The client will not experience falls or burns.	16.a.1. Implement measures *to reduce the risk for trauma*:
	a. perform actions *to prevent falls*:
	  1. keep bed in low position with side rails up when client is in bed
	  2. keep needed items within easy reach and assist client to identify their location
	  3. encourage client to request assistance whenever needed; have call signal within easy reach
	  4. use lap belt when client is in chair if indicated
	  5. instruct client to wear well-fitting slippers/shoes with nonslip soles and low heels when ambulating
	  6. keep floor free of clutter and wipe up spills promptly
	  7. instruct and assist client to get out of bed slowly *in order to reduce dizziness associated with postural hypotension*
	  8. carefully position tubings and equipment so that they will not interfere with ambulation
	  9. accompany client during ambulation and use a transfer safety belt if he/she is weak or dizzy
	  10. provide ambulatory aids (e.g. walker, cane) if client is weak or unsteady on feet
	  11. reinforce instructions from physical therapist on correct ambulation and transfer techniques
	  12. if vision is impaired, orient client to surroundings, room, and arrangement of furniture and identify obstacles during ambulation
	  13. instruct client to move slowly, use wider stance when ambulating, and avoid rapidly turning head or body *in order to prevent loss of balance*
	  14. instruct client to ambulate in well-lit areas and to use handrails if needed
	  15. do not rush client; allow adequate time for ambulation to the bathroom and in hallway
	  16. make sure that shower has a nonslip bottom surface and that shower chair, secure bath mat, call signal, grab bars, and adequate lighting are present
	  17. implement measures to maintain adequate strength and activity tolerance (see Nursing Diagnosis 9, action b) and an optimal level of physical mobility (see Nursing Diagnosis 10, action a)
	b. perform actions *to prevent burns*:
	  1. let hot foods and fluids cool slightly before serving
	  2. supervise client while smoking if indicated
	  3. assess temperature of bath water and direct heat application device (e.g. K-pad, warm compress, hot water bottle) before and during use
	c. administer central nervous system depressants judiciously.
	2. Include client and significant others in planning and implementing measures to prevent falls and burns. Discuss:
	a. the need to evaluate home for environmental hazards (e.g. thick or loose carpets, inadequate or loose railings, insufficient lighting) and make necessary modifications
	b. the importance of continuing appropriate safety precautions after discharge.
	3. If falls or burns occur, initiate appropriate first aid and notify physician.

Desired Outcome	Nursing Actions and *Selected Purposes/Rationales*

16.b. The client will not aspirate foods/fluids as evidenced by:
1. clear breath sounds
2. resonant percussion note over lungs
3. absence of cough, tachypnea, and dyspnea.
	16.b.1. Assess for signs and symptoms of aspiration of foods/fluids (e.g. rhonchi, dull percussion note over affected lung area, cough, tachypnea, dyspnea, tachycardia).
	2. Monitor chest x-ray results. Report findings of pulmonary infiltrate.
	3. Implement measures *to reduce the risk for aspiration*:
	  a. perform actions to reduce gastroesophageal reflux (see Nursing Diagnosis 5, action c.1)
	  b. instruct client to avoid laughing and talking while eating and drinking
	  c. encourage client to concentrate on eating and drinking and allow ample time for meals and snacks
	  d. instruct and assist client to perform oral hygiene after meals *to ensure that food particles do not remain in mouth.*
	4. If signs and symptoms of aspiration occur:
	  a. perform tracheal suctioning
	  b. withhold oral intake
	  c. notify physician
	  d. prepare client for chest x-ray
	  e. prepare client for bronchoscopy if ordered *to remove aspirated food particles.*

16.c. The client will not experience pathologic fractures as evidenced by:
1. usual mobility and range of motion
2. absence of unusual motion, abnormal joint position, and obvious deformity of any body part
3. absence of pain and swelling over skeletal structures
4. x-ray reports showing absence of fractures.
	16.c.1. Assess for and report signs and symptoms of pathologic fractures (e.g. decrease in mobility or range of motion, motion at site where motion does not usually occur, abnormal joint position or obvious deformity, pain or swelling over skeletal structures).
	2. Monitor x-ray reports and notify physician of findings of pathologic fractures.
	3. Implement measures *to prevent pathologic fractures*:
	  a. move client carefully; obtain adequate assistance as needed
	  b. when turning client, logroll and support all extremities
	  c. use smooth movements when moving client; avoid pulling or pushing on body parts
	  d. correctly apply back brace or corset if ordered
	  e. perform actions to prevent falls (see action a.1.a in this diagnosis)
	  f. perform actions *to prevent or delay bone demineralization*:
	    1. assist client to maintain maximum mobility (*weight-bearing reduces bone breakdown*)
	    2. consult physician about use of a tilt table to facilitate weight-bearing if client is immobile
	    3. administer calcium preparations, vitamin D, and medications *that inhibit bone resorption* (e.g. estrogen preparations) if ordered
	    4. emphasize need for client to follow a regular exercise program after discharge.
	4. If fractures occur:
	  a. maintain activity restrictions if ordered
	  b. apply external stabilization device (e.g. cervical collar, brace, splint, sling) if ordered
	  c. prepare client for surgery (e.g. internal fixation) if planned
	  d. administer analgesics, anti-inflammatory agents, and/or muscle relaxants if ordered *to control pain*
	  e. provide emotional support to client and significant others.

16.d. The client will not develop drug toxicity as evidenced by absence of signs and symptoms commonly associated with drug toxicity such as:
1. ataxia, agitation, confusion, and blurred vision
2. anorexia, nausea, vomiting, and diarrhea
	16.d.1. Assess client for signs and symptoms that might be indicative of drug toxicity (e.g. ataxia, agitation, confusion, blurred vision, anorexia, nausea, vomiting, diarrhea, dizziness, arrhythmias, postural hypotension, dyspnea, stridor, rash, urticaria, elevated BUN and creatinine, elevated transaminase levels). Be aware that the signs and symptoms will vary depending on drugs being taken.
	2. Implement measures *to prevent drug toxicity*:
	  a. be alert to possible drug interactions and nursing implications for the elderly; hold dose and consult physician if medication or dose appears contraindicated
	  b. administer central nervous system depressants judiciously

3. dizziness, arrhythmias, and postural hypotension
4. dyspnea and stridor
5. rash and urticaria
6. elevated BUN, creatinine, and transaminase levels.

c. inform client of common adverse effects of drugs being taken and ways to avoid toxicity; encourage him/her to report adverse effects or any other unusual symptoms immediately
d. obtain baseline vital signs and results of laboratory studies indicative of renal and hepatic function *to facilitate assessment of the effects of medications on these systems*
e. monitor blood levels (e.g. peak, trough) of drugs as ordered and report results to physician; be aware that the elderly client may experience toxic effects when drug levels are within the "normal" therapeutic range
f. prior to discharge:
1. provide client and family members with clear, simple, written instructions for taking medications prescribed; include drug name, dose, schedule, route of administration, special precautions such as incompatible foods or drugs, and adverse reactions to observe for
2. assist client to set up a system for remembering to take medication as prescribed (e.g. divided pill container, use of timer)
3. emphasize the importance of taking only those medications that are prescribed, following the directions carefully, and keeping the physician informed of adverse effects experienced.
3. If signs and symptoms of drug toxicity occur, withhold dose and notify physician.

---

17. NURSING DIAGNOSIS:

Altered sexuality patterns

related to:
a. fear of rejection associated with feelings of loss of physical attractiveness;
b. inadequate opportunities for sexual expression associated with lack of available partner;
c. misconceptions about sexual functioning in old age;
d. fear of urinary incontinence;
e. dyspareunia associated with vaginal changes (e.g. decreased vaginal lubrication; thinning of the epithelium; decreased length, width, and size of opening) resulting from decreased estrogen levels;
f. embarrassment associated with possible impotence (erections are usually less intense and slower in the elderly male and may be further affected by certain disease processes [e.g. diabetes, chronic renal failure] and medications [e.g. thiazide diuretics, tricyclic antidepressants, certain antihypertensive agents]).

Desired Outcome	Nursing Actions and *Selected Purposes/Rationales*
17. The client will demonstrate beginning adaptation to changes in sexuality patterns as evidenced by: a. verbalization of a perception of self as sexually acceptable and adequate b. statements reflecting ways to adjust to effects of aging on sexual functioning.	17.a. Assess for symptoms of altered sexuality patterns (e.g. verbalization of sexual concerns, limitations, or difficulties; reports of changes in sexual activities or behaviors). b. Determine client's perception of desired sexuality, usual pattern of sexual expression, recent changes in sexuality patterns, and knowledge of age-related changes in sexual functioning. Be aware that the client may be reluctant to express concerns *because of common stereotype that elderly are not sexually active.* c. Implement measures *to promote an optimal sexuality pattern*: 1. inform client of age-related changes in sexual functioning (e.g. sexual responses are slower and less intense, vaginal secretions are diminished, erections take longer to achieve but can be maintained longer, seminal fluid volume is reduced, erection is rapidly lost after orgasm, refractory time between orgasms is longer); encourage questions and clarify misconceptions

Desired Outcome	Nursing Actions and *Selected Purposes/Rationales*
	2. facilitate communication between client and partner; focus on feelings shared by the couple and assist them to identify changes that may affect their sexual relationship
	3. discuss ways to be creative in expressing sexuality (e.g. massage, fantasies, cuddling)
	4. arrange for uninterrupted privacy during hospital stay if desired by couple
	5. perform actions to improve client's self-concept (see Nursing Diagnosis 19, actions c–p)
	6. if dyspareunia is a problem:
	a. encourage female client to use a water-soluble lubricant before sexual intercourse *to reduce vaginal dryness*
	b. suggest experimentation with different positions during intercourse *to reduce the depth of penetration*
	c. administer estrogen if ordered *to reduce vaginal dryness and thinning of vaginal epithelium*
	7. if impotence is a problem:
	a. encourage client to discuss it with physician (*impotence may be due to reversible factors such as medication therapy, alcohol, smoking, or poorly controlled chronic disease conditions*)
	b. assure client that occasional episodes of impotence are normal
	c. suggest alternative methods of sexual gratification if appropriate
	d. encourage client to discuss various treatment options (e.g. penile prosthesis, external vacuum device) with physician if appropriate
	8. reinforce the importance of rest before sexual activity
	9. if incontinence of urine is a problem, encourage client to void just before intercourse and other sexual activity
	10. include partner in above discussions and encourage continued support of the client.
	d. Consult physician if counseling appears indicated.

---

18. NURSING DIAGNOSIS:

Anxiety

related to unfamiliar environment; signs and symptoms of current diagnosis; lack of understanding of diagnostic tests, diagnosis, and treatment plan; financial concerns; and effects of diagnosis on health status, usual roles, and ability to live independently.

Desired Outcome	Nursing Actions and *Selected Purposes/Rationales*

18. The client will experience a reduction in anxiety as evidenced by:
a. verbalization of feeling less anxious
b. usual sleep pattern
c. relaxed facial expression and body movements
d. stable vital signs
e. usual perceptual ability and interactions with others.
	18.a. Assess client for signs and symptoms of anxiety (e.g. verbalization of feeling anxious, insomnia, tenseness, shakiness, restlessness, diaphoresis, tachycardia, increase in blood pressure, self-focused behaviors). Validate perceptions carefully, remembering that sympathetic nervous system responses are often diminished in the elderly.
	b. Implement measures *to reduce fear and anxiety*:
	  1. orient client to hospital environment, equipment, and routines
	  2. introduce client to staff who will be participating in care; if possible, maintain consistency in staff assigned to his/her care *in order to provide feelings of stability and comfort with the environment*
	  3. assure client that staff members are nearby; respond to call signal as soon as possible
	  4. maintain a calm, supportive, confident manner when interacting with client
	  5. encourage verbalization of fear and anxiety; provide feedback
	  6. explain all diagnostic tests

7. reinforce physician's explanations and clarify misconceptions the client has about his/her diagnosis, treatment plan, and prognosis
8. provide a calm, restful environment
9. instruct client in relaxation techniques and encourage participation in diversional activities
10. assist client to identify specific stressors and ways to cope with them
11. when appropriate, assist client to meet spiritual needs (e.g. arrange for a visit from clergy)
12. encourage significant others to project a caring, concerned attitude without obvious anxiousness
13. include significant others in orientation and teaching sessions and encourage their continued support of the client
14. if surgical intervention is indicated, begin preoperative teaching
15. encourage client to discuss his/her concerns about the cost of health care and about future living situation; obtain a social service consult to assist client with financial planning and finding an alternative living situation if indicated
16. administer prescribed antianxiety agents if indicated; give these agents cautiously *because the metabolism, distribution, and excretion of drugs are often altered in the elderly*
17. provide information based on current needs of client at a level he/she can understand; encourage questions and clarification of information provided.

c. Consult physician if above actions fail to control fear and anxiety.

---

19. NURSING DIAGNOSIS:

Self-concept disturbance*

related to:
a. changes in appearance and body functioning (e.g. graying and thinning of hair; sagginess of eyelids, earlobes, and breasts; dry, wrinkled skin; reduced height; increase in and change in distribution of body fat; reduction in lean body mass; impotence; decreased bladder control; diminished visual acuity and hearing);
b. increased dependence on others to meet basic needs;
c. feelings of powerlessness;
d. changes in usual life style and roles associated with decreased strength and endurance and sensory/perceptual alterations.

---

*This diagnostic label includes the nursing diagnoses of body image disturbance, self-esteem disturbance, and altered role performance.

Desired Outcome	Nursing Actions and *Selected Purposes/Rationales*
19. The client will demonstrate beginning adaptation to changes in appearance, body functioning, level of independence, life style, and roles as evidenced by: a. verbalization of feelings of self-worth and sexual adequacy b. maintenance of relationships with significant others c. active participation in activities of daily living d. verbalization of a	19.a. Assess for signs and symptoms of a self-concept disturbance (e.g. verbalization of negative feelings about self, withdrawal from significant others, lack of participation in activities of daily living, lack of plan for adapting to necessary changes in life style). b. Determine the meaning of changes in appearance, body functioning, life style, and roles to the client by encouraging him/her to verbalize feelings and by noting nonverbal responses to the changes experienced. c. Implement measures *to assist client to increase self-esteem* (e.g. limit negative self-assessment, encourage positive comments about self, assist to identify strengths, give positive feedback about accomplishments and behaviors that are indicative of high self-esteem). d. Assist client to identify and utilize coping techniques that have been helpful in the past. e. Reinforce measures to promote an optimal sexuality pattern (see Nursing Diagnosis 17, action c).

Desired Outcome	Nursing Actions and *Selected Purposes/Rationales*
beginning plan for adapting life style to changes associated with the aging process and current diagnosis.	f. Implement measures to assist client to adapt to sensory/perceptual alterations (see Nursing Diagnosis 6, actions b–f). g. If client is incontinent, instruct in ways to minimize the problem *so that socialization is possible* (e.g. placing disposable liners in underwear, wearing absorbent undergarments such as Attends). h. Assist client with usual grooming and makeup habits if necessary. i. Implement measures *to assist the client to maintain his/her sense of dignity and feeling of well-being about appearance* (e.g. do not expose client unnecessarily during assessments, procedures, and care; do not discuss incontinence episodes in front of client's visitors; assist client with bathing, makeup, hair-styling, and shaving before visitors arrive). j. Implement measures to reduce client's feelings of powerlessness (see Nursing Diagnosis 20, actions c–n). k. Demonstrate acceptance of client using techniques such as touch and frequent visits. Encourage significant others to do the same. l. Support behaviors suggesting positive adaptation to changes that have occurred (e.g. interest in personal appearance, verbalization of feelings of self-worth, maintenance of relationships with significant others). m. Encourage visits and support from significant others. n. Encourage client to pursue usual roles and interests and continue involvement in social activities. If previous roles, interests, and hobbies cannot be pursued, encourage development of new ones. o. Instruct client in ways to promote and maintain optimal body functioning after discharge (e.g. maintain good nutritional status, participate in an active exercise program). p. Provide information about and encourage use of community agencies and support groups (e.g. senior centers; family, individual, and/or financial counseling). q. Consult physician about psychological counseling if client desires or seems unwilling or unable to adapt to changes resulting from the aging process.

---

20. NURSING DIAGNOSIS: **Powerlessness**

related to:
a. increased dependence on others to meet basic needs;
b. inability to pursue usual life activities and roles associated with age-related changes in body functioning, current diagnosis and its treatment, and inadequate financial resources;
c. inability to control many of the changes that occur with aging.

Desired Outcome	Nursing Actions and *Selected Purposes/Rationales*
20. The client will demonstrate increased feelings of control over his/her situation as evidenced by: a. verbalization of same b. active participation in the planning of care c. participation in self-care activities within physical limitations.	20.a. Assess for behaviors that may indicate feelings of powerlessness (e.g. verbalization of lack of control over self-care or current situation, anger, irritability, passivity, lack of participation in care planning or self-care). b. Obtain information from client and significant others regarding client's usual response to situations in which he/she has had limited control (e.g. loss of job, financial stress). c. Evaluate client's perception of current situation, strengths, weaknesses, expectations, and parts of current situation that are under his/her control. Correct misinformation and inaccurate perceptions and encourage discussion of feelings about areas in which he/she perceives a lack of control.

    d. Assist client to establish realistic short- and long-term goals.

    e. Discuss a living will and advanced directives for health care with client and significant others if appropriate; provide assistance if needed to complete necessary documents.

    f. Reinforce physician's explanations about the aging process, disease condition or injury, and treatment plan. Clarify misconceptions.

    g. Support realistic hope about the probability of future independence.

    h. Remind client of the right to ask questions about changes that are occurring, current condition, and plan of care.

    i. Support client's efforts to increase knowledge of and control over condition. Provide relevant pamphlets and audiovisual materials.

    j. Include client in the planning of care, encourage maximum participation in the treatment plan, and allow choices whenever possible *to promote a sense of control.*

    k. Provide information about scheduled procedures and tests *so that client knows what to expect, which promotes a sense of control.*

    l. Consult physician about arranging for physical and occupational therapists to perform a physical functional assessment. Implement recommendations about assistive devices and environmental modifications that would allow client more independence in performing activities of daily living.

    m. Encourage significant others to allow client to do as much as he/she is able *so that a feeling of independence can be maintained.*

    n. Encourage client to be as active as possible in making decisions about his/her living situation.

    o. Encourage client's participation in self-help groups if indicated.

---

21. NURSING DIAGNOSIS: **Social isolation**

related to:

a. decreased sensory and motor functioning;

b. reduced opportunities for socialization associated with inadequate financial resources, death or disability of friends and family members, reluctance of others to include the elderly in activities, reluctance to establish new relationships and try new activities, and/or placement in a long-term care facility;

c. decreased desire to communicate with others associated with an imbalance between the effort required to interact with others and the anticipated rewards of the interaction;

d. fear of injury such as falls in unfamiliar surroundings;

e. withdrawal from others associated with fear of embarrassment resulting from functional changes such as incontinence or hearing loss.

Desired Outcome	Nursing Actions and *Selected Purposes/Rationales*

21. The client will experience a decreased sense of isolation as evidenced by:
  a. maintenance of relationships with significant others
  b. verbalization of decreasing feelings of aloneness and rejection.
	21.a. Ascertain client's usual degree of social interaction.
	    b. Assess for indications of social isolation (e.g. absence of supportive significant others; uncommunicative and withdrawn; expression of feelings of rejection, being different from others, or aloneness imposed by others; hostility; sad, dull affect).
	    c. Implement measures *to decrease social isolation*:
	      1. assist client to identify reasons for feeling isolated and alone; aid him/her in developing a plan of action to reduce these feelings
	      2. use touch to demonstrate acceptance of client
	      3. encourage significant others to visit
	      4. encourage client to maintain telephone contact with others
	      5. schedule time each day to sit and talk with client

Desired Outcome	Nursing Actions and *Selected Purposes/Rationales*
	6. assist client to identify a few persons he/she feels comfortable with and encourage interactions with them
	7. make objects such as telephone, TV, radio, newspapers, and greeting cards accessible to client
	8. have significant others bring client's favorite objects from home and place in room
	9. change room assignments as feasible *to provide client with roommate with similar interests*; encourage their interaction
	10. emphasize the importance of maintaining active friendships and seeking out new relationships; encourage participation in support groups if appropriate
	11. encourage client to participate in structured activity programs following discharge; provide information about community senior centers and the programs they offer.

---

22. NURSING DIAGNOSIS: **Ineffective management of therapeutic regimen**

related to:
a. lack of motivation, inadequate support and supervision, and insufficient financial resources;
b. confusion about appropriate health care practices and a decreased level of trust associated with conflicting advice from multiple health care providers;
c. conflicting values between client and health care providers;
d. knowledge deficit regarding current diagnosis, medications and treatments prescribed, and consequences of failure to comply with treatment plan.

Desired Outcome	Nursing Actions and *Selected Purposes/Rationales*
22. The client will demonstrate the probability of effective management of therapeutic regimen as evidenced by: a. willingness to learn about and participate in treatments and care b. statements reflecting ways to modify personal habits and integrate treatments into life style c. statements reflecting an understanding of the implications of not following the prescribed treatment plan.	22.a. Assess for indications that the client may be unable to effectively manage the therapeutic regimen: 　1. statements reflecting inability to manage care at home 　2. failure to adhere to treatment plan while in hospital (e.g. not adhering to dietary modifications, refusing medications, refusing to ambulate) 　3. statements reflecting a lack of understanding of the factors that will cause further progression of current illness and/or accelerate aging process 　4. statements reflecting an unwillingness or inability to modify personal habits and integrate necessary treatments into life style 　5. statements reflecting view that situation is hopeless and that efforts to comply are useless. b. Implement measures *to promote effective management of the therapeutic regimen*: 　1. discuss with client the specific factors that may interfere with management of care (e.g. inadequate financial resources, religious or cultural conflicts, lack of support systems) 　2. explain the aging process and current diagnosis in terms the client can understand; stress the fact that adherence to the treatment plan is necessary in order to delay and/or prevent complications associated with the diagnosis and minimize some of the changes that occur with aging 　3. assist client to clarify values and to identify ways to incorporate the therapeutic goals and priorities into value system 　4. encourage questions and clarify misconceptions the client has about aging and his/her diagnosis and effects of each

5. perform actions to promote trust in caregivers (e.g. validate conflicting advice, explain reasons for treatment plan)
6. encourage client to participate in treatment plan (e.g. take medications as prescribed, perform recommended exercises)
7. provide instruction regarding medications and treatments prescribed; allow time for return demonstration of procedures; determine areas of difficulty and misunderstanding and reinforce teaching as necessary
8. provide client with written instructions about medications and treatments
9. assist client to identify ways to incorporate treatments into life style; focus on modifications of life style rather than complete change if possible
10. encourage client to discuss financial concerns; obtain a social service consult to assist client with financial planning and to obtain financial aid if indicated
11. provide information about and encourage utilization of community resources that can assist client to make necessary life style changes if appropriate
12. encourage client to attend follow-up educational classes if appropriate
13. reinforce behaviors suggesting future compliance with the therapeutic regimen (e.g. statements reflecting plans for integrating treatments into life style, active participation in exercise program, changes in personal habits)
14. include significant others in explanations and teaching sessions and encourage their support; reinforce the need for client to assume responsibility for managing as much of care as possible.

c. Consult physician about referrals to community health agencies if continued instruction, support, or supervision is needed.

---

23. NURSING DIAGNOSIS:

Altered family processes

related to:
a. financial, physical, and psychological stresses associated with family member's illness and/or progressive disability;
b. inadequate knowledge about the normal aging process, client's current diagnosis, and necessary care;
c. inadequate support services;
d. decreased ability of client to fulfill usual family roles;
e. guilt associated with need to change client's living situation resulting from family's inability to provide necessary care.

Desired Outcome	Nursing Actions and *Selected Purposes/Rationales*
23. The family members* will demonstrate beginning adjustment to changes in functioning of family member and family roles and structure as evidenced by: a. meeting client's needs b. verbalization of ways to adapt to required role and life-style changes	23.a. Assess for signs and symptoms of altered family processes (e.g. inability to meet client's needs, statements of not being able to accept client's disabilities or make necessary role and life-style changes, inability to make decisions, inability or refusal to participate in client's care and/or rehabilitation, negative family interactions). b. Identify components of the family and their patterns of communication and role expectations. c. Implement measures *to facilitate family members' adjustment to age- or diagnosis-related changes in client and resultant changes in family roles and structure:* 1. encourage family members to verbalize feelings about changes in

*The term *family members* is being used here to include client's significant others.

Desired Outcome	Nursing Actions and *Selected Purposes/Rationales*
c. active participation in decision making and client's rehabilitation d. positive interactions with one another.	client and the effect of these on family structure; actively listen to each family member and maintain a nonjudgmental attitude about feelings shared 2. instruct client and family about normal aging processes (e.g. sensory deficits, decreased muscle strength, reduced coordination) 3. reinforce physician's explanation of the effects of the current diagnosis and planned treatment and rehabilitation 4. assist family members to gain a realistic perspective of client's situation, conveying as much hope as appropriate 5. provide privacy *so that family members can share their feelings with one another*; stress the importance of and facilitate the use of good communication techniques 6. assist family members to progress through their own grieving processes; explain that they may encounter times when they need to focus on meeting their own rather than the client's needs 7. emphasize the need for family members to obtain adequate rest and nutrition and to identify and utilize stress management techniques *so they are better able to emotionally and physically deal with changes experienced* 8. encourage and assist family members to identify coping strategies for dealing with client's age-related changes and changes in health status and their effect on the family 9. assist family members to identify realistic goals and ways of reaching these goals 10. include family members in decision making about client and his/her care; convey appreciation for their input and continued support of client 11. encourage and allow family members to participate in client's care and rehabilitation; instruct family in any special procedures and allow them to practice with supervision in the hospital prior to discharge of the client 12. assist family members to identify resources that could assist them in coping with their feelings and meeting their immediate and long-term needs (e.g. counseling and social services; pastoral care; service, church, and support groups); initiate a referral if indicated. d. Consult physician if family members continue to demonstrate difficulty adapting to changes in client's functioning, roles, and family structure.

Bibliography

See pages 897–898.

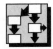

UNIT FOUR

NURSING CARE OF THE CLIENT HAVING SURGERY

PREOPERATIVE CARE

This care plan focuses on the adult client who is scheduled for a surgical procedure. The goals of preoperative care are to prepare the client physically and psychologically for the surgery and the postoperative period. Thorough preoperative preparation reduces the client's postoperative fear and anxiety and the risk of postoperative complications. Basic preoperative care is discussed here. In order to individualize this care plan, the client's psychological and physiological status, the length of time before the surgical procedure, the type of anesthesia to be used, and the planned surgical procedure must be considered. **This care plan is to be used in conjunction with each surgical care plan.**

PREOPERATIVE GOALS

Prior to surgery, the client will:

- share thoughts and feelings about the impending surgery and its anticipated effects
- verbalize an understanding of the surgical procedure, preoperative care, and postoperative sensations and care
- demonstrate the ability to perform activities designed to prevent postoperative complications.

NURSING DIAGNOSES
1. Anxiety △ 96
2. Sleep pattern disturbance △ 97
3. Anticipatory grieving △ 98

CLIENT TEACHING
4. Knowledge deficit △ 99

1. NURSING DIAGNOSIS:

Anxiety

related to:
a. unfamiliar environment and separation from significant others;
b. anticipated loss of control associated with effects of anesthesia;
c. lack of understanding of diagnostic tests and planned surgical procedure;
d. financial concerns associated with hospitalization;
e. potential embarrassment or loss of dignity associated with body exposure;
f. risk of disease if blood transfusions are necessary;
g. anticipated discomfort; surgical findings; and changes in appearance, body functioning, and usual life style and roles;
h. possibility of death.

Desired Outcome	Nursing Actions and *Selected Purposes/Rationales*

1. The client will experience a reduction in anxiety as evidenced by:
a. verbalization of feeling less anxious
	1.a. Gather the following data from the client during the preoperative period:
	   1. level of understanding of planned surgical procedure
	   2. perceptions about the surgery and its anticipated results
	   3. significance of the surgical procedure and hospitalization
	   4. previous surgical and hospital experiences

b. usual sleep pattern
c. relaxed facial expression and body movements
d. stable vital signs
e. usual perceptual ability and interactions with others.

5. availability of adequate support systems.
b. Assess client for signs and symptoms of anxiety (e.g. verbalization of feeling anxious, insomnia, tenseness, shakiness, restlessness, diaphoresis, tachycardia, elevated blood pressure, facial pallor, self-focused behaviors).
c. Implement measures *to reduce fear and anxiety:*
   1. orient client to hospital environment, equipment, and routines
   2. introduce client to staff who will be participating in care; if possible maintain consistency in staff assigned to his/her care *to provide feelings of stability and comfort with the environment*
   3. assure client that staff members are nearby; respond to call signal as soon as possible
   4. maintain a calm, supportive, confident manner when interacting with client
   5. encourage verbalization of fear and anxiety; provide feedback
   6. reinforce physician's explanations and clarify misconceptions the client has about the surgical procedure (e.g. purpose, size and location of incision, anticipated outcome)
   7. explain all presurgical diagnostic tests
   8. instruct client regarding preoperative routines and postoperative care (see Nursing Diagnosis 4, actions a.1–4 and b.1)
   9. enable client *to maintain a sense of control by:*
      a. including him/her in planning of preoperative care and allowing choices whenever possible
      b. explaining purpose of the written consent form (e.g. indicates voluntary and informed consent, protects against unsanctioned surgery)
   10. provide a calm, restful environment
   11. instruct client in relaxation techniques and encourage participation in diversional activities
   12. assist client to identify specific stressors and ways to cope with them
   13. provide information based on current needs of client at a level he/she can understand; encourage questions and clarification of information provided
   14. perform actions *to help client maintain a sense of dignity* (e.g. provide privacy when appropriate; avoid unnecessary body exposure during preoperative procedures; allow client to wear dentures, glasses, wig, etc. into the operating room suite if possible)
   15. assure client that pain relief needs will be met postoperatively
   16. assure client that blood is screened carefully and that the risk for contracting blood-borne disease is minimal
   17. initiate financial and/or social service referrals if indicated
   18. encourage significant others to project a caring, concerned attitude without obvious anxiousness
   19. include significant others in orientation and teaching sessions and encourage their continued support of client
   20. when appropriate, assist client to meet spiritual needs (e.g. arrange for a visit from clergy)
   21. administer prescribed antianxiety agents if indicated.
d. Consult physician if above actions fail to control fear and anxiety.

2. NURSING DIAGNOSIS: Sleep pattern disturbance

related to fear, anxiety, activities to prepare client for the surgical experience, and unfamiliar environment.

Desired Outcome	Nursing Actions and *Selected Purposes/Rationales*

2. The client will attain optimal amounts of sleep as evidenced by:
  a. statements of feeling well rested
  b. usual mental status
  c. absence of frequent yawning, dark circles under eyes, and hand tremors.
	2.a. Assess for signs and symptoms of a sleep pattern disturbance (e.g. statements of difficulty falling asleep, sleep interruptions, or not feeling well rested; irritability; lethargy; disorientation; frequent yawning; dark circles under eyes; slight hand tremors).
	  b. Determine the client's usual sleep habits.
	  c. Implement measures *to promote sleep:*
	    1. perform actions to reduce fear and anxiety (see Nursing Diagnosis 1, action c)
	    2. encourage participation in relaxing diversional activities during the evening
	    3. discourage intake of fluids high in caffeine (e.g. coffee, tea, colas), especially in the evening
	    4. offer client an evening snack that includes milk or cheese unless contraindicated (*the L-tryptophan in milk and cheese helps induce and maintain sleep*)
	    5. allow client to continue usual sleep practices (e.g. position; time; presleep routines such as reading, watching television, listening to music, and meditating) unless contraindicated
	    6. satisfy basic needs such as comfort and warmth before sleep
	    7. encourage client to urinate just before bedtime
	    8. reduce environmental distractions (e.g. close door to client's room, use night light rather than overhead light whenever possible, lower volume of paging system, keep staff conversations at a low level and away from client's room, close curtains between clients in a semi-private room or ward, keep beepers and alarms on low volume, have earplugs available for client if needed)
	    9. administer prescribed sedative-hypnotics if indicated
	    10. perform actions *to reduce interruptions during sleep (80–100 minutes of uninterrupted sleep is usually needed to complete one sleep cycle)*:
	      a. restrict visitors
	      b. group care (e.g. medications, treatments, physical care, assessments) whenever possible.

---

3. NURSING DIAGNOSIS: **Anticipatory grieving**

related to potential loss of or change in a body part and/or usual body functioning.

Desired Outcome	Nursing Actions and *Selected Purposes/Rationales*

3. The client will demonstrate beginning progression through the grieving process as evidenced by:
  a. verbalization of feelings about anticipated change in body image and usual body functioning
  b. usual sleep pattern
  c. participation in
	3.a. Assess for signs and symptoms of anticipatory grieving (e.g. expression of distress about potential loss, change in eating habits, inability to concentrate, insomnia, anger, sadness, withdrawal from significant others).
	  b. Implement measures *to facilitate the grieving process:*
	    1. assist client to acknowledge the anticipated loss *so grief work can begin*; assess for factors that may hinder and facilitate acknowledgment
	    2. discuss the grieving process and assist client to accept the phases of grieving (phases vary among theorists but progress from shock and alarm to acceptance) as an expected response to anticipated loss

preoperative care and self-care activities
d. use of available support systems.

3. provide an atmosphere of care and concern (e.g. provide privacy, be available and nonjudgmental, display empathy and respect) *so client will feel free to express feelings*
4. perform actions *to promote trust* (e.g. answer questions honestly, provide requested information)
5. encourage the verbal expression of anger and sadness about the anticipated loss; recognize displacement of anger and assist client to see the actual cause of angry feelings and resentment
6. encourage client to express feelings in whatever ways are comfortable (e.g. writing, drawing, conversation)
7. assist client to identify and utilize techniques that have helped him/her cope in previous situations of loss
8. support realistic hope about changes that may result from surgery
9. support behaviors suggesting successful grief work (e.g. verbalizing feelings about anticipated loss, expressing sorrow, focusing on ways to adapt to anticipated loss)
10. explain the phases of the grieving process to significant others; encourage their support and understanding
11. provide information about counseling services and support groups that might assist client in working through grief
12. when appropriate, assist client to meet spiritual needs (e.g. arrange for a visit from clergy).
c. Consult physician regarding a referral for counseling if signs of dysfunctional grieving (e.g. persistent denial of the anticipated loss, excessive anger or sadness, emotional lability) occur.

Client Teaching

4. NURSING DIAGNOSIS: **Knowledge deficit**

regarding the surgical procedure, hospital routines associated with surgery, physical preparation for the surgical procedure, sensations that normally occur following surgery and anesthesia, and postoperative care.

Desired Outcomes	Nursing Actions and *Selected Purposes/Rationales*

4.a. The client will verbalize an understanding of the surgical procedure, preoperative care, and postoperative sensations and care.

4.a.1. Provide information about usual preoperative routines for the surgery to be performed (e.g. blood work, ECG, urinalysis, chest x-ray, insertion of urinary catheter and/or nasogastric tube, bowel and skin preparation, removal of prosthetic devices).
2. Provide information about:
a. scheduled time and estimated length of surgery
b. food and fluid restrictions before surgery
c. preoperative medications and planned anesthesia
d. body position during surgical procedure
e. purpose for and estimated length of stay in preoperative holding area and postanesthesia care unit (PACU)
f. sensations that can occur after surgery (e.g. dryness of mouth, sore throat following endotracheal intubation, pain at surgical site).
3. Reinforce information provided by the anesthesiologist and surgeon about the surgery.
4. Inform client of the anticipated postoperative care:
a. equipment (e.g. dressings, intravenous lines, drainage tubes, traction devices, antiembolism stockings, sequential compression device)
b. activity limitations and expectations
c. dietary modifications
d. treatments (e.g. respiratory care, circulatory management, wound care) and expected frequency

Desired Outcomes	Nursing Actions and *Selected Purposes/Rationales*
	e. assessments (e.g. intake and output, lung sounds, vital signs, neurological checks, bowel sounds) and expected frequency
	f. medications (e.g. antiemetics, analgesics, antimicrobials)
	g. pain management methods (e.g. oral, parenteral, and/or intravenous medications; epidural analgesia; patient-controlled analgesia [PCA]; positioning; relaxation techniques).
	5. Allow time for questions and clarification. Provide feedback.
4.b. The client will demonstrate the ability to perform activities designed to prevent postoperative complications.	4.b.1. Provide instructions about activities the client will be expected to perform postoperatively. These may include:
	a. effective coughing and deep breathing techniques
	b. correct use of incentive spirometer
	c. active foot and leg exercises
	d. correct methods for moving in bed, getting out of bed, and ambulating.
	2. Allow time for questions, clarification, and return demonstration.

Bibliography

See pages 897–898.

POSTOPERATIVE CARE

The postoperative phase begins when the client is transferred from surgery to a postanesthesia care unit (PACU) and ends when he/she has recovered from the surgical intervention. The length of the postoperative phase varies depending on factors such as the client's age and preoperative health status, type of anesthesia used, length and type of surgery, and the client's physiological and psychological responses postoperatively.

This care plan focuses on postoperative care of an adult client who has received general anesthesia and has been transferred from the recovery area to the clinical care unit. The goals of care are to prevent complications and to assist the client to attain an optimal health status postoperatively. **This care plan should be used in conjunction with all surgical care plans.**

DISCHARGE CRITERIA

Prior to discharge, the client will:

- tolerate prescribed diet
- tolerate expected level of activity
- have surgical pain controlled
- have clear, audible breath sounds throughout lungs
- have evidence of normal wound healing
- have no signs and symptoms of infection or postoperative complications
- identify ways to prevent postoperative infection
- demonstrate the ability to perform wound care
- state signs and symptoms to report to the health care provider
- share thoughts and feelings about the surgery, diagnosis, prognosis, and treatment plan
- verbalize an understanding of and a plan for adhering to recommended follow-up care including future appointments with health care provider, dietary modifications, activity level, treatments, and medications prescribed.

NURSING/ COLLABORATIVE DIAGNOSES

1. Altered tissue perfusion △ 101
2. Ineffective breathing pattern △ 102
3. Ineffective airway clearance △ 103
4. Altered fluid and electrolyte balance:

1. NURSING DIAGNOSIS:

Altered tissue perfusion

related to:
a. hypovolemia associated with fluid loss and decreased fluid intake;
b. peripheral pooling of blood associated with decreased activity and diminished vasomotor responses resulting from the effects of anesthesia and some medications (e.g. narcotic [opioid] analgesics, central-acting muscle relaxants).

Desired Outcome	Nursing Actions and *Selected Purposes/Rationales*

1. The client will maintain adequate tissue perfusion as evidenced by:
  a. B/P within normal range for client and stable with position change
  b. usual mental status
  c. extremities warm with absence of pallor and cyanosis
  d. palpable peripheral pulses
	1.a. Assess for and report signs and symptoms of diminished tissue perfusion (e.g. significant decrease in B/P, postural hypotension, syncope when changing to an upright position, restlessness, confusion, cool extremities, pallor or cyanosis of extremities, diminished or absent peripheral pulses, slow capillary refill, oliguria).
	  b. Implement measures *to maintain adequate tissue perfusion:*
	    1. maintain a minimum fluid intake of 2500 ml/day unless contraindicated; if oral intake is inadequate or contraindicated, maintain intravenous fluid therapy as ordered
	    2. administer blood and blood products as ordered
	    3. instruct client to change from a supine to an upright position slowly *in*

Desired Outcome	Nursing Actions and *Selected Purposes/Rationales*

e. capillary refill time less than 3 seconds
f. urine output at least 30 ml/hour.
	order to allow time for autoregulatory mechanisms to adjust to upright position
	4. perform actions *to prevent peripheral pooling of blood and increase venous return:*
	  a. instruct and assist client to perform active foot and leg exercises every 1–2 hours while awake
	  b. encourage and assist with ambulation as soon as allowed and tolerated (client should be instructed to pick up feet instead of shuffling *in order to promote contractions of the leg muscles*)
	  c. discourage positions that compromise blood flow in lower extremities (e.g. crossing legs, pillows under knees, sitting for long periods)
	  d. consult physician regarding order for elastic stockings or a sequential compression device if prolonged activity restriction is expected
	5. perform actions *to prevent vasoconstriction:*
	  a. implement measures to reduce stress
	  b. discourage smoking
	  c. implement measures *to keep client from getting cold* (e.g. maintain a comfortable room temperature, provide adequate clothing and blankets).
	c. Consult physician if signs and symptoms of diminished tissue perfusion persist or worsen.

---

2. NURSING DIAGNOSIS: **Ineffective breathing pattern**

related to:
a. increased rate and decreased depth of respirations associated with fear and anxiety;
b. decreased rate and depth of respirations associated with the depressant effect of anesthesia and some medications (e.g. narcotic [opioid] analgesics, central-acting muscle relaxants);
c. diminished lung/chest wall expansion associated with positioning, weakness, fatigue, abdominal distention, and reluctance to breathe deeply because of pain.

Desired Outcome	Nursing Actions and *Selected Purposes/Rationales*

2. The client will maintain an effective breathing pattern as evidenced by:
  a. normal rate and depth of respirations
  b. absence of dyspnea
  c. blood gases within normal range.
	2.a. Assess for signs and symptoms of an ineffective breathing pattern (e.g. shallow or slow respirations, tachypnea, dyspnea, use of accessory muscles when breathing).
	b. Monitor for and report the following:
	  1. abnormal blood gases
	  2. significant decrease in oximetry results.
	c. Implement measures *to improve breathing pattern:*
	  1. perform actions to reduce fear and anxiety (see Nursing Diagnosis 20, action b)
	  2. perform actions to reduce pain (see Nursing Diagnosis 6, action e)
	  3. perform actions to reduce the accumulation of gastrointestinal gas and fluid (see Nursing Diagnosis 7.A, action 3) *in order to decrease pressure on the diaphragm*
	  4. perform actions to increase strength and improve activity tolerance (see Nursing Diagnosis 10, action b) *in order to decrease weakness and fatigue*
	  5. instruct client to deep breathe or use incentive spirometer every 1–2 hours

6. assist with positive airway pressure techniques (e.g. IPPB, continuous positive airway pressure [CPAP], biphasic positive airway pressure [BiPAP], expiratory positive airway pressure [EPAP]) if ordered
7. instruct client to breathe slowly if hyperventilating
8. place client in a semi- to high Fowler's position unless contraindicated; position with pillows *to prevent slumping*
9. assist client to turn from side to side at least every 2 hours while in bed
10. increase activity as allowed and tolerated
11. administer central nervous system depressants judiciously; hold medication and consult physician if respiratory rate is less than 12/ minute.
   d. Consult physician if:
   1. ineffective breathing pattern continues
   2. signs and symptoms of impaired gas exchange (e.g. restlessness, irritability, confusion, decreased PaO_2 and increased $PaCO_2$ levels) are present.

---

3. NURSING DIAGNOSIS: **Ineffective airway clearance**

related to:
a. occlusion of the pharynx associated with relaxation of the tongue resulting from effect of anesthesia and some medications (e.g. narcotic [opioid] analgesics, central-acting muscle relaxants);
b. stasis of secretions associated with:
   1. decreased activity
   2. depressed ciliary function resulting from effects of anesthesia
   3. difficulty coughing up secretions resulting from the depressant effect of anesthesia and some medications (e.g. narcotic [opioid] analgesics, central-acting muscle relaxants), pain, weakness, fatigue, and presence of tenacious secretions (can occur as a result of fluid volume deficit);
c. increased secretions associated with irritation of the respiratory tract (can result from inhalation anesthetics and endotracheal intubation).

Desired Outcome	Nursing Actions and *Selected Purposes/Rationales*

3. The client will maintain clear, open airways as evidenced by:
a. normal breath sounds
b. normal rate and depth of respirations
c. absence of dyspnea.
	3.a. Assess for signs and symptoms of ineffective airway clearance (e.g. abnormal breath sounds; rapid, shallow respirations; dyspnea; cough).
	b. Implement measures *to promote effective airway clearance:*
	  1. position client on side and/or insert an artificial airway if necessary *to prevent obstruction of airway by tongue*
	  2. perform actions to reduce pain (see Nursing Diagnosis 6, action e)
	  3. instruct and assist client to turn, deep breathe, and cough or "huff" every 1–2 hours
	  4. increase activity as allowed and tolerated
	  5. perform actions *to facilitate removal of secretions:*
	    a. implement measures *to thin tenacious secretions and reduce drying of the respiratory mucous membrane:*
	      1. maintain a fluid intake of at least 2500 ml/day unless contraindicated
	      2. humidify inspired air as ordered
	    b. assist with administration of mucolytics and diluent or hydrating agents via nebulizer if ordered
	    c. perform suctioning if needed
	  6. discourage smoking (*irritants present in smoke increase mucus production, impair ciliary function, and can cause inflammation and damage to the bronchial walls*)

Desired Outcome | Nursing Actions and *Selected Purposes/Rationales*

7. administer central nervous system depressants judiciously.
   c. Consult physician if:
   1. signs and symptoms of ineffective airway clearance persist
   2. signs and symptoms of impaired gas exchange (e.g. restlessness, irritability, confusion, decreased PaO_2 and increased $PaCO_2$ levels) are present.

---

4. NURSING/COLLABORATIVE DIAGNOSIS:

Altered fluid and electrolyte balance:

a. **fluid volume deficit** related to restricted oral fluid intake before, during, and after surgery; blood loss; loss of fluid associated with vomiting, nasogastric tube drainage, and/or profuse wound drainage; and inadequate fluid replacement;

b. **hypokalemia, hypochloremia, and metabolic alkalosis** related to loss of electrolytes and hydrochloric acid associated with vomiting and nasogastric tube drainage;

c. **fluid volume excess or water intoxication** related to vigorous fluid therapy during and immediately following surgery and an increased secretion of antidiuretic hormone (output of ADH is stimulated by trauma, pain, and anesthetic agents).

Desired Outcome | Nursing Actions and *Selected Purposes/Rationales*

4.a. The client will not experience fluid volume deficit, hypokalemia, hypochloremia, or metabolic alkalosis as evidenced by:
1. normal skin turgor
2. moist mucous membranes
3. stable weight
4. B/P and pulse within normal range for client and stable with position change
5. hand vein filling time less than 3–5 seconds
6. usual mental status
7. balanced intake and output within 48 hours after surgery
8. urine specific gravity within normal range
9. return of peristalsis within expected time
10. absence of cardiac dysrhythmias, muscle weakness, paresthesias, twitching, spasms, and dizziness
11. BUN, serum electrolytes, and blood gases within normal range.

4.a.1. Assess for and report signs and symptoms of:
   a. fluid volume deficit:
      1. decreased skin turgor, dry mucous membranes, thirst
      2. sudden weight loss of 2% or greater
      3. postural hypotension and/or low B/P
      4. weak, rapid pulse
      5. delayed hand vein filling time (longer than 3–5 seconds)
      6. change in mental status
      7. continued low urine output 48 hours after surgery with a change in specific gravity (the specific gravity will usually increase with an actual fluid volume deficit but may be decreased depending on the cause of the deficit)
      8. elevated BUN
   b. hypokalemia (e.g. cardiac dysrhythmias, postural hypotension, muscle weakness, nausea and vomiting, continued abdominal distention and hypoactive or absent bowel sounds)
   c. hypochloremia and metabolic alkalosis (e.g. dizziness, irritability, paresthesias, muscle twitching or spasms, hypoventilation).
2. Monitor serum electrolyte and blood gas results. Report abnormal values.
3. Implement measures *to prevent or treat fluid volume deficit, hypokalemia, hypochloremia, and metabolic alkalosis:*
   a. perform actions to prevent nausea and vomiting (see Nursing Diagnosis 7.B, action 2)
   b. if a nasogastric tube is present, irrigate it with normal saline rather than water
   c. perform actions to reduce fever if present (e.g. administer antipyretics as ordered, sponge client with tepid water, remove excessive clothing or bedcovers) *in order to prevent diaphoresis and subsequent loss of fluid*
   d. administer fluid and electrolyte replacements if ordered
   e. maintain a fluid intake of at least 2500 ml/day unless contraindicated
   f. when oral intake is allowed and tolerated, assist client to select foods/fluids high in potassium (e.g. bananas, orange juice, potatoes, raisins, apricots, cantaloupe, tomato juice).

4. Consult physician if signs and symptoms of fluid volume deficit and electrolyte imbalances persist or worsen.

4.b. The client will not experience fluid volume excess or water intoxication as evidenced by:
  1. stable weight
  2. stable B/P
  3. absence of an S₃ heart sound
  4. normal pulse volume
  5. balanced intake and output within 48 hours following surgery
  6. usual mental status
  7. normal breath sounds
  8. BUN, Hct, and serum sodium and osmolality levels within normal range
  9. absence of dyspnea, orthopnea, edema, and distended neck veins
  10. hand vein emptying time less than 3–5 seconds
  11. CVP within normal range.

4.b.1. Assess for and report signs and symptoms of fluid volume excess and water intoxication:
  a. weight gain of 2% or greater over a short period
  b. elevated B/P (B/P may not be elevated if fluid has shifted out of vascular space)
  c. presence of an S_3 heart sound
  d. full, bounding pulse
  e. intake that continues to be greater than output 48 hours postoperatively (for the first 48 hours after surgery, output is expected to be less than intake *due to increased secretion of ADH*)
  f. change in mental status
  g. crackles (rales), diminished or absent breath sounds
  h. low serum sodium and osmolality (indicates water intoxication)
  i. decreased BUN and Hct (low Hct could also indicate blood loss)
  j. dyspnea, orthopnea
  k. edema (peripheral edema reflects fluid volume excess; cellular edema reflects water intoxication)
  l. distended neck veins
  m. delayed hand vein emptying time (longer than 3–5 seconds)
  n. elevated CVP (use internal jugular vein pulsation method to estimate CVP if monitoring device not present).
  2. Monitor chest x-ray results. Report findings of pulmonary vascular congestion, pleural effusion, or pulmonary edema.
  3. Implement measures *to prevent or treat fluid volume excess and water intoxication:*
    a. administer fluid replacement therapy judiciously, especially within first 48 hours after surgery
    b. maintain fluid restrictions if ordered
    c. administer diuretics if ordered.
  4. Consult physician if signs and symptoms of fluid volume excess or water intoxication persist or worsen.

---

5. **NURSING DIAGNOSIS:**

Altered nutrition: less than body requirements

related to:
a. decreased oral intake associated with prescribed dietary modifications, pain, weakness, fatigue, nausea, dislike of prescribed diet, and feeling of fullness (can occur as a result of abdominal distention);
b. inadequate nutritional replacement therapy;
c. loss of nutrients associated with vomiting;
d. increased nutritional needs associated with the increased metabolic rate that occurs during wound healing.

Desired Outcome

Nursing Actions and *Selected Purposes/Rationales*

5. The client will maintain an adequate nutritional status as evidenced by:
  a. weight within normal range for client's age, height, and body frame
  b. normal BUN and serum albumin, Hct, Hb,

5.a. Assess for and report signs and symptoms of malnutrition:
  1. weight below normal for client's age, height, and body frame
  2. abnormal BUN and low serum albumin, Hct, Hb, transferrin, and lymphocyte levels (decreased Hct and Hb may also result from blood loss)
  3. weakness and fatigue
  4. sore, inflamed oral mucous membrane
  5. pale conjunctiva.

Desired Outcome	Nursing Actions and *Selected Purposes/Rationales*

transferrin, and lymphocyte levels
c. usual strength and activity tolerance
d. healthy oral mucous membrane.
	b. Assess for return of bowel function every 2–4 hours. Notify physician when client has normal bowel sounds and is expelling flatus *so that oral intake can be resumed as soon as possible.*
	c. When oral intake is allowed, monitor percentage of meals and snacks client consumes. Report pattern of inadequate intake.
	d. Implement measures *to maintain an adequate nutritional status:*
	   1. when food or oral fluids are allowed, perform actions *to improve oral intake:*
	     a. implement measures to prevent nausea and vomiting (see Nursing Diagnosis 7.B, action 2)
	     b. implement measures to reduce pain (see Nursing Diagnosis 6, action e)
	     c. implement measures to reduce the accumulation of gastrointestinal gas and fluid (see Nursing Diagnosis 7.A, action 3)
	     d. increase activity as allowed and tolerated (*activity usually promotes a sense of well-being and improves appetite*)
	     e. encourage a rest period before meals *to minimize fatigue*
	     f. obtain a dietary consult if necessary to assist client in selecting foods/fluids that meet nutritional needs, are appealing, and adhere to personal and cultural preferences as well as the prescribed dietary modifications
	     g. maintain a clean environment and a relaxed, pleasant atmosphere
	     h. provide oral hygiene before meals
	     i. serve frequent, small meals rather than large ones if client is weak, fatigues easily, and/or has a poor appetite
	     j. encourage significant others to bring in client's favorite foods unless contraindicated
	     k. allow adequate time for meals; reheat foods/fluids if necessary
	     l. limit fluid intake with meals (unless the fluid has high nutritional value) *to reduce early satiety and subsequent decreased food intake*
	   2. ensure that meals are well balanced and high in essential nutrients; offer dietary supplements if indicated
	   3. administer vitamins and minerals if ordered.
	e. Perform a calorie count if ordered. Report information to dietitian and physician.
	f. Consult physician about an alternative method of providing nutrition (e.g. parenteral nutrition, tube feedings) if client does not consume enough food or fluids to meet nutritional needs.

---

6. NURSING DIAGNOSIS: **Pain**

related to tissue trauma and reflex muscle spasms associated with the surgery; irritation from drainage tubes; and stress on surgical area associated with deep breathing, coughing, and/or movement.

Desired Outcome	Nursing Actions and *Selected Purposes/Rationales*
6. The client will experience diminished pain as evidenced by: a. verbalization of a decrease in or absence of pain b. relaxed facial expression and body positioning c. increased participation in activities	6.a. Assess for signs and symptoms of pain (e.g. verbalization of pain, grimacing, reluctance to move, restlessness, diaphoresis, facial pallor, increased B/P, tachycardia). b. Assess client's perception of the severity of pain using a pain intensity rating scale. c. Assess the client's pain pattern (e.g. location, quality, onset, duration, precipitating factors, aggravating factors, alleviating factors). d. Ask the client to describe previous pain experiences and methods used to manage pain effectively.

d. stable vital signs.

e. Implement measures *to reduce pain:*
  1. perform actions *to reduce fear and anxiety about the pain experience* (e.g. assure client that his/her need for pain relief is understood, plan methods for achieving pain control with client)
  2. perform actions to reduce fear and anxiety (see Nursing Diagnosis 20, action b) *in order to promote relaxation and subsequently increase the client's threshold and tolerance for pain*
  3. administer analgesics before activities and procedures that can cause pain and before pain becomes severe
  4. perform actions to promote rest (e.g. minimize environmental activity and noise) *in order to reduce fatigue and subsequently increase the client's threshold and tolerance for pain*
  5. provide or assist with nonpharmacologic methods for pain relief (e.g. massage; position change; progressive relaxation exercises; restful environment; diversional activities such watching television, reading, or conversing)
  6. instruct and assist client to support abdominal or chest incision with a pillow or hands when turning, coughing, and deep breathing
  7. if client has an abdominal incision, instruct him/her to bend knees while coughing and deep breathing *in order to reduce tension on abdominal muscles and incision*
  8. securely anchor drainage tubes *to decrease tissue irritation resulting from movement of tubes*
  9. encourage client to use patient-controlled analgesia (PCA) device as instructed
  10. if client is receiving epidural analgesia, perform actions *to maintain patency of the system* (e.g. keep tubing free of kinks, tape catheter securely, and use caution when moving client *to avoid dislodging catheter*)
  11. administer analgesics, anti-inflammatory agents, and muscle relaxants if ordered.

f. Consult physician if above measures fail to provide adequate pain relief.

7.A. NURSING DIAGNOSIS:

Altered comfort: abdominal distention and gas pain

related to accumulation of gas and fluid associated with:
1. decreased peristalsis resulting from manipulation of the bowel during abdominal surgery and depressant effect of anesthesia and some medications (e.g. narcotic [opioid] analgesics, central-acting muscle relaxants);
2. decreased activity.

Desired Outcome	Nursing Actions and *Selected Purposes/Rationales*

7.A. The client will experience diminished abdominal distention and gas pain as evidenced by:
1. verbalization of decreased abdominal fullness and pain
2. relaxed facial expression and body positioning
3. decrease in abdominal girth.
	7.A.1. Assess for verbal reports of abdominal fullness or gas pain.
	2. Assess for nonverbal signs of abdominal distention or gas pain (e.g. clutching or guarding of abdomen, restlessness, reluctance to move, grimacing, increasing abdominal girth).
	3. Implement measures *to reduce the accumulation of gastrointestinal gas and fluid:*
	  a. encourage and assist client with frequent position changes and ambulation as soon as allowed and tolerated (*activity stimulates peristalsis and expulsion of flatus*)
	  b. instruct the client to avoid activities such as chewing gum and smoking *in order to reduce air swallowing*
	  c. maintain patency of nasogastric, gastric, or intestinal tube if present
	  d. maintain food and oral fluid restrictions as ordered

Desired Outcome	Nursing Actions and *Selected Purposes/Rationales*
	e. when oral intake is allowed, instruct client to avoid intake of carbonated beverages and gas-producing foods (e.g. cabbage, onions, beans) f. encourage client to expel flatus whenever the urge is felt g. consult physician regarding insertion of a rectal tube or administration of a return flow enema if indicated h. encourage use of nonnarcotic analgesics once the period of severe pain has subsided (*narcotic [opioid] analgesics depress gastrointestinal activity*) i. administer gastrointestinal stimulants (e.g. metoclopramide, cisapride, bisacodyl) if ordered *to increase gastrointestinal motility.* 4. Consult physician if signs and symptoms of abdominal distention and gas pain persist or worsen.

■━━━

7.B. NURSING DIAGNOSIS: **Altered comfort: nausea and vomiting**

related to stimulation of the vomiting center associated with:
1. stimulation of visceral afferent pathways resulting from abdominal distention and/or irritating effect of some medications on the gastric mucosa;
2. stimulation of the cerebral cortex resulting from pain, stress, and/or noxious environmental stimuli;
3. stimulation of the chemoreceptor trigger zone resulting from rapid movement and the effect of some medications (e.g. morphine).

Desired Outcome	Nursing Actions and *Selected Purposes/Rationales*

7.B. The client will experience relief of nausea and vomiting as evidenced by:
1. verbalization of relief of nausea
2. absence of vomiting.
	7.B.1. Assess client for nausea and vomiting.
	2. Implement measures *to prevent nausea and vomiting:*
	  a. perform actions to reduce the accumulation of gastrointestinal gas and fluid (see Nursing Diagnosis 7.A, action 3)
	  b. perform actions to reduce pain (see Nursing Diagnosis 6, action e)
	  c. perform actions to reduce fear and anxiety (see Nursing Diagnosis 20, action b)
	  d. eliminate noxious sights and odors from the environment (*noxious stimuli can cause stimulation of the vomiting center*)
	  e. encourage client to take deep, slow breaths when nauseated
	  f. instruct client to change positions slowly (*rapid movement can result in chemoreceptor trigger zone stimulation and subsequent excitation of the vomiting center*)
	  g. provide oral hygiene after each emesis
	  h. when oral intake is allowed:
	    1. advance diet slowly (usually beginning with clear liquids and progressing to solid food)
	    2. avoid serving foods with an overpowering aroma; remove lids from hot foods before entering room
	    3. provide small, frequent meals rather than 3 large ones
	    4. instruct client to ingest foods and fluids slowly
	    5. instruct client to avoid foods/fluids that irritate the gastric mucosa (e.g. spicy foods; caffeine-containing beverages such as coffee, tea, and colas)
	    6. encourage client to eat dry foods (e.g. toast, crackers) and avoid drinking liquids with meals if nauseated
	    7. instruct client to avoid foods high in fat (*fat delays gastric emptying*)
	    8. instruct client to rest after eating with head of bed elevated

9. administer medications known to cause gastric irritation (e.g. aspirin and aspirin-containing products, corticosteroids, ibuprofen) with or immediately after meals unless contraindicated

i. administer antiemetics and gastrointestinal stimulants (e.g. metoclopramide, cisapride) if ordered.

3. Consult physician if above measures fail to control nausea and vomiting.

---

8. NURSING DIAGNOSIS: **Altered oral mucous membrane: dryness**

related to:
a. fluid volume deficit associated with restricted oral intake and fluid loss;
b. decreased salivation associated with food and fluid restrictions and the effect of some medications (e.g. anesthetic agents, narcotic [opioid] analgesics).

Desired Outcome	Nursing Actions and *Selected Purposes/Rationales*

8. The client will maintain a moist, intact oral mucous membrane.	8.a. Assess client for dryness of the oral mucosa.
	b. Implement measures *to relieve dryness of the oral mucous membrane:*
	  1. instruct and assist client to perform oral hygiene as often as needed; avoid use of products that contain lemon and glycerin and use of mouthwashes containing alcohol (*these products have a drying and irritating effect on the oral mucous membrane*)
	  2. encourage client to rinse mouth frequently with water
	  3. lubricate client's lips frequently
	  4. encourage client to breathe through nose rather than mouth
	  5. encourage client not to smoke (*smoking irritates and dries the mucosa*)
	  6. maintain intravenous fluid therapy as ordered *to improve hydration*
	  7. encourage client to suck on hard candy unless contraindicated *in order to stimulate salivation*
	  8. increase oral fluid intake as soon as allowed and tolerated *to improve hydration and stimulate salivation.*
	c. Consult physician if signs and symptoms of parotitis (e.g. pain, tenderness, and swelling at the angle of the jaw; fever) occur.

---

9. NURSING DIAGNOSIS: **Actual/Risk for impaired tissue integrity**

related to:
a. disruption of tissue associated with the surgical procedure;
b. delayed wound healing associated with factors such as decreased nutritional status and inadequate blood supply to wound area;
c. irritation of skin associated with contact with wound drainage, pressure from tubes, and use of tape.

Desired Outcomes	Nursing Actions and *Selected Purposes/Rationales*
9.a. The client will experience normal healing of surgical wound(s) as evidenced by:	9.a.1. Assess for and report signs and symptoms of impaired wound healing (e.g. increasing periwound swelling and redness, pale or necrotic tissue in wounds healing by secondary intention, separation of wound edges in wounds healing by primary intention).

Desired Outcomes	Nursing Actions and *Selected Purposes/Rationales*

1. gradual reduction in periwound swelling and redness
2. presence of granulation tissue if healing is by secondary intention
3. intact, approximated wound edges if healing is by primary intention.

2. Implement measures *to promote wound healing:*
   a. perform actions to maintain an adequate nutritional status (see Nursing Diagnosis 5, action d)
   b. perform actions *to maintain adequate circulation to wound area:*
      1. implement measures to maintain adequate tissue perfusion (see Nursing Diagnosis 1, action b)
      2. do not apply dressings tightly unless ordered (*excessive pressure impairs circulation to the area*)
   c. perform actions *to protect the wound from mechanical injury:*
      1. ensure that dressings are secure enough to keep them from rubbing and irritating wound
      2. carefully remove tape and dressings when performing wound care
      3. remind client to keep hands away from wound area
      4. implement measures to prevent falls (see Nursing Diagnosis 17, action a)
   d. perform actions *to decrease stress on wound area:*
      1. instruct and assist client to support the involved area when moving
      2. instruct and assist client to splint abdominal and chest wounds when coughing
      3. apply an abdominal binder during periods of activity if ordered *for additional support following abdominal surgery*
      4. implement measures to reduce the accumulation of gastrointestinal gas and fluid (see Nursing Diagnosis 7.A, action 3) in clients who have had abdominal surgery
      5. implement measures to prevent nausea and vomiting (see Nursing Diagnosis 7.B, action 2) in clients who have had chest, back, or abdominal surgery
   e. perform actions to prevent wound infection (see Nursing Diagnosis 16, action b.4).
3. If signs and symptoms of impaired wound healing occur:
   a. perform or assist with wound care (e.g. debridement, packing, irrigation) as ordered
   b. prepare client for surgical revision of the wound if planned.

9.b. The client will maintain tissue integrity in areas in contact with wound drainage, tape, and tubings as evidenced by:
1. absence of redness and irritation
2. no skin breakdown.

9.b.1. Inspect skin areas that are in contact with wound drainage, tape, and tubings for signs of irritation and breakdown.
2. Implement measures *to prevent tissue irritation and breakdown in areas in contact with wound drainage, tape, and tubings:*
   a. perform actions *to prevent wound drainage from contacting or remaining on skin:*
      1. inspect dressings, wounds, and areas around drains and puncture sites; cleanse skin and change dressings when appropriate
      2. maintain patency of drainage tubes *to decrease risk of leakage around the tubes*
      3. apply a collection device over drains and incisions that are draining continuously and/or copiously
      4. apply a protective barrier product to skin that is likely to be in frequent contact with drainage
   b. when positioning client, ensure that he/she is not lying on tubings (*pressure on the skin can compromise circulation to that area; in addition, if a drainage tubing is occluded, there is an increased risk for leakage of drainage around the tube*)
   c. anchor all tubings securely *to prevent excessive movement of tubes against tissues*
   d. apply a water-soluble lubricant to external nares every 2–4 hours *to decrease irritation from nasogastric tube and nasal airway or cannula*
   e. perform actions *to decrease skin irritation resulting from the use of tape:*
      1. use only necessary amount of tape
      2. use hypoallergenic tape whenever possible

3. use Montgomery straps or tubular netting *to avoid repeated application and removal of tape if frequent dressing changes are anticipated*
4. when removing tape, pull it in the direction of hair growth; use adhesive solvents if necessary.

3. If tissue breakdown occurs:
   a. notify physician
   b. continue with above measures to prevent further irritation and breakdown
   c. perform care of involved areas as ordered or per standard hospital procedure
   d. assess client closely and report signs and symptoms of infection (e.g. elevated temperature; redness, heat, increased pain, and swelling around area of breakdown; unusual drainage from site).

---

10. NURSING DIAGNOSIS: Activity intolerance

related to:
a. tissue hypoxia associated with diminished tissue perfusion and anemia if present;
b. inadequate nutritional status;
c. difficulty resting and sleeping associated with discomfort, fear, and anxiety.

Desired Outcome	Nursing Actions and *Selected Purposes/Rationales*

10. The client will demonstrate an increased tolerance for activity as evidenced by:
a. verbalization of feeling less fatigued and weak
b. ability to perform activities of daily living without exertional dyspnea, chest pain, diaphoresis, dizziness, and a significant change in vital signs.
	10.a. Assess for signs and symptoms of activity intolerance:
	1. statements of fatigue or weakness
	2. exertional dyspnea, chest pain, diaphoresis, or dizziness
	3. abnormal heart rate response to activity (e.g. increase in rate of 20 beats/minute above resting rate, rate not returning to preactivity level within 3 minutes after stopping activity, change from regular to irregular rate)
	4. decreased systolic B/P or a significant increase (10–15 mm Hg) in diastolic pressure with activity.
	b. Implement measures *to improve activity tolerance:*
	1. perform actions *to promote rest and/or conserve energy:*
	  a. maintain activity restrictions as ordered
	  b. minimize environmental activity and noise
	  c. organize nursing care to allow for periods of uninterrupted rest
	  d. limit number of visitors and their length of stay
	  e. assist client with self-care activities as needed
	  f. keep supplies and personal articles within easy reach
	  g. instruct client in energy-saving techniques (e.g. using shower chair when showering, sitting to brush teeth or comb hair)
	  h. implement measures to reduce fear and anxiety (see Nursing Diagnosis 20, action b)
	  i. implement measures to promote sleep (see Nursing Diagnosis 15, action c)
	  j. implement measures to reduce discomfort (see Nursing Diagnoses 6, action e; 7.A, action 3; and 7.B, action 2)
	2. perform actions to maintain adequate tissue perfusion (see Nursing Diagnosis 1, action b)
	3. perform actions to improve breathing pattern and facilitate airway clearance (see Nursing Diagnoses 2, action c and 3, action b) *in order to promote maximum tissue oxygenation*
	4. maintain oxygen therapy as ordered

Desired Outcome	Nursing Actions and **Selected Purposes/Rationales**

5. perform actions to maintain an adequate nutritional status (see
    Nursing Diagnosis 5, action d)
6. administer packed red cells if ordered
7. increase client's activity gradually as allowed and tolerated.
c. Instruct client to:
    1. report a decreased tolerance for activity
    2. stop any activity that causes chest pain, shortness of breath, dizziness,
        or extreme fatigue or weakness.
d. Consult physician if signs and symptoms of activity intolerance persist or
    worsen.

---

11. NURSING DIAGNOSIS: **Ineffective breathing pattern**

related to:
a. weakness and fatigue associated with tissue hypoxia, inadequate nutritional
    status, and difficulty resting and sleeping;
b. pain and nausea;
c. depressant effect of anesthesia and some medications (e.g. narcotic [opioid]
    analgesics, central-acting muscle relaxants);
d. fear of falling, dislodging tubes, and compromising surgical wound;
e. activity restrictions imposed by the treatment plan.

Desired Outcome	Nursing Actions and **Selected Purposes/Rationales**

11. The client will achieve
maximum physical mobility
within the limitations
imposed by the surgical
procedure and postoperative
treatment plan.

11.a. Implement measures *to increase mobility:*
1. perform actions to improve activity tolerance (see Nursing Diagnosis
    10, action b) *in order to reduce weakness and fatigue*
2. perform actions to reduce pain (see Nursing Diagnosis 6, action e)
3. perform actions to prevent nausea and vomiting (see Nursing
    Diagnosis 7.B, action 2)
4. schedule attempts to increase activity when analgesics and/or
    antiemetics are at peak effect
5. encourage use of nonnarcotic analgesics once severe pain has subsided
6. perform actions *to decrease client's fear of injury:*
    a. implement measures to prevent falls (see Nursing Diagnosis 17,
        action a)
    b. anchor all dressings and tubings securely *to decrease risk of
        inadvertent removal during activity*
7. assure client that level of activity ordered is expected to facilitate
    rather than compromise wound healing and postoperative recovery
8. encourage activity and participation in self-care as allowed and
    tolerated; put side rails up and provide overhead trapeze if
    appropriate *to promote independent movement.*
b. Provide praise and encouragement for all efforts to increase physical
    mobility.
c. Encourage the support of significant others. Allow them to assist client
    with activity if desired.
d. Consult physician if client is unable to achieve expected level of mobility.

---

12. NURSING DIAGNOSIS: **Self-care deficit**

related to impaired physical mobility associated with activity intolerance, pain,
nausea, depressant effect of some medications, fear of dislodging tubes and
compromising surgical wound, and activity restrictions.

Desired Outcome	Nursing Actions and *Selected Purposes/Rationales*

12. The client will perform self-care activities within physical limitations and postoperative activity restrictions.	12.a. With client, develop a realistic plan for meeting daily physical needs.
	b. Implement measures *to facilitate the client's ability to perform self-care activities:*
	  1. schedule care at time when client is most likely to be able to participate (e.g. when analgesics are at peak effect, after rest periods, not immediately after meals or treatments)
	  2. keep needed objects within easy reach
	  3. allow adequate time for accomplishment of self-care activities
	  4. perform actions to increase physical mobility (see Nursing Diagnosis 11, action a).
	c. Encourage maximum independence within physical limitations and postoperative activity restrictions. Provide positive feedback for all efforts and accomplishments of self-care.
	d. Assist the client with activities he/she is unable to perform independently.
	e. Inform significant others of client's abilities to perform own care. Explain the importance of encouraging and allowing client to maintain an optimal level of independence.

■——

13. NURSING DIAGNOSIS: **Urinary retention**

related to:
a. increased tone of the urinary sphincters associated with sympathetic nervous system stimulation resulting from pain, fear, and anxiety;
b. decreased perception of bladder fullness associated with depressant effect of some medications (e.g. anesthetic agents, narcotic [opioid] analgesics, central-acting muscle relaxants);
c. relaxation of the bladder muscle associated with depressant effect of some medications (e.g. anesthetic agents, narcotic [opioid] analgesics, central-acting muscle relaxants) and stimulation of the sympathetic nervous system (can result from pain, fear, and anxiety).

Desired Outcome	Nursing Actions and *Selected Purposes/Rationales*

13. The client will not experience urinary retention as evidenced by:
a. voiding at normal intervals
b. no reports of bladder fullness and suprapubic discomfort
c. absence of bladder distention and dribbling of urine
d. balanced intake and output within 48 hours following surgery.
	13.a. Determine client's usual urinary elimination pattern.
	b. Assess for signs and symptoms of urinary retention:
	  1. frequent voiding of small amounts (25–60 ml) of urine
	  2. reports of bladder fullness or suprapubic discomfort
	  3. bladder distention
	  4. dribbling of urine.
	c. Monitor intake and output. Consult physician if there is no urine output within 6–8 hours after surgery or if intake and output are not balanced within 48 hours after surgery (for first 48 hours postoperatively, urine output is expected to be less than intake *due to factors such as blood loss and increased secretion of ADH*).
	d. Implement measures *to prevent urinary retention:*
	  1. instruct client to urinate when the urge is first felt
	  2. perform actions *to promote relaxation during voiding attempts* (e.g. provide privacy, hold a warm blanket against abdomen, encourage client to read)
	  3. perform actions *that may help trigger the micturition reflex and promote a sense of relaxation during voiding attempts* (e.g. run water, place client's hands in warm water, pour warm water over perineum)

Desired Outcome	Nursing Actions and *Selected Purposes/Rationales*

4. allow client to assume a normal position for voiding unless contraindicated
5. instruct client to lean his/her upper body forward and/or gently press downward on lower abdomen during voiding attempts unless contraindicated *in order to put pressure on the bladder (pressure helps create a sensation of bladder fullness, which stimulates the micturition reflex)*
6. perform actions to reduce postoperative pain (see Nursing Diagnosis 6, action e)
7. encourage use of nonnarcotic analgesics once period of severe pain has subsided
8. administer cholinergic drugs (e.g. bethanechol) if ordered *to stimulate bladder contraction.*

  e. Consult physician regarding intermittent catheterization or insertion of an indwelling catheter if above actions fail to alleviate urinary retention.

  f. If urinary catheter is present, prevent urinary retention by maintaining patency of the catheter (e.g. keep tubing free of kinks, irrigate as ordered).

---

14. NURSING DIAGNOSIS:

Constipation

related to:
a. decreased gastrointestinal motility associated with manipulation of bowel during abdominal surgery, depressant effect of anesthesia and narcotic (opioid) analgesics, and decreased activity;
b. decreased fluid intake;
c. decreased intake of foods high in fiber.

Desired Outcome	Nursing Actions and *Selected Purposes/Rationales*

14. The client will not experience constipation as evidenced by:
  a. usual frequency of bowel movements about two days after usual oral intake is resumed
  b. passage of soft, formed stool
  c. absence of increasing abdominal distention and pain, feeling of rectal fullness or pressure, and straining during defecation.

14.a. Ascertain client's usual bowel elimination habits.
  b. Assess for signs and symptoms of constipation (e.g. decrease in frequency of bowel movements; passage of hard, formed stools; anorexia; increasing abdominal distention and pain; feeling of fullness or pressure in rectum; straining during defecation).
  c. Assess bowel sounds. Report diminishing sounds or sounds that do not return to normal when expected.
  d. Implement measures *to prevent constipation:*
    1. increase activity as allowed and tolerated
    2. encourage client to defecate whenever the urge is felt
    3. assist client to the bathroom or bedside commode or place in high Fowler's position on bedpan for bowel movements unless contraindicated
    4. encourage client to relax, provide privacy, and have call signal within reach during attempts to defecate (*measures to promote relaxation enable client to relax the levator ani muscle and external anal sphincter, which facilitates evacuation of stool*)
    5. encourage client to establish a regular time for defecation, preferably an hour after a meal
    6. encourage use of nonnarcotic analgesics once period of severe pain has subsided
    7. when oral intake is allowed:
      a. instruct client to maintain a minimum fluid intake of 2500 ml/day unless contraindicated
      b. encourage client to drink hot liquids upon arising in the morning *in order to stimulate peristalsis*

    c. when diet advances, instruct client to increase intake of foods high in fiber (e.g. bran, whole-grain breads and cereals, fresh fruits and vegetables) unless contraindicated

  8. administer laxatives or cathartics and/or enemas if ordered.

e. Consult physician if signs and symptoms of constipation persist.

---

15. NURSING DIAGNOSIS: **Sleep pattern disturbance**

related to fear, anxiety, discomfort, inability to assume usual sleep position, and frequent assessments and treatments.

Desired Outcome	Nursing Actions and *Selected Purposes/Rationales*

15. The client will attain optimal amounts of sleep as evidenced by:
  a. statements of feeling well rested
  b. usual mental status
  c. absence of frequent yawning, dark circles under eyes, and hand tremors.
	15.a. Assess for signs and symptoms of a sleep pattern disturbance (e.g. statements of difficulty falling asleep, sleep interruptions, or not feeling well rested; irritability; lethargy; disorientation; frequent yawning; dark circles under eyes; slight hand tremors).
	b. Determine the client's usual sleep habits.
	c. Implement measures *to promote sleep:*
	  1. discourage long periods of sleep during the day unless signs and symptoms of sleep deprivation exist or daytime sleep is usual for client
	  2. perform actions to reduce fear and anxiety (see Nursing Diagnosis 20, action b)
	  3. perform actions to reduce discomfort (see Nursing Diagnoses 6, action e; 7.A, action 3; and 7.B, action 2)
	  4. encourage participation in relaxing diversional activities during the evening
	  5. when oral intake is allowed:
	    a. discourage intake of fluids high in caffeine (e.g. coffee, tea, colas), especially in the evening
	    b. offer client an evening snack that includes milk or cheese unless contraindicated (*the L-tryptophan in milk and cheese helps induce and maintain sleep*)
	  6. allow client to continue usual sleep practices (e.g. position; time; presleep routines such as reading, watching television, listening to music, and meditating) unless contraindicated
	  7. satisfy basic needs such as comfort and warmth before sleep
	  8. encourage client to urinate just before bedtime
	  9. reduce environmental distractions (e.g. close door to client's room; use night light rather than overhead light whenever possible; lower volume of paging system; keep staff conversations at a low level and away from client's room; close curtains between clients in a semi-private room or ward; keep beepers and alarms on low volume; provide client with "white noise" such as fan, soft music, or tape-recorded sounds of the ocean or rain; have earplugs available for client if needed)
	  10. administer prescribed sedative-hypnotics if indicated
	  11. perform actions *to reduce interruptions during sleep (80–100 minutes of uninterrupted sleep is usually needed to complete one sleep cycle):*
	    a. restrict visitors
	    b. group care (e.g. medications, treatments, physical care, assessments) whenever possible.
	d. Consult physician if signs and symptoms of sleep deprivation persist or worsen.

---

16. NURSING DIAGNOSIS: **Risk for infection:**

    a. **pneumonia** related to stasis of pulmonary secretions and aspiration (if it occurs);

    b. **wound infection** related to:

      1. wound contamination associated with introduction of pathogens during or following surgery

      2. decreased resistance to infection associated with factors such as diminished tissue perfusion of wound area and inadequate nutritional status;

    c. **urinary tract infection** related to:

      1. increased growth and colonization of microorganisms associated with urinary stasis

      2. introduction of pathogens associated with an indwelling catheter if present.

Desired Outcomes	Nursing Actions and *Selected Purposes/Rationales*

16.a. The client will not develop pneumonia as evidenced by:
1. normal breath sounds
2. resonant percussion note over lungs
3. absence of tachypnea
4. cough productive of clear mucus only
5. afebrile status
6. absence of pleuritic pain
7. WBC count declining toward normal
8. blood gases within normal range for client
9. negative sputum culture.
	16.a.1. Assess for and report signs and symptoms of pneumonia:
	  a. abnormal breath sounds (e.g. crackles [rales], pleural friction rub, bronchial breath sounds, diminished or absent breath sounds)
	  b. dull percussion note over affected lung area
	  c. increase in respiratory rate
	  d. cough productive of purulent, green, or rust-colored sputum
	  e. chills and fever
	  f. pleuritic pain
	  g. persistent elevation of or increase in WBC count.
	2. Monitor oximetry and blood gas results. Report abnormal findings.
	3. Monitor chest x-ray results. Report findings indicative of pneumonia.
	4. Obtain sputum specimen for culture if ordered. Report abnormal results.
	5. Implement measures *to prevent pneumonia:*
	  a. perform actions to maintain an effective breathing pattern and airway clearance (see Nursing Diagnoses 2, action c and 3, action b)
	  b. perform actions to reduce risk for aspiration (see Nursing Diagnosis 18, action c)
	  c. encourage and assist client to perform frequent oral hygiene *in order to reduce the colonization of bacteria in the oropharynx and subsequent aspiration of these microorganisms*
	  d. protect client from persons with respiratory tract infections.
	6. If signs and symptoms of pneumonia occur:
	  a. continue with above measures
	  b. administer oxygen as ordered
	  c. administer antimicrobials if ordered
	  d. perform or assist with postural drainage therapy (PDT) if ordered
	  e. refer to Care Plan on Pneumonia for additional care measures.

16.b. The client will remain free of wound infection as evidenced by: 1. absence of chills and fever 2. absence of redness, heat, swelling, and increased pain in wound area	**16.b.1.** Assess for and report signs and symptoms of wound infection (e.g. chills; fever; redness, heat, swelling, and increased pain in wound area; unusual wound drainage; foul odor from wound area). 2. Monitor for and report persistent elevation of WBC count and significant change in differential. 3. Obtain cultures of wound drainage as ordered. Report positive results. 4. Implement measures *to prevent wound infection:* a. perform actions to promote wound healing (see Nursing Diagnosis 9, actions a.2.a–d)

3. usual drainage from wounds
4. WBC and differential counts returning toward normal
5. negative cultures of wound drainage.

b. perform actions *to reduce the introduction of pathogens into the wound:*
   1. use good handwashing technique and encourage client to do the same
   2. instruct client to avoid touching incisions, dressings, drainage tubings, and open wounds
   3. use sterile technique during all dressing changes and wound care
   4. replace equipment and solutions used for wound care according to hospital policy *in order to reduce the risk of colonization of microorganisms*
   5. anchor wound drainage tubings securely *to reduce in-and-out movement of the tubes*
   6. maintain a closed system for wound drains whenever possible
   7. protect client from others with infections
c. administer antimicrobials if ordered.

5. If signs and symptoms of infection are present, continue with above actions.

16.c. The client will remain free of urinary tract infection as evidenced by:
   1. clear urine
   2. no unusual odor to urine
   3. absence of frequency, urgency, and burning on urination
   4. absence of chills and fever
   5. absence of nitrites, bacteria, and WBCs in urine
   6. negative urine culture.

16.c.1. Assess for and report signs and symptoms of urinary tract infection (e.g. cloudy, foul-smelling urine; reports of frequency, urgency, or burning on urination; chills; elevated temperature).

2. Monitor urinalysis and report presence of nitrites, bacteria, and/or WBCs.

3. Obtain a urine specimen for culture and sensitivity if ordered. Report abnormal results.

4. Implement measures *to prevent urinary tract infection:*
   a. perform actions to prevent urinary retention (see Nursing Diagnosis 13, actions d and f)
   b. instruct female client to wipe from front to back after urinating or defecating
   c. assist client with perineal care routinely and after each bowel movement
   d. maintain fluid intake of at least 2500 ml/day unless contraindicated *to promote urine formation and subsequent voiding, which flushes pathogens from the bladder and urethra*
   e. increase activity as allowed and tolerated *to decrease urinary stasis*
   f. maintain sterile technique during urinary catheterizations and irrigations
   g. if an indwelling urinary catheter is present:
      1. secure the catheter tubing to lower abdomen or thigh on males or to thigh on females *to minimize risk of accidental traction on the catheter and subsequent trauma to the bladder and urethra*
      2. perform catheter care as often as needed *to prevent accumulation of mucus around the meatus*
      3. anchor tubing securely *to reduce the amount of in-and-out movement of the catheter* (*this movement can result in the introduction of pathogens into the urinary tract and can cause tissue trauma, which can result in colonization of microorganisms*)
      4. maintain a closed drainage system whenever possible *to reduce the risk of the introduction of pathogens into the urinary tract*
      5. keep urine collection container lower than level of the bladder at all times *to prevent reflux or stasis of urine*
      6. remove catheter as soon as allowed (*the risk for urinary tract infection increases the longer the catheter is in place*).

5. If signs and symptoms of urinary tract infection are present:
   a. continue with the above actions
   b. administer antimicrobials if ordered.

17. NURSING DIAGNOSIS: **Risk for trauma: falls**

related to:
a. weakness and fatigue;
b. dizziness or syncope associated with postural hypotension resulting from peripheral pooling of blood and blood loss during surgery;
c. central nervous system depressant effect of some medications (e.g. narcotic [opioid] analgesics, central-acting muscle relaxants);
d. presence of tubings or equipment.

Desired Outcome	Nursing Actions and *Selected Purposes/Rationales*
17. The client will not experience falls.	17.a. Implement measures *to prevent falls*:

    1. keep bed in low position with side rails up when client is in bed
    2. keep needed items within easy reach
    3. encourage client to request assistance whenever needed; have call signal within easy reach
    4. use lap belt when client is in chair if indicated
    5. instruct client to wear well-fitting slippers/shoes with nonslip soles and low heels when ambulating
    6. keep floor free of clutter and wipe up spills promptly
    7. instruct and assist client to get out of bed slowly *in order to reduce dizziness or syncope associated with postural hypotension*
    8. carefully position tubings and equipment so that they will not interfere with ambulation
    9. provide ambulatory aids (e.g. walker, cane) if client is weak or unsteady on feet
    10. accompany client during ambulation and use a transfer safety belt if he/she is weak or dizzy
    11. instruct client to ambulate in well-lit areas and to utilize handrails if needed
    12. do not rush client; allow adequate time for ambulation to the bathroom and in hallway
    13. make sure that shower area has a nonslip bottom surface and that shower chair, secure bath mat, call signal, grab bars, and adequate lighting are present
    14. perform actions to increase strength and improve activity tolerance (see Nursing Diagnosis 10, action b).
  b. Include client and significant others in planning and implementing measures to prevent falls.
  c. If client falls, initiate first aid measures if appropriate and notify physician.

18. NURSING DIAGNOSIS: **Risk for aspiration**

related to:
a. decreased level of consciousness and absent or diminished gag reflex associated with depressant effect of anesthesia and narcotic (opioid) analgesics;
b. supine positioning;
c. increased risk for gastroesophageal reflux associated with increased gastric pressure resulting from decreased gastrointestinal motility.

Desired Outcome	Nursing Actions and *Selected Purposes/Rationales*

18. The client will not aspirate secretions, vomitus, or foods/fluids as evidenced by:
   a. clear breath sounds
   b. resonant percussion note over lungs
   c. absence of cough, tachypnea, and dyspnea.

18.a. Assess for signs and symptoms of aspiration of secretions, vomitus, or foods/fluids (e.g. rhonchi, dull percussion note over affected lung area, cough, tachypnea, dyspnea, tachycardia).
   b. Monitor chest x-ray results. Report findings of pulmonary infiltrate.
   c. Implement measures *to reduce the risk for aspiration:*
      1. withhold oral foods/fluids and place client in a side-lying position unless contraindicated if gag reflex is absent or client is not alert
      2. have suction equipment readily available for use
      3. perform oropharyngeal suctioning and provide oral hygiene as often as needed *to remove secretions, vomitus, and/or food particles*
      4. perform actions to prevent nausea and vomiting (see Nursing Diagnosis 7.B, action 2)
      5. perform actions to reduce accumulation of gastrointestinal gas and fluid (see Nursing Diagnosis 7.A, action 3) *in order to prevent gastric distention and gastroesophageal reflux*
      6. place client in high Fowler's position during and for at least 30 minutes after eating or drinking unless contraindicated.
   d. If signs and symptoms of aspiration occur:
      1. perform tracheal suctioning
      2. withhold oral intake
      3. notify physician
      4. prepare client for chest x-ray.

---

19. **COLLABORATIVE DIAGNOSES:**

Potential complications following surgery:
   a. **hypovolemic shock** related to:
      1. hemorrhage associated with opening of wound (can occur as a result of inadequate wound closure, stress on incision line, and/or poor wound healing), slippage of closures on ligated vessels, and/or disruption of clots at incision site
      2. fluid volume deficit associated with excessive fluid loss and inadequate fluid replacement;
   b. **atelectasis** related to shallow respirations, stasis of secretions in the alveoli and bronchioles, and decreased surfactant production (results from inadequate deep breathing and changes in regional blood flow in the lungs);
   c. **thromboembolism** related to:
      1. venous stasis associated with decreased activity, positioning during and following surgery, increased blood viscosity (can result from fluid volume deficit), and abdominal distention (the distended intestine may put pressure on the abdominal vessels)
      2. hypercoagulability associated with increased release of tissue thromboplastin into the blood (occurs as a result of surgical trauma) and hemoconcentration and increased blood viscosity (can occur as a result of fluid volume deficit)
      3. trauma to vein walls during surgery;
   d. **paralytic ileus** related to manipulation of intestines during abdominal surgery, effect of anesthesia and some medications (e.g. central nervous system depressants), hypokalemia, and hypovolemia (can cause decreased blood supply to the intestine);
   e. **dehiscence** related to:
      1. inadequate wound closure
      2. stress on incision line associated with persistent coughing, distention, or vomiting
      3. poor wound healing associated with decreased tissue perfusion of wound area, inadequate nutritional status, and infection.

Desired Outcomes	Nursing Actions and *Selected Purposes/Rationales*

19.a. The client will not develop hypovolemic shock as evidenced by:
1. usual mental status
2. stable vital signs
3. skin warm, dry, and usual color
4. palpable peripheral pulses
5. urine output at least 30 ml/hour.
	19.a.1. Assess for and report excessive bleeding and gastrointestinal and wound drainage, persistent vomiting, and/or difficulty maintaining intravenous or oral fluid intake as ordered.
	2. Monitor RBC, Hct, and Hb levels. Report decreasing values.
	3. Assess for and report signs and symptoms of hypovolemic shock:
	  a. restlessness, agitation, confusion, or other change in mental status
	  b. significant decrease in B/P
	  c. postural hypotension
	  d. rapid, weak pulse
	  e. rapid respirations
	  f. cool, moist skin
	  g. pallor, cyanosis
	  h. diminished or absent peripheral pulses
	  i. urine output less than 30 ml/hour.
	4. Implement measures *to prevent hypovolemic shock:*
	  a. if bleeding occurs, apply firm, prolonged pressure to area if possible
	  b. perform actions to prevent fluid volume deficit (see Nursing Diagnosis 4, actions a.3.a–e).
	5. If signs and symptoms of hypovolemic shock occur:
	  a. continue with above measures to control bleeding and prevent fluid volume deficit
	  b. place client flat in bed with legs elevated unless contraindicated
	  c. monitor vital signs frequently
	  d. administer oxygen as ordered
	  e. administer blood and/or volume expanders if ordered
	  f. prepare client for insertion of hemodynamic monitoring devices (e.g. central venous catheter, intra-arterial catheter) if indicated
	  g. provide emotional support to client and significant others.

19.b. The client will not develop atelectasis as evidenced by:
1. clear, audible breath sounds
2. resonant percussion note over lungs
3. unlabored respirations at 14–20/minute
4. pulse rate within normal range for client
5. afebrile status.
	19.b.1. Assess for and report signs and symptoms of atelectasis (e.g. diminished or absent breath sounds, dull percussion note over affected area, increased respiratory rate, dyspnea, tachycardia, elevated temperature).
	2. Monitor chest x-ray results. Report findings of atelectasis.
	3. Implement measures *to prevent atelectasis:*
	  a. perform actions to improve breathing pattern (see Nursing Diagnosis 2, action c)
	  b. perform actions to promote effective airway clearance (see Nursing Diagnosis 3, action b).
	4. If signs and symptoms of atelectasis occur:
	  a. increase frequency of turning, coughing or "huffing," deep breathing, and use of incentive spirometer
	  b. consult physician if signs and symptoms of atelectasis persist or worsen.

19.c.1. The client will not develop a deep vein thrombus as evidenced by:
a. absence of pain, tenderness, swelling, and distended superficial vessels in extremities
b. usual temperature of extremities
c. negative Homans' sign.
	19.c.1.a. Assess for and report signs and symptoms of a deep vein thrombus:
	  1. pain or tenderness in extremity
	  2. increase in circumference of extremity
	  3. distention of superficial vessels in extremity
	  4. unusual warmth of extremity
	  5. positive Homans' sign (not always a reliable indicator).
	  b. Implement measures *to prevent thrombus formation:*
	    1. perform actions to prevent peripheral pooling of blood (see Nursing Diagnosis 1, action b.4)
	    2. maintain a minimum fluid intake of 2500 ml/day (unless contraindicated) *to prevent increased blood viscosity*
	    3. administer anticoagulants (e.g. low- or adjusted-dose heparin, warfarin, low-molecular-weight heparin) or antiplatelet agents (e.g. low-dose aspirin) if ordered.
	  c. If signs and symptoms of a deep vein thrombus occur:
	    1. maintain client on bed rest until activity orders received
	    2. elevate foot of bed 15–20° above heart level if ordered

3. discourage positions that compromise blood flow (e.g. pillows under knees, crossing legs, sitting for long periods)
4. prepare client for diagnostic studies (e.g. venography, duplex ultrasound, impedance plethysmography) if indicated
5. administer anticoagulants (e.g. heparin, warfarin) if ordered
6. refer to Care Plan on Deep Vein Thrombosis for additional care measures.

19.c.2. The client will not experience a pulmonary embolism as evidenced by:
    a. absence of sudden chest pain
    b. unlabored respirations at 14–20/minute
    c. pulse 60–100 beats/minute
    d. blood gases within normal range.

19.c.2.a. Assess for and report signs and symptoms of a pulmonary embolism (e.g. sudden chest pain, dyspnea, tachypnea, tachycardia, apprehension, low PaO_2).
    b. Implement measures *to prevent a pulmonary embolism:*
      1. perform actions to prevent and treat a deep vein thrombus (see actions c.1.b and c.1.c in this diagnosis)
      2. do not exercise, check for Homans' sign in, or massage any extremity known to have a thrombus
      3. caution client to avoid activities that create a Valsalva response (e.g. straining to have bowel movement, holding breath while moving up in bed) *in order to prevent dislodgment of existing thrombi*
      4. prepare client for a vena caval interruption (e.g. insertion of an intracaval filtering device) if planned.
    c. If signs and symptoms of a pulmonary embolism occur:
      1. maintain client on strict bed rest in a semi- to high Fowler's position
      2. maintain oxygen therapy as ordered
      3. prepare client for diagnostic tests (e.g. blood gases, ventilation-perfusion lung scan, pulmonary angiography)
      4. administer anticoagulants (e.g. continuous intravenous heparin, warfarin) if ordered
      5. prepare client for a vena caval interruption (e.g. insertion of an intracaval filtering device) if planned *to prevent further pulmonary emboli*
      6. provide emotional support to client and significant others
      7. refer to Care Plan on Pulmonary Embolism for additional care measures.

19.d. The client will not develop a paralytic ileus as evidenced by:
    1. absence or resolution of abdominal pain and cramping
    2. soft, nondistended abdomen
    3. gradual return of bowel sounds
    4. passage of flatus.

19.d.1. Assess for and report signs and symptoms of paralytic ileus (e.g. development of or persistent abdominal pain and cramping; firm, distended abdomen; absent bowel sounds; failure to pass flatus).
    2. Implement measures *to prevent paralytic ileus:*
      a. increase activity as soon as allowed and tolerated
      b. perform actions to prevent hypokalemia (see Nursing Diagnosis 4, action a.3) in order *to prevent the resultant decrease in peristalsis*
      c. perform actions to maintain adequate tissue perfusion (see Nursing Diagnosis 1, action b) in order *to maintain adequate blood supply to the bowel*
      d. administer gastrointestinal stimulants (e.g. metoclopramide, cisapride) if ordered.
    3. If signs and symptoms of paralytic ileus occur:
      a. continue with above measures
      b. withhold all oral intake
      c. insert nasogastric tube and maintain suction as ordered
      d. assess for and report signs of bowel necrosis (e.g. fever, increased or persistent elevation of WBCs, significant decrease in B/P and increase in pulse).

19.e. The client will not experience dehiscence as evidenced by intact, approximated wound edges.

19.e.1. Assess for and report evidence of dehiscence (separation of edges of the wound).
    2. Implement measures to promote wound healing (see Nursing Diagnosis 9, action a.2) *in order to decrease the risk of dehiscence.*
    3. If dehiscence occurs:
      a. apply skin closures (e.g. butterfly tape, Steri-Strips) to the incision line if appropriate

Desired Outcomes	Nursing Actions and *Selected Purposes/Rationales*

b. cover wound with a sterile, nonadherent dressing
c. assist with resuturing the wound if indicated
d. if client has an abdominal incision, assess for and immediately report signs and symptoms of evisceration (e.g. client statements that "something popped" or "gave way," sudden drainage of serosanguineous peritoneal fluid from wound, protrusion of intestinal contents).

---

20. NURSING DIAGNOSIS: **Anxiety**

related to unfamiliar environment; pain; lack of understanding of surgical procedure performed, diagnosis, and postoperative treatment plan; changes in body image and roles; and financial concerns.

Desired Outcome	Nursing Actions and *Selected Purposes/Rationales*

20. The client will experience a reduction in anxiety as evidenced by:
   a. verbalization of feeling less anxious
   b. usual sleep pattern
   c. relaxed facial expression and body movements
   d. stable vital signs
   e. usual perceptual ability and interactions with others.

20.a. Assess client for signs and symptoms of anxiety (e.g. verbalization of feeling anxious, insomnia, tenseness, shakiness, restlessness, diaphoresis, tachycardia, elevated blood pressure, facial pallor, self-focused behaviors). Validate perceptions carefully, remembering that some behavior may result from factors such as pain, fluid and electrolyte imbalances, and infection.
   b. Implement measures *to reduce fear and anxiety:*
      1. orient client to hospital environment, equipment, and routines
      2. introduce client to staff who will be participating in care; if possible, maintain consistency in staff assigned to his/her care *to provide feelings of stability and comfort with the environment*
      3. assure client that staff members are nearby; respond to call signal as soon as possible
      4. maintain a calm, supportive, confident manner when interacting with client
      5. encourage verbalization of fear and anxiety; provide feedback
      6. reinforce the physician's explanations and clarify any misconceptions the client has about the diagnosis, surgical procedure performed, treatment plan, and prognosis
      7. perform actions to reduce pain (see Nursing Diagnosis 6, action e)
      8. provide a calm, restful environment
      9. instruct client in relaxation techniques and encourage participation in diversional activities
      10. assist client to identify specific stressors and ways to cope with them
      11. provide information based on current needs of client at a level he/she can understand; encourage questions and clarification of information provided
      12. when appropriate, assist client to meet spiritual needs (e.g. arrange for a visit from clergy)
      13. initiate financial and/or social service referrals if indicated
      14. encourage significant others to project a caring, concerned attitude without obvious anxiousness
      15. include significant others in orientation and teaching sessions and encourage their continued support of the client
      16. administer prescribed antianxiety agents if indicated.
   c. Consult physician if above actions fail to control fear and anxiety.

Discharge Teaching

■

21. NURSING DIAGNOSIS:	**Knowledge deficit, Ineffective management of therapeutic regimen, or Altered health maintenance***

*The nurse should select the diagnostic label that is most appropriate for the client's discharge teaching needs.

Desired Outcomes	Nursing Actions and *Selected Purposes/Rationales*
21.a. The client will identify ways to prevent postoperative infection.	21.a. Instruct client in ways to prevent postoperative infection: 1. continue with coughing (if allowed) and deep breathing every 2 hours while awake 2. reinforce continued use of incentive spirometer if indicated 3. increase activity as ordered 4. avoid contact with persons who have infections 5. avoid crowds during flu and cold seasons 6. decrease or stop smoking 7. drink at least 10 glasses of liquid/day unless contraindicated 8. maintain a balanced nutritional intake 9. maintain proper balance of rest and activity 10. maintain good personal hygiene (especially oral care, handwashing, and perineal care) 11. avoid touching any wound unless it is completely healed 12. maintain sterile or clean technique as ordered during wound care.
21.b. The client will demonstrate the ability to perform wound care.	21.b.1. Discuss the rationale for, frequency of, and equipment necessary for the prescribed wound care. 2. Provide client with the necessary supplies (e.g. dressings, irrigating solution, tape) for wound care and with names and addresses of places where additional supplies can be obtained. 3. Demonstrate wound care and proper cleansing of any reusable equipment. Allow time for questions, clarification, and return demonstration.
21.c. The client will state signs and symptoms to report to the health care provider.	21.c. Instruct the client to report the following signs and symptoms: 1. persistent low-grade or significantly elevated (38.3° C [101° F]) temperature 2. difficulty breathing 3. chest pain 4. cough productive of purulent, green, or rust-colored sputum 5. increasing weakness or inability to tolerate prescribed activity level 6. increasing discomfort or discomfort not controlled by prescribed medications and treatments 7. continued nausea or vomiting 8. increasing abdominal distention and/or discomfort 9. separation of wound edges 10. increasing redness, warmth, pain, or swelling around wound 11. unusual or excessive drainage from any wound site 12. pain or swelling in calf of one or both legs 13. urine retention 14. frequency, urgency, or burning on urination 15. cloudy, foul-smelling urine.
21.d. The client will verbalize an understanding of and a plan for adhering to recommended follow-up care including future appointments with health	21.d.1. Reinforce importance of keeping scheduled follow-up appointments with the health care provider. 2. Reinforce physician's instructions about dietary modifications. Obtain a dietary consult for client if needed. 3. Reinforce physician's instructions on suggested activity level and treatment plan.

Desired Outcomes	Nursing Actions and *Selected Purposes/Rationales*

care provider, dietary modifications, activity level, treatments, and medications prescribed.	4. Explain the rationale for, side effects of, and importance of taking medications prescribed. Inform client of pertinent food and drug interactions.
	5. Implement measures to improve client compliance:
	   a. include significant others in teaching sessions if possible
	   b. encourage questions and allow time for reinforcement and clarification of information provided
	   c. provide written instructions on scheduled appointments with health care provider, dietary modifications, activity level, treatment plan, medications prescribed, and signs and symptoms to report.

Bibliography

See pages 897–898.

NURSING CARE
OF THE
IMMOBILE CLIENT

▤ IMMOBILITY

Immobility refers to a limitation of physical activity as a result of a disease process, trauma, or therapeutic intervention. Immobility for periods greater than 48 to 72 hours will result in changes in all body systems. **This care plan focuses on the adult client who is on complete bed rest for a prolonged period during hospitalization.**

Goals of care are to maintain comfort, prevent complications, and educate the client regarding follow-up care. **Many of the actions included in the care plan will help prevent disuse syndrome, which is a deterioration of body systems as a result of prescribed or unavoidable musculoskeletal inactivity.**

DISCHARGE CRITERIA

Prior to discharge, the client will:

- have no signs or symptoms of complications of immobility
- have no evidence of tissue irritation or breakdown
- have clear, audible breath sounds throughout lungs
- have an adequate nutritional status
- verbalize an understanding of ways to prevent complications associated with continued decreased mobility
- demonstrate techniques for meeting self-care needs
- state signs and symptoms to report to the health care provider
- identify community agencies that can provide assistance with home care and transportation
- verbalize an understanding of and a plan for adhering to recommended follow-up care including future appointments with health care provider and physical therapist, exercise regimen, and medications prescribed.

1. NURSING DIAGNOSIS: **Ineffective breathing pattern**

related to:
a. decreased rate and depth of respirations associated with the depressant effect of some medications (e.g. narcotic [opioid] analgesics, sedatives, central-acting muscle relaxants) that may be given for treatment of current diagnosis;
b. diminished lung/chest wall expansion associated with:
   1. recumbent positioning (in this position, full expansion of the lungs is restricted by the bed surface and by the abdominal contents pushing up against the diaphragm)
   2. weakness.

Desired Outcome	Nursing Actions and *Selected Purposes/Rationales*

1. The client will maintain an effective breathing pattern as evidenced by:
a. normal rate and depth of respirations
b. blood gases within normal range.
	1.a. Assess for signs and symptoms of an ineffective breathing pattern (e.g. shallow or slow respirations).
	b. Monitor for and report the following:
	  1. abnormal blood gases
	  2. significant decrease in oximetry results.
	c. Implement measures *to improve breathing pattern:*
	  1. place client in a semi- to high Fowler's position unless contraindicated; position client with pillows *to prevent slumping*
	  2. turn client at least every 2 hours
	  3. instruct client to deep breathe or use incentive spirometer every 1–2 hours
	  4. assist with positive airway pressure techniques (e.g. IPPB, continuous positive airway pressure [CPAP], biphasic positive airway pressure [BiPAP], expiratory positive airway pressure [EPAP]) if ordered
	  5. instruct client to avoid intake of gas-forming foods (e.g. beans, cauliflower, cabbage, onions), carbonated beverages, and large meals *in order to prevent gastric distention and additional pressure on the diaphragm*
	  6. increase activity as allowed
	  7. administer central nervous system depressants judiciously; hold medication and consult physician if respiratory rate is less than 12/minute.
	d. Consult physician if:
	  1. ineffective breathing pattern continues
	  2. signs and symptoms of impaired gas exchange (e.g. restlessness, irritability, confusion, decreased PaO_2 and increased $PaCO_2$ levels) are present.

2. NURSING DIAGNOSIS: **Ineffective airway clearance**

related to stasis of secretions associated with:
a. decreased mobility;
b. decreased effectiveness of cough resulting from diminished lung/chest wall expansion, depressant effect of certain medications (e.g. narcotic [opioid] analgesics, central-acting muscle relaxants, sedatives), and possible tenacious secretions if fluid intake is inadequate.

Desired Outcome	Nursing Actions and *Selected Purposes/Rationales*

2. The client will maintain clear, open airways as evidenced by:
   a. normal breath sounds
   b. normal rate and depth of respirations
   c. absence of dyspnea.

2.a. Assess for signs and symptoms of ineffective airway clearance (e.g. abnormal breath sounds; rapid, shallow respirations; dyspnea; cough).
   b. Implement measures *to promote effective airway clearance:*
   1. instruct and assist client to turn, deep breathe, and cough or "huff" every 1–2 hours
   2. perform actions *to facilitate removal of secretions:*
      a. implement measures *to thin tenacious secretions and reduce drying of the respiratory mucous membrane:*
         1. maintain a fluid intake of at least 2500 ml/day unless contraindicated
         2. humidify inspired air as ordered
      b. assist with administration of mucolytics and diluent or hydrating agents via nebulizer if ordered
      c. assist with or perform postural drainage therapy (PDT) if ordered
      d. perform suctioning if needed
   3. discourage smoking (*irritants present in smoke increase mucus production, impair ciliary function, and can cause inflammation and damage to the bronchial walls*)
   4. administer central nervous system depressants judiciously
   5. increase activity as allowed.
   c. Consult physician if:
   1. signs and symptoms of ineffective airway clearance persist
   2. signs and symptoms of impaired gas exchange (e.g. restlessness, irritability, confusion, decreased PaO_2 and increased $PaCO_2$ levels) are present.

---

3. NURSING DIAGNOSIS:

Altered nutrition: less than body requirements

related to:
a. decreased oral intake associated with:
   1. anorexia resulting from boredom, depression, a slowed metabolic rate, and early satiety that occurs with decreased gastrointestinal motility
   2. difficulty feeding self as a result of impaired or limited physical mobility;
b. increased nutritional needs associated with an imbalance in the rate of catabolism and anabolism (in the immobilized person, catabolic processes occur at a faster rate than anabolic processes).

Desired Outcome	Nursing Actions and *Selected Purposes/Rationales*

3. The client will maintain an adequate nutritional status as evidenced by:
   a. weight within normal range for client's age, height, and body frame
   b. normal BUN and serum albumin, Hct, Hb, transferrin, and lymphocyte levels
   c. no further decline in strength and activity tolerance
   d. healthy oral mucous membrane.

3.a. Assess for and report signs and symptoms of malnutrition:
   1. weight below normal for client's age, height, and body frame
   2. abnormal BUN and low serum albumin, Hct, Hb, transferrin, and lymphocyte levels
   3. weakness and fatigue
   4. sore, inflamed oral mucous membrane
   5. pale conjunctiva.
   b. Monitor percentage of meals and snacks client consumes. Report a pattern of inadequate intake.
   c. Implement measures *to maintain an adequate nutritional status:*
   1. perform actions *to improve oral intake:*
      a. obtain a dietary consult if necessary to assist client in selecting foods/fluids that meet nutritional needs, are appealing, and adhere to personal and cultural preferences
      b. encourage a rest period before meals *to minimize fatigue*

    c. maintain a clean environment and relaxed, pleasant atmosphere
    d. provide oral hygiene before meals
    e. serve frequent, small meals rather than large ones if client is weak, fatigues easily, and/or has a poor appetite
    f. implement measures to prevent constipation (see Nursing Diagnosis 9, action d) *in order to reduce feeling of fullness*
    g. encourage significant others to bring in client's favorite foods unless contraindicated and eat with him/her *to make eating more of a familiar social experience*
    h. encourage significant others to be present to assist client with meals if needed
    i. allow adequate time for meals; reheat foods/fluids if necessary
    j. limit fluid intake with meals (unless the fluid has high nutritional value) *to reduce early satiety and subsequent decreased food intake*
    k. enable client to feed self if possible; if client needs to be fed, offer foods/fluids in the order he/she prefers
    l. increase activity as allowed (*activity usually promotes a sense of well-being and improves appetite*)
  2. ensure that meals are well balanced and high in essential nutrients; offer high-protein, high-calorie dietary supplements if indicated
  3. administer vitamins and minerals if ordered.
d. Perform a calorie count if ordered. Report information to dietitian and physician.
e. Consult physician about an alternative method of providing nutrition (e.g. parenteral nutrition, tube feedings) if client does not consume enough food or fluids to meet nutritional needs.

---

4. NURSING DIAGNOSIS: **Risk for impaired tissue integrity**

related to:
a. accumulation of waste products and decreased oxygen and nutrient supply to the skin and subcutaneous tissue associated with reduced blood flow resulting from prolonged pressure on the tissues;
b. damage to the skin and/or subcutaneous tissue associated with friction or shearing;
c. increased fragility of the skin associated with dependent edema and inadequate nutritional status.

Desired Outcome	Nursing Actions and *Selected Purposes/Rationales*

4. The client will maintain tissue integrity as evidenced by:
  a. absence of redness and irritation
  b. no skin breakdown.
	4.a. Inspect the skin, especially bony prominences and dependent areas, for pallor, redness, and breakdown.
	  b. Implement measures *to prevent tissue breakdown:*
	    1. assist client to turn at least every 2 hours unless contraindicated
	    2. position client properly; use pressure-reducing or pressure-relieving devices (e.g. pillows, gel or foam cushions, alternating pressure mattress, air-fluidized bed) if indicated
	    3. gently massage around reddened areas at least every 2 hours
	    4. apply a thin layer of powder or cornstarch to bottom sheet or skin and to opposing skin surfaces (e.g. axillae, beneath breasts) if indicated *to absorb moisture and/or reduce friction*
	    5. lift and move client carefully using a turn sheet and adequate assistance
	    6. limit length of time client is in semi-Fowler's position to 30 minutes (*in this position, client tends to slide down in bed, which can cause skin surface abrasion and shearing*)

Desired Outcome	Nursing Actions and *Selected Purposes/Rationales*

7. instruct or assist client to shift weight at least every 30 minutes
8. keep skin clean and dry
9. keep bed linens dry and wrinkle-free
10. ensure that external devices such as braces, casts, and restraints are applied properly
11. protect the skin from contact with urine and feces (e.g. keep perineal area clean and dry, apply a protective ointment or cream to perineal area)
12. perform actions *to prevent drying of the skin:*
    a. encourage a fluid intake of 2500 ml/day unless contraindicated
    b. provide a mild soap for bathing
    c. apply moisturizing lotion and/or emollient to skin at least once a day
13. perform actions to maintain an adequate nutritional status (see Nursing Diagnosis 3, action c)
14. if edema is present:
    a. perform actions *to reduce fluid accumulation in dependent areas:*
       1. instruct client in and assist with range of motion exercises
       2. elevate affected extremities whenever possible
    b. handle edematous areas carefully
15. increase activity as allowed.

c. If tissue breakdown occurs:
   1. notify physician
   2. continue with above measures to prevent further irritation and breakdown
   3. perform care of involved areas as ordered or per standard hospital procedure
   4. assess client closely and report signs and symptoms of infection (e.g. elevated temperature; redness, heat, pain, and swelling around area of breakdown; unusual drainage from site).

---

5. NURSING DIAGNOSIS: **Risk for activity intolerance**

related to:
a. decrease in available energy associated with slowed metabolic rate;
b. loss of muscle mass, tone, and strength associated with disuse and inadequate nutritional status;
c. eventual decrease in cardiac reserve associated with:
   1. increased cardiac workload resulting from the increased venous return in a recumbent position
   2. decreased coronary blood flow resulting from a shortened diastolic filling time (a result of the progressive increase in heart rate that occurs when a person is immobile)
   3. weakening of the myocardium (not usually a factor until client has been immobilized for 3 weeks or longer);
d. difficulty resting and sleeping associated with inability to assume usual sleep position, frequent assessments and treatments, fear, anxiety, and unfamiliar environment.

Desired Outcome	Nursing Actions and *Selected Purposes/Rationales*

5. The client will not experience activity intolerance as evidenced by:
   a. no reports of fatigue and weakness

5.a. Assess for signs and symptoms of activity intolerance:
   1. statements of fatigue or weakness
   2. exertional dyspnea, chest pain, diaphoresis, or dizziness
   3. abnormal heart rate response to activity (e.g. increase in rate of 20 beats/minute above resting rate, rate not returning to preactivity level

b. ability to perform activities of daily living within physical limitations/restrictions without exertional dyspnea, chest pain, diaphoresis, dizziness, and a significant change in vital signs.

within 3 minutes after stopping activity, change from regular to irregular rate)

4. decreased systolic B/P or a significant increase (10–15 mm Hg) in diastolic pressure with activity.

b. Implement measures *to prevent activity intolerance:*

1. perform actions *to promote rest and/or conserve energy:*
   a. minimize environmental activity and noise
   b. organize nursing care to allow for periods of uninterrupted rest
   c. limit the number of visitors and their length of stay
   d. assist client with self-care activities as needed
   e. keep supplies and personal articles within easy reach
   f. implement measures to reduce fear and anxiety (see Nursing Diagnosis 13, action b)
   g. implement measures to promote sleep (see Nursing Diagnosis 10, action c)

2. perform additional actions *to reduce cardiac workload and help maintain adequate cardiac reserve:*
   a. place client in a semi- to high Fowler's position periodically if allowed
   b. instruct client to avoid activities that create a Valsalva response (e.g. straining to have a bowel movement, holding breath while moving up in bed)
   c. implement measures to improve breathing pattern and airway clearance (see Nursing Diagnoses 1, action c and 2, action b) *in order to promote adequate tissue oxygenation*
   d. discourage smoking and excessive intake of beverages high in caffeine such as coffee, tea, and colas

3. perform actions to help maintain muscle strength (see Nursing Diagnosis 6, actions a.1–4)

4. perform actions to maintain an adequate nutritional status (see Nursing Diagnosis 3, action c)

5. when activity can be increased:
   a. increase activity gradually
   b. instruct client in energy-saving techniques (e.g. using shower chair when showering, sitting to brush teeth or comb hair).

c. Instruct client to:
   1. report a decreased tolerance for activity
   2. stop any activity that causes chest pain, shortness of breath, dizziness, or extreme fatigue or weakness.

d. Consult physician if signs and symptoms of activity intolerance develop and persist or worsen.

6. NURSING DIAGNOSIS:

Impaired physical mobility

related to:
a. activity limitations imposed by current diagnosis and/or treatment plan;
b. loss of muscle mass, tone, and strength associated with prolonged disuse and inadequate nutritional status.

Desired Outcome	Nursing Actions and *Selected Purposes/Rationales*
6. The client will maintain maximum physical mobility within limitations imposed by the disease or injury and treatment plan.	6.a. Implement measures *to maintain optimal joint mobility and muscle function during period of immobility:* 1. instruct client in and assist with range of motion exercises at least 3 times/day unless contraindicated 2. reinforce instructions, activities, and exercise plan recommended by physical and occupational therapists

Desired Outcome	Nursing Actions and ***Selected Purposes/Rationales***

3. assist with use of electrical stimulation devices that promote muscle strengthening if ordered
4. encourage participation in self-care as allowed; put side rails up and provide overhead trapeze unless contraindicated *to promote independent movement*
5. perform actions to reduce the risk of contractures (see Collaborative Diagnosis 12, actions d.2–6)
6. perform actions to maintain an adequate nutritional status (see Nursing Diagnosis 3, action c) *in order to help maintain muscle mass, tone, and strength.*

  b. Encourage the support of significant others. Allow them to assist with range of motion exercises and positioning if desired.

---

7. NURSING DIAGNOSIS: **Self-care deficit**

related to:
a. activity limitations imposed by current diagnosis and/or treatment plan;
b. possible activity intolerance associated with decreased metabolic rate, cardiac deconditioning, loss of muscle strength, and difficulty resting and sleeping.

Desired Outcome	Nursing Actions and ***Selected Purposes/Rationales***

7. The client will perform self-care activities within physical limitations and activity restrictions imposed by treatment plan.

7.a. With client, develop a realistic plan for meeting daily physical needs.
  b. Implement measures *to facilitate client's ability to perform self-care activities:*
1. schedule care at a time when client is most likely to be able to participate (e.g. when analgesics are at peak effect, after rest periods, not immediately after meals or treatments)
2. keep needed objects within easy reach
3. perform actions to prevent activity intolerance (see Nursing Diagnosis 5, action b)
4. perform actions to maintain optimal joint mobility and muscle function (see Nursing Diagnosis 6, action a)
5. consult occupational therapist about assistive devices available if indicated
6. allow adequate time for accomplishment of self-care activities.

  c. Encourage client to perform as much of self-care as possible within physical limitations and activity restrictions imposed by the treatment plan. Provide positive feedback for all efforts and accomplishments of self-care.
  d. Assist the client with activities he/she is unable to perform independently.
  e. Inform significant others of client's abilities to perform own care. Explain importance of encouraging and allowing client to maintain an optimal level of independence within prescribed activity restrictions and physical capabilities.

---

8. NURSING DIAGNOSIS: **Urinary retention**

related to:
a. stasis of urine in kidney and bladder associated with prolonged horizontal positioning;

b. difficulty urinating associated with anxiety regarding use of bedpan or urinal;
c. incomplete bladder emptying associated with:
    1. horizontal positioning (the gravity needed for complete bladder emptying is lost)
    2. decreased bladder muscle tone resulting from the generalized loss of muscle tone that occurs with prolonged immobility.

Desired Outcome	Nursing Actions and *Selected Purposes/Rationales*

8. The client will not experience urinary retention as evidenced by:
    a. voiding at normal intervals
    b. no reports of bladder fullness and suprapubic discomfort
    c. absence of bladder distention and dribbling of urine
    d. balanced intake and output.

8.a. Determine client's usual urinary elimination pattern.
  b. Assess for signs and symptoms of urinary retention:
      1. frequent voiding of small amounts (25–60 ml) of urine
      2. reports of bladder fullness or suprapubic discomfort
      3. bladder distention
      4. dribbling of urine
      5. output less than intake.
  c. Catheterize client if ordered *to determine the amount of residual urine.*
  d. Implement measures *to prevent urinary retention:*
      1. instruct client to urinate when the urge is first felt
      2. perform actions *to promote relaxation during voiding attempts* (e.g. provide privacy, hold a warm blanket against abdomen, encourage client to read)
      3. perform actions *that may help trigger the micturition reflex and promote a sense of relaxation during voiding attempts* (e.g. run water, place client's hands in warm water, pour warm water over perineum)
      4. allow client to assume a normal position for voiding unless contraindicated
      5. instruct and/or assist client to lean his/her upper body forward and/or gently press downward on lower abdomen during voiding attempts unless contraindicated *in order to put pressure on the bladder area (pressure helps create a sensation of bladder fullness, which stimulates the micturition reflex)*
      6. administer cholinergic drugs (e.g. bethanechol) if ordered *to stimulate bladder contraction.*
  e. Consult physician about intermittent catheterization or insertion of an indwelling catheter if above actions fail to alleviate urinary retention.

9. NURSING DIAGNOSIS: Constipation

related to:
a. diminished defecation reflex associated with:
    1. suppression of urge to defecate because of reluctance to use bedpan
    2. decreased gravity filling of lower rectum resulting from horizontal positioning;
b. weakened abdominal muscles associated with generalized loss of muscle tone resulting from prolonged immobility;
c. decreased gastrointestinal motility associated with decreased activity and the increased sympathetic nervous system activity that occurs with anxiety.

Desired Outcome	Nursing Actions and *Selected Purposes/Rationales*

9. The client will not experience constipation as evidenced by:

9.a. Ascertain client's usual bowel elimination habits.
  b. Assess for signs and symptoms of constipation (e.g. decrease in frequency of bowel movements; passage of hard, formed stools; anorexia; abdominal

Desired Outcome	Nursing Actions and *Selected Purposes/Rationales*

a. usual frequency of bowel movements
b. passage of soft, formed stool
c. absence of abdominal distention and pain, feeling of rectal fullness or pressure, and straining during defecation.
	distention and pain; feeling of fullness or pressure in rectum; straining during defecation).
	c. Assess bowel sounds. Report a pattern of decreasing bowel sounds.
	d. Implement measures *to prevent constipation:*
	  1. encourage client to defecate whenever the urge is felt
	  2. place client in high Fowler's position for bowel movements unless contraindicated
	  3. encourage client to relax, provide privacy, and have call signal within reach during attempts to defecate (*measures to promote relaxation enable client to relax the levator ani muscle and external anal sphincter, which facilitates evacuation of stool*)
	  4. encourage client to establish a regular time for defecation, preferably an hour after a meal
	  5. instruct client to increase intake of foods high in fiber (e.g. bran, whole-grain breads and cereals, fresh fruits and vegetables) unless contraindicated.
	  6. instruct client to maintain a minimum fluid intake of 2500 ml/day unless contraindicated
	  7. encourage client to drink hot liquids upon arising in the morning *in order to stimulate peristalsis*
	  8. encourage client to perform isometric abdominal strengthening exercises unless contraindicated
	  9. increase activity as allowed
	  10. administer laxatives or cathartics and/or enemas if ordered.
	e. Consult physician about checking for an impaction and digitally removing stool if client has not had a bowel movement in 3 days, if he/she is passing liquid stool, or if other signs and symptoms of constipation are present.

---

10. NURSING DIAGNOSIS: **Sleep pattern disturbance**

related to current illness/injury, decreased physical activity, fear, anxiety, inability to assume usual sleep position, frequent assessments or treatments, and unfamiliar environment.

Desired Outcome	Nursing Actions and *Selected Purposes/Rationales*

10. The client will attain optimal amounts of sleep as evidenced by:
a. statements of feeling well rested
b. usual mental status
c. absence of frequent yawning, dark circles under eyes, and hand tremors.
	10.a. Assess for signs and symptoms of a sleep pattern disturbance (e.g. statements of difficulty falling asleep, not feeling well rested, or sleep interruptions; irritability; disorientation; lethargy; frequent yawning; dark circles under eyes; slight hand tremors).
	b. Determine the client's usual sleep habits.
	c. Implement measures *to promote sleep:*
	  1. perform actions to reduce fear and anxiety (see Nursing Diagnosis 13, action b)
	  2. discourage long periods of sleep during the day unless signs and symptoms of sleep deprivation exist or daytime sleep is usual for client
	  3. encourage participation in relaxing diversional activities during the evening
	  4. discourage intake of fluids high in caffeine (e.g. coffee, tea, colas), especially in the evening
	  5. offer client an evening snack that includes milk or cheese unless contraindicated (the *L-tryptophan in milk and cheese helps induce and maintain sleep*)

6. allow client to continue usual sleep practices (e.g. position; time; presleep routines such as reading, watching television, listening to music, and meditating) unless contraindicated
7. satisfy basic needs such as comfort and warmth before sleep
8. encourage client to urinate just before bedtime
9. reduce environmental distractions (e.g. close door to client's room; use night light rather than overhead light whenever possible; lower volume of paging system; keep staff conversations at a low level and away from client's room; close curtains between clients in a semi-private room or ward; keep beepers and alarms on low volume; provide client with "white noise" such as a fan, soft music, or tape-recorded sounds of the ocean or rain; have sleep mask and earplugs available for client if needed)
10. ensure good room ventilation
11. administer prescribed sedative-hypnotics if indicated
12. perform actions *to reduce interruptions during sleep (80–100 minutes of uninterrupted sleep is usually needed to complete one sleep cycle)*
    a. restrict visitors
    b. group care (e.g. medications, treatments, physical care, assessments) whenever possible.
d. Consult physician if signs and symptoms of sleep deprivation persist or worsen.

---

11. NURSING DIAGNOSIS:

Risk for infection:

a. **pneumonia** related to stasis of secretions in the lungs (secretions provide a good medium for bacterial growth);
b. **urinary tract infection** related to:
   1. increased growth and colonization of microorganisms associated with urinary stasis and the increased urine alkalinity that results from hypercalciuria (with prolonged immobility, excess calcium is released from the bones and excreted in the urine)
   2. introduction of pathogens into the urinary tract associated with the presence of an indwelling catheter and/or difficulty maintaining good perineal hygiene during period of immobility.

Desired Outcomes	Nursing Actions and *Selected Purposes/Rationales*
11.a. The client will not develop pneumonia as evidenced by: 1. normal breath sounds 2. resonant percussion note over lungs 3. absence of tachypnea 4. cough productive of clear mucus only 5. afebrile status 6. absence of pleuritic pain 7. blood gases and WBC count within normal range for client 8. negative sputum culture.	11.a.1. Assess for and report signs and symptoms of pneumonia: a. abnormal breath sounds (e.g. crackles [rales], pleural friction rub, bronchial breath sounds, diminished or absent breath sounds) b. dull percussion note over affected lung area c. tachypnea d. cough productive of purulent, green, or rust-colored sputum e. chills and fever f. pleuritic pain g. elevated WBC count. 2. Monitor oximetry and blood gas results. Report abnormal findings. 3. Obtain sputum specimen for culture if ordered. Report abnormal results. 4. Monitor chest x-ray results. Report findings indicative of pneumonia. 5. Implement measures *to prevent pneumonia:* a. perform actions to promote effective airway clearance (see Nursing Diagnosis 2, action b) b. protect client from persons with respiratory tract infections

Desired Outcomes	Nursing Actions and *Selected Purposes/Rationales*

        c. encourage and assist client to perform frequent oral care *in order to reduce the colonization of bacteria in the oropharynx and subsequent aspiration of these microorganisms.*

   6. If signs and symptoms of pneumonia occur:
      a. continue with above measures
      b. administer oxygen as ordered
      c. administer antimicrobials if ordered
      d. refer to Care Plan on Pneumonia for additional care measures.

11.b. The client will remain free of urinary tract infection as evidenced by:
1. clear urine
2. no unusual odor to urine
3. absence of frequency, urgency, and burning on urination
4. absence of chills and fever
5. absence of nitrites, bacteria, and WBCs in urine
6. negative urine culture.

11.b.1. Assess for and report signs and symptoms of urinary tract infection (e.g. cloudy, foul-smelling urine; reports of frequency, urgency, or burning on urination; chills; elevated temperature).
   2. Monitor urinalysis and report presence of nitrites, bacteria, and/or WBCs.
   3. Obtain a urine specimen for culture and sensitivity if ordered. Report abnormal results.
   4. Implement measures *to prevent urinary tract infection:*
      a. perform actions to prevent urinary stasis (see Collaborative Diagnosis 12, action c.2.a)
      b. maintain a fluid intake of at least 2500 ml/day unless contraindicated *to promote urine formation and subsequent voiding, which flushes pathogens from the urethra and bladder*
      c. instruct female client to wipe from front to back after urinating or defecating
      d. assist client with perineal care routinely and after each bowel movement
      e. maintain sterile technique during urinary catheterization and irrigations
      f. if an indwelling urinary catheter is present:
         1. secure the catheter tubing to lower abdomen or thigh on males or to thigh on females *to minimize risk of accidental traction on the catheter and subsequent trauma to the bladder and urethra;* anchor tubing securely *to reduce the amount of in-and-out movement of the catheter* (*this movement can result in introduction of pathogens into the urinary tract and cause tissue trauma, which can result in colonization of microorganisms*)
         2. perform catheter care as often as needed *to prevent accumulation of mucus around the meatus*
         3. maintain a closed drainage system whenever possible *to reduce the risk of introduction of pathogens into the urinary tract*
         4. keep urine collection container below bladder level at all times *to prevent reflux or stasis of urine*
         5. change catheter according to hospital policy.
   5. If signs and symptoms of urinary tract infection are present:
      a. continue with above actions
      b. administer antimicrobials if ordered.

---

12. COLLABORATIVE DIAGNOSES:

Potential complications of immobility:
  a. **thromboembolism** related to:
    1. venous stasis associated with decreased mobility and increased blood viscosity if fluid intake is inadequate
    2. injury to the vessel wall associated with external pressure on the calf vessels from the mattress, pillows, or knee gatch when in a recumbent position
    3. hypercoagulability associated with:
      a. hemoconcentration and increased blood viscosity if fluid intake is inadequate

b. increased levels of certain clotting factors (e.g. calcium, fibrinogen) in the blood after approximately 8 days of bed rest;

b. **atelectasis** related to shallow respirations, stasis of secretions in the alveoli and bronchioles, and decreased surfactant production (can result from inadequate deep breathing and changes in regional blood flow in the lungs) associated with prolonged recumbent positioning;

c. **renal calculi** related to crystallization and precipitation of calcium salts in the urine associated with:
1. urinary stasis that occurs in a recumbent position
2. change in the calcium/citrate ratio and urine pH (results primarily from the increased urinary excretion of calcium that occurs with bone demineralization)
3. decreased flushing of calcium salts from the urinary tract if urine formation is reduced because of inadequate fluid intake;

d. **contractures** related to lack of joint movement associated with prolonged immobility;

e. **pathologic fractures** related to the osteoporosis that can develop with prolonged immobility.

Desired Outcomes	Nursing Actions and *Selected Purposes/Rationales*
12.a.1. The client will not develop a deep vein thrombus as evidenced by: a. absence of pain, tenderness, swelling, and distended superficial vessels in extremities b. usual temperature of extremities c. negative Homans' sign.	12.a.1.a. Assess for and report signs and symptoms of a deep vein thrombus: 1. pain or tenderness in extremity 2. increase in circumference of extremity 3. distention of superficial vessels in extremity 4. unusual warmth of extremity 5. positive Homans' sign (not always a reliable indicator). b. Implement measures *to prevent thrombus formation:* 1. encourage and assist client to perform active foot and leg exercises every 1–2 hours while awake 2. instruct client to avoid positions that compromise blood flow (e.g. pillows under knees, crossing legs, sitting for long periods) 3. elevate foot of bed for 20-minute intervals several times a shift unless contraindicated 4. consult physician about an order for antiembolism stockings or a sequential compression device 5. maintain a minimum fluid intake of 2500 ml/day unless contraindicated *to prevent increased blood viscosity* 6. administer anticoagulants (e.g. low- or adjusted-dose heparin, warfarin, low-molecular-weight heparin) or antiplatelet agents (e.g. low-dose aspirin) if ordered 7. progress activity as allowed. c. If signs and symptoms of a deep vein thrombus occur: 1. maintain client on bed rest until activity orders are received 2. elevate foot of bed 15–20° above heart level if ordered 3. discourage positions that compromise blood flow (e.g. pillows under knees, crossing legs, sitting for long periods) 4. prepare client for diagnostic studies (e.g. venography, duplex ultrasound, impedance plethysmography) if indicated 5. administer anticoagulants (e.g. heparin, warfarin) as ordered 6. prepare client for injection of a thrombolytic agent (e.g. streptokinase) if planned 7. refer to Care Plan on Deep Vein Thrombosis for additional care measures.
12.a.2. The client will not experience a pulmonary embolism as evidenced by: a. absence of sudden chest pain	12.a.2.a. Assess for and report signs and symptoms of pulmonary embolism (e.g. sudden chest pain, dyspnea, tachypnea, tachycardia, apprehension, low PaO$_2$). b. Implement measures *to prevent a pulmonary embolism:* 1. perform actions to prevent and treat a deep vein thrombus (see actions a.1.b and c in this diagnosis)

Desired Outcomes | Nursing Actions and *Selected **Purposes/Rationales***

b. unlabored respirations at 14–20/minute
c. pulse 60–100 beats/minute
d. blood gases within normal range.

2. do not exercise, check for Homans' sign in, or massage any extremity known to have a thrombus
3. caution client to avoid activities that create a Valsalva response (e.g. straining to have a bowel movement, holding breath while moving up in bed) *in order to prevent dislodgment of existing thrombi*
4. prepare client for a vena caval interruption (e.g. insertion of an intracaval filtering device) if planned.

c. If signs and symptoms of a pulmonary embolism occur:
1. maintain client on strict bed rest in a semi- to high Fowler's position
2. maintain oxygen therapy as ordered
3. prepare client for diagnostic tests (e.g. blood gases, ventilation-perfusion lung scan, pulmonary angiography)
4. administer anticoagulants (e.g. continuous intravenous heparin, warfarin) as ordered
5. prepare client for the following if planned:
   a. injection of a thrombolytic agent (e.g. streptokinase, urokinase, tissue plasminogen activator [tPA])
   b. vena caval interruption (e.g. insertion of an intracaval filtering device) *to prevent further pulmonary emboli*
6. provide emotional support to client and significant others
7. refer to Care Plan on Pulmonary Embolism for additional care measures.

12.b. The client will not develop atelectasis as evidenced by:
1. clear, audible breath sounds
2. resonant percussion note over lungs
3. unlabored respirations at 14–20/minute
4. pulse rate within normal range for client
5. afebrile status.

12.b.1. Assess for and report signs and symptoms of atelectasis (e.g. diminished or absent breath sounds, dull percussion note over affected area, increased respiratory rate, dyspnea, tachycardia, elevated temperature).
2. Monitor chest x-ray results. Report findings of atelectasis.
3. Implement measures *to prevent atelectasis:*
   a. perform actions to maintain an effective breathing pattern (see Nursing Diagnosis 1, action c)
   b. perform actions to maintain effective airway clearance (see Nursing Diagnosis 2, action b).
4. If signs and symptoms of atelectasis occur:
   a. increase frequency of turning, coughing or "huffing," deep breathing, and use of incentive spirometer
   b. consult physician if signs and symptoms of atelectasis persist or worsen.

12.c. The client will not develop renal calculi as evidenced by:
1. absence of flank pain, hematuria, nausea, and vomiting
2. clear urine without calculi.

12.c.1. Assess for and report signs and symptoms of renal calculi (e.g. dull, aching or severe, colicky flank pain; hematuria; nausea; vomiting).
2. Implement measures *to prevent calcium stone formation:*
   a. perform actions *to prevent urinary stasis:*
      1. assist client to change positions at least every 2 hours; elevate head of bed periodically unless contraindicated
      2. progress activity as allowed
      3. implement measures to prevent urinary retention (see Nursing Diagnosis 8, action d)
      4. maintain patency of urinary catheter if present
   b. encourage a minimum fluid intake of 2500 ml/day unless contraindicated *to promote adequate urine formation* and the subsequent flushing of calcium salts from the urinary tract
   c. perform actions to prevent or delay bone demineralization (see action e.3.a in this diagnosis) *in order to reduce the amount of calcium present in the urine*
   d. instruct client to avoid excessive intake of foods/fluids high in calcium (e.g. dairy products)
   e. perform actions to prevent urinary tract infections (see Nursing Diagnosis 11, action b.4) *in order to prevent an increase in urine alkalinity*

    f. instruct client to reduce intake of foods/fluids high in oxalate (e.g. tea, chocolate, nuts, rhubarb, spinach) *in order to help prevent precipitation of calcium oxalate stones.*

3. If signs and symptoms of renal calculi occur:
    a. strain all urine carefully and save any calculi for analysis; report finding to physician
    b. encourage maximum fluid intake allowed
    c. administer analgesics as ordered
    d. prepare client for removal of calculi (e.g. extracorporeal shock wave lithotripsy [ESWL], percutaneous ultrasonic lithotripsy; pyelolithotomy) if planned.

12.d. The client will regain or maintain normal range of motion.

12.d.1. Assess for reports of joint stiffness and limitations in range of motion.
2. Implement general measures *to prevent contractures:*
    a. maintain proper body alignment at all times
    b. perform actions to maintain optimal joint mobility and muscle function during period of immobility (see Nursing Diagnosis 6, actions a.1–4).
3. Implement measures *to prevent hip and knee contractures:*
    a. place client in a flat, supine position at least every 4 hours
    b. limit length of time client is in high Fowler's position (usually no longer than 1 hour at a time)
    c. avoid use of knee gatch and pillows under knees
    d. instruct client to do quadriceps- and gluteal-setting exercises if able *in order to maintain muscle strength and tone and improve ability to perform range of motion exercises of hips and knees*
    e. when client is in a supine or Fowler's position, place trochanter roll or sandbag along outer aspect of each thigh *to prevent external rotation of the hips.*
4. Implement measures *to prevent footdrop:*
    a. instruct and assist client to perform active foot exercises every 1–2 hours while awake
    b. if necessary, use devices to keep feet in a neutral or slightly dorsiflexed position (e.g. high-topped tennis shoes, foam boots)
    c. keep bed linen from exerting excessive pressure on toes and feet.
5. Implement measures *to prevent contractures in upper extremities:*
    a. encourage client to use upper extremities to perform self-care and assist in moving unless contraindicated
    b. reposition upper extremities at least every 2 hours
    c. use handroll and wrist splints if indicated.
6. Use a small rather than large pillow to support client's head and shoulders *in order to prevent a neck flexion contracture.*
7. Consult physician if range of motion becomes restricted.

12.e. The client will not experience pathologic fractures as evidenced by:
1. usual mobility and range of motion
2. absence of unusual motion, abnormal joint position, and obvious deformity of any body part
3. absence of pain and swelling over skeletal structures
4. x-ray reports showing absence of fractures.

12.e.1. Assess for and report signs and symptoms of pathologic fractures (e.g. further decrease in mobility or range of motion, motion at site where motion does not usually occur, abnormal joint position or obvious deformity, pain or swelling over skeletal structures).
2. Monitor x-ray reports and notify physician of findings of pathologic fractures.
3. Implement measures *to prevent pathologic fractures:*
    a. perform actions *to prevent or delay bone demineralization:*
        1. consult physician about the use of a tilt table while client is immobile
        2. assist client with weight-bearing activities as soon as allowed (*weight-bearing reduces bone breakdown*)
        3. administer medications *that inhibit bone resorption* (e.g. estrogen, calcitonin) if ordered
        4. encourage client to consume a diet that has adequate amounts of protein, vitamins, and calcium and to avoid smoking and excessive caffeine intake
    b. if evidence of osteoporosis exists:
        1. move client carefully; obtain adequate assistance as needed

Desired Outcomes	Nursing Actions and *Selected Purposes/Rationales*

        2. when turning client, logroll and support all extremities

        3. use smooth movements when moving client; avoid pulling or pushing on body parts

        4. correctly apply back brace or corset if ordered.

    4. If fractures occur:

       a. apply external stabilization device (e.g. cervical collar, brace, splint, sling) if ordered

       b. administer analgesics, anti-inflammatory agents, and/or muscle relaxants if ordered *to control pain*

       c. prepare client for surgery (e.g. internal fixation) if planned

       d. provide emotional support to client and significant others.

---

13. NURSING DIAGNOSIS: **Anxiety**

related to unfamiliar environment; lack of understanding of diagnosis, diagnostic tests, and treatments; financial concerns; and feelings of confinement.

Desired Outcome	Nursing Actions and *Selected Purposes/Rationales*

13. The client will experience a reduction in anxiety as evidenced by:
    a. verbalization of feeling less anxious
    b. usual sleep pattern
    c. relaxed facial expression and body movements
    d. stable vital signs
    e. usual perceptual ability and interactions with others.

13.a. Assess client for signs and symptoms of anxiety (e.g. verbalization of feeling anxious, insomnia, tenseness, shakiness, restlessness, diaphoresis, tachycardia, elevated blood pressure, facial pallor, self-focused behaviors).

   b. Implement measures *to reduce fear and anxiety:*

     1. orient client to hospital environment, equipment, and routines; explain the purpose for and operation of a kinetic bed if indicated

     2. introduce client to staff who will be participating in care; if possible, maintain consistency in staff assigned to his/her care *to provide feelings of stability and comfort with the environment*

     3. assure client that staff members are nearby; respond to call signal as soon as possible

     4. keep door and curtains open as much as possible *to reduce feeling of confinement*

     5. maintain a calm, supportive, confident manner when interacting with client

     6. encourage verbalization of fear and anxiety; provide feedback

     7. reinforce physician's explanations and clarify misconceptions client has about his/her diagnosis, treatment plan, and prognosis

     8. explain all diagnostic tests

     9. provide a calm, restful environment

     10. instruct client in relaxation techniques and encourage participation in diversional activities

     11. assist client to identify specific stressors and ways to cope with them

     12. initiate financial and/or social service referrals if indicated

     13. provide information based on current needs of client at a level he/she can understand; encourage questions and clarification of information provided

     14. encourage significant others to project a caring, concerned attitude without obvious anxiousness

     15. include significant others in orientation and teaching sessions and encourage their continued support of the client

     16. administer prescribed antianxiety agents if indicated.

   c. Consult physician if above actions fail to control fear and anxiety.

14. NURSING DIAGNOSIS:

Self-concept disturbance*

related to dependence on others to meet basic needs, feelings of powerlessness, and change in body functioning and usual roles and life style associated with physical limitations and/or prescribed activity restrictions.

*This diagnostic label includes the nursing diagnoses of body image disturbance, self-esteem disturbance, and altered role performance.

Desired Outcome	Nursing Actions and *Selected Purposes/Rationales*
14. The client will demonstrate beginning adaptation to changes in body functioning, life style, roles, and level of independence as evidenced by: a. verbalization of feelings of self-worth b. maintenance of relationships with significant others c. active participation in activities of daily living d. verbalization of a beginning plan for adapting life style to changes resulting from the injury or disease and/or its treatment.	14.a. Assess for signs and symptoms of a self-concept disturbance (e.g. verbalization of negative feelings about self, withdrawal from significant others, lack of participation in activities of daily living, lack of plan for adapting to necessary changes in life style). b. Determine the meaning of feelings of dependency and changes in body functioning, life style, and roles to the client by encouraging the verbalization of feelings and by noting nonverbal responses to the changes experienced. c. Discuss with client improvements in body functioning and ability to resume usual roles and life style that can realistically be expected. d. Implement measures *to assist client to increase self-esteem* (e.g. limit negative self-assessment, encourage positive comments about self, assist to identify strengths, give positive feedback about accomplishments). e. Assist client to identify and use coping techniques that have been helpful in the past. f. Assist client with usual grooming and makeup habits if necessary. g. Implement measures to reduce client's feelings of powerlessness (see Nursing Diagnosis 15, actions c–n). h. Support behaviors suggesting positive adaptation to changes that have occurred (e.g. verbalization of feelings of self-worth, maintenance of relationships with significant others). i. Assist client's and significant others' adjustment by listening, facilitating communication, and providing information. j. Encourage visits and support from significant others. k. Encourage client to continue involvement in interests and hobbies if possible. If previous interests and hobbies cannot be pursued, encourage development of new ones. l. Provide information about and encourage use of community agencies and support groups (e.g. vocational rehabilitation; family, individual, and/or financial counseling). m. Consult physician about psychological counseling if client desires or seems unwilling or unable to adapt to changes that have occurred as a result of the disease or injury and its treatment.

15. NURSING DIAGNOSIS:

Powerlessness

related to:
a. physical limitations and/or prescribed activity restrictions;
b. dependence on others to meet basic needs;
c. alterations in roles, relationships, and future plans.

Desired Outcome	Nursing Actions and *Selected Purposes/Rationales*
15. The client will demonstrate increased feelings of control over his/her situation as evidenced by: a. verbalization of same b. active participation in planning of care c. participation in self-care activities within physical limitations and prescribed activity restrictions.	15.a. Assess for behaviors that may indicate feelings of powerlessness (e.g. verbalization of lack of control over self-care or current situation, anger, irritability, passivity, lack of participation in self-care or care planning). b. Obtain information from client and significant others regarding client's usual response to situations in which he/she has had limited control (e.g. loss of job, financial stress). c. Evaluate client's perception of current situation, strengths, weaknesses, expectations, and parts of current situation that are under his/her control. Correct misinformation and inaccurate perceptions and encourage discussion of feelings about areas in which he/she perceives a lack of control. d. Reinforce physician's explanations about the disease or injury and treatment plan. Clarify misconceptions. e. Support realistic hope about probability of future independence and ability to resume usual roles and life style. f. Assist client to meet spiritual needs (e.g. arrange for a visit from clergy if desired by client). g. Remind client of the right to ask questions about condition and treatment regimen. h. Support client's efforts to increase knowledge of and control over condition. Provide relevant pamphlets and audiovisual materials. i. Include client in the planning of care, encourage maximum participation in the treatment plan, and allow choices whenever possible *to promote a sense of control.* j. Consult occupational therapist if indicated about assistive devices and environmental modifications that would allow client more independence in performing activities of daily living. k. Inform client of scheduled procedures and tests *so that he/she knows what to expect, which promotes a sense of control.* l. Encourage significant others to allow client to do as much as he/she is able *so that a feeling of independence can be maintained.* m. Assist client to establish realistic short- and long-term goals. n. Encourage client's participation in self-help groups if indicated.

---

16. NURSING DIAGNOSIS: Social isolation

related to inability to participate in usual activities, limited contact with significant others, and decreased exposure to events in the outside world associated with prolonged immobility.

Desired Outcome	Nursing Actions and *Selected Purposes/Rationales*
16. The client will experience a decreased sense of isolation as evidenced by: a. maintenance of relationships with significant others b. verbalization of decreasing feelings of aloneness and rejection.	16.a. Ascertain client's usual degree of social interaction. b. Assess for indications of social isolation (e.g. absence of supportive significant others; uncommunicative and withdrawn; expression of feelings of rejection, being different from others, or aloneness imposed by others; sad, dull affect). c. Implement measures *to decrease social isolation:* 1. assist client to identify reasons for feeling isolated and alone; aid him/her in developing a plan of action to reduce these feelings 2. encourage significant others to visit 3. encourage client to maintain telephone contact with others 4. schedule time each day to sit and talk with client

5. make objects such as clock, TV, radio, newspapers, and greeting cards accessible to client
6. have significant others bring client's favorite objects from home and place in room
7. move client periodically to a more stimulating environment (e.g. hall, lounge, garden) when condition allows
8. change room assignments as feasible *to provide client with roommate with similar interests.*

Discharge Teaching

17. NURSING DIAGNOSIS: **Knowledge deficit, Ineffective management of therapeutic regimen, or Altered health maintenance***

---

*The nurse should select the diagnostic label that is most appropriate for the client's discharge teaching needs.

Desired Outcomes	Nursing Actions and *Selected Purposes/Rationales*
17.a. The client will verbalize an understanding of ways to prevent complications associated with continued decreased mobility.	17.a.1. Provide instructions regarding ways to prevent respiratory tract infection: 　a. avoid contact with persons having respiratory tract infections 　b. drink at least 10 glasses of liquid/day unless contraindicated 　c. continue with respiratory care (e.g. incentive spirometer, coughing and deep breathing) as long as mobility is impaired 　d. avoid smoking. 2. Provide instructions regarding ways to prevent urinary tract infection: 　a. drink at least 10 glasses of liquid/day unless contraindicated 　b. void whenever the urge is felt 　c. wipe from front to back after urinating or defecating (if female) and keep perineal area clean. 3. Provide instructions regarding ways to prevent urinary calcium stone formation: 　a. drink at least 10 glasses of liquid/day unless contraindicated 　b. void whenever the urge is felt 　c. avoid excessive intake of foods high in calcium (e.g. dairy products) and oxalate (e.g. tea, chocolate, nuts, rhubarb, spinach). 4. Provide instructions regarding ways to prevent a thromboembolism: 　a. drink at least 10 glasses of liquid/day unless contraindicated 　b. avoid placing pillows under knees, crossing legs, and prolonged sitting 　c. perform active foot and leg exercises every 1–2 hours during periods of inactivity 　d. wear elastic stockings as prescribed 　e. do not massage extremities. 5. Provide instructions regarding ways to prevent fainting spells associated with position change: 　a. wear elastic stockings as prescribed 　b. change from a lying to sitting or standing position slowly. 6. Provide instructions regarding ways to prevent skin breakdown: 　a. change positions at least every 2 hours 　b. avoid pressure on any reddened or irritated area 　c. keep skin clean and dry 　d. place an alternating pressure pad or foam or gel cushion on bed and chair if prone to skin breakdown or if activity is severely limited. 7. Provide instructions regarding ways to prevent constipation: 　a. drink at least 10 glasses of liquid/day unless contraindicated

Desired Outcomes	Nursing Actions and *Selected Purposes/Rationales*
	b. increase intake of foods high in fiber (e.g. bran, whole-grain breads and cereals, fresh fruits and vegetables) c. defecate whenever the urge is felt d. assume a sitting position for defecation if possible.
17.b. The client will demonstrate techniques for meeting self-care needs.	17.b.1. Assist the client to identify techniques that will allow him/her to perform as much self-care as possible. 2. Reinforce occupational therapist's instructions about use of assistive devices. 3. Allow time for return demonstration of self-care techniques and use of assistive devices.
17.c. The client will state signs and symptoms to report to the health care provider.	17.c. Instruct client to report the following signs and symptoms: 1. temperature elevation lasting longer than 2 days 2. skin breakdown 3. cough productive of purulent, green, or rust-colored sputum 4. pain or swelling in any extremity 5. chest pain 6. flank pain 7. nausea and vomiting 8. frequency, urgency, or burning on urination 9. cloudy, foul-smelling urine 10. increased restriction of any joint motion.
17.d. The client will identify community agencies that can provide assistance with home care and transportation.	17.d.1. Provide information about community agencies that can provide assistance to client with home care or transportation (e.g. home health agencies, Meals on Wheels, church groups, transportation agencies). 2. Initiate a referral if indicated.
17.e. The client will verbalize an understanding of and a plan for adhering to recommended follow-up care including future appointments with health care provider and physical therapist, exercise regimen, and medications prescribed.	17.e.1. Reinforce the importance of keeping follow-up appointments with health care provider and physical therapist. 2. Reinforce physician's instructions regarding exercises and activity limitations. 3. Explain the rationale for, side effects of, and importance of taking medications prescribed. 4. Implement measures to improve client compliance: a. include significant others in teaching sessions if possible b. encourage questions and allow time for reinforcement and clarification of information provided c. provide written instructions regarding scheduled appointments with health care provider and physical therapist, medications prescribed, and signs and symptoms to report.

Bibliography

See pages 897–898.

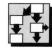

NURSING CARE OF THE CLIENT WHO IS DYING

▤ TERMINAL CARE

This care plan focuses on care of the hospitalized adult client who is facing death in the very near future. The major goals of nursing care are to prevent or control physiological problems that could reduce the quality of the client's remaining life; facilitate the client's psychological adjustment to his/her imminent death; and assist the client to experience a peaceful, dignified death. The nurse also assists the significant others to understand the dying process, support the dying person, meet their own physical and emotional needs, and adjust to their loss of the client.

This care plan does not deal with any particular medical diagnosis. The nursing diagnoses included are those that are relatively common to all persons facing death. Care plans that pertain to the client's specific medical diagnosis will provide additional guidelines for nursing care during the terminal stages of that illness.

Use in conjunction with the Care Plan on Immobility and care plans that pertain to the client's medical diagnosis.

Refer to Care Plan on Immobility and care plans that pertain to the client's medical diagnosis for additional diagnoses.

---

1. NURSING DIAGNOSIS: **Impaired respiratory function:***

a. **ineffective breathing pattern** related to:

---

*This diagnostic label includes the following nursing diagnoses: ineffective breathing pattern, ineffective airway clearance, and impaired gas exchange.

1. increased rate and decreased depth of respirations associated with fear, anxiety, and pain
2. the depressant effect of some medications (e.g. narcotic [opioid] analgesics, central-acting muscle relaxants)
3. diminished lung/chest wall expansion associated with recumbent positioning (in this position, full expansion of the lungs is restricted by the bed surface and by the abdominal contents pushing up against the diaphragm), weakness, fatigue, and/or abdominal distention
4. altered function of the respiratory center (can occur as a result of the underlying disease process);

b. **ineffective airway clearance** related to:
   1. stasis of secretions associated with:
      a. decreased mobility
      b. difficulty coughing up secretions resulting from impaired lung/chest wall expansion and presence of tenacious secretions if fluid intake is inadequate
   2. fluid accumulation in the alveoli and bronchioles associated with pulmonary edema if present
   3. airway obstruction associated with the underlying disease process and/or relaxation of the tongue (can occur with decreased level of consciousness and as a result of administration of central nervous system depressant medications);

c. **impaired gas exchange** related to:
   1. loss of effective lung tissue (can occur as a result of the underlying disease process)
   2. a thickened alveolar-capillary membrane associated with stasis of pulmonary secretions and pulmonary edema if present
   3. decreased oxygen availability associated with anemia (can result from decreased nutritional status and/or the underlying disease process).

Desired Outcome	Nursing Actions and *Selected Purposes/Rationales*

1. The client will experience adequate respiratory function as evidenced by:
a. usual rate, rhythm, and depth of respirations
b. absence of dyspnea
c. usual breath sounds
d. usual mental status
e. usual skin color
f. blood gases within normal range for client.
	1.a. Assess for signs and symptoms of impaired respiratory function:
	   1. rapid, shallow, slow, or irregular respirations
	   2. dyspnea, orthopnea
	   3. use of accessory muscles when breathing
	   4. adventitious breath sounds (e.g. crackles [rales], rhonchi)
	   5. diminished or absent breath sounds
	   6. restlessness, irritability
	   7. cough
	   8. confusion, somnolence
	   9. central cyanosis (a late sign).
	b. Monitor for and report the following:
	   1. abnormal blood gases
	   2. significant decrease in oximetry results
	   3. abnormal chest x-ray results.
	c. Implement measures *to maintain an adequate respiratory status and prevent respiratory distress:*
	   1. perform actions to reduce pain (see Nursing Diagnosis 4, action e)
	   2. perform actions to decrease accumulation of gastrointestinal gas and fluid (see Nursing Diagnosis 5.B, action 3) *in order to decrease pressure on the diaphragm*
	   3. perform actions to decrease fear and anxiety (see Nursing Diagnosis 16)
	   4. perform actions to reduce the risk for aspiration (see Nursing Diagnosis 3, action d)
	   5. place client in a semi- to high Fowler's position unless contraindicated; position client with pillows *to prevent slumping*
	   6. instruct client to breathe slowly if hyperventilating
	   7. assist client to turn from side to side at least every 2 hours

Desired Outcome	Nursing Actions and *Selected Purposes/Rationales*

8. encourage client to deep breathe or use incentive spirometer every 1–2 hours
9. encourage and assist client to use diaphragmatic and pursed-lip breathing techniques if appropriate
10. perform actions *to facilitate removal of secretions:*
    a. instruct and assist client to cough or "huff" every 1–2 hours
    b. implement measures *to thin secretions and reduce drying of the respiratory mucous membrane:*
        1. encourage maximum fluid intake allowed and tolerated
        2. humidify inspired air as ordered
    c. assist with administration of mucolytics and diluent or hydrating agents via nebulizer if ordered
    d. perform oral, pharyngeal, and/or tracheal suctioning if necessary (deep suctioning should be avoided during the final stage of dying)
11. maintain oxygen therapy as ordered
12. discourage smoking (*smoke increases mucus production, impairs ciliary function, decreases oxygen availability, and can cause inflammation and damage to the bronchial walls*)
13. encourage activity as tolerated
14. administer the following medications if ordered:
    a. diuretics *to decrease pulmonary fluid accumulation*
    b. morphine sulfate *to reduce apprehension associated with dyspnea and decrease pulmonary vascular congestion* (*the vasodilatory action of morphine sulfate reduces cardiac workload and improves left ventricular emptying, which results in increased blood return from the pulmonary veins*)
    c. bronchodilators (e.g. theophylline)
15. prepare client for thoracentesis or paracentesis if performed *to facilitate lung expansion.*
d. Consult physician about an order for an anticholinergic medication (e.g. atropine) *to reduce bronchial secretions if frequent suctioning is necessary or the sound of excessive secretions is disturbing to significant others.*
e. Consult physician if the client is experiencing respiratory distress.

■

2. NURSING DIAGNOSIS:

Fluid volume deficit

related to:
a. decreased oral intake associated with:
    1. anorexia, weakness, fatigue, and decreased level of consciousness
    2. nausea, dysphagia, pain, and/or dyspnea if present;
b. increased fluid loss associated with vomiting and/or diaphoresis if client has a fever.

Desired Outcome	Nursing Actions and *Selected Purposes/Rationales*

2. The client will maintain adequate fluid volume as evidenced by:
   a. normal skin turgor
   b. moist mucous membranes
   c. stable weight
   d. B/P and pulse within normal range for client and stable with position change

2.a. Assess for signs and symptoms of fluid volume deficit:
   1. decreased skin turgor
   2. dry mucous membranes, thirst
   3. sudden weight loss of 2% or greater
   4. postural hypotension and/or low B/P
   5. weak, rapid pulse
   6. delayed hand vein filling time (longer than 3–5 seconds)
   7. change in mental status
   8. decreased urine output (reflects an actual rather than potential fluid volume deficit).

e. hand vein filling time less than 3–5 seconds
f. usual mental status
g. balanced intake and output.

b. Implement measures *to prevent or treat fluid volume deficit:*
  1. perform actions to prevent nausea and vomiting if present (see Nursing Diagnosis 5.A, action 2)
  2. perform actions to reduce fever if present (e.g. administer antipyretics if ordered, sponge client with tepid water, remove excessive clothing or bedcovers) *in order to prevent diaphoresis and subsequent loss of fluid*
  3. encourage the maximum fluid intake allowed and tolerated; if client has difficulty drinking from a glass or through a straw:
     a. give frequent sips of water or juice using a syringe
     b. use a spoon to provide small amounts of ice chips
     c. provide popsicles if client desires.
c. Consult physician if signs and symptoms of fluid volume deficit worsen or create discomfort for the client. Encourage significant others and client to discuss the positive and negative aspects of intravenous therapy with physician.

---

3. NURSING DIAGNOSIS: **Risk for aspiration**

related to:
a. decreased level of consciousness;
b. absent or diminished gag reflex associated with the underlying disease process and/or the depressant effect of some medications (e.g. narcotic [opioid] analgesics, central-acting muscle relaxants);
c. supine positioning;
d. increased risk for gastroesophageal reflux associated with increased gastric pressure resulting from decreased gastrointestinal motility;
e. impaired swallowing associated with dry mouth and absent or diminished swallowing reflex (can occur as a result of the underlying disease process).

Desired Outcome	Nursing Actions and *Selected Purposes/Rationales*

3. The client will not aspirate secretions or foods/fluids as evidenced by:
a. clear or usual breath sounds
b. resonant percussion note over lungs
c. absence of cough and tachypnea
d. absence of or no increase in dyspnea.

3.a. Assess for signs and symptoms of aspiration of secretions, vomitus, or foods/fluids (e.g. rhonchi, dull percussion note over affected lung area, cough, tachypnea, tachycardia, development of or increase in dyspnea, presence of tube feeding in tracheal aspirate).
b. Monitor chest x-ray results. Report findings of pulmonary infiltrate.
c. If client is receiving tube feedings, add food coloring to the solution *so that it can be readily identified in tracheal aspirate.*
d. Implement measures *to reduce the risk for aspiration:*
  1. position client in side-lying or semi- to high Fowler's position at all times
  2. have suction equipment readily available for use
  3. perform oropharyngeal suctioning and oral hygiene as often as needed *to remove excess secretions, vomitus, and food particles*
  4. perform actions to prevent nausea and vomiting (see Nursing Diagnosis 5.A, action 2)
  5. perform actions to reduce the accumulation of gastrointestinal gas and fluid (see Nursing Diagnosis 5.B, action 3) *in order to reduce the risk of gastric distention and gastroesophageal reflux*
  6. withhold oral food/fluids if gag reflex is depressed or absent, client is not alert, or he/she is experiencing severe dysphagia
  7. if client is receiving tube feedings:
     a. check tube placement before each feeding or on a routine basis if continuous feeding
     b. do not increase continuous tube feeding unless allowed and tolerated; administer intermittent tube feedings slowly

Desired Outcome	Nursing Actions and *Selected Purposes/Rationales*

c. maintain client in semi- to high Fowler's position during and for at least 30 minutes after feeding
d. stop tube feeding and notify physician if residuals exceed established parameters
8. if client is taking foods/fluids orally:
   a. offer foods/fluids that promote an effective swallow (e.g. thick rather than thin fluids, moist rather than dry foods)
   b. allow ample time for meals
   c. instruct client to avoid talking or laughing when swallowing
   d. maintain client in high Fowler's position during and for at least 30 minutes after meals and snacks.
   e. If signs and symptoms of aspiration occur:
      1. perform tracheal suctioning
      2. withhold oral intake
      3. notify physician
      4. prepare client for chest x-ray if ordered.

---

4. NURSING DIAGNOSIS: **Pain**

related to:
a. the underlying disease process;
b. reluctance to take pain medication associated with fear of loss of control and/or oversedation, feeling that pain is a sign of weakness or has redemptive qualities, and/or need to be stoic.

Desired Outcome	Nursing Actions and *Selected Purposes/Rationales*

4. The client will experience diminished pain as evidenced by:
   a. verbalization of decrease in or absence of pain
   b. relaxed facial expression and body positioning
   c. stable vital signs.

4.a. Assess for signs and symptoms of pain (e.g. verbalization of pain, grimacing, reluctance to move, restlessness, diaphoresis, facial pallor, increased B/P, tachycardia).
b. Assess client's perception of the severity of pain using a pain intensity rating scale.
c. Assess the client's pain pattern (e.g. location, quality, onset, duration, precipitating factors, aggravating factors, alleviating factors).
d. Ask the client to describe previous pain experiences and methods used to manage pain effectively.
e. Implement measures *to reduce pain:*
   1. perform actions *to reduce fear and anxiety about the pain experience* (e.g. assure client that his/her need for pain relief is understood, plan methods for achieving pain control with client)
   2. perform actions to reduce fear and anxiety (see Nursing Diagnosis 16) *in order to promote relaxation and subsequently increase the client's threshold and tolerance for pain*
   3. administer analgesics before activities and procedures that can cause pain and before pain becomes severe
   4. perform actions to promote rest (e.g. minimize environmental activity and noise) *in order to reduce fatigue, which can decrease the client's threshold and tolerance for pain*
   5. plan methods for achieving pain control with client *in order to assist him/her to maintain a sense of control over the pain experience*
   6. provide or assist with nonpharmacologic methods for pain relief (e.g. massage; position change; progressive relaxation exercise; restful environment; diversional activities such as watching television, reading, or conversing)
   7. encourage client to use patient-controlled analgesia (PCA) device as instructed

8. administer the following medications as ordered *to provide maximum pain relief with minimal side effects:*
   a. narcotic (opioid) analgesics (route of administration may include intermittent intravenous doses; continuous intravenous or subcutaneous infusion; or epidural, intrathecal, or intraspinal infusion *since medication absorption via the oral and intramuscular routes is less predictable*)
   b. nonnarcotic (nonopioid) analgesics such as nonsteroidal anti-inflammatory agents, salicylates, or acetaminophen.
   f. Consult physician or pain management nurse specialist if above measures fail to provide adequate pain relief.

5.A. NURSING DIAGNOSIS: **Altered comfort: nausea and vomiting**

related to stimulation of the vomiting center associated with:
1. stimulation of the visceral afferent pathways resulting from abdominal distention if present;
2. stimulation of the cerebral cortex resulting from pain and stress;
3. stimulation of the chemoreceptor trigger zone by some medications (e.g. morphine sulfate, meperidine hydrochloride).

Desired Outcome	Nursing Actions and *Selected Purposes/Rationales*

5.A. The client will experience relief of nausea and vomiting as evidenced by:
1. verbalization of relief of nausea
2. absence of vomiting.
	5.A.1. Assess client for nausea and vomiting.
	    2. Implement measures *to prevent nausea and vomiting:*
	        a. perform actions to reduce accumulation of gastrointestinal gas and fluid (see Nursing Diagnosis 5.B, action 3)
	        b. perform actions to reduce pain (see Nursing Diagnosis 4, action e)
	        c. perform actions to reduce fear and anxiety (see Nursing Diagnosis 16)
	        d. eliminate noxious sights and odors from the environment (*noxious stimuli can cause stimulation of the vomiting center*)
	        e. encourage client to take deep, slow breaths when nauseated
	        f. instruct client to change positions slowly (*rapid movement can result in stimulation of the chemoreceptor trigger zone and subsequent excitation of the vomiting center*)
	        g. provide oral hygiene after each emesis
	        h. if oral intake is allowed and tolerated:
	            1. avoid serving foods with an overpowering aroma; remove lids from hot foods before entering room
	            2. provide small, frequent meals; instruct client to ingest foods and fluids slowly
	            3. encourage client to eat dry foods (e.g. toast, crackers) and avoid drinking liquids with meals if nauseated
	            4. instruct client to avoid foods/fluids that irritate gastric mucosa (e.g. spicy foods; caffeine-containing beverages such as coffee, tea, and colas)
	            5. instruct client to avoid foods high in fat (*fat delays gastric emptying*)
	            6. instruct client to rest after eating with head of bed elevated
	            7. administer medications known to cause gastric irritation (e.g. aspirin and aspirin-containing products, corticosteroids, ibuprofen) with or immediately after meals or snacks unless contraindicated
	        i. administer antiemetics and gastrointestinal stimulants (e.g. metoclopramide, cisapride) if ordered.

Desired Outcome	Nursing Actions and *Selected Purposes/Rationales*
	3. If above measures fail to control nausea and vomiting: a. consult physician b. be prepared to insert a nasogastric tube and maintain suction as ordered.

5.B. NURSING DIAGNOSIS: **Altered comfort: abdominal distention and gas pain**

related to an accumulation of gas and fluid associated with decreased gastrointestinal motility resulting from depressant effect of some medications (e.g. narcotic [opioid] analgesics, central-acting muscle relaxants) and decreased activity.

Desired Outcome	Nursing Actions and *Selected Purposes/Rationales*

5.B. The client will experience diminished abdominal distention and gas pain as evidenced by:
1. verbalization of decreased abdominal fullness and pain
2. relaxed facial expression and body positioning
3. decrease in abdominal girth.
	5.B.1. Assess for verbal reports of abdominal fullness or gas pain.
	2. Assess for nonverbal signs of abdominal distention or gas pain (e.g. clutching or guarding of abdomen, restlessness, reluctance to move, grimacing, increasing abdominal girth).
	3. Implement measures *to reduce the accumulation of gastrointestinal gas and fluid:*
	a. encourage and assist client with frequent position changes and ambulation as tolerated (*activity stimulates peristalsis and expulsion of flatus*)
	b. instruct client to avoid activities such as chewing gum and smoking *in order to reduce air swallowing*
	c. maintain patency of nasogastric or intestinal tube if present
	d. maintain food and oral fluid restrictions if ordered
	e. instruct client to avoid intake of carbonated beverages and gas-producing foods (e.g. cabbage, onions, beans)
	f. encourage client to eructate and expel flatus whenever the urge is felt
	g. consult physician about insertion of a rectal tube or administration of a return flow enema if indicated
	h. encourage use of nonnarcotic analgesics if possible (*narcotic [opioid] analgesics depress gastrointestinal activity*)
	i. administer the following medications if ordered:
	  1. antiflatulents (e.g. simethicone) *to reduce gas accumulation*
	  2. gastrointestinal stimulants (e.g. metoclopramide, cisapride, bisacodyl) *to increase gastrointestinal motility.*
	4. Consult physician if signs and symptoms of abdominal distention or gas pain persist or worsen.

---

6. NURSING DIAGNOSIS: **Risk for impaired tissue integrity**

related to:
a. accumulation of waste products and decreased oxygen and nutrient supply to the skin and subcutaneous tissue associated with reduced blood flow from prolonged pressure on the tissues resulting from decreased mobility;
b. damage to the skin and/or subcutaneous tissue associated with friction or shearing;
c. frequent contact with irritants associated with incontinence of urine or stool;
d. increased fragility of skin associated with inadequate nutritional status, dryness, and dependent edema.

Desired Outcome	Nursing Actions and *Selected Purposes/Rationales*

6. The client will maintain tissue integrity as evidenced by:
  a. absence of redness and irritation
  b. no skin breakdown.
	6.a. Inspect the skin (especially bony prominences; dependent, edematous, and pruritic areas; and perianal area) for pallor, redness, and breakdown.
	  b. Refer to Care Plan on Immobility, Nursing Diagnosis 4, action b (pp. 129–130), for measures to prevent tissue breakdown.
	  c. Implement additional measures *to maintain tissue integrity:*
	    1. perform actions *to prevent skin irritation resulting from incontinence of urine or stool:*
	      a. implement measures to reduce the episodes of urinary and bowel incontinence (see Nursing Diagnoses 10, actions b and c.1 and 12, action b)
	      b. assist client to thoroughly cleanse and dry perineal area with soft tissue or cloth after each episode of incontinence; apply a protective ointment or cream
	      c. apply a fecal incontinence pouch if bowel incontinence is a persistent problem
	      d. provide incontinence pads if needed to absorb moisture; do not allow skin to come in contact with plastic portion of the pads
	    2. perform actions to prevent or treat fluid volume deficit (see Nursing Diagnosis 2, action b) *in order to reduce risk of skin breakdown associated with dryness.*
	  d. If tissue breakdown occurs:
	    1. notify physician
	    2. continue with above measures to prevent further irritation and breakdown
	    3. perform pressure ulcer care as ordered or per standard hospital procedure (extensiveness of treatment is usually limited to that necessary to maintain comfort)
	    4. assess client closely and report signs and symptoms of infection (e.g. elevated temperature; redness, heat, pain, and swelling around area of breakdown; unusual drainage from site).

■━━━

7. NURSING DIAGNOSIS: **Altered oral mucous membrane: dryness**

related to:
a. decreased salivation associated with decreased oral intake and some medications (e.g. tricyclic antidepressants, anticholinergics, narcotic [opioid] analgesics, phenothiazines);
b. fluid volume deficit associated with decreased fluid intake and increased fluid loss;
c. prolonged oxygen therapy (especially if administered by mask);
d. mouth breathing.

Desired Outcome	Nursing Actions and *Selected Purposes/Rationales*

7. The client will maintain a moist, intact oral mucous membrane.	7.a. Assess client frequently for dryness of the oral mucosa.
	  b. Implement measures *to relieve dryness of the oral mucous membrane:*
	    1. assist client to perform oral hygiene as often as needed; avoid use of products that contain lemon and glycerin and mouthwashes containing alcohol (*these have a drying and irritating effect on the oral mucous membrane*)
	    2. assist client to rinse mouth frequently with water
	    3. lubricate client's lips frequently

Desired Outcome	Nursing Actions and *Selected Purposes/Rationales*
	4. encourage client to breathe through nose rather than mouth
	5. encourage client not to smoke (*smoking irritates and dries the mucosa*)
	6. perform actions to prevent or treat fluid volume deficit (see Nursing Diagnosis 2, action b)
	7. encourage client to suck on hard candy if allowed *in order to stimulate salivation*
	8. encourage client to use artificial saliva if needed *to lubricate the mucous membrane.*
	c. If oral mucosa is irritated or cracked, implement measures *to relieve discomfort and promote healing:*
	1. if client is alert and able to take nourishment by mouth, assist him/her to select soft, bland foods
	2. instruct client to avoid foods/fluids that are extremely hot
	3. use a soft bristle brush, gauze-wrapped tongue blade, sponge-tipped applicator, or low-pressure power spray for oral hygiene
	4. administer topical anesthetics, oral protective agents, and analgesics if ordered.
	d. Consult physician if dryness, irritation, and/or discomfort persist.

---

8. NURSING DIAGNOSIS: **Impaired physical mobility**

related to:
a. weakness and fatigue;
b. dyspnea and/or sensory and motor deficits (can occur as a result of the underlying disease process);
c. reluctance to move associated with pain and nausea if present;
d. decreased level of consciousness.

Desired Outcome	Nursing Actions and *Selected Purposes/Rationales*
8. The client will maintain maximum physical mobility within limitations imposed by terminal state.	8.a. Implement measures *to maintain mobility for as long as possible:*
	1. perform actions to reduce pain and prevent nausea (see Nursing Diagnoses 4, action e and 5.A, action 2)
	2. perform actions to improve respiratory status (see Nursing Diagnosis 1, action c) *in order to relieve dyspnea*
	3. provide adequate rest periods before activity sessions
	4. instruct client in and assist with active and/or passive range of motion exercises at least 3 times/day unless contraindicated
	5. put side rails up and provide overhead trapeze unless contraindicated *to promote independent movement*
	6. instruct client in and assist with use of mobility aids (e.g. cane, walker) if appropriate
	7. provide assistive devices appropriate for client's specific sensory and motor deficits if indicated
	8. consult with occupational and/or physical therapists about ways to facilitate client's mobility if appropriate.
	b. Provide praise and encouragement for all efforts to maintain physical mobility.
	c. Encourage the support of significant others. Allow them to assist with range of motion exercises, positioning, and activity if desired.

9. NURSING DIAGNOSIS: **Self-care deficit**

related to:
a. weakness and fatigue;
b. activity limitations associated with the underlying disease process;
c. pain, nausea, dyspnea, and/or altered thought processes if present;
d. decreased level of consciousness.

Desired Outcome	Nursing Actions and *Selected Purposes/Rationales*
9. The client will perform self-care activities within cognitive and physical limitations.	9.a. Refer to Care Plan on Immobility, Nursing Diagnosis 7 (p. 132), for measures related to planning for and meeting client's self-care needs. b. Implement measures to maintain mobility (see Nursing Diagnosis 8, action a) *in order to further facilitate client's ability to perform self-care.*

10. NURSING DIAGNOSIS: **Altered urinary elimination: incontinence**

related to:
a. decreased ability to respond to the urge to urinate associated with decreased level of consciousness and impaired physical mobility;
b. decreased awareness of full bladder and poor urinary sphincter control associated with decreased level of consciousness and/or the underlying disease process.

Desired Outcome	Nursing Actions and *Selected Purposes/Rationales*
10. The client will experience urinary continence.	10.a. Assess for urinary incontinence. b. Implement measures *to maintain or regain urinary continence:* 1. offer bedpan or urinal or assist client to bedside commode or bathroom every 2–3 hours 2. allow client to assume a normal position for voiding unless contraindicated *in order to promote complete bladder emptying* 3. perform actions *to reduce delays in toileting* (e.g. have call signal within client's reach and respond promptly to requests for assistance; have bedpan, urinal, or bedside commode readily available to client; provide client with easy-to-remove clothing such as pajamas with Velcro closures or an elastic waistband) 4. if client has a good fluid intake, encourage him/her to space fluids evenly throughout the day rather than drinking a large quantity at one time (*rapid filling of bladder can result in incontinence if client has decreased urinary sphincter control*) 5. encourage intake of beverages that are decaffeinated or caffeine-free rather than caffeinated (*caffeine is a mild diuretic and a bladder irritant; both effects may make urinary control more difficult*). c. If urinary incontinence persists: 1. consult physician about intermittent catheterization, insertion of indwelling catheter, or use of external catheter 2. provide client with or apply disposable undergarments (e.g. Depends, Attends) if indicated.

11. NURSING DIAGNOSIS: **Constipation**

related to:
a. diminished defecation reflex associated with decreased nervous system responses in terminal state, suppression of the urge to defecate because of reluctance to use bedpan, and decreased gravity filling of lower rectum resulting from horizontal positioning;
b. decreased ability to respond to the urge to defecate associated with weakened abdominal muscles, impaired physical mobility, and decreased level of consciousness;
c. decreased gastrointestinal motility associated with decreased activity, increased sympathetic nervous system activity that occurs with anxiety, and use of some medications (e.g. narcotic [opioid] analgesics, antacids containing aluminum or calcium);
d. decreased intake of fluid and foods high in fiber.

Desired Outcome	Nursing Actions and *Selected Purposes/Rationales*

11. The client will maintain a bowel routine that provides optimal comfort.	11.a. Refer to Care Plan on Immobility, Nursing Diagnosis 9 (pp. 133–134), for measures related to assessment, prevention, and management of constipation.
	b. Implement additional measures *to prevent constipation:*
	    1. assist client to toilet or place in high Fowler's position or on bedside commode for bowel movements unless contraindicated
	    2. if client is taking antacids containing aluminum or calcium, consult physician about alternating them with antacids containing magnesium.

12. NURSING DIAGNOSIS: **Bowel incontinence**

related to:
a. decreased ability to respond to the urge to defecate associated with decreased level of consciousness and impaired physical mobility;
b. decreased awareness of urge to defecate and poor anal sphincter control associated with decreased level of consciousness;
c. fecal impaction if present (continuous stimulation of the defecation reflex by the fecal mass inhibits the internal anal sphincter and results in loss of ability to retain the mucus and fluid that collect proximal to and leak around the fecal mass).

Desired Outcome	Nursing Actions and *Selected Purposes/Rationales*

12. The client will maintain optimal bowel control as evidenced by absence of or decrease in episodes of incontinence.	12.a. Monitor for episodes of bowel incontinence.
	b. Implement measures *to reduce the risk of bowel incontinence:*
	    1. perform bowel care routinely *to promote emptying of the lower colon*
	    2. perform actions *to reduce delays in toileting* (e.g. have call signal within client's reach and respond promptly to requests for assistance; have bedpan or bedside commode readily available to client; provide client with easy-to-remove clothing such as pajamas with Velcro closures or an elastic waistband)
	    3. consult physician regarding measures to remove fecal impaction if present (e.g. digital removal of stool, oil retention enema).

c. If bowel incontinence persists:
    1. consult physician about use of a fecal incontinence pouch
    2. provide client with disposable liners for underwear or disposable undergarments such as Attends
    3. use room deodorants as necessary.

---

13. NURSING DIAGNOSIS: **Altered thought processes***

related to:
a. drug toxicity associated with organ failure;
b. fluid volume deficit and electrolyte imbalances associated with decreased oral intake, increased fluid loss, and the underlying disease process;
c. cerebral hypoxia, cerebral tissue damage, and/or metabolic changes associated with the underlying disease process;
d. uncontrolled pain.

---

*The diagnostic label of acute or chronic confusion may be more appropriate depending on the client's symptoms.

Desired Outcome	Nursing Actions and *Selected Purposes/Rationales*

13. The client will maintain optimal thought processes.	13.a. Assess client for altered thought processes (e.g. impaired memory, shortened attention span, slowed verbal response time, confusion).
	b. Ascertain from significant others client's usual level of cognitive functioning.
	c. If client shows evidence of altered thought processes:
	  1. assess for possible causes (e.g. drug toxicity, pain, hypoxia, fluid and electrolyte imbalances) and implement measures to treat them if appropriate
	  2. reorient client to person, place, time, and others as necessary
	  3. address client by name
	  4. encourage significant others to bring in client's favorite items and place them within client's view
	  5. approach client in a slow, calm manner; allow adequate time for communication
	  6. repeat instructions as necessary using clear, simple language and short sentences
	  7. keep environmental stimuli to a minimum
	  8. have client perform only one activity at a time and allow adequate time for performance of activities
	  9. encourage significant others to spend time with and to be supportive of client; instruct them in methods of dealing with client's altered thought processes
	  10. leave light on at night *to facilitate client's orientation to surroundings.*

---

14. NURSING DIAGNOSIS: **Sleep pattern disturbance**

related to decreased physical activity, fear, anxiety, unfamiliar environment, discomfort, and inability to assume usual sleep position associated with orthopnea if present.

Desired Outcome	Nursing Actions and *Selected Purposes/Rationales*
14. The client will attain optimal amounts of sleep (see Care Plan on Immobility, Nursing Diagnosis 10 [p. 134], for outcome criteria).	14.a. Refer to Care Plan on Immobility Nursing Diagnosis 10 (pp. 134–135), for measures related to assessment and promotion of sleep. b. Implement additional measures *to promote sleep:* 1. perform actions to reduce fear and anxiety (see Nursing Diagnosis 16) 2. perform actions to reduce discomfort (see Nursing Diagnoses 4, action e; 5.A, action 2; and 5.B, action 3) 3. if client has orthopnea, assist him/her to assume a position *that will facilitate breathing* (e.g. head of bed elevated with arms supported on pillows, resting forward on overbed table with good pillow support, sitting in a chair) 4. maintain oxygen therapy during sleep if indicated.

---

15. NURSING DIAGNOSIS: **Risk for trauma: falls, burns, and lacerations**

related to weakness, fatigue, confusion if present, and decreased level of consciousness.

Desired Outcome	Nursing Actions and *Selected Purposes/Rationales*
15. The client will not experience falls, burns, or lacerations.	15.a. Implement measures *to prevent trauma:* 1. perform actions *to prevent falls:* a. keep bed in low position with side rails up when client is in bed b. keep needed items within easy reach c. encourage client to request assistance whenever needed; have call signal within easy reach d. use lap belt when client is in chair if indicated e. instruct client to wear well-fitting slippers/shoes with nonslip soles and low heels when ambulating f. keep floor free of clutter and wipe up spills promptly g. instruct and assist client to get out of bed slowly *in order to reduce dizziness associated with postural hypotension* h. carefully position tubing and equipment so that they will not interfere with ambulation i. accompany client during ambulation and use transfer safety belt if he/she is weak or dizzy j. provide ambulatory aids (e.g. walker, cane) if client is weak or unsteady on feet k. reinforce instructions from physical therapist on correct transfer and ambulation techniques l. instruct client to ambulate in well-lit areas and to use handrails if needed m. do not rush client; allow adequate time for ambulation to the bathroom and in hallway n. make sure that shower has a nonslip bottom surface and that shower chair, secure bath mat, call signal, grab bars, and adequate lighting are present 2. perform actions *to prevent burns:* a. let hot foods and fluids cool slightly before serving b. supervise client while smoking if indicated c. assess temperature of bath water and direct heat application device (e.g. K-pad, warm compress, hot water bottle) before and during use 3. assist client with tasks that require fine motor skills (e.g. shaving) *in order to prevent lacerations*

4. if client is confused:
   a. reorient frequently to surroundings and necessity of adhering to safety precautions
   b. provide appropriate level of supervision
   c. consult physician about the temporary use of a bed alarm or jacket or wrist restraints if necessary
   d. administer prescribed antianxiety and antipsychotic medications if indicated.
   b. Include client and significant others in planning and implementing measures to prevent trauma.
   c. If injury does occur, initiate appropriate first aid and notify physician.

---

16. NURSING DIAGNOSIS: **Anxiety**

related to:
a. unfamiliar environment and separation from significant others;
b. feelings of hopelessness, abandonment, loneliness, and that life has been meaningless;
c. the unknown;
d. pain, dyspnea, and loss of control over life and body functioning;
e. concern about the welfare of significant others and loss of loved ones;
f. unfinished business, unresolved conflicts, and recognition of nonbeing.

Desired Outcome	Nursing Actions and *Selected Purposes/Rationales*
16. The client will experience a reduction in anxiety as evidenced by: a. verbalization of feeling less anxious b. usual sleep pattern c. relaxed facial expression and body movements d. stable vital signs e. statements reflecting resolution of unfinished business, conflicts, and concerns.	16.a. Refer to Care Plan on Immobility, Nursing Diagnosis 13 (p. 140), for measures related to assessment and reduction of fear and anxiety. b. Implement additional measures *to reduce fear and anxiety:* 1. perform actions to reduce discomfort (see Nursing Diagnoses 4, action e; 5.A, action 2; and 5.B, action 3) 2. perform actions to improve respiratory status (see Nursing Diagnosis 1, action c) *in order to relieve dyspnea if present* 3. perform actions to reduce feelings of hopelessness (see Nursing Diagnosis 18, action b) 4. spend time with client *to reduce feelings of loneliness and isolation* 5. encourage reminiscence about life experiences if he/she desires *to promote feelings of meaningfulness about the life he/she has lived* 6. assist client to formulate plans for completing unfinished business and providing for care of significant others if appropriate 7. encourage significant others to stay with client and participate in care if their presence seems to relieve the client's fear and anxiety 8. when appropriate, assist client to meet spiritual needs (e.g. arrange for a visit with clergy).

---

17. NURSING DIAGNOSIS: **Grieving***

related to loss of control over life and body functioning, changes in body image, loss of significant others, and imminent death.

---

*This diagnostic label includes anticipatory grieving and grieving following the actual losses.

Desired Outcome	Nursing Actions and *Selected Purposes/Rationales*

17. The client will demonstrate progression through the grieving process as evidenced by:
    a. verbalization of feelings about dying
    b. usual sleep pattern
    c. use of available support systems.

17.a. Assess for signs and symptoms of grieving (e.g. change in eating habits, inability to concentrate, insomnia, anger, sadness, withdrawal from significant others, denial of loss).
  b. Implement measures *to facilitate the grieving process:*
    1. assist client to acknowledge that death is imminent *so that grief work can progress*; assess for factors that may hinder and facilitate acknowledgment
    2. discuss the grieving process and assist client to accept the phases of grieving as an expected response to actual and/or anticipated losses
    3. allow time for client to progress through the phases of grieving (phases vary among theorists, but progress from shock and alarm to acceptance); be aware that not every phase is expressed by all individuals, that phases do not necessarily occur in sequential order, and that recurrence of phases is common during the course of an illness and the dying process
    4. provide an atmosphere of care and concern (e.g. provide privacy, be available and nonjudgmental, display empathy and respect) *so client will feel free to express feelings*
    5. perform actions *to promote trust* (e.g. answer questions honestly, provide requested information)
    6. encourage the verbal expression of anger and sadness about the losses experienced; recognize displacement of anger and assist client to see the actual cause of angry feelings and resentment; establish limits on abusive behavior if demonstrated
    7. encourage client to express feelings in whatever ways are comfortable (e.g. writing, drawing, conversation)
    8. assist client to identify and utilize techniques that have helped him/her cope in previous situations of loss
    9. if desired by client, assist with after-death arrangements (e.g. funeral, religious service, who should be called)
    10. perform actions *to assist the client to maintain a positive self-concept and feel good about the life he/she has experienced:*
      a. visit frequently and encourage verbalization about past events, life accomplishments, interests, and feelings
      b. help client to focus on positive rather than negative aspects of his/her life experience
      c. maintain a nonjudgmental attitude about the kind of life client has led and his/her beliefs
      d. encourage participation in decisions about care
      e. encourage and assist client with good physical hygiene and grooming; suggest use of personal rather than hospital clothing *to assist client to maintain his/her identity*
    11. support behaviors suggesting successful grief work (e.g. verbalizing feelings about losses, use of available support systems)
    12. explain the phases of the grieving process to significant others; encourage their support and understanding
    13. facilitate communication between the client and significant others; be aware that they may be in different phases of the grieving process
    14. provide information about counseling services and support groups that might assist client and significant others in working through grief
    15. when appropriate, assist client to meet spiritual needs (e.g. arrange for visit from clergy).
  c. Consult physician regarding referral for counseling if signs of dysfunctional grieving (e.g. persistent denial of losses, excessive anger or sadness, emotional lability) occur.

18. NURSING DIAGNOSIS:

Hopelessness

related to deteriorating physical condition, feelings of abandonment, and inability to reach self-fulfillment associated with terminal state.

Desired Outcome	Nursing Actions and *Selected Purposes/Rationales*

18. The client will maintain hope as evidenced by:
 a. verbal expression of same
 b. maintenance of satisfying relationships with others
 c. participation in self-care and decision making as able
 d. identification of realistic goals.
	18.a. Assess client for signs and symptoms of hopelessness (e.g. statements of feeling hopeless, decreased response to significant others, decreased participation in self-care and decision making, decreased verbalization, flat affect).
	 b. Implement measures *to assist client to reduce feelings of hopelessness:*
	   1. perform actions to facilitate the grieving process (see Nursing Diagnosis 17, action b)
	   2. if client has religious beliefs, encourage the use of them as a support system; support his/her renewal of spiritual being by creating an environment in which these beliefs can be openly acknowledged and practiced
	   3. allow client to retain as much control as possible over activities of daily living; involve him/her in as much self-care and decision making as feasible
	   4. assist client to identify goals that are achievable in the time that he/she has left, ways to continue working toward goals previously set even if not possible to achieve them totally, and the purpose remaining in his/her life such as role model or advisor to significant others.
	 c. Consult physician if client demonstrates increased feelings of hopelessness.

19. NURSING DIAGNOSIS:

Altered family processes

related to excessive anxiety, grief, disorganization and role changes within the family unit, inadequate support systems, and fatigue.

Desired Outcome	Nursing Actions and *Selected Purposes/Rationales*
19. The family members* will demonstrate beginning adjustment to loss of client and changes in family roles and structure as evidenced by: a. meeting client's needs b. verbalization of ways to adapt to required role and life-style changes	19.a. Assess for signs and symptoms of altered family processes (e.g. inability to meet client's needs, statements of not being able to accept client's imminent death or to make necessary role and life-style changes, inability to make decisions, infrequent visits, inappropriate response to client's situation, verbalization of guilt, preoccupation with other aspects of life, negative family interactions). b. Identify components of the family and their patterns of communication and role expectations. c. Implement measures *to facilitate family members' adjustment to imminent loss of client and altered family roles and structure:*

*The term "family members" is being used here to include client's significant others.

Desired Outcome	Nursing Actions and *Selected Purposes/Rationales*

c. active participation in decision making and client's care
d. positive interactions with one another.
	1. encourage and assist family members to verbalize feelings about the death of the client and the effect of it on their life style and family structure; actively listen to each family member and maintain a nonjudgmental attitude about feelings shared
	2. assist family members to confront the reality of the client's imminent death when they are ready; encourage them to imagine life after death of the client and to set some personal goals if appropriate
	3. provide privacy *so that family members can share their feelings and grief with one another*; stress the importance of and facilitate the use of good communication techniques
	4. explain the phases of grieving and assist family members to progress through their own grieving process; explain that they may encounter times when they need to focus on meeting their own rather than the client's needs
	5. emphasize the need for family members to obtain adequate rest and nutrition and to identify and use stress management techniques *so that they are better able to emotionally and physically deal with the death of the client*; assure them that the client will be well cared for in their absence
	6. encourage and assist family members to identify coping strategies for dealing with the client's death and its effect on those left behind
	7. include family members in decision making about client and his/her care; convey appreciation of their input and continued support of the client
	8. encourage and allow family members to participate in client's care if desired by both client and family members
	9. assist family members to make necessary postmortem arrangements for or with the client (e.g. funeral home, burial place, clergy visitation)
	10. provide information to family members about:
	  a. the current status of client
	  b. behaviors to expect as the client progresses through terminal stages of disease and his/her own grieving
	  c. physical signs and symptoms of approaching death (e.g. lack of interest in environment; withdrawal from relationships; disorientation; vision-like experiences; "out-of-character" statements or requests; increased sleeping; incontinence; decreased level of consciousness; reduced urine output; cool, mottled extremities; respiratory sounds such as gurgling or rattling, labored breathing, or periods of no breathing)
	  d. ways they can best assist in meeting client's needs
	11. when appropriate, help and encourage family members to "let go" of client and say goodbye
	12. assist family members to identify resources that can assist them in coping with their feelings and in meeting their immediate and long-term needs (e.g. counseling and social services; pastoral care; service, bereavement, and church groups; Hospice); initiate a referral if indicated
	13. assist family members to contact appropriate persons (e.g. funeral home director, clergy) when death occurs.
	d. Consult physician if family members continue to demonstrate difficulty adjusting to the loss of the client and role changes within the family unit.

Bibliography

See pages 897–899.

UNIT SEVEN

NURSING CARE OF THE CLIENT RECEIVING TREATMENT FOR NEOPLASTIC DISORDERS

BRACHYTHERAPY

Brachytherapy is the continuous delivery of radiation to a malignancy at a specific body site by placing the radioactive source close to or within the tumor. Brachytherapy can deliver a higher dose of radiation than is possible with external radiation therapy (teletherapy) and does so with minimal damage occurring to the surrounding healthy tissue because of the rapid fall in dose outside the implanted area. It can be used as a primary treatment or in combination with external radiation therapy and/or surgery. Brachytherapy can be sealed or unsealed, temporary or permanent, and local or systemic. The method of application selected depends on the type, location, and size of the tumor; its radiocurability; the sensitivity of surrounding normal tissue; and the age and physical condition of the client. The radioactive isotope used depends on the site to be treated, lesion size, availability and half-life of the isotope, and financial and safety concerns.

The most common types of brachytherapy are interstitial implants using iridium 192 (^{192}Ir) seeds or wire or iodine 125 (^{125}I) seeds and intracavitary implants using cesium 137 (^{137}Cs). Both types are sealed and temporary. Interstitial implants are used in the treatment of skin, brain, prostate, and oral cavity lesions, whereas intracavitary implants are used primarily in treating gynecological malignancies. With both interstitial and intracavitary implants, varying kinds of applicators (e.g. hollow needles, templates, plastic tubes, Fletcher-Suit) are surgically placed in the tissue or cavity to be treated and the radioactive source is either preloaded or, more commonly, afterloaded when the client returns to his/her room. With brachytherapy using low-dose-rate (LDR) sources, the implant is commonly left in place for 24–72 hours and delivers a dose of 40–60 cGy (centigrays)/hour. High-dose-rate (HDR) brachytherapy is increasingly being used because it can produce the same effect on the tumor cells in a significantly shorter time. With HDR brachytherapy, 500–1000 cGy can be delivered in less than 10 minutes. Remote afterloading systems, which eliminate personnel exposure to the radioactive source during the loading and unloading process, are being used with increasing frequency for intracavity brachytherapy. These systems allow for retraction of the radioactive source by means of a transfer tube into a shielded bedside safe whenever personnel and/or family members enter the client's room.

Brachytherapy using unsealed isotopes is also commonly done. These isotopes can be ingested, injected, or implanted permanently in a body part. Unsealed interstitial implants using ^{125}I or gold 198 (^{198}Au) typically have been used in the treatment of pancreatic, prostate, and neck cancers. Iodine 131 (^{131}I) is commonly used to treat thyroid cancer and Graves' disease. It is ingested and metabolized by the body before being concentrated in the thyroid gland in 3–5 days. Although not in common use, colloidal forms of phosphorus 32 (^{32}P) can be injected into the pleural or peritoneal cavity to treat local disease or related effusions and/or ascites.

Another type of brachytherapy, surface brachytherapy, is accomplished by placing a radioactive source in a mold, which is then placed on or adjacent to an external body surface. It is used to treat sites such as small surface lesions that are difficult to access in other ways.

This care plan focuses on the adult client hospitalized for brachytherapy. The nursing care required will depend on the isotope used, its method of administration, and the physiological condition of the client. Before the initiation of brachytherapy, the goals of care are to reduce fear and anxiety and to educate the client regarding the therapy and expected side effects. During and following the treatment, the goals of care are to maintain comfort, prevent complications, and educate the client regarding follow-up care.

DISCHARGE CRITERIA

Prior to discharge, the client will:

- have implant site pain at a manageable level
- verbalize appropriate safety precautions related to brachytherapy
- identify measures to increase comfort and prevent complications associated with vaginal irradiation
- share thoughts and feelings about the diagnosis of cancer and need for radiation therapy
- state signs and symptoms to report to the health care provider
- identify community resources that can assist with adjustment to the effects of the diagnosis and its treatment
- verbalize an understanding of and a plan for adhering to recommended follow-up care including future appointments with health care provider and radiologist and medications prescribed.

NURSING DIAGNOSES   **Pre-radiation**
1. Anxiety △   165
2. Knowledge deficit △   165

See Standardized Preoperative Care Plan for additional diagnoses.

Radiation and Postradiation
1. Pain:
   a. muscle aches
   b. pain at or around implant site △   168
2. Impaired physical mobility △   169
3. Self-care deficit △   169

DISCHARGE TEACHING
4. Knowledge deficit, Ineffective management of therapeutic regimen, or Altered health maintenance △   170

PRERADIATION

Use in conjunction with the Standardized Preoperative Care Plan.

---

1. NURSING DIAGNOSIS:

Anxiety

related to:
a. lack of knowledge and preconceived ideas about treatment with radiation and its effect on physiological functioning;
b. unfamiliar environment and separation from significant others;
c. potential embarrassment or loss of dignity associated with body exposure;
d. anticipated loss of control associated with the effects of anesthesia if a general anesthetic will be used;
e. anticipated discomfort;
f. financial concerns;
g. diagnosis of cancer.

Desired Outcome	Nursing Actions and *Selected Purposes/Rationales*

1. The client will experience a reduction in anxiety (see Standardized Preoperative Care Plan, Nursing Diagnosis 1 [pp. 96–97], for outcome criteria).	1. Refer to Standardized Preoperative Care Plan, Nursing Diagnosis 1 (pp. 96–97), for measures related to assessment and reduction of fear and anxiety.
	2. Implement additional measures *to reduce fear and anxiety:*
	  a. reinforce physician's explanations and clarify misconceptions client has about the diagnosis of cancer, treatment plan and its effects, and prognosis
	  b. provide information related to the specific type of brachytherapy the client will be receiving (see Preradiation Nursing Diagnosis 2, action b).

Client Teaching

---

2. NURSING DIAGNOSIS:

Knowledge deficit

regarding:
a. hospital routines associated with brachytherapy;
b. physical preparation for implant of the radioactive source and sensations to expect following the implant;
c. the procedure for placement of the radioactive source;
d. precautions necessary to protect staff and significant others from exposure to radiation and prevent dislodgment of the radioactive source.

Desired Outcome	Nursing Actions and *Selected Purposes/Rationales*

2. The client will verbalize an understanding of the procedure for placement of the radioactive source and usual preradiation and postradiation care.	2.a. Refer to Standardized Preoperative Care Plan, Nursing Diagnosis 4, actions a.1–4 (pp. 99–100), for teaching related to routine preoperative and postoperative care.
	b. Provide additional information regarding care associated with the type of brachytherapy the client will be receiving:
	1. if the client is to receive a sealed, temporary interstitial or intracavitary implant:
	  a. reinforce preoperative teaching
	  b. explain that localization x-rays will be done following insertion of the applicator(s) in order to determine accuracy of placement
	  c. explain the manual loading procedure; reassure client that it is not painful
	  d. if a remote afterloading system will be used:
	    1. explain the process and indications for loading and unloading the radioactive source
	    2. explain that only essential care will be given (e.g. basic hygiene, change of soiled linen) by staff and visiting hours will be restricted so that radioactive source will not be unloaded for extended periods
	  e. if the radioactive source will be manually loaded and unloaded, explain the precautions that will be taken while the radioactive source is in place:
	    1. time and distance requirements should be followed by all who come in contact with the client
	    2. only essential care will be given (e.g. basic hygiene, change of soiled linen) in order to minimize staff exposure to radiation
	    3. each visitor will be limited to 30 minutes/day, children under 18 and women who may be or are pregnant will not be permitted to visit, and visitors must maintain a distance of 6 feet from the radioactive source
	  f. assure client that redness and edema around applicator insertion sites are normal
	  g. explain that a minimum fluid intake of 2500 ml/day will be encouraged to promote elimination of the by-products of tumor breakdown
	  h. assure client that personal belongings will not be contaminated
	  i. explain that body fluids will not be contaminated
	  j. if a perineal or vaginal implant is planned:
	    1. inform client that sensations of rectal fullness, lower abdominal pressure, and low back pain may be experienced due to pressure of applicator and vaginal packing (vaginal packing is inserted to separate the bladder and rectum from the radioactive source and to maintain applicator position)
	    2. encourage client to do active foot exercises at regular intervals while on bed rest
	    3. explain purpose for antiembolism stockings the client will wear while on bed rest
	    4. inform client that applicator will be checked for correct positioning routinely
	    5. explain precautions that will be taken to prevent dislodgment of the implant:
	      a. complete bed rest will be required with head of bed slightly elevated
	      b. only minimal movement will be allowed (some physicians allow client to logroll from side to side 3–4 times/day)
	      c. a urinary catheter will be inserted to reduce the need for frequent use of bedpan (the catheter also maintains bladder decompression and inhibits close contact of bladder with radioactive source)

        d. an enema will be given and a liquid or low-residue diet may be prescribed preoperatively to cleanse the bowel and decrease the chance that the client will have a bowel movement after implant insertion; a fracture pan will be used if bowel movement is necessary

        e. no perineal care will be given unless absolutely necessary

    k. if a brain implant is planned:

      1. reinforce physician's explanation about the stereotactic equipment that will be used to implant radioactive source:

        a. describe the stereotactic frame using pictures or diagrams and explain how it will be applied

        b. discuss the use of computed tomography (CT) in conjunction with the stereotactic frame (this is done to facilitate precise placement of the radioactive source)

        c. explain that local anesthesia will be used during the procedure

        d. explain that while the frame is being applied, pressure from the ear bars may cause temporary discomfort; emphasize that the bars will be removed once the frame is in place

      2. clarify the physician's explanation about the amount of scalp hair that will be removed for the procedure

      3. explain the safety precautions that will be followed while the radioactive source is in place (these will vary depending on the isotope used)

      4. explain that self-care will be encouraged to minimize staff exposure to the radioactive source

      5. arrange for a visit to the intensive care unit if client is expected to be there following implant insertion

2. if the client is to receive oral ^{131}I:

    a. explain that the isotope will be mixed with water and that he/she should drink it through a straw (may also be given in capsule form)

    b. instruct client to notify staff if he/she is nauseous; emphasize the importance of not vomiting, particularly during first 4 hours after ingestion of the isotope, in order to retain it and prevent contamination of others

    c. reinforce physician's explanation that stool, urine, sweat, saliva, and other body fluids will be highly contaminated for about 4 days

    d. emphasize the need to wear hospital clothing to prevent contamination of personal articles

    e. explain that articles in the room and on the floor will be covered with plastic to prevent contamination

    f. instruct client in good handwashing technique; stress the need to wash hands carefully, particularly after contact with urine, for 14 days after ingestion of the isotope

    g. instruct client to flush toilet at least 2 times after each voiding for 14 days after ingestion of the isotope to dilute the excreted isotope

    h. instruct male client to sit while urinating to prevent splashing of urine

    i. assure client that body fluids are no longer contaminated once the isotope is metabolized and excreted (usually 2 weeks after discharge)

3. if the client is to receive an intracavitary injection of colloidal ^{32}P or ^{198}Au:

    a. explain that there are no isolation requirements (the isotope emits beta particles and is hazardous only if the colloidal substance leaks from body) but that staff will wear gloves when handling dressings or linens in case leakage has occurred

    b. explain that he/she will be assisted to turn frequently to ensure equal distribution of the colloidal substance within the body cavity

    c. explain that the colloidal substance is dyed so that leakage is easily recognized by stains on dressings or linens

Desired Outcome	Nursing Actions and *Selected Purposes/Rationales*

4. if the client is receiving a permanent implant of ^{125}I in a tumor or body part (e.g. prostate, neck, pancreas):
   a. explain that because the range for radiation of ^{125}I is only about 2 cm, body fluids are not contaminated but that some time and distance precautions will still need to be followed
   b. caution client to notify staff immediately if a seed is found in urine or wound dressing
5. if client is receiving a permanent implant of ^{198}Au seeds into the prostate:
   a. explain that ^{198}Au seeds have a very short half-life (2.7 days) and safety precautions will be necessary during that time
   b. inform client that his urine will need to be filtered before being disposed of in the toilet to monitor for seed dislodgment.
c. Allow adequate time for questions and clarification of information provided.

RADIATION AND POSTRADIATION

■──────────────────────────────────────

1. NURSING DIAGNOSIS:	**Pain**

a. **muscle aches** related to prescribed activity restrictions (required for some intracavitary and interstitial implants);
b. **pain at or around implant site** related to:
   1. contractions of hollow organ into which an intracavitary implant has been placed
   2. tissue trauma associated with placement of applicator(s) used to hold the radioactive source in place.

Desired Outcome	Nursing Actions and *Selected Purposes/Rationales*

1. The client will experience diminished pain as evidenced by:
   a. verbalization of same
   b. relaxed facial expression and body positioning
   c. stable vital signs.

1.a. Assess for signs and symptoms of pain (e.g. verbalization of pain; grimacing; reluctance to move; guarding of implant site; rubbing hips, shoulders, or lower back; restlessness; diaphoresis; facial pallor; increased blood pressure; tachycardia).
b. Assess client's perception of the severity of pain using a pain intensity rating scale.
c. Assess the client's pain pattern (e.g. location, quality, onset, duration, precipitating factors, aggravating factors, alleviating factors).
d. Ask the client to describe previous pain experiences and methods used to manage pain effectively.
e. Implement measures *to reduce pain:*
   1. perform actions *to reduce fear and anxiety about the pain experience* (e.g. assure client that his/her need for pain relief is understood, plan methods for achieving pain control with client)
   2. perform actions to reduce fear and anxiety (e.g. reinforce preradiation teaching; provide care in a calm, confident manner) *in order to promote relaxation and subsequently increase the client's threshold and tolerance for pain*
   3. perform actions to promote rest (e.g. minimize environmental activity and noise, limit the number of visitors and their length of stay) *in order to reduce fatigue and subsequently increase the client's threshold and tolerance for pain*
   4. support body with pillows if a particular position needs to be maintained

5. provide or assist with nonpharmacologic measures for relief of pain (e.g. massage, position change as allowed, relaxation exercises, restful environment, diversional activities such as watching television or reading), being careful to adhere to time and distance requirements
6. place an alternating pressure mattress or pad on bed *to reduce discomfort associated with restricted body movement*
7. administer analgesics if ordered.
   f. Consult physician if above measures fail to provide adequate relief of pain.

---

2. NURSING DIAGNOSIS: **Impaired physical mobility**

related to:
a. prescribed activity restrictions associated with the need to maintain accurate placement of the radioactive source;
b. reluctance to move associated with pain and/or fear of dislodging applicator(s).

Desired Outcome	Nursing Actions and *Selected Purposes/Rationales*
2. The client will achieve maximum physical mobility within prescribed activity restrictions.	2.a. Implement measures *to increase mobility if allowed:* 1. perform actions to reduce pain (see Radiation and Postradiation Nursing Diagnosis 1, action e) 2. assure client that the risk of displacement of the device containing the radioactive source will be minimized if activity restrictions are adhered to (mobility restrictions will depend on the type of applicator and/or location of the implant) 3. instruct client in exercises that can be performed in bed without affecting applicator or implant placement and encourage him/her to do them frequently 4. encourage activity and participation in self-care activities as allowed. b. Provide praise and encouragement for all efforts to maintain level of mobility allowed.

---

3. NURSING DIAGNOSIS: **Self-care deficit**

related to:
a. reluctance to move associated with pain and/or fear of dislodging applicator(s);
b. prescribed activity restrictions during the time the radioactive source is in place.

Desired Outcome	Nursing Actions and *Selected Purposes/Rationales*
3. The client will perform self-care activities within restrictions imposed by the treatment plan.	3.a. With client, develop a realistic plan for meeting daily physical needs. b. Implement measures *to facilitate client's ability to perform self-care activities:* 1. schedule care at a time when client is most likely to be able to participate (e.g. when analgesics are at peak effect, after rest periods) 2. keep needed objects within easy reach. c. Encourage maximum independence within prescribed activity restrictions. Provide positive feedback for all efforts and accomplishments of self-care.

Desired Outcome	Nursing Actions and *Selected Purposes/Rationales*
	d. Reinforce preradiation teaching that the nursing staff will assist only with necessary hygiene activities that the client is unable to perform independently.

Discharge Teaching

4. NURSING DIAGNOSIS: **Knowledge deficit, Ineffective management of therapeutic regimen, or Altered health maintenance***

---

*The nurse should select the diagnostic label that is most appropriate for the client's discharge teaching needs.

Desired Outcomes	Nursing Actions and *Selected Purposes/Rationales*
4.a. The client will verbalize appropriate safety precautions related to brachytherapy.	4.a.1. If client has received systemic ^{131}I, provide the following instructions: a. use separate toilet facilities if possible, flush toilet at least twice after urinating, and sit when urinating to prevent splashing of urine (urine contains the highest levels of radioactive iodine) b. wash hands several times a day, particularly after urinating or having a bowel movement, to minimize contamination of any objects touched c. take a bath or shower daily; rinse the bath tub or shower stall well after use d. avoid shared use of items such as soap, comb, brush, toothbrush, makeup, clothing, linen, dishes, and eating utensils e. launder clothing and wash dishes separately from those of others; rinse sink for at least 2–3 minutes after washing dishes f. minimize physical contact with others, particularly pregnant women and children (perspiration and saliva contain small amounts of radioactive iodine) g. adhere to radiologist's guidelines regarding distance requirements and limitations on time spent with others h. if breastfeeding, stop until permission to resume is given by radiologist (radioactive iodine is excreted in breast milk) i. sleep alone for the first week after hospital discharge j. strictly adhere to contraceptive measures for 6 weeks following discharge k. continue to adhere to these precautions for the length of time specified by the radiologist. 2. Notify radiologist if a medical emergency occurs or if unexpected medical procedures need to be done in the 6 week period following discharge. 3. If client has had a temporary interstitial or intracavitary implant, reinforce the fact that no precautions are necessary after discharge. 4. If client has received a permanent implant of ^{125}I into the prostate, provide the following information: a. distance requirements need to be adhered to for 2 months following insertion of the implant (i.e. 6 feet should be maintained from women who are or may be pregnant, children under 4 years should not sit on client's lap) b. seed loss can occur during urination, particularly for 1 month postimplant; if this occurs, the seed should be retrieved if possible using tweezers or pliers, wrapped in foil, and returned to the Radiation Oncology Unit for disposal (the seeds are the size of a grain of rice)

c. a condom needs to be used during intercourse for 2 months following the implant insertion.

4.b. The client will identify measures to increase comfort and prevent complications associated with vaginal irradiation.

4.b.1. If client has received vaginal irradiation:
  a. explain that a pink to tan vaginal discharge is normal for 7–10 days after removal of the implant
  b. instruct client to abstain from using tampons and to change sanitary napkins every 4 hours
  c. reinforce physician's explanation about the possibility of vaginal stenosis occurring and ways to prevent permanent sealing of vaginal walls (e.g. intercourse 3 times/week as soon as allowed, use of vaginal dilator [obturator] for 5–10 minutes 3 times/week)
  d. if client is sexually active:
    1. explain that intercourse can be resumed in 2–3 weeks
    2. encourage her to try various positions for intercourse to compensate for shortening and narrowing of vagina (some clients may lose the upper ⅔ of the vaginal vault)
    3. explain that having male partner use a condom will prevent the burning sensation that may result when semen comes in contact with the fragile vaginal tissue
    4. explain that a water-soluble lubricant can be used to reduce discomfort if dryness associated with decreased vaginal secretions is problematic.
  2. Allow time for questions and clarification of information provided.

4.c. The client will state signs and symptoms to report to the health care provider.

4.c. Instruct client to report the following:
  1. unusual discharge, odor, or excessive bleeding from irradiated area
  2. signs and symptoms of radiation cystitis (e.g. blood in urine, pain on urination, urinary frequency or urgency)
  3. signs and symptoms of tissue fibrosis within the treatment area (e.g. **BOWEL**: inability to move bowels, distended abdomen, loss of appetite, alternating diarrhea and constipation; **SKIN**: uneven texture, changes in appearance of surface blood vessels; **VAGINA**: pain or difficulty with sexual intercourse)
  4. increasing pain in irradiated area
  5. significant, unexplained weight loss
  6. excessive depression or difficulty coping
  7. persistent urgency, frequency, or burning on urination and/or increased temperature after removal of a gynecological implant (these symptoms are an expected response to the inflammation that occurs 8–10 days after removal of the radioactive source but the health care provider should be notified if symptoms do not diminish by day 15).

4.d. The client will identify community resources that can assist with adjustment to the effects of the diagnosis and its treatment.

4.d.1. Provide information about and encourage use of community resources that can assist the client and significant others with adjustment to effects of the diagnosis and radiation therapy (e.g. local support groups, American Cancer Society, counselors, social service agencies, Make Today Count, Hospice).
  2. Initiate a referral if indicated.

4.e. The client will verbalize an understanding of and a plan for adhering to recommended follow-up care including future appointments with health care provider and radiologist and medications prescribed.

4.e.1. Reinforce the importance of keeping follow-up appointments with the health care provider and radiologist.
  2. Teach the client the rationale for, side effects of, and importance of taking prescribed medications (e.g. antimicrobials). Inform client of pertinent food and drug interactions.
  3. Implement measures to improve client compliance:
    a. include significant others in teaching sessions if possible
    b. encourage questions and allow time for reinforcement and clarification of information provided
    c. provide written instructions on future appointments with health care provider and radiologist, medications prescribed, and signs and symptoms to report.

Bibliography

See pages 897–898 and 899.

CHEMOTHERAPY

This care plan focuses on the use of cytotoxic drugs (chemotherapeutic agents) in the treatment of cancer. The drugs are used alone or with surgery and/or radiation therapy to achieve a cure or to control or relieve symptoms associated with advanced disease. Success of the therapy depends on the size, type, and location of the tumor in addition to the client's physiological and psychological condition.

Cytotoxic drugs are classified according to their chemical structure (e.g. antimetabolites, plant alkaloids, alkylating agents), their primary mode of action (e.g. interfere with folic acid synthesis, produce cross-links of DNA strands), or their effect on the cell life cycle. Some drugs are more effective during a specific phase of the cell cycle and are called cell cycle–specific (e.g. plant alkaloids, antimetabolites), whereas other drugs may interrupt the cell replication process without regard to the phase of the cell cycle and are classified as cell cycle–nonspecific (e.g. alkylating agents, antibiotics).

The primary effect of cytotoxic drugs is to interrupt cell replication. It is believed that cytotoxic drugs kill a fixed percentage, rather than a specific number, of tumor cells with each dose and that tumors with a large percentage of growing cells will experience greater cell death than tumors with a smaller percentage of growing cells. Cells in the resting phase are less responsive to chemotherapeutic agents and are better able to repair themselves if damaged during treatment.

The finding that tumor cells may develop resistance to chemotherapeutic agents has resulted in the development of multiple drug protocols in which a combination of drugs are given simultaneously or in a particular sequence. The additive and sometimes synergistic effects that occur when drugs are used together allow an increased percentage of tumor cell kill without a concomitant increase in drug-induced toxicities. Drugs are selected for combination based on their effectiveness, action on the cell cycle, toxic effects, and nadir.

Cytotoxic drugs do not discriminate between the normal and the cancerous cell and, as a result, the client may experience certain side effects and/or toxic effects following their administration. The drugs have the greatest effect on rapidly dividing cancerous and normal cells (e.g. bone marrow, skin, hair follicles, lining of the gastrointestinal tract). Because of this lack of selectivity between the cancerous and the normal cell, nursing care of the recipient of the drugs is indeed a challenge.

This care plan focuses on the adult client hospitalized for an initial or subsequent cycle of chemotherapy and/or management of side effects of treatment with cytotoxic agents. The major goals of care are to maintain comfort; prevent complications; and educate the client about chemotherapy, expected side effects, and toxic effects to be reported. The nurse also plays a major role in assisting the client and significant others to cope with actual and anticipated changes in body image, life style, and roles as a result of cancer and chemotherapy.

DISCHARGE CRITERIA

Prior to discharge, the client will:

- have no signs and symptoms of toxic effects of cytotoxic agents
- have side effects of cytotoxic agents under control
- have fatigue at a manageable level
- have an adequate or improved nutritional status
- identify ways to prevent infection during periods of lowered immunity
- demonstrate the ability to take an oral and an axillary temperature correctly
- demonstrate appropriate oral hygiene techniques
- identify techniques to control nausea and vomiting
- verbalize ways to improve appetite and nutritional status
- verbalize ways to manage and cope with persistent fatigue
- verbalize ways to prevent bleeding when platelet counts are low
- verbalize ways to adjust to alterations in reproductive and sexual functioning
- demonstrate the ability to care for a central venous catheter, a peritoneal catheter, or an implanted infusion device if in place
- verbalize an understanding of the care and precautions necessary if an Ommaya reservoir is in place
- verbalize an understanding of an implanted infusion pump and precautions necessary if one is in place
- state signs and symptoms of complications to report to the health care provider
- share thoughts and feelings about changes in body image resulting from chemotherapy

- identify community resources that can assist with home management and adjustment to the diagnosis of cancer and chemotherapy and its effects
- verbalize an understanding of and a plan for adhering to recommended follow-up care including medications prescribed and schedule for chemotherapy, laboratory studies, and future appointments with health care provider.

1. NURSING DIAGNOSIS: **Anxiety**

related to:
a. unfamiliar environment;
b. lack of knowledge about chemotherapy including administration procedure, expected side effects, and impact on usual life style and roles if admitted for chemotherapy;
c. need for hospitalization to manage current side effects and/or toxic effects of chemotherapy and expectation that additional untoward effects will occur with a subsequent cycle of chemotherapy;
d. financial concerns;
e. diagnosis of cancer with potential for premature death.

Desired Outcome	Nursing Actions and *Selected Purposes/Rationales*
1. The client will experience a reduction in anxiety as evidenced by: a. verbalization of feeling less anxious b. usual sleep pattern c. relaxed facial expression and body movements d. stable vital signs e. usual perceptual ability and interactions with others.	1.a. Assess client on admission for: 　1. fears, misconceptions, and level of understanding of chemotherapy and its effects on body functioning, life style, and roles 　2. perception of anticipated results of planned chemotherapeutic regimen 　3. feelings about past experiences with chemotherapy or other treatments for cancer 　4. availability of an adequate support system 　5. signs and symptoms of anxiety (e.g. verbalization of feeling anxious, insomnia, tenseness, shakiness, restlessness, diaphoresis, tachycardia, elevated blood pressure, facial pallor, self-focused behaviors). b. Implement measures *to reduce fear and anxiety:* 　1. orient client to hospital environment, equipment, and routines 　2. introduce client to staff who will be participating in care; if possible, maintain consistency in staff assigned to his/her care *to provide feelings of stability and comfort with the environment* 　3. assure client that staff members are nearby; respond to call signal as soon as possible 　4. maintain a calm, supportive, confident manner when interacting with client 　5. encourage verbalization of fear and anxiety; provide feedback 　6. explain all tests that may be done before the initiation of chemotherapy (e.g. blood and urine studies, ECG, echocardiography, pulmonary function studies) 　7. reinforce physician's explanations and clarify misconceptions the client has about how prescribed drugs work, expected side effects, and potential drug toxicities 　8. provide a calm, restful environment 　9. instruct client in relaxation techniques (e.g. listening to music, exercise, yoga, guided imagery) and encourage participation in diversional activities 　10. perform actions to assist the client to cope with the diagnosis of cancer and chemotherapy and its effects (see Nursing Diagnosis 14, action c) 　11. initiate financial and/or social service referrals if indicated 　12. provide information based on current needs of client at a level he/she can understand; encourage questions and clarification of information provided 　13. encourage significant others to project a caring, concerned attitude without obvious anxiousness 　14. include significant others in orientation and teaching sessions and encourage their continued support of the client 　15. initiate preoperative teaching if placement of a peritoneal or central venous catheter, Ommaya reservoir, or implanted infusion device is planned 　16. administer prescribed antianxiety agents if indicated. c. Consult physician if above actions fail to control fear and anxiety.

---

2. NURSING DIAGNOSIS:　**Altered nutrition: less than body requirements**

related to:
a. decreased oral intake associated with:
　1. oral, pharyngeal, and esophageal pain and difficulty swallowing resulting from mucositis if it has developed
　2. anorexia resulting from factors such as depression, fear, anxiety, fatigue, discomfort, early satiety, and an altered sense of taste (an altered sense of taste is often reported by persons with cancer);
b. loss of nutrients associated with vomiting and diarrhea if present;

c. impaired utilization of nutrients associated with:
1. accelerated and inefficient metabolism of proteins, carbohydrates, and fats resulting from the disease process
2. decreased absorption of nutrients resulting from loss of intestinal absorptive surface if mucositis has developed;
d. utilization of available nutrients by the malignant cells rather than the host.

Desired Outcome	Nursing Actions and *Selected Purposes/Rationales*

2. The client will have or attain an adequate nutritional status as evidenced by:
   a. weight within or returning toward normal range for client's age, height, and body frame
   b. normal BUN and serum albumin, Hct, Hb, and transferrin levels
   c. usual strength and activity tolerance
   d. healthy oral mucous membrane.

2.a. Assess for and report signs and symptoms of malnutrition:
1. weight below normal for client's age, height, and body frame
2. abnormal BUN and low serum albumin, Hct, Hb, and transferrin levels
3. weakness and fatigue
4. sore, inflamed oral mucous membrane
5. pale conjunctiva.
b. Monitor percentage of meals and snacks client consumes. Report a pattern of inadequate intake.
c. Implement measures *to maintain or promote an adequate nutritional status:*
1. perform actions *to improve oral intake:*
   a. implement measures to reduce nausea and vomiting (see Nursing Diagnosis 4, action b)
   b. implement measures to reduce oral, pharyngeal, esophageal, and abdominal pain (see Nursing Diagnosis 3, action e.4)
   c. implement measures to assist client to adjust psychologically to the diagnosis of cancer and treatment with chemotherapy (see Nursing Diagnoses 13, actions d–n; 14, action c; 15, action b; and 16, actions c–m)
   d. implement measures *to compensate for taste alterations that might be present:*
      1. encourage the client to select fish, cold chicken, eggs, and cheese as protein sources if beef or pork tastes bitter or rancid
      2. provide meat for breakfast if aversion to meat tends to increase as day progresses
      3. add extra sweeteners to foods if acceptable to client
      4. experiment with different flavorings, seasonings, and textures
      5. serve food warm *to stimulate sense of smell*
   e. if client is having difficulty swallowing:
      1. implement measures to reduce the severity of stomatitis and/or relieve dryness of the oral mucous membrane (see Nursing Diagnosis 6, actions d and e)
      2. assist client to select foods that require little or no chewing and are easily swallowed (e.g. custard, eggs, canned fruit, mashed potatoes)
      3. avoid serving foods that are sticky (e.g. peanut butter, soft bread, honey)
      4. moisten dry foods with gravy or sauces
   f. increase activity as tolerated (*activity usually promotes a sense of well-being and improves appetite*)
   g. obtain a dietary consult if necessary to assist client in selecting foods/fluids that are appealing and adhere to personal and cultural preferences
   h. encourage a rest period before meals *to minimize fatigue*
   i. maintain a clean environment and a relaxed, pleasant atmosphere
   j. provide oral hygiene before meals
   k. provide largest amount of calories and protein when appetite is the best (usually at breakfast)
   l. serve frequent, small meals rather than large ones if client is weak, fatigues easily, and/or has a poor appetite

Desired Outcome	Nursing Actions and *Selected Purposes/Rationales*

m. encourage significant others to bring in client's favorite foods and eat with him/her *to make eating more of a familiar social experience*

n. limit fluid intake with meals (unless the fluid has high nutritional value) *to reduce early satiety and subsequent decreased food intake*

o. allow adequate time for meals; reheat foods/fluids if necessary

2. ensure that meals are well balanced and high in essential nutrients; offer high-calorie, high-protein dietary supplements (e.g. milk shakes, puddings, or eggnog made with cream or powdered milk reconstituted with whole milk; commercially-prepared dietary supplements) if indicated

3. perform actions to control diarrhea (see Nursing Diagnosis 9, action c)

4. administer vitamins and minerals if ordered.

d. Perform a calorie count if ordered. Report information to dietitian and physician.

e. Consult physician regarding an alternative method of providing nutrition (e.g. parenteral nutrition, tube feedings) if client does not consume enough food or fluids to meet nutritional needs.

■━━

3. NURSING DIAGNOSIS:

Pain:

a. **oral, pharyngeal, esophageal, and/or abdominal pain** related to mucositis associated with the effects of cytotoxic drugs on the rapidly dividing cells of the gastrointestinal mucosa;

b. **muscle and bone pain** (the cause is not known but it sometimes occurs in persons receiving paclitaxel and high doses of vinblastine or etoposide).

Desired Outcome	Nursing Actions and *Selected Purposes/Rationales*

3. The client will experience diminished pain as evidenced by:
a. verbalization of a decrease in or absence of pain
b. relaxed facial expression and body positioning
c. increased participation in activities.

3.a. Assess client for:

1. reports of oral, pharyngeal, esophageal, and/or abdominal pain
2. statements of painful swallowing
3. reports of gastric pain induced by spicy or acidic foods
4. reports of achiness (usually in lower extremities)
5. grimacing, reluctance to move, clutching abdomen, or restlessness.

b. Assess client's perception of the severity of pain using a pain intensity rating scale.

c. Assess the client's pain pattern (e.g. location, quality, onset, duration, precipitating factors, alleviating factors).

d. Ask the client to describe previous pain experiences and methods used to manage pain effectively.

e. Implement measures *to reduce pain:*

1. perform actions to reduce fatigue (see Nursing Diagnosis 7, action e) *in order to increase the client's threshold and tolerance for pain*

2. perform actions to reduce fear and anxiety (see Nursing Diagnosis 1, action b) *in order to promote relaxation and subsequently increase the client's threshold and tolerance for pain*

3. provide or assist with nonpharmacologic methods for pain relief (e.g. massage; position change; progressive relaxation exercises; guided imagery; restful environment; diversional activities such as watching television, reading, or conversing)

4. if client has oral, pharyngeal, esophageal, or abdominal pain:

a. perform actions to reduce the severity of stomatitis (see Nursing Diagnosis 6, actions d and e)

b. instruct client to avoid substances that might further irritate the

gastrointestinal mucosa (e.g. extremely hot, spicy, or acidic foods/ fluids; dry or hard foods; raw vegetables)
   c. offer cool, soothing liquids such as nonacidic juices and ices
   d. instruct client to gargle with a saline solution every 2 hours or spray mouth with a solution containing diphenhydramine and water (1 oz diphenhydramine and 1 qt water) if ordered *to soothe the oral mucous membrane*
   e. administer topical anesthetics and oral protective agents (e.g. mixture of diphenhydramine, antacid, and viscous xylocaine; sucralfate oral suspension; Zilactin) if ordered
   5. if client has muscle or bone pain, administer the following medications if ordered:
      a. nonsteroidal anti-inflammatory agents (NSAIDs)
      b. opioid (narcotic) analgesics.
   f. Consult physician or pain management nurse specialist if pain persists or worsens.

---

4. NURSING DIAGNOSIS: **Altered comfort: nausea and vomiting**

related to stimulation of the vomiting center associated with:
a. stimulation by cytotoxic drugs, the by-products of cellular destruction, and the foul taste created by some cytotoxic agents;
b. stimulation of the visceral afferent pathways resulting from inflammation of the gastrointestinal mucosa if mucositis is present;
c. stimulation of the cerebral cortex resulting from stress and a learned conditioned response to previous experience with nausea and vomiting after the administration of cytotoxic drugs.

Desired Outcome	Nursing Actions and *Selected Purposes/Rationales*

4. The client will experience a reduction in nausea and vomiting as evidenced by:
a. verbalization of decreased nausea
b. reduction in the number of episodes of vomiting.
	4.a. Assess client for nausea and vomiting.
	b. Implement measures *to reduce nausea and vomiting:*
	  1. perform actions to promote psychological adjustment to the diagnosis of cancer and treatment with chemotherapy (see Nursing Diagnoses 1, action b; 13, actions d–n; 14, action c; 15, action b; and 16, actions c–m) *in order to reduce stress*
	  2. convey an attitude that nausea and vomiting might not occur (*not every client experiences nausea and vomiting every time*)
	  3. administer the following medications as ordered 1–24 hours before initiating chemotherapy and routinely for the expected period of nausea and vomiting for the specific chemotherapeutic agents being administered:
	    a. phenothiazines (e.g. prochlorperazine)
	    b. butyrophenones (e.g. droperidol, haloperidol)
	    c. gastrointestinal stimulants (e.g. metoclopramide)
	    d. benzodiazepines (e.g. lorazepam, diazepam) *to decrease anxiety and/or induce amnesia in order to lessen the possibility of client's developing a conditioned response to chemotherapy*
	    e. corticosteroids (e.g. dexamethasone)
	    f. serotonin antagonists (e.g. ondansetron)
	  4. administer intravenous cytotoxic drugs slowly unless contraindicated *to decrease stimulation of the vomiting center*
	  5. if feasible, administer the cytotoxic drugs at night *so client will sleep and experience less nausea*
	  6. provide sour, hard candy for client to suck on if he/she can taste the drug

Desired Outcome	Nursing Actions and *Selected Purposes/Rationales*

7. eliminate noxious sights and odors from the environment (*noxious stimuli can cause stimulation of the vomiting center*)
8. encourage client to take deep, slow breaths when nauseated
9. encourage client to change positions slowly (*rapid movement can result in chemoreceptor trigger zone stimulation and subsequent excitation of the vomiting center*)
10. provide oral hygiene every two hours and after each emesis
11. provide carbonated beverages for client to sip if nauseated
12. avoid serving foods with an overpowering aroma; remove lids from hot foods before entering room
13. provide small, frequent meals; instruct client to ingest foods and fluids slowly
14. encourage client to eat dry foods (e.g. toast, crackers) and avoid drinking liquids with meals if nauseated
15. instruct client to avoid foods/fluids that irritate the gastric mucosa (e.g. spicy foods; caffeine-containing beverages such as coffee, tea, and colas)
16. instruct client to rest after eating.

   c. Consult physician if above measures fail to control nausea and vomiting.

---

5. NURSING DIAGNOSIS:

Risk for impaired tissue integrity

related to:
a. increased skin fragility associated with malnutrition and dryness (a result of the effects of cytotoxic drugs on sebaceous and sweat glands);
b. frequent contact of the skin with irritants associated with diarrhea if present;
c. damage to the skin and/or subcutaneous tissue associated with prolonged pressure on tissues, friction, or shearing if mobility is decreased.

Desired Outcome	Nursing Actions and *Selected Purposes/Rationales*

5. The client will maintain skin integrity as evidenced by:
   a. absence of redness and irritation
   b. no skin breakdown.

5.a. Inspect the skin, especially bony prominences and dependent areas, for pallor, redness, and breakdown.
   b. Implement measures *to prevent tissue breakdown*:
     1. assist client to turn at least every 2 hours if activity is limited
     2. gently massage around reddened areas at least every 2 hours
     3. position client properly; use pressure-reducing or pressure-relieving devices (e.g. pillows, gel or foam cushions, alternating pressure mattress, air-fluidized bed) if indicated
     4. apply a thin layer of powder or cornstarch to bottom sheet or skin and opposing skin surfaces (e.g. axillae, beneath breasts) if indicated *to absorb moisture and reduce friction*
     5. lift and move client carefully using a turn sheet and adequate assistance
     6. limit length of time client is in semi-Fowler's position to 30 minutes (*in this position, client tends to slide down in bed, which can cause skin surface abrasion and shearing*)
     7. instruct or assist client to shift weight every 30 minutes
     8. keep skin clean and dry
     9. keep bed linens dry and wrinkle-free
     10. increase activity as tolerated
     11. perform actions *to prevent drying of the skin*:
       a. encourage a fluid intake of 2500 ml/day unless contraindicated
       b. provide a mild soap for bathing
       c. apply moisturizing lotion and/or emollient to skin at least once a day

12. perform actions *to prevent skin irritation resulting from diarrhea:*
    a. implement measures to control diarrhea (see Nursing Diagnosis 9, action c)
    b. assist client to thoroughly cleanse and dry perineal area with soft tissue or cloth after each bowel movement; apply a protective ointment or cream
13. perform actions to promote an adequate nutritional status (see Nursing Diagnosis 2, action c).
c. If tissue breakdown occurs:
    1. notify physician
    2. continue with above measures to prevent further irritation and breakdown
    3. perform care of involved area(s) as ordered or per standard hospital procedure
    4. assess client closely and report signs and symptoms of infection (e.g. elevated temperature; redness, heat, pain, and swelling around area of breakdown; unusual drainage from site).

---

6. NURSING DIAGNOSIS:

Altered oral mucous membrane:

a. **dryness** related to reduced oral intake;
b. **stomatitis** related to:
    1. malnutrition and inadequate oral hygiene
    2. disruption in the renewal process of mucosal epithelial cells associated with toxic effects of cytotoxic drugs (particularly antimetabolites, antibiotics, plant alkaloids, and paclitaxel)
    3. infection, particularly gingival, during the period of myelosuppression.

Desired Outcome	Nursing Actions and *Selected Purposes/Rationales*

6. The client will maintain a healthy oral cavity as evidenced by:
a. absence of inflammation
b. pink, moist, intact mucosa
c. no reports of oral dryness and burning
d. ability to swallow without discomfort.
	6.a. Assess client for dryness of the oral mucosa.
	b. Assess for and report signs and symptoms of stomatitis (e.g. inflamed and/or ulcerated oral mucosa, reports of burning pain in mouth, dysphagia, viscous saliva).
	c. Culture oral lesions as ordered. Report positive results.
	d. Implement measures *to prevent or reduce the severity of stomatitis and/or relieve dryness of the oral mucous membrane:*
	  1. reinforce importance of and assist client with oral hygiene after meals and snacks; avoid use of products that contain lemon and glycerin and commercial mouthwashes containing alcohol (*these products have a drying and irritating effect on the oral mucous membrane*)
	  2. have client rinse mouth frequently (warm saline is recommended for rinsing; however, the frequency and consistency of performing oral hygiene is more important than the product used)
	  3. use a soft-bristle brush, sponge-tipped applicator, or low-pressure power spray for oral hygiene
	  4. lubricate client's lips frequently
	  5. encourage client to breathe through nose rather than mouth *in order to reduce mouth dryness*
	  6. encourage a fluid intake of at least 2500 ml/day unless contraindicated
	  7. encourage client not to smoke (*smoking irritates and dries the mucosa*)
	  8. if stomatitis is not severe, encourage client to use artificial saliva *to lubricate the oral mucous membrane*
	  9. instruct client to avoid substances that might further irritate the oral mucosa (e.g. extremely hot, spicy, or acidic foods/fluids)

Desired Outcome	Nursing Actions and **Selected Purposes/Rationales**
	10. perform actions to promote an adequate nutritional status (see Nursing Diagnosis 2, action c)
	11. consult physician regarding an order for a prophylactic antimicrobial agent.
	e. If stomatitis is not controlled:
	1. increase frequency of oral hygiene
	2. if client has dentures, remove and replace only for meals.
	f. Consult physician if signs and symptoms of dryness and stomatitis persist or worsen.

---

7. NURSING DIAGNOSIS: **Fatigue**

related to:*
a. a build up of cellular waste products associated with rapid lysis of cancerous and normal cells exposed to cytotoxic drugs;
b. difficulty resting and sleeping associated with fear, anxiety, and discomfort;
c. tissue hypoxia associated with anemia (a result of malnutrition and chemotherapy-induced bone marrow suppression);
d. overwhelming emotional demands associated with the diagnosis of cancer and treatment with chemotherapy;
e. increased energy expenditure associated with an increase in the metabolic rate resulting from continuous, active tumor growth and the energy needed to repair damaged cells;
f. malnutrition.

---

*Some of the etiological factors presented here are under investigation.

Desired Outcome	Nursing Actions and **Selected Purposes/Rationales**

7. The client will experience a reduction in fatigue as evidenced by:
a. verbalization of feelings of increased energy
b. ability to perform usual activities of daily living
c. increased interest in surroundings and ability to concentrate
d. decreased emotional lability.
	7.a. Assess for signs and symptoms of fatigue (e.g. verbalization of unremitting, overwhelming lack of energy and inability to maintain usual routines; lack of interest in surroundings; decreased ability to concentrate; increased emotional lability).
	b. Assess client's perception of the severity of fatigue using a fatigue rating scale.
	c. Inform client that a feeling of persistent fatigue is not unusual and is a result of the disease itself as well as a side effect of chemotherapy.
	d. Assist client to identify personal patterns of fatigue (e.g. time of day, after certain activities) and to plan activities so that times of greatest fatigue are avoided.
	e. Implement measures *to reduce fatigue:*
	  1. perform actions *to promote rest and/or conserve energy:*
	    a. schedule several short rest periods during the day
	    b. minimize environmental activity and noise
	    c. limit the number of visitors and their length of stay
	    d. assist client with self-care activities as needed
	    e. keep supplies and personal articles within easy reach
	    f. implement measures to reduce fear and anxiety (see Nursing Diagnosis 1, action b)
	    g. implement measures to promote sleep (see Nursing Diagnosis 10, action c)
	    h. implement measures to reduce discomfort (see Nursing Diagnosis 3, action e and 4, action b)
	    i. instruct client in energy-saving techniques (e.g. using shower chair when showering, sitting to brush teeth or comb hair)

2. perform actions to promote an adequate nutritional status (see Nursing Diagnosis 2, action c)
3. encourage client to maintain a fluid intake of at least 2500 ml/day *to promote elimination of the by-products of cellular breakdown*
4. administer the following if ordered for treatment of anemia:
   a. epoetin alfa (EPO)
   b. blood transfusions (e.g. packed red blood cells)
   c. peripheral blood stem cell transplantation
5. increase activity gradually as tolerated
6. perform actions to facilitate client's psychological adjustment to the diagnosis of cancer and the treatment regimen and its effects (see Nursing Diagnoses 13, actions d–n; 14, action c; 15, action b; and 16, actions c–m).
   f. Consult physician if signs and symptoms of fatigue worsen.

---

8. NURSING DIAGNOSIS: Self-care deficit

related to:
a. fatigue, weakness, and discomfort;
b. sedation associated with effects of some medications administered to control nausea and vomiting;
c. tactile and proprioceptive impairments associated with neurotoxic effects of some cytotoxic agents (particularly the vinca alkaloids, platinum, procarbazine, paclitaxel, or etoposide).

Desired Outcome	Nursing Actions and *Selected Purposes/Rationales*

8. The client will perform self-care activities within physical limitations.	8.a. With client, develop a realistic plan for meeting daily physical needs.
	b. Implement measures *to facilitate client's ability to perform self-care activities:*
	  1. perform actions to reduce fatigue (see Nursing Diagnosis 7, action e)
	  2. schedule care at a time when client is most likely to be able to participate (e.g. following rest periods, before chemotherapy administration)
	  3. allow adequate time for accomplishment of self-care activities
	  4. consult occupational therapist about assistive devices available (e.g. ring pulls for zippers, built-up eating utensils) if indicated.
	c. Encourage maximum independence within limitations imposed by fatigue, weakness, and discomfort. Provide positive feedback for all efforts and accomplishments of self-care.
	d. Assist the client with those activities he/she is unable to perform independently.

---

9. NURSING DIAGNOSIS: Diarrhea

related to increased intestinal motility associated with extreme fear and anxiety and inflammation and ulceration of the gastrointestinal mucosa resulting from effects of cytotoxic drugs (particularly fluorouracil, actinomycin D, doxorubicin, daunorubicin, and methotrexate) on rapidly dividing epithelial cells.

Desired Outcome	Nursing Actions and *Selected Purposes/Rationales*

9. The client will have fewer bowel movements and more formed stool if diarrhea occurs.	9.a. Ascertain client's usual bowel elimination habits.
	  b. Assess for signs and symptoms of diarrhea (e.g. frequent, loose stools; urgency; abdominal pain and cramping; hyperactive bowel sounds).
	  c. Implement measures *to control diarrhea:*
	   1. perform actions *to rest the bowel:*
	    a. restrict oral intake if ordered
	    b. when oral intake is allowed:
	     1. gradually progress from fluids to small meals
	     2. instruct client to avoid foods/fluids that may stimulate or irritate the inflamed bowel:
	      a. those high in fiber (e.g. whole-grain cereals, raw fruits and vegetables)
	      b. those that are spicy or extremely hot or cold
	      c. those high in lactose (e.g. milk, milk products)
	    c. implement measures to reduce fear and anxiety (see Nursing Diagnosis 1, action b)
	    d. encourage client to rest
	    e. discourage smoking (*nicotine has a stimulant effect on the gastrointestinal tract*)
	   2. administer the following medications if ordered *to control diarrhea:*
	    a. opiates or opiate derivatives (e.g. paregoric, loperamide, diphenoxylate hydrochloride) *to decrease gastrointestinal motility*
	    b. bulk-forming agents (e.g. methylcellulose, psyllium hydrophilic mucilloid, calcium polycarbophil) *to absorb water in the bowel, which results in a more formed stool*
	    c. adsorbents (e.g. kaolin, pectin, attapulgite [Kaopectate], bismuth subsalicylate [Pepto-Bismol])
	    d. octreotide acetate (Sandostatin) *to suppress the output of motilin and subsequently slow gastrointestinal activity.*
	  d. Consult physician if diarrhea persists or worsens.

---

10. NURSING DIAGNOSIS: **Sleep pattern disturbance**

related to:
a. nausea, vomiting, and pain;
b. anxiety, fear, and grief;
c. frequent need to defecate associated with diarrhea if present.

Desired Outcome	Nursing Actions and *Selected Purposes/Rationales*

10. The client will attain optimal amounts of sleep as evidenced by:
a. statements of feeling well rested
b. usual mental status
c. absence of frequent yawning, dark circles under eyes, and hand tremors.
	10.a. Assess for signs and symptoms of a sleep pattern disturbance (e.g. statements of difficulty falling asleep, not feeling well rested, or sleep interruptions; irritability; lethargy; disorientation; frequent yawning; dark circles under eyes; slight hand tremors).
	  b. Determine the client's usual sleep habits.
	  c. Implement measures *to promote sleep:*
	   1. discourage long periods of sleep during the day unless signs and symptoms of sleep deprivation exist or daytime sleep is usual for client
	   2. perform actions to reduce discomfort (see Nursing Diagnoses 3, action e and 4, action b)
	   3. perform actions to control diarrhea (see Nursing Diagnosis 9, action c)
	   4. perform actions to reduce fear and anxiety (see Nursing Diagnosis 1, action b) and assist the client to adjust psychologically to the

diagnosis of cancer and treatment with chemotherapy (see Nursing Diagnoses 13, actions d–n; 14, action c; 15, action b; and 16, actions c–m)

5. encourage participation in relaxing diversional activities during the evening
6. discourage intake of fluids high in caffeine (e.g. coffee, tea, colas), especially in the evening
7. allow client to continue usual sleep practices (e.g. position; time; presleep routines such as reading, watching television, listening to music, and meditating) unless contraindicated
8. satisfy basic needs such as comfort and warmth before sleep
9. encourage client to urinate just before bedtime
10. reduce environmental distractions (e.g. close door to client's room; use night light rather than overhead light whenever possible; lower volume of paging system; keep staff conversations at a low level and away from client's room; close curtains between clients in a semi-private room or ward; provide client with 'white noise' such as fan, soft music, or tape-recorded sounds of the ocean or rain; have earplugs available for client if needed)
11. administer prescribed sedative-hypnotics if indicated
12. perform actions *to reduce interruptions during sleep (80–100 minutes of uninterrupted sleep is usually needed to complete one sleep cycle)*:
    a. restrict visitors
    b. group care (e.g. medications, treatments, physical care, assessments) whenever possible.
d. Consult physician if signs and symptoms of sleep deprivation persist or worsen.

---

11. NURSING DIAGNOSIS: **Risk for infection**

related to:
a. lowered natural resistance associated with:
   1. malnutrition
   2. chemotherapy-induced bone marrow suppression
   3. long-term treatment with corticosteroids (may be used in treatment of certain types of cancer)
   4. disruption in normal, endogenous microbial flora resulting from antimicrobial therapy
   5. impaired immune system functioning resulting from certain malignancies (e.g. Hodgkin's disease, lymphoma, multiple myeloma, leukemia);
b. break in mucosal surfaces associated with delayed cellular renewal resulting from effects of cytotoxic agents;
c. break in integrity of the skin associated with placement of a central venous catheter (e.g. Groshong), implanted infusion device (e.g. Port-a-Cath), or peritoneal catheter (e.g. Tenckhoff);
d. stasis of secretions in lungs and urinary stasis if mobility is decreased.

Desired Outcome	Nursing Actions and *Selected Purposes/Rationales*
11. The client will remain free of infection as evidenced by: a. absence of fever and chills b. pulse within normal limits c. normal breath sounds d. usual mental status	11.a. Assess for and report signs and symptoms of infection (be alert to subtle changes in the client since the signs of infection may be minimal as a result of immunosuppression; also be aware that some signs and symptoms vary depending on the site of the infection, the causative organism, and the age of the client): 1. increase in client's usual temperature 2. chills 3. increased pulse

Desired Outcome	Nursing Actions and *Selected Purposes/Rationales*

e. cough productive of clear mucus only

f. voiding clear urine without reports of frequency, urgency, and burning

g. absence of heat, pain, redness, swelling, and unusual drainage in any area

h. no reports of increased weakness and fatigue

i. WBC and differential counts within normal range for client

j. negative results of cultured specimens.

    4. abnormal breath sounds

    5. development of or increased malaise

    6. lethargy, acute confusion

    7. further loss of appetite

    8. cough productive of purulent, green, or rust-colored sputum

    9. cloudy, foul-smelling urine

   10. reports of frequency, urgency, or burning when urinating

   11. presence of WBCs, bacteria, and/or nitrites in urine

   12. heat, pain, redness, swelling, or unusual drainage in any area

   13. reports of increased weakness or fatigue

   14. increase in WBC count and/or significant change in differential.

b. Monitor absolute neutrophil count (WBC count multiplied by the percentage of neutrophils). Report values below 1000/mm³.

c. Obtain specimens (e.g. urine, vaginal drainage, mouth, sputum, stool, blood) for culture as ordered. Report positive results.

d. Implement measures *to reduce the risk for infection:*

    1. protect client from others with infections and those who have recently been vaccinated (*a person may have a subclinical infection after a vaccination*)

    2. use good handwashing technique and encourage client to do the same

    3. maintain a fluid intake of at least 2500 ml/day unless contraindicated

    4. perform actions to promote an adequate nutritional status (see Nursing Diagnosis 2, action c); encourage intake of foods high in vitamins C and E (*it is theorized that antioxidant vitamins promote phagocytosis of organisms*)

    5. encourage a low-microbial diet (e.g. cooked foods, no unwashed fresh fruits and vegetables) if the client is likely to be immunosuppressed

    6. perform actions to prevent or reduce severity of stomatitis and relieve dryness of the oral mucous membrane (see Nursing Diagnosis 6, actions d and e)

    7. perform actions to prevent tissue breakdown (see Nursing Diagnosis 5, action b)

    8. avoid invasive procedures (e.g. urinary catheterizations, arterial and venous punctures, injections) whenever possible; if such procedures are necessary, perform them using sterile technique

    9. rotate intravenous insertion sites according to hospital policy

   10. anchor catheters/tubings (e.g. urinary, intravenous) securely *in order to reduce trauma to the tissues and the risk for introduction of pathogens associated with the in-and-out movement of the tubing*

   11. maintain a closed system for drains (e.g. urinary catheter) and intravenous infusions whenever possible

   12. change equipment, tubings, and solutions used for treatments such as intravenous infusions, respiratory care, irrigations, and enteral feedings according to hospital policy

   13. initiate measures to prevent constipation (e.g. offer client a daily fiber supplement such as a mixture of bran, applesauce, and prune juice; encourage a minimum fluid intake of 2500 ml/day; encourage increased intake of foods high in fiber; administer laxatives as ordered) *in order to prevent damage to the bowel mucosa from hard stool*

   14. avoid unnecessary rectal invasion (e.g. temperature taking, enemas, suppositories, rectal tube) *to prevent trauma to rectal mucosa and possible abscess formation*

   15. perform actions to reduce stress and discomfort (see Nursing Diagnoses 1, action b; 3, action e; and 4, action b) *in order to prevent excessive secretion of cortisol (cortisol inhibits the immune response)*

   16. perform actions *to prevent stasis of respiratory secretions* (e.g. assist client to turn, cough, and deep breathe; increase activity as tolerated)

   17. perform actions to prevent urinary retention (e.g. instruct client to void when the urge is first felt, promote relaxation during voiding attempts) *in order to prevent urinary stasis*

18. instruct and assist client to perform good perineal care routinely and after every bowel movement
19. instruct and assist client in proper care of the exit site of a central venous catheter or insertion site of an implanted infusion device or peritoneal catheter (see Nursing Diagnosis 17, actions i.1–3)
20. administer the following as ordered:
    a. antimicrobial agents (usually initiated when the neutropenic client becomes febrile or may be administered prophylactically if the neutrophil count is less than 500/mm^3)
    b. colony-stimulating factors (e.g. filgrastim) *to stimulate granulocyte production.*

---

12. COLLABORATIVE DIAGNOSES:

Potential complications of chemotherapy:

a. **bleeding** related to thrombocytopenia associated with chemotherapy-induced bone marrow suppression;
b. **impaired renal function** related to:
   1. direct toxic effects of some cytotoxic agents (e.g. cisplatin, high-dose methotrexate and mithramycin, streptozocin) on renal cells
   2. nephropathy associated with:
      a. excessive uric acid accumulation resulting from the rapid lysis of large numbers of tumor cells
      b. precipitation of certain drugs (e.g. high doses of methotrexate) in the renal tubules and collecting ducts as a result of low urinary pH and inadequate hydration before, during, and after drug administration;
c. **hemorrhagic cystitis** related to irritation of the bladder mucosa by toxic metabolites of certain cytotoxic agents, particularly cyclophosphamide and ifosfamide;
d. **local tissue irritation and sloughing** related to excessive vein irritation and the subsequent extravasation of vesicant drugs (e.g. doxorubicin, daunorubicin, vinblastine, vincristine, paclitaxel);
e. **cardiac dysrhythmias** related to cardiotoxic effects of certain cytotoxic drugs (primarily doxorubicin, daunorubicin, and paclitaxel);
f. **inflammation and fibrosis of lung tissue** related to toxic effects of some cytotoxic agents on the lung (particularly bleomycin, carmustine, and mitomycin);
g. **neurotoxicity** related to the toxic effects of certain cytotoxic agents (e.g. vinca alkaloids, cisplatin, paclitaxel, ifosfamide, high-dose methotrexate or cytarabine) on the nerves;
h. **anaphylactic reaction** related to a hypersensitivity response to a cytotoxic drug (occurs primarily with cisplatin, L-asparaginase, and paclitaxel).

Desired Outcomes	Nursing Actions and *Selected Purposes/Rationales*

12.a. The client will not experience unusual bleeding as evidenced by:
1. skin and mucous membranes free of petechiae, purpura, ecchymoses, and active bleeding
2. absence of unusual joint pain
3. absence of frank and occult blood in stool, urine, and vomitus
	12.a.1. Assess client for and report signs and symptoms of unusual bleeding:
	  a. petechiae, purpura, or ecchymoses
	  b. gingival bleeding
	  c. prolonged bleeding from puncture sites
	  d. epistaxis, hemoptysis
	  e. unusual joint pain
	  f. frank or occult blood in stool, urine, or vomitus
	  g. increase in abdominal girth
	  h. menorrhagia
	  i. restlessness, confusion
	  j. decreasing B/P and increased pulse rate
	  k. decrease in Hct and Hb levels.
	  2. Monitor platelet count and coagulation test results (e.g. bleeding time).

Desired Outcomes	Nursing Actions and *Selected Purposes/Rationales*

4. no increase in abdominal girth
5. usual menstrual flow
6. usual mental status
7. vital signs within normal range for client
8. stable or improved Hct and Hb.

Report abnormal values.

3. If platelet count is low, coagulation test results are abnormal, or Hct and Hb levels decrease, test all stools, urine, and vomitus for occult blood. Report positive results.

4. Implement measures *to prevent bleeding:*
   a. avoid giving injections whenever possible; consult physician about prescribing an alternative route for medications ordered to be given intramuscularly or subcutaneously
   b. when giving injections or performing venous and arterial punctures, use the smallest gauge needle possible
   c. apply gentle, prolonged pressure to puncture sites after injections, venous and arterial punctures, and diagnostic tests such as bone marrow aspiration
   d. take B/P only when necessary and avoid overinflating the cuff
   e. caution client to avoid activities that increase the risk for trauma (e.g. shaving with a straight-edge razor, using stiff-bristle toothbrush or dental floss)
   f. whenever possible, avoid intubations (e.g. nasogastric) and procedures that can cause injury to rectal mucosa (e.g. taking temperatures rectally, inserting a rectal suppository or tube, administering an enema)
   g. pad side rails if client is confused or restless
   h. perform actions *to reduce the risk for falls* (e.g. keep bed in low position with side rails up when client is in bed, avoid unnecessary clutter in room, instruct client to wear slippers/shoes with nonslip soles when ambulating)
   i. instruct client to avoid blowing nose forcefully or straining to have a bowel movement; consult physician about an order for a decongestant and/or laxative if indicated
   j. administer the following if ordered:
      1. estrogen-progestin preparations *to suppress menses*
      2. platelets.

5. If bleeding occurs and does not subside spontaneously:
   a. apply firm, prolonged pressure to bleeding area(s) if possible
   b. if epistaxis occurs, place client in high Fowler's position and apply pressure and ice pack to nasal area
   c. maintain oxygen therapy as ordered
   d. perform gastric lavage as ordered *to control gastric bleeding*
   e. administer whole blood or blood products (e.g. platelets) as ordered
   f. assess for and report signs and symptoms of hypovolemic shock (e.g. restlessness; confusion; significant decrease in B/P; rapid, weak pulse; rapid respirations; cool, pale skin; urine output less than 30 ml/hour).

12.b. The client will maintain adequate renal function as evidenced by:
1. urine output at least 30 ml/hour
2. BUN, serum creatinine, and creatinine clearance within normal range.

12.b.1. Assess for and report a urine output below 100 ml/hour during and for 24 hours after administration of nephrotoxic drugs (consult physician about insertion of a urinary catheter if output cannot be monitored accurately).

2. Assess for and report signs and symptoms of impaired renal function (e.g. urine output less than 30 ml/hour, urine specific gravity fixed at or less than 1.010, elevated BUN and serum creatinine levels).

3. Collect a 24-hour urine specimen if ordered. Report decreased creatinine clearance.

4. Implement measures *to maintain adequate renal function:*
   a. hydrate client with at least 150 ml fluid/hour unless contraindicated for 6–24 hours before administration of drugs known to be nephrotoxic (e.g. cisplatin, high-dose methotrexate and mithramycin, streptozocin)
   b. administer intravenous fluids as ordered during administration of nephrotoxic drugs and for 24 hours after therapy *to maintain a high rate of glomerular blood flow*
   c. administer the following medications as ordered:

1. diuretics (e.g. furosemide, mannitol) *to promote more rapid plasma clearance of the cytotoxic agent*
2. xanthine oxidase inhibitor (e.g. allopurinol) *to decrease the formation of uric acid*
3. sodium bicarbonate *to alkalinize the urine and subsequently increase the solubility of uric acid in the urine and prevent the precipitation of methotrexate in renal tubules and collecting ducts*
4. leucovorin calcium (folinic acid) *to diminish the toxic effects of methotrexate on the renal cells*
5. chemoprotectant agents (e.g. WR 2721, diethyldithiocarbamate) *to protect the renal cells against toxicity from some cytotoxic agents* (*e.g. cisplatin*).

5. If signs and symptoms of impaired renal function occur:
  a. continue with above actions
  b. assess for and report signs of acute renal failure (e.g. oliguria or anuria; weight gain; edema; elevated B/P; lethargy and confusion; increasing BUN and serum creatinine, phosphorus, and potassium levels)
  c. prepare client for dialysis if indicated
  d. refer to Care Plan on Renal Failure for additional care measures.

12.c. The client will not develop hemorrhagic cystitis as evidenced by absence of dysuria, urinary frequency and urgency, suprapubic pain, and hematuria.

12.c.1. Assess for and report signs and symptoms of hemorrhagic cystitis (e.g. dysuria, urinary frequency and/or urgency, suprapubic pain, frank or occult blood in urine).

2. Implement measures *to prevent hemorrhagic cystitis*:
  a. ensure that client is vigorously hydrated; maintain intravenous fluids at the rate ordered (often as high as 200 ml/hr during chemotherapy) *in order to reduce the concentration of toxic drug metabolites in the bladder*
  b. administer cyclophosphamide early in the day and encourage client to void every 2 hours and before going to bed *in order to prevent stasis of toxic drug metabolites in the bladder*
  c. administer mesna (Mesnex) if ordered *to interact with and inactivate the toxic drug metabolites of ifosfamide*
  d. maintain continuous bladder irrigation before and after administration of cyclophosphamide or ifosfamide if ordered.

3. If signs and symptoms of hemorrhagic cystitis occur:
  a. discontinue cytotoxic drug administration and notify physician
  b. continue with fluid administration as ordered
  c. administer diuretics as ordered *to increase urine output and thereby decrease the concentration of toxic drug metabolites in the urine*
  d. assist with or perform bladder irrigations as ordered *to facilitate removal of drug metabolites and flush clots from the bladder*
  e. maintain continuous bladder irrigation with silver nitrate or alum solution if ordered *to stop bleeding*
  f. administer aminocaproic acid if ordered *to stop bleeding*
  g. prepare client for the following if planned:
    1. cystoscopy to cauterize bleeding vessels
    2. intravesical instillation of formalin *to control persistent, severe bleeding.*

12.d. The client will not experience drug extravasation as evidenced by:
1. absence of swelling and erythema at drug infusion site
2. no complaints of stinging or burning pain at infusion site.

12.d.1. Assess for signs and symptoms of drug extravasation (e.g. swelling around drug infusion site, erythema at infusion site during and for several hours after drug administration, client complaints of stinging or burning pain at infusion site).

2. Differentiate between a flare reaction (an expected reaction to doxorubicin) and extravasation if giving doxorubicin. (With a flare reaction, swelling and erythema occur within minutes, usually extend along vein line, and disappear in 60–90 minutes. The client experiences itching rather than pain at the infusion site.)

3. Ensure that the infusion site and surrounding tissue are visible at all times.

Desired Outcomes	Nursing Actions and *Selected Purposes/Rationales*

	4. Implement measures *to prevent drug extravasation:*
	  a. select the best vein possible for vesicant drug administration:
	    1. do not use a vein that has been previously used for vesicant agents
	    2. use a site in forearm if possible; avoid the antecubital fossa and small veins in the hand
	    3. do not use an existing intravenous site that is more than 24 hours old
	    4. avoid extremities with compromised circulation
	  b. do not perform multiple punctures in the same vein *in order to prevent leakage from the vessel after infusion has begun*
	  c. tape needle securely
	  d. perform actions *to ensure that the drug is infusing into the vein:*
	    1. test patency of vein with a minimum of 5 ml of normal saline before administration of cytotoxic drug
	    2. stay with client while a vesicant drug is infusing; check site every 2–3 minutes
	  e. perform actions *to prevent increased irritation of the vein:*
	    1. dilute drug according to manufacturer's recommendations
	    2. administer drug at recommended rate of infusion
	  f. stop infusion if there is any indication that the drug is not infusing properly
	  g. when the drug infusion is complete, flush needle with a minimum of 30 ml of normal saline; apply pressure to site for at least 4 minutes after needle removal *to minimize oozing.*
	5. If signs and symptoms of drug extravasation occur:
	  a. stop infusion immediately
	  b. treat area of extravasation as ordered (treatment varies depending on drug used) or per standard hospital procedure
	  c. assess the site closely every shift for signs of increased inflammation and necrosis.

12.e. The client will experience resolution of cardiac dysrhythmias if they occur as evidenced by:
  1. regular apical pulse at 60–100 beats/minute
  2. equal apical and radial pulse rates
  3. absence of syncope and palpitations
  4. ECG reading showing normal sinus rhythm.
	12.e.1. Assess for and report signs and symptoms of cardiac dysrhythmias (e.g. irregular apical pulse; pulse rate below 60 or above 100 beats/minute; apical-radial pulse deficit; syncope; palpitations; abnormal rate, rhythm, or configurations on ECG).
	  2. Monitor liver and kidney function studies and report abnormal results (*cardiotoxicity can result from delayed metabolism or excretion of cytotoxic drugs by the liver or kidneys*).
	  3. If cardiac dysrhythmias occur:
	    a. initiate cardiac monitoring if ordered
	    b. prepare client for ECG if ordered
	    c. administer antidysrhythmic agents (e.g. lidocaine, quinidine, procainamide, propranolol, amiodarone, atropine) if ordered
	    d. restrict client's activity based on his/her tolerance and severity of the dysrhythmia
	    e. maintain oxygen therapy as ordered
	    f. assess cardiovascular status frequently and report signs and symptoms of inadequate tissue perfusion (e.g. decrease in B/P; cool, moist skin; cyanosis; diminished peripheral pulses; declining urine output; restlessness and agitation; shortness of breath)
	    g. have emergency cart readily available for defibrillation, cardioversion, or cardiopulmonary resuscitation.

12.f. The client will experience decreased signs and symptoms of pulmonary inflammation and fibrosis if they occur as evidenced by:
  1. decreased coughing
  2. afebrile status
  3. decreased dyspnea
	12.f.1. Assess for signs and symptoms of pulmonary inflammation and fibrosis (e.g. dry, hacking, persistent cough; fever; tachypnea; dyspnea on exertion; crackles) particularly if client is reaching total allowable cumulative dose of cytotoxic agent(s) known to cause pulmonary toxicity.
	  2. Monitor for and report significant decrease in oximetry results.
	  3. Monitor for and report changes in chest x-ray reports and pulmonary function studies.

4. improved breath
   sounds
5. improved chest x-ray
   and pulmonary
   function studies.

4. If signs and symptoms of pulmonary inflammation and fibrosis occur:
   a. discontinue infusion of cytotoxic agent as ordered
   b. prepare client for diagnostic studies (e.g. CT or gallium scan,
      fiberoptic bronchoscopy, open lung biopsy) if planned
   c. implement measures *to improve respiratory function:*
      1. place client in a semi- to high Fowler's position unless
         contraindicated
      2. instruct and assist client to turn, cough, and deep breathe every
         1–2 hours
      3. reinforce correct use of incentive spirometer every 1–2 hours
      4. assist with positive airway pressure techniques (e.g. IPPB,
         continuous positive airway pressure [CPAP], biphasic positive
         airway pressure [BiPAP], expiratory positive airway pressure
         [EPAP]) if ordered
      5. maintain oxygen therapy as ordered
      6. administer the following medications if ordered:
         a. corticosteroids *to reduce inflammatory response*
         b. bronchodilators
   d. consult physician if signs and symptoms of pulmonary inflammation
      and fibrosis worsen or signs and symptoms of impaired gas exchange
      (e.g. restlessness, irritability, confusion, decreased PaO_2 and
      increased $PaCO_2$) develop.

12.g. The client will adapt to
the signs and symptoms of
neurotoxicity if it occurs
and not experience injury
associated with those
signs and symptoms.

12.g.1. Assess for and report signs and symptoms of neurotoxicity (e.g.
constipation, ataxia, numbness and tingling of extremities, burning pain
in extremity, unusual muscle weakness, gait disturbances, difficulty with
fine motor movements, footdrop or wristdrop, hearing loss, blurred
vision, nystagmus, memory loss, confusion, expressive aphasia, seizures).

2. Assure client that most changes in neurological function may be
   reversible if reported immediately and the neurotoxic drug is
   discontinued.
3. If signs and symptoms of neurotoxicity occur:
   a. implement measures *to prevent falls* (e.g. keep bed in low position
      with side rails up when client is in bed, avoid unnecessary clutter in
      room, instruct client to wear slippers/shoes with nonslip soles when
      ambulating, encourage client to use sight to monitor placement of
      feet)
   b. implement measures *to prevent burns* (e.g. let hot foods/fluids cool
      slightly before serving, assess temperature of bath water before and
      during bathing) *and cuts* (e.g. assist with shaving)
   c. institute seizure precautions if client has a history of seizures and/or
      any symptoms of central nervous system toxicity are present
   d. implement measures *to assist client to adapt to the following if
      present:*
      1. constipation (e.g. encourage a fluid intake of 2500 ml/day,
         increase fiber intake, administer prescribed laxatives)
      2. pain in extremities (e.g. assist with nonpharmacologic methods
         such as distraction, position change, and guided imagery;
         administer carbamazepine, phenytoin, or amitriptyline if
         prescribed)
      3. footdrop (e.g. instruct client to perform active foot exercises every
         1–2 hours while awake, use high-topped tennis shoes or foam
         boots to keep feet in a neutral or slightly dorsiflexed position)
      4. wristdrop (e.g. instruct client to perform active wrist exercises
         every 1–2 hours while awake, provide a wrist splint if necessary)
      5. impaired hearing (e.g. face client when speaking, use gestures,
         respond to client's call signal in person rather than over the
         intercommunication system)
      6. impaired vision (e.g. identify yourself when entering room and
         before any physical contact, describe activities and reasons for
         various noises in room, assist client with personal hygiene he/she
         is unable to perform independently)

Desired Outcomes | Nursing Actions and *Selected Purposes/Rationales*

7. memory loss (e.g. assist to make lists, assist with word association)
8. confusion (e.g. decrease environmental stimuli, keep daily routines consistent and simple if possible, maintain consistency in staff assigned to care for client)
9. expressive aphasia (e.g. encourage client to use short words or phrases, provide an alphabet or word board, encourage client to use gestures)
   e. consult physician if signs and symptoms of neurotoxicity persist or worsen.

12.h. The client will not develop an anaphylactic reaction as evidenced by:
1. usual mental status
2. usual skin color
3. absence of urticaria and pruritus
4. no complaints of abdominal cramps
5. absence of dyspnea, wheezing, and stridor
6. stable vital signs
7. absence of facial and peripheral edema
8. usual speaking ability.

12.h.1. Assess for and report signs and symptoms of an anaphylactic reaction (usually some or all of the signs and symptoms will occur within minutes of drug administration):
a. anxiety, agitation
b. flushing of skin
c. generalized urticaria and pruritus
d. abdominal cramps
e. dyspnea, wheezing, stridor
f. irregular and/or increased pulse rate, decline in B/P
g. edema of face, hands, and feet
h. inability to speak.
2. Implement measures *to prevent an anaphylactic reaction:*
a. consult physician before giving any drug that is the same as or similar to one the client has reacted to previously
b. administer a test dose before giving drug if appropriate
c. administer the following medications if ordered *to reduce sensitivity to the cytotoxic agent:*
   1. corticosteroids (e.g. dexamethasone)
   2. histamine$_1$ receptor antagonists (e.g. diphenhydramine) alone or in combination with histamine$_2$ receptor antagonists (e.g. cimetidine, ranitidine).
3. If signs and symptoms of an anaphylactic reaction occur:
a. discontinue the cytotoxic drug but keep intravenous line open with a normal saline solution
b. administer oxygen as ordered
c. administer the following medications if ordered:
   1. sympathomimetics (e.g. epinephrine) *to relieve bronchospasm and stimulate peripheral vasoconstriction*
   2. antihistamines (e.g. diphenhydramine) *to reduce the sensitivity reaction and control pruritus and urticaria*
   3. bronchodilators (e.g. theophylline) *to relieve bronchospasm*
   4. corticosteroids *to reduce the allergic response and maintain usual vascular wall permeability*
d. assess for and report signs and symptoms of anaphylactic shock (e.g. increased restlessness; significant decrease in B/P; rapid, weak pulse; increased dyspnea; cool, pale skin)
e. provide emotional support to client and significant others.

---

13. NURSING DIAGNOSIS:

Self-concept disturbance*

related to:
a. changes in appearance associated with the side effects of chemotherapy (e.g. alopecia, excessive weight loss, skin and nail changes) and external drug infusion catheter if present;

---

*This diagnostic label includes the nursing diagnoses of body image disturbance, self-esteem disturbance, and altered role performance.

b. possible alteration in usual sexual activities associated with weakness, fatigue, reduced levels of testosterone (can occur with chemotherapy for prostate or testicular cancer or lymphoma), psychological factors, and vaginal discomfort (may result from mucositis and premature menopause if ovarian failure occurs);

c. possible temporary or permanent infertility associated with gonadal dysfunction resulting from extensive therapy with cytotoxic drugs (particularly alkylating agents and nitrosoureas);

d. increased dependence on others to meet self-care needs;

e. changes in life style and roles associated with effects of the disease process and its treatment.

Desired Outcome	Nursing Actions and *Selected Purposes/Rationales*

13. The client will demonstrate beginning adaptation to changes in appearance, body functioning, life style, and roles as evidenced by:
    a. verbalization of feelings of self-worth and sexual adequacy
    b. maintenance of relationships with significant others
    c. active participation in activities of daily living
    d. verbalization of a beginning plan for adapting life style to changes resulting from the disease process and residual effects of chemotherapy.

13.a. Assess for signs and symptoms of a self-concept disturbance (e.g. verbalization of negative feelings about self, withdrawal from significant others, lack of participation in activities of daily living, lack of a plan for adapting to necessary changes in life style).

b. Determine the meaning of the changes in appearance, body functioning, life style, and roles to the client by encouraging him/her to verbalize feelings and by noting nonverbal responses to changes experienced.

c. Implement measures to facilitate the grieving process (see Nursing Diagnosis 15, action b).

d. Discuss with client improvements in appearance and functioning that can realistically be expected.

e. Implement measures *to assist client to increase self-esteem* (e.g. limit negative self-assessment, encourage positive comments about self, assist to identify strengths, give positive feedback about accomplishments and behaviors that are indicative of high self-esteem).

f. Reinforce actions to assist client to cope with effects of chemotherapy (see Nursing Diagnosis 14, action c).

g. Implement measures *to assist client to adapt to the following changes in body functioning and appearance if appropriate:*
   1. alopecia:
      a. inform client that hair loss can be expected approximately 2 weeks after initiation of chemotherapy; may be sudden, gradual, partial, or complete; and can include scalp hair, pubic hair, beard, eyebrows, and eyelashes
      b. reassure client that hair loss is temporary (regrowth sometimes occurs before cessation of treatment but usually occurs 2–3 months after it)
      c. inform client that hair regrowth may be a different color, texture, and consistency
      d. encourage client to cut hair very short *to decrease the anxiety related to seeing large quantities of hair fall out*
      e. inform client that he/she can reduce rate of scalp hair loss by:
         1. brushing hair gently using a soft-bristle brush
         2. shampooing hair only once or twice a week and using a gentle shampoo and lukewarm water
         3. avoiding use of equipment/products that dry hair (e.g. hot rollers, hair dryers, curling iron, dyes)
         4. avoiding hair styles that create tension on hair (e.g. ponytails, braids)
      f. encourage client to wear a wig, scarf, false eyelashes, or makeup if desired *to camouflage hair loss*
      g. inform client of community resources that can provide information and assistance with ways to facilitate adjustment to changes in appearance (e.g. American Cancer Society, Look Good–Feel Better Program)

Desired Outcome | Nursing Actions and *Selected Purposes/Rationales*

2. skin and vein hyperpigmentation:
    a. inform client that skin and vein hyperpigmentation may occur if he/she is receiving cytotoxic drugs such as bleomycin, busulfan, methotrexate, and fluorouracil
    b. inform client that skin and vein discoloration is usually temporary
    c. instruct client to avoid exposure to sunlight and to use sun screen to prevent an increase in hyperpigmentation and photosensitivity reactions
    d. assist client to identify types of clothing that can be worn to camouflage hyperpigmented areas
3. nail changes:
    a. inform client that his/her nails may thicken and stop growing, develop ridges, darken, and detach from nail bed during treatment with certain cytotoxic drugs (e.g. cyclophosphamide, doxorubicin, bleomycin, fluorouracil)
    b. reassure client that normal nail growth will resume when chemotherapy is completed
4. infertility:
    a. clarify physician's explanation that infertility is a possible permanent effect of chemotherapy
    b. discuss alternative methods of becoming a parent (e.g. artificial insemination, adoption) if of concern to client
5. impotence:
    a. encourage client to discuss it with physician (impotence usually resolves after cessation of therapy)
    b. suggest alternative methods of sexual gratification if appropriate
    c. discuss ways to be creative in expressing sexuality (e.g. massage, fantasies, cuddling).
h. Assist client with usual grooming and makeup habits if necessary.
i. Support behaviors suggesting positive adaptation to changes that have occurred (e.g. interest in personal appearance, maintenance of relationships with significant others).
j. Assist client's and significant others' adjustment to changes by listening, facilitating communication, and providing information.
k. Encourage significant others to allow client to do what he/she is able *so that independence can be re-established and/or self-esteem redeveloped.*
l. Encourage client contact with others *so that he/she can test and establish a new self-image.*
m. Encourage visits and support from significant others.
n. Encourage client to pursue usual roles and interests and continue involvement in social activities. If previous roles, interests, and hobbies cannot be pursued, encourage development of new ones.
o. Consult physician about psychological counseling if client desires or if he/she seems unwilling or unable to adapt to changes that have occurred as a result of cancer and its treatment.

---

14. NURSING DIAGNOSIS: **Ineffective individual coping**

related to persistent discomfort associated with the side effects of chemotherapy, fear, anxiety, chronic fatigue, feeling of powerlessness, and uncertainty of the effectiveness of chemotherapy.

Desired Outcome	Nursing Actions and *Selected Purposes/Rationales*

14. The client will demonstrate effective coping as evidenced by:
    a. verbalization of ability to cope with diagnosis of cancer and chemotherapy and its effects
    b. use of appropriate problem-solving techniques
    c. willingness to participate in treatment plan and meet basic needs
    d. absence of destructive behavior toward self and others
    e. appropriate use of defense mechanisms
    f. use of available support systems.

14.a. Assess for and report signs and symptoms of ineffective individual coping (e.g. verbalization of inability to cope; inability to ask for help, problem solve, or meet basic needs; insomnia; withdrawal; reluctance to participate in treatment plan; destructive behavior toward self or others; inappropriate use of defense mechanisms; inability to meet role expectations).
   b. Assess client's perception of current situation.
   c. Implement measures *to promote effective coping:*
      1. allow time for client to begin to adjust to the diagnosis, need for chemotherapy, side effects of drugs administered, and anticipated changes in life style and roles
      2. assist client to recognize and manage inappropriate denial if it is present
      3. perform actions to reduce fear and anxiety (see Nursing Diagnosis 1, action b)
      4. perform actions to reduce discomfort (see Nursing Diagnoses 3, action e and 4, action b)
      5. perform actions to reduce fatigue (see Nursing Diagnosis 7, action e)
      6. encourage verbalization about current situation and ways comparable situations have been handled in the past
      7. assist client to identify personal strengths and resources that can be used to facilitate coping with the current situation
      8. demonstrate acceptance of client but set limits on inappropriate behavior
      9. create an atmosphere of trust and support
      10. if acceptable to client, arrange for a visit with another individual who has been successfully treated for cancer with cytotoxic drugs
      11. perform actions to reduce feeling of powerlessness (see Nursing Diagnosis 16, actions c–m)
      12. instruct client in effective problem-solving techniques (e.g. accurate identification of stressors, determination of various options to solve problem)
      13. assist client to maintain usual daily routines whenever possible
      14. assist client to identify priorities and attainable goals as he/she starts to plan for necessary life-style and role changes
      15. assist client and significant others to identify ways that personal and family goals can be adjusted rather than abandoned
      16. administer antianxiety and/or antidepressant agents if ordered
      17. assist client to identify and use available support systems; provide information regarding available community resources that can assist client and significant others in coping with effects of chemotherapy and diagnosis of cancer (e.g. American Cancer Society; support groups; individual, family, and financial counselors)
      18. encourage client to share with significant others the kind of support that would be most beneficial (e.g. listening, inspiring hope, providing reassurance and accurate information)
      19. support behaviors indicative of effective coping (e.g. willingness to care for central venous catheter, compliance with treatment plan, verbalization of the ability to cope, use of effective problem-solving strategies).
   d. Consult physician about psychological counseling if appropriate. Initiate a referral if necessary.

15. NURSING DIAGNOSIS:

Grieving*

related to:
a. changes in body image and usual roles and life style;
b. diagnosis of cancer with potential for premature death.

*This diagnostic label includes anticipatory grieving and grieving following the actual losses.

Desired Outcome	Nursing Actions and *Selected Purposes/Rationales*

15. The client will demonstrate beginning progression through the grieving process as evidenced by:
   a. verbalization of feelings about the diagnosis of cancer and chemotherapy
   b. usual sleep pattern
   c. participation in the treatment plan and self-care activities
   d. use of available support systems
   e. verbalization of a plan for integrating prescribed follow-up care into life style.

15.a. Assess for signs and symptoms of grieving (e.g. change in eating habits, inability to concentrate, insomnia, anger, sadness, withdrawal from significant others, denial of losses).
   b. Implement measures *to facilitate the grieving process:*
   1. assist client to acknowledge the losses *so grief work can begin*; assess for factors that may hinder and facilitate acknowledgment
   2. discuss the grieving process and assist client to accept the phases of grieving as an expected response to actual and/or anticipated losses
   3. allow time for client to progress through the phases of grieving (phases vary among theorists but progress from shock and alarm to acceptance); be aware that not every phase is expressed by all individuals, that recurrence of phases is common, and that the grieving process may take months to years
   4. provide an atmosphere of care and concern (e.g. provide privacy, be available and nonjudgmental, display empathy and respect) *so client will feel free to express feelings*
   5. perform actions *to promote trust* (e.g. answer questions honestly, provide requested information)
   6. encourage the verbal expression of anger and sadness about the diagnosis and losses; recognize displacement of anger and assist client to see the actual cause of angry feelings and resentment
   7. encourage client to express feelings in whatever ways are comfortable (e.g. writing, drawing, conversation)
   8. perform actions to promote effective coping (see Nursing Diagnosis 14, action c)
   9. support realistic hope about the prognosis and the temporary nature of most of the physical changes
   10. support behaviors suggesting successful grief work (e.g. verbalizing feelings about the diagnosis and losses, focusing on ways to adapt to losses)
   11. explain the phases of the grieving process to significant others; encourage their support and understanding
   12. facilitate communication between the client and significant others; be aware that they may be in different phases of the grieving process
   13. provide information regarding counseling services and support groups that might assist client in working through grief
   14. when appropriate, assist client to meet spiritual needs (e.g. arrange for visit from clergy).
   c. Consult physician regarding referral for counseling if signs of dysfunctional grieving (e.g. persistent denial of diagnosis or losses, excessive anger or sadness, emotional lability) occur.

16. NURSING DIAGNOSIS: Powerlessness

related to:
a. the possibility of disease progression and death despite treatment;
b. dependence on others to assist with basic needs as a result of fatigue, weakness, and discomfort;
c. possible alterations in roles, relationships, and future plans associated with changes that can occur as a result of the cancer and the side effects/toxic effects of the cytotoxic drugs.

Desired Outcome	Nursing Actions and *Selected Purposes/Rationales*
16. The client will demonstrate increased feelings of control over his/her situation as evidenced by: a. verbalization of same b. active participation in planning of care c. participation in self-care activities within physical limitations.	16.a. Assess for behaviors that may indicate feelings of powerlessness (e.g. verbalization of lack of control over self-care or current situation, anger, irritability, passivity, lack of participation in care planning or self-care). b. Obtain information from client and significant others regarding client's usual response to situations in which he/she has had limited control (e.g. loss of job, financial stress). c. Evaluate client's perception of current situation, strengths, weaknesses, expectations, and parts of current situation that are under his/her control. Correct misinformation and inaccurate perceptions and encourage discussion of feelings about areas in which there is a perceived lack of control. d. Assist client to establish realistic short- and long-term goals. e. Reinforce physician's explanations about the type of cancer client has, the prognosis, and the chemotherapy regimen planned. Clarify misconceptions. f. Implement measures to promote effective coping (see Nursing Diagnosis 14, action c) *in order to promote an increased sense of control over his/her situation.* g. Support realistic hope about the effects of chemotherapy on the disease progression and about the management of side effects/toxic effects of chemotherapy. h. Remind client of the right to ask questions about the cancer, the treatment regimen, current status, and prognosis. i. Support client's efforts to increase knowledge and control over condition. Suggest resources available on self-help techniques such as visualization (e.g. guided imagery) that may assist client to gain a sense of control over the disease process and the side effects of chemotherapy. j. Inform client of scheduled procedures/treatments *so that he/she knows what to expect, which promotes a sense of control.* k. Include client in the planning of care, encourage maximum participation in the treatment plan, and allow choices whenever possible *to promote a sense of control.* l. Encourage significant others to allow client to do as much as he/she is able *so that a feeling of independence can be maintained.* m. Encourage client to participate in self-help and support groups.

Discharge Teaching

17. NURSING DIAGNOSIS: Knowledge deficit, Ineffective management of therapeutic regimen, or Altered health maintenance*

---

*The nurse should select the diagnostic label that is most appropriate for the client's discharge teaching needs.

Desired Outcomes	Nursing Actions and *Selected Purposes/Rationales*

17.a. The client will identify ways to prevent infection during periods of lowered immunity.

17.a.1. Explain to client that his/her resistance to infection is reduced when WBC counts are low. Emphasize need to adhere closely to recommended techniques to prevent infection.

2. Instruct the client in ways to prevent infection:
   a. avoid crowds, persons with any sign of infection, and persons who have recently been vaccinated
   b. avoid trauma to the skin and mucous membranes
   c. take axillary rather than oral temperature if stomatitis is present
   d. lubricate skin frequently to prevent dryness and subsequent cracking
   e. use excellent handwashing technique
   f. maintain sterile technique when caring for a central venous or peritoneal catheter, Ommaya reservoir, or implanted infusion device (e.g. MediPort) if in place
   g. avoid unnecessary rectal invasion (e.g. temperature taking, enemas, suppositories, sexual activity) to prevent rectal trauma
   h. avoid constipation to prevent damage to the bowel mucosa from hard or impacted stool
   i. wash perianal area thoroughly with soap and water after each bowel movement and after sexual activity; instruct female client to always wipe from front to back after urination and defecation
   j. drink at least 10 glasses of liquid/day unless contraindicated
   k. cough and deep breathe or use incentive spirometer every 2 hours until usual activity is resumed
   l. stop smoking
   m. perform meticulous oral hygiene after meals and at bedtime
   n. avoid douching unless ordered (douching disturbs normal vaginal flora and may cause trauma to the vaginal mucosa)
   o. maintain an optimal nutritional status (e.g. diet high in protein, calories, vitamins, and minerals)
   p. avoid intake of foods with a high microorganism content (e.g. unwashed fruits and vegetables; undercooked meat, poultry, or seafood)
   q. avoid sharing eating utensils
   r. maintain an adequate balance between activity and rest.

17.b. The client will demonstrate the ability to take an oral and axillary temperature correctly.

17.b.1. Demonstrate the correct way to take an oral and axillary temperature.
2. Allow time for questions, clarification, and return demonstration.

17.c. The client will demonstrate appropriate oral hygiene techniques.

17.c.1. Explain the rationale for and importance of frequent oral hygiene.
2. Provide instructions regarding oral hygiene techniques:
   a. cleanse mouth after eating and at bedtime; increase frequency to every 2 hours if stomatitis is present
   b. use a soft-bristle toothbrush to prevent trauma to fragile mucous membranes
   c. rinse mouth with the following solutions as prescribed:
      1. salt and water (1 tsp:1 quart)
      2. hydrogen peroxide and normal saline or water (1:4) or baking soda and water (1 T:1 quart) if crusting, debris, and/or tenacious mucus are present (solutions containing hydrogen peroxide should be mixed just before using and mouth should be rinsed thoroughly with a saline solution after use to avoid further damage to the oral mucous membrane)
   d. avoid commercial mouthwashes that have an alcohol base (these are drying to oral mucosa).

17.d. The client will identify techniques to control nausea and vomiting.

17.d. Instruct client in methods to control nausea and vomiting:
1. eat foods that are cool or room temperature (hot foods frequently have an overpowering aroma that stimulates nausea)
2. eat dry foods (e.g. toast, crackers) or sip cold carbonated beverages if nausea is present

3. eat several small meals per day instead of 3 large ones
4. avoid drinking liquids with meals
5. select bland foods (e.g. mashed potatoes, cottage cheese) rather than fatty, spicy foods (e.g. fried potatoes, chili)
6. rest after eating
7. if feasible, have someone else prepare the food
8. avoid offensive odors and sights
9. cleanse mouth frequently
10. take deep, slow breaths when nauseated
11. take antiemetics on a regular basis for prescribed length of time and if nausea is persistent.

17.e. The client will verbalize ways to improve appetite and nutritional status.

17.e. Instruct client in ways to improve appetite and maintain an adequate nutritional status:
1. try fish, cheese, chicken, and eggs as protein sources instead of beef and pork if taste distortion is a problem
2. increase amount of sugar or sweeteners and seasonings usually used in foods and beverages
3. eat in a pleasant environment with company if possible
4. perform frequent meticulous oral hygiene to eliminate disagreeable tastes in mouth
5. try recommended methods of controlling nausea (see action d in this diagnosis)
6. eat several high-calorie, high-protein, nutritious small meals/day rather than 3 large ones
7. take vitamins and minerals as prescribed.

17.f. The client will verbalize ways to manage and cope with persistent fatigue.

17.f. Instruct client in ways to manage and cope with persistent fatigue:
1. view fatigue as a protective mechanism rather than a problematic limitation
2. determine ways in which daily patterns of activity can be modified to conserve energy and prevent excessive fatigue (e.g. spread light and heavy tasks throughout the day, take short rests during an activity whenever possible, sit during an activity whenever possible, take several short rest periods during the day instead of one long one)
3. determine if life demands are realistic in light of physical state and adjust short- and long-term goals accordingly
4. avoid situations that are particularly fatiguing such as those that are boring, frustrating, or require prolonged or strenuous physical activity
5. participate in a regular aerobic exercise program that is approved by physician to improve cardiovascular and respiratory fitness, reduce anxiety and stress, and build up tolerance for activity.

17.g. The client will verbalize ways to prevent bleeding when platelet counts are low.

17.g.1. Instruct client in ways to minimize risk of bleeding:
a. avoid taking aspirin and other nonsteroidal anti-inflammatory agents (e.g. ibuprofen) on a regular basis
b. use an electric rather than a straight-edge razor
c. floss and brush teeth gently
d. cut nails and cuticles carefully
e. avoid putting sharp objects (e.g. toothpicks) in mouth
f. use caution when ambulating to prevent falls or bumps and do not walk barefoot
g. avoid situations that could result in injury (e.g. contact sports)
h. avoid straining to have a bowel movement
i. avoid blowing nose forcefully
j. avoid wearing constrictive clothing (e.g. garters, knee-high stockings)
k. use an ample amount of water-soluble lubricant prior to sexual intercourse and avoid anal sexual activity, douching, use of rectal suppositories, and enemas in order to prevent trauma to the vaginal and rectal mucosa
l. avoid heavy lifting.
2. Instruct client to control any bleeding by applying firm, prolonged pressure to the area if possible.

Desired Outcomes	Nursing Actions and *Selected Purposes/Rationales*

17.h. The client will verbalize ways to adjust to alterations in reproductive and sexual functioning.

17.h.1. Assure client that many of the side effects of chemotherapy (e.g. decreased libido, impotence) are temporary or can be treated.

    2. Explain to the female client that ovarian failure during chemotherapy may result in irritability, hot flashes, and other symptoms of premature menopause.

    3. Instruct client in the childbearing years to use contraception (many cytotoxic drugs cause genetic abnormalities in the developing fetus).

    4. Encourage client to rest before sexual activity if fatigue is a problem.

    5. Instruct client in measures to decrease discomfort associated with decreased vaginal secretions and mucositis:
- a. use an ample amount of water-soluble lubricant prior to intercourse
- b. use vaginal steroid cream if prescribed to ease dryness and inflammation if present
- c. take a sitz bath 2–3 times a day
- d. avoid intercourse until mucositis of the vaginal canal resolves.

    6. Instruct client to take hormone replacements (e.g. estrogen, testosterone) as prescribed.

17.i. The client will demonstrate the ability to care for a central venous catheter, a peritoneal catheter, or an implanted infusion device if in place.

17.i.1. Provide instructions related to care of a central venous catheter (e.g. Groshong) if appropriate:
- a. change dressing if present according to protocol using aseptic technique
- b. observe exit site for changes in appearance, redness, swelling, and unusual drainage
- c. flush catheter according to protocol to maintain patency
- d. replace injection cap as directed
- e. tape catheter securely to the chest wall to prevent accidental dislodgment
- f. notify physician if unable to flush catheter, if signs and symptoms of infection occur at exit site, or if catheter appears to be leaking.

    2. Provide instructions related to care of a peritoneal catheter if in place:
- a. change dressing daily according to protocol utilizing aseptic technique
- b. keep catheter capped between treatments
- c. keep water below the level of the catheter when taking a tub bath (a tub bath may be taken 7–10 days after catheter insertion)
- d. observe for and notify physician if any of the following occur:
  1. redness, swelling, or change in appearance of insertion site
  2. unusual drainage from exit site
  3. increasing abdominal pain
  4. chills or fever
  5. increased abdominal distention between treatments
  6. persistent nausea or vomiting
  7. dyspnea.

    3. Provide instructions related to care of an implanted infusion device (e.g. MediPort, Port-a-Cath) if in place:
- a. keep appointment to have device flushed or flush as instructed
- b. avoid trauma to insertion site
- c. notify physician if area around infusion device becomes reddened or painful.

    4. Allow time for questions, clarification, and return demonstration of procedures.

17.j. The client will verbalize an understanding of the care and precautions necessary if an Ommaya reservoir is in place.

17.j. Provide instructions related to care and precautions necessary if an Ommaya reservoir is in place:
1. wash site daily with soap and water
2. observe for and report redness, drainage, or discomfort at insertion site; stiff neck; or persistent headache
3. avoid activities that could result in trauma to the head and damage to the reservoir (e.g. contact sports).

17.k. The client will verbalize an understanding of an implanted infusion pump and precautions necessary if one is in place.

17.k.1. Reinforce physician's explanation about the purpose of the pump and how it works.
2. Instruct client to avoid activities that could result in abdominal trauma and dislodgment of pump.
3. Caution client to notify physician if:
   a. air travel is planned (client should carry an explanatory letter since pump may trigger airport weapon security devices; flow rate of pump may also need to be adjusted if the flight time is lengthy)
   b. body temperature is elevated more than 2° F for more than 24 hours (an increase in vapor pressure in the pump can increase flow rate)
   c. he/she plans to move to an area of greater or lesser altitude (alterations in the pump's flow rate may need to be made)
   d. redness, swelling, or drainage occurs at incisional or refilling site.
4. Emphasize importance of keeping appointments to have pump refilled (permanent blockage of the catheter can occur if pump is allowed to empty completely).

17.l. The client will state signs and symptoms of complications to report to the health care provider.

17.l. Instruct client to observe for and report the following:
1. signs and symptoms of infection (stress that usual signs of infection are diminished in people with altered bone marrow function and/or a suppressed immune system and that it is necessary to monitor closely for the following signs and symptoms):
   a. temperature above 38° C (100.4° F)
   b. changes in odor, color, or consistency of urine or pain on urination
   c. white patches in mouth
   d. crusted ulcerations around or in oral cavity
   e. swollen, reddened, coated tongue
   f. painful rectal or vaginal area
   g. unusual vaginal drainage
   h. changes in the appearance or temperature of skin, particularly around puncture sites
   i. persistent productive or nonproductive cough
2. signs and symptoms of bleeding (e.g. excessive bruising, black stools, persistent nosebleeds or bleeding from gums, sudden swelling in joints, red or smoke-colored urine, blood in vomitus)
3. signs and symptoms of hemorrhagic cystitis (e.g. blood in urine, pain on urination, urinary frequency or urgency)
4. signs and symptoms of extravasation (e.g. redness, pain, swelling, and/or skin changes at infusion site)
5. signs and symptoms of pulmonary dysfunction (e.g. shortness of breath; persistent, dry, hacking cough; fever)
6. signs and symptoms of dehydration (e.g. dry mouth, significant weight loss, concentrated urine, lightheadedness)
7. signs and symptoms of cardiotoxicity (e.g. irregular or rapid heart rate, increased weakness and fatigue, shortness of breath, unexplained weight gain, swelling of extremities); emphasize that cardiotoxicity can occur several days to months after administration of drugs known to cause it
8. signs and symptoms of neurotoxicity (e.g. numbness and tingling of extremities, change in hearing acuity, blurred vision, constipation, change in motor function and coordination, burning pain in extremity, impaired memory or ability to communicate)
9. persistent diarrhea, nausea, vomiting, and/or decreased oral intake
10. significant weight loss
11. inability to cope with the effects of the diagnosis and treatment.

Desired Outcomes	Nursing Actions and *Selected Purposes/Rationales*
17.m. The client will identify community resources that can assist with home management and adjustment to the diagnosis of cancer and chemotherapy and its effects.	17.m.1. Provide information about and encourage use of community resources that can assist client and significant others with home management and adjustment to diagnosis of cancer and chemotherapy and its effects (e.g. American Cancer Society, counselors, social service agencies, Meals on Wheels, Make Today Count, Look Good–Feel Better Program, Hospice, local community support groups). 2. Initiate a referral if indicated.

17.n. The client will verbalize an understanding of and a plan for adhering to recommended follow-up care including medications prescribed and schedule for chemotherapy, laboratory studies, and future appointments with health care provider.	17.n.1. Thoroughly explain rationale for, side effects of, and importance of taking medications prescribed. Inform client of pertinent food and drug interactions.
	 2. Reinforce physician's explanation of planned chemotherapy schedule.
	 3. Discuss with client any difficulties he/she might have adhering to the schedule and assist in planning ways to overcome these.
	 4. Reinforce importance of keeping appointments for chemotherapy and laboratory studies.
	 5. Reinforce importance of keeping follow-up appointments with health care provider.
	 6. Implement measures to improve client compliance:
	   a. include significant others in teaching sessions
	   b. encourage questions and allow time for reinforcement and clarification of information provided
	   c. provide written instructions regarding ways to maintain nutritional status, future appointments with health care provider and laboratory, medications prescribed, and signs and symptoms to report.

Bibliography

See pages 897–898 and 899–900.

EXTERNAL RADIATION THERAPY (TELETHERAPY)

Radiation therapy is one of the four major modes of treatment for cancer. It can be either external (teletherapy) or internal (brachytherapy) and is a local treatment in which cellular destruction occurs only at the treatment site. It is most effective on well-oxygenated tumors with a high growth fraction. Unfortunately, radiation therapy is not a selective process, and changes in cellular structure and function occur in both cancerous and normal cells within the treatment field. The normal cells, however, have a greater capacity for self-repair.

The effect of radiation therapy on the cell begins immediately and continues through several reproductive cycles of the cell. The time of cellular death and the side effects experienced by the client depend on the number of grays (Gy) or centigrays (cGy) received, the volume of tissue irradiated, whether or not both strands of DNA are broken, the extent of the damage to the cell's reproductive abilities, and the cell's ability to repair damage. The side effects that all clients receiving external radiation may experience are a skin reaction at the radiation treatment site, fatigue, malaise, and anorexia. Other side effects experienced depend on the anatomic site being radiated, the mitotic rate of the cells within the treatment field, fractionation of the dose, total dose delivered, and the general condition of the client.

Although it may be used alone, radiation therapy is increasingly being used in combination with surgery, chemotherapy, biotherapy, or hyperthermia to achieve palliation, control, or cure of cancer. External beam radiation is also being combined with brachytherapy to treat certain cancers (e.g. prostate, endometrial) more effectively. Radiation therapy in combination with surgical treatment of some cancers has also resulted in the need for less extensive surgery.

Minimization of damage to normal tissue with maximum tumor kill is a primary goal of radiation therapy. This goal is being accomplished more frequently with changes in technology and techniques. Computerized three-dimensional treatment planning provides more accurate targeting of tumor tissue while the use of equipment that contains multiple, computer-operated shields results in preservation of a greater amount of the normal tissue surrounding the tumor. Radiosensitizers that increase the sensitivity of tumor cells to radiation or radioprotectants that help protect normal cells from radiation damage may be used during teletherapy for some patients to achieve this same goal. Adaptation of standard radiation protocols, such as more frequent but smaller doses of radiation, may also be done to increase tumor cell kill and decrease damage to normal cells.

This care plan focuses on the adult client hospitalized for initiation of external radiation therapy or the adult client who is currently undergoing treatment on an outpatient basis and is admitted because of difficulty tolerating certain side effects. The major goals of care are to maintain comfort; promote an optimal nutritional status; maintain or regain skin integrity; prevent compli- cations; and educate the client about radiation therapy, expected side effects, and toxic effects to be reported. The nurse also plays a major role in assisting the client and significant others to cope with actual and antici- pated changes in body image, life style, and roles as a result of cancer and radiation therapy.

DISCHARGE CRITERIA

Prior to discharge, the client will:

- have an adequate or improved nutritional status
- have fatigue at a manageable level
- have evidence of normal healing of skin at site of irradiation
- have no signs and symptoms of complications of radiation therapy
- verbalize an understanding of appropriate skin care for site of irradiation
- identify techniques to control nausea and vomiting
- verbalize ways to improve appetite and nutritional status
- identify ways to reduce the risk of dental caries and periodontal disease and manage stomatitis if present
- identify ways to prevent bleeding if platelet counts are low
- identify ways to prevent infection if WBC counts are low
- verbalize an understanding of and ways to manage the effects of radiation therapy on sexual and reproductive functioning
- verbalize ways to manage and cope with persistent fatigue
- verbalize an understanding of the signs and symptoms of lymphedema and ways to manage it if it occurs
- state signs and symptoms to report to the health care provider
- share feelings and thoughts about the diagnosis of cancer and the effects of radiation therapy on body image
- identify community resources that can assist with home management and adjustment to the diagnosis of cancer and radiation therapy and its effects
- verbalize an understanding of and a plan for adhering to recommended follow-up care including medications prescribed and future appointments with health care provider, radiation department, and laboratory.

NURSING/ COLLABORATIVE DIAGNOSES

1. Anxiety △ 202
2. Altered nutrition: less than body requirements △ 203
3. Impaired swallowing △ 205
4. Pain △ 205
5A. Altered comfort: nausea and vomiting △ 206
5B. Altered comfort: pruritus △ 207
6. Actual/Risk for impaired skin integrity △ 208
7. Altered oral mucous membrane:
   a. dryness
   b. stomatitis △ 210
8. Fatigue △ 211
9. Diarrhea △ 212
10. Sleep pattern disturbance △ 213
11. Risk for infection △ 214
12. Potential complications:
    a. bleeding
    b. radiation cystitis
    c. radiation pneumonitis
    d. lymphedema △ 216
13. Self-concept disturbance △ 218
14. Ineffective individual coping △ 220
15. Grieving △ 221

DISCHARGE TEACHING

16. Knowledge deficit, Ineffective management of therapeutic regimen, or Altered health maintenance △ 222

1. NURSING DIAGNOSIS: **Anxiety**

related to:
a. unfamiliar environment;
b. lack of knowledge about radiation therapy if admitted to initiate therapy
c. need for hospitalization to manage existing side effects of radiation therapy and concern that additional untoward effects will occur with subsequent radiation treatments;
d. financial concerns;
e. diagnosis of cancer with potential for premature death.

Desired Outcome	Nursing Actions and *Selected Purposes/Rationales*

1. The client will experience a reduction in anxiety as evidenced by:
a. verbalization of feeling less anxious
b. usual sleep pattern
c. relaxed facial expression and body movements
d. stable vital signs
e. usual perceptual ability and interactions with others.
	1.a. Assess client on admission for:
	  1. fears, misconceptions, and level of understanding of radiation therapy and its therapeutic and nontherapeutic effects
	  2. concerns about particular side effects of radiation and their effect on life style
	  3. significance to client of the site to be irradiated
	  4. perception of the impact of daily radiation therapy for several weeks on usual life style, roles, and personal relationships
	  5. availability of an adequate support system
	  6. past experience with radiation therapy or other treatments for cancer
	  7. signs and symptoms of anxiety (e.g. verbalization of feeling anxious, insomnia, tenseness, shakiness, restlessness, diaphoresis, tachycardia, elevated blood pressure, facial pallor, self-focused behaviors); validate perceptions carefully, remembering that some behavior may be a result of the disease process.

b. Implement measures *to reduce fear and anxiety:*
1. orient client to hospital environment, equipment, and routines
2. introduce client to staff who will be participating in care; if possible, maintain consistency in staff assigned to his/her care *to provide feelings of stability and comfort with the environment*
3. assure client that staff members are nearby; respond to call signal as soon as possible
4. maintain a calm, supportive, confident manner when interacting with client
5. encourage verbalization of fear and anxiety; provide feedback
6. provide information about radiation therapy:
   a. explain how radiation therapy works and why the total radiation dose prescribed is fractionated
   b. inform client that he/she will be alone in the room during the few minutes of therapy but will be observed continuously via a television monitor; explain that communication will be possible by means of an intercommunication system
   c. inform client that the machine may click or make a whirring noise but that no discomfort will be felt during treatment
   d. instruct client about the expected general side effects of radiation therapy (e.g. fatigue; anorexia; itchy, dry, reddened skin; dry or moist desquamation and increase in skin pigmentation at radiation site) and anticipated side effects for the particular site being irradiated; explain when they can be expected to occur and resolve
   e. explain the treatment simulation process the client will experience before initiation of therapy (the simulation process is done to accurately determine the treatment field and design devices such as molds, plaster casts, or lead blocks that will be used to immobilize or position client and/or shield vital body organs within the treatment field)

     f. inform client that vital organs within the radiation treatment field are shielded during treatment to prevent unnecessary exposure to radiation; assure client that the treatment field will include the smallest amount of normal tissue possible and that the field may be changed or reduced as the tumor shrinks in size

     g. explain how the treatment field will be outlined (e.g. skin markings with an indelible dye, ink, or felt tip marker); inform client that the markings will be replaced by pinpoint tattoos once the reproducibility of the field is ensured

  7. arrange for client and significant others to visit the radiation department and meet those individuals responsible for his/her care

  8. prepare client for waiting room experiences with others receiving therapy; emphasize that each individual has a different treatment plan, response, and prognosis and that comparison should be avoided

  9. reinforce physician's explanations and clarify misconceptions client has about the diagnosis of cancer, treatment plan and its effects, and prognosis

  10. provide a calm, restful environment

  11. instruct client in relaxation techniques (e.g. listening to music, exercise, yoga, guided imagery) and encourage participation in diversional activities

  12. encourage appropriate use of humor

  13. perform actions to assist client to cope with radiation therapy and its effects (see Nursing Diagnosis 14, action c)

  14. initiate financial and/or social service referrals if indicated

  15. provide information based on current needs of client at a level he/she can understand; encourage questions and clarification of information provided

  16. encourage significant others to project a caring, concerned attitude without obvious anxiousness

  17. include significant others in orientation and teaching sessions and encourage their continued support of client

  18. administer prescribed antianxiety agents if indicated.

  c. Consult physician if above actions fail to control fear and anxiety.

---

2. NURSING DIAGNOSIS:

Altered nutrition: less than body requirements

related to:

a. decreased oral intake associated with:

  1. anorexia resulting from factors such as depression, fear, anxiety, fatigue, discomfort, early satiety, and altered sense of taste (an altered sense of taste is often reported by persons with cancer; it can also result from damage to the taste buds and salivary glands following administration of 1000–2000 cGy to the head and neck area)

  2. impaired swallowing resulting from pharyngitis, esophagitis, dry mouth, and/or viscous oral secretions if present as a result of treatment to the head, neck, or mediastinum;

b. loss of nutrients associated with vomiting and diarrhea if present;

c. impaired utilization of nutrients associated with:

  1. accelerated and inefficient metabolism of proteins, carbohydrates, and fats resulting from the disease process

  2. decreased absorption of nutrients resulting from loss of intestinal absorptive surface if mucositis has developed (can occur with treatment to the abdomen or lower back);

d. utilization of available nutrients by the malignant cells rather than the host.

Desired Outcome	Nursing Actions and *Selected Purposes/Rationales*

2. The client will have or attain an adequate nutritional status as evidenced by:
  a. weight within or returning toward normal range for client's age, height, and body frame
  b. normal BUN and serum albumin, Hct, Hb, and transferrin levels
  c. usual strength and activity tolerance
  d. healthy oral mucous membrane.
	2.a. Assess for and report signs and symptoms of malnutrition:
	  1. weight below normal for client's age, height, and body frame
	  2. abnormal BUN and low serum albumin, Hct, Hb, and transferrin levels
	  3. weakness and fatigue
	  4. sore, inflamed oral mucous membrane
	  5. pale conjunctiva.
	  b. Monitor percentage of meals and snacks client consumes. Report a pattern of inadequate intake.
	  c. Implement measures *to maintain or promote an adequate nutritional status:*
	    1. perform actions *to improve oral intake:*
	      a. implement measures to control nausea and vomiting (see Nursing Diagnosis 5.A, action 2)
	      b. implement measures to reduce pain (see Nursing Diagnosis 4, action e)
	      c. implement measures to assist client to adjust psychologically to the diagnosis of cancer and treatment with radiation therapy (see Nursing Diagnoses 13, actions d–n; 14, action c; and 15, action b)
	      d. implement measures to improve client's ability to swallow (see Nursing Diagnosis 3, action b)
	      e. implement measures *to compensate for taste alteration* (loss of sense of taste occurs within 2 weeks of initiation of radiation treatment to head and neck, persists for 4–6 weeks after completion of therapy, and usually is not permanent):
	        1. encourage client to select fish, cold cooked chicken, eggs, and cheese as protein sources if beef or pork tastes bitter or rancid
	        2. provide meat for breakfast if aversion to meat tends to increase during day
	        3. add extra sweeteners to foods if acceptable to client
	        4. experiment with different flavorings, seasonings, and textures
	        5. serve food warm *to stimulate the sense of smell*
	      f. increase activity as tolerated (*activity usually promotes a sense of well-being and improves appetite*)
	      g. obtain a dietary consult if necessary to assist client in selecting foods/fluids that meet nutritional needs, are appealing, and adhere to personal and cultural preferences
	      h. encourage a rest period before meals *to minimize fatigue*
	      i. maintain a clean environment and a relaxed, pleasant atmosphere
	      j. provide oral hygiene before meals
	      k. provide largest amount of calories and protein when appetite is best (usually at breakfast)
	      l. serve frequent, small meals rather than large ones if client is weak, fatigues easily, and/or has a poor appetite
	      m. encourage significant others to bring in client's favorite foods and eat with him/her *to make eating more of a familiar social experience*
	      n. limit fluid intake with meals (unless the fluid has high nutritional value) *to reduce early satiety and subsequent decreased food intake*
	      o. allow adequate time for meals; reheat foods/fluids if necessary
	    2. ensure that meals are well balanced and high in essential nutrients; offer high-protein, high-calorie dietary supplements if indicated
	    3. perform activities to control diarrhea (see Nursing Diagnosis 9, action c)
	    4. administer vitamins and minerals if ordered.
	  d. Perform a calorie count if ordered. Report information to dietitian and physician.
	  e. Consult physician about an alternative method of providing nutrition (e.g. parenteral nutrition, tube feedings) if client does not consume enough food or fluids to meet nutritional needs.

3. **NURSING DIAGNOSIS:**   **Impaired swallowing**

related to:
a. oral, pharyngeal, or esophageal pain associated with inflammation and/or ulceration of the mucosa if the treatment field includes the head, neck, or mediastinum;
b. dry mouth and viscous oral secretions associated with:
    1. destruction of the salivary glands (particularly the parotids) if the treatment field includes the head and neck area
    2. decreased oral intake.

Desired Outcome	Nursing Actions and *Selected Purposes/Rationales*

3. The client will experience an improvement in swallowing as evidenced by:
  a. verbalization of same
  b. absence of food in oral cavity after swallowing
  c. absence of coughing and choking when eating and drinking.
	3.a. Assess for signs and symptoms of impaired swallowing (e.g. statements of difficulty swallowing, stasis of food in oral cavity, coughing or choking when eating or drinking).
	  b. Implement measures *to improve ability to swallow:*
	    1. perform actions to reduce oral, pharyngeal, and esophageal pain (see Nursing Diagnosis 4, action e.7)
	    2. perform actions to decrease dryness of the oral mucous membrane (see Nursing Diagnosis 7, action a.2)
	    3. assist client to select foods that require little or no chewing and are easily swallowed (e.g. custard, eggs, canned fruit, mashed potatoes)
	    4. avoid serving foods that are sticky (e.g. peanut butter, soft bread, honey)
	    5. moisten dry foods with gravy or sauces (e.g. sour cream, salad dressing)
	    6. perform actions *to stimulate salivation at meal time:*
	      a. provide oral hygiene before meals
	      b. provide a piece of hard candy for client to suck on just before meals unless contraindicated
	      c. serve foods that are visually pleasing
	      d. place a piece of lemon or sour pickle on client's plate
	    7. perform actions *to reduce and/or liquefy viscous oral secretions:*
	      a. encourage a fluid intake of 2500 ml/day unless contraindicated
	      b. encourage client to avoid milk, milk products, and chocolate (*when combined with saliva, they produce very thick secretions*).
	  c. If swallowing difficulties persist or worsen:
	    1. withhold oral intake
	    2. consult physician
	    3. assess for and report signs and symptoms of aspiration (e.g. rhonchi, dull percussion note over affected lung area, cough, tachypnea, dyspnea).

4. **NURSING DIAGNOSIS:**   **Pain**

related to inflammation and/or moist desquamation (if it occurs) in irradiated area.

Desired Outcome	Nursing Actions and *Selected Purposes/Rationales*

4. The client will experience diminished pain as evidenced by:
  a. verbalization of decreased pain
	4.a. Assess for signs and symptoms of pain (e.g. verbalization of pain, grimacing, reluctance to move, restlessness, diaphoresis, facial pallor, increased B/P, tachycardia).
	  b. Assess client's perception of the severity of pain using a pain intensity rating scale.

Desired Outcome	Nursing Actions and **Selected Purposes/Rationales**
b. relaxed facial expression and body positioning	c. Assess the client's pain pattern (e.g. location, quality, onset, duration, precipitating factors, aggravating factors, alleviating factors).
c. increased participation in activities	d. Ask the client to describe previous pain experiences and methods used to manage pain effectively.
d. stable vital signs.	e. Implement measures *to reduce pain:*

    1. perform actions *to reduce fear and anxiety about the pain experience* (e.g. assure client that his/her need for pain relief is understood, plan methods of achieving pain control with client)

    2. perform actions to reduce fear and anxiety (see Nursing Diagnosis 1, action b) *in order to promote relaxation and subsequently increase the client's threshold and tolerance for pain*

    3. administer analgesics before activities and procedures that can cause pain and before pain becomes severe

    4. perform actions to reduce fatigue (see Nursing Diagnosis 8, action e) *in order to increase the client's threshold and tolerance for pain*

    5. perform actions *to reduce pain associated with moist desquamation:*

        a. implement measures identified in Nursing Diagnosis 6, action b.1.h. to treat a moist desquamation reaction

        b. if open method of treatment is being used, position a covered bed cradle over affected area *to reduce airflow over exposed nerve endings*

    6. perform actions *to reduce perianal pain* (can occur if the perineum is in the treatment field or if diarrhea is present):

        a. provide a foam pad for client to sit on

        b. consult physician about an order for sitz baths unless contraindicated

        c. implement measures to decrease skin irritation and prevent breakdown associated with diarrhea (see Nursing Diagnosis 6, action b.3)

        d. avoid taking temperature rectally or administering rectal suppositories

        e. apply a topical anesthetic–corticosteroid cream (e.g. Corticaine) if ordered

    7. perform actions *to reduce oral, pharyngeal, and esophageal pain* (can occur with radiation exposure of approximately 3000 cGy to the head, neck, and mediastinum):

        a. implement measures to reduce severity of stomatitis (see Nursing Diagnosis 7, actions b.3 and 4)

        b. offer cool, soothing liquids such as nonacidic juices and ices

        c. instruct client to gargle with a saline solution every 2 hours or spray mouth with a solution containing diphenhydramine and water (1 oz diphenhydramine and 1 qt water) *to soothe the oral mucous membrane*

        d. administer topical anesthetics and oral protective agents (e.g. mixture of diphenhydramine, antacid, and viscous xylocaine; sucralfate oral suspension) if ordered

    8. provide or assist with nonpharmacologic measures for pain relief (e.g. massage; position change; relaxation exercises; guided imagery; restful environment; diversional activities such as watching television, reading, or conversing)

    9. administer analgesics if ordered.

  f. Consult physician if above measures fail to provide adequate pain relief.

5.A. NURSING DIAGNOSIS: **Altered comfort: nausea and vomiting**

related to stimulation of the vomiting center associated with:
1. presence of by-products of cellular destruction if client is receiving a large daily fraction of radiation or daily treatments over a period of several weeks;

2. stimulation of the visceral afferent pathways resulting from inflammation of the gastrointestinal mucosa (occurs when areas of the chest, back, abdomen, or pelvis are irradiated);
3. stimulation of the cerebral cortex resulting from cerebral inflammation (if client is receiving whole brain irradiation) and stress.

Desired Outcome	Nursing Actions and *Selected Purposes/Rationales*

5.A. The client will experience relief of nausea and vomiting as evidenced by:
1. verbalization of relief of nausea
2. absence of vomiting.

5.A.1. Assess client for nausea and vomiting (tends to occur within 1–3 hours after treatment).
   2. Implement measures *to control nausea and vomiting*:
      a. perform actions to reduce fear and anxiety (see Nursing Diagnosis 1, action b) and promote psychological adjustment to the diagnosis of cancer and treatment with external radiation (see Nursing Diagnoses 13, actions d–n; 14, action c; and 15, action b)
      b. eliminate noxious sights and odors from the environment (*noxious stimuli can cause stimulation of the vomiting center*)
      c. encourage client to take deep, slow breaths when nauseated
      d. encourage client to change positions slowly (*rapid movement can result in stimulation of the chemoreceptor trigger zone and subsequent excitation of the vomiting center*)
      e. provide oral hygiene after each emesis and before meals
      f. maintain food and fluid restrictions if ordered (client may be placed on a clear liquid or bland diet for short periods if nausea is severe)
      g. provide carbonated beverages for client to sip if nauseated
      h. avoid serving foods with an overpowering aroma; remove lids from hot foods before entering room
      i. provide small, frequent meals; instruct client to ingest foods and fluids slowly
      j. if nausea tends to peak after each treatment, instruct client to eat his/her major meal of the day at least 3 hours before treatment if possible and to eat lightly for 3–4 hours after the treatment
      k. encourage client to eat dry foods (e.g. toast, crackers) and avoid drinking liquids with meals if nauseated
      l. instruct client to avoid foods/fluids that irritate the gastric mucosa (e.g. spicy foods; caffeine-containing beverages such as coffee, tea, and colas)
      m. instruct client to avoid foods high in fat (*fat delays gastric emptying*)
      n. instruct client to rest after eating
      o. administer antiemetics as ordered (these are often given on a regular schedule 1–2 hours before radiation therapy and every 4–6 hours for 12 hours after treatment).
   3. Consult physician if above measures fail to control nausea and vomiting.

5.B. NURSING DIAGNOSIS: **Altered comfort: pruritus**

related to dry skin associated with decreased function of sebaceous and sweat glands within the treatment field.

Desired Outcome	Nursing Actions and *Selected Purposes/Rationales*

5.B. The client will experience relief of pruritus as evidenced by:
1. verbalization of same

5.B.1. Assess for the following:
   a. reports of itchiness
   b. persistent scratching or rubbing of skin
   c. dryness and redness or excoriation of skin within the treatment field.

Desired Outcome	Nursing Actions and *Selected Purposes/Rationales*

2. no scratching and rubbing of skin.	2. Instruct client in and/or implement measures *to relieve pruritus in the treatment area*:
	  a. perform actions *to promote capillary constriction*:
	    1. apply cool, moist compresses to pruritic areas
	    2. maintain a cool environment
	  b. perform actions *to reduce skin dryness*:
	    1. use tepid water and mild soaps for bathing, being careful not to remove skin markings
	    2. apply water-based lubricant lotions (e.g. Lubriderm, Eucerin) 2–3 times daily and after bath (avoid lotions that contain lanolin or petrolatum *because they must be removed before treatments*)
	    3. limit bathing to every other day
	    4. encourage a fluid intake of 2500 ml/day unless contraindicated
	    5. utilize a room humidifier *to increase moisture in the air*
	  c. add emollients, cornstarch, or baking soda to bath water
	  d. apply cornstarch to areas of dry desquamation (cornstarch should not be used if moist desquamation is present)
	  e. pat skin dry after bathing, making sure to dry thoroughly
	  f. encourage participation in diversional activities
	  g. use relaxation techniques
	  h. use cutaneous stimulation techniques (e.g. stroking with a soft brush) at sites of itching or acupressure points (skin within the treatment field should never be rubbed or massaged)
	  i. encourage client to wear loose cotton garments
	  j. administer antihistamines if ordered.
	3. Consult physician if above measures fail to relieve pruritus or if the skin becomes more excoriated.

---

6. NURSING DIAGNOSIS:

Actual/Risk for impaired skin integrity

related to:
a. dry desquamation of irradiated site associated with increased sensitivity of skin in certain areas (e.g. opposing skin surfaces, face, perineum) and destruction of rapidly dividing epithelial cells of the skin (occurs with a cumulative dose of 3000–4000 cGy);
b. moist desquamation of irradiated area (particularly if client is receiving electron beam therapy) associated with damage to the basal cells of the skin (occurs with doses above 4500 cGy or lower cumulative doses if client is receiving concurrent chemotherapy);
c. increased skin fragility associated with:
  1. tissue edema resulting from vascular changes in irradiated area
  2. malnutrition;
d. excessive scratching associated with pruritus;
e. damage to the skin and/or subcutaneous tissue associated with prolonged pressure on the tissues, friction, or shearing if mobility is decreased;
f. frequent contact of the skin with irritants associated with diarrhea if present.

Desired Outcome	Nursing Actions and *Selected Purposes/Rationales*

6. The client will maintain or regain skin integrity as evidenced by:
  a. minimal redness and irritation within the treatment field
	6.a. Inspect the following areas for pallor, redness, and breakdown:
	  1. treatment field and area on the body surface opposite to it
	  2. opposing skin surfaces
	  3. bony prominences
	  4. dependent, pruritic, and edematous areas
	  5. perineum.

b. absence of redness and irritation in body areas not in treatment field

c. no skin breakdown.

b. Implement measures *to maintain or regain skin integrity*:

1. perform actions *to prevent or treat skin irritation or breakdown within the treatment field*:

   a. cleanse irradiated area gently each shift with tepid water and mild soap (may be contraindicated initially when skin markings rather than tattoos are used)

   b. pat skin dry using soft materials, paying particular attention to opposing skin surfaces within the treatment field

   c. expose irradiated area to the air as much as possible, avoiding extremes in temperature

   d. avoid use of tape within irradiated area

   e. instruct client to:

      1. wear loose cotton clothing

      2. avoid use of perfumed lotions or soaps, cosmetics, and deodorants *to prevent chemical irritation* (*many of these products contain heavy metals that will augment effects of radiation on the skin*)

      3. apply cornstarch to areas of dry desquamation *to reduce friction*

      4. use water-based (hydrophilic), mild, lubricant lotion (e.g. Lubriderm, Eucerin) *to reduce skin dryness and subsequent cracking*

      5. avoid use of hydrophobic products (e.g. Vaseline) *because they are difficult to remove*

      6. use an electric rather than a straight-edge razor if it is absolutely necessary to shave in irradiated area

   f. avoid applications of heat and cold to irradiated area

   g. implement measures *to prevent skin breakdown associated with scratching*:

      1. perform actions to relieve pruritus (see Nursing Diagnosis 5.B, action 2)

      2. keep nails trimmed and/or apply mittens if necessary

      3. instruct client to apply firm pressure to pruritic areas rather than scratching

   h. implement measures *to treat a moist desquamation reaction if it has occurred*:

      1. if open method of treatment is prescribed:

         a. cleanse area well with warm saline, water, or a dilute solution of chlorhexidine gluconate 3 times/day; apply an astringent soak if ordered

         b. keep involved area exposed to the air as much as possible

      2. if semi-open method of treatment is prescribed:

         a. apply a weak astringent soak (e.g. dilute Domeboro solution) for 15 minutes 3 times/day

         b. apply a hydrogel primary wound dressing (e.g. Vigilon, Geliperm) or a nonadherent dressing (e.g. Adaptic) as ordered

      3. if closed method of treatment is prescribed, apply occlusive dressings *to maintain a moist environment*

      4. apply a topical antimicrobial agent as ordered if signs and symptoms of a localized infection occur

2. perform actions *to prevent skin breakdown resulting from decreased mobility*:

   a. assist client to turn at least every 2 hours if activity is limited

   b. gently massage around reddened areas at least every 2 hours

   c. position client properly; use pressure-reducing or pressure-relieving devices (e.g. pillows, gel or foam cushions, alternating pressure mattress, air-fluidized bed) if indicated

   d. apply a thin layer of powder or cornstarch to bottom sheet or skin and opposing skin surfaces (e.g. axillae, beneath breasts) if indicated *to absorb moisture and reduce friction*

Desired Outcome	Nursing Actions and *Selected Purposes/Rationales*

      e. lift and move client carefully using a turn sheet and adequate assistance

      f. limit length of time client is in semi-Fowler's position to 30 minutes (*in this position, client tends to slide down in bed, which can cause skin surface abrasion and shearing*)

      g. instruct or assist client to shift weight at least every 30 minutes

      h. keep skin clean and dry

      i. keep bed linens dry and wrinkle-free

      j. increase activity as tolerated

   3. perform actions *to decrease skin irritation and prevent breakdown associated with diarrhea*:

      a. implement measures to control diarrhea (see Nursing Diagnosis 9, action c)

      b. assist client to thoroughly cleanse and dry perineal area with soft tissue or cloth after each bowel movement; apply a protective ointment or cream, being sure to remove it before treatments if rectal area is within treatment field

      c. provide incontinence pads if needed to absorb moisture; do not allow skin to come in contact with plastic portion of pads

   4. if edema is present:

      a. perform actions *to reduce fluid accumulation in dependent areas*:

         1. instruct client in and assist with range of motion exercises

         2. elevate affected extremities whenever possible

      b. handle edematous areas carefully

   5. perform actions to promote an adequate nutritional status (see Nursing Diagnosis 2, action c).

 c. If unexpected skin irritation or breakdown occurs:

   1. notify physician

   2. continue with above measures to prevent further irritation and breakdown

   3. perform care of involved areas as ordered or per standard hospital procedure

   4. assess client closely and report signs and symptoms of infection (e.g. elevated temperature; redness, heat, pain, and swelling around area of breakdown; unusual drainage from site).

---

7. NURSING DIAGNOSIS:

Altered oral mucous membrane:

a. **dryness** related to decreased oral intake and destruction of salivary glands if the treatment field includes the head and neck;

b. **stomatitis** related to malnutrition, inadequate oral hygiene, and disruption in the renewal process of mucosal epithelial cells if the oral cavity is irradiated.

Desired Outcomes	Nursing Actions and *Selected Purposes/Rationales*

7.a. The client will maintain a moist, intact oral mucous membrane.

   7.a.1. Assess client for dryness of the oral mucosa (reduction in salivary flow may occur after a cumulative dose of as little as 1000 cGy to the head and neck area and may persist for many months after treatment; dryness will be permanent after a radiation exposure of over 6000 cGy).

      2. Implement measures *to decrease dryness of oral mucous membrane*:

        a. instruct and assist client to perform oral hygiene after eating and as often as needed; avoid use of products that contain lemon and glycerin and mouthwashes containing alcohol (*these products have a drying and irritating effect on the oral mucous membrane*)

b. encourage client to rinse or spray mouth frequently with water
c. lubricate client's lips frequently
d. encourage client to breathe through nose rather than mouth
e. encourage client not to smoke (*smoking irritates and dries the mucosa*)
f. encourage a fluid intake of at least 2500 ml/day unless contraindicated
g. perform actions *to stimulate salivation*:
  1. encourage client to suck on hard candy unless contraindicated
  2. provide beverages containing lemon (e.g. tea with lemon, lemonade)
  3. administer sialagogues (e.g. oral pilocarpine [Salagen]) if ordered
h. if stomatitis is not severe, encourage client to use artificial saliva *to lubricate the mucous membrane.*

7.b. The client will maintain a healthy oral cavity as evidenced by:
1. absence of inflammation
2. pink, intact mucosa
3. no reports of oral dryness and burning
4. ability to swallow without discomfort
5. usual consistency of saliva.

7.b.1. Assess client for and report signs and symptoms of stomatitis such as inflamed and/or ulcerated oral mucosa, reports of burning pain in mouth, dysphagia, and viscous saliva. (Stomatitis usually begins by the end of the second week of therapy and persists for up to 4 weeks following the cessation of treatment. Signs and symptoms initially appear on the buccal surfaces and/or palate.)
2. Culture oral lesions as ordered. Report positive results.
3. Implement measures *to prevent or reduce the severity of stomatitis*:
  a. perform actions to reduce dryness of the oral mucous membrane (see action a.2 in this diagnosis)
  b. have client rinse mouth every 1–2 hours with warm saline; baking soda and water; or a solution of salt, baking soda, and water
  c. use a soft-bristle brush, sponge-tipped applicator, or low-pressure power spray for oral hygiene
  d. instruct client to avoid substances that might further irritate the oral mucosa (e.g. extremely hot, spicy, or acidic foods/fluids)
  e. perform actions to promote an adequate nutritional status (see Nursing Diagnosis 2, action c)
  f. consult physician regarding an order for a prophylactic antimicrobial agent.
4. If stomatitis is not controlled:
  a. increase frequency of oral hygiene
  b. if client has dentures, remove and replace only for meals.
5. Consult physician if signs and symptoms of stomatitis persist or worsen.

---

8. NURSING DIAGNOSIS: **Fatigue**

related to:*
a. a build up of cellular waste products associated with rapid lysis of cancerous and normal cells exposed to radiation;
b. tissue hypoxia associated with anemia (can result from malnutrition or depression of bone marrow activity if large amounts of active bone marrow are included in the treatment field);
c. difficulty resting and sleeping associated with fear, anxiety, and discomfort;
d. overwhelming emotional demands associated with the diagnosis of cancer and treatment with radiation;
e. increased energy expenditure associated with an increase in the metabolic rate resulting from continuous active tumor growth and the energy needed to repair damaged cells;
f. malnutrition.

---

*Some of the etiological factors presented here are under investigation.

Desired Outcome	Nursing Actions and **Selected Purposes/Rationales**

8. The client will experience a reduction in fatigue as evidenced by:
  a. verbalization of feelings of increased energy
  b. ability to perform usual activities of daily living
  c. increased interest in surroundings and ability to concentrate
  d. decreased emotional lability.
	8.a. Assess for signs and symptoms of fatigue (e.g. verbalization of unremitting, overwhelming lack of energy and inability to maintain usual routines; lack of interest in surroundings; decreased ability to concentrate; increased emotional lability).
	  b. Assess client's perception of the severity of fatigue using a fatigue rating scale.
	  c. Inform client that a feeling of persistent fatigue is not unusual and is a result of the disease itself as well as an expected effect of cell breakdown that occurs with radiation therapy.
	  d. Assist client to identify personal patterns of fatigue (e.g. time of day, after treatments or certain activities) and to plan activities so that times of greatest fatigue are avoided.
	  e. Implement measures *to reduce fatigue*:
	    1. perform actions *to promote rest and/or conserve energy*:
	      a. schedule several short rest periods during the day
	      b. minimize environmental activity and noise
	      c. limit the number of visitors and their length of stay
	      d. assist client with self-care activities as needed
	      e. keep supplies and personal articles within easy reach
	      f. implement measures to reduce fear and anxiety (see Nursing Diagnosis 1, action b)
	      g. implement measures to promote sleep (see Nursing Diagnosis 10, action c)
	      h. implement measures to reduce discomfort (see Nursing Diagnoses 4, action e; 5.A, action 2; and 5.B, action 2)
	      i. instruct client in energy-saving techniques (e.g. using shower chair when showering, sitting to brush teeth or comb hair)
	    2. perform actions to promote an adequate nutritional status (see Nursing Diagnosis 2, action c)
	    3. encourage client to maintain a fluid intake of at least 2500 ml/day *to promote elimination of the by-products of cellular breakdown*
	    4. administer the following if ordered *to treat anemia*:
	      a. epoetin alfa (EPO)
	      b. blood transfusions (e.g. packed red blood cells)
	    5. increase activity gradually as tolerated
	    6. perform actions to facilitate client's psychological adjustment to the diagnosis of cancer and the treatment regimen and its effects (see Nursing Diagnoses 13, actions d–n; 14, action c; and 15, action b).
	  f. Consult physician if signs and symptoms of fatigue worsen.

■ ──

9. NURSING DIAGNOSIS: **Diarrhea**

related to increased peristalsis and disorders of intestinal secretion and absorption associated with damage to the intestinal mucosa if the treatment field includes the pelvis, abdomen, or lower back.

Desired Outcome	Nursing Actions and **Selected Purposes/Rationales**
9. The client will have fewer bowel movements and more formed stool if diarrhea occurs.	9.a. Ascertain client's usual bowel elimination habits. b. Assess for signs and symptoms of diarrhea (e.g. frequent, loose stools; urgency; abdominal pain and cramping; hyperactive bowel sounds). Diarrhea will usually begin after 1500–3000 cGy have been received and end 2–3 weeks after cessation of treatment.

    c. Implement measures *to control diarrhea*:
      1. perform actions *to rest the bowel*:
        a. restrict oral intake if ordered
        b. when oral intake is allowed:
          1. gradually progress from fluids to small meals
          2. instruct client to avoid foods/fluids that may stimulate or irritate the inflamed bowel:
            a. those high in fiber (e.g. whole-grain cereals, raw fruits and vegetables)
            b. those that are spicy or extremely hot or cold
            c. those high in lactose (e.g. milk, milk products)
            d. those high in fat (e.g. butter, cream, fried foods)
        c. implement measures to reduce fear and anxiety (see Nursing Diagnosis 1, action b)
        d. encourage client to rest
        e. discourage smoking (*nicotine has a stimulant effect on the gastrointestinal tract*)
      2. administer the following medications if ordered *to control diarrhea*:
        a. opiates or opiate derivatives (e.g. paregoric, loperamide, diphenoxylate hydrochloride) *to decrease gastrointestinal motility*
        b. bulk-forming agents (e.g. methylcellulose, psyllium hydrophilic mucilloid, calcium polycarbophil) *to absorb water in the bowel, which results in a more formed stool*
        c. adsorbents (e.g. kaolin, pectin, attapulgite [Kaopectate], bismuth subsalicylate [Pepto-Bismol]).
    d. Consult physician if diarrhea persists.

---

10. NURSING DIAGNOSIS: **Sleep pattern disturbance**

related to:
a. pain, nausea, vomiting, pruritus, and severe xerostomia;
b. anxiety, fear, and grief;
c. frequent need to defecate associated with diarrhea if present.

Desired Outcome	Nursing Actions and *Selected Purposes/Rationales*

10. The client will attain optimal amounts of sleep as evidenced by:
  a. statements of feeling well rested
  b. usual mental status
  c. absence of frequent yawning, dark circles under eyes, and hand tremors.
	10.a. Assess for signs and symptoms of a sleep pattern disturbance (e.g. statements of difficulty falling asleep, not feeling well rested, or sleep interruptions; irritability; lethargy; disorientation; frequent yawning; dark circles under eyes; slight hand tremors).
	   b. Determine the client's usual sleep habits.
	   c. Implement measures *to promote sleep*:
	    1. discourage long periods of sleep during the day unless signs and symptoms of sleep deprivation exist or daytime sleep is usual for client
	    2. perform actions to reduce fear and anxiety (see Nursing Diagnosis 1, action b) and assist client to adjust psychologically to the diagnosis of cancer and treatment with radiation (see Nursing Diagnoses 13, actions d–n; 14, action c; and 15, action b)
	    3. perform actions to reduce discomfort (see Nursing Diagnoses 4, action e; 5.A, action 2; and 5.B, action 2)
	    4. perform actions to control diarrhea (see Nursing Diagnosis 9, action c)
	    5. if client has xerostomia, instruct him/her to use artificial saliva before sleep *to prevent the dry, choking sensation that often occurs during sleep*

Desired Outcome	Nursing Actions and *Selected Purposes/Rationales*

6. encourage participation in relaxing diversional activities during the evening
7. discourage intake of fluids high in caffeine (e.g. coffee, tea, colas), especially in the evening
8. allow client to continue usual sleep practices (e.g. position; time; presleep routines such as reading, watching television, listening to music, and meditating) unless contraindicated
9. satisfy basic needs such as comfort and warmth before sleep
10. encourage client to urinate just before bedtime
11. reduce environmental distractions (e.g. close door to client's room; use night light rather than overhead light whenever possible; lower volume of paging system; keep staff conversations at a low level and away from client's room; close curtains between clients in a semi-private room or ward; provide client with 'white noise' such as fan, soft music, or tape-recorded sounds of the ocean or rain; have earplugs available for client if needed)
12. administer prescribed sedative-hypnotics if indicated
13. perform actions *to reduce interruptions during sleep (80–100 minutes of uninterrupted sleep is usually needed to complete one sleep cycle)*:
    a. restrict visitors
    b. group care (e.g. medications, treatments, physical care, assessments) whenever possible.
d. Consult physician if signs and symptoms of sleep deprivation persist or worsen.

---

11. NURSING DIAGNOSIS: **Risk for infection**

related to:
a. break in the integrity of the skin associated with dry or moist desquamation;
b. lowered natural resistance associated with:
   1. malnutrition
   2. neutropenia resulting from bone marrow suppression if large amounts of active bone marrow are included in the treatment field
   3. impaired immune system functioning resulting from certain malignancies (e.g. Hodgkin's disease, lymphoma);
c. stasis of respiratory secretions and urinary stasis if mobility is decreased.

Desired Outcome	Nursing Actions and *Selected Purposes/Rationales*

11. The client will remain free of infection as evidenced by:
    a. absence of fever and chills
    b. pulse within normal limits
    c. normal breath sounds
    d. usual mental status
    e. cough productive of clear mucus only
    f. voiding clear urine without reports of frequency, urgency, and burning
    g. absence of redness, heat, pain, swelling, and

11.a. Assess for and report signs and symptoms of infection (be alert to subtle changes in the client since the signs of infection may be minimal as a result of immunosuppression; also be aware that some signs and symptoms vary depending on the site of the infection, the causative organism, and the age of the client):
1. elevated temperature
2. chills
3. increased pulse
4. abnormal breath sounds
5. development of or increased malaise
6. lethargy, acute confusion
7. further loss of appetite
8. cough productive of purulent, green, or rust-colored sputum
9. cloudy, foul-smelling urine
10. reports of frequency, urgency, or burning when urinating
11. presence of WBCs, bacteria, and/or nitrites in urine

unusual drainage in any area
h. no reports of increased weakness and fatigue
i. WBC and differential counts within normal range for client
j. negative results of cultured specimens.

12. redness, heat, pain, swelling, or unusual drainage in any area
13. reports of increased weakness or fatigue
14. elevated WBC count and/or significant change in differential.
b. Obtain specimens (e.g. urine, vaginal drainage, mouth, sputum, blood, moist desquamation sites) for culture as ordered. Report positive results.
c. Implement measures *to reduce the risk for infection:*
   1. protect client from others with infections and those who have recently been vaccinated (*a person may have a subclinical infection after a vaccination*)
   2. use good handwashing technique and encourage client to do the same
   3. maintain a fluid intake of at least 2500 ml/day unless contraindicated
   4. perform actions to promote an adequate nutritional status (see Nursing Diagnosis 2, action c); encourage intake of foods high in vitamins C and E (*it is theorized that antioxidant vitamins promote phagocytosis of organisms*)
   5. encourage a low-microbial diet (e.g. cooked foods, no unwashed fresh fruits and vegetables) if client is immunosuppressed
   6. perform actions to prevent or reduce the severity of stomatitis (see Nursing Diagnosis 7, actions b.3 and 4)
   7. perform actions to maintain or regain skin integrity (see Nursing Diagnosis 6, actions b and c)
   8. avoid invasive procedures (e.g. urinary catheterizations, arterial and venous punctures, injections) whenever possible; if such procedures are necessary, perform them using sterile technique
   9. rotate intravenous insertion sites according to hospital policy
   10. anchor catheters/tubings (e.g. urinary, intravenous) securely *in order to reduce trauma to the tissues and the risk for introduction of pathogens associated with the in-and-out movement of the tubing*
   11. maintain a closed system for drains (e.g. urinary catheter) and intravenous infusions whenever possible
   12. change equipment, tubings, and solutions used for treatments such as intravenous infusions, respiratory care, irrigations, and enteral feedings according to hospital policy
   13. initiate measures to prevent constipation (e.g. offer client a daily fiber supplement such as a mixture of bran, applesauce, and prune juice; encourage a minimum fluid intake of 2500 ml/day; administer laxatives as ordered) *in order to prevent damage to the bowel mucosa from hard stool*
   14. avoid unnecessary rectal invasion (e.g. temperature taking, enemas, suppositories, rectal tube) *to prevent trauma to rectal mucosa and possible abscess formation*
   15. perform actions to reduce stress and discomfort (see Nursing Diagnoses 1, action b; 4, action e; 5.A, action 2; and 5.B, action 2) *in order to prevent excessive secretion of cortisol (cortisol inhibits the immune response)*
   16. perform actions *to prevent stasis of respiratory secretions* (e.g. assist client to turn, cough, and deep breathe; increase activity as tolerated)
   17. perform actions to prevent urinary retention (e.g. instruct client to urinate when the urge is first felt, promote relaxation during voiding attempts) *in order to prevent urinary stasis*
   18. instruct and assist client to perform good perineal care routinely and after each bowel movement
   19. administer the following if ordered:
       a. antimicrobial agents (usually initiated when the neutropenic client becomes febrile or may be administered prophylactically if the neutrophil count is less than 500/mm^3)
       b. colony-stimulating factors (e.g. filgrastim) *to stimulate granulocyte production.*

12. COLLABORATIVE DIAGNOSES:

Potential complications of external radiation therapy:

a. **bleeding** related to thrombocytopenia associated with bone marrow suppression if large amounts of active bone marrow are included in the treatment field;

b. **radiation cystitis** related to irritation of the bladder mucosa (occurs after radiation exposure of the bladder to 3000–4000 cGy);

c. **radiation pneumonitis** related to inflammation of lung tissue resulting from radiation to the chest;

d. **lymphedema** related to damage to and subsequent obstruction of lymphatic vessels in the area being irradiated (seen most frequently in persons having radiation for breast cancer, melanoma in an upper or lower extremity, or gynecologic cancer or whole pelvic irradiation for prostate cancer).

Desired Outcomes	Nursing Actions and *Selected Purposes/Rationales*

12.a. The client will not experience unusual bleeding as evidenced by:

1. skin and mucous membranes free of petechiae, purpura, ecchymoses, and active bleeding
2. absence of unusual joint pain
3. no increase in abdominal girth
4. absence of frank and occult blood in stool, urine, and vomitus
5. usual menstrual flow
6. usual mental status
7. vital signs within normal range for client
8. stable or improved Hct and Hb.

12.a.1. Assess client for and report signs and symptoms of unusual bleeding:
   a. petechiae, purpura, or ecchymoses
   b. gingival bleeding
   c. prolonged bleeding from puncture sites
   d. epistaxis, hemoptysis
   e. unusual joint pain
   f. increase in abdominal girth
   g. frank or occult blood in stool, urine, or vomitus
   h. menorrhagia
   i. restlessness, confusion
   j. decreasing B/P and increased pulse rate
   k. decrease in Hct and Hb levels.

2. Monitor platelet count and coagulation test results (e.g. bleeding time). Report abnormal values.

3. If platelet count is low, coagulation test results are abnormal, or Hct and Hb levels decrease, test all stools, urine, and vomitus for occult blood. Report positive results.

4. Implement measures *to prevent bleeding*:
   a. avoid giving injections whenever possible; consult physician about prescribing an alternative route for medications ordered to be given intramuscularly or subcutaneously
   b. when giving injections or performing venous or arterial punctures, use the smallest gauge needle possible and apply gentle, prolonged pressure to the site after the needle is removed
   c. take B/P only when necessary and avoid overinflating the cuff
   d. caution client to avoid activities that increase the risk for trauma (e.g. shaving with a straight-edge razor, using stiff-bristle toothbrush or dental floss)
   e. whenever possible, avoid intubations (e.g. nasogastric) and procedures that can cause injury to rectal mucosa (e.g. taking temperature rectally, inserting a rectal suppository, administering an enema)
   f. pad side rails if client is confused or restless
   g. perform actions *to reduce the risk for falls* (e.g. keep bed in low position with side rails up when client is in bed, avoid unnecessary clutter in room, instruct client to wear slippers/shoes with nonslip soles when ambulating)
   h. instruct client to avoid blowing nose forcefully or straining to have a bowel movement; consult physician regarding an order for a decongestant and/or laxative if indicated
   i. administer the following if ordered:
      1. estrogen-progestin preparations *to suppress menses*
      2. platelets.

5. If bleeding occurs and does not subside spontaneously:
   a. apply firm, prolonged pressure to bleeding area(s) if possible
   b. if epistaxis occurs, place client in a high Fowler's position and apply pressure and ice pack to nasal area
   c. maintain oxygen therapy as ordered
   d. perform gastric lavage as ordered *to control gastric bleeding*
   e. administer whole blood or blood products (e.g. platelets) as ordered
   f. assess for and report signs and symptoms of hypovolemic shock (e.g. restlessness; confusion; significant decrease in B/P; rapid, weak pulse; rapid respirations; cool, pale skin; urine output less than 30 ml/hour)
   g. provide emotional support to client and significant others.

12.b. The client will experience resolution of radiation cystitis if it occurs as evidenced by:
1. reports of decreasing dysuria, urinary frequency and urgency, and suprapubic discomfort
2. absence of hematuria.

12.b.1. Assess for and report signs and symptoms of radiation cystitis (e.g. reports of dysuria, urinary frequency and/or urgency, or suprapubic discomfort; frank or occult blood in the urine). Symptoms of acute cystitis may appear 2–3 weeks after radiation therapy is initiated and persist for 1 month following the completion of treatment.
2. If signs and symptoms of radiation cystitis occur:
   a. implement measures *to reduce discomfort associated with cystitis:*
      1. encourage a minimum fluid intake of 2500 ml/day *to keep urine dilute and thereby reduce further irritation of the bladder lining*
      2. instruct client to avoid substances that can cause bladder irritation (e.g. caffeinated beverages, alcohol, tobacco, spicy foods)
      3. administer urinary tract analgesic/anesthetic agents (e.g. phenazopyridine) and antispasmodics (e.g. oxybutynin, flavoxate hydrochloride) if ordered
   b. assist with measures *to control bleeding* (e.g. continuous bladder irrigation with silver nitrate, cystoscopy to cauterize bleeding vessels, instillation of formalin into the bladder) if bleeding occurs and is persistent or severe.

12.c. The client will have improvement of radiation pneumonitis if it occurs as evidenced by:
1. decreased dyspnea and coughing
2. temperature declining toward normal
3. fewer reports of night sweats.

12.c.1. Assess for and report signs and symptoms of radiation pneumonitis (e.g. dyspnea, cough, fever, night sweats, finding of infiltrates on chest x-ray results).
2. If signs and symptoms of radiation pneumonitis occur:
   a. implement measures *to improve respiratory function:*
      1. instruct and assist client to turn, cough, and deep breathe every 1–2 hours
      2. reinforce correct use of incentive spirometer every 1–2 hours
      3. maintain oxygen therapy if ordered
      4. assist with positive airway pressure techniques (e.g. IPPB, continuous positive airway pressure [CPAP], biphasic positive airway pressure [BiPAP], expiratory positive airway pressure [EPAP]) if ordered
   b. administer the following medications if ordered:
      1. corticosteroids *to reduce pulmonary inflammation*
      2. bronchodilators
   c. consult physician if signs and symptoms of pneumonitis worsen or signs and symptoms of impaired gas exchange (e.g. restlessness, irritability, confusion, decreased PaO_2 and increased $PaCO_2$) develop.

12.d. The client will have decreasing signs and symptoms of lymphedema if it occurs as evidenced by:
1. decreased pain and feeling of heaviness and tightness in involved extremity
2. reduction in size of involved extremity

12.d.1. Assess extremities in or near the treatment field for signs and symptoms of lymphedema (e.g. pain or feeling of heaviness, fullness, or tightness in extremity; increase in size of extremity [determined by daily measurement of limb circumference]; sensory or motor deficits in extremity).
2. If signs and symptoms of lymphedema occur:
   a. elevate the involved extremity
   b. avoid use of involved extremity for B/P measurements, injections, and venipunctures
   c. apply a graded-pressure or sequential compression device to involved extremity if ordered

Desired Outcomes	Nursing Actions and *Selected Purposes/Rationales*

3. improved motor and sensory function in involved extremity.	d. encourage client to eat a well-balanced, protein-rich, low-sodium diet
	e. administer the following medications if ordered:
	   1. antimicrobial agents *to prevent or treat cellulitis and lymphangitis*
	   2. analgesics
	f. consult physician if signs and symptoms of lymphedema persist or worsen or if signs and symptoms of infection (e.g. redness or unusual warmth in extremity, fever) develop.

---

13. NURSING DIAGNOSIS: **Self-concept disturbance***

related to:

a. changes in appearance (e.g. temporary or permanent hair loss within the treatment field; skin changes such as erythema, uneven skin texture, or hyperpigmentation within the treatment field; excessive weight loss);

b. possible alteration in usual sexual activities associated with:
  1. fatigue, decreased levels of testosterone (if testes are in the treatment field), psychological factors, and vaginal and/or urethral discomfort (if the lower abdomen, pelvis, or perineal area is irradiated)
  2. temporary or permanent impotence resulting from psychological factors, decreased levels of testosterone (if testes are in the treatment field), and/or injury to pelvic nerves and blood vessels if included within the treatment field;

c. altered reproductive function:
  1. sterility associated with exposure of testes or ovaries to radiation
  2. potential for genetic mutations associated with sperm or ova chromosomal damage resulting from irradiation of the gonads (oophoropexy is frequently done in a woman of childbearing age to prevent ovarian exposure);

d. increased dependence on others to meet self-care needs;

e. changes in life style and roles associated with the effects of the disease process and its treatment.

---

*This diagnostic label includes the nursing diagnoses of body image disturbance, self-esteem disturbance, and altered role performance.

Desired Outcome	Nursing Actions and *Selected Purposes/Rationales*

13. The client will demonstrate beginning adaptation to changes in appearance, body functioning, life style, and roles as evidenced by:
  a. verbalization of feelings of self-worth and sexual adequacy
  b. maintenance of relationships with significant others
  c. active participation in activities of daily living
  d. verbalization of a beginning plan for adapting life style to changes resulting from
	13.a. Assess for signs and symptoms of a self-concept disturbance (e.g. verbalization of negative feelings about self, withdrawal from significant others, lack of participation in activities of daily living, lack of a plan for adapting to necessary changes in life style).
	b. Determine the meaning of the changes in appearance, body functioning, life style, and roles to the client by encouraging verbalization of feelings and by noting nonverbal responses to changes experienced.
	c. Implement measures to facilitate the grieving process (see Nursing Diagnosis 15, action b).
	d. Discuss with client improvements in appearance and functioning that can realistically be expected.
	e. Implement measures *to assist client to increase self-esteem* (e.g. limit negative self-assessment, encourage positive comments about self, assist to identify strengths, give positive feedback about accomplishments and behaviors that are indicative of high self-esteem).
	f. Reinforce actions to assist client to cope with effects of radiation therapy (see Nursing Diagnosis 14, action c).

the disease process and
the residual effects of
radiation therapy.

g. Implement measures *to assist client to adapt to the following changes in appearance and body functioning if appropriate:*
   1. alopecia:
      a. inform client that hair loss usually begins 2–3 weeks after initiation of therapy
      b. reassure client that regrowth of hair within the treatment field will occur within 2–3 months after cessation of therapy if the loss is temporary (temporary or patchy loss will usually occur with a radiation dose of 1500–3000 cGy; delayed hair growth or complete, permanent hair loss within the treatment field may result from a radiation exposure above 5000 cGy); explain that regrowth may be a different color, texture, and thickness
      c. instruct the client in ways *to minimize scalp hair loss if thinning or partial hair loss is anticipated:*
         1. brush and comb hair gently
         2. wash hair only when necessary and avoid harsh shampoo, cream rinse, and other hair care products
         3. do not use hair dryer, curling iron, curlers, or constrictive decorations (e.g. clips, rubber bands) on hair
      d. encourage the client to wear a wig, scarf, or turban if desired to conceal hair loss; contact the American Cancer Society for a wig if client is unable to obtain one but desires to do so
      e. encourage use of the wig before hair loss *to facilitate adjustment to wig and its integration into body image*; caution client to remove wig several times/day to allow for exposure of treatment area to the air
   2. skin changes within the treatment field:
      a. reinforce physician's explanation about skin changes that will occur and when they can be expected
      b. suggest possible clothing styles that will make changes in skin texture and pigmentation less obvious
   3. sterility or chromosomal damage:
      a. clarify physician's explanation about probable effects of radiation therapy on the gonads if they are in the treatment field
      b. discuss alternative methods of becoming a parent (e.g. artificial insemination, adoption) if of concern to client
   4. impotence:
      a. reinforce physician's explanation about the temporary or permanent nature of impotence; if it will be permanent, encourage client to discuss various treatment options (e.g. vacuum erection aids, penile prosthesis) with physician
      b. suggest alternative methods of sexual gratification if appropriate
      c. discuss ways to be creative in expressing sexuality (e.g. massage, fantasies, cuddling).
h. Assist client with usual grooming and makeup habits if necessary.
i. Support behaviors suggesting positive adaptation to changes that have occurred (e.g. interest in personal appearance, maintenance of relationships with significant others).
j. Encourage significant others to allow client to do what he/she is able *so that independence can be re-established and/or self-esteem redeveloped.*
k. Assist client's and significant others' adjustment by listening, facilitating communication, and providing information.
l. Encourage visits and support from significant others.
m. Encourage client to pursue usual roles and interests and to continue involvement in social activities. If previous roles, interests, and hobbies cannot be pursued, encourage development of new ones.
n. Provide information about and encourage use of community agencies and support groups (e.g. vocational rehabilitation; sexual, family, individual, and/or financial counseling).

Desired Outcome	Nursing Actions and *Selected Purposes/Rationales*
	o. Consult physician about psychological counseling if client desires or seems unwilling or unable to adapt to changes resulting from cancer and radiation therapy.

---

14. NURSING DIAGNOSIS: **Ineffective individual coping**

related to persistent discomfort associated with side effects of radiation therapy, chronic fatigue, fear, anxiety, uncertainty of the effectiveness of radiation therapy, and feeling of powerlessness.

Desired Outcome	Nursing Actions and *Selected Purposes/Rationales*

14. The client will demonstrate effective coping as evidenced by:
a. verbalization of ability to cope with the diagnosis of cancer and radiation therapy and its effects
b. use of appropriate problem-solving techniques
c. willingness to participate in treatment plan and meet basic needs
d. absence of destructive behavior toward self and others
e. appropriate use of defense mechanisms
f. use of available support systems.
	14.a. Assess for and report signs and symptoms of ineffective individual coping (e.g. verbalization of inability to cope; inability to ask for help, problem solve, or meet basic needs; insomnia; withdrawal; reluctance to participate in treatment plan; destructive behavior toward self or others; inappropriate use of defense mechanisms; inability to meet role expectations).
	b. Assess client's perception of current situation.
	c. Implement measures *to promote effective coping:*
	  1. allow time for client to begin to adjust to the diagnosis, radiation therapy and possible side effects, and anticipated changes in life style and roles
	  2. assist client to recognize and manage inappropriate denial if it is present
	  3. perform actions to reduce discomfort (see Nursing Diagnoses 4, action e; 5.A, action 2; and 5.B, action 2)
	  4. perform actions to reduce fear and anxiety (see Nursing Diagnosis 1, action b)
	  5. perform actions to reduce fatigue (see Nursing Diagnosis 8, action e)
	  6. encourage verbalization about current situation and ways comparable situations have been handled in the past
	  7. assist client to identify personal strengths and resources that can be used to facilitate coping with the current situation
	  8. demonstrate acceptance of client but set limits on inappropriate behavior
	  9. create an atmosphere of trust and support
	  10. arrange for a visit with another individual who has been successfully treated for cancer with radiation therapy
	  11. include client in planning of care, encourage maximum participation in treatment plan, and allow choices when possible *to enable him/ her to maintain a sense of control*
	  12. instruct client in effective problem-solving techniques (e.g. accurate identification of stressors, determination of various options to solve problem)
	  13. assist client to maintain usual daily routines whenever possible
	  14. assist client to identify priorities and attainable goals as he/she starts to plan for necessary life-style and role changes
	  15. assist client and significant others to identify ways that personal and family goals can be adjusted rather than abandoned
	  16. administer antianxiety and/or antidepressant agents if ordered
	  17. assist client to identify and use available support systems; provide information regarding available community resources that can assist client and significant others in coping with effects of radiation therapy and the diagnosis of cancer (e.g. American Cancer Society; support groups; individual, family, and/or financial counseling)

18. discuss any difficulties client may have in meeting the schedule for radiation treatments (usually 5 days/week for 3–8 weeks depending on site, dose, and desired therapeutic effect); refer to community agencies and/or support groups if transportation is a problem
19. encourage the client to share with significant others the kind of support that would be most beneficial (e.g. listening, inspiring hope, providing reassurance and accurate information)
20. support behaviors indicative of effective coping (e.g. compliance with treatment plan, maintenance of personal appearance, verbalization of the ability to cope, use of effective problem-solving strategies).
   d. Consult physician about psychological counseling if appropriate. Initiate a referral if necessary.

---

15. NURSING DIAGNOSIS: **Grieving***

related to:
a. changes in body image and usual life style and roles;
b. diagnosis of cancer with potential for premature death.

---

*This diagnostic label includes anticipatory grieving and grieving following the actual losses.

Desired Outcome	Nursing Actions and *Selected Purposes/Rationales*

15. The client will demonstrate beginning progression through the grieving process as evidenced by:
a. verbalization of feelings about the diagnosis of cancer and radiation therapy and its effects
b. usual sleep pattern
c. participation in treatment plan and self-care activities
d. use of available support systems
e. verbalization of a plan for integrating prescribed follow-up care into life style.
	15.a. Assess for signs and symptoms of grieving (e.g. change in eating habits, inability to concentrate, insomnia, anger, sadness, withdrawal from significant others, denial of losses).
	b. Implement measures *to facilitate the grieving process:*
	  1. assist client to acknowledge the losses *so grief work can begin*; assess for factors that may hinder and facilitate acknowledgment
	  2. discuss the grieving process and assist client to accept the phases of grieving as an expected response to actual and/or anticipated losses
	  3. allow time for client to progress through the phases of grieving (phases vary among theorists but progress from shock and alarm to acceptance); be aware that not every phase is expressed by all individuals, that recurrence of phases is common, and that the grieving process may take months to years
	  4. provide an atmosphere of care and concern (e.g. provide privacy, be available and nonjudgmental, display empathy and respect) *so client will feel free to express feelings*
	  5. perform actions *to promote trust* (e.g. answer questions honestly, provide requested information)
	  6. encourage the verbal expression of anger and sadness about the diagnosis and losses experienced; recognize displacement of anger and assist client to see the actual cause of angry feelings and resentment
	  7. encourage client to express feelings in whatever ways are comfortable (e.g. writing, drawing, conversation)
	  8. perform actions to promote effective coping (see Nursing Diagnosis 14, action c)
	  9. support realistic hope about the prognosis and the temporary nature of most of the changes in appearance
	  10. support behaviors suggesting successful grief work (e.g. verbalizing feelings about the diagnosis, expressing sorrow, focusing on ways to adapt to losses)
	  11. explain the phases of the grieving process to significant others; encourage their support and understanding

Desired Outcome	Nursing Actions and *Selected Purposes/Rationales*
	12. facilitate communication between the client and significant others; be aware that they may be in different phases of the grieving process 13. provide information regarding counseling services and support groups that might assist client in working through grief 14. when appropriate, assist client to meet spiritual needs (e.g. arrange for visit from clergy). c. Consult physician about referral for counseling if signs of dysfunctional grieving (e.g. persistent denial of losses, excessive anger or sadness, emotional lability) occur.

Discharge Teaching

▬▬▬▬▬▬▬▬▬▬▬▬▬▬▬▬▬▬▬▬▬▬▬▬▬▬▬▬▬▬▬▬▬▬▬▬▬

16. NURSING DIAGNOSIS: **Knowledge deficit, Ineffective management of therapeutic regimen, or Altered health maintenance***

*The nurse should select the diagnostic label that is most appropriate for the client's discharge teaching needs.

Desired Outcomes	Nursing Actions and *Selected Purposes/Rationales*

16.a. The client will verbalize an understanding of appropriate skin care for site of irradiation.	16.a.1. Reinforce teaching about the expected skin reaction at the site of irradiation (e.g. redness, tanned appearance, peeling, itching, loss of hair, decreased perspiration).
	2. Instruct the client to:
	  a. cleanse irradiated area gently using a mild soap and tepid water, being careful not to wash off skin markings
	  b. pat skin dry with a soft cotton towel
	  c. avoid rubbing, scratching, and massaging irradiated skin
	  d. relieve itching by:
	    1. applying cornstarch to area of dry desquamation
	    2. adding emollients, cornstarch, or baking soda to bath water
	  e. relieve dryness by applying a water-based lubricant lotion (e.g. Lubriderm, Eucerin)
	  f. avoid use of deodorant if treatment field includes axilla
	  g. check with physician before using cosmetics or perfumed lotions or creams in treatment area
	  h. protect irradiated skin from exposure to temperature extremes and wind
	  i. avoid exposure of treated area to direct sunlight during treatment period and for at least 1 month after therapy is complete (burns can occur easily because melanin production in new epidermal cells is slowed)
	  j. wear soft cotton garments next to treatment area; use a gentle detergent to launder clothing and add a mixture of vinegar and water (1 tsp vinegar per qt of water) to rinse water to neutralize the detergent residue
	  k. avoid wearing tight or constrictive clothing over irradiated area in order to reduce mechanical irritation
	  l. avoid shaving and using tape within treatment field; use an electric razor if shaving is absolutely necessary
	  m. care for a moist desquamation reaction by:
	    1. performing wound care and applying sterile dressings as prescribed (stretchable netting should be used instead of tape to hold dressings in place)
	    2. exposing area to the air as much as possible.
	3. Demonstrate care of treatment site.

4. Allow time for questions, clarification, and return demonstration of skin and wound care.

16.b. The client will identify techniques to control nausea and vomiting.

16.b. Instruct client in the following techniques to control nausea and vomiting:
1. cleanse mouth frequently
2. avoid offensive odors and sights
3. eat several small meals/day instead of 3 large ones
4. eat the largest meal 3–4 hours before treatments and eat lightly for at least 3–4 hours after a treatment
5. eat foods that are cool or at room temperature (hot foods frequently have an overpowering aroma that stimulates nausea)
6. eat dry foods (e.g. toast, crackers) or sip cold carbonated beverages if nausea is present
7. select bland foods (e.g. mashed potatoes, cottage cheese) rather than fatty, spicy foods (e.g. fried potatoes, chili)
8. if feasible, have someone else prepare the food
9. avoid drinking liquids with meals
10. rest after eating
11. take deep, slow breaths when nauseated
12. follow prescribed antiemetic regimen if nausea is persistent.

16.c. The client will verbalize ways to improve appetite and nutritional status.

16.c. Instruct client in ways to improve appetite and maintain an adequate nutritional status:
1. try chicken, fish, cheese, and eggs as protein sources instead of beef and pork if taste distortion is a problem
2. increase the amount of sweeteners and seasonings usually used in foods or beverages
3. cook foods in glass or plastic containers rather than metal ones, if possible, to help reduce the metallic taste of foods
4. moisten dry foods with sauces, salad dressing, or sour cream
5. eat in a pleasant environment with company if possible
6. perform frequent oral hygiene to eliminate disagreeable tastes in mouth
7. try recommended methods of controlling nausea (see action b in this diagnosis)
8. eat several high-calorie, high-protein, nutritious small meals/day rather than 3 large ones
9. take vitamins and minerals as prescribed.

16.d. The client will identify ways to reduce the risk of dental caries and periodontal disease and manage stomatitis if present.

16.d.1. Inform client that dental caries and periodontal disease can occur months to years after irradiation of the jaw, neck, or oral cavity. Emphasize that a meticulous daily oral hygiene program is essential, particularly if salivary flow is permanently reduced.
2. Instruct client in ways to reduce the risk of dental caries and periodontal disease:
a. use appropriate technique for cleansing teeth
b. brush teeth with a fluoridated toothpaste or fluoride gel several times a day for 3–4 minutes, particularly after eating
c. use a small, soft, flexible toothbrush to brush teeth
d. rinse with a topical fluoride solution after brushing.
3. If stomatitis is present, instruct client to:
a. irrigate mouth and cleanse teeth frequently with a gentle power spray using a salt water solution or water instead of brushing
b. rinse mouth every 4 hours with a baking soda and water solution followed by a thorough rinsing with salt water if tenacious mucus, crusting, and/or debris are present
c. consult physician about use of preparations to soothe the oral mucous membrane (e.g. diphenhydramine and water mixture) if mouth is painful
d. wear dentures only at mealtime
e. eat soft, bland foods and avoid substances that might further irritate the mouth (e.g. extremely hot, spicy, or acidic foods/fluids).

Desired Outcomes	Nursing Actions and *Selected Purposes/Rationales*
	4. Allow time for questions, clarification, and practice of oral hygiene techniques.
	5. Instruct client to discuss any planned dental care with the radiologist and to inform the dentist that he/she is receiving or has had radiation to the oral cavity.

16.e. The client will identify ways to prevent bleeding if platelet counts are low.	16.e.1. Instruct client in ways to minimize the risk of bleeding:
	   a. avoid taking aspirin and other nonsteroidal anti-inflammatory agents (e.g. ibuprofen) on a regular basis
	   b. use an electric rather than a straight-edge razor
	   c. floss and brush teeth gently
	   d. cut nails and cuticles carefully
	   e. use caution when ambulating to prevent falls or bumps and do not walk barefoot
	   f. avoid blowing nose forcefully
	   g. avoid situations that could result in injury (e.g. contact sports)
	   h. avoid straining to have a bowel movement
	   i. avoid wearing constrictive clothing (e.g. garters, knee-high stockings)
	   j. avoid putting sharp objects (e.g. toothpicks) in mouth
	   k. use an ample amount of water-soluble lubricant prior to sexual intercourse and avoid anal sexual activity, douching, use of rectal suppositories, and enemas in order to prevent trauma to the vaginal and rectal mucosa
	   l. avoid heavy lifting.
	2. Instruct client to control any bleeding by applying firm, prolonged pressure to the area(s) if possible.

16.f. The client will identify ways to prevent infection if WBC counts are low.	16.f.1. Explain to client that his/her resistance to infection is reduced when WBC counts are low. Emphasize the need to adhere closely to recommended techniques to prevent infection.
	2. Instruct client in ways to prevent infection:
	   a. avoid crowds, persons with any sign of infection, and persons who have recently been vaccinated
	   b. avoid trauma to the skin and mucous membranes
	   c. take an axillary rather than an oral temperature if stomatitis is present
	   d. lubricate the skin outside irradiated area frequently to prevent dryness and subsequent cracking
	   e. cleanse and care for skin within treatment field as recommended (see action a.2 in this diagnosis)
	   f. use excellent handwashing technique
	   g. avoid unnecessary rectal invasion (e.g. temperature taking, enemas, suppositories, sexual activity) to prevent trauma to the rectal mucosa
	   h. avoid constipation to prevent trauma to the bowel mucosa from hard or impacted stool
	   i. wash perianal area thoroughly with soap and water after each bowel movement; inform female client to always wipe from front to back after defecating and urinating
	   j. avoid douching unless ordered (douching disturbs the normal vaginal flora and may cause trauma to the vaginal mucosa)
	   k. drink at least 10 glasses of liquid/day unless contraindicated
	   l. cough and deep breathe or use incentive spirometer every 2 hours until usual activity level is resumed
	   m. stop smoking
	   n. perform meticulous oral hygiene after meals and at bedtime or more often if directed
	   o. maintain an optimal nutritional status (e.g. diet high in protein, calories, vitamins, and minerals)
	   p. avoid intake of foods with a high microorganism content (e.g. unwashed fresh fruits and vegetables; undercooked meat, poultry, or seafood)

q. avoid sharing eating utensils

r. maintain an adequate balance between activity and rest.

16.g. The client will verbalize an understanding of and ways to manage the effects of radiation therapy on sexual and reproductive functioning.

16.g.1. Clarify physician's explanation about the possible effects of irradiation on the gonads if included in the treatment field.

2. Explain that a temporary decrease in libido may occur as a result of radiation treatment.

3. Encourage client to rest before sexual activity if fatigue is a problem.

4. Instruct client in measures to reduce discomfort associated with decreased vaginal secretions and mucositis:

a. use an ample amount of water-soluble lubricant to prevent trauma to the vaginal mucosa and increase lubrication during intercourse

b. use a vaginal steroid cream, if prescribed, to ease dryness and inflammation

c. avoid intercourse until mucositis of the vaginal canal and/or urethra resolves

d. have male partner use a condom during intercourse to prevent contact of vaginal area with semen (semen can cause a burning sensation in the early months after vaginal irradiation).

5. Emphasize the need for frequent intercourse or vaginal dilatation once mucositis has resolved to prevent stenosis of the vaginal canal (stenosis may develop several weeks or months after cessation of treatment that includes the vaginal area).

6. Explain to the female client that ovarian failure during therapy may result in decreased libido, irritability, hot flashes, and other symptoms of premature menopause.

7. Inform the female client that her usual menstrual cycle will resume within 6 months to 1 year after treatment if sterility is temporary.

8. Emphasize the need for both male and female clients to practice birth control during treatment and for at least 2 years after it. Encourage both male and female clients to seek genetic counseling before attempting conception to ascertain the risk of chromosomal anomalies.

9. Instruct client to take hormone replacements (e.g. estrogen, testosterone) as prescribed.

16.h. The client will verbalize ways to manage and cope with persistent fatigue.

16.h. Instruct client in ways to manage and cope with persistent fatigue:

1. view fatigue as a protective mechanism rather than a problematic limitation

2. determine ways that daily patterns of activity can be modified to conserve energy and prevent excessive fatigue (e.g. spread light and heavy tasks throughout the day, take short rests during an activity whenever possible, take several short rest periods during the day instead of one long one)

3. determine whether life demands are realistic in light of physical state and adjust short- and long-term goals accordingly

4. avoid situations that are particularly fatiguing such as those that are boring, frustrating, or require prolonged or strenuous physical activity

5. participate in a regular aerobic exercise program that is approved by physician to improve cardiovascular and respiratory fitness, reduce anxiety and stress, and build up tolerance for activity.

16.i. The client will verbalize an understanding of the signs and symptoms of lymphedema and ways to manage it if it occurs.

16.i.1. Instruct the client at risk for lymphedema (e.g. person receiving radiation for breast cancer, melanoma in an extremity, or gynecologic cancer; person receiving whole pelvic irradiation for prostate cancer) to:

a. monitor for and report signs and symptoms of lymphedema (e.g. pain or a feeling of heaviness or tightness in involved extremity)

b. measure the circumference of involved arm or leg daily if the extremity appears swollen and report a sudden increase in size to the physician.

2. Provide the following instructions about ways to manage lymphedema if it occurs:

a. avoid wearing items that put pressure on the involved extremity (e.g. tight jewelry, clothes with constricting bands, elastic stockings with constricting bands)

Desired Outcomes	Nursing Actions and *Selected Purposes/Rationales*
	b. keep involved extremity elevated as much as possible c. avoid injury to the involved extremity (e.g. do not allow finger sticks or venipunctures in involved extremity, use an electric rather than straight-edge razor when shaving involved extremity, wear gardening and cooking gloves and use a thimble for sewing if upper extremity is affected, do not walk barefoot if lower extremity is affected, do not cut cuticles on hand or foot of involved extremity).

16.j. The client will state signs and symptoms to report to the health care provider.	16.j. Instruct the client to observe for and report the following:
	  1. signs and symptoms of infection (stress that the usual signs of infection are diminished in people with a suppressed immune system and that it is necessary to monitor closely for the following signs and symptoms):
	    a. temperature above 38° C (100.4° F)
	    b. changes in odor, color, or consistency of urine or pain on urination
	    c. white patches in mouth
	    d. crusted ulcerations around or in oral cavity
	    e. swollen, reddened, coated tongue
	    f. painful rectal or vaginal area
	    g. unusual vaginal drainage
	    h. persistent or productive cough
	    i. redness, heat, swelling, or unusual drainage in any area, particularly site being irradiated or venipuncture sites
	  2. signs and symptoms of bleeding (e.g. excessive bruising, black stools, persistent nosebleeds or bleeding from gums, sudden swelling in joints, red or smoke-colored urine, blood in vomitus)
	  3. signs and symptoms of radiation cystitis (e.g. blood in the urine, pain on urination, urinary frequency or urgency)
	  4. signs and symptoms of radiation pneumonitis (e.g. shortness of breath, persistent cough, night sweats, fever); radiation pneumonitis can occur 2–3 months after cessation of treatment depending on total dose of radiation received, fractionation of dose, and volume of lung tissue within the treatment field
	  5. signs and symptoms of tissue fibrosis within treatment field (e.g. LUNG: increasing shortness of breath, cough; BOWEL: inability to move bowels, distended abdomen, loss of appetite, alternating diarrhea and constipation; ESOPHAGUS: difficulty swallowing; SKIN: uneven texture; VAGINA: pain during intercourse)
	  6. excessive tooth decay
	  7. signs and symptoms of dehydration (e.g. dry mouth, significant weight loss, concentrated urine, persistent thirst)
	  8. persistent nausea, vomiting, or decreased oral intake
	  9. significant weight loss
	  10. persistent diarrhea
	  11. excessive depression or difficulty coping with the effects of the diagnosis and treatment.

16.k. The client will identify community resources that can assist with home management and adjustment to the diagnosis of cancer and radiation therapy and its effects.	16.k.1. Provide information about and encourage use of community resources that can assist the client and significant others with home management and adjustment to cancer and the effects of radiation therapy (e.g. local support groups, American Cancer Society, home health agencies, counselors, social service agencies, Meals on Wheels, Make Today Count, Hospice). 2. Initiate a referral if indicated.

16.l. The client will verbalize an understanding of and a plan for adhering to recommended follow-up care including medications prescribed and future appointments	16.l.1. Explain the rationale for, side effects of, and importance of taking medications prescribed. Inform client of pertinent food and drug interactions.
	  2. Reinforce physician's explanation of planned radiation therapy schedule.
	  3. Discuss with client any difficulties he/she might have adhering to the schedule and assist in planning ways to overcome these.

with health care provider, radiation department, and laboratory.

4. Reinforce the importance of keeping appointments for radiation treatments and follow-up laboratory studies.
5. Reinforce the importance of keeping follow-up appointments with health care provider.
6. Implement measures to improve client compliance:
   a. include significant others in teaching sessions
   b. encourage questions and allow time for reinforcement and clarification of information provided
   c. provide written instructions regarding future appointments with health care provider, radiation department, and laboratory; medications prescribed; and signs and symptoms to report.

Bibliography

See pages 897–898 and 900–901.

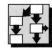

UNIT EIGHT

NURSING CARE OF THE CLIENT WITH DISTURBANCES OF NEUROLOGICAL FUNCTION

CEREBROVASCULAR ACCIDENT

A cerebrovascular accident (CVA), or stroke, is the result of an interruption in the blood supply to certain areas of the brain and is characterized by the sudden development of focal neurological deficits that last for at least 24 hours. These deficits range from mild symptoms such as tingling, weakness, and slight speech impairment to more severe symptoms such as hemiplegia, aphasia, dysphagia, loss of portions of visual field, spatial-perceptual changes, altered cognitive function, and loss of consciousness. Clinical manifestations depend on factors such as the area(s) of the brain affected, the adequacy of collateral cerebral circulation, and the extensiveness of subsequent cerebral edema.

Cerebrovascular accidents are classified according to etiology. The most common cause of a CVA is a thrombosis that is associated with atherosclerosis. Other causes include an embolus, cerebral hemorrhage (which is often associated with extreme hypertension or a cerebral an-eurysm), and cerebral hypoperfusion associated with hypotension. Treatment following a CVA is determined by the etiology and the neurological deficits that are present.

This care plan focuses on the adult client hospitalized with signs and symptoms of a CVA. During the acute phase, the goals of care are to improve cerebral tissue perfusion, prevent life-threatening complications, and perform or assist the client with those activities he/she is unable to accomplish independently. When the client's condition stabilizes, goals of care are to prevent complications of immobility and assist the client to attain an optimal level of functioning. This care plan focuses on the more common problems that occur as a result of a CVA. The reader should refer to neurological texts for additional information about specific speech, motor, and sensory deficits that can occur.

DIAGNOSTIC TESTS

Computed tomography (CT)
Magnetic resonance imaging (MRI)
Cerebral vessel and transcranial ultrasound
Electroencephalogram (EEG)
Cerebral angiography
Positron emission tomography (PET)

DISCHARGE CRITERIA

Prior to discharge, the client will:

- have improved cerebral tissue perfusion
- have improved or stable neurological function
- have an adequate nutritional status
- have clear, audible breath sounds throughout lungs
- have no evidence of tissue irritation or breakdown
- experience optimal control of urinary and bowel elimination
- have no signs or symptoms of complications
- communicate an awareness of ways to decrease the risk of a recurrent CVA
- identify ways to manage sensory and verbal communication impairments and altered thought processes
- identify ways to manage urinary and bowel incontinence
- demonstrate measures to facilitate the performance of activities of daily living and increase physical mobility
- communicate an awareness of signs and symptoms to report to the health care provider
- share thoughts and feelings about the effects of the CVA on life style, roles, and self-concept
- communicate knowledge of community resources that can assist with home management and adjustment to changes resulting from the CVA
- communicate an understanding of and a plan for adhering to recommended follow-up care including future appointments with health care provider and therapists and medications prescribed.

Use in conjunction with the Care Plan on Immobility.

NURSING/ COLLABORATIVE DIAGNOSES	**1.** Altered cerebral tissue perfusion △ 231
	2. Altered nutrition: less than body requirements △ 232
	3. Impaired swallowing △ 232
	4. Sensory/perceptual alterations:
	a. visual
	b. kinesthetic △ 233
	5. Unilateral neglect △ 234
	6. Impaired verbal communication △ 235
	7. Impaired physical mobility △ 236
	8. Self-care deficit △ 236
	9. Altered urinary elimination: incontinence △ 237
	10. Constipation △ 238
	11. Bowel incontinence △ 238
	12. Altered thought processes △ 239
	13. Risk for infection: pneumonia △ 240
	14. Risk for trauma: falls, burns, and lacerations △ 240
	15. Risk for aspiration △ 242
	16. Potential complications:
	a. increased intracranial pressure (IICP)
	b. corneal irritation and abrasion
	c. subluxation of shoulder △ 243
	17. Sexual dysfunction △ 245
	18. Anxiety △ 245
	19. Self-concept disturbance △ 246
	20. Ineffective individual coping △ 247
	21. Grieving △ 248
	22. Altered family processes △ 249
DISCHARGE TEACHING	**23.** Knowledge deficit, Ineffective management of therapeutic regimen, or Altered health maintenance △ 250

See Care Plan on Immobility for additional diagnoses.

---

1. NURSING DIAGNOSIS:

Altered cerebral tissue perfusion

related to decreased cerebral blood flow associated with thrombus, embolus, cerebral hemorrhage, hypotension, and/or subsequent spasm or compression of cerebral vessel(s).

Desired Outcome	Nursing Actions and *Selected Purposes/Rationales*
1. The client will experience improved cerebral tissue perfusion as evidenced by: a. absence of or reduction in dizziness, visual disturbances, and speech impairments b. improved mental status c. improved sensory and motor function.	1.a. Assess the client for signs and symptoms of decreased cerebral tissue perfusion: 1. dizziness 2. visual disturbances (e.g. blurred or dimmed vision, diplopia, change in visual field) 3. aphasia 4. irritability and restlessness 5. decreased level of consciousness 6. paresthesias, weakness, paralysis. b. Implement measures *to improve cerebral tissue perfusion:* 1. if a thrombus or embolus is present: a. assist with administration of a thrombolytic agent (e.g. tissue plasminogen activator [tPA]) if ordered b. administer anticoagulants (e.g. heparin, warfarin) or platelet aggregation inhibitors (e.g. aspirin, ticlopidine) if ordered

Desired Outcome	Nursing Actions and *Selected Purposes/Rationales*
	2. if intracerebral hemorrhage occurred as a result of cerebral aneurysm rupture, administer a hemostatic agent (e.g. aminocaproic acid) if ordered *to prevent the lysis of formed clots and subsequent rebleeding* 3. if intracerebral hemorrhage occurred as a result of extreme hypertension, perform actions *to control high blood pressure* (e.g. administer prescribed antihypertensive agents, reduce stress) 4. if client is hypotensive, perform actions *to improve cerebral blood flow* (e.g. administer prescribed sympathomimetic agents, maintain intravenous fluid therapy as ordered) 5. administer calcium-channel blockers (e.g. nimodipine) if ordered *to reduce cerebral vasospasm* (*the calcium that is released by the injured neural cells can cause vasospasm*) 6. perform actions to prevent and treat increased intracranial pressure (see Collaborative Diagnosis 16, actions a.2 and 3) 7. prepare client for surgery (e.g. evacuation of hematoma, repair of ruptured aneurysm) if planned. c. Consult physician if signs and symptoms of decreased cerebral tissue perfusion worsen.

■━━

2. NURSING DIAGNOSIS: **Altered nutrition: less than body requirements**

related to decreased oral intake associated with:
a. anorexia resulting from fear, anxiety, depression, and early satiety that occurs with decreased gastrointestinal motility (can result from decreased activity and anxiety);
b. difficulty feeding self as a result of impaired motor function of the affected arm, visual impairments, and/or spatial-perceptual difficulties;
c. difficulty chewing resulting from weakness or paralysis of the muscles of mastication on the affected side;
d. dysphagia.

Desired Outcome	Nursing Actions and *Selected Purposes/Rationales*
2. The client will maintain an adequate nutritional status (see Care Plan on Immobility, Nursing Diagnosis 3 [p. 128], for outcome criteria).	2.a. Refer to Care Plan on Immobility, Nursing Diagnosis 3 (pp. 128–129), for measures related to assessment and maintenance of an adequate nutritional status. b. Implement additional measures *to improve oral intake and maintain an adequate nutritional status:* 1. perform actions to reduce fear and anxiety (see Nursing Diagnosis 18, actions b and c) 2. perform actions to facilitate client's psychological adjustment to the effects of the CVA (see Nursing Diagnoses 19; 20, action c; and 21, action b) 3. perform actions to improve ability to swallow (see Nursing Diagnosis 3, action c) 4. perform actions to enable client to feed self (see Nursing Diagnosis 8, action b.3).

■━━

3. NURSING DIAGNOSIS: **Impaired swallowing**

related to weakness or paralysis of the swallowing muscles on the affected side and diminished or absent swallowing reflex.

Desired Outcome	Nursing Actions and *Selected Purposes/Rationales*

3. The client will experience an improvement in swallowing as evidenced by:
a. communication of same
b. absence of food in oral cavity after swallowing
c. absence of coughing and choking when eating and drinking.
	3.a. Assess for signs and symptoms of impaired swallowing (e.g. communication of difficulty swallowing, stasis of food in oral cavity, coughing or choking when eating or drinking).
	b. Assist with studies that evaluate client's ability to swallow (e.g. videofluoroscopy, manometry) if indicated.
	c. Implement measures *to improve ability to swallow:*
	  1. place client in high Fowler's position for meals and snacks; head and neck should be tilted forward slightly *to facilitate elevation of the larynx and posterior movement of the tongue*
	  2. assist client to select foods that require little or no chewing and are easily swallowed (e.g. custard, eggs, canned fruit, mashed potatoes)
	  3. instruct client to avoid mixing foods of different texture in his/her mouth at the same time
	  4. avoid serving foods that are sticky (e.g. peanut butter, soft bread, honey)
	  5. serve foods/fluids that are hot or cold instead of room temperature (*the more extreme temperatures stimulate the sensory receptors and swallowing reflex*)
	  6. serve thick rather than thin fluids or add a thickening agent (e.g. "Thick-it," gelatin, baby cereal) to thin fluids
	  7. moisten dry foods with gravy or sauces (e.g. catsup, salad dressing, sour cream)
	  8. utilize assistive devices (e.g. long-handled spoon) to place food that does not need to be chewed (e.g. gelatin, mashed potatoes, custard) in the back of mouth on unaffected side if tongue movement is impaired
	  9. instruct client to avoid putting too much food/fluid in mouth at one time
	  10. encourage client to concentrate on the act of swallowing
	  11. if client has decreased lip control, instruct him/her to gently hold lips closed with fingers after putting food in mouth
	  12. gently stroke client's throat when he/she is swallowing if indicated
	  13. consult speech pathologist or therapist about methods for dealing with impaired swallowing; reinforce recommended exercises and techniques.
	d. Consult physician if swallowing difficulties persist or worsen.

---

4. NURSING DIAGNOSIS:

Sensory/perceptual alterations:

a. **visual** related to ischemia of portions of the visual pathways in the occipital lobe and the parieto-occipitotemporal interpretative (association) area;
b. **kinesthetic** related to visual deficits and ischemia of portions of the parietal lobe (primarily of the nondominant hemisphere) and the cerebellum.

Desired Outcome	Nursing Actions and *Selected Purposes/Rationales*

4. The client will experience a reduction in and/or demonstrate beginning adaptation to sensory/perceptual alterations as evidenced by:
a. communication of same
b. increased participation in activities.
	4.a. Assess for signs and symptoms of:
	  1. visual impairments such as homonymous hemianopsia and/or diplopia (e.g. lack of response to visual stimuli on side of hemiplegia, reports of double vision, decreased participation in activities)
	  2. kinesthetic impairment (e.g. difficulty maintaining balance, determining body position, buttoning clothing, or locating mouth when trying to feed self; decreased participation in activities).
	b. Implement measures to improve cerebral tissue perfusion (see Nursing Diagnosis 1, action b) *in order to reduce cerebral ischemia.*

Desired Outcome	Nursing Actions and **Selected Purposes/Rationales**

	c. Implement measures *to assist client to adapt to changes in visual and/or kinesthetic functioning:*
	1. provide an eyepatch or opaque lens for client to wear if diplopia is present
	2. if client is experiencing homonymous hemianopsia:
	   a. perform actions *to decrease the risk of startling client* (e.g. approach client from unaffected side whenever possible, verbally acknowledge client before touching him/her if approaching on affected side)
	   b. perform actions *to ensure client receives visual stimuli* (e.g. position client's bed and chair so that window or door to hall rather than blank wall is within visual field, instruct visitors to sit or stand on client's unaffected side)
	   c. after condition has stabilized, place some items (e.g. television, clock, calendar, pictures) on affected side *to promote environmental scanning*
	3. if client is experiencing kinesthetic impairments, place him/her in front of a full-length mirror during activities when possible after condition has stabilized (*viewing his/her reflection may help the client to identify body position and vertical and horizontal planes*)
	4. perform actions to facilitate performance of self-care activities (see Nursing Diagnosis 8, actions b.3 and 4)
	5. consult physical and occupational therapists about additional ways to facilitate client's adaptation to sensory/perceptual impairments
	6. inform significant others and health care personnel of approaches being used to increase client's awareness of affected side; encourage their use of these techniques.
	d. Consult physician if sensory/perceptual alterations worsen or client is unable to adapt to the ones he/she is experiencing.

---

5. NURSING DIAGNOSIS: **Unilateral neglect**

related to ischemia of portions of the brain (primarily the parietal lobe of the nondominant cerebral hemisphere).

Desired Outcome	Nursing Actions and **Selected Purposes/Rationales**

5. The client will experience a gradual reduction in and/or demonstrate beginning adaptation to unilateral neglect as evidenced by:
a. awareness of stimuli on affected side
b. awareness of the affected side of body.
	5.a. Assess client for presence of unilateral neglect (e.g. not looking toward affected side, no response to stimuli on affected side, lack of awareness of affected extremities).
	b. Implement measures to improve cerebral tissue perfusion (see Nursing Diagnosis 1, action b) *in order to reduce cerebral ischemia.*
	c. If unilateral neglect is present:
	1. ensure that affected extremities are positioned properly at all times
	2. protect affected extremities from injury
	3. after client's condition stabilizes, implement measures *to increase client's awareness of affected side:*
	   a. encourage client to handle affected extremities when bathing, dressing, and repositioning self
	   b. place some items (e.g. television, clock, calendar, pictures) on affected side *to increase the likelihood of the client viewing his/her affected extremities*
	   c. place familiar items (e.g. favorite bracelet or watch, frequently worn shoe or slipper) on affected extremities *to assist client to recognize that the extremities are a part of his/her body*

4. consult physical and occupational therapists about additional ways to facilitate client's adaptation to unilateral neglect
5. inform significant others and health care personnel of approaches being used to increase client's awareness of affected side; encourage their use of these techniques
6. consult physician if client is unable to begin to adapt to unilateral neglect.

---

6. NURSING DIAGNOSIS: **Impaired verbal communication**

related to:
a. impaired function of the muscles that are used to produce speech;
b. ischemia in the dominant cerebral hemisphere (ischemia of Wernicke's area in the temporoparietal cortex will result in receptive aphasia; ischemia of Broca's area in the frontal cortex will result in expressive aphasia).

Desired Outcome	Nursing Actions and *Selected Purposes/Rationales*
6. The client will communicate needs and desires effectively.	6.a. Assess client for impaired verbal communication (e.g. inability to speak, difficulty forming words or sentences, difficulty expressing thoughts verbally, inappropriate verbalization). Validate verbal responses with an assessment of nonverbal behavior *in order to determine if client is experiencing receptive aphasia.*

b. Implement measures *to facilitate communication:*
1. answer call signal in person rather than using the intercommunication system
2. maintain a patient, calm approach; listen attentively and allow ample time for communication
3. maintain a calm, quiet environment *so that client can concentrate on communication efforts, does not have to speak loudly, and is able to hear others clearly*
4. ask questions that require short answers, eyeblinks, or nod of head if client is having difficulty speaking and/or is frustrated or fatigued
5. schedule rest periods before visiting hours and speech therapy sessions *to maximize communication ability during those times*
6. when speaking to client, face him/her; speak slowly; use direct, short statements; repeat key words; and avoid using unrelated gestures
7. provide materials such as magic slate, pad and pencil, word cards, and/or picture board if appropriate; try to ensure that placement of intravenous line does not interfere with client's use of these communication aids
8. consult speech pathologist or therapist regarding methods for dealing with speech impairments; reinforce exercises and techniques recommended.
c. Inform significant others and health care personnel of techniques being used to facilitate client's ability to communicate. Stress the importance of consistent use of these techniques.
d. Encourage significant others and staff to talk to client even if he/she is unresponsive or unable to communicate.
e. Consult physician if client experiences increasing impairment of verbal communication.

7. NURSING DIAGNOSIS: **Impaired physical mobility**

related to:
a. activity limitations associated with decreased motor function and spatial-perceptual impairments;
b. loss of muscle tone during period of flaccidity of affected extremities (flaccid paralysis may be present during the first few days following a CVA);
c. hypertonia of affected extremities (as muscle tone returns after period of flaccidity, it often progresses to spasticity);
d. reluctance to move associated with fear of injuring self (occurs mainly with ischemia of the dominant hemisphere);
e. loss of muscle mass, tone, and strength associated with prolonged disuse and inadequate nutritional status.

Desired Outcome	Nursing Actions and *Selected Purposes/Rationales*

7. The client will achieve maximum physical mobility within limitations imposed by the CVA.	7.a. Refer to Care Plan on Immobility, Nursing Diagnosis 6 (pp. 131–132), for measures related to ways to maintain optimal joint mobility and muscle function in order to increase mobility.
	b. Implement additional measures *to increase mobility:*
	1. provide adequate rest periods before activity sessions
	2. administer muscle relaxants (e.g. baclofen, dantrolene) if ordered *to relieve spasticity in affected extremities*
	3. perform actions to prevent falls (see Nursing Diagnosis 14, action a.1) *in order to decrease client's fear of injury*
	4. instruct client in and assist with use of mobility aids (e.g. cane, walker) if appropriate
	5. after client's condition has stabilized, assist with and reinforce the following if appropriate:
	  a. neurodevelopmental treatment (e.g. Bobath approach) *to promote more normal movement of the affected extremities*
	  b. neuromuscular re-education techniques (e.g. electromyographic biofeedback) *to improve muscle strength and reduce spasticity of the affected extremities*
	6. perform actions to maintain an adequate nutritional status (see Nursing Diagnosis 2) *in order to help maintain muscle mass, tone, and strength.*
	c. Provide praise and encouragement for all efforts to increase physical mobility.
	d. Encourage the support of significant others. Allow them to assist with range of motion exercises, positioning, and activity if desired.
	e. Consult physician if client is unable to achieve expected level of mobility or if range of motion becomes restricted.

8. NURSING DIAGNOSIS: **Self-care deficit**

related to impaired physical mobility, visual and spatial-perceptual impairments, apraxia, unilateral neglect, and altered thought processes.

Desired Outcome	Nursing Actions and *Selected Purposes/Rationales*
8. The client will perform self-care activities within	8.a. Refer to Care Plan on Immobility, Nursing Diagnosis 7 (p. 132), for measures to facilitate client's ability to perform self-care activities.

cognitive and physical limitations.

 b. Implement additional measures *to facilitate client's ability to perform self-care activities:*
  1. if apraxia is present, explain and demonstrate use of items such as toothbrush, comb, and washcloth as often as necessary
  2. encourage client to wear eyepatch or opaque lens if diplopia is present
  3. perform actions *to enable client to feed self:*
   a. place foods/fluids within client's visual field until he/she learns to effectively utilize scanning techniques
   b. place only a few items on the tray at one time if spatial-perceptual deficits are present
   c. identify where items are placed on the plate and tray and open containers, cut meat, and butter bread as indicated
   d. consult with occupational therapist about assistive devices available (e.g. broad-handled utensils, rocker knife, nonslip tray mat, plate guard); reinforce use of these devices
  4. perform actions *to enable client to dress self:*
   a. encourage use of assistive devices such as button hooks, long-handled shoehorns, and pull loops for pants
   b. encourage client to select clothing that is easy to put on and remove (e.g. clothing with zippers rather than buttons, loose-fitting clothing, shoes with Velcro fasteners or elastic laces)
   c. if client has difficulty distinguishing right from left, mark outer aspect of shoes with tape
  5. perform actions to increase mobility (see Nursing Diagnosis 7) *in order to further facilitate the client's ability to perform self-care activities*
  6. reinforce exercises and activities recommended by the occupational therapist to improve fine motor skills.
 c. After client's condition stabilizes, encourage him/her to perform as much of self-care as possible. Provide positive feedback for all efforts and accomplishments of self-care.
 d. Assist the client with activities he/she is unable to perform independently.
 e. Inform significant others of client's abilities to perform own care. Explain importance of encouraging and allowing client to maintain an optimal level of independence.

---

9. NURSING DIAGNOSIS:

Altered urinary elimination: incontinence

related to:
a. increased reflex activity of the bladder and loss of voluntary control of urinary elimination associated with upper motor neuron involvement if it has occurred;
b. decreased ability to control urination associated with decreased level of consciousness or inability to recognize sensation of bladder fullness;
c. inability to get to bedside commode or bathroom in a timely manner associated with:
 1. delay in obtaining assistance resulting from inability to communicate the urge to urinate
 2. impaired physical mobility.

Desired Outcome	Nursing Actions and *Selected Purposes/Rationales*
9. The client will experience urinary continence.	9.a. Assess for and report urinary incontinence. b. Monitor client's pattern of fluid intake and urination (e.g. times and amounts of fluid intake, types of fluids consumed, times and amounts of

Desired Outcome	Nursing Actions and *Selected Purposes/Rationales*
	voluntary and involuntary voiding, reports of sensation of need to void, activities preceding incontinence).

c. Implement measures *to reduce the risk of urinary incontinence:*
   1. offer bedpan or urinal or assist client to bedside commode or bathroom every 2–3 hours
   2. allow client to assume a normal position for voiding unless contraindicated *in order to promote complete bladder emptying*
   3. perform actions *to reduce delays in toileting* (e.g. have call signal within client's reach and respond promptly to requests for assistance; have bedpan, urinal, or bedside commode readily available to client; provide client with easy-to-remove clothing such as pajamas with Velcro closures or an elastic waistband)
   4. if client is aphasic, establish an effective method for him/her to communicate the urge to urinate
   5. instruct client to space fluids evenly throughout the day rather than drinking a large quantity at one time (*rapid filling of bladder can result in incontinence if client has decreased urinary sphincter control*)
   6. limit oral fluid intake in the evening *to decrease possibility of nighttime incontinence*
   7. instruct client to avoid drinking beverages containing caffeine (*caffeine is a mild diuretic and a bladder irritant; both effects may make urinary control more difficult*).

d. If urinary incontinence persists, consult physician about intermittent catheterization, insertion of indwelling catheter, or use of external catheter.

---

10. NURSING DIAGNOSIS: Constipation

related to:
a. decreased gastrointestinal motility associated with decreased activity and the increased sympathetic nervous system activity that occurs with anxiety;
b. decreased intake of fluids and foods high in fiber associated with difficulty feeding self, chewing, and swallowing;
c. failure to respond to the urge to defecate associated with decreased level of consciousness or inability to recognize sensation of rectal fullness;
d. weakened abdominal muscles associated with generalized loss of muscle tone resulting from prolonged immobility.

Desired Outcome	Nursing Actions and *Selected Purposes/Rationales*

10. The client will not experience constipation (see Care Plan on Immobility, Nursing Diagnosis 9 [pp. 133–134], for outcome criteria).	10.a. Refer to Care Plan on Immobility, Nursing Diagnosis 9 (pp. 133–134), for measures related to assessment, prevention, and management of constipation.
	b. Implement additional measures *to prevent constipation:*
	  1. perform actions to increase mobility (see Nursing Diagnosis 7)
	  2. initiate a bowel training program *so that client will have a bowel movement at regularly scheduled intervals*
	  3. perform actions to improve oral intake (see Nursing Diagnosis 2) *in order to increase intake of fluids and foods high in fiber.*

---

10. NURSING DIAGNOSIS: Bowel incontinence

related to:
a. increased reflex activity of the bowel and loss of voluntary control of bowel

elimination associated with upper motor neuron involvement if it has occurred;
b. decreased ability to control defecation associated with decreased level of consciousness or inability to recognize sensation of rectal fullness;
c. inability to get to bedside commode or bathroom in a timely manner associated with:
1. delay in obtaining assistance resulting from inability to communicate need to defecate
2. impaired physical mobility;
d. fecal impaction if present (continuous stimulation of the defecation reflex by the fecal mass inhibits the internal anal sphincter and results in loss of ability to retain the mucus and fluid that collect proximal to and leak around the fecal mass).

Desired Outcome	Nursing Actions and *Selected Purposes/Rationales*
11. The client will not experience bowel incontinence.	11.a. Monitor for episodes of bowel incontinence. b. Implement measures *to reduce the risk of bowel incontinence:* 1. initiate a bowel training program *so that the client will evacuate the lower colon at regularly scheduled intervals* 2. perform actions *to reduce delays in toileting* (e.g. have call signal within client's reach and respond promptly to requests for assistance; have bedpan or bedside commode readily available to client; provide client with easy-to-remove clothing such as pajamas with Velcro closures or an elastic waistband) 3. if client is aphasic, establish an effective method for him/her to communicate the urge to defecate 4. if client has a fecal impaction: a. consult physician regarding measures to remove the impaction (e.g. digital removal of stool, oil retention enema) b. perform actions to prevent constipation (see Nursing Diagnosis 10) *in order to prevent recurrent impactions.* c. If bowel incontinence persists, consult physician about revision of bowel training program.

12. NURSING DIAGNOSIS:

Altered thought processes*

related to damage to cerebral tissue associated with cerebral ischemia.

*The diagnostic label of acute or chronic confusion may be more appropriate depending on the client's symptoms.

Desired Outcome	Nursing Actions and *Selected Purposes/Rationales*
12. The client will experience improvement in thought processes as evidenced by: a. improved attention span, memory, and problem-solving abilities b. improved level of orientation c. reduction in instances of inappropriate responses.	12.a. Assess client for altered thought processes (e.g. shortened attention span, impaired memory, decreased ability to problem solve, confusion, inappropriate responses). b. Ascertain from significant others client's usual level of cognitive and emotional functioning. c. Implement measures to improve cerebral tissue perfusion (see Nursing Diagnosis 1, action b) *in order to reduce cerebral ischemia and subsequently improve thought processes.* d. If client shows evidence of altered thought processes: 1. reorient to person, place, and time as necessary

Desired Outcome	Nursing Actions and *Selected Purposes/Rationales*
	2. address client by name
	3. place familiar objects, clock, and calendar within client's view
	4. face client when conversing with him/her
	5. approach client in a slow, calm manner; allow adequate time for communication
	6. repeat instructions as necessary using clear, simple language and short sentences
	7. keep environmental stimuli to a minimum but avoid sensory deprivation
	8. maintain a consistent and fairly structured routine
	9. provide written or taped information whenever possible for client to review as often as necessary
	10. have client perform only one activity at a time and allow adequate time for performance of activities
	11. encourage client to make lists of planned activities, questions, and concerns
	12. assist client to problem solve if necessary
	13. implement measures *to stop emotional outbursts and inappropriate responses if they occur* (e.g. provide distraction by clapping hands, handing client an object to look at or hold, or turning on the radio or television)
	14. maintain realistic expectations of client's ability to learn, comprehend, and remember information provided
	15. encourage significant others to be supportive of client; instruct them in methods of dealing with client's altered thought processes
	16. discuss physiological basis for altered thought processes with client and significant others; inform them that cognitive and emotional functioning may improve gradually during the next 6–12 months
	17. consult physician if altered thought processes worsen.

■━━

13. NURSING DIAGNOSIS: **Risk for infection: pneumonia**

related to:
a. aspiration associated with difficulty swallowing, depressed cough and gag reflexes, and decreased level of consciousness;
b. stasis of secretions in the lungs associated with poor cough effort and decreased mobility (secretions provide a good medium for bacterial growth).

Desired Outcome	Nursing Actions and *Selected Purposes/Rationales*
13. The client will not develop pneumonia (see Care Plan on Immobility, Nursing Diagnosis 11, outcome a [p. 135], for outcome criteria).	13.a. Refer to Care Plan on Immobility, Nursing Diagnosis 11, action a (pp. 135–136), for measures related to assessment, prevention, and treatment of pneumonia. b. Implement measures to reduce the risk for aspiration (see Nursing Diagnosis 15, action d) *in order to further reduce the risk for pneumonia.*

■━━

14. NURSING DIAGNOSIS: **Risk for trauma: falls, burns, and lacerations**

related to:
a. motor, visual, and spatial-perceptual impairments;
b. weakness;

c. spasticity if present;

d. quick, impulsive behavior (occurs primarily with ischemia of the nondominant cerebral hemisphere);

e. altered thought processes (e.g. impaired memory, shortened attention span, confusion).

Desired Outcome	Nursing Actions and *Selected Purposes/Rationales*

14. The client will not experience falls, burns, or lacerations.

14.a. Implement measures *to reduce the risk for trauma:*

1. perform actions *to prevent falls:*

   a. keep bed in low position with side rails up when client is in bed

   b. keep needed items within easy reach and within client's visual field

   c. encourage client to request assistance whenever needed; have call signal within easy reach

   d. if vision is impaired:

      1. orient client to surroundings, room, and arrangement of furniture and identify obstacles during ambulation

      2. provide an eyepatch or opaque lens for client to wear if diplopia is present

      3. encourage visual scanning if homonymous hemianopsia is present

   e. use lap belt when client is in chair if indicated

   f. instruct client to wear well-fitting slippers/shoes with nonslip soles and low heels when ambulating

   g. keep floor free of clutter and wipe up spills promptly

   h. accompany client during ambulation utilizing a transfer safety belt

   i. provide ambulatory aids (e.g. walker, cane) if client is weak or unsteady on feet

   j. reinforce instructions from physical therapist on correct transfer and ambulation techniques

   k. instruct client to ambulate in well-lit areas and to utilize handrails if needed

   l. do not rush client; allow adequate time for ambulation to the bathroom and in hallway

   m. make sure that shower has a nonslip bottom surface and that shower chair, secure bath mat, call signal, grab bars, and adequate lighting are present

   n. implement measures *to reduce weakness:*

      1. maintain an adequate nutritional status (see Nursing Diagnosis 2)

      2. perform actions to prevent activity intolerance (see Care Plan on Immobility, Nursing Diagnosis 5, action b [pp. 130–131])

   o. stabilize client's affected arm with a sling when he/she is out of bed *in order to improve balance*

2. perform actions *to prevent burns:*

   a. let hot foods/fluids cool slightly before serving

   b. supervise client while smoking if indicated

   c. assess temperature of bath water and direct heat application device (e.g. K-pad, warm compress, hot water bottle) before and during use

3. assist client with tasks that require fine motor skills (e.g. shaving) *in order to prevent lacerations*

4. if client is confused or irrational:

   a. reorient frequently to surroundings and necessity of adhering to safety precautions

   b. provide appropriate level of supervision

   c. consult physician about the temporary use of a bed alarm or jacket or wrist restraints if necessary

Desired Outcome	Nursing Actions and *Selected Purposes/Rationales*

         d. administer prescribed antianxiety and antipsychotic medications if indicated

      5. administer muscle relaxants if ordered *to reduce spasticity of affected muscles.*

   b. Include client and significant others in planning and implementing measures to prevent trauma.

   c. If injury does occur, initiate appropriate first aid and notify physician.

---

15. NURSING DIAGNOSIS: **Risk for aspiration**

related to impaired swallowing, depressed cough and gag reflexes, and decreased level of consciousness.

Desired Outcome	Nursing Actions and *Selected Purposes/Rationales*

15. The client will not aspirate secretions or foods/fluids as evidenced by:
   a. clear breath sounds
   b. resonant percussion note over lungs
   c. absence of cough, tachypnea, and dyspnea.

15.a. Assess for signs and symptoms of aspiration of secretions or foods/fluids (e.g. rhonchi, dull percussion note over affected lung area, cough, tachypnea, tachycardia, dyspnea, presence of tube feeding in tracheal aspirate).

   b. Monitor chest x-ray results. Report findings of pulmonary infiltrate.

   c. If client is receiving tube feedings, add food coloring to the solution *so that it can readily be identified in tracheal aspirate.*

   d. Implement measures *to reduce the risk for aspiration:*
     1. withhold oral foods/fluids and place client in side-lying position if he/she has a depressed or absent gag reflex, severe dysphagia, and/or is not alert
     2. have suction equipment readily available for use
     3. perform oropharyngeal suctioning, encourage client to use tonsil-tip suction, and provide oral hygiene as often as needed *to remove excess secretions*
     4. if client is receiving tube feedings:
       a. check tube placement before each feeding or on a routine basis if feeding is continuous
       b. maintain continuous tube feeding infusion rate as ordered; administer intermittent tube feedings slowly
       c. maintain client in a semi- to high Fowler's position during and for at least 30 minutes after feeding
       d. stop tube feeding and notify physician if residuals exceed established parameters
     5. if oral intake is allowed:
       a. perform actions to improve ability to swallow (see Nursing Diagnosis 3, action c)
       b. allow ample time for meals
       c. instruct client to avoid laughing and talking while eating and drinking
       d. maintain client in high Fowler's position during and for at least 30 minutes after meals and snacks
       e. assist client with oral hygiene after eating *to ensure that food particles do not remain in mouth.*

   e. If signs and symptoms of aspiration occur:
     1. perform tracheal suctioning
     2. withhold oral intake
     3. notify physician
     4. prepare client for chest x-ray
     5. prepare client for bronchoscopy if ordered *to remove aspirated food particles.*

16. COLLABORATIVE DIAGNOSES:

Potential complications of cerebrovascular accident:

a. **increased intracranial pressure (IICP)** related to:
1. accumulation of blood in the cerebral tissue (can occur if CVA resulted from conditions such as ruptured cerebral aneurysm)
2. cerebral edema associated with increased capillary permeability of cerebral vessels and disruption of the sodium pump within the cells (both occur as a result of cerebral hypoxia)
3. increase in cerebral vascular volume associated with vasodilation of the cerebral vessels (a compensatory response to cerebral hypoxia);

b. **corneal irritation and abrasion** related to inability to close eye on affected side if facial nerve paresis or paralysis has occurred;

c. **subluxation of shoulder** related to muscle weakness in affected upper arm and shoulder and gravity pull on affected arm.

Desired Outcomes	Nursing Actions and *Selected Purposes/Rationales*

16.a. The client will not develop IICP as evidenced by:
1. usual or improved level of consciousness
2. no reports of headache
3. stable or improved motor and sensory function
4. absence of vomiting, papilledema, and seizure activity
5. usual pupillary size and reactivity
6. stable vital signs.

16.a.1. Assess for and report signs and symptoms of IICP:
a. restlessness, agitation, confusion, lethargy
b. reports of headache
c. decreasing motor and sensory function
d. abnormal posturing (e.g. extension [decerebrate], flexion [decorticate])
e. vomiting (usually without nausea)
f. papilledema
g. seizures
h. change in pupil size or reactivity
i. altered respiratory pattern (e.g. Cheyne-Stokes, central neurogenic hyperventilation)
j. full, bounding, slow pulse
k. rise in systolic B/P with widening pulse pressure.

2. Implement measures *to prevent IICP:*
a. maintain fluid restrictions as ordered
b. administer the following medications if ordered *to reduce cerebral edema:*
1. osmotic diuretics (e.g. mannitol)
2. loop diuretics (e.g. furosemide)
3. corticosteroids (e.g. dexamethasone)
c. perform actions *to promote adequate cerebral venous drainage:*
1. elevate head of bed 30° unless contraindicated
2. keep client's head and neck in neutral position; avoid flexion, extension, and rotation of head and neck
3. administer a laxative, antitussive, and antiemetic if ordered *to prevent straining to have a bowel movement, coughing, and vomiting (these conditions cause an increase in intrathoracic pressure that subsequently impedes venous return from the brain)*
d. perform actions *to prevent further cerebral hypoxia and the subsequent cerebral edema and vasodilation:*
1. implement measures to improve cerebral tissue perfusion (see Nursing Diagnosis 1, action b)
2. implement measures *to maintain a patent airway* (e.g. position client on side, suction if necessary)
3. administer oxygen as ordered and before and after tracheal suctioning
e. perform additional actions *to prevent further dilation of the cerebral vessels:*
1. implement measures *to prevent an increase in blood pressure:*
a. observe for and control conditions that can cause agitation (e.g. fear, anxiety, distended bladder)

Desired Outcomes	Nursing Actions and *Selected Purposes/Rationales*

b. instruct client to avoid activities that result in isometric muscle contractions (e.g. pushing feet against footboard, tightly gripping side rails)

    2. assist with mechanical hyperventilation (*may be done to lower arterial CO_2 and prevent the vasodilation that occurs with high levels of CO_2*)

  f. schedule care so activities that could raise intracranial pressure (e.g. suctioning, bathing, repositioning) are not grouped together.

3. If signs and symptoms of IICP are present:
  a. continue with above actions
  b. initiate seizure precautions
  c. prepare client for the following if planned:
    1. insertion of an intracranial pressure monitoring device (e.g. intraventricular catheter, subarachnoid screw or bolt, epidural fiberoptic catheter or transducer, intraparenchymal catheter)
    2. surgical intervention (e.g. ligation of bleeding vessel, evacuation of expanding hematoma)
  d. provide emotional support to client and significant others.

16.b. The client will not experience corneal irritation or abrasion as evidenced by:
1. absence of excessive tearing and eye redness
2. no reports of eye discomfort
3. usual visual acuity.

16.b.1. Assess for and report signs and symptoms of corneal irritation and abrasion (e.g. excessive tearing; reddened eye; reports of sensation of foreign body in eye, eye pain, itchy eye, or blurred vision).

2. Implement measures *to prevent corneal irritation and abrasion of eye on affected side:*
  a. reduce client's exposure to irritants such as powder, dust, and smoke
  b. have client wear his/her glasses *to protect eye*
  c. lubricate conjunctiva with isotonic eyedrops frequently
  d. tape eyelid shut if client is unable to close eye
  e. instruct client to avoid rubbing eye.

3. If signs and symptoms of corneal irritation or abrasion occur:
  a. continue with above measures
  b. assist with removal of any foreign body in the eye
  c. administer antimicrobial and anti-inflammatory ophthalmic ointments or solutions if ordered.

16.c. The client will not experience subluxation of shoulder as evidenced by:
1. absence of shoulder pain, tenderness, and swelling
2. maintenance of full range of motion of shoulder.

16.c.1. Assess for and report signs and symptoms of subluxation of the shoulder (e.g. shoulder pain, tenderness, or swelling; decreased range of motion of shoulder).

2. Implement measures *to prevent subluxation of the shoulder on the affected side:*
  a. perform actions *to improve muscle tone in affected shoulder and upper arm:*
    1. instruct client in and assist with range of motion exercises of affected shoulder and arm
    2. encourage client to use affected upper extremity to perform self-care and to assist in moving whenever possible
  b. when client is in bed or chair, position arm in correct alignment using pillows or lap board for support if necessary
  c. assist client with application of an arm support before sitting up in bed or getting out of bed
  d. use turn sheet or transfer belt when assisting client to move; never pull on his/her shoulder or arm.

3. If signs and symptoms of shoulder subluxation occur:
  a. continue with above actions
  b. apply heat or cold to area as ordered
  c. administer anti-inflammatory medications and analgesics if ordered.

17. NURSING DIAGNOSIS: **Sexual dysfunction**

related to:
a. alteration in usual sexual activities associated with impaired motor function and lengthy hospitalization;
b. decreased libido and/or impotence associated with depression, impaired motor and sensory function, fear of urinary and bowel incontinence, self-concept disturbance, and fear of rejection by partner.

Desired Outcome	Nursing Actions and *Selected Purposes/Rationales*

17. The client will perceive self as sexually adequate and acceptable as evidenced by:
a. communication of same
b. maintenance of relationship with significant other.
	17.a. Assess for signs and symptoms of sexual dysfunction (e.g. communication of sexual concerns or inability to achieve sexual satisfaction, alteration in relationship with significant other, physical limitations imposed by CVA).
	  b. Provide accurate information about the possible effects of the CVA on sexual functioning. Encourage questions and clarify misconceptions.
	  c. Implement measures *to promote optimal sexual functioning:*
	    1. facilitate communication between client and partner; focus on the feelings the couple share and assist them to identify changes that may affect their sexual relationship
	    2. discuss ways to be creative in expressing sexuality (e.g. massage, fantasies, cuddling)
	    3. arrange for uninterrupted privacy during hospital stay if desired by the couple
	    4. perform actions to improve client's self-concept (see Nursing Diagnosis 19)
	    5. if impotence is a problem:
	      a. encourage client to discuss it and various treatment options (e.g. vacuum erection aids, penile prosthesis) with physician
	      b. suggest alternative methods of sexual gratification if appropriate
	      c. discuss alternative methods of becoming a parent (e.g. adoption) if of concern to client
	    6. if appropriate, involve partner in care of client *to facilitate partner's adjustment to the changes in client's appearance and/or body functioning and subsequently decrease the possibility of partner's rejection of client*
	    7. if client is experiencing incontinence, reinforce adherence to bowel and bladder training programs and encourage him/her to void and/or defecate just before intercourse and other sexual activity
	    8. encourage client to rest before sexual activity
	    9. discuss positions that may facilitate sexual activity (e.g. lying on affected side, client in supine position)
	    10. include partner in above discussions and encourage continued support of the client.
	  d. Consult physician if counseling appears indicated.

18. NURSING DIAGNOSIS: **Anxiety**

related to impaired verbal communication and/or motor and sensory function; unfamiliar environment; lack of understanding of diagnosis, diagnostic tests, and treatments; uncertain prognosis; altered thought processes; financial concerns; and anticipated effect of the CVA on future life style and roles.

Desired Outcome	Nursing Actions and *Selected Purposes/Rationales*

18. The client will experience a reduction in anxiety (see Care Plan on Immobility, Nursing Diagnosis 13 [p. 140], for outcome criteria).	18.a. Assess client for signs and symptoms of anxiety (e.g. communication of feeling anxious, insomnia, tenseness, shakiness, restlessness, diaphoresis, elevated blood pressure, tachycardia, facial pallor, self-focused behaviors). Validate perceptions carefully, remembering that some behaviors may result from neurological changes.
	b. Refer to Care Plan on Immobility, Nursing Diagnosis 13, action b (p. 140), for measures to reduce fear and anxiety.
	c. Implement additional measures *to reduce fear and anxiety:*
	  1. if speech or comprehension is impaired, establish an effective communication system (e.g. paper and pencil, word or picture board, magic slate, gestures) as soon as possible
	  2. if client is experiencing homonymous hemianopsia, approach on unaffected side within his/her visual field
	  3. simplify the client's environment as much as possible
	  4. explain that motor, sensory, and speech impairments and altered thought processes are often more extensive initially and may gradually improve
	  5. perform actions to assist client to cope with the diagnosis and its effects (see Nursing Diagnosis 20, action c).

■━━

19. NURSING DIAGNOSIS: **Self-concept disturbance***

related to:
a. change in appearance (e.g. hemiplegia, facial droop, ptosis) and sexual functioning;
b. life-style and role changes associated with motor and spatial-perceptual impairments and altered thought processes;
c. impaired verbal communication;
d. loss of self-control (e.g. automatic speech, emotional lability, inappropriate behavior);
e. urinary and bowel incontinence;
f. dependence on others to meet basic needs.

---

*This diagnostic label includes the nursing diagnoses of body image disturbance, self-esteem disturbance, and altered role performance.

Desired Outcome	Nursing Actions and *Selected Purposes/Rationales*

19. The client will demonstrate beginning adaptation to changes in appearance, physical and cognitive functioning, level of independence, life style, and roles (see Care Plan on Immobility, Nursing Diagnosis 14 [p. 141], for outcome criteria).	19.a. Refer to Care Plan on Immobility, Nursing Diagnosis 14 (p. 141), for measures related to assessment and promotion of a positive self-concept.
	b. Implement additional measures *to assist client to adapt to changes in appearance, physical and cognitive functioning, level of independence, life style, and roles:*
	  1. perform actions to facilitate the grieving process (see Nursing Diagnosis 21, action b)
	  2. reinforce measures to assist client to cope with effects of CVA (see Nursing Diagnosis 20, action c)
	  3. reinforce measures to promote optimal sexual functioning (see Nursing Diagnosis 17, action c)
	  4. discuss techniques the client can utilize *to adapt to altered thought processes:*
	    a. encourage client to make lists and jot down messages and refer to these notes rather than relying on memory
	    b. instruct client to place self in a calm environment when making decisions

    c. encourage client to validate decisions, clarify information, and seek assistance problem-solving if indicated

5. instruct significant others in ways to manage client's emotional lability and inappropriate laughing, crying, or swearing (e.g. provide privacy; distract client by clapping hands, turning on television, or handing him/her an object)

6. perform actions to reduce the risk of urinary and bowel incontinence (see Nursing Diagnoses 9, action c and 11, action b)

7. instruct and assist client to position self with affected extremities well supported and in proper alignment (*if extremities are positioned awkwardly, the impairment is more obvious*)

8. demonstrate acceptance of client using techniques such as touch and frequent visits; encourage significant others to do the same

9. perform actions to facilitate communication (see Nursing Diagnosis 6, action b)

10. reinforce use of assistive devices (e.g. plate guards, broad-handled utensils, universal cuff, button hook, long-handled shoehorn) and mobility aids (e.g. walker, cane) *to increase client's independence*

11. encourage significant others to allow client to do what he/she is able *so that independence can be re-established and/or self-esteem redeveloped*

12. use adjectives such as weak, affected, or right- or left-sided rather than "bad" when referring to side of hemiplegia

13. assist client and significant others to have similar expectations and understanding of future life style.

---

20. NURSING DIAGNOSIS: **Ineffective individual coping**

related to fear; anxiety; decreased ability to communicate verbally; changes in motor and sensory function, thought processes, and future life style and roles; and need for lengthy rehabilitation.

Desired Outcome	Nursing Actions and *Selected Purposes/Rationales*

20. The client will demonstrate effective coping as evidenced by:
  a. communication of ability to cope with the effects of the CVA
  b. utilization of appropriate problem-solving techniques
  c. willingness to participate in treatment plan and meet basic needs
  d. appropriate use of defense mechanisms
  e. utilization of available support systems.
	20.a. Assess for and report signs and symptoms of ineffective individual coping (e.g. communication of inability to cope; inability to ask for help, problem solve, or meet basic needs; insomnia; withdrawal; reluctance to participate in treatment plan; inappropriate use of defense mechanisms; inability to meet role expectations). Validate perceptions carefully, remembering that some behaviors may be a result of neurological changes.
	  b. Assess client's perception of current situation.
	  c. Implement measures *to promote effective coping:*
	    1. allow time for client to begin to adjust to the diagnosis and planned treatment, residual effects of the CVA, and anticipated life-style and role changes
	    2. perform actions to facilitate communication (see Nursing Diagnosis 6, action b)
	    3. perform actions to reduce fear and anxiety (see Nursing Diagnosis 18, actions b and c)
	    4. assist client to recognize and manage inappropriate denial if it is present
	    5. encourage communication about current situation
	    6. assist client to identify personal strengths and resources that can be utilized to facilitate coping with the current situation
	    7. create an atmosphere of trust and support

Desired Outcome	Nursing Actions and *Selected Purposes/Rationales*
	8. if acceptable to client, arrange for a visit with another individual who has successfully adjusted to the effects of a CVA
	9. include client in the planning of care, encourage maximum participation in treatment plan, and allow choices when possible *to enable him/her to maintain a sense of control*
	10. instruct client in effective problem-solving techniques (e.g. accurate identification of stressors, determination of various options to solve problem)
	11. assist client to maintain usual daily routines whenever possible
	12. assist client to identify priorities and attainable goals as he/she starts to plan for necessary life-style and role changes
	13. assist client through methods such as role playing to prepare for negative reactions of others to his/her altered appearance and other neurological impairments
	14. if client is incontinent, instruct in ways to minimize the problem *so that socialization with others is possible* (e.g. placing disposable liners in underwear, wearing absorbent undergarments such as Depends)
	15. set up a home evaluation appointment with occupational and physical therapists before client's discharge *so that changes in home environment* (*e.g. installation of ramps and handrails, widening doorways, altering kitchen facilities*) *can be completed by discharge*
	16. assist client and significant others to identify ways that personal and family goals can be adjusted rather than abandoned
	17. inform client that he/she may have times when impairments worsen; assure client that this is usually temporary and the result of physical and/or emotional stress or fatigue rather than an indication of deteriorating neurological status
	18. administer antianxiety and/or antidepressant agents if ordered
	19. assist client to identify and utilize available support systems; provide information regarding available community resources that can assist client and significant others in coping with effects of the CVA (e.g. stroke support groups, local chapter of the American Heart Association)
	20. encourage the client to share with significant others the kind of support that would be most beneficial (e.g. listening, inspiring hope, providing reassurance and accurate information)
	21. support behaviors indicative of effective coping (e.g. participation in treatment plan and self-care activities, communication of ability to cope, utilization of effective problem-solving strategies).
	d. Consult physician about psychological and vocational counseling if appropriate. Initiate a referral if necessary.

■

21. NURSING DIAGNOSIS: **Grieving***

related to changes in motor and sensory function and thought processes and the effect of these changes on future life style and roles.

---

*This diagnostic label includes anticipatory grieving and grieving following the actual losses.

Desired Outcome	Nursing Actions and *Selected Purposes/Rationales*
21. The client will demonstrate beginning progression through the grieving process as evidenced by:	21.a. Assess for signs and symptoms of grieving (e.g. change in eating habits, inability to concentrate, insomnia, anger, sadness, withdrawal from significant others, denial of loss).
	b. Implement measures *to facilitate the grieving process:*

a. communication of feelings about the CVA and its effects
b. usual sleep pattern
c. participation in treatment plan and self-care activities
d. utilization of available support systems
e. communication of a plan for integrating prescribed follow-up care into life style.

1. assist client to acknowledge the losses *so grief work can begin*; assess for factors that may hinder and facilitate acknowledgment
2. discuss the grieving process and assist client to accept the phases of grieving as an expected response to changes that have occurred
3. allow time for client to progress through the phases of grieving (phases vary among theorists but progress from shock and alarm to acceptance); be aware that not every phase is expressed by all individuals, that recurrence of phases is common, and that the grieving process may take months to years
4. provide an atmosphere of care and concern (e.g. provide privacy, be available and nonjudgmental, display empathy and respect) *so client will feel free to express feelings*
5. perform actions *to promote trust* (e.g. answer questions honestly, provide requested information)
6. encourage the communication of anger and sadness about the losses experienced; recognize displacement of anger and assist client to see the actual cause of angry feelings and resentment if demonstrated
7. encourage client to express feelings in whatever ways are comfortable (e.g. writing, drawing, conversation)
8. perform actions to promote effective coping (see Nursing Diagnosis 20, action c)
9. perform actions *to support realistic hope about the effects of treatment on the residual impairments:*
   a. focus on what the client is able to accomplish independently and with the use of assistive devices
   b. reinforce knowledge that impairments may improve with time
   c. reinforce positive effects of speech, physical, and occupational therapies and control of underlying cause of the CVA (e.g. hypertension, diabetes)
10. support behaviors suggesting successful grief work (e.g. communicating feelings about losses, focusing on ways to adapt to losses, developing or renewing relationships)
11. explain the phases of the grieving process to significant others; encourage their support and understanding
12. facilitate communication between client and significant others; be aware that they may be in different phases of the grieving process
13. provide information regarding counseling services and support groups that might assist client in working through grief
14. when appropriate, assist client to meet spiritual needs (e.g. arrange for visit from clergy).
c. Consult physician regarding referral for counseling if signs of dysfunctional grieving (e.g. persistent denial of losses, excessive anger or sadness, emotional lability) occur.

■———

22. NURSING DIAGNOSIS: **Altered family processes**

related to change in family roles and structure associated with a family member's verbal, motor, and sensory impairments; altered thought processes; and need for lengthy rehabilitation.

Desired Outcome	Nursing Actions and *Selected Purposes/Rationales*
22. The family members* will demonstrate beginning	22.a. Assess for signs and symptoms of altered family processes (e.g. inability to meet client's needs, statements of not being able to accept client's

---
*The term "family members" is being used here to include client's significant others.

Desired Outcome	Nursing Actions and *Selected Purposes/Rationales*

adjustment to changes in functioning of family member and family roles and structure as evidenced by:
a. meeting client's needs
b. verbalization of ways to adapt to required role and life-style changes
c. active participation in decision making and client's rehabilitation
d. positive interactions with one another.
	diagnosis of CVA and its effects or make necessary role and life-style changes, inability to make decisions, inability or refusal to participate in client's rehabilitation, negative family interactions).
	b. Identify components of the family and their patterns of communication and role expectations.
	c. Implement measures *to facilitate family members' adjustment to client's diagnosis, changes in client's functioning within the family system, and altered family roles and structure:*
	   1. encourage verbalization of feelings about the CVA and its effects on family structure; actively listen to each family member and maintain a nonjudgmental attitude about feelings shared
	   2. reinforce physician's explanation about the CVA and planned treatment and rehabilitation
	   3. assist family members to gain a realistic perspective of client's situation, conveying as much hope as appropriate
	   4. provide privacy *so that family members and client can share their feelings with one another*; stress the importance of and facilitate the use of good communication techniques
	   5. assist family members to progress through their own grieving process; explain that they may encounter times when they need to focus on meeting their own rather than the client's needs
	   6. emphasize the need for family members to obtain adequate rest and nutrition and to identify and utilize stress management techniques *so that they are better able to emotionally and physically deal with the changes and losses experienced and the physical care of the client*
	   7. encourage and assist family members to identify coping strategies for dealing with the client's impairments and their effects on the family
	   8. assist family members to identify realistic goals and ways of reaching these goals
	   9. include family members in decision making about client and his/her care; convey appreciation for their input and continued support of client
	   10. encourage and allow family members to participate in client's care and rehabilitation as appropriate
	   11. assist family members to identify resources that could assist them in coping with their feelings and meeting their immediate and long-term needs (e.g. counseling and social services; pastoral care; service, church, and stroke support groups); initiate a referral if indicated.
	d. Consult physician if family members continue to demonstrate difficulty adapting to changes in client's functioning, roles, and family structure.

Discharge Teaching

■━━━

23. NURSING DIAGNOSIS: **Knowledge deficit, Ineffective management of therapeutic regimen, or Altered health maintenance***

---

   *The nurse should select the diagnostic label that is most appropriate for the client's discharge teaching needs.

Desired Outcomes	Nursing Actions and *Selected Purposes/Rationales*
23.a. The client will communicate an awareness of ways to decrease the risk of a recurrent CVA.	23.a.1. Assist client to recognize factors that may have contributed to the CVA (e.g. hypertension, elevated serum lipids, diabetes, obesity, atrial fibrillation, use of oral contraceptives). 2. Identify appropriate actions client can take to decrease risk of a recurrent CVA (e.g. take medications as prescribed, decrease stress, lose weight, stop smoking, modify diet, adhere to medical treatment plan to

control hypertension and/or diabetes, use another form of birth control if taking oral contraceptives).

3. Provide information about resources that can help client to control risk factors (e.g. National Stroke Association; American Heart Association; smoking cessation, weight reduction, and stress management programs). Initiate a referral if indicated.

23.b. The client will identify ways to manage sensory and verbal communication impairments and altered thought processes.

23.b.1. Reinforce instructions regarding ways to adapt to visual impairments if present:
  a. utilize scanning techniques if visual field cut is present
  b. arrange home setting so that when in favorite chair or in bed, stimuli other than wall or furniture are within visual field
  c. wear eyepatch or opaque lens if double vision persists.
2. Reinforce use of established communication techniques and continuation with speech therapy if indicated.
3. If spatial-perceptual deficits and/or unilateral neglect is present, stress need for assistance with usual daily activities and strict adherence to safety measures to prevent injury.
4. Reinforce methods of adapting to impaired memory and shortened attention span (e.g. make lists of planned activities, review taped or written instructions frequently).
5. Instruct client to request assistance when problem-solving and setting priorities and to seek validation of decisions if reasoning ability is impaired.

23.c. The client will identify ways to manage urinary and bowel incontinence.

23.c.1. Reinforce instructions regarding client's bladder and bowel training programs. Stress the importance of adhering to the programs in order to reduce the risk of incontinence.
2. Demonstrate procedures that are included in client's bladder training program (e.g. intermittent catheterization, application of an external catheter) and bowel training program (e.g. insertion of a rectal suppository, administration of an enema). Allow time for questions, clarification, and return demonstration.

23.d. The client will demonstrate measures to facilitate the performance of activities of daily living and increase physical mobility.

23.d.1. Reinforce measures that the client is using to improve his/her ability to perform activities of daily living and increase physical mobility (e.g. participation in exercise program; use of assistive devices and mobility aids; continued concentration on body positioning, balance, and movement).
2. Allow time for questions, clarification, and return demonstration.

23.e. The client will communicate an awareness of signs and symptoms to report to the health care provider.

23.e.1. Refer to Care Plan on Immobility, Nursing Diagnosis 17, action c (p. 144), for signs and symptoms to report to health care provider.
2. Instruct client to report these additional signs and symptoms:
  a. increased weakness or loss of sensation in extremities
  b. increase in or development of visual disturbances such as tunnel vision, blurred vision, or transient blindness
  c. increased lethargy, irritability, or confusion
  d. increased difficulty chewing or swallowing
  e. increased difficulty speaking or understanding verbal and nonverbal communication
  f. increased difficulty maintaining balance
  g. seizures (can develop months after the CVA as scar tissue forms in the ischemic area).

23.f. The client will communicate knowledge of community resources that can assist with home management and adjustment to changes resulting from the CVA.

23.f.1. Provide information about community resources that can assist client and significant others with home management and adjustment to impairments in motor and sensory function and altered thought processes resulting from the CVA (e.g. home health agencies, stroke support groups, Meals on Wheels, social and financial services, local chapter of the American Heart Association, local service groups that can help obtain assistive devices, individual and family counselors).
2. Initiate a referral if indicated.

23.g. The client will communicate an understanding of and a

23.g.1. Reinforce the importance of keeping follow-up appointments with health care provider and physical, occupational, and speech therapists.

Desired Outcomes	Nursing Actions and *Selected Purposes/Rationales*
plan for adhering to recommended follow-up care including future appointments with health care provider and therapists and medications prescribed.	2. Teach client the rationale for, side effects of, and importance of taking prescribed medications (e.g. anticoagulants, antihypertensives). Inform client of pertinent food and drug interactions. 3. Implement measures to improve client compliance: 　a. include significant others in teaching sessions if possible 　b. encourage questions and allow time for reinforcement and clarification of information provided 　c. provide written instructions on scheduled appointments with health care provider and occupational, physical, and speech therapists; medications prescribed; signs and symptoms to report; and exercise program.

Bibliography

See pages 897–898 and 901.

CRANIOCEREBRAL TRAUMA

The leading causes of craniocerebral trauma (head injury, traumatic brain injury [TBI]) are motor vehicle accidents, falls, sports/recreational injuries, and assaults. Examples of skull and brain injury that can occur include skull fracture; dural tear; cerebral contusion, concussion, and laceration; brain stem damage; and intracranial hemorrhage.

Brain damage can occur during the initial injury and as a result of subsequent cerebral damage resulting from factors such as cerebral hematoma, infection, and edema; diffuse axonal injury (DAI); seizure activity; and/or obstruction in the flow of cerebral spinal fluid (CSF). Following craniocerebral trauma, a person may have a disturbance in consciousness ranging from a brief loss of contact with the environment to persistent coma. As the state of consciousness improves, clients often experience posttraumatic syndrome (postconcussional state), which can include headache, dizziness, and alterations in thought processes (e.g. irritability, posttraumatic amnesia, bewilderment, decreased ability to concentrate, personality changes). The signs and symptoms of posttraumatic syndrome tend to subside gradually but often persist for weeks to years. Additional signs and symptoms following craniocerebral trauma vary depending on the area of the brain that has been affected. For example, tissue damage in the frontal lobe could result in loss of voluntary motor control, personality changes, and/or expressive aphasia; damage to the occipital lobe could cause visual disturbances; and damage to the temporal lobe could result in receptive aphasia and/or hearing impairment.

Craniocerebral trauma is classified according to location (e.g. skull, epidural area, brain stem), effect (e.g. concussion, diffuse axonal injury, depressed fracture of the skull, contusion, subdural hematoma), and severity. The severity of trauma ranges from minor (usually a concussion with no alteration in consciousness or a loss of consciousness lasting 5 minutes or less) to severe, in which extensive contusion and/or laceration of brain tissue and possible brain stem injury occurs. Severe craniocerebral trauma usually involves a period of prolonged unconsciousness and results in permanent neurological impairments that require extensive rehabilitation and long-term care.

This care plan focuses on the adult client hospitalized following craniocerebral trauma. It deals mainly with nursing and collaborative diagnoses appropriate for a client who has regained consciousness after sustaining a moderate brain injury. Goals of care during the acute phase are to prevent life-threatening complications and perform or assist the client with those activities he/she is unable to perform independently. After the client's condition has stabilized, care is focused on assisting him/her to adapt to residual neurological impairments. Nursing care and discharge teaching need to be individualized according to the areas of the brain affected and the extensiveness of the tissue damage. If the client has sustained more severe craniocerebral trauma, refer also to the Care Plans on Immobility and Cerebrovascular Accident.

DIAGNOSTIC TESTS

Computed tomography (CT)
Magnetic resonance imaging (MRI)
Skull x-rays
Cerebral angiography
Brain scan
Positron emission tomography (PET)
Electroencephalogram (EEG)
Transcranial ultrasound
Evoked potentials (auditory, visual, and/or somatosensory)

DISCHARGE CRITERIA

Prior to discharge, the client will:

- have improved cerebral tissue perfusion
- have improved or stable neurological function
- have an adequate nutritional status
- have no signs or symptoms of complications
- identify ways to adapt to neurological deficits that may persist following craniocerebral trauma
- identify ways to reduce headache
- state signs and symptoms to report to the health care provider
- share thoughts and feelings about residual neurological impairments
- identify community resources that can assist with home management and adjustment to changes resulting from craniocerebral trauma
- verbalize an understanding of and a plan for adhering to recommended follow-up care including future appointments with health care provider and therapists and medications prescribed.

NURSING/ COLLABORATIVE DIAGNOSES

1. Altered cerebral tissue perfusion △   253
2. Altered nutrition: less than body requirements △   254
3. Pain: headache △   255
4. Impaired physical mobility △   256
5. Self-care deficit △   257
6. Altered thought processes △   258
7. Risk for trauma: falls, burns, and lacerations △   259
8. Risk for altered body temperature: increased △   260
9. Potential complications:
    a. increased intracranial pressure (IICP)
    b. meningitis
    c. seizures
    d. cranial nerve damage
    e. diabetes insipidus
    f. syndrome of inappropriate antidiuretic hormone (SIADH)
    g. gastrointestinal (GI) bleeding △   260
10. Anxiety △   266
11. Self-concept disturbance △   267
12. Ineffective individual coping △   268
13. Altered family processes △   269

DISCHARGE TEACHING

14. Knowledge deficit, Ineffective management of therapeutic regimen, or Altered health maintenance △   270

1. NURSING DIAGNOSIS:

Altered cerebral tissue perfusion

related to decreased cerebral blood flow associated with:
a. cerebral hemorrhage resulting from laceration of blood vessels at the time of injury;
b. pressure on cerebral vessels resulting from hematoma formation and/or edema;
c. vascular spasm (can occur in response to damage to and stretching of cerebral vessels).

Desired Outcome	Nursing Actions and *Selected Purposes/Rationales*
1. The client will experience improved cerebral tissue perfusion as evidenced by: a. decrease in or absence of dizziness, visual disturbances, and speech impairments b. improved mental status c. improved or usual sensory and motor function.	1.a. Assess client for signs and symptoms of decreased cerebral tissue perfusion: 1. dizziness 2. visual disturbances (e.g. blurred or dimmed vision, diplopia, change in visual field) 3. aphasia 4. irritability and restlessness 5. decreased level of consciousness 6. paresthesias, weakness, paralysis. b. Implement measures *to improve cerebral tissue perfusion:* 1. perform actions to prevent and treat increased intracranial pressure (see Collaborative Diagnosis 9, actions a.2 and 3) 2. if client is hypotensive, perform actions *to improve cerebral blood flow* (e.g. administer prescribed sympathomimetic agents, maintain intravenous fluid therapy as ordered) 3. administer calcium-channel blockers (e.g. nimodipine) if ordered *to reduce cerebral vasospasm* (*the calcium that is released by the injured neural cells can cause vasospasm*) 4. prepare client for surgery (e.g. evacuation of hematoma, ligation of bleeding vessels) if planned. c. Consult physician if signs and symptoms of decreased cerebral tissue perfusion worsen.

---

2. NURSING DIAGNOSIS:

Altered nutrition: less than body requirements

related to:
a. decreased oral intake associated with:
  1. anorexia resulting from fear, anxiety, depression, headache, and impaired sense of taste (can occur with damage to the facial nerve[s] and/or as a result of loss of sense of smell [the olfactory nerves are often impaired because they are extremely sensitive to pressure])
  2. dysphagia (can occur with damage to cranial nerves IX [glossopharyngeal] and X [vagus])
  3. difficulty feeding self if visual disturbances are present (can occur as a result of damage to cranial nerves II [optic], III [oculomotor], IV [trochlear], and/or VI [abducens]) or if motor function is impaired
  4. prescribed dietary restrictions (may be necessary if client has a decreased level of consciousness or if damage to cranial nerves has resulted in a depressed or absent gag reflex or severe dysphagia)
  5. restlessness, agitation, and/or shortened attention span;
b. the increased metabolic rate that occurs following craniocerebral trauma.

Desired Outcome	Nursing Actions and *Selected Purposes/Rationales*
2. The client will maintain an adequate nutritional status as evidenced by: a. weight within normal range for client's age, height, and body frame b. normal BUN and serum albumin, Hct, Hb, transferrin, and lymphocyte levels	2.a. Assess the client for signs and symptoms of malnutrition: 1. weight below normal for client's age, height, and body frame 2. abnormal BUN and low serum albumin, Hct, Hb, transferrin, and lymphocyte levels 3. weakness and fatigue 4. sore, inflamed oral mucous membrane 5. pale conjunctiva. b. Monitor percentage of meals and snacks client consumes. Report a pattern of inadequate intake. c. Implement measures *to maintain an adequate nutritional status:*

c. usual strength and activity tolerance
d. healthy oral mucous membrane.

1. when food or oral fluids are allowed, perform actions *to improve oral intake*:
   a. implement measures to reduce headache (see Nursing Diagnosis 3, action e)
   b. implement measures to reduce fear and anxiety and facilitate client's psychological adjustment to the effects of craniocerebral trauma (see Nursing Diagnoses 10, action b; 11, actions c–s; and 12, action c)
   c. implement measures to assist client to adapt to loss of or diminished sense of smell, visual impairments, impaired swallowing ability, and/or altered sense of taste if present (see Collaborative Diagnosis 9, actions d.3.a and b; d.3.d.2.b; and d.3.e)
   d. increase activity as allowed and tolerated (*activity usually promotes a sense of well-being and improves appetite*)
   e. obtain a dietary consult if necessary to assist client in selecting foods/fluids that meet nutritional needs, are appealing, and adhere to personal and cultural preferences
   f. maintain a clean environment and a relaxed, quiet, pleasant atmosphere
   g. provide oral hygiene before meals
   h. serve frequent, small meals rather than large ones if client is weak, quickly loses interest in eating, and/or has a poor appetite
   i. encourage significant others to bring in client's favorite foods unless contraindicated and eat with him/her *to make eating more of a familiar social experience*
   j. allow adequate time for meals; reheat foods/fluids if necessary
   k. implement measures to enable client to feed self (see Nursing Diagnosis 5, action b.6); if client needs to be fed, offer foods/fluids in the order he/she prefers
2. ensure that meals are well balanced and high in essential nutrients; offer dietary supplements if indicated
3. administer vitamins and minerals if ordered.

d. Perform a calorie count if ordered. Report information to dietitian and physician.
e. Consult physician regarding an alternative method of providing nutrition (e.g. parenteral nutrition, tube feedings) if client does not consume enough food or fluids to meet nutritional needs.

■

3. NURSING DIAGNOSIS:

Pain: headache

related to:
a. trauma to the scalp, dura, and cerebral vessels and tissue;
b. stretching or compression of cerebral vessels and tissue associated with increased intracranial pressure if it occurs;
c. irritation of the meninges (occurs primarily if blood is present in the cerebrospinal fluid or meningitis develops).

Desired Outcome	Nursing Actions and *Selected Purposes/Rationales*

3. The client will experience diminished headache as evidenced by:
  a. verbalization of same
  b. relaxed facial expression and body positioning
	3.a. Assess for signs and symptoms of headache (e.g. statement of same, new or increased restlessness or irritability, grimacing, rubbing head, avoidance of bright lights and noises, reluctance to move).
	b. Assess client's perception of the severity of the headache using a pain intensity rating scale.
	c. Assess the client's pain pattern (e.g. location, quality, onset, duration,

Desired Outcome	Nursing Actions and *Selected Purposes/Rationales*

c. increased participation in activities.	precipitating factors, aggravating factors, alleviating factors).
	d. Ask the client to describe previous experiences with headaches and methods used to relieve them effectively.
	e. Implement measures *to reduce headache:*
	  1. perform actions *to reduce fear and anxiety about the pain experience* (e.g. assure client that his/her need for headache relief is understood, plan methods for relieving headache with client)
	  2. perform actions to reduce fear and anxiety (see Nursing Diagnosis 10, action b) *in order to promote relaxation and subsequently increase the client's threshold and tolerance for pain*
	  3. administer analgesics before activities and procedures that can cause headache and before headache becomes severe
	  4. perform actions *to minimize environmental stimuli* (e.g. provide a quiet environment, limit number of visitors and their length of stay, dim lights)
	  5. avoid jarring bed or startling client *to minimize risk of sudden movements*
	  6. perform actions to prevent and treat increased intracranial pressure and meningitis (see Collaborative Diagnosis 9, actions a.2 and 3 and b.5 and 6)
	  7. provide or assist with nonpharmacologic measures to reduce headache (e.g. cool cloth to forehead, progressive relaxation exercises)
	  8. administer nonnarcotic analgesics or codeine (other narcotic [opioid] analgesics are usually contraindicated *because they have a greater depressant effect on the central nervous system*) if ordered.
	f. Consult physician if above actions fail to reduce headache.

■━━━

4. NURSING DIAGNOSIS: **Impaired physical mobility**

related to:
a. motor and spatial-perceptual impairments if present;
b. activity restrictions imposed by the treatment plan;
c. reluctance to move because of headache.

Desired Outcome	Nursing Actions and *Selected Purposes/Rationales*

4. The client will achieve maximum physical mobility within limitations imposed by the treatment plan and effects of craniocerebral trauma.	4.a. Implement measures *to increase mobility when allowed:*
	  1. instruct client in and assist with range of motion exercises at least 3 times/day unless contraindicated
	  2. instruct client in and assist with correct use of mobility aids (e.g. cane, walker) if appropriate
	  3. reinforce instructions, activities, and exercise plan recommended by physical and occupational therapists
	  4. perform actions to reduce headache (see Nursing Diagnosis 3, action e)
	  5. increase activity and participation in self-care as allowed and tolerated.
	b. Provide praise and encouragement for all efforts to increase physical mobility.
	c. Encourage the support of significant others. Allow them to assist with range of motion exercises, positioning, and activity if desired.
	d. Consult physician if client is unable to achieve expected level of mobility or range of motion becomes restricted.

5. NURSING DIAGNOSIS: **Self-care deficit**

related to impaired physical mobility, altered thought processes, and/or visual impairments if present.

Desired Outcome	Nursing Actions and *Selected Purposes/Rationales*

5. The client will perform self-care activities within cognitive and physical limitations and prescribed activity restrictions.	5.a. With client, develop a realistic plan for meeting daily physical needs.
	b. Implement measures *to facilitate client's ability to perform self-care activities:*
	  1. perform actions to increase mobility when allowed (see Nursing Diagnosis 4, action a)
	  2. schedule care at a time when client is most likely to be able to participate (e.g. when analgesics are at peak effect, after rest periods, not immediately after meals or treatments)
	  3. keep needed objects within easy reach
	  4. allow adequate time for accomplishment of self-care activities
	  5. if vision is impaired:
	    a. orient client to surroundings and location of items needed for self-care
	    b. instruct client to visually scan his/her environment to locate needed items if visual field cut is present
	    c. encourage client to wear an eyepatch or opaque lens if diplopia is present
	  6. perform actions *to enable client to feed self:*
	    a. place only a few items on the tray at one time if spatial-perceptual deficits are present
	    b. consult with occupational therapist about assistive devices available (e.g. broad-handled utensils, rocker knives, plate guards); reinforce use of these devices
	  7. perform actions *to enable client to dress self when condition stabilizes:*
	    a. encourage use of assistive devices such as button hooks, long-handled shoehorns, and pull loops for pants
	    b. encourage client to select clothing that is easy to put on and remove (e.g. clothing with zippers rather than buttons, loose-fitting clothing, shoes with Velcro fasteners rather than laces)
	    c. if client has difficulty distinguishing right from left, mark outer aspect of shoes with tape
	  8. reinforce exercises and activities recommended by the occupational therapist to improve fine motor skills.
	c. Encourage client to perform as much of self-care as possible within cognitive and physical limitations and activity restrictions imposed by the treatment plan. Provide positive feedback for all efforts and accomplishments of self-care.
	d. Assist the client with activities he/she is unable to perform independently.
	e. Inform significant others of client's abilities to perform own care. Explain importance of encouraging and allowing client to maintain an optimal level of independence.

■ ━━

6. NURSING DIAGNOSIS: **Altered thought processes***

related to impaired cerebral functioning associated with cerebral tissue irritation and ischemia resulting from craniocerebral trauma.

───────────

*The diagnostic label of acute or chronic confusion may be more appropriate depending on the client's symptoms.

Desired Outcome	Nursing Actions and *Selected Purposes/Rationales*

6. The client will experience improvement in thought processes as evidenced by:
  a. improved attention span, memory, reasoning ability, and judgment
  b. decreased irritability and instances of inappropriate responses
  c. improved level of orientation.
	6.a. Assess client for altered thought processes (e.g. shortened attention span, impaired memory, decreased ability to concentrate, slow response time, poor reasoning ability or judgment, irritability, inappropriate responses, confusion).
	  b. Ascertain from significant others client's usual level of cognitive and emotional functioning.
	  c. Implement measures to improve cerebral tissue perfusion (see Nursing Diagnosis 1, action b) *in order to reduce cerebral ischemia and subsequently improve thought processes.*
	  d. If client shows evidence of altered thought processes:
	    1. reorient client to person, place, and time as necessary
	    2. address client by name
	    3. place familiar objects, clock, and calendar within client's view
	    4. face client when conversing with him/her
	    5. approach client in a slow, calm manner; allow adequate time for communication
	    6. repeat instructions as necessary using clear, simple language and short sentences
	    7. keep environmental stimuli to a minimum but avoid sensory deprivation
	    8. maintain a consistent and fairly structured routine
	    9. provide written or taped information whenever possible for client to review as often as necessary
	    10. have client perform only one activity at a time and allow adequate time for performance of activities
	    11. encourage client to make lists of planned activities, questions, and concerns
	    12. assist client to problem solve if necessary
	    13. implement measures *to stop emotional outbursts and inappropriate responses if they occur* (e.g. provide distraction by taking client for a walk, decrease environmental stimuli by turning off television or radio and/or requesting that visitors leave for short while)
	    14. maintain realistic expectations of client's ability to learn, comprehend, and remember information provided
	    15. encourage significant others to be supportive of client; instruct them in methods of dealing with client's altered thought processes
	    16. discuss physiological basis for altered thought processes with client and significant others; inform them that cognitive and emotional functioning usually improve gradually but caution them that posttraumatic syndrome (a postconcussion state manifested in part by altered thought processes) may persist for a few weeks to a year or more depending on the severity of the head injury
	    17. assist with neuropsychological testing if indicated
	    18. consult physician if altered thought processes worsen.

7. NURSING DIAGNOSIS: **Risk for trauma: falls, burns, and lacerations**

related to:
a. dizziness;
b. motor, visual, and/or spatial-perceptual impairments if present;
c. quick, impulsive behavior (can occur with injury involving the nondominant cerebral hemisphere);
d. ataxia (can occur with cerebellar injury);
e. altered thought processes (e.g. impaired memory, shortened attention span, confusion, slow response time).

Desired Outcome	Nursing Actions and *Selected Purposes/Rationales*

7. The client will not experience falls, burns, or lacerations.	7.a. Implement measures *to reduce the risk for trauma:*
	1. perform actions *to prevent falls:*
	  a. keep bed in low position with side rails up when client is in bed; consult physician about use of a floor bed or cubicle bed (large mattress on floor with surrounding "wall" of mattresses or padding) if indicated
	  b. keep needed items within easy reach
	  c. encourage client to request assistance whenever needed; have call signal within easy reach
	  d. use lap belt when client is in chair if indicated
	  e. instruct client to wear well-fitting slippers/shoes with nonslip soles and low heels when ambulating
	  f. keep floor free of clutter and wipe up spills promptly
	  g. accompany client during ambulation utilizing a transfer safety belt
	  h. provide ambulatory aids (e.g. walker, cane) if client is weak or unsteady on feet
	  i. reinforce instructions from physical therapist on correct transfer and ambulation techniques
	  j. instruct client to ambulate in well-lit areas, utilize handrails if needed, and avoid sudden movements
	  k. do not rush client; allow adequate time for ambulation to the bathroom and in hallway
	  l. if vision is impaired:
	    1. orient client to surroundings, room, and arrangement of furniture and identify obstacles during ambulation
	    2. instruct client to wear an eyepatch or opaque lens if diplopia is present
	    3. encourage visual scanning if a visual field cut is present
	  m. make sure that shower has a nonslip bottom surface and that shower chair, secure bath mat, call signal, grab bars, and adequate lighting are present
	2. perform actions *to prevent burns:*
	  a. let hot foods and fluids cool slightly before serving
	  b. supervise client while smoking if indicated
	3. assist client with tasks that require fine motor skills (e.g. shaving) *in order to prevent lacerations*
	4. administer central nervous system depressants judiciously
	5. if client is confused or irrational:
	  a. reorient frequently to surroundings and necessity of adhering to safety precautions
	  b. provide appropriate level of supervision
	  c. consult physician about the temporary use of a bed alarm or jacket or wrist restraints if necessary
	  d. administer prescribed antianxiety and antipsychotic medications if indicated.

Desired Outcome	Nursing Actions and *Selected Purposes/Rationales*

    b. Include client and significant others in planning and implementing measures to prevent trauma.

    c. If injury does occur, initiate appropriate first aid and notify physician.

---

8. NURSING DIAGNOSIS:

Risk for altered body temperature: increased

related to direct trauma to the hypothalamus and/or pressure on the hypothalamus associated with hematoma formation or edema of the surrounding tissue.

Desired Outcome	Nursing Actions and *Selected Purposes/Rationales*

8. The client will maintain a normal body temperature.

8.a. Assess for and report signs and symptoms of increased body temperature resulting from trauma to the hypothalamus (e.g. elevated temperature; pale, hot, dry skin).

    b. Implement measures *to reduce pressure on the hypothalamus in order to reduce the risk for increased body temperature:*

      1. administer osmotic diuretics (e.g. mannitol), loop diuretics (e.g. furosemide), and/or corticosteroids (e.g. dexamethasone) if ordered *to decrease edema of the hypothalamus and surrounding tissue*

      2. prepare client for surgery (e.g. evacuation of hematoma, ligation of bleeding vessels) if planned.

    c. If increased body temperature occurs:

      1. implement external cooling measures (e.g. apply a hypothermia blanket if ordered, reduce room temperature, bathe client with tepid water)

      2. administer antipyretics if ordered (antipyretics are often not ordered *because they have little, if any, effect on temperature elevation resulting from failure of central regulatory structures*).

---

9. COLLABORATIVE DIAGNOSES:

Potential complications of craniocerebral trauma:

  a. **increased intracranial pressure (IICP)** related to:

    1. accumulation of blood in the cerebral tissue associated with trauma to the cerebral vessels

    2. cerebral edema associated with:

      a. increased capillary permeability of cerebral vessels (occurs with cerebral hypoxia)

      b. an increase in cellular volume resulting from disruption of the sodium pump within the cells (occurs as a result of cerebral hypoxia) and syndrome of inappropriate antidiuretic hormone (SIADH) if it occurs

    3. hydrocephalus associated with obstruction of normal cerebrospinal fluid (CSF) flow resulting from edema, hematoma, and/or presence of blood in the subarachnoid space

    4. increase in cerebral vascular volume associated with vasodilation of the cerebral vessels (a compensatory response to cerebral hypoxia);

  b. **meningitis** related to:

    1. irritation of the meninges associated with trauma to the meningeal vessels or presence of blood in the CSF

    2. introduction of pathogens into the meninges or CSF associated with a tear in the dura (more likely to occur with a compound fracture of the skull, a linear fracture of the frontal or temporal bone, and/or penetration of the skull by an object such as a bullet);

c. **seizures** related to altered activity of the cerebral neurons associated with irritation of the brain tissue resulting from the initial injury and IICP and meningitis if they occur;

d. **cranial nerve damage** related to trauma to the nerves during the initial injury and/or compression of the nerves associated with the development of cerebral hematoma or edema;

e. **diabetes insipidus** related to decreased production and/or impaired release of antidiuretic hormone (ADH) associated with trauma to the hypothalamus and/or the posterior lobe of the pituitary gland;

f. **syndrome of inappropriate antidiuretic hormone (SIADH)** related to:
   1. increased production and/or release of ADH associated with trauma to the hypothalamus and/or the posterior lobe of the pituitary gland
   2. stimulation of ADH output associated with pain, trauma, and stress;

g. **gastrointestinal (GI) bleeding** related to the development of an ulcer (stress-induced ulcer, stress-erosive gastritis, Cushing's ulcer) associated with:
   1. gastric ischemia resulting from vasoconstriction (occurs with sympathetic nervous system stimulation that can result from cerebral injury)
   2. hypersecretion of hydrochloric acid resulting from parasympathetic nervous system stimulation that can occur with cerebral injury and stress.

Desired Outcomes	Nursing Actions and *Selected Purposes/Rationales*

9.a. The client will not develop IICP as evidenced by:
1. usual or improved level of consciousness
2. no reports of increased headache
3. stable or improved motor and sensory function
4. absence of vomiting, papilledema, and seizure activity
5. usual pupillary size and reactivity
6. stable vital signs.
	9.a.1. Assess for and report signs and symptoms of IICP:
	a. increased restlessness, agitation, confusion, or lethargy
	b. reports of increased headache
	c. decreasing motor and sensory function
	d. abnormal posturing (e.g. extension [decerebrate], flexion [decorticate])
	e. vomiting (usually without nausea)
	f. papilledema
	g. seizures
	h. change in pupil size or reactivity
	i. altered respiratory pattern (e.g. Cheyne-Stokes, central neurogenic hyperventilation)
	j. full, bounding, slow pulse
	k. rise in systolic B/P with widening pulse pressure.
	2. Implement measures *to prevent IICP:*
	a. maintain fluid restrictions as ordered
	b. administer the following medications if ordered *to reduce cerebral edema:*
	  1. osmotic diuretics (e.g. mannitol)
	  2. loop diuretics (e.g. furosemide)
	  3. corticosteroids (e.g. dexamethasone)
	c. perform actions *to promote adequate cerebral venous drainage:*
	  1. elevate head of bed 30° unless contraindicated
	  2. keep head and neck in neutral position; avoid flexion, extension, and rotation of head and neck
	  3. administer a laxative, antitussive, and antiemetic if ordered *to prevent straining to have a bowel movement, coughing, and vomiting (these conditions cause an increase in intrathoracic pressure, which subsequently impedes venous return from the brain)*
	d. perform actions *to prevent cerebral hypoxia and the subsequent cerebral edema and vasodilation:*
	  1. implement measures to improve cerebral tissue perfusion (see Nursing Diagnosis 1, action b)
	  2. implement measures *to maintain a patent airway* (e.g. position client on side, suction if necessary)
	  3. administer central nervous system depressants judiciously; hold medication and consult physician if respiratory rate is less than 12/minute

Desired Outcomes | Nursing Actions and **Selected Purposes/Rationales**

4. administer oxygen as ordered and before and after tracheal suctioning
e. perform actions to prevent and treat SIADH (see actions f.2 and 3 in this diagnosis) *in order to further reduce the risk for cerebral edema*
f. perform additional actions *to prevent dilation of cerebral vessels:*
   1. implement measures *to prevent an increase in blood pressure:*
      a. observe for and control conditions that can cause agitation (e.g. fear, anxiety, distended bladder)
      b. instruct client to avoid activities that result in isometric muscle contractions (e.g. pushing feet against footboard, tightly gripping side rails)
   2. implement measures *to prevent an increase in metabolic rate:*
      a. administer anticonvulsants (e.g. phenytoin) if ordered *to prevent seizure activity*
      b. perform actions to prevent and treat increased body temperature (see Nursing Diagnosis 8, actions b and c)
      c. perform actions to prevent and treat meningitis (see actions b.5 and 6 in this diagnosis)
   3. assist with mechanical hyperventilation (may be done *to lower arterial CO_2 and prevent the vasodilation that occurs with high levels of CO_2*)
g. schedule care so activities that could raise intracranial pressure (e.g. suctioning, bathing, repositioning) are not grouped together.
3. If signs and symptoms of IICP are present:
   a. continue with above actions
   b. initiate seizure precautions
   c. prepare client for the following if planned:
      1. insertion of an intracranial pressure monitoring device (e.g. intraventricular catheter, subarachnoid screw or bolt, epidural fiberoptic catheter or transducer, intraparenchymal catheter)
      2. lumbar or ventricular puncture *to remove excess CSF*
      3. surgical intervention (e.g. ligation of bleeding vessel, aspiration of hematoma, elevation of depressed bone, removal of bone fragments)
      4. barbiturate coma therapy (may be indicated if other measures fail to control IICP)
   d. provide emotional support to client and significant others.

9.b. The client will not develop meningitis as evidenced by:
1. absence of fever and chills
2. gradual resolution of headache
3. absence of nuchal rigidity and photophobia
4. negative Kernig's and Brudzinski's signs
5. normal CSF analysis.

9.b.1. Assess for and report signs and symptoms of a CSF leak (*indicates a tear in the dura*):
   a. presence of glucose in nasal, ear, or wound drainage as shown by positive results on a glucose reagent strip; be aware that any drainage containing blood will also test positive for glucose
   b. yellowish ring ("halo") around clear, bloody, or serosanguineous drainage on dressing or pillowcase
   c. reports of postnasal drip
   d. constant swallowing.
2. Assess for and report signs and symptoms of meningitis:
   a. fever, chills
   b. increasing or persistent headache
   c. nuchal rigidity
   d. photophobia
   e. positive Kernig's sign (inability to straighten knee when hip is flexed)
   f. positive Brudzinski's sign (flexion of hip and knee in response to forward flexion of the neck).
3. Assist with lumbar puncture if indicated. Document appearance of CSF (a cloudy appearance can indicate elevated WBC levels) and CSF pressure (pressure is often elevated with meningitis).
4. Monitor results of the CSF analysis and report increased WBC and protein levels.

5. Implement measures *to prevent meningitis:*
   a. assist with thorough cleansing and debridement of head wound if indicated
   b. use sterile technique when changing dressings and working with intracranial pressure monitoring device and ventricular drain
   c. instruct client to keep hands away from head wound, drainage tube(s), and dressing; apply wrist restraints or mittens if necessary
   d. if a CSF leak is present:
      1. instruct client to avoid excessive movement and activity (bed rest is usually ordered *to prevent further stress on the torn dura*)
      2. instruct client to avoid coughing, sneezing, blowing nose, or straining to have a bowel movement (*these activities raise intracranial pressure and can cause extension of the dural tear*); consult physician regarding an order for an antitussive, decongestant, and laxative if indicated
      3. if CSF is leaking from nose:
         a. position client with head of bed elevated at least 20° unless contraindicated *to allow the fluid to drain*
         b. instruct client to avoid putting finger in nose
         c. do not perform nasal suctioning or insert a nasogastric tube
         d. do not attempt to clean nose unless ordered by physician
      4. if CSF is leaking from ear:
         a. position client on side of CSF leakage unless contraindicated *to allow the fluid to drain*
         b. instruct client to avoid putting finger in ear
         c. do not attempt to clean ear unless ordered by physician
      5. do not pack dressing into area of CSF leakage (nose, ear, or wound) *because it will interfere with the drainage of fluid*; place a sterile pad over area of CSF leakage to absorb drainage and change pad as soon as it becomes damp
      6. prepare client for surgical repair of the torn dura if the leak does not heal spontaneously
   e. administer antimicrobials if ordered.
6. If signs and symptoms of meningitis occur:
   a. continue with above measures
   b. initiate seizure precautions (*cerebral irritation can cause seizures*)
   c. provide a quiet environment with dim lighting *to reduce discomfort associated with headache and photophobia*
   d. provide emotional support to client and significant others.

9.c. The client will not experience seizure activity or injury if seizure occurs.

9.c.1. Assess for and report signs and symptoms of seizure activity (e.g. twitching [usually of face or hands], clonic-tonic movements).
2. Implement measures *to prevent seizures:*
   a. perform actions to prevent and treat IICP and meningitis (see actions a.2 and 3 and b.5 and 6 in this diagnosis)
   b. administer anticonvulsants (e.g. phenytoin) if ordered.
3. Initiate and maintain seizure precautions:
   a. have oral airway and suction equipment readily available
   b. pad side rails with blankets or soft pads
   c. keep bed in low position with side rails up when client is in bed.
4. If seizures do occur:
   a. implement measures *to decrease risk of injury:*
      1. ease client to the floor if he/she is sitting in chair or ambulating at onset of seizure
      2. remain with but do not restrain client during seizure activity
      3. do not force any object between clenched teeth or try to pry mouth open
      4. clear area of objects that may cause injury
      5. place towel under client's head if he/she is on floor
      6. as seizure activity subsides, perform actions *to maintain a patent airway* (e.g. turn client on side, insert an oral airway, suction as needed)

Desired Outcomes	Nursing Actions and *Selected Purposes/Rationales*

<table>
<tr><td></td><td>b. observe for and report characteristics of seizures (e.g. progression, time elapsed)
c. administer intravenous anticonvulsants (e.g. phenytoin, phenobarbital) if ordered
d. provide emotional support to client and significant others.</td></tr>
<tr><td>9.d. The client will not experience cranial nerve damage or will adapt to cranial nerve damage if it occurs.</td><td>9.d.1. Assess for signs and symptoms of damage to the following cranial nerves:
a. olfactory (e.g. decreased or absent sense of smell)
b. optic, oculomotor, trochlear, or abducens (e.g. diplopia, visual field cut, decreased visual acuity, abnormal extraocular movements)
c. trigeminal (e.g. decreased or absent corneal reflex, difficulty chewing, pain when chewing)
d. vagus or glossopharyngeal (e.g. loss of gag reflex, difficulty swallowing, hoarseness, inability to speak clearly)
e. hypoglossal (e.g. difficulty chewing, swallowing, or speaking)
f. facial (e.g. facial ptosis, impaired sense of taste).
2. Implement measures to prevent IICP (see actions a.2 and 3 in this diagnosis) *in order to reduce the risk for compression of and subsequent damage to the cranial nerves.*
3. Implement measures *to help the client compensate for cranial nerve damage if it has occurred:*
a. if the olfactory nerve is affected, provide meals that are visually appealing *to help stimulate appetite*
b. if vision is impaired, provide an eyepatch or opaque lens (*helps reduce double vision*), instruct client in visual scanning techniques (if experiencing visual field cut), and assist client with self-care and ambulation if indicated
c. if the corneal reflex is absent or the client is unable to close his/her eye, perform actions *to protect the cornea from irritation and abrasion* (e.g. instruct client to avoid rubbing eye; reduce exposure to dust, powder, and smoke; instill isotonic eyedrops frequently)
d. if the trigeminal, hypoglossal, vagus, and/or glossopharyngeal nerves are affected:
  1. withhold oral foods/fluids until gag reflex returns and client is better able to chew and swallow *in order to reduce the risk for aspiration*; provide parenteral nutrition or tube feedings if indicated
  2. when oral intake is allowed:
    a. perform actions *to prevent aspiration* (e.g. place client in high Fowler's position during and for at least 30 minutes after meals and snacks, assist client with oral hygiene after eating *to ensure that food particles do not remain in mouth,* instruct client to avoid laughing and talking while eating and drinking)
    b. perform actions *to improve client's ability to swallow* (e.g. avoid serving sticky foods such as peanut butter and bananas, assist client to select foods that require little or no chewing and are easily swallowed, serve thick fluids or thicken thin fluids with substances such as "Thick-it" or gelatin)
  3. perform actions *to facilitate communication* (e.g. maintain quiet environment; provide pad and pencil, magic slate, or word cards; listen carefully when client speaks)
  4. consult speech pathologist about additional ways to facilitate swallowing and communication
e. if the sensory component of the facial nerve is affected, instruct client to add extra sweeteners or seasonings to food/fluids if desired *in order to compensate for impaired sense of taste.*</td></tr>
<tr><td>9.e. The client will not experience diabetes insipidus as evidenced by:
1. absence of polyuria
2. absence of intense thirst (polydipsia).</td><td>9.e.1. Assess for and report signs and symptoms of diabetes insipidus:
a. polyuria (urine output can range from 4–10 or more liters/day)
b. reports of intense thirst (usually with a craving for ice-cold beverages); if the client is able to tolerate oral liquids, he/she may drink 4–10 or more liters of fluid/day
c. a decrease in urine specific gravity (often 1.005 or less).</td></tr>
</table>

2. Administer osmotic diuretics (e.g. mannitol), loop diuretics (e.g. furosemide), and/or corticosteroids (e.g. dexamethasone) if ordered *to decrease edema of the hypothalamus, pituitary gland, and surrounding tissue and subsequently reduce the risk for the development of diabetes insipidus.*

3. If signs and symptoms of diabetes insipidus occur:
   a. maintain fluid intake equal to output *in order to prevent water deficit*
   b. administer an ADH replacement (e.g. vasopressin, desmopressin [DDAVP]) if ordered
   c. assess for and report signs and symptoms of water deficit (e.g. decreased skin turgor; dry mucous membranes; sudden weight loss of 2% or greater; postural hypotension and/or low B/P; weak, rapid pulse; elevated serum sodium and osmolality).

9.f. The client will not develop SIADH as evidenced by:
1. stable weight
2. balanced intake and output
3. stable or improved mental status
4. stable or improved muscle strength
5. decreased reports of headache
6. absence of cellular edema, abdominal cramping, nausea, vomiting, and seizure activity
7. urine and serum sodium and osmolality levels within normal limits.

9.f.1. Assess for and report signs and symptoms of SIADH:
   a. sudden weight gain
   b. intake greater than output
   c. increased irritability or confusion
   d. increasing muscle weakness
   e. reports of persistent or increased headache
   f. fingerprint edema over sternum (reflects cellular edema)
   g. abdominal cramping, nausea, or vomiting
   h. seizures
   i. elevated urine sodium and osmolality levels
   j. low serum sodium and osmolality levels.

2. Implement measures *to reduce the risk for the development of SIADH:*
   a. perform actions to reduce pain (see Nursing Diagnosis 3, action e)
   b. perform actions to reduce fear and anxiety (see Nursing Diagnosis 10, action b)
   c. administer osmotic diuretics (e.g. mannitol), loop diuretics (e.g. furosemide), and/or corticosteroids (e.g. dexamethasone) if ordered *to decrease edema of the hypothalamus, pituitary gland, and surrounding tissue.*

3. If signs and symptoms of SIADH occur:
   a. maintain fluid restrictions if ordered (usually 500–700 ml/day) *to prevent further fluid retention*
   b. encourage intake of foods/fluids high in sodium (e.g. tomato juice, cured meats, processed cheese, canned soups, catsup, canned vegetables, dill pickles, bouillon) if oral intake is allowed and tolerated
   c. initiate seizure precautions
   d. administer the following if ordered:
      1. diuretics (usually furosemide) *to promote water excretion*
      2. intravenous infusion of a hypertonic saline solution *to treat hyponatremia*
      3. demeclocycline *to promote water excretion* (*inhibits the effect of ADH on the renal tubules*).

9.g. The client will not experience GI bleeding as evidenced by:
1. no reports of epigastric discomfort and fullness
2. absence of frank and occult blood in stool and gastric contents
3. B/P and pulse within normal range for client
4. RBC, Hct, and Hb levels within normal range.

9.g.1. Assess for and report signs and symptoms of GI bleeding (e.g. reports of epigastric discomfort or fullness, frank or occult blood in stool or gastric contents, decreased B/P, increased pulse).

2. Monitor RBC, Hct, and Hb levels. Report decreasing values.

3. Implement measures *to prevent ulceration of the gastric and duodenal mucosa:*
   a. perform actions to decrease fear and anxiety (see Nursing Diagnosis 10, action b)
   b. when oral intake is allowed:
      1. administer ulcerogenic medications (e.g. corticosteroids, phenytoin) with meals or snacks *to decrease gastric irritation*
      2. instruct client to avoid foods/fluids that stimulate hydrochloric acid secretion or irritate the gastric mucosa (e.g. coffee; caffeine-containing tea and colas; spices such as black pepper, chili powder, and nutmeg)

Desired Outcomes | Nursing Actions and *Selected Purposes/Rationales*

    c. administer histamine₂ receptor antagonists (e.g. cimetidine, ranitidine, famotidine), antacids, and cytoprotective agents (e.g. sucralfate) if ordered.

4. If signs and symptoms of GI bleeding occur:
    a. continue with above actions
    b. withhold oral foods/fluids as ordered
    c. insert nasogastric tube and maintain suction as ordered
    d. administer blood products and/or volume expanders if ordered
    e. assist with measures to control bleeding (e.g. gastric lavage, endoscopic electrocoagulation) if planned
    f. if bleeding is not controlled, refer to Care Plan on Peptic Ulcer for additional care measures.

---

10. NURSING DIAGNOSIS: Anxiety

related to impaired motor and/or sensory function; altered thought processes; uncertainty as to permanence of neurological deficits; unfamiliar environment; and lack of understanding of diagnostic tests, diagnosis, and treatments.

Desired Outcome | Nursing Actions and *Selected Purposes/Rationales*

10. The client will experience a reduction in anxiety as evidenced by:
    a. verbalization of feeling less anxious
    b. usual sleep pattern
    c. relaxed facial expression and body movements
    d. stable vital signs
    e. usual perceptual ability and interactions with others.

10.a. Assess client for signs and symptoms of anxiety (e.g. verbalization of feeling anxious, insomnia, tenseness, shakiness, restlessness, diaphoresis, elevated blood pressure, tachycardia, facial pallor, self-focused behaviors). Validate perceptions carefully, remembering that some behaviors may result from neurological changes.

b. Implement measures *to reduce fear and anxiety:*
  1. orient client to hospital environment, equipment, and routines
  2. introduce client to staff who will be participating in care; if possible, maintain consistency in staff assigned to his/her care *to provide feelings of stability and comfort with the environment*
  3. assure client that staff members are nearby; respond to call signal as soon as possible
  4. maintain a calm, supportive, confident manner when interacting with client
  5. encourage verbalization of fear and anxiety; provide feedback and assure client that posttraumatic amnesia and feelings of nervousness and bewilderment are common
  6. reinforce physician's explanations and clarify misconceptions client has about the injury, treatment plan, and prognosis
  7. explain all diagnostic tests
  8. provide a calm, restful environment
  9. instruct client in relaxation techniques and encourage participation in diversional activities
  10. perform actions to assist the client to cope with the effects of the injury (see Nursing Diagnosis 12, action c)
  11. provide information based on current needs of client at a level he/she can understand; encourage questions and clarification of information provided
  12. encourage significant others to project a caring, concerned attitude without obvious anxiousness
  13. if surgical intervention is indicated, begin preoperative teaching
  14. include significant others in orientation and teaching sessions and encourage their continued support of the client
  15. administer prescribed antianxiety agents if indicated.

c. Consult physician if above actions fail to control fear and anxiety.

11. NURSING DIAGNOSIS: **Self-concept disturbance***

related to:
a. change in appearance (e.g. periocular edema and ecchymosis, loss of hair on head if an area was shaved to repair lacerations);
b. changes in motor and sensory function;
c. dependence on others to meet basic needs;
d. anticipated changes in life style and roles associated with sensory and motor impairments and altered thought processes.

---

*This diagnostic label includes the nursing diagnoses of body image disturbance, self-esteem disturbance, and altered role performance.

Desired Outcome	Nursing Actions and *Selected Purposes/Rationales*

11. The client will demonstrate beginning adaptation to changes in appearance, physical and cognitive functioning, life style, roles, and level of independence as evidenced by:
a. verbalization of feelings of self-worth
b. maintenance of relationships with significant others
c. active participation in activities of daily living
d. verbalization of a beginning plan for adapting life style to changes resulting from craniocerebral trauma.
	11.a. Assess for signs and symptoms of a self-concept disturbance (e.g. verbalization of negative feelings about self, withdrawal from significant others, lack of participation in activities of daily living, lack of plan for adapting to necessary changes in life style).
	b. Determine the meaning of changes in appearance, physical and cognitive functioning, life style, roles, and level of independence to the client by encouraging verbalization of feelings and by noting nonverbal responses to the changes experienced.
	c. Discuss with client improvements in appearance and neurological function that can realistically be expected.
	d. Implement measures *to assist client to increase self-esteem* (e.g. limit negative self-assessment, encourage positive comments about self, give positive feedback about accomplishments and behaviors that are indicative of high self-esteem).
	e. Implement measures to assist the client to cope with the effects of craniocerebral trauma (see Nursing Diagnosis 12, action c).
	f. If periocular edema and ecchymosis are present:
	  1. reinforce that they are temporary (edema usually begins to subside 48–72 hours after the injury and ecchymosis usually disappears in 10–14 days)
	  2. instruct and assist client with measures *to reduce swelling* (e.g. cold compresses to affected area, lying on unaffected side, keeping head of bed elevated 30° unless contraindicated).
	g. Implement measures *to reduce client's embarrassment about loss of hair* (e.g. assist with hair styling that makes shaved area less obvious, provide a scarf or surgical cap if desired). Reinforce the fact that the hair will grow back.
	h. Assist client with usual grooming and makeup habits if necessary.
	i. Discuss techniques the client can utilize *to adapt to altered thought processes:*
	  1. encourage client to make lists and jot down messages and to refer to these rather than relying on memory
	  2. instruct the client to place self in a calm environment when making decisions
	  3. encourage client to validate decisions, clarify information, and seek assistance to problem solve if indicated
	  4. encourage client to schedule adequate rest periods and reduce stressors *in order to decrease irritability.*
	j. Instruct significant others in ways to manage client's emotional lability and inappropriate behavior (e.g. provide privacy, reduce environmental stimuli, distract client by clapping hands).

Desired Outcome	Nursing Actions and *Selected Purposes/Rationales*

k. Reinforce use of assistive devices (e.g. plate guard, nonslip tray mat, broad-handled utensils, universal cuff, button hook, long-handled shoehorn) and mobility aids (e.g. walker, cane) *to increase client's independence.*

l. Encourage significant others to allow client to do what he/she is able *so that independence can be re-established and/or self-esteem redeveloped.*

m. Demonstrate acceptance of client using techniques such as touch and frequent visits. Encourage significant others to do the same.

n. Assist client's and significant others' adjustment by listening, facilitating communication, and providing information.

o. Support behaviors suggesting positive adaptation to changes that have occurred (e.g. use of assistive devices to perform self-care, verbalization of feelings of self-worth, maintenance of relationships with significant others).

p. Assist client and significant others to have similar expectations and understanding of future life style.

q. Encourage visits and support from significant others.

r. Encourage client to continue involvement in social activities and to pursue usual roles and interests. If previous roles, interests, and hobbies cannot be pursued, encourage development of new ones.

s. Provide information about and encourage utilization of community agencies and support groups (e.g. brain injury support groups, vocational rehabilitation, family and individual counseling) if appropriate.

t. Consult physician about psychological counseling if client desires or seems unwilling or unable to adapt to changes resulting from craniocerebral trauma.

---

12. NURSING DIAGNOSIS: **Ineffective individual coping**

related to fear, anxiety, persistent headache, changes in motor and sensory function and thought processes, and possibility of lengthy rehabilitation and changes in future life style and roles.

Desired Outcome	Nursing Actions and *Selected Purposes/Rationales*

12. The client will demonstrate effective coping as evidenced by:
   a. verbalization of ability to cope with the effects of craniocerebral trauma
   b. utilization of appropriate problem-solving techniques
   c. willingness to participate in treatment plan and meet basic needs
   d. absence of destructive behavior toward self and others
   e. appropriate use of defense mechanisms
   f. utilization of available support systems.

12.a. Assess for and report signs and symptoms of ineffective individual coping (e.g. verbalization of inability to cope; inability to ask for help, problem solve, or meet basic needs; insomnia; withdrawal; reluctance to participate in treatment plan; destructive behavior toward self or others; inappropriate use of defense mechanisms; inability to meet role expectations). Validate perceptions carefully, remembering that some behaviors may be the result of neurological changes.

b. Assess client's perception of current situation.

c. Implement measures *to promote effective coping:*
   1. allow time for client to begin to adjust to planned treatment, residual effects of craniocerebral trauma, and anticipated life-style and role changes
   2. perform actions to reduce fear and anxiety (see Nursing Diagnosis 10, action b)
   3. perform actions to reduce headache (see Nursing Diagnosis 3, action e)
   4. assist client to recognize and manage inappropriate denial if it is present
   5. encourage verbalization about current situation

6. assist client to identify personal strengths and resources that can be utilized to facilitate coping with the current situation
7. demonstrate acceptance of client but set limits on inappropriate behavior
8. create an atmosphere of trust and support
9. if acceptable to client, arrange for a visit with another individual who has successfully recovered from craniocerebral trauma
10. include client in the planning of care, encourage maximum participation in treatment plan, and allow choices when possible *to enable him/her to maintain a sense of control*
11. instruct client in effective problem-solving techniques (e.g. accurate identification of stressors, determination of various options to solve problem)
12. assist client to maintain usual daily routines whenever possible
13. assist client to identify priorities and attainable goals as he/she starts to plan for necessary life-style and role changes
14. set up a home evaluation appointment with occupational and physical therapists before client's discharge if indicated *so that changes in the home environment (e.g. installation of ramps and handrails, widening doorways, altering kitchen facilities) can be completed by discharge*
15. assist client and significant others to identify ways that personal and family goals can be adjusted rather than abandoned
16. inform client that he/she may have days when impairments worsen; assure client that this is usually temporary and the result of physical and/or emotional stress or fatigue rather than an indication of deteriorating neurological status
17. administer antianxiety and/or antidepressant agents if ordered
18. assist client to identify and utilize available support systems; provide information regarding available community resources that can assist client and significant others in coping with effects of craniocerebral trauma (e.g. brain injury support groups; individual, family, and financial counseling services)
19. encourage client to share with significant others the kind of support that would be most beneficial (e.g. listening, inspiring hope, providing reassurance and accurate information)
20. support behaviors indicative of effective coping (e.g. participation in treatment plan and self-care activities, communication of ability to cope, utilization of effective problem-solving strategies).
   d. Consult physician about psychological and vocational counseling if appropriate. Initiate a referral if necessary.

---

13. NURSING DIAGNOSIS: **Altered family processes**

related to change in family roles and structure associated with a family member's motor and sensory impairments, altered thought processes, and possible need for lengthy rehabilitation.

Desired Outcome	Nursing Actions and *Selected Purposes/Rationales*
13. The family members* will demonstrate beginning adjustment to changes in functioning of family	13.a. Assess for signs and symptoms of altered family processes (e.g. inability to meet client's needs, statements of not being able to accept client's physical impairments and changes in thought processes or make necessary role and life-style changes, inability to make decisions,

*The term "family members" is being used here to include client's significant others.

Desired Outcome	Nursing Actions and *Selected Purposes/Rationales*

member and family roles and structure as evidenced by:
a. meeting client's needs
b. verbalization of ways to adapt to required role and life-style changes
c. active participation in decision making and client's rehabilitation
d. positive interactions with one another.
	inability or refusal to participate in client's rehabilitation, negative family interactions).
	b. Identify components of the family and their patterns of communication and role expectations.
	c. Implement measures *to facilitate family members' adjustment to client's diagnosis, changes in client's functioning within the family system, and altered family roles and structure:*
	  1. encourage verbalization of feelings about client's disabilities and the effect of these on their family structure; actively listen to each member and maintain a nonjudgmental attitude about feelings shared
	  2. reinforce physician's explanation about the effects of craniocerebral trauma and planned treatment and rehabilitation
	  3. assist family members to gain a realistic perspective of client's situation, conveying as much hope as appropriate
	  4. provide privacy *so that family members and client can share their feelings with one another;* stress the importance of and facilitate the use of good communication techniques
	  5. assist family members to progress through their own grieving process; explain that they may encounter times when they need to focus on meeting their own rather than the client's needs
	  6. emphasize the need for family members to obtain adequate rest and nutrition and to identify and utilize stress management techniques *so that they are better able to emotionally and physically deal with the changes and losses experienced*
	  7. encourage and assist family members to identify coping strategies for dealing with the client's disabilities and the effects on the family
	  8. assist family members to identify realistic goals and ways of reaching these goals
	  9. include family members in decision making about client and his/her care; convey appreciation for their input and continued support of client
	  10. encourage and allow family members to participate in client's care and rehabilitation
	  11. assist family members to identify resources that could assist them in coping with their feelings and meeting their immediate and long-term needs (e.g. counseling and social services; pastoral care; service, church, and brain injury support groups); initiate a referral if indicated.
	d. Consult physician if family members continue to demonstrate difficulty adapting to changes in client's functioning, roles, and family structure.

Discharge Teaching

---

14. NURSING DIAGNOSIS:	**Knowledge deficit, Ineffective management of therapeutic regimen, or Altered health maintenance***

    *The nurse should select the diagnostic label that is most appropriate for the client's discharge teaching needs.

Desired Outcomes	Nursing Actions and *Selected Purposes/Rationales*
14.a. The client will identify ways to adapt to	14.a.1. Instruct client in ways to adapt to neurological deficits* resulting from craniocerebral trauma:

    *Neurological deficits can range from a temporary increase in irritability or a slight facial droop to hemiplegia, aphasia, or severely altered thought processes depending on the areas of the brain that have been affected. Ways of adapting to a few of the more common deficits are included here. For more specific rehabilitative measures and a more extensive discussion of deficits, refer to textbooks on neurological nursing and the Care Plan on Cerebrovascular Accident.

neurological deficits that may persist following craniocerebral trauma.

    a. wear an eyepatch or opaque lens if double vision is a problem

    b. utilize scanning techniques if visual field cut is present

    c. utilize paper and pencil, magic slate, computer, pictures, and gestures to express self if verbal communication is impaired

    d. write down messages and reminders and refer to written instructions repeatedly if experiencing difficulty concentrating or remembering

    e. request assistance when problem solving and setting priorities and seek validation of decisions if reasoning ability is impaired

    f. continue with techniques and exercises to improve swallowing if indicated

    g. prepare meals that are visually appealing to help stimulate appetite if senses of smell and/or taste are impaired

    h. utilize assistive devices (e.g. wheelchair, cane, walker, broad-handled eating utensils, plate guard) if motor function is impaired

    i. plan daily activities to allow for adequate rest periods in order to reduce irritability that often occurs after craniocerebral trauma.

  2. Allow time for questions, clarification, and return demonstration of techniques.

14.b. The client will identify ways to reduce headache.

14.b. Instruct client in ways to reduce headache (headache may persist for months following injury):

  1. dim environmental lighting if possible or wear sunglasses when light is bright

  2. reduce environmental noise whenever possible (e.g. lower volume on TV and radio)

  3. avoid situations that increase stress

  4. take analgesics as prescribed.

14.c. The client will state signs and symptoms to report to the health care provider.

14.c. Instruct client to report the following signs and symptoms:

  1. increased drowsiness unrelated to a significant increase in activity or decrease in amount of sleep obtained

  2. increased irritability or restlessness

  3. changes in behavior, increased difficulty remembering or concentrating

  4. new or increased weakness of extremities

  5. decreased sensation in extremities

  6. severe headache

  7. new or increased difficulty speaking or understanding what others are saying

  8. new or increased difficulty chewing or swallowing

  9. increase in or development of changes in vision (e.g. double vision, blurred vision, visual field cuts)

  10. new or increased dizziness, difficulty maintaining balance

  11. bloody, yellowish, or clear drainage from nose or ears

  12. stiff neck

  13. sudden weight gain or loss

  14. excessive thirst

  15. unusual increase or decrease in amount of urination

  16. unexplained fever

  17. seizures.

14.d. The client will identify community resources that can assist with home management and adjustment to changes resulting from craniocerebral trauma.

14.d.1. Inform client and significant others of community resources that can assist with home management and adjustment to changes resulting from craniocerebral trauma (e.g. home health agencies, Meals on Wheels, social and financial services, brain injury support groups, local service groups that can help obtain assistive devices, individual and family counseling services).

  2. Initiate a referral if indicated.

14.e. The client will verbalize an understanding of and a plan for adhering to recommended follow-up care including future

14.e.1. Reinforce the importance of keeping follow-up appointments with health care provider and physical, occupational, and speech therapists.

  2. Teach client the rationale for, side effects of, schedule for taking, and importance of taking medications prescribed (e.g. phenytoin, antimicrobials). Inform client of pertinent food and drug interactions.

Desired Outcomes	Nursing Actions and *Selected Purposes/Rationales*
appointments with health care provider and therapists and medications prescribed.	3. Implement measures to improve client compliance: a. include significant others in teaching sessions if possible b. encourage questions and allow time for reinforcement and clarification of information provided c. provide written instructions on scheduled appointments with health care provider and occupational, physical, and speech therapists; medications prescribed; and signs and symptoms to report.

Bibliography

See pages 897–898 and 901.

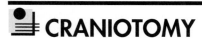

CRANIOTOMY

A craniotomy is a surgical opening into the skull to gain access to the brain. Reasons for the surgery include removing a tumor, abscess, hematoma, bone fragments, or foreign object (e.g. bullet); controlling bleeding; repairing a vascular abnormality (e.g. aneurysm, arteriovenous malformation); and improving ventricular drainage. A craniectomy (excision of a portion of the skull) is the usual method of entering the brain. If this portion of the skull is replaced (using the preserved bone or a synthetic substance), it can be done on completion of the surgery or sometime in the future after there are no longer concerns about increased intracranial pressure and/or cerebral infection.

A craniotomy is described in relation to the approach (i.e. supratentorial, infratentorial) and the location of the pathology (e.g. temporal, occipital, parietal). The neurological deficits that can occur following the surgical procedure depend primarily on the areas of the brain that are disrupted to gain access to the desired area (e.g. speech may be impaired following a temporal approach, ataxia is expected after a cerebellar approach) and the amount and location of the brain tissue that is excised or traumatized at the site of the pathology.

This care plan focuses on the adult client hospitalized for a craniotomy. Preoperative goals of care are to decrease fear and anxiety and educate the client about postoperative expectations and management. Postoperatively, goals of care are to reduce pain, prevent complications, assist the client to adjust to any neurological impairments, and educate the client regarding follow-up care. Client care and discharge teaching need to be individualized based on the diagnosis and the neurological deficits he/she is experiencing. For more detailed coverage of nursing care measures for various neurological deficits, refer to the Care Plan on Cerebrovascular Accident.

DIAGNOSTIC TESTS

Computed tomography (CT)
Magnetic resonance imaging (MRI)
Skull x-rays
Cerebral angiography
Brain scan
Positron emission tomography (PET)
Transcranial ultrasound

DISCHARGE CRITERIA

Prior to discharge, the client will:

- have adequate cerebral tissue perfusion

- have improved or stable neurological function

- have no signs and symptoms of complications

- have surgical pain controlled

- have evidence of normal wound healing

- identify ways to adapt to neurological deficits resulting from the underlying disease condition and/or surgical procedure

- identify ways to protect the surgical site from injury

- state signs and symptoms to report to the health care provider

- share thoughts and feelings about the diagnosis and neurological deficits resulting from the underlying disease process and/or the surgery
- identify community resources that can assist with home management and adjustment to changes resulting from the diagnosis and/or the surgery
- verbalize an understanding of and a plan for adhering to recommended follow-up care including future appointments with health care provider, activity level, pain management, and medications prescribed.

NURSING/ COLLABORATIVE DIAGNOSES	**Preoperative** 1. Anxiety △ 273 **Postoperative** 1. Pain: headache △ 274 2. Risk for altered body temperature: increased △ 275 3. Potential complications: a. increased intracranial pressure (IICP) b. meningitis c. seizures d. diabetes insipidus e. cranial nerve damage △ 275 4. Self-concept disturbance △ 280
DISCHARGE TEACHING	5. Knowledge deficit, Ineffective management of therapeutic regimen, or Altered health maintenance △ 282

See Standardized Preoperative and Postoperative Care Plans for additional diagnoses.

PREOPERATIVE

Use in conjunction with the Standardized Preoperative Care Plan.

1. NURSING DIAGNOSIS:

Anxiety

related to:
a. unfamiliar environment and separation from significant others;
b. lack of understanding of diagnostic tests and planned surgical procedure;
c. anticipated loss of control associated with effects of anesthesia;
d. financial concerns associated with hospitalization;
e. possibility of continued and/or new neurological impairments;
f. anticipated discomfort, surgical findings, and changes in appearance (e.g. shaved head, skull indentation) and usual life style and roles;
g. possibility of death.

Desired Outcome	Nursing Actions and *Selected Purposes/Rationales*
1. The client will experience a reduction in anxiety (see Standardized Preoperative Care Plan, Nursing Diagnosis 1 [pp. 96–97], for outcome criteria).	1.a. Refer to Standardized Preoperative Care Plan, Nursing Diagnosis 1 (pp. 96–97), for measures related to assessment and reduction of fear and anxiety. b. Implement additional measures *to reduce fear and anxiety:* 1. explain the necessity for intensive care monitoring after most craniotomies; orient client to the critical care unit if appropriate 2. describe and explain the rationale for equipment and tubes that may be present postoperatively (e.g. intracranial pressure monitoring device, ventilator, ventricular drain, wound drain, intravenous lines) 3. establish an effective method of communicating (e.g. magic slate, word

Desired Outcome	Nursing Actions and *Selected Purposes/Rationales*

cards and/or picture board, hand signals) if client is expected to be intubated or speech impairment is anticipated following surgery

4. perform actions *to reduce fear and anxiety about anticipated changes in physical appearance:*
   a. if the surgical site is shaved before anesthesia induction, cover client's head with a surgical cap, stockinette, or clean scarf (helps keep the client warm and reduce embarrassment)
   b. inform client that the incision line is usually made behind the hairline (with a supratentorial approach) or just above the nape of the neck (with an infratentorial approach) and should not be apparent when hair grows back
   c. assure client that when head dressing is removed, he/she can wear a surgical cap or scarf if desired (most physicians advise clients to avoid wearing a wig or hairpiece until incision has healed)
   d. discuss alternative hair styles that might make incision, skull indentation, and/or shaved portion of scalp less apparent
   e. assure client that the swollen eyes and facial bruising that can occur after surgery are temporary (these are usually the result of prone positioning and/or pressure from devices used to immobilize the head during surgery)
5. reinforce physician's explanations about anticipated effects of the surgery on neurological function; discuss resources available to assist client to adapt to anticipated impairments (e.g. speech, occupational, and physical therapists).

POSTOPERATIVE

Use in conjunction with the Standardized Postoperative Care Plan.

---

1. NURSING DIAGNOSIS: **Pain: headache**

related to:
a. trauma to the cerebral tissue associated with the surgical procedure;
b. stretching or compression of cerebral vessels and tissue associated with increased intracranial pressure if it occurs;
c. irritation of the meninges associated with bleeding from meningeal vessels, leakage of blood into the cerebrospinal fluid (CSF), and/or inflammation of the meninges.

Desired Outcome	Nursing Actions and *Selected Purposes/Rationales*

1. The client will obtain relief from headache as evidenced by:
   a. verbalization of same
   b. relaxed facial expression and body positioning.

1.a. Assess for signs and symptoms of headache (e.g. statements of same, restlessness, irritability, grimacing, rubbing head, avoidance of bright lights and noises, reluctance to move).
b. Assess client's perception of the severity of the headache using a pain intensity rating scale.
c. Assess the client's pain pattern (e.g. location, quality, onset, duration, precipitating factors, aggravating factors, alleviating factors).
d. Ask the client to describe previous experiences with headaches and methods used to manage them effectively.
e. Implement measures *to relieve headache:*
   1. perform actions *to reduce fear and anxiety about the pain experience* (e.g. assure client that his/her need for headache relief is understood, plan methods for relieving headache with client)
   2. perform actions to reduce fear and anxiety (see Standardized Postoperative Care Plan, Nursing Diagnosis 20, action b [p. 122]) *in*

order to promote relaxation and subsequently increase the client's threshold and tolerance for pain

3. administer analgesics before activities and procedures that can cause headache and before headache becomes severe

4. perform actions *to minimize environmental stimuli* (e.g. provide a quiet environment, limit number of visitors and their length of stay, dim lights)

5. avoid jarring bed or startling client *to minimize risk of sudden movements*

6. perform actions to prevent and treat increased intracranial pressure and meningitis (see Postoperative Collaborative Diagnosis 3, actions a.2 and 3 and b.5 and 6)

7. provide or assist with nonpharmacologic measures for headache relief (e.g. cool cloth to forehead, progressive relaxation exercises)

8. administer nonnarcotic analgesics or codeine (other narcotic [opioid] analgesics are usually contraindicated *because they have a greater depressant effect on the central nervous system*) if ordered.

f. Consult physician if above actions fail to relieve headache.

---

2. NURSING DIAGNOSIS:

Risk for altered body temperature: increased

related to:
a. pressure on the hypothalamus associated with the underlying disease process and/or development of a hematoma or cerebral edema postoperatively;
b. trauma to the hypothalamus during surgery.

Desired Outcome	Nursing Actions and *Selected Purposes/Rationales*

2. The client will maintain a normal body temperature.	2.a. Assess for and report signs and symptoms of increased body temperature resulting from impaired function of the hypothalamus (e.g. elevated temperature; pale, hot, dry skin).
	b. Implement measures *to reduce pressure on the hypothalamus:*
	  1. administer osmotic diuretics (e.g. mannitol), loop diuretics (e.g. furosemide), and/or corticosteroids (e.g. dexamethasone) if ordered *to decrease edema of the hypothalamus and surrounding tissue*
	  2. prepare client for removal of bone flap, evacuation of hematoma, or ligation of bleeding vessels if planned.
	c. If increased body temperature occurs:
	  1. implement external cooling measures (e.g. apply a hypothermia blanket if ordered, reduce room temperature, bathe client with tepid water)
	  2. administer antipyretics if ordered (antipyretics are often not ordered *because they have little, if any, effect on temperature elevation resulting from failure of central regulatory structures*).

---

3. COLLABORATIVE DIAGNOSES:

Potential complications of craniotomy:

a. **increased intracranial pressure (IICP)** related to:
1. accumulation of blood in the cerebral tissue associated with surgical trauma to the cerebral vessels
2. cerebral edema associated with increased capillary permeability of cerebral vessels and an increase in cellular volume resulting from

disruption of the sodium pump within the cells (both can occur as a result of cerebral hypoxia)

3. hydrocephalus associated with obstruction of normal CSF flow resulting from edema, hematoma, presence of blood in the subarachnoid space, and/or occlusion of ventricular shunt if present

4. increase in cerebral vascular volume associated with vasodilation of the cerebral vessels (a compensatory response to cerebral hypoxia);

b. **meningitis** related to:

1. irritation of the meninges associated with trauma to the meningeal vessels or presence of blood in the CSF

2. introduction of pathogens into the meninges or CSF associated with an interruption in the dura, which is incised to gain access to the brain tissue;

c. **seizures** related to altered activity of the cerebral neurons associated with irritation of the brain tissue during surgery (especially if a supratentorial approach was used) or IICP and meningitis if they occur;

d. **diabetes insipidus** related to decreased production and/or impaired release of antidiuretic hormone (ADH) associated with altered function of the hypothalamus or posterior lobe of the pituitary gland (can occur because of surgical trauma or postoperative edema or hematoma in that area);

e. **cranial nerve damage** related to trauma to the nerves prior to or during surgery and/or compression of the nerves associated with postoperative cerebral hematoma or edema.

Desired Outcomes	Nursing Actions and *Selected Purposes/Rationales*

3.a. The client will not develop IICP as evidenced by:
1. usual or improved level of consciousness
2. no reports of increased headache
3. stable or improved motor and sensory function
4. absence of vomiting, papilledema, and seizure activity
5. usual pupillary size and reactivity
6. stable vital signs.
	3.a.1. Assess for and report signs and symptoms of IICP:
	  a. restlessness, agitation, confusion, lethargy
	  b. reports of increased headache
	  c. decreasing motor and sensory function
	  d. abnormal posturing (e.g. extension [decerebrate], flexion [decorticate])
	  e. vomiting (usually without nausea)
	  f. elevation of bone flap or bulging in area where bone was removed
	  g. papilledema
	  h. seizures
	  i. change in pupil size or reactivity
	  j. altered respiratory pattern (e.g. Cheyne-Stokes, central neurogenic hyperventilation)
	  k. full, bounding, slow pulse
	  l. rise in systolic B/P with widening pulse pressure.
	  2. Implement measures *to prevent IICP:*
	    a. maintain fluid restrictions as ordered
	    b. administer the following medications if ordered *to reduce cerebral edema:*
	      1. osmotic diuretics (e.g. mannitol)
	      2. loop diuretics (e.g. furosemide)
	      3. corticosteroids (e.g. dexamethasone)
	    c. perform actions *to promote adequate cerebral venous drainage:*
	      1. elevate head of bed 30° unless contraindicated (if surgery was performed using the infratentorial approach, head of bed is usually kept flat postoperatively *to reduce pressure on the brain stem*)
	      2. keep head and neck in neutral position; avoid flexion, extension, and rotation of head and neck
	      3. administer a laxative, antitussive, and antiemetic if ordered *to prevent straining to have a bowel movement, coughing, and vomiting (these conditions cause an increase in intrathoracic pressure, which subsequently impedes venous return from the brain)*
	    d. perform actions *to prevent cerebral hypoxia and the subsequent cerebral edema and vasodilation:*

1. implement measures *to maintain a patent airway* (e.g. position client on side, suction if necessary)
2. administer central nervous system depressants judiciously; hold medication and consult physician if respiratory rate is less than 12/minute
3. administer oxygen as ordered and before and after tracheal suctioning

  e. perform additional actions *to prevent dilation of cerebral vessels:*

1. implement measures *to prevent an increase in blood pressure:*
   a. observe for and control conditions that can cause agitation (e.g. fear, anxiety, distended bladder)
   b. instruct client to avoid activities that result in isometric muscle contractions (e.g. pushing feet against footboard, tightly gripping side rails)
2. implement measures *to prevent an increase in metabolic rate:*
   a. administer anticonvulsants (e.g. phenytoin) if ordered *to prevent seizure activity*
   b. perform actions to prevent and treat increased body temperature (see Postoperative Nursing Diagnosis 2, actions b and c)
   c. perform actions to prevent and treat meningitis (see actions b.5 and 6 in this diagnosis)
3. assist with mechanical hyperventilation (may be done *to lower arterial CO_2 and prevent the vasodilation that occurs with high levels of CO_2*)

  f. schedule care so activities that could raise intracranial pressure (e.g. suctioning, bathing, repositioning) are not grouped together

  g. position client on unoperative side if bone flap and/or large mass was removed (*helps prevent increased pressure and venous congestion in the operative area*)

  h. if client has a wound drain, perform actions *to maintain its patency* (e.g. keep tubing free of kinks, empty drainage collection device when appropriate, maintain wound suction as ordered)

  i. if client has an internal shunt, perform actions *to maintain its patency* (e.g. avoid pressure on the skin over the shunt, tubing, and reservoir site; pump shunt as ordered)

  j. if client has an external shunt, perform actions *to maintain its patency* (e.g. avoid kinks in tubing, keep client's head and drainage collection device at the prescribed levels).

3. If signs and symptoms of IICP are present:
   a. continue with above actions
   b. initiate seizure precautions
   c. prepare client for the following if planned:
      1. insertion of an intracranial pressure monitoring device (e.g. intraventricular catheter, subarachnoid screw or bolt, epidural fiberoptic catheter or transducer, intraparenchymal catheter)
      2. lumbar or ventricular puncture *to remove excess CSF*
      3. surgical intervention (e.g. ligation of bleeding vessel, repair of blocked shunt, removal of bone flap or hematoma)
   d. provide emotional support to client and significant others.

3.b. The client will not develop meningitis as evidenced by:
1. absence of fever and chills
2. absence of nuchal rigidity and photophobia
3. gradual resolution of headache
4. negative Kernig's and Brudzinski's signs
5. normal CSF analysis.

3.b.1. Assess for and report signs and symptoms of a CSF leak (*indicates an opening in the dura*):
   a. presence of glucose in nasal, ear, or wound drainage as shown by positive results on a glucose reagent strip; be aware that any drainage containing blood will also test positive for glucose
   b. yellowish ring ("halo") around clear, bloody, or serosanguineous drainage on dressing or pillowcase
   c. reports of postnasal drip
   d. constant swallowing.

2. Assess for and report signs and symptoms of meningitis:
   a. fever, chills

Desired Outcomes	Nursing Actions and *Selected Purposes/Rationales*

       b. nuchal rigidity

       c. photophobia

       d. increasing or persistent headache

       e. positive Kernig's sign (inability to straighten knee when hip is flexed)

       f. positive Brudzinski's sign (flexion of hip and knee in response to forward flexion of the neck).

3. Assist with lumbar puncture if indicated. Document appearance of CSF (a cloudy appearance can indicate elevated WBC levels) and CSF pressure (pressure is often elevated with meningitis).

4. Monitor results of CSF analysis and report increased WBC and protein levels.

5. Implement measures *to prevent meningitis:*

       a. use sterile technique when changing dressings and working with an external ventricular shunt, wound drain, and intracranial pressure monitoring device

       b. instruct client to keep hands away from drains and dressings; apply wrist restraints or mittens if necessary

       c. if a CSF leak is present:

          1. instruct client to avoid excessive movement and activity (bed rest is usually ordered *to prevent further stress on the incised dura*)

          2. instruct client to avoid coughing, sneezing, blowing nose, and straining to have a bowel movement (*these activities raise intracranial pressure and can cause extension of the dural tear*); consult physician about an order for an antitussive, decongestant, and laxative if indicated

          3. if CSF is leaking from nose:

             a. position client with head of bed elevated at least 20° unless contraindicated *to allow the fluid to drain*

             b. instruct client to avoid putting finger in nose

             c. do not perform nasal suctioning or insert a nasogastric tube

             d. do not attempt to clean nose unless ordered by physician

          4. if CSF is leaking from ear:

             a. position client on side of CSF leakage unless contraindicated *to allow the fluid to drain*

             b. instruct client to avoid putting finger in ear

             c. do not attempt to clean ear unless ordered by physician

          5. do not pack dressing into area of CSF leakage (nose, ear, or wound) *because it will interfere with the drainage of fluid*; place a sterile pad over area of CSF leakage to absorb drainage and change pad as soon as it becomes damp

          6. prepare client for surgical repair of the dura if leak does not heal spontaneously (the area usually heals without surgical intervention within 7–10 days)

       d. administer antimicrobials if ordered.

6. If signs and symptoms of meningitis occur:

       a. continue with above measures

       b. initiate seizure precautions (*cerebral irritation can cause seizures*)

       c. provide a quiet environment with dim lighting *to reduce discomfort associated with headache and photophobia*

       d. provide emotional support to client and significant others.

3.c. The client will not experience seizure activity or injury if seizure occurs.

3.c.1. Assess for and report signs and symptoms of seizure activity (e.g. twitching [usually of face or hands], clonic-tonic movements).

2. Implement measures *to prevent seizures:*

       a. perform actions to prevent and treat IICP and meningitis (see actions a.2 and 3 and b.5 and 6 in this diagnosis)

       b. administer anticonvulsants (e.g. phenytoin) if ordered.

3. Initiate and maintain seizure precautions:

       a. have an oral airway and suction equipment readily available

       b. pad side rails with blankets or soft pads

       c. keep bed in low position with side rails up when client is in bed.

4. If seizures do occur:
  a. implement measures *to decrease risk of injury:*
    1. ease client to the floor if he/she is sitting in chair or ambulating at onset of seizure
    2. remain with but do not restrain client during seizure activity
    3. do not force any object between clenched teeth or try to pry mouth open
    4. clear area of objects that may cause injury
    5. place towel under client's head if he/she is on the floor
    6. as seizure activity subsides, perform actions *to maintain a patent airway* (e.g. turn client on side, insert an oral airway, suction as needed)
  b. observe for and report characteristics of seizures (e.g. progression, time elapsed)
  c. administer intravenous anticonvulsants (e.g. phenytoin, phenobarbital) if ordered
  d. provide emotional support to client and significant others.

3.d. The client will not experience diabetes insipidus as evidenced by:
1. absence of polyuria
2. absence of intense thirst (polydipsia).
	3.d.1. Assess for and report signs and symptoms of diabetes insipidus:
	  a. polyuria (urine output can range from 4–10 or more liters/day)
	  b. reports of intense thirst (usually with a craving for ice-cold beverages);
	  c. low urine specific gravity (often 1.005 or less).
	2. Administer osmotic diuretics (e.g. mannitol), loop diuretics (e.g. furosemide), and/or corticosteroids (e.g. dexamethasone) if ordered *to reduce edema of the hypothalamus, pituitary gland, and surrounding tissue and subsequently reduce the risk for the development of diabetes insipidus.*
	3. If signs and symptoms of diabetes insipidus occur:
	  a. maintain fluid intake equal to output *in order to prevent water deficit*
	  b. administer an ADH replacement (e.g. vasopressin, desmopressin [DDAVP]) as ordered
	  c. assess for and report signs and symptoms of water deficit (e.g. decreased skin turgor; dry mucous membranes; sudden weight loss of 2% or greater; postural hypotension and/or low B/P; weak, rapid pulse; elevated serum sodium and osmolality).

3.e. The client will not experience cranial nerve damage or will adapt to cranial nerve damage if it occurs.	**3.e.1.** Assess for signs and symptoms of damage to the following cranial nerves:
	  a. olfactory (e.g. decreased or absent sense of smell)
	  b. optic, oculomotor, trochlear, or abducens (e.g. diplopia, visual field cut, decreased visual acuity, abnormal extraocular movements)
	  c. trigeminal (e.g. decreased or absent corneal reflex, difficulty chewing, pain when chewing)
	  d. vagus or glossopharyngeal (e.g. loss of gag reflex, difficulty swallowing, hoarseness, inability to speak clearly)
	  e. hypoglossal (e.g. difficulty chewing, swallowing, or speaking)
	  f. facial (e.g. facial ptosis, impaired sense of taste).
	2. Implement measures to prevent IICP (see actions a.2 and 3 in this diagnosis) *in order to reduce the risk for compression of and subsequent damage to the cranial nerves.*
	3. Implement measures *to assist the client to adapt to cranial nerve damage if it has occurred:*
	  a. if the olfactory nerve is affected, provide meals that are visually appealing *to help stimulate appetite*
	  b. if vision is affected, provide an eyepatch or opaque lens (*helps reduce double vision*), instruct client in visual scanning techniques if experiencing visual field cut, and assist client with self-care and ambulation if indicated
	  c. if the corneal reflex is absent or the client is unable to close his/her eye, perform actions *to protect the cornea from irritation and abrasion* (e.g. instruct client to avoid rubbing eye; reduce exposure to dust, powder, and smoke; instill isotonic eyedrops frequently)
	  d. if the trigeminal, hypoglossal, vagus, and/or glossopharyngeal nerves are affected:

Desired Outcomes	Nursing Actions and *Selected Purposes/Rationales*

1. withhold oral foods/fluids until gag reflex returns and client is better able to chew and swallow *in order to reduce the risk for aspiration*; provide parenteral nutrition or tube feedings if indicated
2. when oral intake is allowed:
   a. perform actions *to prevent aspiration* (e.g. place client in high Fowler's position during and for at least 30 minutes after meals and snacks unless contraindicated, assist client with oral hygiene after eating *to ensure that food particles do not remain in mouth*, instruct client to avoid laughing and talking while eating and drinking)
   b. perform actions *to improve client's ability to swallow* (e.g. avoid serving sticky foods such as peanut butter and bananas, assist client to select foods that require little or no chewing and are easily swallowed, serve thick fluids or thicken thin fluids with substances such as "Thick-it" or gelatin)
3. perform actions *to facilitate communication* (e.g. maintain quiet environment; provide pad and pencil, magic slate, or word cards; listen carefully when client speaks)
4. consult speech pathologist about additional ways to facilitate swallowing and communication
   e. if the sensory component of the facial nerve is affected, instruct client to add extra sweeteners or seasonings to foods/fluids if desired *in order to compensate for impaired sense of taste.*

---

4. NURSING DIAGNOSIS: **Self-concept disturbance***

related to:
a. changes in appearance (e.g. periocular edema and ecchymosis, skull indentation, loss of scalp hair);
b. dependence on others to meet basic needs;
c. anticipated changes in life style and roles associated with impaired motor and sensory function (e.g. hemiplegia, visual disturbances, speech impairment) and altered thought processes (these changes can occur as a result of cerebral tissue damage).

---

*This diagnostic label includes the nursing diagnoses of body image disturbance, self-esteem disturbance, and altered role performance.

Desired Outcome	Nursing Actions and *Selected Purposes/Rationales*

4. The client will demonstrate beginning adaptation to changes in appearance, physical and cognitive functioning, life style, and roles as evidenced by:
   a. verbalization of feelings of self-worth
   b. maintenance of relationships with significant others
   c. active participation in activities of daily living

4.a. Assess for signs and symptoms of a self-concept disturbance (e.g. verbalization of negative feelings about self, withdrawal from significant others, lack of participation in activities of daily living, lack of plan for adapting to necessary changes in life style).
  b. Determine the meaning of the changes in appearance, physical and cognitive functioning, life style, and roles to the client by encouraging verbalization of feelings and by noting nonverbal responses to the changes experienced.
  c. Be aware that client may recognize and grieve for the losses experienced. Provide support during the grieving process.
  d. Discuss with client improvements in appearance and neurological function that can realistically be expected.
  e. Implement measures *to assist client to increase self-esteem* (e.g. limit

d. verbalization of a beginning plan for adapting life style to changes resulting from the underlying disease process and/or residual effects of the surgery.

negative self-assessment, encourage positive comments about self, give positive feedback about accomplishments and behaviors that are indicative of high self-esteem, assist to identify strengths).

f. Assist the client to identify and utilize coping techniques that have been helpful in the past.

g. If periocular edema and ecchymosis are present:
   1. reinforce that they are temporary (edema usually begins to subside 48–72 hours after surgery and ecchymosis usually disappears in 10–14 days)
   2. instruct client in and assist with measures *to reduce swelling* (e.g. cold compresses to affected area, lying on unoperative side unless contraindicated, keeping head of bed elevated 30° unless contraindicated).

h. Implement measures *to reduce client's embarrassment about partial or total loss of hair and misshapen skull if bone flap was not replaced* (e.g. provide client with a surgical cap or scarf, assist client to obtain a wig or hairpiece to wear after the incision has healed). Reinforce the fact that the hair will grow back and encourage client to discuss with physician the possibility of a cranioplasty in the future to restore the original shape of the skull.

i. Assist client with usual grooming and makeup habits if necessary.

j. Discuss techniques the client can utilize *to adapt to altered thought processes if present:*
   1. encourage client to make lists and jot down messages and to refer to these rather than relying on memory
   2. instruct the client to place self in a calm environment when making decisions
   3. encourage client to validate decisions, clarify information, and seek assistance to problem-solve if indicated
   4. encourage client to schedule adequate rest periods and reduce stressors *in order to decrease irritability.*

k. Demonstrate acceptance of client using techniques such as touch and frequent visits. Encourage significant others to do the same.

l. Support behaviors suggesting positive adaptation to changes that have occurred (e.g. scanning environment or wearing eyepatch if visual disturbances are present, utilizing alternative methods of communicating if speech is impaired, utilizing assistive devices to perform self-care activities).

m. Encourage significant others to allow client to do what he/she is able *so that independence can be re-established and/or self-esteem redeveloped.*

n. Encourage client contact with others *so that he/she can test and establish a new self-image.*

o. Assist client's and significant others' adjustment by listening, facilitating communication, and providing information.

p. Assist client and significant others to have similar expectations and understanding of future life style and to identify ways that personal and family goals can be adjusted rather than abandoned.

q. Teach client the rationale for treatments, encourage maximum participation in treatment regimen, and allow choices whenever possible *to enable him/her to maintain a sense of control over life.*

r. Encourage visits and support from significant others.

s. Encourage client to continue involvement in social activities and to pursue usual roles and interests. If previous roles, interests, and hobbies cannot be pursued, encourage development of new ones.

t. Provide information about and encourage utilization of community agencies and support groups (e.g. brain injury support groups; vocational rehabilitation; American Cancer Society; family, individual, and/or financial counseling) if appropriate.

u. Consult physician about psychological counseling if client desires or seems unwilling or unable to adapt to changes resulting from the disease and/or the surgery.

Discharge Teaching

---

5. NURSING DIAGNOSIS: **Knowledge deficit, Ineffective management of therapeutic regimen, or Altered health maintenance***

> *The nurse should select the diagnostic label that is most appropriate for the client's discharge teaching needs.

Desired Outcomes	Nursing Actions and *Selected Purposes/Rationales*

5.a. The client will identify ways to adapt to neurological deficits resulting from the underlying disease condition and/or surgical procedure.

5.a.1. Instruct client in ways to adapt to neurological deficits* resulting from the underlying disease condition and/or surgical procedure:
  a. wear an eyepatch or opaque lens if double vision is a problem
  b. utilize scanning techniques if visual field cut is present
  c. utilize pencil and paper, magic slate, computer, pictures, and gestures to express self if verbal communication is impaired
  d. write down messages and reminders and refer to written instructions repeatedly if experiencing difficulty concentrating or memory is impaired
  e. request assistance when problem-solving and setting priorities and seek validation of decisions if reasoning ability is impaired
  f. prepare meals that are visually appealing to help stimulate appetite if sense of smell and/or taste is diminished
  g. utilize assistive devices (e.g. wheelchair, cane, walker, broad-handled eating utensils, plate guard) if motor function is impaired
  h. plan daily activities to allow for adequate rest periods in order to reduce the irritability that can occur after cerebral tissue trauma.
  2. Allow time for questions, clarification, and return demonstration of techniques.

5.b. The client will identify ways to protect the surgical site from injury.

5.b. Instruct the client in ways to protect the surgical site from injury:
  1. wear a scarf, hat, or cap until hair has grown back
  2. do not shampoo hair until the incision has healed (usually 7–10 days following surgery)
  3. when shampooing hair, avoid vigorous scrubbing; pat surgical site dry rather than rubbing
  4. avoid use of hair dryer on hot setting, curling iron, and hot curlers at or near surgical site until hair has grown back (the direct heat can burn the unprotected scalp)
  5. avoid scratching the surgical site; if it itches as the incision heals and the hair grows back, apply light pressure to the surgical site or distract self with activities like taking a walk or watching television
  6. if the bone flap was not replaced, avoid bumping or putting excessive pressure on the surgical site (if the skull depression is large, client may need to wear a protective helmet as level of activity increases).

5.c. The client will state signs and symptoms to report to the health care provider.

5.c.1. Refer to Standardized Postoperative Care Plan, Nursing Diagnosis 21, action c (p. 123), for signs and symptoms to report to the health care provider.
  2. Instruct client to report these additional signs and symptoms:

> *Neurological deficits can range from a temporary increase in irritability or a slight facial droop to hemiplegia, aphasia, or severely altered thought processes depending on the area(s) of the brain that have been affected. Ways of adapting to a few of the more common deficits are included here. For more specific rehabilitative measures and a more extensive discussion of deficits, refer to textbooks on neurological and neurosurgical nursing and the Care Plan on Cerebrovascular Accident.

a. increased drowsiness unrelated to a significant increase in activity or a decrease in amount of sleep obtained
b. increased irritability or restlessness
c. changes in behavior, decreased ability to concentrate
d. decreased sensation in extremities
e. new or increased weakness of extremities
f. difficulty speaking or understanding what others are saying
g. change in vision (e.g. double vision, blurred vision, visual field cuts)
h. increased difficulty chewing or swallowing
i. dizziness, difficulty maintaining balance
j. increased swelling at wound site
k. bloody, yellowish, or clear drainage from ears, nose, or incision
l. stiff neck
m. excessive thirst
n. excessive urination
o. severe or persistent headache
p. seizures.

5.d. The client will identify community resources that can assist with home management and adjustment to changes resulting from the diagnosis and/or the surgery.	5.d.1. Inform client and significant others of community resources that can assist with home management and adjustment to neurological changes resulting from the diagnosis and/or surgery (e.g. physical, occupational, and speech therapists; Meals on Wheels; social services; home health agencies; American Cancer Society; brain injury support groups). 2. Initiate a referral if indicated.
5.e. The client will verbalize an understanding of and a plan for adhering to recommended follow-up care including future appointments with health care provider, activity level, pain management, and medications prescribed.	5.e.1. Refer to Standardized Postoperative Care Plan, Nursing Diagnosis 21 (pp. 123–124), for routine postoperative instructions and measures to improve client compliance. 2. Instruct client in ways to reduce headache if present (e.g. reduce environmental lighting and noise whenever possible, avoid situations that increase stress, take analgesics as prescribed). 3. Explain the rationale for, side effects of, schedule for taking, and importance of taking the prescribed medications (e.g. phenytoin, antimicrobials). Inform client of pertinent food and drug interactions.

Bibliography

See pages 897–898 and 901–902.

SPINAL CORD INJURY

Spinal cord injury (spinal cord trauma) can result from a motor vehicle accident, fall, sports or recreational injury, or act of violence. It is classified according to the cause of cord injury (e.g. contusion, compression, transection), direction of movement of the vertebrae or mechanism of injury (e.g. flexion, hyperextension, rotation), level of injury (e.g. cervical, sacral), stability of the vertebral column (i.e. stable, unstable), and/or degree of cord involvement (i.e. complete, incomplete).

Immediately following spinal cord injury, spinal shock (complete loss of motor, sensory, autonomic, and reflex activity below the level of the injury) usually occurs. Spinal shock usually lasts between 1 and 6 weeks but can persist for months. The neurological impairments that remain following the period of spinal shock depend upon the level of the cord injury (the higher the level, the greater the loss of body function) and the degree of cord involvement (if complete, there is total loss of sensory function and voluntary motor function below the level of the injury; if incomplete, some of the motor and/or sensory fibers below the level of injury are able to function).

This care plan focuses on the adult client hospitalized with a complete injury of the spinal cord at the level of the fifth cervical vertebra (C5). After the period of spinal shock, a client with a complete cord injury at the C5 level experiences loss of voluntary motor function below the clavicles; however, full neck, upper shoulder, and some biceps control and elbow flexion are retained. Sensory function is intact above the clavicles and in certain areas of the deltoids and forearms. With rehabilitation, the client should be able to do things such as operate an electric wheelchair and a manual wheelchair with hand rim projections (quad pegs), feed self using assistive devices, utilize reflex activity to achieve an erection and stimulate bowel and bladder elimination, accomplish some change in body position, and operate some equipment (e.g. typewriter, computer, telephone) using assistive devices.

Initially, goals of care are to sustain life and prevent further cord damage by stabilizing the vertebral column and reducing spinal cord ischemia. Subsequently, goals of care are to mobilize the client, prevent complications, assist him/her to regain as much independence as possible, and facilitate psychological adjustment to the effects of the injury.

DIAGNOSTIC TESTS

Cervical spine x-rays
Computed tomography (CT)
Magnetic resonance imaging (MRI)
Somatosensory-evoked potentials

DISCHARGE CRITERIA

Prior to discharge, the client will:

- have clear, audible breath sounds throughout lungs
- have no evidence of tissue irritation or breakdown
- have an adequate nutritional status
- experience optimal control of urinary and bowel elimination
- direct own care and perform or participate in self-care when possible
- have adequate tissue perfusion and thermoregulation
- have no signs and symptoms of complications resulting from the spinal cord injury and decreased mobility
- identify ways to prevent complications associated with spinal cord injury and decreased mobility
- demonstrate the ability to correctly use and maintain assistive devices
- identify ways to manage altered bowel and bladder function
- state signs and symptoms to report to the health care provider
- identify community resources that can assist with home management and adjustment to changes resulting from spinal cord injury
- share thoughts and feelings about the effects of spinal cord injury on self-concept, life style, and roles
- verbalize an understanding of and a plan for adhering to recommended follow-up care including future appointments with health care provider and occupational and physical therapists and medications prescribed.

Use in conjunction with the Care Plan on Immobility.

**NURSING/
COLLABORATIVE
DIAGNOSES**

1. Anxiety △ 285
2. Altered tissue perfusion △ 287
3. Ineffective breathing pattern △ 288
4. Ineffective airway clearance △ 288
5. Altered nutrition: less than body requirements △ 289
6. Pain:
   a. headache
   b. neck pain
   c. upper arm and shoulder pain △ 289
7. Ineffective thermoregulation △ 291
8. Sensory/perceptual alterations:
   a. visual
   b. tactile △ 291

See Care Plan on Immobility for additional diagnoses.

---

1. NURSING DIAGNOSIS:	**Anxiety**

related to extensive loss of motor and sensory function; application of immobilization device to stabilize and align the cervical spine; lack of understanding of diagnostic tests, diagnosis, and treatment; unfamiliar environment; financial concerns; and anticipated effect of the spinal cord injury on life style and roles.

Desired Outcome	Nursing Actions and *Selected Purposes/Rationales*

1. The client will experience a reduction in anxiety as evidenced by:
a. verbalization of feeling less anxious
b. usual sleep pattern
	1.a. Assess client for signs and symptoms of anxiety (e.g. verbalization of feeling anxious, insomnia, tenseness, facial pallor, self-focused behaviors).
	b. Implement measures *to reduce fear and anxiety:*
	  1. remain with client while immobilization device is being applied
	  2. explain necessity of frequent neurological checks
	  3. provide information about the insertion of skull pins:

Desired Outcome	Nursing Actions and *Selected Purposes/Rationales*

c. relaxed facial expression
d. usual perceptual ability and interactions with others.

a. assure client that the pins penetrate only the outer table of the skull, not the brain
b. assure client that very little pain is associated with the insertion but that the procedure will be quite loud since bone is such a good sound conductor
c. assure client that only a small amount of hair is clipped at each insertion site
d. explain that tongs and traction or a halo ring and traction or body jacket will be attached to the pins in order to keep the cervical spine immobilized and in correct alignment

4. explain the purpose and safety features of the turning frame or kinetic bed if appropriate
5. assure client that measures have been taken to keep him/her from falling off bed/frame (e.g. side rails up, safety straps securely fastened)
6. if client is placed on a turning frame (e.g. Stryker frame), explain the sensations that may be experienced when the frame is turned (e.g. closed-in feeling, momentary dizziness); assure client that these sensations disappear when the turn is completed
7. if client is placed on a kinetic bed (e.g. Roto Rest bed), explain the sensations that may be experienced as the bed continually rotates from side-to-side (e.g. motion sickness, fear of falling); assure client that these sensations usually disappear after being on the bed for a day or two
8. once cervical spine immobilization is accomplished:
   a. orient client to hospital environment, equipment, and routines
   b. assure client that staff members are nearby; provide call signal that has been adapted to meet client's needs (e.g. voice-activated call light) and respond to call signal as soon as possible
   c. introduce client to staff who will be participating in care; if possible, maintain consistency in staff assigned to his/her care *to provide feelings of stability and comfort with the environment*
   d. maintain a calm, supportive, confident manner when interacting with client
   e. avoid startling client (e.g. speak client's name and identify yourself when entering room and before physical contact, place self in client's visual field whenever possible during care and conversation)
   f. encourage verbalization of fear and anxiety; provide feedback
   g. reinforce physician's explanations and clarify misconceptions client has about spinal cord injury, treatment plan, and prognosis
   h. explain all diagnostic tests
   i. explain that the flaccid paralysis and lack of reflex activity below the level of the cord injury that occurs immediately following the injury is a result of spinal shock; emphasize that some reflex activity will return after spinal shock subsides
   j. provide a calm, restful environment
   k. instruct client in relaxation techniques and encourage participation in diversional activities
   l. initiate financial and/or social service referrals if indicated
   m. perform actions to assist client to cope with effects of the injury (see Nursing Diagnosis 23, action c)
   n. provide information based on current needs of client at a level he/she can understand; encourage questions and clarification of information provided
   o. when appropriate, assist client to meet spiritual needs (e.g. arrange for a visit from clergy)
   p. encourage significant others to project a caring, concerned attitude without obvious anxiousness

q. include significant others in orientation and teaching sessions and encourage their continued support of the client

r. if comfortable for nurse and client, reinforce verbal messages of caring by touching areas where client has sensation (e.g. shoulders, head, neck); encourage significant others to do the same.

c. Consult physician if above actions fail to control fear and anxiety.

---

2. NURSING DIAGNOSIS: **Altered tissue perfusion**

related to:

a. decreased cardiac output associated with:
1. bradycardia resulting from loss of sympathetic nervous system activity and subsequent unopposed action of the parasympathetic nervous system on the heart
2. decreased venous return resulting from vasodilation below the level of the injury (the vasodilation occurs because of loss of sympathetic nervous system activity below the level of cord injury);

b. peripheral pooling of blood associated with vasodilation below the level of the injury and loss of muscle tone in extremities resulting from paralysis of extremities and decreased mobility.

Desired Outcome	Nursing Actions and *Selected Purposes/Rationales*
2. The client will maintain adequate tissue perfusion as evidenced by: a. B/P within normal range for client b. usual mental status c. extremities warm with absence of pallor and cyanosis d. palpable peripheral pulses e. capillary refill time less than 3 seconds f. absence of edema g. urine output at least 30 ml/hour.	2.a. Assess for and report signs and symptoms of diminished tissue perfusion (e.g. hypotension, restlessness, confusion, cool extremities, pallor or cyanosis of extremities, diminished or absent peripheral pulses, slow capillary refill, edema, oliguria). b. Implement measures *to maintain adequate tissue perfusion:* 　1. avoid activities that cause vagal stimulation (e.g. suctioning) unless absolutely necessary *in order to prevent a further reduction in pulse rate* 　2. administer the following medications if ordered: 　　a. anticholinergics (e.g. atropine) *to increase heart rate* 　　b. sympathomimetics (e.g. dopamine) *to increase cardiac output and maintain arterial pressure* 　3. perform actions *to prevent peripheral pooling of blood and/or increase venous return:* 　　a. perform passive range of motion exercises at least 3 times/day 　　b. avoid positions that compromise blood flow in the lower extremities (e.g. crossing legs, pillows under knees, sitting for long periods) 　　c. apply thigh-high elastic stockings as ordered 　　d. apply/maintain a sequential compression device to lower extremities if ordered 　　e. elevate lower extremities for 20-minute intervals several times a shift unless contraindicated 　　f. apply an abdominal binder if ordered before placing client in a sitting or upright position (*the binder reduces pooling of blood in the abdominal/pelvic vessels*) 　4. perform actions *to allow time for remaining autoregulatory mechanisms to adjust to position changes:* 　　a. change client's position slowly 　　b. gradually progress client to a sitting or upright position using a recliner wheelchair or tilt table when allowed and tolerated. c. Consult physician if signs and symptoms of decreased tissue perfusion persist or worsen.

3. NURSING DIAGNOSIS:

Ineffective breathing pattern

related to:
a. diminished lung/chest wall expansion associated with:
  1. loss of abdominal and intercostal muscle function (innervation of these muscles occurs at the thoracic level)
  2. impaired function of the diaphragm (the diaphragm is innervated by the phrenic nerve, which travels through segments 3–5 of the cervical spine)
  3. weakness and fatigue
  4. upward pressure on the diaphragm resulting from gastric distention (can occur if paralytic ileus develops during period of spinal shock)
  5. decreased activity and recumbent positioning (in this position, full expansion of the lungs is restricted by the bed or turning frame surface and by the abdominal contents pushing up against the diaphragm)
  6. pressure on the chest wall associated with improper fit or application of halo device body jacket or abdominal binder;
b. decreased rate and depth of respirations associated with the depressant effect of some medications (e.g. narcotic [opioid] analgesics, central-acting muscle relaxants).

Desired Outcome	Nursing Actions and *Selected Purposes/Rationales*

3. The client will maintain an effective breathing pattern (see Care Plan on Immobility, Nursing Diagnosis 1 [p. 127], for outcome criteria).	3.a. Refer to Care Plan on Immobility, Nursing Diagnosis 1 (p. 127), for measures related to assessment and improvement of breathing pattern.
	 b. Assist with pulmonary function studies (e.g. tidal volume, vital capacity, inspiratory force) if done to evaluate respiratory status and effectiveness of treatment measures.
	 c. Implement additional measures *to promote lung/chest wall expansion in order to improve breathing pattern:*
	   1. perform actions to treat paralytic ileus if it develops (see Collaborative Diagnosis 20, action b.2) *in order to reduce gastric distention and upward pressure on diaphragm*
	   2. if client needs an abdominal binder, make sure it is positioned below the rib cage
	   3. limit the length of time client remains in prone position on turning frame
	   4. progress client to a sitting or upright position when allowed and tolerated
	   5. if client is wearing a halo device body jacket, consult physician and orthotist about having it readjusted if it appears too tight
	   6. encourage and assist client to perform exercises that strengthen the accessory muscles used in breathing (e.g. shoulder shrugs *to strengthen the trapezius muscles*) when allowed and tolerated.

4. NURSING DIAGNOSIS:

Ineffective airway clearance

related to stasis of secretions associated with:
a. decreased mobility;
b. decreased effectiveness of cough resulting from diminished lung/chest wall expansion, depressant effect of certain medications (e.g. narcotic [opioid] analgesics, central-acting muscle relaxants), and possible tenacious secretions if fluid intake is inadequate.

Desired Outcome	Nursing Actions and *Selected Purposes/Rationales*

4. The client will maintain clear, open airways (see Care Plan on Immobility, Nursing Diagnosis 2 [p. 128], for outcome criteria).	4.a. Refer to Care Plan on Immobility, Nursing Diagnosis 2 (p. 128), for measures related to assessment and promotion of effective airway clearance.
	b. Implement measures *to facilitate the client's cough efforts in order to further promote effective airway clearance:*
	  1. place client in a horizontal position during cough efforts unless contraindicated (*this position promotes a more effective forced expiration by decreasing the effect of gravity on the diaphragm*)
	  2. use an assisted coughing technique (e.g. place palm of hand below diaphragm and push upward as client exhales).

---

5. NURSING DIAGNOSIS: **Altered nutrition: less than body requirements**

related to:
a. decreased oral intake associated with:
  1. dietary restrictions during period of spinal shock if paralytic ileus develops
  2. anorexia resulting from boredom, fatigue, depression, a slowed metabolic rate (occurs with decreased activity), and early satiety that occurs with decreased gastrointestinal activity
  3. difficulty swallowing resulting from neck hyperextension and/or horizontal body position during the time that the cervical spine is immobilized
  4. difficulty feeding self resulting from loss of most of upper extremity motor function;
b. imbalance in rate of catabolism and anabolism (catabolic processes occur at a faster rate than anabolic processes in persons who have sustained a spinal cord injury and in those who are immobile).

Desired Outcome	Nursing Actions and *Selected Purposes/Rationales*

5. The client will maintain an adequate nutritional status (see Care Plan on Immobility, Nursing Diagnosis 3 [p. 128], for outcome criteria).	5.a. Refer to Care Plan on Immobility, Nursing Diagnosis 3 (pp. 128–129), for measures related to assessment and maintenance of an adequate nutritional status.
	b. Implement additional measures *to improve oral intake and maintain an adequate nutritional status:*
	  1. facilitate client's psychological adjustment to effects of spinal cord injury (see Nursing Diagnoses 22; 23, action c; 24; and 25, action b)
	  2. perform actions *to facilitate swallowing if client is on a turning frame* (e.g. place in prone position during meals, use a straw for all liquids)
	  3. perform actions *to facilitate swallowing if client's neck is in a hyperextended position while the cervical spine is being immobilized* (e.g. place in side-lying position during meals unless contraindicated, use a straw for all liquids)
	  4. feed client until he/she is able to feed self using assistive devices.

---

6. NURSING DIAGNOSIS: **Pain:**

a. **headache** related to contractions of the neck muscles (can occur in response to stress and/or neck pain);

b. **neck pain** related to nerve root irritation at the site of spinal cord injury, muscle stiffness while immobilization device is in place, and muscle strain associated with increased use of neck muscles following removal of immobilization device;

c. **upper arm and shoulder pain** related to muscle strain associated with increased use of biceps and shoulders as activity progresses.

Desired Outcome	Nursing Actions and *Selected Purposes/Rationales*

6. The client will experience diminished pain as evidenced by:
   a. verbalization of same
   b. relaxed facial expression
   c. increased participation in activities when allowed.

6.a. Assess for signs and symptoms of pain (e.g. verbalization of pain, grimacing or tense facial expression, reluctance to turn head or move shoulders when increased activity is allowed, restlessness, facial pallor).

b. Assess client's perception of the severity of pain using a pain intensity rating scale.

c. Assess the client's pain pattern (e.g. location, quality, onset, duration, precipitating factors, aggravating factors, alleviating factors).

d. Ask the client to describe previous pain experiences and methods used to manage pain effectively.

e. Implement measures *to reduce pain:*
   1. perform actions *to reduce fear and anxiety about the pain experience* (e.g. assure client that his/her need for pain relief is understood, plan methods for achieving pain control with client)
   2. perform actions to promote rest (e.g. schedule uninterrupted rest periods, minimize environmental activity and noise, limit number of visitors and their length of stay) *in order to reduce fatigue and subsequently increase the client's threshold and tolerance for pain*
   3. perform actions *to prevent or relieve headache:*
      a. minimize environmental stimuli (e.g. provide a calm environment, dim lights)
      b. implement measures to reduce psychological stress (see Nursing Diagnoses 1, action b; 22; 23, action c; 24; and 25, action b)
      c. avoid letting any object hit the skull pins, tongs, traction weights, and/or halo frame (*sound transmitted through these objects is intensified by their contact with the skull and loud noise is a noxious stimulus that can cause or intensify headache*)
      d. apply cool cloth to forehead if client desires
   4. perform actions *to prevent or relieve neck, upper arm, and/or shoulder pain:*
      a. maintain immobilization of the cervical spine as ordered *to reduce nerve root irritation*
      b. when moving client, provide support to neck and utilize turn sheet rather than pushing or pulling on shoulders and arms
      c. apply neck support (e.g. soft cervical collar) if ordered following removal of immobilization device
      d. massage client's upper arms and shoulders, being careful to avoid area around or over cervical spine until the injury has stabilized
      e. consult physician about application of heat and/or cold to upper arms, shoulders, and neck
   5. provide or assist with additional nonpharmacologic measures for pain relief (e.g. position change if allowed, progressive relaxation exercises, guided imagery, diversional activities such as watching television or conversing)
   6. administer analgesics if ordered (narcotic [opioid] analgesics are usually contraindicated *because of their respiratory depressant effect*).

f. Consult physician if above measures fail to provide adequate relief of pain.

7. NURSING DIAGNOSIS:

Ineffective thermoregulation

related to:
a. interruption in the feedback system between the area below the level of cord injury and the hypothalamus and loss of vasomotor tone below the level of the injury (these conditions result in the loss of compensatory responses to temperature changes [i.e. vasodilation, sweating, vasoconstriction, shivering, and piloerection]);
b. reduction in heat generation associated with limited body movement (especially during period of spinal shock).

Desired Outcome	Nursing Actions and *Selected Purposes/Rationales*

7. The client will experience effective thermoregulation as evidenced by:
a. verbalization of comfortable body temperature
b. absence of excessively warm or cool skin below the level of the injury
c. temperature between 36–38° C.
	7.a. Assess for signs and symptoms of ineffective thermoregulation (e.g. reports of feeling too warm or too cold, excessively warm or cool skin below the level of the injury).
	b. Monitor client's temperature. Report if less than 36° C or greater than 38° C.
	c. Implement measures *to maintain effective thermoregulation:*
	  1. perform actions *to prevent hypothermia:*
	    a. maintain room temperature at 70° F
	    b. provide extra clothing and bedding as necessary
	    c. protect client from drafts
	    d. apply warming blanket as ordered
	    e. provide warm liquids for client to drink
	    f. avoid taking client outdoors when it is very cold
	  2. perform actions *to prevent hyperthermia:*
	    a. maintain room temperature at 70° F
	    b. avoid use of excessive clothing and bedding
	    c. apply cooling blanket as ordered
	    d. remove extra clothing during physical and occupational therapy sessions
	    e. avoid taking client outdoors when it is very hot (especially if the humidity is high).
	d. Consult physician if above measures fail to maintain effective thermoregulation.

8. NURSING DIAGNOSIS:

Sensory/perceptual alterations:

a. **visual** related to decreased ability to move head associated with immobilization device used to stabilize and align the cervical spine;
b. **tactile** related to loss of integrity of ascending spinal pathways at the level of the cord injury.

Desired Outcomes	Nursing Actions and *Selected Purposes/Rationales*

8.a. The client will experience adequate visual stimulation as evidenced by verbalization of same.	8.a. Implement measures *to provide visual stimulation if the client's head movement or visual field is limited by the immobilization device:*
	  1. provide prism glasses for client's use
	  2. position mirrors in strategic places *to provide increased visualization of surroundings*

Desired Outcomes	Nursing Actions and *Selected Purposes/Rationales*
	3. place self within client's visual field when talking with him/her; instruct others to do the same
	4. put posters, pictures, and cards on the ceiling and suspend objects such as mobiles from ceiling (these will be within client's visual field when supine)
	5. if client is on a turning frame, place objects of interest (e.g. posters, clock, flowers, cards, small TV, pictures) on the floor within client's visual field when in prone position.

8.b. The client will experience adequate tactile stimulation as evidenced by verbalization of same.	8.b.1. Ascertain areas of body where client can perceive tactile sensation (mainly head, neck, and shoulders).
	2. Implement measures *to provide tactile stimulation:*
	  a. touch client on shoulders, head, and neck when appropriate; encourage significant others to do the same
	  b. obtain materials of various textures (e.g. cotton, leather) to rub gently on areas of sensation
	  c. consult occupational therapist for additional ways to provide tactile stimulation.

---

9. NURSING DIAGNOSIS:

Risk for impaired tissue integrity

related to:
a. accumulation of waste products and decreased oxygen and nutrient supply to the skin and subcutaneous tissue associated with reduced blood flow from prolonged pressure on the tissues as a result of decreased mobility and/or presence of an external device (e.g. halo device body jacket, wrist splint) that is improperly applied or does not fit properly;
b. damage to the skin or subcutaneous tissue associated with friction or shearing;
c. increased fragility of the skin associated with dependent edema, decreased tissue perfusion, and inadequate nutritional status;
d. frequent contact with irritants if client is incontinent of urine or stool.

Desired Outcome	Nursing Actions and *Selected Purposes/Rationales*

9. The client will maintain tissue integrity as evidenced by:
a. absence of redness and irritation
b. no skin breakdown.
	9.a. Inspect the skin (especially bony prominences, dependent and/or edematous areas, perineum, area underneath halo device body jacket, and areas of sensory loss) for pallor, redness, and breakdown.
	b. Refer to Care Plan on Immobility, Nursing Diagnosis 4, action b (pp. 129–130) for measures to prevent tissue breakdown associated with decreased mobility.
	c. Implement additional measures *to prevent tissue breakdown:*
	  1. perform actions to maintain adequate tissue perfusion (see Nursing Diagnosis 2, action b)
	  2. perform actions to maintain an adequate nutritional status (see Nursing Diagnosis 5)
	  3. if client is wearing a halo device body jacket:
	    a. ensure that jacket lining and skin beneath it are kept clean and dry
	    b. make sure that clothing worn under the jacket is clean, dry, wrinkle-free, and made of cotton (some physicians allow client to wear a T-shirt under the jacket; others do not because they feel the shirt promotes slippage of the jacket)
	    c. cover all rough jacket edges with foam tape
	    d. consult physician and orthotist about having the jacket readjusted if it is placing excessive pressure on any skin area
	  4. perform actions to prevent urinary and bowel incontinence (see Nursing Diagnoses 12, actions e. 2–4 and f; and 14, action b)

5. perform actions to decrease spasticity (see Nursing Diagnosis 10, action a.8) *because spasms can cause movement and subsequent friction and make it difficult to keep client positioned properly*
6. ensure that wheelchair is not too small for client and that it is adequately cushioned
7. ensure that shoes, jewelry, clothing, and straps that secure assistive devices are not too tight
8. be sure that client wears shoes or sturdy slippers when in wheelchair *to protect feet from trauma*
9. if fade time (length of time it takes for reddened area to fade after pressure is removed) is greater than 15 minutes, increase frequency of position changes and/or provide more effective methods of cushioning, padding, and positioning.
d. If skin breakdown occurs:
1. notify physician
2. continue with above measures to prevent further irritation and breakdown
3. perform care of involved area(s) as ordered or per standard hospital procedure
4. assess client closely and report signs and symptoms of infection (e.g. elevated temperature; redness, heat, and swelling around area of breakdown; unusual drainage from site).

---

10. NURSING DIAGNOSIS:	**Impaired physical mobility**

related to:
a. activity limitations associated with quadriplegia and immobilization of the spine;
b. spasticity following the period of spinal shock associated with stimulation of the reflex arcs below the level of the injury;
c. decreased motivation associated with fatigue and the psychological response to the extensive motor and sensory losses that have occurred;
d. pain;
e. loss of muscle mass, tone, and strength in areas of existing motor function (biceps, upper shoulders, and neck) associated with prolonged disuse (more likely to occur when client is in skeletal traction and confined to a turning frame or bed) and inadequate nutritional status;
f. contractures (if they develop).

Desired Outcome	Nursing Actions and *Selected Purposes/Rationales*
10. The client will achieve maximum physical mobility within limitations imposed by the injury and the treatment plan.	10.a. Implement measures *to increase mobility*: 1. facilitate client's psychological adjustment to the effects of the spinal cord injury (see Nursing Diagnoses 22; 23, action c; 24; and 25, action b) 2. perform actions to reduce pain (see Nursing Diagnosis 6, action e) 3. instruct client in and assist with active and active-resistive exercises of neck, shoulders, and biceps when allowed by physician 4. perform actions to prevent contractures (see Collaborative Diagnosis 20, actions e.2 and 3) *in order to maintain joint mobility* 5. when activity is allowed, instruct client in ways to move body (e.g. hook arm over side rail to assist in turning self, trigger flexor spasm of knees to help swing legs over side of bed during transfer to and from wheelchair) 6. instruct client in and assist with use of mobility aids (e.g. sliding board, electric wheelchair) as activity progresses

Desired Outcome	Nursing Actions and *Selected Purposes/Rationales* ·

      7. reinforce instructions, activities, and exercise plan recommended by physical and occupational therapists

      8. perform actions *to reduce spasticity* (*spasms can interfere with attempts to increase mobility*):

        a. avoid stimulating extremities or muscle groups (e.g. do not jar bed; use slow, steady movements when repositioning client; do not touch easily stimulated areas unnecessarily)

        b. implement measures to prevent conditions such as urinary tract infection, fecal impaction, pressure ulcers, fatigue, and chills (*these conditions can result in the stimulation of various muscle groups*)

        c. assist client to change position frequently and perform range of motion exercises *in order to keep muscles stretched* (*when muscles tighten, spasms are more likely to occur*)

        d. if planned, assist with functional electrical stimulation of muscles that spasm most often or most severely (*it is believed that repeated contraction fatigues the muscle and reduces its spasticity*)

        e. administer muscle relaxants (e.g. baclofen, dantrolene, diazepam) if ordered

        f. if undesired muscle spasms occur while moving client, hold the affected area firmly until the spasm subsides

      9. provide adequate rest periods before activity sessions.

    b. Provide praise and encouragement for all efforts to increase physical mobility.

    c. Encourage the support of significant others. Allow them to assist with range of motion exercises, positioning, and activity if desired.

    d. Consult physician if client is unable to achieve expected level of mobility or if range of motion becomes restricted.

---

11. NURSING DIAGNOSIS: **Self-care deficit**

related to impaired physical mobility associated with quadriplegia, spasticity, decreased motivation, pain, weakness, and activity restrictions imposed by treatment plan.

Desired Outcome	Nursing Actions and *Selected Purposes/Rationales*

11. The client will demonstrate increased participation in self-care activities within the limitations imposed by the treatment plan and effects of the spinal cord injury.

11.a. With client, develop a realistic plan for meeting daily physical needs. Inform client that with rehabilitation and use of assistive devices, he/she should be able to accomplish activities such as:

    1. feeding self once meal has been set up

    2. washing face and chest

    3. combing front and sides of hair, brushing teeth, and shaving with an electric razor

    4. participating in dressing upper body.

  b. When condition stabilizes and physician allows, implement measures *to facilitate client's ability to perform self-care activities*:

    1. perform actions to increase mobility (see Nursing Diagnosis 10, action a)

    2. consult occupational therapist regarding assistive devices available; reinforce use of these devices, which may include:

      a. rocker feeder, overhead sling, plate guard, sandwich holder, and broad-handled and/or swivel utensils for feeding self

      b. flexor-hinge splint or universal cuff to aid in brushing teeth, combing hair, and shaving with electric razor

      c. bath mitt for bathing face and chest

      d. Velcro fasteners to facilitate dressing upper body

3. schedule care at a time when client is most likely to be able to participate (e.g. when analgesics are at peak effect, after rest periods, not immediately after physical therapy sessions or meals)
4. keep objects client can use independently within easy reach
5. allow adequate time for accomplishment of self-care activities.
c. Encourage client to perform as much of self-care as possible within physical limitations and activity restrictions imposed by the treatment plan; provide positive feedback for all efforts and accomplishments of self-care.
d. Perform for client the self-care activities that he/she is unable to accomplish.
e. Inform significant others of client's abilities to participate in own care. Explain the importance of encouraging and allowing client to achieve an optimal level of independence.

---

12. NURSING DIAGNOSIS: **Altered urinary elimination:**

a. **retention** related to:
1. atony of bladder wall and contraction of external urinary sphincter during period of spinal shock
2. spasticity of the external urinary sphincter and/or loss of ability to coordinate bladder contraction and relaxation of the external urinary sphincter following period of spinal shock
3. incomplete bladder emptying associated with horizontal positioning (in this position, the gravity needed for complete bladder emptying is lost);
b. **incontinence** related to:
1. spasticity of the bladder following period of spinal shock and loss of ability to contract the external urinary sphincter voluntarily (incontinence can occur if the bladder contracts strongly when the external urinary sphincter is relaxed)
2. inadvertent stimulation of the voiding reflex.

Desired Outcome	Nursing Actions and *Selected Purposes/Rationales*
12. The client will experience an optimal pattern of urinary elimination as evidenced by: a. absence of bladder distention b. balanced intake and output c. absence of urinary incontinence.	12.a. Assess for and report signs and symptoms of altered urinary elimination: 1. urinary retention (e.g. bladder distention, intake greater than output) 2. urinary incontinence. b. Catheterize client if ordered *to determine amount of residual urine.* c. Assist with urodynamic studies (e.g. cystometrogram) if ordered. d. Monitor client's pattern of fluid intake and urinary elimination (e.g. times and amounts of fluid intake, types of fluids consumed, amount of triggered and involuntary voidings, times of and amount of urine obtained from intermittent catheterizations, activities preceding incontinence). e. Implement measures *to promote optimal urinary elimination:* 1. perform actions *to prevent urinary retention during period of spinal shock:* a. perform intermittent catheterizations or insert indwelling urinary catheter as ordered b. implement measures *to maintain patency of urinary catheter if present* (e.g. keep tubing free of kinks) 2. following the period of spinal shock, perform actions *to promote complete bladder emptying and/or reduce the risk of incontinence:* a. attempt to initiate voiding periodically by stimulating the trigger zones of the reflex sacral arc (e.g. tap suprapubic area, stroke or massage abdomen, stroke inner thigh, perform anal sphincter

Desired Outcome	Nursing Actions and *Selected Purposes/Rationales*

stretching, pull pubic hair); if voiding occurs, repeat stimulus as necessary *to empty the bladder*

b. if possible, place client on bedside commode or toilet when triggering voiding reflex or performing intermittent catheterization (*gravity facilitates complete bladder emptying*)

c. instruct client to space fluid intake evenly throughout the day rather than drinking a large quantity at one time (*if the bladder fills rapidly and frequency of emptying is not increased, bladder distention occurs*)

d. instruct client to limit intake of beverages containing caffeine such as colas, coffee, and tea (*caffeine is a mild diuretic and a bladder irritant; the increased urine production can result in bladder distention if the frequency of bladder emptying is not also increased and the bladder irritation can trigger bladder spasms and subsequent incontinence*)

e. limit oral fluid intake in the evening *so that the bladder does not become overdistended during the night* (as rehabilitation progresses, most clients do not perform intermittent catheterization or attempt to trigger voiding during the night)

3. instruct client and others to avoid stimulating the voiding reflex trigger zones at times other than during bladder care *in order to reduce the risk of incontinence*

4. administer central-acting muscle relaxants (e.g. baclofen) or urinary antispasmodic agents (e.g. oxybutynin) if ordered *to decrease spastic contraction of the bladder and the subsequent risk of incontinence and to decrease tone of the external urinary sphincter* (*decreased sphincter tone allows for more complete bladder emptying during reflex voiding attempts*).

f. If urinary retention or incontinence persists:
   1. carefully review bladder training program
   2. prepare client for insertion of an indwelling catheter (urethral or suprapubic) if indicated.

---

13. NURSING DIAGNOSIS:

Constipation

related to:

a. decreased gastrointestinal motility associated with:
   1. loss of autonomic nervous system function below the level of the injury during period of spinal shock
   2. decreased activity;

b. lack of awareness of stool in rectum associated with sensory loss below the level of the injury;

c. loss of central nervous system control over defecation reflex;

d. decreased gravity filling of lower rectum associated with horizontal positioning;

e. decreased intake of fluids and foods high in fiber.

Desired Outcome	Nursing Actions and *Selected Purposes/Rationales*

13. The client will not experience constipation as evidenced by:
   a. usual frequency of bowel movements
   b. passage of soft, formed stool

13.a. Ascertain client's usual bowel elimination habits.

b. Assess for signs and symptoms of constipation (e.g. decrease in frequency of bowel movements; passage of hard, formed stools; abdominal distention).

c. Assess bowel sounds. Report a pattern of decreasing bowel sounds.

d. Implement measures *to prevent constipation* (the following are usually included in a bowel training program):

c. absence of abdominal distention.

1. instruct client to increase intake of foods high in fiber (e.g. bran, whole-grain breads and cereals, fresh fruits and vegetables) unless contraindicated
2. assist client to maintain a minimum fluid intake of 2500 ml/day unless contraindicated
3. encourage client to drink hot liquids before scheduled bowel evacuation *in order to stimulate peristalsis*
4. assist client to eat at scheduled times and adhere to a routine time for defecation; follow client's preinjury pattern if possible
5. increase activity as allowed and tolerated
6. perform digital stimulation and/or insert rectal suppository *to stimulate peristalsis and reflex emptying of rectum*
7. place client on toilet or bedside commode or place in high Fowler's position on bedpan for bowel movements unless contraindicated
8. allow ample time for bowel evacuation (may take up to an hour after rectal stimulation)
9. if an analgesic is needed, encourage use of nonnarcotics rather than narcotics (opioids) *to prevent further decrease in bowel activity*
10. administer laxatives or cathartics and/or enemas if ordered.

e. Consult physician about checking for an impaction and digitally removing stool if client has not had a bowel movement in 3 days, if he/she is passing liquid stool, or if other signs and symptoms of constipation are present.

f. If constipation occurs, review bowel training program and revise it as needed.

---

14. NURSING DIAGNOSIS:

Bowel incontinence

related to:
a. increased reflex activity of the bowel and loss of voluntary control of bowel elimination associated with upper motor neuron damage;
b. lack of awareness of stool in rectum associated with sensory loss below the level of the injury;
c. fecal impaction if present (continuous stimulation of the defecation reflex by the fecal mass inhibits the internal anal sphincter and results in loss of ability to retain the mucus and fluid that collect proximal to and leak around the fecal mass).

Desired Outcome	Nursing Actions and *Selected Purposes/Rationales*

14. The client will not experience bowel incontinence.

14.a. Monitor for episodes of bowel incontinence.
    b. Implement measures *to reduce the risk of bowel incontinence:*
      1. initiate a bowel training program *so that client will evacuate the lower colon at regularly scheduled intervals*
      2. avoid inserting a rectal suppository (unless it is part of the bowel care program) or taking client's temperature rectally *in order to avoid stimulation of reflex bowel activity and subsequent incontinence*
      3. if client has a fecal impaction:
        a. consult physician regarding measures to remove the impaction (e.g. digital removal of stool, oil retention enema)
        b. perform actions to prevent constipation (see Nursing Diagnosis 13, action d) *in order to prevent recurrent impactions*
      4. administer central-acting muscle relaxants (e.g. baclofen) if ordered *to decrease the risk for spontaneous spastic contractions of the bowel.*
    c. If bowel incontinence persists, consult physician about revision of bowel training program.

15. NURSING DIAGNOSIS:

Sleep pattern disturbance

related to:
a. inability to assume usual sleep position associated with loss of motor function and use of devices to immobilize the spine (e.g. halo device, turning frame);
b. frequent assessments and treatments;
c. fear and anxiety;
d. unfamiliar environment;
e. sudden, uncontrolled movement associated with spasticity following period of spinal shock.

Desired Outcome	Nursing Actions and *Selected Purposes/Rationales*

15. The client will attain optimal amounts of sleep (see Care Plan on Immobility, Nursing Diagnosis 10 [p. 134], for outcome criteria).	15.a. Refer to Care Plan on Immobility, Nursing Diagnosis 10 (pp. 134–135), for measures related to assessment and promotion of sleep.
	b. Implement additional measures *to promote sleep:*
	  1. assist client to assume a comfortable sleep position within limits of treatment plan (e.g. if client is on a turning frame and is more comfortable prone than supine, it may be possible to alter turning schedule to allow prone position for longer periods during the night)
	  2. perform actions to decrease fear and anxiety (see Nursing Diagnosis 1, action b)
	  3. perform actions to reduce spasticity (see Nursing Diagnosis 10, action a.8).

16. NURSING DIAGNOSIS:

Risk for infection:

a. **pneumonia** related to stasis of secretions in the lungs (secretions provide a good medium for bacterial growth) and aspiration if it occurs;
b. **urinary tract infection** related to:
  1. growth and colonization of pathogens associated with urinary stasis and the increased urine alkalinity that results from hypercalciuria (with prolonged immobility, excess calcium is released from the bones and excreted in the urine)
  2. introduction of pathogens associated with presence of an indwelling catheter, performance of intermittent catheterizations, and/or difficulty maintaining good perineal hygiene;
c. **skull pin site infection** related to introduction of pathogens during or following insertion of skull pins.

Desired Outcomes	Nursing Actions and *Selected Purposes/Rationales*

16.a. The client will not develop pneumonia (see Care Plan on Immobility, Nursing Diagnosis 11, outcome a [p. 135], for outcome criteria).	16.a.1. Refer to Care Plan on Immobility, Nursing Diagnosis 11, action a (pp. 135–136), for measures related to assessment, prevention, and treatment of pneumonia.
	  2. Implement additional measures *to prevent pneumonia:*
	    a. perform actions to improve breathing pattern and promote effective airway clearance (see Nursing Diagnoses 3 and 4)
	    b. perform actions to reduce the risk for aspiration (see Nursing Diagnosis 18, action c).

16.b. The client will remain free of urinary tract infection as evidenced by:
1. clear urine
2. no unusual odor to urine
3. afebrile status
4. no increase in spasticity
5. absence of WBCs, bacteria, and nitrites in urine
6. negative urine culture.

16.c. The client will remain free of skull pin site infection as evidenced by:
1. afebrile status
2. absence of redness, heat, swelling, and pain around pin sites
3. absence of unusual drainage from pin sites
4. WBC and differential counts within normal range
5. negative cultures of pin site drainage.

16.b.1. Assess for and report signs and symptoms of urinary tract infection (e.g. cloudy, foul-smelling urine; elevated temperature; increase in spasticity [bladder mucosal irritation triggers muscle spasms]).
2. Monitor urinalysis and report presence of WBCs, bacteria, and/or nitrites.
3. Obtain a urine specimen for culture and sensitivity if ordered. Report abnormal results.
4. Refer to Care Plan on Immobility, Nursing Diagnosis 11, actions b.4 and 5 (p. 136), for measures related to prevention and treatment of urinary tract infection.
5. Implement measures to prevent urinary retention (see Nursing Diagnosis 12, actions e.1, 2, and 4 and f) *in order to further reduce the risk of urinary tract infection.*

16.c.1. Assess for and report signs and symptoms of skull pin site infection (e.g. fever; redness, heat, swelling, and pain around pin sites; unusual drainage around pin; foul odor from pin site).
2. Monitor for and report an elevated WBC count and significant change in differential.
3. Obtain cultures of pin site drainage as ordered. Report positive results.
4. Implement measures *to prevent skull pin site infection:*
   a. use good handwashing technique
   b. keep client's hair clean
   c. keep hair around pin sites trimmed *so the tissues are not traumatized when hair is combed and hair does not get tangled around the pins*
   d. instruct persons coming in contact with client to avoid touching pins, tongs, weights, and/or halo ring *in order to reduce movement of the pins and subsequent tissue trauma*
   e. clean pin sites according to physician's order or standard hospital procedure (usual recommendation is a twice daily cleaning using cotton-tipped applicators and a hydrogen peroxide or antiseptic solution)
   f. use sterile technique when performing pin site care
   g. replace equipment and solutions used for pin site care according to hospital policy.
5. If signs and symptoms of skull pin site infection are present:
   a. continue with above actions
   b. administer antimicrobials if ordered
   c. apply antimicrobial ointment to pin site(s) if ordered.

---

17. NURSING DIAGNOSIS:

Risk for trauma:
a. **falls** related to loss of motor function, use of turning frame, loss of sitting balance if wearing a halo device (the structure and weight of the device alter the client's center of gravity), and unexpected body movements resulting from spasticity;
b. **burns** related to loss of motor and sensory function and unexpected body movements resulting from spasticity.

Desired Outcome	Nursing Actions and *Selected Purposes/Rationales*

17. The client will not experience falls or burns.

17.a. Implement measures *to reduce the risk for trauma:*
1. perform actions *to prevent falls:*
   a. if client is in a standard hospital bed, keep bed in low position with side rails up

Desired Outcome	Nursing Actions and **Selected Purposes/Rationales**
	b. if client is in a kinetic bed, utilize safety measures such as safety straps and padded side pieces
	c. keep safety belts securely fastened when client is on a turning frame or stretcher or in a wheelchair
	d. obtain adequate assistance when moving client; utilize instructions from physical therapist on correct transfer techniques
	e. implement measures *to increase client's stability when in a wheelchair* (e.g. use wheelchair equipped with an anti-tipping device, fasten safety belt around upper body and chair to stabilize trunk, use H-straps to keep legs positioned properly)
	f. do not rush client; allow adequate time for the accomplishment of transfers and position changes
	2. perform actions *to prevent burns:*
	a. let hot foods and fluids cool slightly before serving
	b. supervise client while smoking
	c. assess temperature of bath water before and during use
	d. when client is in a wheelchair, instruct him/her to avoid placing self next to sources of heat (e.g. heater, stove)
	3. encourage client to request assistance whenever needed; have a specially adapted call signal available to client at all times
	4. perform actions to decrease spasticity (see Nursing Diagnosis 10, action a.8) *in order to reduce the risk of unexpected body movements.*
	b. Include client and significant others in planning and implementing measures to prevent trauma.
	c. If injury does occur, initiate appropriate first aid and notify physician.

---

18. NURSING DIAGNOSIS: **Risk for aspiration**

related to:
a. decreased ability to clear tracheobronchial passages associated with inability to cough forcefully resulting from weakness of the diaphragm and paralysis of the abdominal and intercostal muscles;
b. reflux of gastric contents associated with accumulation of gas and fluid in the stomach as a result of decreased or absent gastrointestinal motility (especially during period of spinal shock);
c. difficulty swallowing associated with neck hyperextension and/or horizontal body positioning during the time that the cervical spine is immobilized.

Desired Outcome	Nursing Actions and **Selected Purposes/Rationales**

18. The client will not aspirate secretions or foods/fluids as evidenced by:
 a. clear breath sounds
 b. resonant percussion note over lungs
 c. absence of cough, tachypnea, and dyspnea.
	18.a. Assess for signs and symptoms of aspiration of secretions or foods/fluids (e.g. rhonchi, dull percussion note over affected lung area, cough, tachypnea, dyspnea).
	 b. Monitor chest x-ray results. Report findings of pulmonary infiltrate.
	 c. Implement measures *to reduce the risk for aspiration:*
	   1. if client has absent bowel sounds, withhold oral foods/fluids and consult physician about insertion of a nasogastric tube for gastric decompression *to reduce the possibility of gastric reflux or vomiting and subsequent aspiration*
	   2. place client in a prone position (if on turning frame) or a side-lying position as often as possible during period of spinal shock when client's ability to clear upper airways is most severely compromised
	   3. have suction equipment readily available for use
	   4. perform oropharyngeal suctioning and provide oral hygiene as often as needed *to remove excess secretions and food particles*
	   5. when oral intake is allowed:

a. maintain client in the following position during and for at least 30 minutes after meals and snacks:
1. prone position if on turning frame
2. high Fowler's or side-lying position if in halo device
b. decrease environmental stimuli during meals and snacks *so client can concentrate on chewing and swallowing*
c. encourage client to use a straw for all liquids and to take small sips and sip slowly when drinking
d. provide small, frequent meals rather than 3 large ones *to decrease risk of gastric distention and gastroesophageal reflux*
e. cut food in bite-size pieces and remind client to chew food thoroughly
f. allow ample time for meals
g. instruct client to avoid laughing and talking while eating and drinking
h. assist client with oral hygiene after eating *to ensure that food particles do not remain in mouth*
i. administer upper gastrointestinal stimulants (e.g. metoclopramide) if ordered *to promote gastric emptying, which decreases the risk of gastric distention and subsequent regurgitation.*
d. If signs and symptoms of aspiration occur:
1. perform the assisted coughing maneuver if client begins to choke on food particles
2. withhold oral intake
3. notify physician
4. prepare client for chest x-ray
5. prepare client for bronchoscopy if ordered *to remove aspirated food particles.*

---

19. NURSING DIAGNOSIS: **Dysreflexia**

related to loss of autonomic nervous system control below the level of the cord injury (can occur once reflex activity returns following period of spinal shock).

Desired Outcome	Nursing Actions and *Selected Purposes/Rationales*

19. The client will not experience dysreflexia as evidenced by:
a. vital signs within normal range for client
b. skin dry and usual color above the level of the injury
c. no reports of pounding headache, nasal congestion, and blurred vision.
	19.a. Assess for signs and symptoms of dysreflexia:
	  1. sudden rise in B/P (systolic pressure may go as high as 300 mm Hg)
	  2. bradycardia
	  3. flushing and profuse diaphoresis above level of injury
	  4. pounding headache
	  5. nasal congestion
	  6. blurred vision.
	b. Implement measures *to prevent stimulation of the sympathetic nervous system below the level of the cord injury in order to prevent dysreflexia:*
	  1. perform actions to prevent distention of the bladder and bowel (see Nursing Diagnoses 12, actions e.1, 2, and 4 and f and 13, action d)
	  2. perform actions *to prevent pressure on any area of the client's body below the level of the cord injury:*
	    a. instruct and assist client to change position frequently
	    b. ensure that overbed tray is not resting on client
	    c. ensure that clothing is not constrictive and shoes are not too tight
	  3. perform good nail care (*ingrown nails can stimulate the sympathetic nervous system*)
	  4. perform actions to prevent and treat urinary tract infection (see Nursing Diagnosis 16, actions b.4 and 5)

Desired Outcome | Nursing Actions and **Selected Purposes/Rationales**

5. apply a topical anesthetic agent to any existing pressure ulcer
6. apply a local anesthetic (e.g. Nupercainal ointment) if ordered before performing actions that can result in an exaggerated sympathetic response (e.g. urinary catheterization, removal of a fecal impaction, administration of an enema, care of any wound below the level of the injury).
   c. If signs and symptoms of dysreflexia occur:
      1. immediately raise head of bed and lower client's legs unless contraindicated (*this will usually decrease B/P significantly*)
      2. monitor B/P and pulse frequently
      3. assess for and, if possible, alleviate the condition causing sympathetic stimulation; if client needs to be catheterized or have a fecal impaction removed, be sure to use an anesthetic ointment when performing the procedure *in order to decrease the risk of aggravating the dysreflexia*
      4. notify physician immediately if signs and symptoms persist or if complications resulting from severe hypertension (e.g. seizures, intraocular hemorrhage, cerebrovascular accident, myocardial infarction) occur
      5. administer antihypertensives (e.g. diazoxide, hydralazine, trimethaphan, nitroprusside) if ordered
      6. notify all persons participating in client's care of the episode of dysreflexia *since such episodes can recur.*
   d. Consult physician about the administration of a ganglionic blocking agent (e.g. mecamylamine) on a routine basis if dysreflexia recurs frequently.

20. **COLLABORATIVE DIAGNOSES:**

Potential complications of spinal cord injury:

   a. **ascending spinal cord injury** related to further damage to and/or ischemia of the cord above the C5 level associated with vasospasm of damaged vessels, progressive edema, bleeding, compression of cord by hematoma or bone fragments, and/or ineffective immobilization of an unstable cord injury;
   b. **paralytic ileus** related to absence of neural stimulation of the intestine associated with absence of autonomic nervous system and reflex activity below the level of the spinal cord injury during period of spinal shock;
   c. **thromboembolism** related to:
      1. venous stasis associated with decreased mobility and decreased vasomotor tone below the level of the injury
      2. hypercoagulability associated with:
         a. hemoconcentration and increased blood viscosity if fluid intake is inadequate
         b. increased levels of certain clotting factors (e.g. calcium, fibrinogen) in the blood after approximately 8 days of bed rest;
   d. **gastrointestinal (GI) bleeding** related to:
      1. erosions of the gastric and duodenal mucosa (can develop as a result of the increased output of hydrochloric acid that occurs with stress)
      2. irritation of the gastric mucosa associated with side effect of certain medications (e.g. corticosteroids, some muscle relaxants);
   e. **contractures** related to:
      1. lack of joint movement associated with prolonged immobility and quadriplegia
      2. prolonged periods of hip flexion associated with use of wheelchair
      3. difficulty putting joints through full range of motion associated with severe spasticity if it occurs and/or heterotopic ossification (excessive bone formation that can develop around joints of paralyzed limbs as early as 1 month after the spinal cord injury).

Desired Outcomes	Nursing Actions and *Selected Purposes/Rationales*
20.a. The client will not experience spinal cord injury above the level of C5 as evidenced by: 1. stable respiratory status 2. stable B/P and pulse 3. no further loss of motor and sensory function.	20.a.1. Assess for and report signs and symptoms of ascending spinal cord injury: a. respiratory failure (e.g. rapid, shallow respirations; dusky or cyanotic skin color; drowsiness; confusion) b. significant decrease in B/P and pulse c. further loss of motor and sensory function. 2. Implement measures *to prevent spinal cord injury above the level of C5:* a. perform actions *to maintain immobilization of the spine until stabilization has been accomplished:* 1. do not release or adjust skeletal traction or halo device unless ordered 2. if skeletal traction is present, keep traction rope and weights hanging freely 3. always use turn sheet and adequate assistance when repositioning client; never use the rods of the halo device as handles 4. check pin sites of halo or traction device every shift; notify physician if pins are loose 5. if immobilization device fails (e.g. pins fall out, traction weights drop, rods on halo device disconnect): a. stabilize client's head, neck, and shoulders with hands, sandbags, or cervical collar b. notify physician immediately b. remind staff to utilize the jaw thrust method rather than hyperextending client's neck if respiratory distress occurs c. perform actions *to prevent ascending spinal cord ischemia:* 1. implement measures to maintain adequate tissue perfusion (see Nursing Diagnosis 2, action b) 2. implement measures to maintain an adequate respiratory status (see Nursing Diagnoses 3 and 4) *in order to promote adequate tissue oxygenation* 3. administer the following medications if ordered: a. corticosteroids (the administration of high doses of methylprednisolone within the first 8 hours following spinal cord injury appears to be the most effective way of slowing the development of ischemia above the level of the injury) b. calcium-channel blockers (e.g. nimodipine) *to decrease vasospasm* d. prepare client for decompression of the spinal cord (e.g. removal of hematoma or bone fragments) or surgical stabilization (e.g. fusion) if planned. 3. If signs and symptoms of ascending spinal cord injury occur: a. continue with above actions b. assist with intubation or tracheostomy and mechanical ventilation c. provide emotional support to client and significant others.
20.b. The client will have resolution of paralytic ileus if it occurs as evidenced by: 1. soft, nondistended abdomen 2. gradual return of bowel sounds 3. passage of flatus.	20.b.1. Assess for and report signs and symptoms of paralytic ileus (e.g. firm, distended abdomen; absent bowel sounds; failure to pass flatus). 2. If signs and symptoms of paralytic ileus occur: a. withhold all oral intake b. insert nasogastric tube and maintain suction as ordered c. assess for and report signs of bowel necrosis (e.g. fever, increased WBCs, significant decrease in B/P).
20.c.1. The client will not develop a deep vein thrombus as evidenced by:	20.c.1.a. Assess for and report signs and symptoms of a deep vein thrombus (e.g. increase in circumference of extremity, distention of superficial vessels in extremity, unusual warmth of extremity). b. Refer to Care Plan on Immobility, Nursing Diagnosis 12, actions a.1.b

Desired Outcomes	Nursing Actions and *Selected Purposes/Rationales*

<table>
<tr><td>

a. absence of swelling and distended superficial vessels in extremities
b. usual temperature of extremities.

</td><td>

and c (p. 137), for measures related to prevention and treatment of a deep vein thrombus.
c. Implement additional measures *to maintain adequate blood flow in legs and subsequently reduce the risk for thrombus formation:*
  1. position firm pillow between client's legs if spasms tend to cause legs to cross
  2. instruct client to obtain assistance to reposition legs properly if they cross.

</td></tr>
<tr><td>

20.c.2. The client will not experience a pulmonary embolism as evidenced by:
a. absence of sudden shoulder pain
b. unlabored respirations at 14–20/minute
c. pulse within normal range for client
d. blood gases within normal range.

</td><td>

20.c.2.a. Assess for and report signs and symptoms of pulmonary embolism (e.g. sudden shoulder pain [this is a referred pain], dyspnea, tachypnea, increase in pulse, apprehension, low PaO$_2$).
b. Refer to Care Plan on Immobility, Nursing Diagnosis 12, actions a.2.b and c (pp. 137–138), for measures related to prevention and treatment of a pulmonary embolism.
c. Implement additional measures *to prevent a pulmonary embolism:*
  1. perform actions to prevent and treat a deep vein thrombus (see actions c.1.b and c in this diagnosis)
  2. perform actions to prevent dysreflexia (see Nursing Diagnosis 19, action b) *in order to prevent a sudden increase in blood pressure and subsequent dislodgment of a thrombus if present.*

</td></tr>
<tr><td>

20.d. The client will not experience GI bleeding as evidenced by:
1. no reports of shoulder pain
2. absence of frank and occult blood in stool and gastric contents
3. B/P and pulse within normal range for client
4. RBC, Hct, and Hb levels within normal range.

</td><td>

20.d.1. Assess for and report signs and symptoms of GI bleeding (e.g. reports of shoulder pain [this is a referred pain], frank or occult blood in stool or gastric contents, decreased B/P, increased pulse).
2. Monitor RBC, Hct, and Hb levels. Report decreasing values.
3. Implement measures *to prevent ulceration of the gastric and duodenal mucosa:*
  a. perform actions to decrease fear and anxiety (see Nursing Diagnosis 1, action b)
  b. when oral intake is allowed:
    1. administer ulcerogenic medications (e.g. corticosteroids, some muscle relaxants) with meals or snacks *to decrease gastric irritation*
    2. instruct client to avoid foods/fluids that stimulate hydrochloric acid secretion or irritate the gastric mucosa (e.g. coffee; caffeine-containing tea and colas; spices such as black pepper, chili powder, and nutmeg)
  c. administer histamine$_2$ receptor antagonists (e.g. cimetidine, ranitidine, famotidine), antacids, and cytoprotective agents (e.g. sucralfate) if ordered.
4. If signs and symptoms of GI bleeding occur:
  a. continue with above actions
  b. withhold oral foods/fluids as ordered
  c. insert nasogastric tube and maintain suction as ordered
  d. administer blood products and/or volume expanders if ordered
  e. assist with measures to control bleeding (e.g. gastric lavage, endoscopic electrocoagulation) if planned
  f. if bleeding is not controlled, refer to Care Plan on Peptic Ulcer for additional care measures.

</td></tr>
<tr><td>

20.e. The client will maintain normal range of motion.

</td><td>

20.e.1. Assess for and report:
  a. statements of shoulder joint stiffness
  b. limitations in range of motion
  c. redness, unusual warmth, and swelling of joints in paralyzed limbs (can be indicative of heterotopic ossification, which can cause restricted movement of the involved joint).
2. Refer to Care Plan on Immobility, Collaborative Diagnosis 12, actions d.2–6 (p. 139), for measures to prevent contractures.
3. Implement additional measures *to reduce the risk of contractures:*
  a. perform actions to reduce spasticity (see Nursing Diagnosis 10, action a.8)

</td></tr>
</table>

b. position client in prone or supine position routinely unless contraindicated *to counteract prolonged periods of hip flexion resulting from wheelchair use*

c. administer etidronate (e.g. Didronel) if ordered *to prevent or treat heterotopic ossification*

d. prepare client for surgical removal of abnormal bone formation around joints if planned *in order to maintain joint mobility.*

---

21. NURSING DIAGNOSIS: **Sexual dysfunction**

related to:
a. decreased libido associated with:
   1. loss of sensory and voluntary motor function below the level of spinal cord injury
   2. presence of a urinary catheter and/or fear of urinary and bowel incontinence
   3. depression, altered self-concept
   4. fear of rejection by partner
   5. fear of dysreflexia (genital stimulation can cause dysreflexia);
b. decreased ability to control and maintain an erection associated with loss of ability to have a psychogenic erection (only reflexogenic erection is possible);
c. altered ejaculatory flow associated with impaired nerve function in the bladder neck (can result in retrograde rather than antegrade ejaculation).

Desired Outcome	Nursing Actions and *Selected Purposes/Rationales*

21. The client will demonstrate beginning acceptance of changes in sexual functioning as evidenced by:
a. verbalization of a perception of self as sexually acceptable and adequate
b. statements reflecting beginning adjustment to the effects of the spinal cord injury on sexual functioning
c. maintenance of relationship with significant other.
	21.a. Assess for signs and symptoms of sexual dysfunction (e.g. verbalization of sexual concerns or inability to achieve sexual satisfaction, alteration in relationship with significant other, limitations imposed by quadriplegia).
	b. Provide accurate information about the effects of the spinal cord injury on sexual functioning. Encourage questions and clarify misconceptions.
	c. Implement measures *to promote optimal sexual functioning:*
	  1. facilitate communication between client and partner; focus on the feelings the couple share and assist them to identify changes that affect their sexual relationship
	  2. discuss ways to be creative in expressing sexuality (e.g. massage, fantasies, cuddling)
	  3. arrange for uninterrupted privacy during hospital stay if desired by the couple
	  4. perform actions to improve client's self-concept (see Nursing Diagnosis 22)
	  5. suggest alternative methods of sexual gratification and use of assistive devices if appropriate; encourage partner to explore erogenous areas on the client's lips, neck, and ears
	  6. inform male client and his partner of techniques for eliciting and maintaining reflexogenic erection (e.g. stimulate genitalia, stroke inner thigh, stimulate the rectum, manipulate the urinary catheter)
	  7. if client has difficulty maintaining an erection, encourage him to discuss various treatment options (e.g. vacuum erection aids, penile prosthesis) with physician if desired
	  8. if client experiences episodes of dysreflexia, instruct him/her to consult physician about ways to prevent it during sexual activity (e.g. take a ganglionic blocking agent before sexual activity, have partner apply a local anesthetic to client's genitalia)
	  9. inform female client that vaginal lubrication can occur by local stimulation or can be enhanced by using a water-soluble lubricant

Desired Outcome	Nursing Actions and *Selected Purposes/Rationales*
	10. if client has an indwelling urethral catheter, instruct him/her on ways to fold and secure the catheter tubing prior to sexual intercourse
	11. if incontinence of urine is a concern, instruct client to: a. limit fluid intake 2 hours before sexual activity b. have bladder emptied immediately before sexual activity
	12. instruct client to perform bowel care several hours before sexual activity *in order to reduce the risk of bowel incontinence if anal or rectal stimulation occurs during sexual activity*
	13. if appropriate, involve partner in care of client *to facilitate partner's adjustment to the changes in client's appearance and body functioning and subsequently decrease the possibility of partner's rejection of client*
	14. encourage client to rest before sexual activity
	15. instruct client and partner to establish a relaxed, unhurried atmosphere for sexual activity
	16. discuss positions that may facilitate sexual activity (e.g. lying on side, client in supine position)
	17. provide explicit films and literature if desired by client and/or partner
	18. include partner in above discussions and encourage continued support of the client.
	d. Consult physician when client is ready for sexual counseling and/or sexual counseling appears indicated.

---

22. NURSING DIAGNOSIS: **Self-concept disturbance***

related to:
a. dependence on others to meet self-care needs;
b. feelings of powerlessness;
c. change in appearance associated with temporary presence of devices to immobilize the spine, necessity of wheelchair use, and spasticity following period of spinal shock;
d. infertility (in males) associated with:
   1. possibility of retrograde ejaculation (can result from impaired nerve function in the bladder neck)
   2. decreased sperm formation and viability resulting from testicular atrophy and impaired temperature regulation in the testes;
e. changes in body functioning, life style, and roles.

---

*This diagnostic label includes the nursing diagnoses of body image disturbance, self-esteem disturbance, and altered role performance.

Desired Outcome	Nursing Actions and *Selected Purposes/Rationales*

22. The client will demonstrate beginning adaptation to changes in body functioning, appearance, life style, roles, and level of independence (see Care Plan on Immobility, Nursing Diagnosis 14 [p. 141], for outcome criteria).	22.a. Refer to Care Plan on Immobility, Nursing Diagnosis 14 (p. 141), for measures related to assessment and promotion of a positive self-concept.
	b. Implement additional measures *to promote a positive self-concept:*
	  1. reinforce actions to assist client to cope with effects of the spinal cord injury (see Nursing Diagnosis 23, action c)
	  2. perform actions to prevent urinary and bowel incontinence (see Nursing Diagnoses 12, actions e.2–4 and f and 14, action b)
	  3. perform actions to reduce client's feelings of powerlessness (see Nursing Diagnosis 24)
	  4. perform actions to facilitate the grieving process (see Nursing Diagnosis 25, action b)
	  5. avoid unnecessary exposure of client during care

6. assure client that immobilization device is temporary and will be removed as soon as internal stabilization of the spine occurs; if brace or collar is needed after removal of the skull pins, assist client to select clothing that makes the spinal support less obvious (e.g. high-collared shirts, loose-fitting shirts)

7. demonstrate acceptance of client using techniques such as touch and frequent visits; encourage significant others to do the same

8. promote activities that require client to confront the body changes that have occurred (e.g. exercise, grooming, eating); be aware that the integration of changes in body image may not begin until 2–6 months after the actual physical change has occurred

9. encourage client contact with others *so that he/she can test and establish a new self-image*

10. reinforce actions to assist client to adjust to alterations in sexual functioning (see Nursing Diagnosis 21, action c)

11. discuss alternative methods of becoming a parent (e.g. adoption, sperm recovery, artificial insemination) if of concern to client

12. perform actions to increase the client's ability to perform self-care (see Nursing Diagnosis 11, action b) *in order to increase client's sense of independence*

13. provide privacy during client's attempts at self-care *in order to minimize embarrassment that he/she may feel because of neurological impairments*

14. encourage significant others to allow client to do what he/she is able *so that independence can be re-established and/or self-esteem redeveloped*

15. use the term "disabled" rather than "handicapped," "cripple," or "invalid"; avoid use of slang (e.g. quad, gimp).

---

23. NURSING DIAGNOSIS:	Ineffective individual coping

related to fear and anxiety; changes in body functioning, life style, and roles; feelings of powerlessness; and need for lengthy rehabilitation.

Desired Outcome	Nursing Actions and *Selected Purposes/Rationales*

23. The client will demonstrate effective coping skills as evidenced by:
a. verbalization of ability to cope with the effects of the spinal cord injury
b. utilization of appropriate problem-solving techniques
c. willingness to participate in treatment plan and rehabilitation program
d. absence of destructive behavior toward self
e. appropriate use of defense mechanisms
f. utilization of available support systems.
	23.a. Assess for and report signs and symptoms of ineffective individual coping (e.g. verbalization of inability to cope; inability to ask for help, problem solve, or meet basic needs; insomnia; withdrawal; reluctance to participate in treatment plan; destructive behavior toward self; inappropriate use of defense mechanisms; inability to meet role expectations).
	b. Assess client's perception of current situation.
	c. Implement measures *to promote effective coping*:
	  1. allow time for client to begin to adjust to the diagnosis and planned treatment, residual effects of the spinal cord injury, and anticipated changes in life style and roles
	  2. perform actions to decrease fear and anxiety (see Nursing Diagnosis 1, action b)
	  3. assist client to recognize and manage inappropriate denial if it is present
	  4. encourage verbalization about current situation
	  5. assist client to identify personal strengths and resources that can be utilized to facilitate coping with the current situation
	  6. demonstrate acceptance of client but set limits on inappropriate behavior

Desired Outcome	Nursing Actions and *Selected Purposes/Rationales*

7. create an atmosphere of trust and support
8. if acceptable to client, arrange for a visit with another individual who has successfully adjusted to a similar injury
9. perform actions to reduce client's feelings of powerlessness (see Nursing Diagnosis 24)
10. assist client to maintain usual daily routines whenever possible
11. instruct client in effective problem-solving techniques (e.g. accurate identification of stressors, determination of various options to solve problem)
12. if client is experiencing severe spasticity:
    a. reinforce measures to reduce severity of the spasms (see Nursing Diagnosis 10, action a.8)
    b. reinforce ways that spasms can be beneficial (e.g. help swing legs from bed to wheelchair, initiate arm movements, maintain an erection, evacuate bowels)
    c. inform client that spasticity usually stabilizes in 1–2 years
13. inform client that there will be times when spasticity is worse, bowel and bladder programs are less effective, and efforts at self-care are less successful; assure him/her that these are temporary results of physical and/or emotional stress or fatigue rather than an indication of deteriorating neurological status
14. assist client to identify priorities and attainable goals as he/she starts to plan for necessary life-style and role changes
15. assist client and significant others to identify ways that personal and family goals can be adjusted rather than abandoned
16. assist client through methods such as role playing to prepare for negative reactions of others to his/her quadriplegia
17. administer antianxiety and/or antidepressant agents if ordered
18. assist client to find, hire, and train an attendant before discharge from the rehabilitative care unit
19. set up a home evaluation appointment with occupational and physical therapists before client's discharge *so that changes in the home environment (e.g. installation of ramps, widening doorways, altering bathroom facilities) can be completed by discharge*
20. assist client to identify and utilize available support systems; provide information regarding available community resources that can assist client and significant others in coping with effects of the spinal cord injury (e.g. spinal cord injury groups, recreational programs)
21. encourage the client to share with significant others the kind of support that would be most beneficial (e.g. listening, inspiring hope, providing reassurance and accurate information)
22. support behaviors indicative of effective coping (e.g. verbalization of ability to cope, utilization of available support systems, participation in rehabilitation program).
d. Consult physician about psychological and vocational counseling if appropriate. Initiate a referral if necessary.

---

24. NURSING DIAGNOSIS: **Powerlessness**

related to:
a. quadriplegia;
b. dependence on others to meet basic needs;
c. alterations in roles, relationships, and future plans associated with effects of the injury and need for extensive and lengthy rehabilitation.

Desired Outcome	Nursing Actions and *Selected Purposes/Rationales*
24. The client will demonstrate increasing feelings of control over his/her situation (see Care Plan on Immobility, Nursing Diagnosis 15 [p. 142], for outcome criteria).	24.a. Refer to Care Plan on Immobility, Nursing Diagnosis 15 (p. 142), for measures related to assessment of feelings of powerlessness and measures to promote client's feeling of control over his/her situation. b. Implement additional measures *to reduce client's feelings of powerlessness:* 1. perform actions to promote effective coping (see Nursing Diagnosis 23, action c) *in order to promote an increased sense of control over situation* 2. support realistic hope about the effects of rehabilitation on future independence (within 3–6 months and with the aid of assistive devices, the client should be able to perform many activities including operating an electric wheelchair, feeding self once meal has been set up, washing face and chest, brushing teeth, and using a computer) 3. stress to persons coming in contact with client that an individual has an enormous potential for adjusting to a disability and that they need to avoid being overly sympathetic (*an overly sympathetic attitude can communicate a feeling of hopelessness*) 4. assist client to select wheelchairs (usually a manual and an electric one) that best meet mobility needs and promote a more active life style 5. encourage client to be as active as possible in making decisions about his/her living situation 6. provide client with information about technical advances (e.g. the Environmental Control System [ECS]) that can make independent operation of electronic devices such as lights, radio, television, and specially installed door openers and window shades possible 7. discuss with significant others client's need to maintain as much control over his/her life as possible; stress the necessity of their encouraging and allowing the client to actively participate in the rehabilitation program and discharge planning.

25. NURSING DIAGNOSIS: Grieving*

related to extensive loss of motor and sensory function and the effects of this loss on future life style and roles.

---

*This diagnostic label includes anticipatory grieving and grieving following the actual losses.

Desired Outcome	Nursing Actions and *Selected Purposes/Rationales*
25. The client will demonstrate beginning progression through the grieving process as evidenced by: a. verbalization of feelings about the loss of motor and sensory function and its effects b. usual sleep pattern c. participation in treatment plan and self-care activities d. utilization of available support systems	25.a. Assess for signs and symptoms of grieving (e.g. change in eating habits, inability to concentrate, insomnia, anger, sadness, withdrawal from significant others, denial of loss). b. Implement measures *to facilitate the grieving process:* 1. assist client to acknowledge the losses *so grief work can begin*; assess for factors that may hinder and facilitate acknowledgment 2. discuss the grieving process and assist client to accept the phases of grieving as an expected response to the actual and anticipated losses 3. allow time for client to progress through the phases of grieving (phases vary among theorists but progress from shock and alarm to acceptance); be aware that not every phase is expressed by all individuals, that recurrence of phases is common, and that the grieving process will probably continue in varying degrees throughout the client's life

Desired Outcome	Nursing Actions and *Selected Purposes/Rationales*
e. verbalization of a plan for integrating prescribed follow-up care into life style.	4. provide an atmosphere of care and concern (e.g. provide privacy, be available and nonjudgmental, display empathy and respect) *so client will feel free to express feelings* 5. perform actions *to promote trust* (e.g. answer questions honestly, provide requested information) 6. encourage the verbal expression of anger and sadness about the losses experienced; recognize displacement of anger and assist client to see actual cause of angry feelings and resentment; establish limits on abusive behavior if demonstrated 7. encourage client to express feelings in whatever ways are comfortable (e.g. conversation); provide client with an acceptable outlet for frustration and anger (e.g. punching bag to swing arms against, wheeling outside when able, privacy) 8. perform actions to promote effective coping (see Nursing Diagnosis 23, action c) 9. support realistic hope about effects of rehabilitation on future independence 10. support behaviors suggesting successful grief work (e.g. verbalizing feelings about losses, focusing on ways to adapt to losses, learning needed skills, developing or renewing relationships) 11. explain the phases of the grieving process to significant others; encourage their support and understanding 12. facilitate communication between client and significant others; be aware that they may be in different phases of the grieving process 13. provide information about counseling services and support groups that might assist client in working through grief 14. when appropriate, assist client to meet spiritual needs (e.g. arrange for visit from clergy). c. Consult physician about referral for counseling if signs of dysfunctional grieving (e.g. persistent denial of losses, excessive anger or sadness, emotional lability) occur.

■━━

26. NURSING DIAGNOSIS: **Social isolation**

related to inability to participate in usual activities, depression, limited contact with significant others, and decreased exposure to events in the outside world associated with quadriplegia and prolonged hospitalization.

Desired Outcome	Nursing Actions and *Selected Purposes/Rationales*
26. The client will experience a decreased sense of isolation (see Care Plan on Immobility, Nursing Diagnosis 16 [p. 142], for outcome criteria).	26.a. Refer to Care Plan on Immobility, Nursing Diagnosis 16 (pp. 142–143), for measures related to assessment of and ways to decrease social isolation. b. Implement additional measures *to decrease social isolation:* 1. provide client with an effective method of contacting nurses' station (e.g. pressure-sensitive pad under shoulder or upper arm) 2. perform actions to reduce depression by implementing measures to facilitate client's psychological adjustment to effects of spinal cord injury (see Nursing Diagnoses 22; 23, action c; 24; and 25, action b) 3. set up a schedule of visiting times so that client will not go for long periods of time without visitors 4. assist client to identify a few persons with whom he/she feels comfortable and encourage interactions with them 5. encourage and assist client to maintain telephone contact with others; if possible, provide a speaker phone that has a dialing mechanism the client can activate independently 6. encourage participation in support groups.

■━━━━━━━━━━━━━━━━━━━━━━━━━━━━━━━

27. NURSING DIAGNOSIS: Altered family processes

related to change in family roles and structure associated with a family member's sudden, catastrophic injury; permanent disability; and need for extensive rehabilitation.

Desired Outcome	Nursing Actions and *Selected Purposes/Rationales*
27. The family members* will demonstrate beginning adjustment to changes in functioning of a family member and family roles and structure as evidenced by: a. meeting client's needs b. verbalization of ways to adapt to required role and life-style changes c. active participation in decision making and client's rehabilitation d. positive interactions with one another.	27.a. Assess for signs and symptoms of altered family processes (e.g. inability to meet client's needs, statements of not being able to accept client's quadriplegia or make necessary role and life-style changes, inability to make decisions, inability or refusal to participate in client's rehabilitation, negative family interactions). b. Identify components of the family and their patterns of communication and role expectations. c. Implement measures *to facilitate family members' adjustment to client's diagnosis, changes in client's functioning within the family system, and altered family roles and structure:* 　1. encourage verbalization of feelings about client's quadriplegia and the effect of this on family structure; actively listen to each family member and maintain a nonjudgmental attitude about feelings shared 　2. reinforce physician's explanations of the effects of the injury and planned treatment and rehabilitation 　3. assist family members to gain a realistic perspective of client's situation, conveying as much hope as appropriate 　4. provide privacy *so that family members and client can share their feelings with one another*; stress the importance of and facilitate the use of good communication techniques 　5. assist family members to progress through their own grieving process; explain that they may encounter times when they need to focus on meeting their own rather than the client's needs 　6. emphasize the need for family members to obtain adequate rest and nutrition and to identify and utilize stress management techniques *so that they are better able to emotionally and physically deal with the changes and losses experienced* 　7. encourage and assist family members to identify coping strategies for dealing with the client's quadriplegia and its effects on the family 　8. assist family members to identify realistic goals and ways of reaching these goals 　9. include family members in decision making about client and care; convey appreciation for their input and continued support of client 　10. encourage and allow family members to participate in client's care and rehabilitation 　11. assist family members to identify resources that can assist them in coping with their feelings and meeting their immediate and long-term needs (e.g. counseling and social services; caregiver assistance programs; pastoral care; service, church, and spinal cord injury groups); initiate a referral if indicated. d. Consult physician if family members continue to demonstrate difficulty adapting to changes in client's functioning and family structure.

─────────────

*The term "family members" is being used here to include client's significant others.

Discharge Teaching

■━━━━━━━━━━━━━━━━━━━━━━━━━━━━━━━━━━━━━

28. NURSING DIAGNOSIS: **Knowledge deficit, Ineffective management of therapeutic regimen, or Altered health maintenance*†**

———————————

    *The nurse should select the diagnostic label that is most appropriate for the client's discharge teaching needs.

    †Although the client will not be able to perform many of the following actions independently, he/she must be knowledgeable about them in order to provide proper instruction to significant others and attendant and maintain an active role in the rehabilitation process.

Desired Outcomes	Nursing Actions and *Selected Purposes/Rationales*
28.a. The client will identify ways to prevent complications associated with spinal cord injury and decreased mobility.	28.a.1. Refer to Care Plan on Immobility, Nursing Diagnosis 17, action a (pp. 143–144), for instructions related to ways to prevent complications associated with decreased mobility.

     2. Instruct client in ways to prevent complications associated with spinal cord injury:
      a. position firm pillow between legs if spasms tend to cause legs to cross (helps to prevent thrombus formation and adduction contractures)
      b. wear an abdominal binder when changing from a reclining to a sitting position and take vasoconstrictor drugs if prescribed to prevent dizziness and fainting
      c. elevate legs periodically during the day to promote venous return
      d. implement measures to reduce severe spasticity (e.g. avoid fatigue and chills, change position at least every 2 hours, take muscle relaxants as prescribed) in order to increase mobility and prevent contractures
      e. use full-length and long-handled mirrors to examine all skin surfaces in the morning and the evening
      f. obtain a kinetic bed for home use if possible
      g. wear shoes when in wheelchair to protect feet from injury
      h. avoid putting items such as coins, keys, and wallet in skirt or pant pockets (these items can cause pressure on underlying skin areas)
      i. avoid wearing tight-fitting belts, clothing, shoes, and jewelry
      j. replace wheelchair cushions when they become worn-out
      k. implement measures to prevent hyperthermia (e.g. avoid direct sunlight in hot weather, avoid excessive clothing and bedding)
      l. implement measures to prevent hypothermia (e.g. wear adequate amounts of clothing, wear a hat when in a cold environment, drink warm liquids)
      m. implement measures to prevent falls (e.g. always use safety belt during transfers and when in chair, be certain to have adequate assistance for transfer activity)
      n. implement measures to prevent burns:
        1. always check temperature of shower or bath water before use (can use bath water thermometer or have attendant check water temperature)
        2. never smoke when alone
        3. let hot foods/fluids cool slightly before attempting to feed self
        4. never position self next to a stove, heater, or other major source of heat
        5. never use an electric heating pad or electric blanket
      o. implement measures to prevent dysreflexia:
        1. do not allow bladder or bowel to become distended
        2. change position frequently
        3. seek medical attention at first sign of infection, persistent pressure area, or ingrown toenail

4. apply a topical anesthetic to any area being stimulated or take a ganglionic blocking agent as prescribed (may need to be taken routinely or before activities known to precipitate dysreflexia).

3. Demonstrate the following procedures to client, significant others, and attendant:
   a. assisted coughing technique
   b. skin care
   c. proper positioning and padding
   d. transfer techniques
   e. active and passive range of motion exercises
   f. application of elastic stockings, abdominal binder, and heel and elbow protectors
   g. emergency treatment of dysreflexia (e.g. elevate head of bed and lower client's legs, alleviate causative factor, administer an antihypertensive agent).

4. Allow time for questions, clarification, and return demonstration.

28.b. The client will demonstrate the ability to correctly use and maintain assistive devices.

28.b.1. Reinforce instructions of physical and occupational therapists regarding use of assistive devices. Allow time for questions, clarification, and return demonstration.

2. Instruct client in proper maintenance of assistive devices (e.g. replace parts that are worn-out or broken, clean wheel hubs and crossbars of wheelchairs per manufacturer's instruction, keep wheelchair tires properly inflated).

28.c. The client will identify ways to manage altered bowel and bladder function.

28.c.1. Reinforce bladder and bowel training programs. (Guidelines are included in Nursing Diagnoses 12, action e; 13, action d; and 14, action b, but the specific program will vary for each client.)

2. Demonstrate bowel care (e.g. digital stimulation, insertion of suppositories, administration of enemas) and bladder care (e.g. stimulation techniques, intermittent catheterization, emptying of urinary collection bag). Allow time for questions, clarification, and return demonstration.

28.d. The client will state signs and symptoms to report to the health care provider.

28.d. Instruct the client to report the following:
   1. cloudy, foul-smelling urine
   2. nausea and vomiting
   3. cough productive of purulent, green, or rust-colored sputum
   4. difficulty breathing or increased shortness of breath with activity
   5. sudden or persistent shoulder pain (this can be a referred pain)
   6. fever
   7. chills or profuse sweating (can occur above the level of the injury)
   8. increase in spasticity (could indicate an infection below the level of the injury)
   9. unsuccessful bowel and/or bladder programs
   10. redness in any extremity
   11. swelling that appears suddenly, occurs only in one extremity, or does not subside overnight
   12. increased restriction of any joint motion
   13. persistent swelling over a joint
   14. signs and symptoms of dysreflexia (e.g. pounding headache, sudden rise in blood pressure, blurred vision, slow pulse, flushing and sweating above level of injury, nasal congestion) that do not subside once the stimulus is removed
   15. any area of persistent skin irritation or breakdown
   16. indications of pregnancy (stress that appropriate prenatal care should be initiated as soon as possible).

28.e. The client will identify community resources that can assist with home management and adjustment to changes resulting from spinal cord injury.

28.e.1. Inform client and significant others of community resources that can assist with home management and adjustment to changes resulting from spinal cord injury (e.g. spinal cord injury support and social groups; home health agencies; community health agencies; local service groups; financial, individual, family, and vocational counselors).

2. Initiate a referral if indicated.

Desired Outcomes	Nursing Actions and **Selected Purposes/Rationales**

28.f. The client will verbalize an understanding of and a plan for adhering to recommended follow-up care including future appointments with health care provider and occupational and physical therapists and medications prescribed.	28.f.1. Reinforce the importance of keeping scheduled follow-up visits with health care provider and occupational and physical therapists.
	2. Explain the rationale for, side effects of, and importance of taking prescribed medications. Inform client of pertinent food and drug interactions.
	3. Implement measures designed to improve client compliance:
	  a. include significant others and caregivers in teaching sessions
	  b. encourage questions and allow time for reinforcement and clarification of information provided
	  c. provide written instructions on scheduled appointments with health care provider and occupational and physical therapists, medications prescribed, and signs and symptoms to report.

Bibliography

See pages 897–898 and 902.

UNIT NINE

NURSING CARE OF THE CLIENT WITH DISTURBANCES OF CARDIOVASCULAR FUNCTION

ANGINA PECTORIS

Angina pectoris is a syndrome characterized by transient episodes of retrosternal chest pain that are caused by an imbalance between myocardial oxygen supply and demand. The most common cause of angina pectoris is decreased coronary blood supply due to atherosclerosis of a major coronary artery. The atherosclerosis causes narrowing of the vessel lumen and an inability of the vessel to dilate and supply sufficient blood to the myocardium at times when myocardial oxygen needs are increased. Other conditions that can compromise coronary blood flow are spasm and/or thrombosis of a coronary artery, hypotension, and aortic stenosis. Conditions that reduce oxygen availability and/or increase myocardial workload and oxygen demands (e.g. anemia, smoking, chronic lung disease, exercise, heavy meals, exposure to cold, stress, thyrotoxicosis, hypertension) may precipitate or increase the frequency of angina attacks by widening the gap between oxygen needs and availability.

The three major types of angina pectoris are stable (classic exertional) angina, unstable (crescendo, preinfarction) angina, and variant (Prinzmetal's) angina. These types differ with regard to severity and frequency of attacks, refractoriness of the pain, and typical precipitants of the pain. In all types of angina, the pain usually occurs in the retrosternal area; may or may not radiate; and is described as a tight, heavy, squeezing, burning, or choking sensation. Stable angina, the most common type, is usually precipitated by physical exertion or emotional stress, lasts 3 to 5 minutes, and is relieved by rest and nitroglycerin. Unstable angina is characterized by an increasing frequency and/or severity of attacks that occur with less provocation or at rest. Because thrombus formation frequently complicates unstable angina, the person with unstable angina is usually hospitalized and treated with intravenous heparin while decisions regarding medical versus surgical treatment are made.

This care plan focuses on the adult client hospitalized during an episode of chest pain suspected to be unstable angina. The goals of care are to improve myocardial oxygen supply, relieve pain, prevent complications, and educate the client regarding follow-up care.

DIAGNOSTIC TESTS

Electrocardiogram (ECG)
Cardiac enzymes/isoenzymes
Serum lipid levels
Radionuclide imaging
Exercise stress test
Coronary angiography
Echocardiography

DISCHARGE CRITERIA

Prior to discharge, the client will:

- perform activities of daily living and ambulate without angina
- have angina controlled by oral medication
- have no signs and symptoms of complications
- verbalize a basic understanding of angina pectoris
- identify factors that may precipitate angina attacks and ways to control these factors
- identify modifiable cardiovascular risk factors and ways to alter these factors
- verbalize an understanding of the rationale for and components of a diet low in saturated fat and cholesterol
- demonstrate accuracy in counting pulse
- verbalize an understanding of medications ordered including rationale, food and drug interactions, side effects, schedule for taking, and importance of taking as prescribed
- state signs and symptoms to report to the health care provider
- identify community resources that can assist in making necessary life-style changes and adjusting to the effects of angina pectoris
- verbalize an understanding of and a plan for adhering to recommended follow-up care including future appointments with health care provider.

| NURSING/ COLLABORATIVE DIAGNOSES | **1.** Risk for decreased cardiac output △ 317
 2. Pain: radiating or nonradiating chest pain △ 318
 3. Potential complications:
   a. cardiac dysrhythmias
   b. myocardial infarction △ 319
 4. Anxiety △ 320 |
| DISCHARGE TEACHING | **5.** Knowledge deficit, Ineffective management of therapeutic regimen, or Altered health maintenance △ 321 |

1. NURSING DIAGNOSIS:

Risk for decreased cardiac output

related to mechanical and electrical dysfunction of the heart associated with transient myocardial ischemia.

Desired Outcome	Nursing Actions and *Selected Purposes/Rationales*

1. The client will maintain adequate cardiac output as evidenced by:
   a. B/P within normal range for client
   b. apical pulse regular and between 60–100 beats/minute
   c. absence of gallop rhythms
   d. absence of fatigue and weakness
   e. unlabored respirations at 14–20/minute
   f. clear, audible breath sounds
   g. usual mental status
   h. absence of vertigo and syncope
   i. palpable peripheral pulses
   j. skin warm, dry, and usual color
   k. capillary refill time less than 3 seconds
   l. urine output at least 30 ml/hour
   m. absence of edema and jugular vein distention.

1.a. Assess for and report signs and symptoms of decreased cardiac output:
   1. variations in B/P (may be increased because of pain or a compensatory response to low cardiac output; may be decreased when compensatory mechanisms and pump fail)
   2. tachycardia (may also be a response to pain)
   3. presence of gallop rhythm(s)
   4. fatigue and weakness
   5. dyspnea, tachypnea
   6. crackles (rales)
   7. restlessness, change in mental status
   8. vertigo, syncope
   9. diminished or absent peripheral pulses
   10. cool, moist skin
   11. pallor or cyanosis of skin
   12. capillary refill time greater than 3 seconds
   13. oliguria
   14. edema
   15. jugular vein distention (JVD).
   b. Monitor for and report the following:
   1. ECG readings showing dysrhythmias or findings indicative of ischemia (e.g. ST segment depression or elevation, peaked or inverted T waves)
   2. chest x-ray results showing pulmonary vascular congestion, pulmonary edema, or pleural effusion
   3. abnormal blood gases
   4. a significant decrease in oximetry results.
   c. Implement measures *to help maintain an adequate cardiac output:*
   1. perform actions *to improve myocardial blood flow and oxygenation and subsequently reduce damage to the myocardium:*
      a. maintain oxygen therapy as ordered
      b. administer the following medications if ordered:
         1. nitrates (e.g. nitroglycerin, isosorbide) *to dilate the coronary and peripheral (primarily venous) blood vessels, thereby improving myocardial blood flow and reducing cardiac workload and myocardial oxygen consumption*
         2. beta-adrenergic blocking agents (e.g. atenolol, nadolol, metoprolol, propranolol) *to decrease myocardial contractility and heart rate, thereby reducing myocardial oxygen consumption*

Desired Outcome   Nursing Actions and **Selected Purposes/Rationales**

---

        3. calcium-channel blockers (e.g. verapamil, diltiazem, amlodipine, nicardipine) *to dilate the coronary arteries and reduce cardiac workload by dilating peripheral vessels*

        4. anticoagulants (e.g. intravenous heparin) and antiplatelet agents (e.g. low-dose aspirin) *to prevent obstruction of the coronary artery(ies) by thrombosis*

    c. prepare client for percutaneous coronary revascularization (e.g. balloon angioplasty, atherectomy, intracoronary stenting) or coronary artery bypass grafting (CABG) if planned

  2. perform additional actions *to reduce cardiac workload:*

    a. maintain activity restrictions as ordered

    b. instruct client to avoid activities that create a Valsalva response (e.g. straining to have a bowel movement, holding breath while moving up in bed) *in order to prevent the marked increase in venous return and preload that occurs with exhalation*

    c. implement measures *to promote emotional rest* (e.g. reduce fear and anxiety)

    d. discourage excessive intake of beverages high in caffeine such as coffee, tea, and colas (*caffeine is a myocardial stimulant and can increase myocardial oxygen consumption*)

    e. discourage smoking (*smoke has a cardiostimulatory effect, causes vasoconstriction, and reduces oxygen availability*)

    f. increase activity gradually as allowed and tolerated.

---

2. NURSING DIAGNOSIS: **Pain: radiating or nonradiating chest pain**

related to decreased myocardial oxygenation (an insufficient oxygen supply forces the myocardium to convert to anaerobic metabolism; the end products of anaerobic metabolism act as irritants to myocardial neural receptors).

Desired Outcome   Nursing Actions and **Selected Purposes/Rationales**

---

2. The client will experience relief of pain as evidenced by:
  a. verbalization of same
  b. relaxed facial expression and body positioning
  c. increased participation in activities
  d. stable vital signs.

2.a. Assess for signs and symptoms of pain (e.g. verbalization of pain; grimacing; rubbing neck, jaw, or arm; reluctance to move; clutching chest; restlessness; diaphoresis; facial pallor; increased B/P; tachycardia).

  b. Assess client's perception of the severity of the pain using a pain intensity rating scale.

  c. Assess the client's pain pattern (e.g. location, quality, onset, duration, precipitating factors, aggravating factors, alleviating factors).

  d. Implement measures *to relieve pain:*

    1. administer nitroglycerin if ordered

    2. maintain client on bed rest in a semi- to high Fowler's position

    3. administer a narcotic (opioid) analgesic if ordered if pain is unrelieved by rest and nitroglycerin within 15–20 minutes (narcotic analgesics are usually administered intravenously *because intramuscular injections are poorly absorbed if tissue perfusion is decreased; intramuscular injections also elevate serum enzyme levels, which makes assessment of myocardial damage more difficult*)

    4. provide or assist with nonpharmacologic measures for pain relief (e.g. position change, relaxation exercises, restful environment).

  e. Consult physician if pain persists or worsens.

  f. Implement measures to help maintain an adequate cardiac output (see Nursing Diagnosis 1, action c) *in order to improve myocardial blood flow and oxygenation and subsequently prevent recurrent episodes of angina.*

3. COLLABORATIVE DIAGNOSES:

Potential complications of angina pectoris:

a. **cardiac dysrhythmias** related to myocardial irritability associated with myocardial hypoxia;

b. **myocardial infarction** related to prolonged myocardial ischemia.

Desired Outcomes	Nursing Actions and *Selected Purposes/Rationales*

3.a. The client will maintain normal sinus rhythm as evidenced by:
  1. regular apical pulse at 60–100 beats/minute
  2. equal apical and radial pulse rates
  3. absence of syncope and palpitations
  4. ECG reading showing normal sinus rhythm.

3.a.1. Assess for and report signs and symptoms of cardiac dysrhythmias (e.g. irregular apical pulse; pulse rate below 60 or above 100 beats/minute; apical-radial pulse deficit; syncope; palpitations; abnormal rate, rhythm, or configurations on ECG).
  2. Implement measures to help maintain an adequate cardiac output (see Nursing Diagnosis 1, action c) *in order to improve myocardial blood flow and oxygenation and subsequently reduce the risk for dysrhythmias.*
  3. If cardiac dysrhythmias occur:
    a. initiate cardiac monitoring if not already being done
    b. administer antidysrhythmics (e.g. lidocaine, procainamide, metoprolol, atenolol, esmolol, adenosine, diltiazem, verapamil, atropine) if ordered
    c. restrict client's activity based on his/her tolerance and severity of the dysrhythmia
    d. maintain oxygen therapy as ordered
    e. assess cardiovascular status frequently and report signs and symptoms of inadequate cardiac output (see Nursing Diagnosis 1, action a)
    f. have emergency cart readily available for cardioversion, defibrillation, or cardiopulmonary resuscitation.

3.b. The client will not experience a myocardial infarction as evidenced by:
  1. resolution of chest pain within 15–20 minutes
  2. stable vital signs
  3. cardiac enzymes within normal range
  4. absence of ST segment elevation, peaked T waves or T wave inversion, and abnormal Q waves on ECG reading.

3.b.1. Assess for and report signs and symptoms of a myocardial infarction (e.g. chest pain that lasts longer than 20 minutes; increase in pulse rate; significant change in B/P; labored respirations; elevation of cardiac enzymes [CK-MB is the first to increase]; ST segment elevation, peaked T waves or T wave inversion, and/or abnormal Q waves on ECG [ST segment elevation can also occur in Prinzmetal's angina]).
  2. Implement measures to help maintain an adequate cardiac output (see Nursing Diagnosis 1, action c) *in order to improve myocardial blood flow and oxygenation and subsequently reduce the risk for a myocardial infarction.*
  3. If signs and symptoms of a myocardial infarction occur:
    a. initiate cardiac monitoring if not already being done
    b. maintain client on strict bed rest in a semi- to high Fowler's position
    c. maintain oxygen therapy as ordered
    d. administer the following medications if ordered:
      1. morphine sulfate *to reduce pain and anxiety and decrease cardiac workload*
      2. nitrates *to improve coronary blood flow and reduce myocardial oxygen requirements*
      3. beta-adrenergic blocking agents *to reduce myocardial oxygen requirements by decreasing the heart rate and force of myocardial contractility*
    e. prepare client for the following procedures that may be performed *to improve myocardial blood flow:*
      1. injection of a thrombolytic agent (e.g. streptokinase, tissue plasminogen activator [tPA], anistreplase [APSAC, Eminase])
      2. mechanical revascularization (e.g. percutaneous transluminal coronary angioplasty [PTCA], coronary artery bypass grafting [CABG])
      3. insertion of an intra-aortic balloon pump (IABP)

Desired Outcomes	Nursing Actions and *Selected Purposes/Rationales*

       f. provide emotional support to client and significant others

       g. refer to Care Plan on Myocardial Infarction for additional care measures.

---

4. NURSING DIAGNOSIS: **Anxiety**

related to pain or threat of recurrent pain; lack of understanding of diagnostic tests, diagnosis, and treatment plan; unfamiliar environment; and effect of angina pectoris on future life style and roles.

Desired Outcome	Nursing Actions and *Selected Purposes/Rationales*

4. The client will experience a reduction in anxiety as evidenced by:
   a. verbalization of feeling less anxious
   b. usual sleep pattern
   c. relaxed facial expression and body movements
   d. stable vital signs
   e. usual perceptual ability and interactions with others.

4.a. Assess client for signs and symptoms of anxiety (e.g. verbalization of feeling anxious, insomnia, tenseness, shakiness, restlessness, diaphoresis, tachycardia, elevated blood pressure, facial pallor, self-focused behaviors).

  b. Implement measures *to reduce fear and anxiety:*

    1. provide care in a calm, supportive, confident manner

    2. if client is having severe pain:

      a. do not leave him/her alone during period of acute distress

      b. perform actions to relieve pain (see Nursing Diagnosis 2, action d)

    3. once period of acute distress has subsided:

      a. orient client to hospital environment, equipment, and routines; include an explanation of cardiac monitoring equipment

      b. keep cardiac monitor out of client's view and the sound turned as low as possible

      c. introduce client to staff who will be participating in care; if possible, maintain consistency in staff assigned to his/her care *to provide feelings of stability and comfort with the environment*

      d. assure client that staff members are nearby; respond to call signal as soon as possible

      e. encourage verbalization of fear and anxiety; provide feedback

      f. explain all diagnostic tests

      g. reinforce physician's explanations and clarify misconceptions the client has about angina pectoris, the treatment plan, and prognosis; stress to client that he/she has not had a "heart attack"

      h. reinforce physician's explanation of percutaneous coronary revascularization procedures (e.g. balloon angioplasty, atherectomy, intracoronary stenting) if planned

      i. initiate preoperative teaching if heart surgery is planned

      j. provide a calm, restful environment

      k. instruct client in relaxation techniques and encourage participation in diversional activities

      l. provide information based on current needs of client at a level he/she can understand; encourage questions and clarification of information provided

      m. assist client to identify specific stressors and ways to cope with them

      n. allow client to discuss concerns about future life style and roles; focus on the need for alteration in rather than elimination of activities

      o. encourage significant others to project a caring, concerned attitude without obvious anxiousness

      p. include significant others in orientation and teaching sessions and encourage their continued support of the client

      q. administer prescribed antianxiety agents if indicated.

  c. Consult physician if above actions fail to control fear and anxiety.

Discharge Teaching

■

5. NURSING DIAGNOSIS:	Knowledge deficit, Ineffective management of therapeutic regimen, or Altered health maintenance*

*The nurse should select the diagnostic label that is most appropriate for the client's discharge teaching needs.

Desired Outcomes	Nursing Actions and *Selected Purposes/Rationales*

5.a. The client will verbalize a basic understanding of angina pectoris.

5.a. Explain angina pectoris in terms that client can understand. Utilize teaching aids (e.g. pamphlets, diagrams) whenever possible.

5.b. The client will identify factors that may precipitate angina attacks and ways to control these factors.

5.b.1. Ask client if there is a pattern to angina attacks and precipitating factors.

2. Inform the client of factors that may precipitate angina pectoris (e.g. strenuous or isometric exercises, change in usual sexual habits and/or partner, consumption of a large meal, exposure to extreme cold, strong emotions, smoking).

3. Provide the following instructions regarding ways to reduce risk of precipitating an angina attack:
   a. take sublingual nitroglycerin 5–10 minutes before strenuous activity or sexual intercourse and during times of high emotional stress
   b. gradually increase activity tolerance by engaging in a regular isotonic exercise program (e.g. walking, biking, swimming)
   c. avoid isometric exercises/activities (e.g. weight lifting, pushing, straining)
   d. rest between activities
   e. stop any activity that causes shortness of breath, palpitations, dizziness, or extreme fatigue or weakness
   f. begin a cardiovascular fitness program when approved by physician
   g. adhere to the following precautions regarding sexual activity:
      1. avoid intercourse for at least 1–2 hours after a heavy meal or alcohol consumption and when fatigued or stressed
      2. engage in sexual activity in a familiar environment and in a position that minimizes exertion (e.g. side-lying, partner on top); recognize that a new sexual relationship can be started but may result in greater energy expenditure initially
      3. avoid hot or cold showers just before and after intercourse.

5.c. The client will identify modifiable cardiovascular risk factors and ways to alter these factors.

5.c.1. Inform client that the following modifiable factors have been shown to contribute to cardiovascular disease:
   a. obesity
   b. elevated serum lipids
   c. lack of regular aerobic exercise
   d. cigarette smoking
   e. hypertension
   f. diabetes mellitus
   g. stressful life style.

2. Encourage client to discuss alcohol intake with health care provider. (The health care provider may advise the client to limit alcohol consumption because there is evidence that a daily alcohol intake exceeding 1 oz of ethanol [i.e. 2 oz of 100-proof whiskey, 8 oz of wine, 24 oz of beer] contributes to the development of hypertension and some forms of heart disease.)

3. Assist client to identify ways he/she can make appropriate changes in life style to modify the above factors. Provide information about weight reduction plans; stress management classes; and cardiovascular fitness, smoking cessation, and alcohol rehabilitation programs if appropriate. Initiate a referral if indicated.

Desired Outcomes	Nursing Actions and *Selected Purposes/Rationales*

5.d. The client will verbalize an understanding of the rationale for and components of a diet low in saturated fat and cholesterol.	5.d.1. Explain the rationale for a diet low in saturated fat and cholesterol.
	2. Provide instructions on ways the client can reduce intake of saturated fat and cholesterol:
	  a. reduce intake of red meat
	  b. trim visible fat off meat and remove all skin from poultry
	  c. use vegetable oil rather than coconut or palm oil in cooking and food preparation
	  d. use cooking methods such as steaming, baking, broiling, poaching, microwaving, and grilling rather than frying
	  e. restrict intake of eggs (recommendations about the number of whole eggs allowed per week vary depending on the client's lipid levels)
	  f. avoid commercial baked goods
	  g. avoid dairy products containing more than 1% fat.

5.e. The client will demonstrate accuracy in counting pulse.	5.e.1. Teach client how to count his/her pulse, being alert to the regularity of the rhythm. 2. Allow time for return demonstration and accuracy check.

5.f. The client will verbalize an understanding of medications ordered including rationale, food and drug interactions, side effects, schedule for taking, and importance of taking as prescribed.	5.f.1. Explain the rationale for, side effects of, and importance of taking the medications prescribed. Inform client of pertinent food and drug interactions.
	2. If client is discharged on sublingual or buccal nitroglycerin, instruct to:
	  a. avoid drinking alcoholic beverages
	  b. have tablets readily available at all times
	  c. take a tablet before strenuous activity and in emotionally stressful situations
	  d. take one tablet when chest pain occurs and another every 5 minutes up to a total of 3 times if necessary; notify physician or obtain emergency medical assistance if pain persists
	  e. place tablet under tongue or in the buccal pouch and allow it to dissolve thoroughly before swallowing
	  f. store tablets in a tightly capped, dark-colored glass container away from heat and moisture
	  g. replace tablets every 6 months or sooner if they do not relieve discomfort
	  h. avoid rising to a standing position quickly after taking nitroglycerin in order to reduce dizziness associated with its vasodilatory effect
	  i. recognize that dizziness, flushing, and mild headache may occur after taking nitroglycerin
	  j. report fainting, persistent or severe headache, blurred vision, or dry mouth.
	3. If nitroglycerin skin patches are prescribed:
	  a. provide instructions about correct application, skin care, need to rotate sites and remove old patch, and frequency of change; if physician prescribes the patch be left off for a certain length of time each day, explain that this helps prevent the development of nitrate tolerance
	  b. caution client that activities that increase blood flow to the skin (e.g. hot bath or shower, sauna) can cause a sudden reduction in blood pressure
	  c. instruct client to avoid drinking alcoholic beverages
	  d. instruct client to remove skin patch if faintness, dizziness, or flushing occurs following application and to then notify health care provider
	  e. instruct client to report persistent redness or itching at patch site.
	4. If client is discharged on a beta-adrenergic blocking agent (e.g. propranolol, metoprolol, atenolol, nadolol), instruct to:
	  a. take the medication at the same time every day
	  b. check pulse before taking medication; consult health care provider if pulse rate is unusually slow (it is expected that pulse will be lower than normal)
	  c. avoid skipping doses, trying to make up for missed doses, altering the prescribed dose, and discontinuing medication without first discussing with health care provider

    d. change from a lying to a sitting or standing position slowly if dizziness is a problem

    e. limit intake of alcoholic beverages

    f. monitor blood glucose on a regular basis if a diabetic (beta blockers may affect blood sugar and mask symptoms of hypoglycemia)

    g. wear a medical alert identification bracelet or tag specifying the name of the medication being taken

    h. report the following:

      1. persistent lightheadedness or dizziness

      2. significant weight gain, night cough, difficulty breathing, or swelling of feet or ankles (may be indicative of heart failure)

      3. cold, painful toes or fingers

      4. persistent fatigue or depression.

5. If client is discharged on a calcium-channel blocker (e.g. amlodipine, nicardipine, verapamil, diltiazem), instruct to:

    a. avoid skipping doses, altering the prescribed dose, and discontinuing medication without first discussing it with health care provider

    b. change from a lying to a sitting or standing position slowly in order to prevent dizziness

    c. report any increase in frequency, duration, or severity of angina

    d. keep medication at room temperature in an airtight, light-resistant container

    e. avoid operating dangerous equipment and driving as long as dizziness is present (common in the early treatment period).

6. Instruct client to take lipid-lowering agents (e.g. lovastatin, gemfibrozil, pravastatin, simvastatin) and antiplatelet agents (e.g. aspirin) as prescribed.

7. Instruct client to consult physician before taking other prescription and nonprescription medications.

8. Instruct client to inform all health care providers of medications being taken.

5.g. The client will state signs and symptoms to report to the health care provider.

5.g. Stress the importance of reporting the following signs and symptoms:

1. chest, arm, neck, or jaw pain unrelieved by rest and/or nitroglycerin taken every 5 minutes for 15 minutes

2. shortness of breath

3. irregular pulse or a resting pulse less than 56 or greater than 100 beats/minute (the rate the client should report may vary depending on the medication[s] prescribed, the client's baseline pulse, and physician's preference)

4. fainting spells

5. diminished activity tolerance

6. swelling of feet or ankles

7. increase in severity or frequency of angina attacks.

5.h. The client will identify community resources that can assist in making necessary life-style changes and adjusting to the effects of angina pectoris.

5.h.1. Provide information about community resources that can assist client in making life-style changes and adjusting to effects of angina pectoris (e.g. weight loss, smoking cessation, and stress management programs; American Heart Association; counseling services).

2. Initiate a referral if indicated.

5.i. The client will verbalize an understanding of and a plan for adhering to recommended follow-up care including future appointments with health care provider.

5.i.1. Reinforce the importance of keeping follow-up appointments with health care provider.

2. Implement measures to improve client compliance:

    a. include significant others in teaching sessions if possible

    b. encourage questions and allow time for reinforcement and clarification of information provided

    c. provide written instructions regarding future appointments with health care provider, dietary modifications, activity level, medications prescribed, and signs and symptoms to report.

Bibliography

See pages 897–898 and 902.

▤ HEART FAILURE

Heart failure is a syndrome in which the heart is unable to pump an adequate supply of blood to meet the body's metabolic needs. Inadequate emptying of the ventricles results in increased pressure in the cardiac chambers, which leads to decreased pulmonary and systemic venous return and subsequent vascular congestion. To compensate for decreased cardiac output, there is an increase in sympathetic nervous system activity, ventricular dilation to accommodate the increased volume of blood remaining in the ventricles, stimulation of renin-angiotensin-aldosterone output and ADH release, and eventual ventricular hypertrophy. These compensatory mechanisms temporarily aid in maintaining an adequate cardiac output but eventually have a deleterious effect on the heart.

Numerous conditions can precipitate heart failure including myocardial ischemia or infarction, cardiomyopathy, cardiac valve malfunction, hypertension, dysrhythmias, constrictive pericarditis, and systemic conditions that increase the metabolic rate (e.g. thyrotoxicosis, infection) or cause prolonged or severe hypoxia. Heart failure can be classified in a number of ways. It is often classified as left-sided or right-sided, backward or forward, low-output or high-output, acute or chronic, and/or systolic (classic) or diastolic failure. A functional classification system based on the relationship between symptoms and the amount of activity to provoke the symptoms was developed by the New York Heart Association and may still be utilized by some practitioners. In this system, which has 4 levels or classes, a person is said to have Class I heart failure if no symptoms are experienced with ordinary physical activity and Class IV failure when symptoms occur with any physical activity and possibly at rest.

The types of medications used for treatment of heart failure are primarily dependent on whether failure is systolic (an impaired inotropic state characterized by ventricular dilation and inadequate ventricle emptying) or diastolic (impaired relaxation of the ventricles with decreased ventricular filling). Positive inotropic agents, as well as diuretics and vasodilators, are the mainstay of treatment in systolic (classic) heart failure. In heart failure associated exclusively with diastolic dysfunction, positive inotropic agents are usually contraindicated.

Signs and symptoms of heart failure are dependent on which side of the heart is failing as well as whether there is forward or backward failure. Symptoms of forward failure are caused by low cardiac output. Symptoms of backward failure are associated with the ventricle failing to empty completely, which results in blood flow backup. In left-sided failure, there is reduced emptying of the left ventricle, which results in decreased systemic tissue perfusion as well as blood flow backup in the left atrium and pulmonary vasculature. Pulmonary vascular congestion leads to pulmonary edema with symptoms such as tachypnea, dyspnea, cough, and abnormal breath sounds. In right-sided failure, the effect of reduced function and emptying of the right ventricle is decreased pulmonary blood flow and backup of blood in the right atrium. This results in systemic venous congestion, which is manifested by peripheral edema and signs of major organ enlargement and dysfunction. Initially only one side of the heart may fail (more commonly the left side), but as failure progresses, both sides are usually affected.

As long as the body's compensatory mechanisms and/or treatment measures are able to maintain cardiac output that is sufficient to prevent or relieve symptoms, a state of compensated heart failure exists. If the myocardium is severely damaged and intrinsic compensatory mechanisms and treatment measures fail to maintain adequate cardiac output and tissue perfusion, a state of decompensated heart failure exists. When this state persists and is no longer responsive to medical treatment, it is termed intractable or refractory heart failure.

This care plan focuses on the adult client hospitalized with signs and symptoms of acute classic biventricular heart failure. The goals of care are to improve cardiac output, reduce fluid excess, increase activity tolerance, prevent complications, and educate the client regarding follow-up care.

DIAGNOSTIC TESTS

Chest x-ray
Echocardiography
Radionuclide imaging
Electrocardiogram (ECG)
Cardiac catheterization
Blood studies (e.g. blood gases, electrolytes, bilirubin, liver enzymes, BUN, creatinine)
Oximetry

DISCHARGE CRITERIA

Prior to discharge, the client will:

- have vital signs within a safe range and evidence of adequate peripheral circulation
- tolerate expected level of activity without undue fatigue or dyspnea
- have achieved dry weight and have minimal or no edema
- have clear, audible breath sounds throughout lungs
- have oxygen saturation within normal limits for client's age
- identify modifiable cardiovascular risk factors and ways to alter these factors

- verbalize an understanding of the rationale for and components of a diet low in sodium
- demonstrate accuracy in counting pulse
- verbalize an understanding of medications ordered including rationale, food and drug interactions, side effects, schedule for taking, and importance of taking as prescribed
- state signs and symptoms to report to the health care provider
- identify community resources that can assist with home management and adjustment to changes resulting from heart failure
- share feelings and concerns about changes in body functioning and usual roles and life style
- verbalize an understanding of and a plan for adhering to recommended follow-up care including future appointments with health care provider and activity limitations.

Use in conjunction with the Care Plan on Immobility.

NURSING/COLLABORATIVE DIAGNOSES	1. Decreased cardiac output △ 325
	2. Impaired respiratory function:
	a. ineffective breathing pattern
	b. ineffective airway clearance
	c. impaired gas exchange △ 327
	3. Altered fluid and electrolyte balance:
	a. fluid volume excess
	b. third-spacing of fluid
	c. hyponatremia △ 328
	4. Altered nutrition: less than body requirements △ 330
	5. Altered comfort: nausea and vomiting △ 331
	6. Risk for impaired tissue integrity △ 332
	7. Activity intolerance △ 332
	8. Self-care deficit △ 333
	9. Altered thought processes △ 333
	10. Sleep pattern disturbance △ 334
	11. Risk for trauma: falls △ 335
	12. Potential complications:
	a. renal failure
	b. cardiac dysrhythmias
	c. thromboembolism
	d. cardiogenic shock △ 336
	13. Anxiety △ 338
	14. Ineffective individual coping △ 339
	15. Ineffective management of therapeutic regimen △ 340
DISCHARGE TEACHING	16. Knowledge deficit or Altered health maintenance △ 342

See Immobility Care Plan for additional diagnoses.

1. NURSING DIAGNOSIS:

Decreased cardiac output

related to decreased filling and/or emptying of the ventricles associated with the cardiac condition causing the heart failure (e.g. ischemia of the myocardium, valve malfunction, cardiomyopathy, dysrhythmias, acute structural changes).

Desired Outcome	Nursing Actions and *Selected Purposes/Rationales*

1. The client will have improved cardiac output as evidenced by:
   a. B/P within normal range for client
   b. apical pulse between 60–100 beats/minute and regular
   c. resolution of gallop rhythm
   d. verbalization of feeling less fatigued and weak
   e. unlabored respirations at 14–20/minute
   f. improved breath sounds
   g. usual mental status
   h. absence of vertigo and syncope
   i. palpable peripheral pulses
   j. skin warm, dry, and usual color
   k. capillary refill time less than 3 seconds
   l. urine output at least 30 ml/hour
   m. decrease in edema and jugular vein distention
   n. central venous pressure (CVP) within normal range.
	1.a. Assess for signs and symptoms of heart failure and decreased cardiac output:
	   1. variations in B/P (may be increased because of compensatory vasoconstriction; may be decreased when compensatory mechanisms and pump fail)
	   2. tachycardia
	   3. pulsus alternans
	   4. presence of an S_3 heart sound
	   5. fatigue and weakness
	   6. dyspnea, orthopnea, tachypnea
	   7. dry, hacking cough or cough productive of frothy or blood-tinged sputum
	   8. abnormal breath sounds (e.g. crackles [rales], wheezes, diminished sounds)
	   9. restlessness, change in mental status
	   10. vertigo, syncope
	   11. diminished or absent peripheral pulses
	   12. cool, moist skin
	   13. pallor or cyanosis of skin
	   14. capillary refill time greater than 3 seconds
	   15. decreased urine output
	   16. edema
	   17. jugular vein distention (JVD)
	   18. increased CVP (use internal jugular vein pulsation method to estimate CVP if monitoring device not present).
	  b. Monitor ECG readings and report dysrhythmias.
	  c. Monitor chest x-ray results. Report findings of cardiomegaly, pleural effusion, or pulmonary edema.
	  d. Implement measures *to improve cardiac output:*
	   1. perform actions *to reduce cardiac workload:*
	    a. place client in a semi- to high Fowler's position
	    b. instruct client to avoid activities that create a Valsalva response (e.g. straining to have a bowel movement, holding breath while moving up in bed) *in order to prevent the marked increase in venous return and preload that occurs with exhalation*
	    c. maintain activity restrictions as ordered
	    d. implement measures *to promote emotional rest* (e.g. reduce fear and anxiety)
	    e. implement measures to improve respiratory status (see Nursing Diagnosis 2, action c) *in order to improve alveolar gas exchange and promote adequate tissue oxygenation*
	    f. discourage smoking (*smoke has a cardiostimulatory effect, causes vasoconstriction, and reduces oxygen availability*)
	    g. provide small meals rather than large ones (*large meals require an increase in blood supply to gastrointestinal tract for digestion*)
	    h. discourage excessive intake of beverages high in caffeine such as coffee, tea, and colas (*caffeine is a myocardial stimulant and can increase myocardial oxygen consumption*)
	    i. increase activity gradually as allowed and tolerated
	    j. implement measures to reduce fluid volume excess (see Nursing Diagnosis 3, action a.4.a)
	   2. administer the following medications if ordered:
	    a. positive inotropic agents (e.g. digitalis preparations, dobutamine, dopamine, amrinone) *to improve myocardial contractility*
	    b. vasodilators (e.g. sodium nitroprusside, nitroglycerin, isosorbide, hydralazine, angiotensin-converting enzyme inhibitors such as captopril or enalapril) *to reduce vascular resistance and subsequently decrease cardiac workload*
	    c. diuretics *to reduce sodium and water retention and subsequently reduce cardiac workload.*

e. If signs and symptoms of decreased cardiac output persist or worsen:
1. consult physician
2. prepare client for insertion of intra-aortic balloon pump (IABP) or surgery (e.g. artificial heart or ventricular assist device implant) if indicated.

2. NURSING DIAGNOSIS:

Impaired respiratory function:*

a. **ineffective breathing pattern** related to:
1. increased rate and decreased depth of respirations associated with fear and anxiety
2. decreased lung compliance (distensibility) associated with pleural effusion and accumulation of fluid in the pulmonary interstitium and alveoli
3. diminished lung/chest wall expansion associated with weakness, decreased mobility, and pressure on the diaphragm as a result of peritoneal fluid accumulation (if present)
4. respiratory depressant and/or stimulant effects of hypoxia, hypercapnia, and diminished cerebral blood flow;

b. **ineffective airway clearance** related to:
1. increased airway resistance associated with edema of the bronchial mucosa and pressure on the airways resulting from engorgement of the pulmonary vessels
2. stasis of secretions associated with decreased mobility and poor cough effort;

c. **impaired gas exchange** related to:
1. impaired diffusion of gases associated with accumulation of fluid in the pulmonary interstitium and alveoli
2. decreased pulmonary tissue perfusion associated with decreased cardiac output.

---

*This diagnostic label includes the following nursing diagnoses: ineffective breathing pattern, ineffective airway clearance, and impaired gas exchange.

Desired Outcome	Nursing Actions and *Selected Purposes/Rationales*
2. The client will experience adequate respiratory function as evidenced by: a. normal rate, rhythm, and depth of respirations b. decreased dyspnea c. usual or improved breath sounds d. usual mental status e. usual skin color f. blood gases within normal range.	2.a. Assess for signs and symptoms of impaired respiratory function: 1. rapid, shallow, slow, or irregular respirations 2. dyspnea, orthopnea 3. use of accessory muscles when breathing 4. adventitious breath sounds (e.g. crackles [rales], wheezes) 5. diminished or absent breath sounds 6. dry, hacking cough or cough productive of frothy or blood-tinged sputum 7. restlessness, irritability 8. confusion, somnolence 9. central cyanosis (a late sign). b. Monitor for and report the following: 1. abnormal blood gases 2. significant decrease in oximetry results 3. abnormal chest x-ray results. c. Implement measures *to improve respiratory status:* 1. perform actions to improve cardiac output (see Nursing Diagnosis 1, action d) *in order to improve pulmonary tissue perfusion and reduce fluid accumulation in the lungs* 2. perform actions to reduce fear and anxiety (see Nursing Diagnosis 13, action b) 3. instruct client to breathe slowly if hyperventilating

Desired Outcome	Nursing Actions and *Selected Purposes/Rationales*

4. place client in a semi- to high Fowler's position unless contraindicated; position overbed table so client can lean forward on it if desired
5. assist client to turn at least every 2 hours
6. instruct client to deep breathe or use incentive spirometer every 1–2 hours
7. perform actions to increase strength and activity tolerance (see Nursing Diagnosis 7, action b) *in order to increase client's willingness and ability to move, cough, deep breathe, and use incentive spirometer*
8. perform actions *to facilitate removal of pulmonary secretions:*
   a. instruct and assist client to cough or "huff" every 1–2 hours
   b. humidify inspired air as ordered *to thin tenacious secretions*
   c. assist with administration of mucolytics and diluent or hydrating agents via nebulizer if ordered
   d. perform suctioning if needed
9. maintain oxygen therapy as ordered
10. assist with positive airway pressure techniques (e.g. IPPB, continuous positive airway pressure [CPAP], biphasic positive airway pressure [BiPAP], expiratory positive airway pressure [EPAP]) if ordered
11. instruct client to avoid intake of gas-forming foods (e.g. beans, cauliflower, cabbage, onions), carbonated beverages, and large meals *in order to prevent gastric distention and an increase in pressure on the diaphragm*
12. discourage smoking (*smoke increases mucus production, impairs ciliary function, decreases oxygen availability, and can cause inflammation and damage to the bronchial walls*)
13. maintain activity restrictions; increase activity gradually as allowed and tolerated
14. administer central nervous system depressants judiciously; hold medication and consult physician if respiratory rate is less than 12/minute
15. administer the following medications if ordered:
   a. diuretics *to decrease pulmonary fluid accumulation* (in acute pulmonary edema, intravenous furosemide is often given *because of its potent diuretic effect as well as its venodilator effect*)
   b. theophylline *to dilate the bronchioles* (*it also augments myocardial contractility and increases renal blood flow, which help increase cardiac output and promote diuresis, thereby leading to decreased pulmonary vascular congestion*)
   c. morphine sulfate *to decrease pulmonary vascular congestion in acute pulmonary edema* (*the vasodilatory action of morphine results in peripheral pooling of blood and a resultant decrease in cardiac workload, which improves left ventricular emptying and allows for increased blood return from the pulmonary veins*); *morphine also reduces the apprehension associated with dyspnea*
16. assist with thoracentesis and/or paracentesis if performed *to allow increased lung expansion.*
   d. Consult physician if signs and symptoms of impaired respiratory function persist or worsen.

---

3. NURSING/COLLABORATIVE DIAGNOSIS:

Altered fluid and electrolyte balance:

a. **fluid volume excess** related to:
   1. retention of sodium and water associated with a decreased glomerular filtration rate (GFR) and activation of the renin-angiotensin-aldosterone mechanism (both are a result of the reduced renal blood flow that occurs with decreased cardiac output)

2. decreased excretion of water associated with increased ADH output (a compensatory response to decreased cardiac output);
b. **third-spacing of fluid** related to:
    1. increased intravascular pressure associated with fluid volume excess
    2. low plasma colloid osmotic pressure if serum albumin is decreased as a result of malnutrition or impaired liver function (occurs with hepatic venous congestion);
c. **hyponatremia** related to dietary restriction of sodium, hemodilution associated with fluid volume excess, and sodium loss associated with diuretic therapy.

Desired Outcomes	Nursing Actions and *Selected Purposes/Rationales*

3.a. The client will experience resolution of fluid imbalance as evidenced by:
  1. decline in weight toward client's normal
  2. B/P and pulse within normal range for client and stable with position change
  3. resolution of S₃ heart sound
  4. balanced intake and output
  5. usual mental status
  6. improved breath sounds
  7. Hct returning toward normal range
  8. decreased dyspnea and orthopnea
  9. decrease in edema and ascites
  10. resolution of neck vein distention
  11. hand vein emptying time less than 3–5 seconds
  12. CVP within normal range.

3.a.1. Assess for signs and symptoms of the following:
  a. fluid volume excess:
    1. weight gain of 2% or greater in a short period
    2. elevated B/P (B/P may not be elevated if cardiac output is poor or fluid has shifted out of the vascular space)
    3. presence of an S₃ heart sound
    4. intake greater than output
    5. change in mental status
    6. crackles (rales)
    7. low Hct (may be normal or even increased if fluid has shifted out of the vascular space)
    8. dyspnea, orthopnea
    9. edema
    10. distended neck veins
    11. delayed hand vein emptying time (longer than 3–5 seconds)
    12. elevated CVP (use internal jugular vein pulsation method to estimate CVP if monitoring device not present)
  b. third-spacing:
    1. ascites
    2. increased dyspnea and diminished or absent breath sounds
    3. evidence of vascular depletion (e.g. postural hypotension; weak, rapid pulse; decreased urine output).
2. Monitor chest x-ray results. Report findings of pulmonary vascular congestion, pleural effusion, or pulmonary edema.
3. Monitor serum albumin levels. Report below-normal levels (*low serum albumin levels result in fluid shifting out of the vascular space because albumin normally maintains plasma colloid osmotic pressure*).
4. Implement measures *to restore fluid balance:*
  a. perform actions *to reduce fluid volume excess:*
    1. restrict sodium intake as ordered
    2. maintain fluid restrictions if ordered
    3. administer the following medications if ordered:
      a. diuretics (e.g. furosemide, bumetanide) *to increase excretion of water*
      b. positive inotropic agents and arterial vasodilators *to increase cardiac output and subsequently improve renal blood flow*
  b. perform actions *to prevent further third-spacing and promote mobilization of fluid back into the vascular space:*
    1. implement measures to reduce fluid volume excess (see action a.4.a in this diagnosis)
    2. administer albumin infusions if ordered *to increase colloid osmotic pressure*
  c. assist with thoracentesis or paracentesis if performed *to remove excess fluid from the pleural space or peritoneal cavity.*
5. Consult physician if signs and symptoms of fluid imbalance persist or worsen.

Desired Outcomes	Nursing Actions and *Selected Purposes/Rationales*

3.b. The client will maintain a safe serum sodium level as evidenced by:
  1. absence of nausea, vomiting, and abdominal cramps
  2. usual mental status
  3. usual muscle strength
  4. absence of seizure activity
  5. serum sodium within normal range.
	3.b.1. Assess for and report signs and symptoms of hyponatremia (e.g. nausea, vomiting, abdominal cramps, lethargy, confusion, weakness, seizures, low serum sodium level).
	  2. Implement measures *to treat hyponatremia:*
	    a. maintain fluid restrictions if ordered
	    b. consult physician about temporary cessation of diuretic therapy and dietary sodium restriction if sodium level is significantly reduced.
	  3. Consult physician if signs and symptoms of hyponatremia persist or worsen.

---

4. NURSING DIAGNOSIS:

Altered nutrition: less than body requirements

related to:
a. decreased oral intake associated with:
  1. anorexia and nausea (result from venous congestion in the gastrointestinal tract and can occur if digitalis levels exceed a therapeutic level)
  2. weakness, fatigue, dyspnea, and dislike of prescribed diet;
b. elevated metabolic rate associated with the increased oxygen needs of the heart and the increased work of breathing;
c. impaired absorption of nutrients associated with poor tissue perfusion.

Desired Outcome	Nursing Actions and *Selected Purposes/Rationales*

4. The client will maintain an adequate nutritional status as evidenced by:
a. dry weight within normal range for client's age, height, and body frame (dry weight is achieved after fluid volume excess has been resolved)
b. normal BUN and serum albumin, Hct, Hb, transferrin, and lymphocyte levels
c. improved strength and activity tolerance
d. healthy oral mucous membrane.
	4.a. Assess for and report signs and symptoms of malnutrition:
	  1. dry weight below normal for client's age, height, and body frame
	  2. abnormal BUN and low serum albumin, Hct, Hb, transferrin, and lymphocyte levels
	  3. weakness and fatigue
	  4. sore, inflamed oral mucous membrane
	  5. pale conjunctiva.
	b. Monitor percentage of meals and snacks client consumes. Report a pattern of inadequate intake.
	c. Implement measures *to maintain an adequate nutritional status:*
	  1. perform actions *to improve oral intake:*
	    a. implement measures to prevent nausea and vomiting (see Nursing Diagnosis 5, action b)
	    b. increase activity as allowed and tolerated (*activity usually promotes a sense of well-being and improves appetite*)
	    c. obtain a dietary consult if necessary to assist client in selecting foods/fluids that meet nutritional needs, are appealing, and adhere to personal and cultural preferences as well as the prescribed dietary modifications
	    d. encourage a rest period before meals *to minimize fatigue*
	    e. maintain a clean environment and a relaxed, pleasant atmosphere
	    f. provide oral hygiene before meals
	    g. serve frequent, small meals rather than large ones if client is weak, fatigues easily, and/or has a poor appetite
	    h. place client in a high Fowler's position for meals and provide supplemental oxygen therapy during meals if indicated *to help relieve dyspnea*

    i. instruct client to use herbs, spices, and salt substitutes if approved by physician or dietitian *in order to make low-sodium diet more palatable*

    j. allow adequate time for meals; reheat foods/fluids if necessary

    k. limit fluid intake with meals (unless the fluid has high nutritional value) *to reduce early satiety and subsequent decreased food intake*

  2. perform actions to improve cardiac output (see Nursing Diagnosis 1, action d) *in order to increase the absorption of nutrients and reduce venous congestion in the gastrointestinal tract*

  3. ensure that meals are well balanced and high in essential nutrients; offer dietary supplements if indicated

  4. administer vitamins and minerals if ordered.

  d. Perform a calorie count if ordered. Report information to dietitian and physician.

  e. Consult physician regarding an alternative method of providing nutrition (e.g. parenteral nutrition, tube feedings) if client does not consume enough food or fluids to meet nutritional needs.

---

5. NURSING DIAGNOSIS:

Altered comfort: nausea and vomiting

related to stimulation of the vomiting center associated with:
a. stimulation of visceral afferent pathways resulting from vascular congestion in the heart and gastrointestinal tract;
b. stimulation of the cerebral cortex resulting from stress;
c. stimulation of the chemoreceptor trigger zone by certain medications (e.g. digitalis preparations).

Desired Outcome	Nursing Actions and *Selected Purposes/Rationales*

5. The client will experience relief of nausea and vomiting as evidenced by:
a. verbalization of relief of nausea
b. absence of vomiting.
	5.a. Assess client for nausea and vomiting.
	b. Implement measures *to prevent nausea and vomiting*:
	  1. perform actions to improve cardiac output (see Nursing Diagnosis 1, action d) *in order to reduce vascular congestion in the heart and gastrointestinal tract*
	  2. monitor serum digoxin levels and report elevated values (be alert to a low serum potassium level *because it may precipitate digitalis toxicity*)
	  3. perform actions to reduce fear and anxiety (see Nursing Diagnosis 13, action b)
	  4. eliminate noxious sights and odors from the environment (*noxious stimuli can cause stimulation of the vomiting center*)
	  5. encourage client to take deep, slow breaths when nauseated
	  6. encourage client to change positions slowly (*rapid movement can result in chemoreceptor trigger zone stimulation and subsequent excitation of the vomiting center*)
	  7. provide oral hygiene after each emesis
	  8. provide small, frequent meals; instruct client to ingest foods and fluids slowly
	  9. avoid serving foods with an overpowering aroma; remove lids from hot foods before entering room
	  10. instruct client to avoid foods high in fat (*fat delays gastric emptying*)
	  11. instruct client to avoid foods/fluids that irritate the gastric mucosa (e.g. spicy foods; caffeine-containing beverages such as coffee, tea, and colas)
	  12. instruct client to eat dry foods (e.g. toast, crackers) and avoid drinking liquids with meals if nauseated

Desired Outcome	Nursing Actions and *Selected Purposes/Rationales*
	13. instruct client to rest after eating with head of bed elevated 14. administer antiemetics if ordered. c. Consult physician if above measures fail to control nausea and vomiting.

---

6. NURSING DIAGNOSIS: **Risk for impaired tissue integrity**

related to:
a. damage to the skin and/or subcutaneous tissue associated with prolonged pressure on the tissues, friction, and/or shearing if mobility is decreased;
b. increased fragility of the skin associated with edema, poor tissue perfusion, and inadequate nutritional status.

Desired Outcome	Nursing Actions and *Selected Purposes/Rationales*

6. The client will maintain tissue integrity as evidenced by:
 a. absence of redness and irritation
 b. no skin breakdown.
	6.a. Inspect the skin, especially bony prominences and dependent and edematous areas, for pallor, redness, and breakdown.
	  b. Refer to Care Plan on Immobility, Nursing Diagnosis 4, actions b and c (pp. 129–130), for measures to prevent and treat tissue breakdown associated with decreased mobility.
	  c. Implement additional measures *to prevent tissue breakdown:*
	  1. perform actions *to improve tissue perfusion and reduce edema:*
	  a. implement measures to increase cardiac output (see Nursing Diagnosis 1, action d)
	  b. implement measures to restore fluid balance (see Nursing Diagnosis 3, action a.4)
	  2. perform actions to maintain an adequate nutritional status (see Nursing Diagnosis 4, action c).

---

7. NURSING DIAGNOSIS: **Activity intolerance**

related to:
a. tissue hypoxia associated with impaired alveolar gas exchange and decreased cardiac output;
b. inadequate nutritional status;
c. difficulty resting and sleeping associated with dyspnea, frequent assessments and treatments, fear, and anxiety.

Desired Outcome	Nursing Actions and *Selected Purposes/Rationales*

7. The client will demonstrate an increased tolerance for activity as evidenced by:
 a. verbalization of feeling less fatigued and weak
 b. ability to perform activities of daily living without exertional dyspnea, chest pain, diaphoresis, dizziness, and a significant change in vital signs.
	7.a. Assess for signs and symptoms of activity intolerance:
	  1. statements of fatigue or weakness
	  2. exertional dyspnea, chest pain, diaphoresis, or dizziness
	  3. abnormal heart rate response to activity (e.g. increase in rate of 20 beats/minute above resting rate, rate not returning to preactivity level within 3 minutes after stopping activity, change from regular to irregular rate)
	  4. decreased systolic B/P or a significant increase (10–15 mm Hg) in diastolic pressure with activity.
	  b. Implement measures *to improve activity tolerance:*
	  1. perform actions *to promote rest and/or conserve energy:*
	  a. maintain activity restrictions as ordered
	  b. minimize environmental activity and noise

    c. organize nursing care to allow for periods of uninterrupted rest

    d. limit the number of visitors and their length of stay

    e. assist client with self-care activities as needed

    f. keep supplies and personal articles within easy reach

    g. instruct client in energy-saving techniques (e.g. using shower chair when showering, sitting to brush teeth or comb hair)

    h. implement measures to reduce fear and anxiety (see Nursing Diagnosis 13, action b)

    i. implement measures to promote sleep (see Nursing Diagnosis 10)

  2. perform actions to improve respiratory status (see Nursing Diagnosis 2, action c) *in order to decrease dyspnea and improve tissue oxygenation*

  3. perform actions to increase cardiac output (see Nursing Diagnosis 1, action d)

  4. perform actions to maintain an adequate nutritional status (see Nursing Diagnosis 4, action c)

  5. increase client's activity gradually as allowed and tolerated; explain that activity is increased gradually *to prevent a sudden increase in cardiac workload.*

c. Instruct client to:

  1. report a decreased tolerance for activity

  2. stop any activity that causes chest pain, a marked increase in shortness of breath, dizziness, or extreme fatigue or weakness.

d. Consult physician if signs and symptoms of activity intolerance persist or worsen.

---

8. NURSING DIAGNOSIS: **Self-care deficit**

related to weakness, fatigue, dyspnea, altered thought processes, and activity restrictions imposed by the treatment plan.

Desired Outcome	Nursing Actions and *Selected Purposes/Rationales*

8. The client will perform self-care activities within physical and cognitive limitations and activity restrictions imposed by the treatment plan.	8.a. Refer to Care Plan on Immobility, Nursing Diagnosis 7 (p. 132) for measures related to planning for and meeting client's self-care needs.
	b. Implement additional measures *to facilitate client's ability to perform self-care activities:*
	  1. perform actions to increase strength and activity tolerance (see Nursing Diagnosis 7, action b)
	  2. perform actions to improve respiratory status and relieve dyspnea (see Nursing Diagnosis 2, action c)
	  3. perform actions to improve cardiac output (see Nursing Diagnosis 1, action d) *in order to improve activity tolerance and increase cerebral blood flow and subsequently improve thought processes.*

---

9. NURSING DIAGNOSIS: **Altered thought processes***

related to:

a. cerebral hypoxia associated with impaired alveolar gas exchange and inadequate cerebral tissue perfusion (a result of decreased cardiac output);

b. fluid and electrolyte imbalances.

---

*The diagnostic label of acute or chronic confusion might be more appropriate depending on the client's symptoms.

Desired Outcome	Nursing Actions and *Selected Purposes/Rationales*

9. The client will regain usual thought processes as evidenced by:
a. improved ability to grasp ideas
b. longer attention span
c. improved memory
d. oriented to person, place, and time.
	9.a. Assess client for altered thought processes (e.g. impaired ability to grasp ideas, shortened attention span, impaired memory, confusion).
	b. Ascertain from significant others client's usual level of cognitive functioning.
	c. Implement measures *to improve thought processes:*
	  1. perform actions *to increase cerebral tissue oxygenation:*
	    a. implement measures to improve cardiac output (see Nursing Diagnosis 1, action d)
	    b. implement measures to improve respiratory status (see Nursing Diagnosis 2, action c)
	  2. perform actions to restore fluid and electrolyte balance (see Nursing Diagnosis 3, actions a.4 and b.2).
	d. If client shows evidence of altered thought processes:
	  1. reorient client to person, place, and time as necessary
	  2. address client by name
	  3. place familiar objects, clock, and calendar within client's view
	  4. approach client in a slow, calm manner; allow adequate time for communication
	  5. repeat instructions as necessary using clear, simple language and short sentences
	  6. maintain a consistent and fairly structured routine and write out a schedule of activities for client to refer to if desired
	  7. have client perform only one activity at a time and allow adequate time for performance of activities
	  8. maintain realistic expectations of client's ability to learn, comprehend, and remember information provided; provide client with a written copy of instructions
	  9. encourage significant others to be supportive of client; instruct them in methods of dealing with client's altered thought processes
	  10. discuss physiological basis for altered thought processes with client and significant others; inform them that cognitive functioning is expected to improve as a result of treatment
	  11. consult physician if altered thought processes persist or worsen.

---

10. NURSING DIAGNOSIS: **Sleep pattern disturbance**

related to unfamiliar environment, frequent assessments and treatments, decreased physical activity, fear, anxiety, and inability to assume usual sleep position associated with orthopnea.

Desired Outcome	Nursing Actions and *Selected Purposes/Rationales*

10. The client will attain optimal amounts of sleep (see Care Plan on Immobility, Nursing Diagnosis 10 [p. 134], for outcome criteria).	10.a. Refer to Care Plan on Immobility, Nursing Diagnosis 10 (pp. 134–135), for measures related to assessment and promotion of sleep.
	b. Implement additional measures *to promote sleep:*
	  1. perform actions to improve respiratory status (see Nursing Diagnosis 2, action c) *in order to relieve dyspnea*
	  2. if client has orthopnea, assist him/her to assume a position *that facilitates breathing* (e.g. head of bed elevated with arms supported on pillows, resting forward on overbed table with good pillow support, sitting in chair)
	  3. maintain oxygen therapy during sleep if indicated

4. perform actions to reduce fear and anxiety (see Nursing Diagnosis 13, action b)
5. increase activity as allowed and tolerated during the day and early evening.

---

11. NURSING DIAGNOSIS: **Risk for trauma: falls**

related to:
a. weakness;
b. dizziness and syncope associated with inadequate cerebral blood flow resulting from decreased cardiac output and the hypotensive effect of some medications (e.g. vasodilators, diuretics);
c. getting up without assistance as a result of restlessness, agitation, forgetfulness, and confusion.

Desired Outcome	Nursing Actions and *Selected Purposes/Rationales*

11. The client will not experience falls.

11.a. Implement measures *to prevent falls:*
1. keep bed in low position with side rails up when client is in bed
2. keep needed items within easy reach
3. encourage client to request assistance whenever needed; have call signal within easy reach
4. use lap belt when client is in chair if indicated
5. instruct client to wear well-fitting slippers/shoes with nonslip soles and low heels when ambulating
6. keep floor free of clutter and wipe up spills promptly
7. accompany client during ambulation utilizing a transfer safety belt if he/she is weak or dizzy
8. provide ambulatory aids (e.g. walker, cane) if client is weak or unsteady on feet
9. instruct client to ambulate in well-lit areas and to utilize handrails if needed
10. do not rush client; allow adequate time for ambulation to the bathroom and in hallway
11. instruct and assist client to get out of bed slowly *in order to reduce dizziness associated with postural hypotension*
12. perform actions to improve cardiac output (see Nursing Diagnosis 1, action d) *in order to improve cerebral blood flow and reduce dizziness and syncope*
13. perform actions to improve thought processes (see Nursing Diagnosis 9, action c)
14. perform actions to increase strength and activity tolerance (see Nursing Diagnosis 7, action b)
15. make sure that shower has a nonslip bottom surface and that shower chair, secure bath mat, call signal, grab bars, and adequate lighting are present
16. administer central nervous system depressants judiciously
17. if client is confused or irrational:
    a. reorient frequently to surroundings and necessity of adhering to safety precautions
    b. provide appropriate level of supervision
    c. consult physician about the temporary use of a bed alarm or jacket or wrist restraints if necessary
    d. administer prescribed antianxiety and antipsychotic medications if indicated.

Desired Outcome	Nursing Actions and *Selected Purposes/Rationales*
	b. Include client and significant others in planning and implementing measures to prevent falls. c. If client falls, initiate first aid measures if appropriate and notify physician.

■───

12. COLLABORATIVE DIAGNOSES:

Potential complications of heart failure:

a. **renal failure** related to a prolonged or severe decrease in renal blood flow associated with low cardiac output, volume depletion (a result of third-spacing and/or excessive diuretic use), and vasodilator-induced hypotension;

b. **cardiac dysrhythmias** related to impaired nodal function and/or altered myocardial conductivity associated with hypoxia, sympathetic nervous system stimulation (a compensatory response to low cardiac output), structural changes in the myocardium (e.g. dilation, hypertrophy), and electrolyte imbalances (particularly the magnesium and potassium depletion that can result from diuretic therapy);

c. **thromboembolism** related to:
   1. venous stasis in the periphery associated with decreased cardiac output and decreased mobility
   2. stasis of blood in the heart associated with decreased ventricular emptying (risk increases if dysrhythmias are present);

d. **cardiogenic shock** related to inability of heart, intrinsic compensatory mechanisms, and treatments to maintain adequate tissue perfusion to vital organs.

Desired Outcomes	Nursing Actions and *Selected Purposes/Rationales*

12.a. The client will maintain adequate renal function as evidenced by:
1. urine output at least 30 ml/hour
2. BUN, serum creatinine, and creatinine clearance within normal range.
	12.a.1. Assess for and report signs and symptoms of impaired renal function (e.g. urine output less than 30 ml/hour, urine specific gravity fixed at or less than 1.010, elevated BUN and serum creatinine levels).
	2. Collect a 24-hour urine specimen if ordered. Report decreased creatinine clearance.
	3. Implement measures *to maintain adequate renal blood flow:*
	  a. perform actions to improve cardiac output (see Nursing Diagnosis 1, action d)
	  b. perform actions to reduce third-spacing (see Nursing Diagnosis 3, action a.4.b.) *in order to prevent hypovolemia*
	  c. ensure a minimum fluid intake of 1000 ml/day unless ordered otherwise
	  d. consult physician before giving vasodilators and diuretics if client is hypotensive.
	4. If signs and symptoms of impaired renal function occur:
	  a. continue with above actions
	  b. administer diuretics if ordered *to increase urine output*
	  c. consult physician about possible need to reduce the digitalis dosage (*digitalis is excreted by the kidney and will quickly reach toxic levels when renal function is impaired*)
	  d. consult physician about lowering the dose of or discontinuing angiotensin-converting enzyme inhibitors and furosemide if BUN and serum creatinine continue to rise significantly (ACE inhibitors and furosemide should be used cautiously in persons with impaired renal function *because they can have an adverse effect on renal function*)

e. assess for and report signs of acute renal failure (e.g. oliguria or anuria; further weight gain; increasing edema; increased B/P; lethargy and confusion; increasing BUN and serum creatinine, phosphorus, and potassium levels)

f. prepare client for dialysis if indicated

g. refer to Care Plan on Renal Failure for additional care measures.

12.b. The client will maintain normal sinus rhythm as evidenced by:
1. regular apical pulse at 60–100 beats/minute
2. equal apical and radial pulse rates
3. absence of syncope and palpitations
4. ECG reading showing normal sinus rhythm.

12.b.1. Assess for and report signs and symptoms of cardiac dysrhythmias (e.g. irregular apical pulse; pulse rate below 60 or above 100 beats/minute; apical-radial pulse deficit; syncope; palpitations; abnormal rate, rhythm, or configurations on ECG).

2. Implement measures *to prevent cardiac dysrhythmias:*
   a. perform actions to improve cardiac output (see Nursing Diagnosis 1, action d) *in order to promote adequate myocardial tissue perfusion and oxygenation*
   b. perform actions to improve respiratory status (see Nursing Diagnosis 2, action c) *in order to improve tissue oxygenation*
   c. consult physician regarding an order for a potassium or magnesium replacement if serum levels of either are below normal.

3. If cardiac dysrhythmias occur:
   a. initiate cardiac monitoring if not already being done
   b. administer antidysrhythmics (e.g. digoxin, quinidine, procainamide, lidocaine, tocainide, amiodarone) if ordered
   c. restrict client's activity based on his/her tolerance and severity of the dysrhythmia
   d. maintain oxygen therapy as ordered
   e. assess cardiovascular status frequently and report signs and symptoms of a further decline in cardiac output and tissue perfusion
   f. prepare client for electrophysiological study (EPS), insertion of a pacemaker, or implantation of an automatic implantable cardioverter defibrillator (AICD) if planned
   g. have emergency cart readily available for cardioversion, defibrillation, or cardiopulmonary resuscitation.

12.c. The client will not develop a thromboembolism as evidenced by:
1. absence of pain, tenderness, swelling, and numbness in extremities
2. usual temperature and color of extremities
3. palpable and equal peripheral pulses
4. usual mental status
5. usual sensory and motor function
6. absence of sudden chest pain and increased dyspnea.

12.c.1. Assess for and report signs and symptoms of:
   a. deep vein thrombus (e.g. pain, tenderness, swelling, unusual warmth, and/or positive Homans' sign in extremity)
   b. arterial embolus (e.g. diminished or absent peripheral pulses; pallor, coolness, numbness, and/or pain in extremity)
   c. cerebral ischemia (e.g. decreased level of consciousness, alteration in usual sensory and motor function)
   d. pulmonary embolism (e.g. sudden chest pain, increased dyspnea, increased restlessness and apprehension).

2. Implement measures to prevent and treat a deep vein thrombus and pulmonary embolism (see Care Plan on Immobility, Collaborative Diagnosis 12, actions a.1.b and c and a.2.b and c [pp. 137–138]).

3. Implement additional measures *to prevent the development of thromboemboli:*
   a. perform actions to improve cardiac output (see Nursing Diagnosis 1, action d)
   b. perform actions to treat cardiac dysrhythmias if present (see action b.3 in this diagnosis)
   c. administer anticoagulants (e.g. warfarin, low- or adjusted-dose heparin, low-molecular-weight heparin) or antiplatelet agents (e.g. low-dose aspirin) if ordered.

4. If signs and symptoms of an arterial embolus occur:
   a. maintain client on strict bed rest with affected extremity in a level or slightly dependent position *to improve arterial blood flow*

Desired Outcomes	Nursing Actions and *Selected Purposes/Rationales*

b. prepare client for the following if planned:
    1. diagnostic studies (e.g. Doppler or duplex ultrasound, arteriography)
    2. injection of a thrombolytic agent (e.g. streptokinase)
    3. embolectomy
c. administer anticoagulants (e.g. continuous intravenous heparin, warfarin) as ordered
d. provide emotional support to client and significant others.
5. If signs and symptoms of cerebral ischemia occur:
    a. maintain client on bed rest
    b. administer anticoagulants (e.g. continuous intravenous heparin, warfarin) as ordered
    c. provide emotional support to client and significant others
    d. refer to Care Plan on Cerebrovascular Accident for additional care measures if signs and symptoms persist.

12.d. The client will not develop cardiogenic shock as evidenced by:
1. stable or improved mental status
2. systolic B/P greater than 80 mm Hg
3. palpable peripheral pulses
4. stable or improved skin temperature and color
5. urine output at least 30 ml/hour
6. pulmonary capillary wedge pressure (PCWP) between 15–18 mm Hg.

12.d.1. Assess for and immediately report signs and symptoms of cardiogenic shock:
a. increased restlessness, lethargy, or confusion
b. systolic B/P below 80 mm Hg
c. rapid, weak pulse
d. diminished or absent peripheral pulses
e. increased coolness and duskiness or cyanosis of skin
f. urine output less than 30 ml/hour
g. PCWP greater than 18 mm Hg.
2. Implement measures *to prevent cardiogenic shock:*
a. perform actions to improve cardiac output (see Nursing Diagnosis 1, action d)
b. perform actions to treat cardiac dysrhythmias if present (see action b.3 in this diagnosis).
3. If signs and symptoms of cardiogenic shock occur:
a. continue with above actions
b. maintain oxygen therapy as ordered
c. prepare client for diagnostic studies (e.g. two-dimensional echocardiogram, cardiac catheterization) if planned
d. administer the following medications if ordered:
    1. sympathomimetics (e.g. dopamine, dobutamine, norepinephrine) *to increase cardiac output and maintain arterial pressure*
    2. phosphodiesterase inhibitors (e.g. amrinone) *to increase myocardial contractility and decrease systemic vascular resistance*
    3. vasodilators (e.g. sodium nitroprusside, nitroglycerin) *to decrease cardiac workload* (the use of vasodilators will be determined by the client's blood pressure and usually not be given if the systolic B/P is less than 100 mm Hg)
e. assist with intubation and insertion of hemodynamic monitoring device (e.g. Swan-Ganz catheter) and intra-aortic balloon pump (IABP) if indicated
f. prepare client for surgery (e.g. ventricular assist device implant, heart transplant) if planned
g. provide emotional support to client and significant others.

---

13. NURSING DIAGNOSIS: **Anxiety**

related to unfamiliar environment; difficulty breathing; and lack of understanding of diagnostic tests, the diagnosis, treatments, and prognosis.

Desired Outcome	Nursing Actions and *Selected Purposes/Rationales*

13. The client will experience a reduction in anxiety as evidenced by:
    a. verbalization of feeling less anxious
    b. usual sleep pattern
    c. relaxed facial expression and body movements
    d. stable vital signs
    e. usual perceptual ability and interactions with others.

13.a. Assess client for signs and symptoms of anxiety (e.g. verbalization of feeling anxious, insomnia, tenseness, shakiness, restlessness, increased dyspnea, diaphoresis, tachycardia, elevated blood pressure, facial pallor, self-focused behaviors). Validate perceptions carefully, remembering that some behavior may result from tissue hypoxia or fluid imbalance.

b. Implement measures *to reduce fear and anxiety:*
   1. maintain a calm, supportive, confident manner when interacting with client
   2. if client is in acute respiratory distress:
      a. do not leave him/her alone during this period
      b. perform actions to improve respiratory status (see Nursing Diagnosis 2, action c)
      c. perform actions *to reduce feeling of suffocation:*
         1. open curtains and doors
         2. limit the number of visitors in room at any one time
         3. remove unnecessary equipment from room
         4. administer oxygen via nasal cannula rather than mask if possible
   3. encourage significant others to project a caring, concerned attitude without obvious anxiousness
   4. once the period of acute respiratory distress has subsided:
      a. orient client to hospital environment, equipment, and routines
      b. introduce client to staff who will be participating in care; if possible, maintain consistency in staff assigned to his/her care *to provide feelings of stability and comfort with the environment*
      c. assure client that staff members are nearby; respond to call signal as soon as possible
      d. provide a calm, restful environment
      e. keep cardiac monitor out of client's view and the sound turned as low as possible
      f. encourage verbalization of fear and anxiety; provide feedback
      g. explain all diagnostic tests
      h. reinforce physician's explanations and clarify misconceptions the client has about heart failure, the treatment plan, and prognosis
      i. instruct client in relaxation techniques and encourage participation in diversional activities
      j. assist client to identify specific stressors and ways to cope with them (see Nursing Diagnosis 14, action c)
      k. provide information based on current needs of client at a level he/she can understand; encourage questions and clarification of information provided
      l. include significant others in orientation and teaching sessions and encourage their continued support of the client
      m. administer prescribed antianxiety agents if indicated.

c. Consult physician if above actions fail to control fear and anxiety.

---

14. NURSING DIAGNOSIS: **Ineffective individual coping**

related to fear, anxiety, possible need to alter life style, and knowledge that condition is chronic and will require lifelong medical supervision and medication therapy.

Desired Outcome	Nursing Actions and *Selected Purposes/Rationales*

14. The client will demonstrate effective coping skills as evidenced by:
a. verbalization of ability to cope
b. utilization of appropriate problem-solving techniques
c. willingness to participate in treatment plan and meet basic needs
d. absence of destructive behavior toward self and others
e. appropriate use of defense mechanisms
f. utilization of available support systems.
	14.a. Assess for and report signs and symptoms of ineffective individual coping (e.g. verbalization of inability to cope; inability to ask for help, problem solve, or meet basic needs; insomnia; withdrawal; reluctance to participate in treatment plan; destructive behavior toward self or others; inappropriate use of defense mechanisms; inability to meet role expectations).
	b. Assess client's perception of current situation.
	c. Implement measures *to promote effective coping:*
	  1. allow time for client to begin to adjust to diagnosis and planned treatment and anticipated changes in life style and roles
	  2. assist client to recognize and manage inappropriate denial if it is present
	  3. perform actions to reduce fear and anxiety (see Nursing Diagnosis 13, action b)
	  4. encourage verbalization about current situation and ways comparable situations have been handled in the past
	  5. assist client to identify personal strengths and resources that can be utilized to facilitate coping with the current situation
	  6. create an atmosphere of trust and support
	  7. include client in planning of care, encourage maximum participation in treatment plan, and allow choices when possible *to enable him/her to maintain a sense of control*
	  8. instruct client in effective problem-solving techniques (e.g. accurate identification of stressors, determination of various options to solve problem)
	  9. assist client to maintain usual daily routines whenever possible
	  10. when appropriate, assist client to meet spiritual needs (e.g. arrange for a visit from clergy)
	  11. assist client to identify priorities and attainable goals as he/she starts to plan for necessary life-style and role changes
	  12. assist client and significant others to identify ways that personal and family goals can be adjusted rather than abandoned
	  13. administer antianxiety and/or antidepressant agents if ordered
	  14. assist client to identify and utilize available support systems; provide information about available community resources that can assist client and significant others in coping with the effects of heart failure
	  15. encourage client to share with significant others the kind of support that would be most beneficial (e.g. listening, inspiring hope, providing reassurance and accurate information)
	  16. support behaviors indicative of effective coping (e.g. participation in treatment plan and self-care activities, communication of the ability to cope, utilization of effective problem-solving strategies).
	d. Consult physician about psychological and vocational counseling if appropriate. Initiate a referral if necessary.

■———————————————————————————————————

15. NURSING DIAGNOSIS:

Ineffective management of therapeutic regimen

related to:
a. lack of understanding of the implications of not following the prescribed treatment plan;
b. difficulty modifying personal habits (e.g. smoking, alcohol intake, diet);
c. insufficient financial resources;
d. unpleasant side effects experienced with some medications used to manage heart failure (e.g. vasodilators, diuretics).

Desired Outcome	Nursing Actions and *Selected Purposes/Rationales*

15. The client will demonstrate the probability of effective management of the therapeutic regimen as evidenced by:
   a. willingness to learn about and participate in treatments and care
   b. statements reflecting ways to modify personal habits and integrate treatments into life style
   c. statements reflecting an understanding of the implications of not following the prescribed treatment plan.

15.a. Assess for indications that the client may be unable to effectively manage the therapeutic regimen:
   1. statements reflecting inability to manage care at home
   2. failure to adhere to treatment plan while in hospital (e.g. not adhering to dietary modifications and fluid restrictions, refusing medications)
   3. statements reflecting a lack of understanding of factors that may cause further progression of heart failure
   4. statements reflecting an unwillingness or inability to modify personal habits and integrate necessary treatments into life style
   5. statements reflecting the view that heart failure resolves completely or is hopeless and that efforts to comply with the treatment plan are useless
   6. statements reflecting that medications are too expensive or that their side effects are too unpleasant.

   b. Implement measures *to promote effective management of the therapeutic regimen:*
   1. explain heart failure in terms the client can understand; stress the fact that heart failure is a chronic disease and that adherence to the treatment program is necessary in order to delay and/or prevent complications
   2. encourage questions and clarify misconceptions the client has regarding heart failure and its effects
   3. encourage client to participate in treatment plan
   4. provide instructions on measuring intake and output, weighing self, counting pulse, and calculating dietary sodium content; allow time for return demonstration; determine areas of difficulty and misunderstanding and reinforce teaching as necessary
   5. provide client with written instructions about medications, signs and symptoms to report, measuring intake and output, weighing self, counting pulse, and prescribed diet
   6. assist client to identify ways treatments can be incorporated into life style; focus on modifications of life style rather than complete change
   7. encourage the client to discuss concerns regarding the cost of hospitalization, medications, and lifelong follow-up care; obtain a social service consult to assist the client with financial planning and to obtain financial aid if indicated
   8. perform actions to promote effective coping (see Nursing Diagnosis 14, action c)
   9. initiate and reinforce discharge teaching outlined in Nursing Diagnosis 16 *in order to promote a sense of control and self-reliance*
   10. provide information about and encourage utilization of community resources that can assist client to make necessary life-style changes (e.g. cardiovascular fitness, weight loss, and smoking cessation programs)
   11. reinforce behaviors suggesting future compliance with the therapeutic regimen (e.g. statements reflecting ways to modify personal habits, active interest and participation in treatment plan)
   12. include significant others in explanations and teaching sessions and encourage their support; reinforce need for client to assume responsibility for managing as much of care as possible.

   c. Consult physician regarding referrals to community health agencies if continued instruction, support, or supervision is needed.

Discharge Teaching

■━━━━━━━━━━━━━━━━━━━━━━━━━━━━━━━━━━━━

16. NURSING DIAGNOSIS: **Knowledge deficit or Altered health maintenance***

*The nurse should select the diagnostic label that is most appropriate for the client's discharge teaching needs.

Desired Outcomes	Nursing Actions and *Selected Purposes/Rationales*
16.a. The client will identify modifiable cardiovascular risk factors and ways to alter these factors.	16.a.1. Inform client that the following modifiable factors have been shown to contribute to cardiovascular disease: a. obesity b. elevated serum lipids c. lack of regular aerobic exercise d. cigarette smoking e. hypertension f. diabetes mellitus g. stressful life style. 2. Encourage client to discuss alcohol intake with health care provider. (The health care provider may advise the client to limit alcohol consumption because there is evidence that a daily alcohol intake exceeding 1 oz of ethanol [i.e. 2 oz of 100-proof whiskey, 8 oz of wine, 24 oz of beer] contributes to the development of hypertension and some forms of heart disease.) 3. Assist client to identify ways he/she can make appropriate changes in life style to modify the above factors. Provide information about weight reduction plans; stress management classes; and cardiovascular fitness, smoking cessation, and alcohol rehabilitation programs if appropriate. Initiate a referral if indicated.
16.b. The client will verbalize an understanding of the rationale for and components of a diet low in sodium.	16.b.1. Explain the rationale for a diet low in sodium. 2. Provide the following information about decreasing sodium intake: a. be aware that the terms salt and sodium are often used interchangeably but are not synonymous; there is 40% sodium in table salt b. read labels on foods/fluids and calculate sodium content of items; avoid those products that tend to have a high sodium content (e.g. canned soups and vegetables, tomato juice, commercial baked goods, commercially prepared frozen or canned entrees and sauces) c. do not add salt when cooking foods or to prepared foods; use low-sodium herbs and spices if desired d. avoid cured and smoked foods e. avoid salty snack foods (e.g. crackers, nuts, pretzels, potato chips) f. avoid commercially prepared fast foods g. avoid routine use of over-the-counter medications with a high sodium content (e.g. Alka-Seltzer, some antacids such as Gaviscon). 3. Obtain a dietary consult to assist client in planning meals that will meet prescribed dietary modifications.
16.c. The client will demonstrate accuracy in counting pulse.	16.c.1. Teach the client how to count his/her pulse, being alert to the regularity of the rhythm. 2. Allow time for return demonstration and accuracy check.
16.d. The client will verbalize an understanding of medications ordered including rationale, food and drug interactions, side effects, schedule for	16.d.1. Explain the rationale for, side effects of, and importance of taking the medications prescribed. Inform client of pertinent food and drug interactions. 2. If client is discharged on a digitalis preparation, instruct to: a. take pulse before taking digitalis (should be a resting pulse rate taken at least 5 minutes after any activity); consult physician before

taking, and importance of taking as prescribed.

     taking medication if pulse rate is more irregular than usual or below 60 or above 110 beats/minute
    b. promptly report a loss of usual appetite, nausea, vomiting, diarrhea, or visual disturbances.
  3. If client is discharged on a diuretic, instruct to:
    a. take once-daily dose in the morning or, if diuretic is to be taken twice each day, take the larger dose in the morning and the second dose no later than 3:00 p.m. (scheduling doses in this manner minimizes nighttime urination)
    b. weigh self daily and keep a record of daily weights
    c. change from a lying to standing position slowly if experiencing dizziness or lightheadedness with position change
    d. increase intake of foods/fluids high in potassium (e.g. orange juice, bananas, potatoes, raisins, apricots, cantaloupe) if taking a potassium-depleting diuretic
    e. notify physician if unable to tolerate food or fluids (dehydration can develop rapidly if intake is poor and client continues to take diuretic)
    f. avoid salt substitutes with a high potassium content if discharged on a potassium-sparing diuretic (e.g. triamterene, spironolactone)
    g. report the following signs and symptoms:
      1. weight loss of more than 5 pounds a week
      2. excessive thirst
      3. severe dizziness or episodes of fainting
      4. muscle weakness or cramping, nausea, vomiting, or increased irregularity of pulse.
  4. If client is discharged on a vasodilator, instruct to:
    a. change from a lying to standing position slowly if experiencing dizziness or lightheadedness with position change
    b. avoid strenuous exercise (especially in hot weather), hot baths and showers, steam room, and sauna
    c. limit alcohol intake
    d. report continued dizziness, lightheadedness, or fainting.
  5. Instruct client to take medications on a regular basis and avoid skipping doses, altering prescribed dose, making up for missed doses, and discontinuing medication without permission of health care provider.
  6. Instruct client to consult physician before taking other prescription and nonprescription medications.
  7. Instruct client to inform all health care providers of medications being taken.

16.e. The client will state signs and symptoms to report to the health care provider.

16.e. Instruct client to report:
  1. weight gain of more than 2 pounds in 2 days
  2. increased swelling of ankles, feet, or abdomen
  3. persistent cough
  4. increasing shortness of breath
  5. chest pain
  6. increased weakness and fatigue
  7. frequent nighttime urination
  8. signs and symptoms of digitalis toxicity (see action d.2.b in this diagnosis)
  9. side effects of diuretic therapy (see action d.3.g in this diagnosis).

16.f. The client will identify community resources that can assist with home management and adjustment to changes resulting from heart failure.

16.f.1. Provide information regarding community resources that can assist with home management and adjustment to changes resulting from heart failure (e.g. Meals on Wheels, home health agencies, transportation services, American Heart Association, counseling services).
  2. Initiate a referral if indicated.

16.g. The client will verbalize an understanding of and a plan for adhering to recommended follow-up

16.g.1. Reinforce the importance of keeping follow-up appointments with health care provider.
  2. Provide the following instructions regarding activity:
    a. progress activity gradually and only as tolerated

Desired Outcomes	Nursing Actions and *Selected Purposes/Rationales*

care including future appointments with health care provider and activity limitations.	b. stop any activity that causes chest pain, dizziness, or a significant increase in shortness of breath or fatigue
	c. plan and adhere to rest periods during the day
	d. adhere to physician's recommendations about activities that should be avoided
	e. notify physician if activity tolerance declines
	f. reduce dyspnea and fatigue during sexual activity by:
	  1. avoiding sexual activity when unusually fatigued
	  2. waiting 1–2 hours after a heavy meal or alcohol intake before engaging in sexual activity
	  3. identifying and using positions that minimize energy expenditure (e.g. side-lying, partner on top)
	  4. using portable oxygen during sexual activities.
	3. Refer to Nursing Diagnosis 15, action b, for measures to promote the client's ability to effectively manage the therapeutic regimen.

Bibliography

See pages 897–898 and 902.

 # HEART SURGERY: CORONARY ARTERY BYPASS GRAFTING (CABG) OR VALVE REPLACEMENT

Heart surgery is performed for a variety of reasons including myocardial revascularization, valve repair or replacement, repair of congenital or acquired structural abnormalities, placement of a mechanical assist device, and heart transplantation. Two common heart surgeries are coronary artery bypass grafting (CABG), which is done to treat severe coronary artery disease, and heart valve replacement. CABG involves removing a segment of the saphenous vein or using the internal mammary artery to create an anastomosis between the aorta and a point on the coronary artery distal to the obstruction. Heart valve replacement involves replacing the stenotic or regurgitant valve with a mechanical prosthesis (e.g. Starr-Edwards valve, St. Jude valve) or a biologic (tissue) valve (porcine or bovine valve, homograft).

Both CABG and valve replacement surgeries are performed through a median sternotomy. Cardiopulmonary bypass (extracorporeal circulation) is maintained during surgery by a machine that performs vital gas exchange functions; maintains the desired body temperature; fil-

ters the blood for thrombi, emboli, and impurities; and recirculates the blood into the arterial system. Systemic hypothermia (provided by the cardiopulmonary bypass machine) along with external cardiac cooling and cold cardioplegia (infusion of a cold solution containing potassium into the aortic root) are used to precipitate global myocardial arrest and reduce the metabolic needs for oxygen during surgery. Prior to closing the chest, pacing electrodes are usually placed on the epicardial surface of the heart and brought out through the chest wall to be used for temporary pacing if needed. A chest tube is placed in the mediastinum to drain blood and if needed, one is also placed in the pleural space to promote lung re-expansion.

This care plan focuses on the adult client hospitalized for either coronary artery bypass grafting (CABG) or valve replacement surgery. Preoperatively, a major goal of care is to reduce fear and anxiety. Goals of postoperative care are to maintain adequate cardiac output and respiratory function, maintain comfort, prevent complications, and educate the client regarding follow-up care.

DIAGNOSTIC TESTS

Coronary angiography or cardiac catheterization
Echocardiography
Electrocardiogram (ECG)
Blood studies (e.g. chemistry screen, type and cross match, coagulation screen, complete blood count, cardiac enzymes/isoenzymes)
Chest x-ray
Radionuclide imaging

DISCHARGE CRITERIA

Prior to discharge, the client will:

- have adequate cardiac output and tissue perfusion
- have clear, audible breath sounds throughout lungs
- have oxygen saturation within normal limits for client's age
- tolerate expected level of activity
- have surgical pain controlled
- have no signs and symptoms of complications
- identify modifiable cardiovascular risk factors and ways to alter these factors
- verbalize an understanding of the rationale for and components of a diet restricted in sodium, saturated fat, and cholesterol
- verbalize an understanding of activity restrictions and the rate of activity progression
- verbalize an understanding of medications ordered including rationale, food and drug interactions, side effects, schedule for taking, and importance of taking as prescribed
- state signs and symptoms to report to the health care provider
- identify community resources that can assist with cardiac rehabilitation and adjustment to having had heart surgery
- verbalize an understanding of and a plan for adhering to recommended follow-up care including future appointments with health care provider, wound care, and pain management.

NURSING/ COLLABORATIVE DIAGNOSES

Preoperative
1. Anxiety △   346

Postoperative
1. Decreased cardiac output △   346
2. Impaired respiratory function:
    a. ineffective breathing pattern
    b. ineffective airway clearance
    c. impaired gas exchange △   348
3. Altered fluid and electrolyte balance:
    a. fluid volume excess or water intoxication
    b. fluid volume deficit
    c. hypokalemia, hypochloremia, and/or metabolic alkalosis △   350
4. Activity intolerance △   350
5. Sensory/perceptual alterations △   351
6. Potential complications:
    a. myocardial infarction (MI)
    b. cardiac dysrhythmias
    c. heart failure
    d. cardiac tamponade
    e. bleeding
    f. thromboembolism
    g. cerebral ischemia
    h. impaired renal function
    i. pneumothorax △   352

DISCHARGE TEACHING

7. Knowledge deficit, Ineffective management of therapeutic regimen, or Altered health maintenance △   358

See Standardized Preoperative and Postoperative Care Plans for additional diagnoses

PREOPERATIVE

Use in conjunction with the Standardized Preoperative Care Plan.

---

1. NURSING DIAGNOSIS:

Anxiety

related to:
a. unfamiliar environment and separation from significant others;
b. lack of understanding of diagnostic tests, preoperative procedures/
   preparation, planned surgery, and postoperative course;
c. anticipated loss of control associated with effects of anesthesia;
d. financial concerns associated with surgery and hospitalization;
e. anticipated postoperative discomfort and alterations in life style and roles;
f. risk of disease if blood transfusions are necessary;
g. potential embarrassment or loss of dignity associated with body exposure;
h. possibility of death.

Desired Outcome	Nursing Actions and *Selected Purposes/Rationales*

1. The client will experience a reduction in anxiety (see Standardized Preoperative Care Plan, Nursing Diagnosis 1 [pp. 96–97], for outcome criteria).	1.a. Refer to Standardized Preoperative Care Plan, Nursing Diagnosis 1 (pp. 96–97), for measures related to assessment and reduction of fear and anxiety.
	 b. Implement additional measures *to reduce fear and anxiety:*
	  1. arrange for a visit from a critical care nurse or a visit to the intensive care unit; assure client and significant others that transfer to the intensive care unit after heart surgery is routine
	  2. describe and explain the rationale for equipment and tubes that may be present postoperatively (e.g. cardiac monitoring equipment, endotracheal tube and ventilator, chest tube, arterial and venous lines, nasogastric tube, urinary catheter)
	  3. if bypass grafting is planned, inform client that he/she may have leg incisions as well as a chest incision
	  4. with client, establish an alternative method of communicating (e.g. magic slate, word board, flash cards, signals) to be used while on the ventilator
	  5. focus on postoperative care (*this promotes a feeling in client that he/she will survive surgery*).

POSTOPERATIVE

Use in conjunction with the Standardized Postoperative Care Plan.

---

1. NURSING DIAGNOSIS:

Decreased cardiac output

related to:
a. pre-existing compromise in cardiac function;
b. trauma to the heart during surgery;
c. increased afterload associated with:
   1. vasoconstriction resulting from hypothermia and an increase in catecholamine output and plasma renin levels (these increases occur with cardiopulmonary bypass and the effect of stressors [e.g. pain, anxiety])
   2. fluid overload;
d. decreased preload associated with:
   1. hypovolemia (can result from blood loss, fluid shifting from the intravascular to interstitial space, loss of fluid from nasogastric tube, decreased fluid intake, and excessive diuresis)

2. hypotension (can occur if body is warmed rapidly following surgery and as a result of the effect of anesthesia and certain medications [e.g. narcotic analgesics, vasodilators]);
e. effects of hypothermia, hypoxemia, and acid-base and/or electrolyte imbalances on contractility and conductivity of the heart.

Desired Outcome	Nursing Actions and *Selected Purposes/Rationales*

1. The client will maintain adequate cardiac output as evidenced by:
  a. B/P within range of 130–100/80–60
  b. apical pulse regular and between 60–100 beats/minute
  c. absence of or no increase in intensity of gallop rhythm
  d. increased strength and activity tolerance
  e. unlabored respirations at 14–20/minute
  f. absence of adventitious breath sounds
  g. usual mental status
  h. absence of vertigo and syncope
  i. palpable peripheral pulses
  j. skin warm, dry, and usual color
  k. capillary refill time less than 3 seconds
  l. urine output at least 30 ml/hour
  m. absence of edema and jugular vein distention
  n. central venous pressure (CVP) within normal limits.
	1.a. Assess for and report signs and symptoms of:
	  1. hypovolemia (e.g. low B/P; resting pulse rate greater than 100 beats/minute; postural hypotension; cool, pale, or cyanotic skin; diminished or absent peripheral pulses; urine output less than 30 ml/hour; low CVP)
	  2. hypotension (systolic B/P persistently below 100 mm Hg)
	  3. decreased cardiac output:
	    a. variations in B/P (may be increased because of compensatory vasoconstriction; may be decreased when compensatory mechanisms and pump fail)
	    b. tachycardia
	    c. presence of gallop rhythm
	    d. fatigue and weakness
	    e. dyspnea, tachypnea
	    f. crackles (rales)
	    g. restlessness, change in mental status
	    h. vertigo, syncope
	    i. diminished or absent peripheral pulses
	    j. cool, moist skin
	    k. pallor or cyanosis of skin
	    l. capillary refill time greater than 3 seconds
	    m. oliguria
	    n. edema
	    o. jugular vein distention (JVD)
	    p. increased CVP (use internal jugular vein pulsation method to estimate CVP if monitoring device not present).
	  b. Monitor for and report the following:
	    1. dysrhythmias on ECG reading
	    2. chest x-ray results showing pulmonary vascular congestion, pulmonary edema, or pleural effusion
	    3. abnormal blood gases
	    4. significant decrease in oximetry results.
	  c. Implement measures *to maintain an adequate cardiac output*:
	    1. perform actions *to prevent or treat hypovolemia*:
	      a. administer blood and/or colloid or crystalloid solutions as ordered
	      b. maintain a minimum fluid intake of 1000 ml/day unless ordered otherwise
	      c. implement measures to prevent and control bleeding (see Postoperative Collaborative Diagnosis 6, actions e.4 and 5)
	    2. perform actions *to prevent or treat hypotension*:
	      a. consult physician before giving negative inotropic agents, diuretics, and vasodilating agents if client is hypotensive
	      b. administer narcotic (opioid) analgesics judiciously; in the immediate postoperative period, be alert to the synergistic effect of the narcotic ordered and the anesthetic that was used during surgery
	      c. avoid rapid rewarming; gradually bring client's body temperature to normal if he/she is hypothermic
	      d. administer sympathomimetics (e.g. dopamine) if ordered
	    3. administer positive inotropic agents (e.g. dopamine, dobutamine, digitalis preparations) if ordered *to increase myocardial contractility*
	    4. perform actions *to reduce cardiac workload*:
	      a. place client in a semi- to high Fowler's position

Desired Outcome	Nursing Actions and ***Selected Purposes/Rationales***

    b. perform actions *to prevent or treat hypertension:*
       1. implement measures to warm client (e.g. increase room temperature, apply warm blankets) if he/she is hypothermic (*helps prevent vasoconstriction associated with hypothermia and also prevents shivering, which elevates the metabolic rate and increases cardiac workload*)
       2. implement measures *to reduce stress* (e.g. initiate pain relief measures, reduce fear and anxiety)
       3. administer vasodilators (e.g. sodium nitroprusside, nitroglycerin) if ordered
    c. instruct client to avoid activities that create a Valsalva response (e.g. straining to have a bowel movement, holding breath while moving up in bed) *in order to prevent the marked increase in venous return and preload that occurs with exhalation*
    d. implement measures *to promote rest* (e.g. maintain activity restrictions, administer prescribed pain medications, limit the number of visitors, reduce anxiety)
    e. implement measures to improve respiratory status (see Postoperative Nursing Diagnosis 2, action c) *in order to promote adequate tissue oxygenation*
    f. discourage smoking (*smoke has a cardiostimulatory effect, causes vasoconstriction, and reduces oxygen availability*)
    g. discourage excessive intake of beverages high in caffeine such as coffee, tea, and colas (*caffeine is a myocardial stimulant and can increase myocardial oxygen consumption*)
    h. implement measures to prevent or treat fluid volume excess (see Postoperative Nursing Diagnosis 3, action a)
    i. increase activity gradually as allowed and tolerated.
  d. Consult physician if signs and symptoms of decreased cardiac output persist or worsen.

---

2. NURSING DIAGNOSIS: **Impaired respiratory function:***

  a. **ineffective breathing pattern** related to:
    1. increased rate and decreased depth of respirations associated with fear and anxiety
    2. decreased rate and depth of respirations associated with the depressant effect of anesthesia and some medications (e.g. narcotic [opioid] analgesics)
    3. diminished lung/chest wall expansion associated with weakness, fatigue, reluctance to breathe deeply because of chest incision and fear of dislodging chest tube, and diaphragmatic dysfunction if phrenic nerve was injured during surgery;
  b. **ineffective airway clearance** related to:
    1. stasis of secretions associated with decreased activity, depressed ciliary function resulting from the effect of anesthesia, and a weak cough effort
    2. increased secretions associated with irritation of the respiratory tract (can result from inhalation anesthetics and endotracheal intubation);
  c. **impaired gas exchange** related to ventilation/perfusion imbalances associated with:
    1. atelectasis (can occur as a result of deflation of the alveoli and decreased surfactant production while on the cardiopulmonary bypass machine and/or postoperative hypoventilation or ineffective clearance of secretions)
    2. accumulation of fluid in the pulmonary interstitium and alveoli (can occur as a result of increased capillary permeability and fluid volume excess)
    3. decreased pulmonary blood flow associated with decreased cardiac output.

---

*This diagnostic label includes the following nursing diagnoses: ineffective breathing pattern, ineffective airway clearance, and impaired gas exchange.

Desired Outcome	Nursing Actions and *Selected Purposes/Rationales*
2. The client will experience adequate respiratory function as evidenced by: a. normal rate and depth of respirations b. absence of dyspnea c. normal breath sounds by 3rd–4th postoperative day d. usual mental status e. usual skin color f. blood gases within normal range.	2.a. Assess for and report signs and symptoms of impaired respiratory function: 1. rapid, shallow, or slow respirations 2. dyspnea, orthopnea 3. use of accessory muscles when breathing 4. adventitious breath sounds (e.g. crackles [rales], rhonchi) 5. diminished or absent breath sounds 6. cough 7. restlessness, irritability 8. confusion, somnolence 9. central cyanosis (a late sign). b. Monitor for and report the following: 1. abnormal blood gases 2. significant decrease in oximetry results 3. abnormal chest x-ray results. c. Implement measures *to improve respiratory status:* 1. monitor mechanical ventilation carefully *to ensure that ventilatory rate and pressures are correct* 2. perform actions to decrease pain (see Standardized Postoperative Care Plan, Nursing Diagnosis 6, action e [p. 107]) and increase strength and activity tolerance (see Postoperative Nursing Diagnosis 4) *in order to increase client's willingness and ability to move, cough, deep breathe, and use incentive spirometer* 3. perform actions *to decrease fear and anxiety* (e.g. explain procedures, interact with client in a confident manner, initiate pain relief measures) 4. perform actions to maintain an adequate cardiac output (see Postoperative Nursing Diagnosis 1, action c) *in order to promote adequate pulmonary blood flow* 5. perform actions to prevent or treat fluid volume excess and water intoxication (see Postoperative Nursing Diagnosis 3, action a) *in order to reduce the risk for fluid accumulation in the lungs* 6. place client in a semi- to high Fowler's position unless contraindicated 7. assist with positive airway pressure techniques (e.g. positive end-expiratory pressure [PEEP], continuous positive airway pressure [CPAP]) if ordered 8. instruct and assist client to turn, cough, and deep breathe or use incentive spirometer every 1–2 hours; assure client that chest tube is sutured in place and that these activities should not dislodge the tube 9. maintain the maximum fluid intake allowed and humidify inspired air if ordered *to thin tenacious secretions* 10. maintain oxygen therapy as ordered 11. instruct client to avoid intake of gas-forming foods (e.g. beans, cauliflower, cabbage, onions), carbonated beverages, and large meals *in order to prevent gastric distention and an increase in pressure on the diaphragm* 12. discourage smoking (*smoke increases mucus production, impairs ciliary function, decreases oxygen availability, and can cause inflammation and damage to the bronchial walls*) 13. maintain activity restrictions; increase activity gradually as allowed and tolerated 14. administer central nervous system depressants judiciously; hold medication and consult physician if respiratory rate is less than 12/minute. d. Consult physician if signs and symptoms of impaired respiratory function persist or worsen.

3. NURSING/COLLABORATIVE DIAGNOSIS:

Altered fluid and electrolyte balance:

a. **fluid volume excess or water intoxication** related to:
1. the hemodilution technique used to prime the cardiopulmonary bypass machine
2. increased production of antidiuretic hormone (output of ADH is stimulated by trauma, pain, and anesthetic agents)
3. reshifting of fluid from the interstitial space back into the intravascular space approximately 3 days after surgery
4. decreased glomerular filtration rate and activation of the renin-angiotensin-aldosterone mechanism (a result of nonpulsatile renal perfusion while on the bypass machine and the decreased renal blood flow that can occur with decreased cardiac output);

b. **fluid volume deficit** related to restricted oral intake before, during, and after surgery; blood loss; inadequate fluid replacement; and loss of fluid associated with nasogastric tube drainage and excessive diuresis;

c. **hypokalemia, hypochloremia, and/or metabolic alkalosis** related to loss of electrolytes and hydrochloric acid associated with nasogastric tube drainage (diuretic therapy and the hemodilution created by priming the bypass machine with large amounts of fluid also contribute to the electrolyte imbalances).

Desired Outcomes	Nursing Actions and *Selected Purposes/Rationales*
3.a. The client will not experience fluid volume excess or water intoxication (see Standardized Postoperative Care Plan, Nursing Diagnosis 4, outcome b [p. 105], for outcome criteria).	3.a.1. Refer to Standardized Postoperative Care Plan, Nursing Diagnosis 4, action b (p. 105), for measures related to assessment, prevention, and management of fluid volume excess and water intoxication. 2. Implement additional measures *to prevent or treat fluid volume excess and water intoxication:* a. perform actions to maintain adequate renal blood flow (see Postoperative Collaborative Diagnosis 6, action h.3) b. administer diuretics if ordered c. maintain fluid and sodium restrictions as ordered (2500 ml fluid and 3–4 gm sodium restrictions are common).
3.b. The client will not experience fluid volume deficit, hypokalemia, hypochloremia, or metabolic alkalosis (see Standardized Postoperative Care Plan, Nursing Diagnosis 4, outcome a [p. 104], for outcome criteria).	3.b.1. Refer to Standardized Postoperative Care Plan, Nursing Diagnosis 4, action a (pp. 104–105), for measures related to assessment, prevention, and treatment of fluid volume deficit, hypokalemia, hypochloremia, and metabolic alkalosis. 2. Administer the following if ordered *to treat fluid volume deficit and hypokalemia:* a. blood and/or colloid or crystalloid solutions (colloid solutions are often used rather than crystalloid solutions *because they help maintain colloid osmotic pressure and subsequently reduce shifting of fluid from the intravascular to the interstitial space*) b. potassium supplements (*keeping the serum potassium at 4.0–4.5 reduces the risk for dysrhythmias*).

---

4. NURSING DIAGNOSIS:

Activity intolerance

related to:
a. tissue hypoxia associated with decreased cardiac output, impaired alveolar gas exchange, and anemia (results from hemodilution, blood loss, and red cell hemolysis [red cells are traumatized by the cardiopulmonary bypass machine]);
b. difficulty resting and sleeping associated with frequent assessments and treatments, discomfort, fear, and anxiety.

Desired Outcome	Nursing Actions and *Selected Purposes/Rationales*

4. The client will demonstrate an increased tolerance for activity (see Standardized Postoperative Care Plan, Nursing Diagnosis 10 [p. 111], for outcome criteria).	4.a. Refer to Standardized Postoperative Care Plan, Nursing Diagnosis 10 (pp. 111–112), for measures related to assessment and improvement of activity tolerance.
	b. Implement additional measures *to improve activity tolerance:*
	  1. perform actions to maintain an adequate cardiac output (see Postoperative Nursing Diagnosis 1, action c)
	  2. perform actions to improve respiratory status (see Postoperative Nursing Diagnosis 2, action c)
	  3. encourage client to increase intake of foods high in iron (e.g. organ meats, dried fruit, dark green leafy vegetables, whole-grain or iron-enriched breads and cereals) and vitamin C *(enhances the absorption of iron from plant products) in order to help resolve anemia*
	  4. administer packed red blood cells if ordered
	  5. increase client's activity gradually as allowed and tolerated; explain to client that a progressive and gradual increase in activity is necessary *in order to strengthen the myocardium without causing a sudden increase in cardiac workload.*

▪—————————————————————————————

5. NURSING DIAGNOSIS: **Sensory/perceptual alterations**

related to:
a. cerebral ischemia associated with factors such as inadequate cerebral perfusion while on cardiopulmonary bypass machine, decreased cardiac output, hypotensive episodes, and an embolus;
b. sleep deprivation and/or sensory overload associated with fear, anxiety, pain, and frequent assessments and treatments.

Desired Outcome	Nursing Actions and *Selected Purposes/Rationales*

5. The client will have resolution of sensory/ perceptual alterations as evidenced by:
a. accurate interpretation of environmental stimuli
b. usual behavior pattern
c. usual problem-solving ability
d. oriented to person, place, and time.
	5.a. Assess for signs and symptoms of sensory/perceptual alterations (e.g. inaccurate interpretation of environmental stimuli, inappropriate responses, change in behavior, impaired problem-solving ability, disorientation).
	b. Ascertain from significant others client's usual level of cognitive and emotional functioning.
	c. Implement measures *to reduce the risk for sensory/perceptual alterations:*
	  1. perform actions *to reduce fear and anxiety* (e.g. explain treatments; keep monitor out of client's view; be readily available to client; project a calm, confident manner)
	  2. perform actions to promote sleep (see Standardized Postoperative Care Plan, Nursing Diagnosis 15, action c [p. 115])
	  3. perform actions to promote adequate cerebral blood flow (see Postoperative Collaborative Diagnosis 6, action g.2)
	  4. perform actions *to minimize environmental stimuli:*
	    a. organize care to allow for periods of uninterrupted rest
	    b. dim lights in room
	    c. keep auditory level on monitors as low as possible
	    d. avoid unnecessary conversations in or directly outside of client's room
	    e. restrict the number of visitors and their length of stay.
	d. If client shows evidence of sensory/perceptual alterations:
	  1. initiate appropriate safety precautions (e.g. side rails up, accompany when out of bed)
	  2. reorient client to person, place, and time as necessary

Desired Outcome	Nursing Actions and *Selected Purposes/Rationales*

3. address client by name
4. place familiar objects, clock, and calendar within client's view
5. approach client in a slow, calm manner; allow adequate time for communication
6. repeat instructions as necessary using clear, simple language and short sentences
7. maintain a consistent and fairly structured routine when possible
8. have client perform only one activity at a time and allow adequate time for performance of activities
9. encourage client to make lists of planned activities, questions, and concerns
10. assist client to problem solve if necessary
11. maintain realistic expectations of client's ability to learn, comprehend, and remember information provided; provide client with a written copy of instructions
12. encourage significant others to be supportive of client; instruct them in methods of dealing with client's sensory/perceptual alterations
13. inform client and significant others that symptoms client is experiencing are not unusual and should gradually subside
14. provide appropriate level of supervision
15. consult physician if sensory/perceptual alterations persist or worsen.

---

6. COLLABORATIVE DIAGNOSES:

Potential complications of heart surgery

a. **myocardial infarction (MI)** related to an increased myocardial oxygen demand and/or insufficient coronary blood flow (can result from coronary artery spasm, hypotension, or thrombosis or embolism of a native coronary vessel or bypass grafts);

b. **cardiac dysrhythmias** related to impaired nodal function and/or altered myocardial conductivity associated with trauma to the heart during surgery, hypothermia, hypoxia, sympathetic stimulation (can result from anxiety, volume depletion, and pain), electrolyte and acid-base imbalances, or the effect of certain medications (e.g. dopamine, digoxin);

c. **heart failure** related to pre-existing myocardial dilation or hypertrophy and decreased cardiac output postoperatively associated with damage to and further stress on the heart;

d. **cardiac tamponade** related to accumulation of fluid (usually blood) in the pericardial sac and/or mediastinum associated with excessive bleeding and/or obstructed drainage of the mediastinal tube;

e. **bleeding** related to:
   1. impaired platelet and clotting factor function (can result from mechanical damage to platelets and clotting factors by cardiopulmonary bypass machine, effects of hypothermia, a relative decrease in levels associated with hemodilution, and consumption coagulopathy that can occur with major trauma)
   2. incomplete neutralization of the heparin used to prime the cardiopulmonary bypass machine
   3. anticoagulant therapy (relevant primarily for clients who have had valve replacement)
   4. disruption of suture lines associated with hypertension if it occurs;

f. **thromboembolism** related to:
   1. trauma to the coronary arteries and donor vessels during grafting procedure
   2. thrombi formation at the prosthetic valve site
   3. formation of microemboli associated with incomplete emptying of cardiac chambers if atrial fibrillation or heart failure occurs
   4. venous stasis associated with diminished cardiac output and decreased activity
   5. hypercoagulability associated with increased release of tissue thromboplastin into the blood (occurs as a result of surgical trauma);

g. **cerebral ischemia** related to inadequate cerebral blood flow associated with:

1. decreased systemic arterial pressure while on cardiopulmonary bypass
2. an embolus (can result from dislodgment of atherosclerotic plaque during cannulation, dislodgment of debris from calcified valve, incomplete filtration of air by bypass machine, or cardiac thrombus formation on prosthetic valve or as a result of dysrhythmias)
3. hypotension or low cardiac output postoperatively;

h. **impaired renal function** related to deposit of hemolyzed red blood cell products in renal tubules or inadequate renal blood flow associated with cardiopulmonary bypass, low cardiac output, hypotension, an embolus, or effect of vasopressor drugs;

i. **pneumothorax** related to the accumulation of air in the pleural space if the pleura was opened during surgery.

Desired Outcomes	Nursing Actions and *Selected Purposes/Rationales*

6.a. The client will not experience an MI as evidenced by:
1. no episodes of sudden and persistent chest pain
2. stable vital signs
3. cardiac enzyme levels declining toward normal range
4. absence of new and persistent Q wave and ST-T wave abnormalities on ECG reading.
	6.a.1. Assess for and report signs and symptoms of a myocardial infarction (e.g. sudden and persistent chest pain; significant change in vital signs; further increase in cardiac enzymes; new and persistent ST segment elevation, T wave changes, and/or abnormal Q waves on ECG reading).
	2. Implement measures to maintain adequate cardiac output (see Postoperative Nursing Diagnosis 1, action c) *in order to improve myocardial blood supply and reduce the risk of myocardial infarction.*
	3. If signs and symptoms of a myocardial infarction occur:
	a. initiate cardiac monitoring if not still being done
	b. maintain client on bed rest in a semi- to high Fowler's position
	c. maintain oxygen therapy as ordered
	d. administer the following medications if ordered:
	  1. morphine sulfate *to reduce pain and anxiety and decrease cardiac workload*
	  2. nitrates *to improve coronary blood flow and reduce myocardial oxygen requirements*
	  3. beta-adrenergic blocking agents *to reduce myocardial oxygen requirements by decreasing heart rate and the force of myocardial contractility*
	e. provide emotional support to client and significant others
	f. refer to Care Plan on Myocardial Infarction for additional care measures.

6.b. The client will maintain normal sinus rhythm as evidenced by: 1. regular apical pulse at 60–100 beats/minute 2. equal apical and radial pulse rates 3. absence of syncope and palpitations 4. ECG reading showing normal sinus rhythm.	6.b.1. Assess for and report signs and symptoms of cardiac dysrhythmias (e.g. irregular apical pulse; pulse rate below 60 or above 100 beats/minute; apical-radial pulse deficit; syncope; palpitations; abnormal rate, rhythm, or configurations on ECG). 2. Implement measures *to prevent cardiac dysrhythmias:* a. perform actions to maintain adequate cardiac output and myocardial blood flow (see Postoperative Nursing Diagnosis 1, action c) b. maintain oxygen therapy as ordered c. monitor serum electrolyte levels; consult physician about administration of a potassium or magnesium supplement if serum levels of either are low d. perform actions to improve respiratory status (see Postoperative Nursing Diagnosis 2, action c) *in order to improve tissue oxygenation and prevent respiratory acidosis or alkalosis (myocardial conductivity is altered by hypoxia and acid-base imbalance).* 3. If cardiac dysrhythmias occur: a. initiate cardiac monitoring if not still being done b. administer antidysrhythmics (e.g. digoxin, diltiazem, verapamil, quinidine, procainamide, metoprolol, esmolol, lidocaine, adenosine, atropine) if ordered c. maintain temporary pacemaker function as ordered d. restrict client's activity based on his/her tolerance and severity of the dysrhythmia

Desired Outcomes	Nursing Actions and *Selected Purposes/Rationales*

e. maintain oxygen therapy as ordered

f. assess cardiovascular status frequently and report signs and symptoms of inadequate tissue perfusion (e.g. decrease in B/P; cool, moist skin; cyanosis; diminished peripheral pulses; urine output less than 30 ml/hour; restlessness and agitation; shortness of breath)

g. have emergency cart readily available for cardioversion, defibrillation, or cardiopulmonary resuscitation.

6.c. The client will not develop heart failure as evidenced by:
1. pulse 60–100 beats/ minute
2. absence of an S₃ heart sound
3. usual mental status
4. absence of adventitious breath sounds
5. absence of dyspnea, orthopnea, and cough
6. palpable peripheral pulses
7. increased strength and activity tolerance
8. skin warm and dry
9. urine output at least 30 ml/hour
10. stable weight
11. absence of edema; distended neck veins; and enlarged, tender liver
12. CVP within normal limits.

6.c.1. Assess for and report signs and symptoms of heart failure:
a. significant increase in pulse rate
b. presence of an S₃ heart sound
c. restlessness, anxiousness, confusion, or other change in mental status
d. crackles (rales)
e. dyspnea, orthopnea
f. dry, hacking cough or cough productive of blood-tinged or frothy sputum
g. diminished or absent peripheral pulses
h. increased weakness and fatigue
i. cool, diaphoretic skin
j. decreased urine output
k. weight gain
l. edema
m. distended neck veins
n. enlarged, tender liver
o. increased CVP.

2. Monitor chest x-ray results. Report findings of cardiomegaly, pleural effusion, or pulmonary edema.

3. Implement measures *to prevent heart failure:*
a. perform actions to maintain adequate cardiac output (see Postoperative Nursing Diagnosis 1, action c)
b. perform actions to prevent and treat cardiac dysrhythmias (see actions b.2 and 3 in this diagnosis) *because dysrhythmias contribute to the development of heart failure.*

4. If signs and symptoms of heart failure occur:
a. continue with above actions
b. maintain oxygen therapy as ordered
c. administer the following medications if ordered:
   1. positive inotropic agents (e.g. dobutamine, dopamine, amrinone, digitalis preparations) *to increase myocardial contractility*
   2. diuretics and vasodilators *to decrease cardiac workload*
   3. morphine sulfate *to reduce preload and anxiety* (used primarily in clients with pulmonary edema)
d. refer to Care Plan on Heart Failure for additional care measures.

6.d. The client will not experience cardiac tamponade as evidenced by:
1. stable vital signs
2. audible heart sounds
3. absence of jugular vein distention
4. absence of pulsus paradoxus
5. CVP within normal limits.

6.d.1. Assess for and immediately report:
a. a sudden decrease in chest tube drainage
b. chest x-ray reports showing widening of the mediastinum
c. signs and symptoms of cardiac tamponade (e.g. significant decrease in B/P, narrowed pulse pressure, pulsus paradoxus and distant or muffled heart sounds [may be obscured by mechanical ventilation], jugular vein distention, increased CVP).

2. Implement measures *to reduce the risk of cardiac tamponade:*
a. perform actions to maintain patency and integrity of chest drainage system (see action i.4.a in this diagnosis)
b. if chest tube becomes obstructed, assist with clearing of existing tube and/or insertion of a new tube
c. when removing the pacemaker catheter(s), do it carefully *to avoid trauma to the surrounding vessels and subsequent bleeding.*

3. If signs and symptoms of cardiac tamponade occur:
a. prepare client for echocardiography
b. administer intravenous fluids and/or vasopressors if ordered *to maintain mean arterial pressure*
c. prepare client for surgical drainage of pericardial fluid.

6.e. The client will not experience unusual bleeding as evidenced by:
1. gradual decrease in amount of bloody drainage from chest tube
2. skin and mucous membranes free of active bleeding, petechiae, purpura, and ecchymoses
3. absence of unusual joint pain
4. no increase in abdominal girth
5. absence of frank and occult blood in stool, urine, and vomitus
6. usual menstrual flow
7. usual mental status
8. vital signs within normal range for client
9. stable or improved Hct and Hb.

6.e.1. Assess client for and report signs and symptoms of unusual bleeding:
   a. excessive amount of bloody drainage from chest tube
   b. continuous oozing of blood from incisions
   c. prolonged bleeding from puncture sites
   d. gingival bleeding
   e. petechiae, purpura, ecchymoses
   f. epistaxis, hemoptysis
   g. unusual joint pain
   h. increase in abdominal girth
   i. frank or occult blood in stool, urine, or vomitus
   j. menorrhagia
   k. restlessness, confusion
   l. significant drop in B/P accompanied by an increased pulse rate
   m. decrease in Hct and Hb levels.
2. Monitor platelet count and coagulation test results (e.g. prothrombin time or International Normalized Ratio [INR], activated partial thromboplastin time, bleeding time). Report abnormal values or values that exceed the therapeutic range if client is on anticoagulant therapy.
3. If platelet count is low, coagulation test results are abnormal, or Hct and Hb levels decrease, test all stools, urine, and vomitus for occult blood. Report positive results.
4. Implement measures *to prevent bleeding:*
   a. when giving injections or performing venous and arterial punctures, use the smallest gauge needle possible and apply gentle, prolonged pressure to the site after the needle is removed
   b. when taking B/P, avoid overinflating the cuff
   c. perform actions to prevent and treat hypertension (see Postoperative Nursing Diagnosis 1, action c.4.b) *in order to maintain systolic B/P at a level less than 140 mm Hg and subsequently decrease the risk for disruption of suture lines*
   d. caution client to avoid activities that increase the risk for trauma (e.g. shaving with a straight-edge razor, using stiff-bristle toothbrush or dental floss)
   e. pad side rails if client is confused or restless
   f. perform actions *to reduce the risk for falls* (e.g. keep bed in low position with side rails up when client is in bed, avoid unnecessary clutter in room, instruct client to wear shoes/slippers with nonslip soles when ambulating)
   g. instruct client to avoid blowing nose forcefully or straining to have a bowel movement; consult physician regarding order for a decongestant and/or laxative if indicated
   h. administer the following if ordered:
      1. vitamin K (e.g. phytonadione, menadione) *to counteract the effect of warfarin therapy*
      2. protamine sulfate *to further neutralize the heparin used to prime the bypass machine*
      3. blood products (e.g. platelets, fresh frozen plasma [FFP])
      4. desmopressin (DDAVP) *to increase factor VIII and subsequently increase platelet aggregation.*
5. If bleeding occurs and does not subside spontaneously:
   a. apply firm, prolonged pressure to bleeding area(s) if possible
   b. maintain oxygen therapy as ordered
   c. assist with positive airway pressure techniques (e.g. positive end-expiratory pressure [PEEP]) if ordered *to increase intrathoracic pressure and subsequently slow venous bleeding in the thoracic cavity*
   d. autotransfuse chest tube drainage if ordered
   e. administer the following if ordered:
      1. vitamin K or protamine sulfate
      2. whole blood or packed red blood cells
      3. blood products (e.g. platelets, FFP)

Desired Outcomes	Nursing Actions and **Selected Purposes/Rationales**

f. perform gastric lavage if ordered *to control gastric bleeding*
g. assess for and report signs and symptoms of hypovolemic shock (e.g. restlessness; confusion; significant decrease in B/P; rapid, weak pulse; rapid respirations; cool, pale skin; urine output less than 30 ml/hour)
h. prepare client for return to surgery if planned
i. provide emotional support to client and significant others.

6.f. The client will not develop a thromboembolism as evidenced by:
1. absence of pain, tenderness, swelling, and numbness in extremities
2. usual temperature and color of extremities
3. palpable and equal peripheral pulses
4. usual mental status
5. usual sensory and motor function
6. absence of sudden chest pain and dyspnea.

6.f.1. Assess for and report signs and symptoms of:
   a. deep vein thrombus (e.g. pain, tenderness, swelling, unusual warmth, and/or positive Homans' sign in extremity)
   b. arterial embolus (e.g. diminished or absent peripheral pulses; pallor, coolness, numbness, and/or pain in extremity)
   c. cerebral ischemia (see action g.1 in this diagnosis for a list of signs and symptoms)
   d. pulmonary embolism (e.g. sudden chest pain, dyspnea, restlessness and apprehension).
2. Implement measures to prevent and treat deep vein thrombus and pulmonary embolism (see Standardized Postoperative Care Plan, Collaborative Diagnosis 19, actions c.1.b and c and c.2.b and c [pp. 120–121]).
3. Implement measures *to prevent thrombi and microemboli formation in the heart:*
   a. perform actions *to prevent stasis of blood in the heart:*
      1. implement measures to prevent and treat cardiac dysrhythmias (see actions b.2 and 3 in this diagnosis)
      2. implement measures to improve cardiac output (see Postoperative Nursing Diagnosis 1, action c)
   b. administer anticoagulants (e.g. low- or adjusted-dose heparin, low-molecular-weight heparin, warfarin) and antiplatelet agents (e.g. low-dose aspirin, dipyridamole) if ordered.
4. If signs and symptoms of an arterial embolus occur:
   a. maintain client on strict bed rest with affected extremity in a level or slightly dependent position *to improve arterial blood flow*
   b. prepare client for diagnostic studies (e.g. Doppler or duplex ultrasound, arteriography)
   c. administer anticoagulants (e.g. continuous intravenous heparin, warfarin) if ordered
   d. prepare client for surgical intervention (e.g. embolectomy, revascularization) if planned
   e. refer to action g.3 in this diagnosis for additional care measures if signs and symptoms of cerebral ischemia occur
   f. provide emotional support to client and significant others.

6.g. The client will maintain adequate cerebral blood flow as evidenced by:
1. absence of dizziness, syncope, visual disturbances, and speech impairments
2. mentally alert and oriented
3. normal sensory and motor function.

6.g.1. Assess for and report signs and symptoms of cerebral ischemia:
   a. dizziness, syncope
   b. visual disturbances
   c. slurred speech, expressive or receptive aphasia
   d. decreased level of consciousness
   e. paresthesias, weakness of extremity, facial ptosis, paralysis.
2. Implement measures *to promote adequate cerebral blood flow:*
   a. keep head of bed flat until B/P is stabilized at a satisfactory level (at least 90 mm Hg systolic)
   b. keep head and neck in proper alignment
   c. perform actions to maintain adequate cardiac output (see Postoperative Nursing Diagnosis 1, action c)
   d. perform actions to prevent thrombi and microemboli formation in the heart (see action f.3 in this diagnosis).
3. If signs and symptoms of cerebral ischemia occur:
   a. continue with above measures
   b. administer anticoagulants (e.g. warfarin, continuous intravenous heparin) if ordered
   c. provide emotional support to client and significant others

d. refer to Care Plan on Cerebrovascular Accident for additional care measures if signs and symptoms persist.

6.h. The client will maintain adequate renal function as evidenced by:
1. urine output at least 30 ml/hour
2. BUN, serum creatinine, and creatinine clearance within normal range.

6.h.1. Assess for and report signs and symptoms of impaired renal function (e.g. urine output less than 30 ml/hour, urine specific gravity fixed at or less than 1.010, elevated BUN and serum creatinine levels).
2. Collect a 24-hour urine specimen if ordered. Report decreased creatinine clearance.
3. Implement measures *to maintain adequate renal blood flow:*
 a. maintain a minimum fluid intake of 1000 ml/day unless ordered otherwise
 b. perform actions to maintain adequate cardiac output (see Postoperative Nursing Diagnosis 1, action c)
 c. perform actions to prevent thrombi and microemboli formation in the heart (see action f.3 in this diagnosis) *in order to reduce the risk for occlusion of the renal artery by an embolus.*
4. If signs and symptoms of impaired renal function occur:
 a. continue with above actions
 b. administer diuretics (e.g. furosemide, mannitol) if ordered *to increase urine output and subsequently reduce further accumulation of hemolyzed red blood cell products in the renal tubules*
 c. assess for and report signs of acute renal failure (e.g. oliguria or anuria; weight gain; edema; elevated B/P; lethargy and confusion; increasing BUN and serum creatinine, phosphorus, and potassium levels)
 d. prepare client for dialysis if indicated
 e. refer to Care Plan on Renal Failure for additional care measures.

6.i. The client will experience normal lung re-expansion as evidenced by:
1. audible breath sounds and a resonant percussion note over lungs by 3rd–4th postoperative day
2. unlabored respirations at 14–20/minute
3. blood gases returning toward normal
4. chest x-ray showing lung re-expansion.

6.i.1. Assess for and immediately report signs and symptoms of:
 a. malfunction of chest drainage system (e.g. respiratory distress, excessive bubbling in water seal chamber, significant increase in subcutaneous emphysema)
 b. further lung collapse (e.g. extended area of absent breath sounds with hyperresonant percussion note; further increase in pulse rate; rapid, shallow, and/or labored respirations; restlessness; confusion).
2. Monitor blood gases. Report values that have worsened.
3. Monitor chest x-ray results. Report findings of delayed lung re-expansion or further lung collapse.
4. Implement measures *to promote lung re-expansion and prevent further lung collapse:*
 a. perform actions *to maintain patency and integrity of chest drainage system:*
  1. maintain fluid level in the water seal and suction chambers as ordered
  2. maintain air occlusive dressing over chest tube insertion site
  3. tape all connections securely
  4. tape the tubing close to insertion site to the chest wall *to reduce the risk of inadvertent removal of the tube*
  5. position tubing *to promote optimum drainage* (e.g. coil excess tubing on bed rather than allowing it to hang down below the collection device, keep tubing free of kinks)
  6. drain any fluid that accumulates in tubing into the collection chamber and milk tube gently if indicated *to dislodge clots*
  7. keep drainage collection device below level of client's chest at all times
 b. perform actions *to facilitate the escape of air from the pleural space* (e.g. maintain suction as ordered, ensure that the air vent is open on the drainage collection device if system is to water seal only)
 c. perform actions to improve respiratory status (see Postoperative Nursing Diagnosis 2, action c).
5. If signs and symptoms of further lung collapse occur:
 a. maintain client on bed rest in a semi- to high Fowler's position
 b. maintain oxygen therapy as ordered

Desired Outcomes	Nursing Actions and *Selected Purposes/Rationales*

    c. assess for and immediately report signs and symptoms of tension pneumothorax (e.g. severe dyspnea, increased restlessness and agitation, rapid and/or irregular pulse rate, hypotension, neck vein distention, shift in trachea from midline)

    d. assist with clearing of existing chest tube and/or insertion of a new tube.

Discharge Teaching

7. NURSING DIAGNOSIS: **Knowledge deficit, Ineffective management of therapeutic regimen, or Altered health maintenance***

    *The nurse should select the diagnostic label that is most appropriate for the client's discharge teaching needs.

Desired Outcomes	Nursing Actions and *Selected Purposes/Rationales*

7.a. The client will identify modifiable cardiovascular risk factors and ways to alter these factors.	7.a.1. Inform client that the following modifiable factors have been shown to contribute to cardiovascular disease:
	  a. obesity
	  b. elevated serum lipids
	  c. lack of regular aerobic exercise
	  d. cigarette smoking
	  e. stressful life style
	  f. hypertension
	  g. diabetes mellitus.
	  2. Encourage client to discuss alcohol intake with health care provider. (The health care provider may advise the client to limit alcohol consumption because there is evidence that a daily alcohol intake exceeding 1 oz of ethanol [i.e. 2 oz of 100-proof whiskey, 8 oz of wine, 24 oz of beer] contributes to the development of hypertension and some forms of heart disease.)
	  3. Assist the client to identify ways he/she can make appropriate changes in life style to modify the above factors. Provide information about stress management classes and weight loss, cardiovascular fitness, smoking cessation, and alcohol rehabilitation programs. Initiate a referral if indicated.

7.b. The client will verbalize an understanding of the rationale for and components of a diet restricted in sodium, saturated fat, and cholesterol.	7.b.1. Explain the rationale for a diet restricting sodium, saturated fat, and cholesterol intake.
	  2. Provide the following information about decreasing sodium intake:
	  a. be aware that the terms salt and sodium are often used interchangeably but are not synonymous; there is 40% sodium in table salt
	  b. read labels on foods/fluids and calculate sodium content of items; avoid those products that tend to have a high sodium content (e.g. canned soups and vegetables, tomato juice, commercial baked goods, commercially prepared frozen or canned entrees and sauces)
	  c. do not add salt when cooking foods or to prepared foods; use low-sodium herbs and spices if desired
	  d. avoid cured and smoked foods
	  e. avoid salty snack foods (e.g. crackers, nuts, pretzels, potato chips)
	  f. avoid commercially prepared fast foods
	  g. avoid routine use of over-the-counter medications with a high sodium content (e.g. Alka-Seltzer, some antacids such as Gaviscon).
	  3. Provide instructions on ways the client can reduce intake of saturated fat and cholesterol:
	  a. trim visible fat off meat and remove all skin from poultry

b. use vegetable oil rather than coconut or palm oil in cooking and food preparation

c. use cooking methods such as steaming, baking, broiling, poaching, microwaving, and grilling rather than frying

d. restrict intake of eggs (recommendations about the number of whole eggs allowed per week vary depending on the client's lipid levels)

e. avoid commercial baked goods

f. avoid dairy products containing more than 1% fat

g. reduce intake of red meat once anemia has resolved.

4. Obtain a dietary consult to assist client in planning meals that will meet the prescribed restrictions of sodium, saturated fat, and cholesterol.

7.c. The client will verbalize an understanding of activity restrictions and the rate of activity progression.	7.c. Reinforce physician's instructions regarding activity. Instruct client to: 1. gradually rebuild activity level by adhering to a planned exercise program (often begins with walking and light household activities) 2. take frequent rest periods for 4–6 weeks following surgery 3. avoid lifting heavy objects in order to allow incision to heal and prevent a sudden increase in cardiac workload 4. avoid driving for 4–6 weeks 5. stop any activity that causes chest pain, shortness of breath, palpitations, dizziness, or extreme fatigue or weakness 6. begin a cardiovascular fitness program when allowed by physician.

7.d. The client will verbalize an understanding of medications ordered including rationale, food and drug interactions, side effects, schedule for taking, and importance of taking as prescribed.	7.d.1. Explain the rationale for, side effects of, and importance of taking medications prescribed. Inform client of pertinent food and drug interactions.
	2. If client has had a valve replacement and is discharged on warfarin (e.g. Coumadin), instruct to:
	a. keep scheduled appointments for periodic blood studies to monitor coagulation times
	b. take medication at the same time each day, do not stop taking medication abruptly, and do not attempt to make up for missed doses
	c. avoid regular and/or excessive intake of alcohol (may alter responsiveness to warfarin)
	d. avoid taking over-the-counter products containing aspirin and other nonsteroidal anti-inflammatory agents (these products enhance the action of warfarin)
	e. avoid eating large amounts of foods high in vitamin K (e.g. green leafy vegetables)
	f. take the following precautions to minimize risk of bleeding:
	  1. use an electric rather than a straight-edge razor
	  2. floss and brush teeth gently
	  3. avoid putting sharp objects (e.g. toothpicks) in mouth
	  4. do not walk barefoot
	  5. cut nails carefully
	  6. avoid situations that could result in injury (e.g. contact sports)
	  7. avoid blowing nose forcefully
	  8. avoid straining to have a bowel movement
	g. report prolonged or excessive bleeding from skin, nose, or mouth; blood in urine, vomitus, sputum, or stools; prolonged or excessive menses; excessive bruising; severe headache; or sudden abdominal or back pain
	h. apply firm, prolonged pressure to any bleeding area if possible
	i. wear a medical alert identification bracelet or tag identifying self as being on anticoagulant therapy
	j. inform physician immediately if pregnancy is suspected (warfarin crosses the placental barrier).
	3. Instruct client to inform physician before taking other prescription and nonprescription medications.
	4. Instruct client to inform all health care providers of medications being taken.

7.e. The client will state signs and symptoms to report to the health care provider.	7.e.1. Refer to Standardized Postoperative Care Plan, Nursing Diagnosis 21, action c (p. 123), for signs and symptoms to report to the health care provider.

Desired Outcomes	Nursing Actions and *Selected Purposes/Rationales*
	2. Instruct client to report these additional signs and symptoms: a. chest pain that seems unrelated to incisional discomfort b. development of or increased shortness of breath c. dizziness, fainting d. increased fatigue and weakness e. weight gain of more than 2 pounds in 2 days f. swelling of feet or ankles g. persistent cough, especially if productive of yellow, green, rust-colored, or frothy sputum h. significant change in pulse rate or rhythm (check with physician about client's need to monitor pulse at home) i. persistent low-grade temperature or temperature above 101° F (38.3° C) for more than 1 day j. depression or problems with concentration or memory that last more than 6 weeks.
7.f. The client will identify community resources that can assist with cardiac rehabilitation and adjustment to having had heart surgery.	7.f.1. Provide information about community resources that can assist client with cardiac rehabilitation and adjustment to having had heart surgery (e.g. American Heart Association, Mended Hearts Club, counseling services). 2. Initiate a referral if indicated.
7.g. The client will verbalize an understanding of and a plan for adhering to recommended follow-up care including future appointments with health care provider, wound care, and pain management.	7.g.1. Refer to Standardized Postoperative Care Plan, Nursing Diagnosis 21 (pp. 123–124), for routine postoperative instructions and measures to improve client compliance. 2. If client had a valve replacement, instruct him/her to: a. not have dental work for 6 months b. inform health care providers of valve surgery so prophylactic antimicrobials may be started before any dental work, invasive diagnostic procedures, or surgery c. perform good oral hygiene in order to reduce the risk for infective endocarditis.

Bibliography

See pages 897–898 and 902–903.

HYPERTENSION

Hypertension is defined as a sustained elevation of arterial blood pressure at a level of 140/90 mm Hg or higher. Isolated systolic hypertension (ISH) is technically defined as a systolic blood pressure greater than 140 mm Hg with a diastolic blood pressure less than 90 mm Hg but, because the systolic pressure is elevated in many elderly persons as a result of the progressive large vessel atherosclerosis that accompanies aging, isolated systolic hypertension is considered by many practitioners to be a systolic blood pressure greater than 160 mm Hg with a diastolic blood pressure less than 90 mm Hg.

Hypertension is classified as primary (essential or idiopathic) or secondary. Primary hypertension, which constitutes approximately 95% of the cases, has an unknown etiology. Secondary hypertension has identifiable causes, which include renal parenchymal or vascular disease, Cushing's syndrome, certain neurological disorders, pheochromocytoma, primary hyperaldosteronism, coarctation of the aorta, and use of certain drugs (e.g. oral contraceptives, amphetamines, sympathomimetics). Hypertension is also classified according to severity. The current classification schema for hypertension includes systolic as well as diastolic pressure levels and divides hypertension into four stages. Stage 1 (mild) hypertension is an average blood pressure of 140–159/90–99 mm Hg, whereas stage 4 (very severe) hypertension includes blood pressure readings of 210/120 mm Hg or greater. In addition to classifying the stages of hypertension on the basis of average blood pressure readings, the clinician usually also specifies the presence or absence of target-organ disease and additional risk factors. Hypertensive crisis, urgency, or emergency are terms used to describe a situation in which the pressure elevation poses an immediate threat to the client's life.

The pathological hallmark of hypertension is an increase in systemic vascular resistance. In order to sustain adequate tissue perfusion when vascular resistance is increased, the heart must pump harder. A prolonged increase in cardiac workload eventually leads to ventricular hypertrophy and heart failure. The prolonged increase in vascular pressure causes widespread pathological changes in the blood vessels. The end result of all the changes in the cardiovascular system is a decreased blood supply to the tissues with target-organ damage occurring most often in the eyes, kidneys, brain, and heart. This target-organ damage is often what causes the initial symptoms in the person with hypertension.

Initial treatment of hypertension is usually nonpharmacologic and consists of life-style modifications such as weight reduction, regular aerobic exercise, and moderation of dietary sodium and alcohol intake. If these measures do not achieve the desired control of blood pressure, pharmacologic therapy is initiated utilizing a stepped-care approach. The type of medication used initially in this approach is often a diuretic or a beta-adrenergic blocking agent because they have been shown to reduce morbidity and mortality. Calcium-channel blocking agents, angiotensin-converting enzyme inhibitors, alpha-adrenergic blockers, and combined alpha- and beta-adrenergic blockers are also considered by many practitioners to be first line agents. If the person's hypertension is inadequately controlled by the initial agent, a different agent or a combination of drugs will be tried until the desired control of blood pressure is achieved with a minimum of side effects.

This care plan focuses on the adult client hospitalized with severe hypertension that is either newly diagnosed or uncontrolled. The goals of care are to lower the blood pressure to a safe level, reduce fear and anxiety, prevent complications, and educate the client regarding follow-up care.

DIAGNOSTIC TESTS

Renal arteriography
Renal radionuclide imaging (renal scan, renography)
Intravenous pyelography (IVP)
Chest x-ray
Urine studies (e.g. urinalysis, vanillylmandelic acid [VMA], creatinine clearance, cortisol level)
Blood studies (e.g. chemistry screen, lipid profile, cortisol level, catecholamine level, renin level, aldosterone level)
Electrocardiogram (ECG)

DISCHARGE CRITERIA

Prior to discharge, the client will:

- have blood pressure within a safe range
- have evidence of adequate tissue perfusion
- have no signs and symptoms of complications
- verbalize a basic understanding of hypertension and its effects on the body
- identify modifiable risk factors for hypertension and ways to alter these factors
- verbalize an understanding of medications ordered including rationale, food and drug interactions, side effects, schedule for taking, and importance of taking as prescribed
- verbalize an understanding of the rationale for and components of the recommended diet
- state signs and symptoms to report to the health care provider
- identify community resources that can assist in making life-style changes necessary for effective control of hypertension
- verbalize an understanding of and a plan for adhering to recommended follow-up care including future appointments with health care provider and activity level.

1. NURSING DIAGNOSIS:

Altered tissue perfusion

related to decreased systemic blood flow associated with increased vascular resistance.

Desired Outcome	Nursing Actions and *Selected Purposes/Rationales*

1. The client will maintain adequate tissue perfusion as evidenced by:
  a. B/P declining toward normal range for client
  b. usual mental status
  c. extremities warm with absence of pallor and cyanosis
  d. palpable peripheral pulses
  e. capillary refill time less than 3 seconds
  f. absence of exercise-induced pain
  g. urine output at least 30 ml/hour.
	1.a. Assess for and report the following:
	  1. further increase in B/P or failure of B/P to decline in response to antihypertensive agents
	  2. signs and symptoms of diminished tissue perfusion (e.g. restlessness, confusion, cool extremities, pallor or cyanosis of extremities, diminished or absent peripheral pulses, slow capillary refill, angina, oliguria).
	  b. Implement measures *to reduce blood pressure in order to improve tissue perfusion:*
	  1. administer the following medications if ordered:
	    a. adrenergic inhibiting agents:
	      1. central-acting adrenergic inhibitors (e.g. clonidine, methyldopa, guanabenz, guanfacine)
	      2. alpha-adrenergic blockers (e.g. phentolamine, prazosin, terazosin, doxozosin)
	      3. peripheral-acting adrenergic inhibitors (e.g. reserpine, guanethidine, guanadrel)
	      4. ganglionic blocking agents (e.g. mecamylamine, trimethaphan)
	      5. beta-adrenergic blockers (e.g. propranolol, metoprolol, atenolol, nadolol, acebutolol)
	      6. combined alpha- and beta-adrenergic blockers (e.g. labetalol)
	    b. direct-acting vasodilators (e.g. minoxidil, hydralazine, sodium nitroprusside, nitroglycerin, diazoxide); this group of medications is most often used when immediate reduction of B/P is necessary
	    c. angiotensin-converting enzyme inhibitors (e.g. captopril, lisinopril, enalapril, fosinopril, quinapril, ramipril, benazepril)
	    d. calcium-channel blocking agents (e.g. nifedipine, verapamil, isradipine, nicardipine, diltiazem, amlodipine, felodipine)
	    e. angiotensin II receptor antagonists (e.g. losartan)
	    f. diuretics

2. perform actions *to reduce sympathetic nervous system stimulation:*
   a. implement measures to reduce fear and anxiety (see Nursing Diagnosis 5, action b)
   b. implement measures to relieve headache (see Nursing Diagnosis 2, action e)
   c. implement measures to promote rest (see Nursing Diagnosis 3, action b.1)
3. discourage excessive intake of beverages high in caffeine such as coffee, tea, and colas
4. discourage smoking *(nicotine causes vasoconstriction)*
5. maintain dietary sodium restrictions as ordered *to reduce fluid retention.*
   c. Consult physician if signs and symptoms of diminished tissue perfusion persist or worsen.

---

2. NURSING DIAGNOSIS: **Pain: headache**

related to distention of the cerebral blood vessels associated with increased vascular pressure.

Desired Outcome	Nursing Actions and *Selected Purposes/Rationales*

2. The client will obtain relief of headache as evidenced by:
a. verbalization of same
b. relaxed facial expression and body positioning
c. increased participation in activities.
	2.a. Assess for signs and symptoms of headache (e.g. statements of same, restlessness, irritability, grimacing, rubbing head, avoidance of bright lights and noises, reluctance to move).
	b. Assess client's perception of the severity of the headache using a pain intensity rating scale.
	c. Assess the client's pain pattern (e.g. location, quality, onset, duration, precipitating factors, aggravating factors, alleviating factors).
	d. Ask the client to describe previous experiences with headaches and methods used to manage them effectively.
	e. Implement measures *to relieve headache:*
	  1. perform actions to reduce blood pressure (see Nursing Diagnosis 1, action b)
	  2. perform actions *to reduce fear and anxiety about the pain experience* (e.g. assure client that his/her need for headache relief is understood, plan methods for relieving headache with client)
	  3. perform action to reduce fear and anxiety (see Nursing Diagnosis 5, action b) *in order to promote relaxation and subsequently increase the client's threshold and tolerance for pain*
	  4. administer analgesics before activities and procedures that can cause headache and before headache becomes severe
	  5. perform actions *to minimize environmental stimuli* (e.g. provide a quiet environment, dim lights)
	  6. avoid jarring bed or startling client *to minimize risk of sudden movements*
	  7. provide or assist with nonpharmacologic measures for headache relief (e.g. cool cloth to forehead, back and neck massage, elevation of head, relaxation exercises, diversional activities)
	  8. administer analgesics if ordered.
	f. Consult physician if above measures fail to relieve headache.

3. NURSING DIAGNOSIS: **Activity intolerance**

related to:
a. decreased tissue oxygenation associated with inadequate tissue perfusion;
b. difficulty resting and sleeping associated with fear, anxiety, frequent assessments, and headache.

Desired Outcome	Nursing Actions and *Selected Purposes/Rationales*

3. The client will demonstrate an increased tolerance for activity as evidenced by:
  a. verbalization of feeling less fatigued and weak
  b. ability to perform activities of daily living without exertional dyspnea, chest pain, diaphoresis, dizziness, and a significant change in vital signs.

3.a. Assess for signs and symptoms of activity intolerance:
  1. statements of fatigue or weakness
  2. exertional dyspnea, chest pain, diaphoresis, or dizziness
  3. abnormal heart rate response to activity (e.g. increase in rate of 20 beats/minute above resting rate, rate not returning to preactivity level within 3 minutes after stopping activity, change from regular to irregular rate)
  4. decreased systolic B/P or a significant increase (10–15 mm Hg) in diastolic pressure with activity.
  b. Implement measures *to improve activity tolerance:*
    1. perform actions *to promote rest and/or conserve energy:*
      a. maintain activity restrictions as ordered
      b. minimize environmental activity and noise
      c. organize nursing care to allow for periods of uninterrupted rest
      d. limit the number of visitors and their length of stay
      e. assist client with self-care activities as needed
      f. keep supplies and personal articles within easy reach
      g. instruct client in energy-saving techniques (e.g. using shower chair when showering, sitting to brush teeth or comb hair)
      h. implement measures to reduce fear and anxiety (see Nursing Diagnosis 5, action b)
      i. implement measures to relieve headache (see Nursing Diagnosis 2, action e)
    2. perform actions to reduce blood pressure (see Nursing Diagnosis 1, action b) *in order to improve tissue perfusion and subsequent tissue oxygenation*
    3. increase client's activity gradually as allowed and tolerated.
  c. Instruct client to:
    1. report a decreased tolerance for activity
    2. stop any activity that causes chest pain, shortness of breath, dizziness, or extreme fatigue or weakness.
  d. Consult physician if signs and symptoms of activity intolerance persist or worsen.

4. COLLABORATIVE DIAGNOSES: **Potential complications of hypertension:**

a. **cerebrovascular accident** related to cerebral thrombosis, embolism, or hemorrhage associated with injury to the arterial walls resulting from atherosclerosis and/or a prolonged increase in pressure in the cerebral vessels;
b. **hypertensive encephalopathy** related to excessive cerebral blood flow (results from decompensation of usual autoregulatory mechanisms in response to markedly elevated blood pressure) and the subsequent increase in intracranial pressure;
c. **angina and/or myocardial infarction** related to:
  1. insufficient myocardial blood flow associated with coronary artery disease (a sequela of inadequately controlled hypertension)

2. myocardial oxygen demands exceeding the oxygen supply (a result of the increased cardiac workload that occurs with increased vascular resistance);
d. **impaired renal function** related to vascular changes in the kidneys associated with effects of prolonged or severe hypertension;
e. **heart failure** related to the prolonged increase in cardiac workload associated with increased systemic vascular resistance;
f. **aortic dissection** related to a severe or prolonged increase in pressure in the aorta.

Desired Outcomes	Nursing Actions and *Selected Purposes/Rationales*
4.a. The client will not experience a cerebrovascular accident or hypertensive encephalopathy as evidenced by: 1. absence of dizziness, syncope, visual disturbances, and speech impairments 2. absence or resolution of headache 3. absence of vomiting 4. mentally alert and oriented 5. pupils equal and normally reactive to light 6. normal sensory and motor function.	4.a.1. Assess for and report signs and symptoms of a cerebrovascular accident and/or hypertensive encephalopathy: a. dizziness, syncope b. visual disturbances (e.g. diplopia, scotoma, blurred vision, loss of vision) c. slurred speech, expressive or receptive aphasia d. persistent or increasing headache e. vomiting f. decreased level of consciousness g. unequal pupils or a sluggish or absent pupillary reaction to light h. paresthesias, facial ptosis, weakness of extremity, paralysis i. seizures. 2. Implement measures *to reduce the risk of a cerebrovascular accident and hypertensive encephalopathy:* a. perform actions to reduce blood pressure (see Nursing Diagnosis 1, action b) b. instruct client to avoid activities that create a Valsalva response (e.g. straining to have a bowel movement, holding breath while moving up in bed) *in order to prevent a sudden increase in intracranial pressure* c. keep head of bed elevated at least 30° and encourage client to keep head and neck in proper alignment *in order to promote adequate venous return from the cerebral vessels.* 3. If signs and symptoms of a cerebrovascular accident or hypertensive encephalopathy occur: a. continue with above measures b. administer antihypertensive agents that may be ordered to provide rapid blood pressure reduction (e.g. sodium nitroprusside, labetalol, phentolamine, nifedipine, enalaprilat) c. maintain client on bed rest d. initiate appropriate safety measures (e.g. side rails up, seizure precautions) e. administer osmotic diuretics (e.g. mannitol) and corticosteroids (e.g. dexamethasone) if ordered *to decrease cerebral edema* f. provide emotional support to client and significant others g. refer to Care Plan on Cerebrovascular Accident for additional care measures if signs and symptoms persist.
4.b. The client will not experience episodes of myocardial ischemia as evidenced by: 1. absence of chest pain 2. unlabored respirations at 14–20/minute 3. cardiac enzymes within normal range 4. absence of ST segment elevation, peaked T	4.b.1. Assess for signs and symptoms of myocardial ischemia (e.g. chest pain, dyspnea). 2. Implement measures *to prevent myocardial ischemia:* a. perform actions to reduce blood pressure (see Nursing Diagnosis 1, action b) b. instruct client to avoid activities that create a Valsalva response (e.g. straining to have a bowel movement, holding breath while moving up in bed) c. increase activity gradually as allowed and tolerated. 3. If signs and symptoms of myocardial ischemia occur: a. consult physician about an order for cardiac enzyme/isoenzyme

Desired Outcomes	Nursing Actions and *Selected Purposes/Rationales*

waves or T wave inversion, and abnormal Q waves on ECG readings.	levels and ECG; report significant elevation of cardiac enzymes and ST segment elevation, T wave changes, and/or abnormal Q waves on ECG reading
	b. maintain client on strict bed rest in a semi- to high Fowler's position
	c. maintain oxygen therapy as ordered
	d. administer the following medications if ordered:
	  1. nitrates *to improve coronary blood flow and reduce myocardial oxygen requirements*
	  2. morphine sulfate *to reduce pain and anxiety and decrease cardiac workload*
	  3. beta-adrenergic blocking agents *to reduce myocardial oxygen requirements by decreasing heart rate and the force of myocardial contractility*
	e. provide emotional support to client and significant others
	f. refer to Care Plans on Angina Pectoris and Myocardial Infarction for additional care measures.

4.c. The client will maintain adequate renal function as evidenced by:
  1. urine output at least 30 ml/hour
  2. absence of proteinuria
  3. BUN, serum creatinine, and creatinine clearance within normal range.
	4.c.1. Assess for and report signs and symptoms of impaired renal function (e.g. nocturia, urine output less than 30 ml/hour, urine specific gravity fixed at or less than 1.010, proteinuria, elevated BUN and serum creatinine levels).
	  2. Collect a 24-hour urine specimen if ordered. Report decreased creatinine clearance.
	  3. Implement measures *to maintain adequate renal blood flow:*
	    a. perform actions to reduce blood pressure (see Nursing Diagnosis 1, action b)
	    b. maintain an adequate fluid intake *to reduce risk of dehydration.*
	  4. If signs and symptoms of impaired renal function occur:
	    a. continue with above actions
	    b. consult physician about lowering the dose of or discontinuing angiotensin-converting enzyme inhibitors if BUN and serum creatinine continue to rise significantly (ACE inhibitors should be used cautiously in persons with impaired renal function *because they can have an adverse effect on renal function*)
	    c. assess for and report signs of acute renal failure (e.g. oliguria or anuria; weight gain; edema; increasing B/P; lethargy and confusion; increasing BUN and serum creatinine, phosphorus, and potassium levels)
	    d. prepare client for dialysis if indicated
	    e. refer to Care Plan on Renal Failure for additional care measures.

4.d. The client will not develop heart failure as evidenced by:
  1. pulse 60–100 beats/minute
  2. absence of an S_3 heart sound
  3. usual mental status
  4. clear, audible breath sounds
  5. absence of dyspnea, orthopnea, and cough
  6. increased strength and activity tolerance
  7. skin warm and dry
  8. palpable peripheral pulses
  9. urine output at least 30 ml/hour
  10. stable weight
  11. absence of edema; distended neck veins;
	4.d.1. Assess for and report signs and symptoms of heart failure:
	    a. tachycardia
	    b. presence of an S_3 heart sound
	    c. restlessness, agitation, confusion, or other change in mental status
	    d. crackles (rales)
	    e. dyspnea, orthopnea
	    f. dry, hacking cough or cough productive of frothy or blood-tinged sputum
	    g. development of or increased weakness and fatigue
	    h. cool, diaphoretic skin
	    i. diminished or absent peripheral pulses
	    j. decreased urine output
	    k. weight gain
	    l. edema
	    m. distended neck veins
	    n. enlarged, tender liver.
	  2. Monitor chest x-ray results. Report findings of cardiomegaly, pleural effusion, or pulmonary edema.
	  3. Implement measures to reduce blood pressure (see Nursing Diagnosis 1, action b) *in order to reduce cardiac workload and prevent heart failure.*
	  4. If signs and symptoms of heart failure occur:
	    a. continue with above actions

and enlarged, tender liver.

b. maintain oxygen therapy as ordered
c. administer the following medications if ordered:
1. positive inotropic agents (e.g. digitalis preparations, dobutamine, amrinone) *to increase myocardial contractility*
2. diuretics and vasodilators (e.g. nitroglycerin, captopril) *to decrease cardiac workload*
3. morphine sulfate *to reduce preload and anxiety* (used primarily in clients with pulmonary edema)
d. provide emotional support to client and significant others
e. refer to Care Plan on Heart Failure for additional care measures.

4.e. The client will not experience dissection of the aorta as evidenced by:
1. absence of sudden, severe chest pain
2. palpable peripheral pulses with no change in pulse pattern
3. usual sensory and motor function
4. usual mental status
5. stable vital signs
6. skin warm, dry, and usual color.

4.e.1. Assess for and immediately report the following:
a. signs and symptoms of aortic dissection (e.g. sudden, severe chest pain that may radiate to back; abnormal pulse pattern [discrepancies in character, timing, and magnitude] in extremities; sudden lack of pulse in an extremity; hemianesthesia; hemiplegia; paraplegia)
b. signs and symptoms of hypovolemic shock (e.g. restlessness; agitation; significant decrease in B/P; rapid, weak pulse; cool, moist skin; pallor; diminished or absent pulses).
2. Implement measures *to prevent aortic dissection:*
a. perform actions to reduce blood pressure (see Nursing Diagnosis 1, action b)
b. instruct client to avoid activities that create a Valsalva response (e.g. straining to have a bowel movement, holding breath while moving up in bed).
3. If signs and symptoms of aortic dissection occur:
a. maintain client on strict bed rest
b. monitor vital signs frequently
c. administer oxygen as ordered
d. prepare client for diagnostic studies (e.g. aortogram, echocardiogram, computed tomography) if planned
e. administer antihypertensive agents (e.g. sodium nitroprusside or trimethaphan and a beta-adrenergic blocker) if ordered
f. prepare client for surgery if planned
g. provide emotional support to client and significant others.

5. NURSING DIAGNOSIS:

Anxiety

related to necessity for urgent treatment; possibility of severe disability or sudden death; unfamiliar environment; persistent or severe headache; and lack of understanding of diagnostic tests, diagnosis, and treatment plan.

Desired Outcome	Nursing Actions and *Selected Purposes/Rationales*

5. The client will experience a reduction in anxiety as evidenced by:
a. verbalization of feeling less anxious
b. usual sleep pattern
c. relaxed facial expression and body movements
d. vital signs returning to normal range for client
e. usual perceptual ability and interactions with others.

5.a. Assess client for signs and symptoms of anxiety (e.g. verbalization of feeling anxious, insomnia, tenseness, shakiness, restlessness, diaphoresis, tachycardia, further elevation of blood pressure, facial pallor, self-focused behaviors). Validate perceptions carefully, remembering that some behaviors may result from decreased tissue perfusion and neurological changes.
b. Implement measures *to reduce fear and anxiety:*
1. orient client to hospital environment, equipment, and routines
2. provide a calm, restful environment
3. introduce client to staff who will be participating in care; if possible, maintain consistency in staff assigned to his/her care *to provide feelings of stability and comfort with the environment*
4. assure client that staff members are nearby; respond to call signal as soon as possible

Desired Outcome	Nursing Actions and *Selected Purposes/Rationales*
	5. maintain a calm, supportive, confident manner when interacting with client
	6. encourage verbalization of fear and anxiety; provide feedback
	7. explain all diagnostic tests
	8. reinforce physician's explanations and clarify misconceptions the client has about hypertension, the treatment plan, and prognosis
	9. perform actions to relieve headache (see Nursing Diagnosis 2, action e)
	10. instruct client in relaxation techniques and encourage participation in diversional activities
	11. assist client to identify specific stressors and ways to cope with them
	12. provide information based on current needs of client at a level he/she can understand; encourage questions and clarification of information provided
	13. encourage significant others to project a caring, concerned attitude without obvious anxiousness
	14. include significant others in orientation and teaching sessions and encourage their continued support of client
	15. administer prescribed antianxiety agents if indicated.
	c. Consult physician if above actions fail to control fear and anxiety.

---

6. NURSING DIAGNOSIS: **Ineffective management of therapeutic regimen**

related to:
a. lack of understanding of the implications of not following the prescribed treatment plan;
b. difficulty modifying personal habits (e.g. alcohol intake, dietary preferences);
c. undesirable side effects of some antihypertensive agents;
d. insufficient financial resources.

Desired Outcome	Nursing Actions and *Selected Purposes/Rationales*
6. The client will demonstrate the probability of effective management of the therapeutic regimen as evidenced by: a. willingness to learn about and participate in treatments and care b. statements reflecting ways to modify personal habits c. statements reflecting an understanding of the implications of not following the prescribed treatment plan.	6.a. Assess for indications that the client may be unable to effectively manage the therapeutic regimen: 1. statements reflecting inability to manage care at home 2. failure to adhere to treatment plan while in hospital (e.g. not adhering to dietary modifications, refusing medications) 3. statements reflecting a lack of understanding of factors that may cause progression of hypertension 4. statements reflecting an unwillingness or inability to modify personal habits 5. statements reflecting view that hypertension will reverse itself or that the situation is hopeless and efforts to comply with the therapeutic regimen are useless 6. statements reflecting that the side effects of medications are too uncomfortable and that he/she feels better when not taking medication 7. statements reflecting that medications are too expensive. b. Implement measures *to promote effective management of the therapeutic regimen:* 1. explain hypertension in terms the client can understand; stress the fact that hypertension is a chronic condition and that adherence to the treatment plan is necessary in order to delay and/or prevent complications

2. encourage questions and clarify misconceptions client has about hypertension and its effects and the side effects of medications

3. provide instructions on and encourage client to participate in the treatment plan (e.g. calculating sodium intake, monitoring blood pressure); determine areas of misunderstanding and reinforce teaching as necessary

4. provide client with written instructions about dietary modifications, signs and symptoms to report, medication therapy, blood pressure monitoring, and exercise regimen

5. assist client to identify ways medication regimen, exercise, and dietary modifications can be incorporated into life style; focus on modifications of life style rather than complete change

6. assist client to identify a reward system for self that will assist him/her to effect necessary change(s)

7. initiate and reinforce discharge teaching outlined in Nursing Diagnosis 7 *in order to promote a sense of control*

8. provide information about and encourage utilization of community resources that can assist client to make necessary life-style changes (e.g. cardiovascular fitness, weight loss, and smoking cessation programs; stress management classes)

9. encourage client to discuss concerns about the cost of medications and visits with health care provider; obtain a social service consult to assist with financial planning and to obtain financial aid if indicated

10. encourage client to attend follow-up educational classes

11. reinforce behaviors suggesting future compliance with the therapeutic regimen (e.g. statements reflecting plans for adhering to treatment plan, statements reflecting an understanding of hypertension and its long-term effects)

12. include significant others in explanations and teaching sessions and encourage their support; reinforce the need for client to assume responsibility for managing as much of care as possible.

c. Consult physician regarding referrals to community health agencies if continued instruction or support is needed.

Discharge Teaching

---

7. NURSING DIAGNOSIS: **Knowledge deficit or Altered health maintenance***

*The nurse should select the diagnostic label that is most appropriate for the client's discharge teaching needs.

Desired Outcomes	Nursing Actions and *Selected Purposes/Rationales*
7.a. The client will verbalize a basic understanding of hypertension and its effects on the body.	7.a.1. Explain hypertension and its effects in terms client can understand. Utilize available teaching aids (e.g. pamphlets, videotapes). 2. Inform client that hypertension is often asymptomatic and that absence of symptoms is not a reliable indication that blood pressure is within a safe range.
7.b. The client will identify modifiable risk factors for hypertension and ways to alter these factors.	7.b.1. Inform client that the following modifiable factors have been shown to contribute to hypertension: a. obesity b. lack of regular aerobic exercise c. daily alcohol intake exceeding 1 oz of ethanol (i.e. 2 oz of 100-proof whiskey, 8 oz of wine, 24 oz of beer) on a regular basis d. excessive sodium intake e. stressful life style.

Desired Outcomes	Nursing Actions and *Selected Purposes/Rationales*
	2. Assist the client to identify ways he/she can make appropriate changes in life style to modify the above factors. Provide information about weight reduction plans, stress management classes, and smoking cessation and alcohol rehabilitation programs. Initiate a referral if indicated.
	3. Instruct client to participate in a regular isotonic exercise program (e.g. walking, swimming) and avoid isometric exercise (e.g. weight training). Caution client to consult physician before beginning an exercise program.
	4. If client is taking an oral contraceptive, instruct her to consult physician regarding other methods of birth control.
7.c. The client will verbalize an understanding of medications ordered including rationale, food and drug interactions, side effects, schedule for taking, and importance of taking as prescribed.	7.c.1. Explain the rationale for, side effects of, and importance of taking medications prescribed. Inform client of pertinent food and drug interactions.
	2. If client is discharged on a diuretic, instruct to:
	a. take once-daily dose in the morning or, if diuretic is to be taken twice each day, take the larger dose in the morning and the second dose no later than 3:00 p.m. (scheduling doses in this manner minimizes nighttime urination)
	b. weigh self as often as instructed (e.g. daily, weekly) and keep a record of weights
	c. change from a lying to a standing position slowly if experiencing dizziness or lightheadedness with position change
	d. increase intake of foods/fluids high in potassium (e.g. orange juice, bananas, cantaloupe, potatoes, raisins, apricots) if taking a potassium-depleting diuretic
	e. notify physician if unable to tolerate food or fluids (dehydration can develop rapidly if intake is poor and client continues to take a diuretic)
	f. avoid salt substitutes with a high potassium content if discharged on a potassium-sparing diuretic (e.g. triamterene, spironolactone)
	g. report the following signs and symptoms:
	1. weight loss of more than 5 pounds a week
	2. excessive thirst
	3. severe dizziness or episodes of fainting
	4. muscle weakness or cramping, nausea, vomiting, or an irregular pulse.
	3. If client is discharged on an antihypertensive agent such as an adrenergic inhibiting agent, direct-acting vasodilator, calcium-channel blocker, or angiotensin-converting enzyme inhibitor, instruct to:
	a. change from a lying to standing position slowly if experiencing dizziness or lightheadedness with position change
	b. avoid strenuous exercise (especially in hot weather), hot baths and showers, steam room, and sauna
	c. limit alcohol intake
	d. report continued dizziness, lightheadedness, or fainting
	e. report side effects such as impotence, dry mouth, and unusual mood changes if they persist more than a few weeks.
	4. Instruct client to take medication on a regular basis and avoid skipping doses, altering prescribed dose, making up for missed doses, and discontinuing medication without first discussing with health care provider.
	5. Instruct the client to consult physician before taking other prescription and nonprescription medications.
7.d. The client will verbalize an understanding of the rationale for and components of the recommended diet.	7.d.1. Explain the rationale for the recommended dietary modifications.
	2. Depending on the physician's recommendations:
	a. provide the following information about decreasing sodium intake:
	1. be aware that the terms salt and sodium are often used interchangeably but are not synonymous; there is 40% sodium in table salt

    2. read labels on foods/fluids and calculate sodium content of items; avoid those products that tend to have a high sodium content (e.g. canned soups and vegetables, tomato juice, commercial baked goods, commercially prepared frozen or canned entrees and sauces)

    3. do not add salt when cooking foods or to prepared foods; use low-sodium herbs and spices if desired

    4. avoid cured and smoked foods

    5. avoid salty snack foods (e.g. crackers, nuts, pretzels, potato chips)

    6. avoid commercially prepared fast foods

    7. avoid routine use of over-the-counter medications with a high sodium content (e.g. Alka-Seltzer, some antacids such as Gaviscon)

  b. provide instructions on ways the client can reduce intake of saturated fat and cholesterol:

    1. reduce intake of red meat

    2. trim visible fat off meat and remove all skin from poultry

    3. use vegetable oil rather than coconut or palm oil in cooking and food preparation

    4. use cooking methods such as steaming, baking, broiling, poaching, microwaving, and grilling rather than frying

    5. restrict intake of eggs (recommendations about the number of whole eggs allowed per week vary depending on the client's lipid levels)

    6. avoid commercial baked goods

    7. avoid dairy products containing more than 1% fat.

  3. Instruct client to include the recommended daily allowances of potassium, calcium, and magnesium in diet.

7.e. The client will state signs and symptoms to report to the health care provider.	7.e. Instruct the client to report:
	  1. persistent headache or headache present upon awakening
	  2. sudden and continued increase in B/P (if B/P is monitored at home)
	  3. chest pain
	  4. shortness of breath
	  5. significant weight gain or swelling of feet or ankles
	  6. changes in vision
	  7. frequent or uncontrollable nosebleeds
	  8. severe depression or emotional lability
	  9. persistent dizziness, lightheadedness, or fainting
	  10. persistent side effects experienced from use of antihypertensive medications (e.g. impotence, dry mouth)
	  11. side effects of diuretic therapy (see action c.2.g in this diagnosis).

7.f. The client will identify community resources that can assist in making life-style changes necessary for effective control of hypertension.	7.f.1. Provide information regarding community resources and support groups that can assist client in making life-style changes that are necessary for effective control of hypertension (e.g. cardiovascular fitness, weight loss, and smoking cessation programs; stress management classes). 2. Initiate a referral if indicated.

7.g. The client will verbalize an understanding of and a plan for adhering to recommended follow-up care including future appointments with health care provider and activity level.	7.g.1. Reinforce the importance of keeping follow-up appointments with health care provider and continuing lifelong medical supervision.
	  2. Reinforce the physician's instructions regarding activity level.
	  3. Refer to Nursing Diagnosis 6, action b, for measures to promote client's ability to effectively manage the therapeutic regimen.

Bibliography

See pages 897–898 and 903.

MYOCARDIAL INFARCTION

A myocardial infarction (MI) is a result of prolonged ischemia of the heart muscle and occurs when blood flow to an area of the myocardium is insufficient to meet the myocardial oxygen requirements. Sustained ischemia causes tissue necrosis and irreversible cellular damage, which results in disturbances in mechanical, biochemical, and electrical function in the necrotic or infarcted area. The degree of altered function depends on the area of the heart involved and the size of the infarct.

Infarctions have traditionally been classified as transmural (involving the full thickness of the myocardium) or subendocardial (nontransmural), which involves only a partial thickness of the myocardium. They are now often classified as Q-wave or non-Q-wave infarctions depending on the presence or absence of an abnormal Q wave on the electrocardiogram. With a non-Q-wave infarction, there is early spontaneous restoration of blood flow, whereas with a Q-wave infarction, the coronary occlusion is sustained long enough to cause extensive necrosis. An MI is most frequently caused by thrombosis of an atherosclerotic coronary artery. Other less common causes include spasm of a coronary artery, severe or prolonged hypotension, a rapid ventricular rate, and cocaine use.

The classic symptom of an MI is intense chest pain that is described as a tight, heavy, squeezing, or crushing sensation; may radiate to the left arm, neck, jaw, or back; lasts longer than 20 minutes; and is unrelieved by nitroglycerin and rest. However 15% to 25% of infarctions go unrecognized because clients have only mild or no chest discomfort. Other signs and symptoms may include shortness of breath, diaphoresis, anxiousness, weakness, pallor, nausea, and vomiting.

The extent of myocardial damage can be limited by early (within 4–6 hours of the onset) restoration of coronary blood flow. This can be accomplished by injection of a thrombolytic agent to dissolve the clot obstructing the coronary artery or by a coronary angioplasty. Intravenous magnesium may also be given in the first few hours of the onset of an MI to reduce ventricular dysrhythmias, dilate the coronary arteries, and inhibit platelet aggregation. The prognosis for a client who has had an MI is largely influenced by size and location of the infarct, concurrent cardiovascular status, and promptness and effectiveness of treatment.

This care plan focuses on the adult client hospitalized during an episode of intense chest pain for definitive diagnosis and management of a myocardial infarction. The goals of care are to relieve pain, improve cardiac output, reduce fear and anxiety, prevent complications, and educate the client regarding follow-up care.

DIAGNOSTIC TESTS

Electrocardiogram (ECG)
Cardiac enzymes/isoenzymes
Radionuclide imaging
Coronary angiography or cardiac catheterization
Echocardiography
Blood gases and chemistry
Oximetry
WBC count
Exercise stress testing

DISCHARGE CRITERIA

Prior to discharge, the client will:

- have adequate cardiac output and tissue perfusion
- tolerate prescribed activity without a significant change in vital signs, chest pain, dyspnea, dizziness, or extreme fatigue or weakness
- verbalize a basic understanding of a myocardial infarction
- demonstrate accuracy in counting pulse
- identify modifiable cardiovascular risk factors and ways to alter these factors
- verbalize an understanding of the rationale for and components of a diet restricted in saturated fat and cholesterol
- verbalize an understanding of medications ordered including rationale, food and drug interactions, side effects, schedule for taking, and importance of taking as prescribed
- verbalize an understanding of activity restrictions and the rate at which activity can be progressed
- state signs and symptoms to report to the health care provider
- identify community resources that can assist with cardiac rehabilitation and adjustment to the effects of a myocardial infarction

■ share feelings and concerns about changes in body functioning and usual roles and life style

■ verbalize an understanding of and a plan for adhering to recommended follow-up care including future appointments with health care provider.

NURSING/ COLLABORATIVE DIAGNOSES	**1.** Decreased cardiac output △ 373
	2. Pain: chest pain that may radiate to arm, neck, jaw, or back △ 375
	3. Activity intolerance △ 375
	4. Sleep pattern disturbance △ 376
	5. Potential complications:
	a. cardiac dysrhythmias
	b. heart failure
	c. thromboembolism
	d. rupture of a portion of the heart (e.g. ventricular free wall, interventricular septum, papillary muscle)
	e. pericarditis
	f. infarct extension or recurrence
	g. cardiogenic shock △ 377
	6. Anxiety △ 381
	7. Grieving △ 382
DISCHARGE TEACHING	**8.** Knowledge deficit, Ineffective management of therapeutic regimen, or Altered health maintenance △ 383

1. NURSING DIAGNOSIS:

Decreased cardiac output

related to decreased contractility and altered conductivity of the heart associated with the myocardial damage that has occurred with infarction.

Desired Outcome	Nursing Actions and *Selected Purposes/Rationales*

1. The client will have improved cardiac output as evidenced by:
a. B/P within normal range for client
b. apical pulse between 60–100 beats/minute and regular
c. resolution of gallop rhythm(s)
d. increased strength and activity tolerance
e. unlabored respirations at 14–20/minute
f. clear, audible breath sounds
g. usual mental status
h. absence of vertigo and syncope
i. palpable peripheral pulses
	1.a. Assess for and report the following:
	  1. diagnostic findings indicative of an MI:
	    a. elevated CK (CPK)-MB
	    b. elevated LDH with an LDH_1 level that is higher than the LDH_2 (a reliable indicator of an acute MI)
	    c. elevated WBC count and/or AST (SGOT); these tests are not specific for myocardial injury but support the diagnosis when CK-MB and LDH are elevated
	    d. temperature elevation (reflects tissue destruction and resulting inflammation)
	    e. ECG showing ST segment elevation, peaked T waves or inversion of T waves, and/or presence of abnormal Q waves (there may be no Q waves and the ST segment may be depressed if client has had a subendocardial infarction)
	    f. presence of an S_4 heart sound
	  2. signs and symptoms of decreased cardiac output:
	    a. variations in B/P (may be increased because of pain or compensatory vasoconstriction; may be decreased when compensatory mechanisms and pump fail)
	    b. tachycardia
	    c. presence of gallop rhythm(s)

Desired Outcome	Nursing Actions and *Selected Purposes/Rationales*

j. improved skin temperature and color

k. capillary refill time less than 3 seconds

l. urine output at least 30 ml/hour

m. absence of edema and jugular vein distention.

d. fatigue and weakness

e. dyspnea, orthopnea, tachypnea

f. crackles (rales)

g. restlessness, anxiousness, confusion, or other change in mental status

h. vertigo, syncope

i. diminished or absent peripheral pulses

j. cool, moist skin

k. pallor or cyanosis of skin

l. capillary refill time greater than 3 seconds

m. oliguria

n. edema

o. jugular vein distention (JVD).

b. Monitor for and report the following:

  1. chest x-ray results showing pulmonary vascular congestion, pulmonary edema, or pleural effusion

  2. abnormal blood gases

  3. significant decrease in oximetry results.

c. Implement measures *to improve cardiac output:*

  1. prepare client for procedures that may be performed *to improve coronary blood flow:*

    a. injection of a thrombolytic agent (e.g. streptokinase, tissue plasminogen activator [tPA], anistreplase [APSAC, Eminase])

    b. percutaneous coronary revascularization (e.g. balloon angioplasty, atherectomy, intracoronary stenting)

    c. insertion of an intra-aortic balloon pump (IABP)

  2. perform actions *to reduce cardiac workload:*

    a. maintain activity restrictions as ordered

    b. place client in a semi- to high Fowler's position

    c. instruct client to avoid activities that create a Valsalva response (e.g. straining to have a bowel movement, holding breath while moving up in bed) *in order to prevent the marked increase in venous return and preload that occurs with exhalation*

    d. implement measures to promote rest and conserve energy (see Nursing Diagnosis 3, action b.1)

    e. maintain oxygen therapy as ordered

    f. discourage smoking (*smoke has a cardiostimulatory effect, causes vasoconstriction, and reduces oxygen availability*)

    g. provide small meals rather than large ones (*large meals require an increase in blood supply to gastrointestinal tract for digestion*)

    h. discourage excessive intake of beverages high in caffeine such as coffee, tea, and colas (*caffeine is a myocardial stimulant and can increase myocardial oxygen consumption*)

    i. restrict sodium intake if ordered *to prevent fluid retention*

    j. increase activity gradually as allowed and tolerated

  3. administer the following medications if ordered:

    a. nitrates (e.g. nitroglycerin) *to dilate the coronary and peripheral (primarily venous) blood vessels and subsequently improve coronary blood flow and reduce cardiac workload and myocardial oxygen requirements*

    b. beta-adrenergic blocking agents (e.g. atenolol, metoprolol) *to decrease the incidence of dysrhythmias and to reduce myocardial oxygen requirements by decreasing heart rate and the force of myocardial contractility*

    c. calcium-channel blocking agents (e.g. diltiazem) *to reduce coronary vasospasm and reduce the risk for infarct extension or reinfarction* (primary uses are for treatment of postinfarction angina, to prevent vasospasm following percutaneous transluminal coronary angioplasty [PTCA], and to reduce the risk for reinfarction in persons with non-Q-wave infarctions)

    d. angiotensin-converting enzyme (ACE) inhibitors such as captopril (*have been shown to reduce the incidence of reinfarction and heart failure following myocardial infarction*)

    e. antidysrhythmics (e.g. lidocaine, procainamide, metoprolol, atenolol, diltiazem, atropine) if dysrhythmias are present

    f. anticoagulants (e.g. intravenous heparin) and antiplatelet agents (e.g. low-dose aspirin) *to prevent reocclusion of the coronary artery(ies) by thrombosis.*

d. Consult physician if signs and symptoms of decreased cardiac output persist or worsen.

---

2. NURSING DIAGNOSIS: **Pain: chest pain that may radiate to arm, neck, jaw, or back**

related to myocardial ischemia (a decreased oxygen supply forces the myocardium to convert to anaerobic metabolism; the end products of anaerobic metabolism act as irritants to myocardial neural receptors).

Desired Outcome	Nursing Actions and *Selected Purposes/Rationales*

2. The client will experience pain relief as evidenced by:
  a. verbalization of same
  b. relaxed facial expression and body positioning
  c. increased participation in activities
  d. stable vital signs.
	2.a. Assess for signs and symptoms of pain (e.g. verbalization of pain; grimacing; rubbing neck, jaw, or arm; reluctance to move; clutching chest; restlessness; diaphoresis; facial pallor; increased B/P; tachycardia).
	  b. Assess client's perception of the severity of the pain using a pain intensity rating scale.
	  c. Assess the client's pain pattern (e.g. location, quality, onset, duration, precipitating factors, aggravating factors, alleviating factors).
	  d. Implement measures *to relieve pain:*
	    1. maintain oxygen therapy as ordered *to increase the myocardial oxygen supply*
	    2. maintain client on bed rest in a semi- to high Fowler's position
	    3. administer the following medications if ordered:
	      a. narcotic (opioid) analgesics (an intravenous rather than an intramuscular route should be used *because intramuscular injections are poorly absorbed if tissue perfusion is decreased; intramuscular injections also elevate serum enzyme levels, which may interfere with assessment of myocardial damage*)
	      b. nitrates (e.g. nitroglycerin)
	    4. implement additional measures to improve cardiac output (see Nursing Diagnosis 1, action c) *in order to improve myocardial blood flow and oxygenation*
	    5. provide or assist with nonpharmacologic measures for pain relief (e.g. relaxation exercises, restful environment).
	  e. Consult physician if above measures fail to provide adequate pain relief.

---

3. NURSING DIAGNOSIS: **Activity intolerance**

related to:
a. tissue hypoxia associated with decreased cardiac output;
b. difficulty resting and sleeping associated with pain, frequent assessments and treatments, fear, and anxiety.

Desired Outcome	Nursing Actions and **Selected Purposes/Rationales**

3. The client will demonstrate an increased tolerance for activity as evidenced by:
  a. verbalization of feeling less fatigued and weak
  b. ability to perform activities of daily living without exertional dyspnea, chest pain, diaphoresis, dizziness, and a significant change in vital signs.
	3.a. Assess for signs and symptoms of activity intolerance:
	  1. statements of fatigue or weakness
	  2. exertional dyspnea, chest pain, diaphoresis, or dizziness
	  3. abnormal heart rate response to activity (e.g. increase in rate of 20 beats/minute above resting rate, rate not returning to preactivity level within 3 minutes after stopping activity, change from regular to irregular rate)
	  4. decreased systolic B/P or a significant increase (10–15 mm Hg) in diastolic pressure with activity.
	  b. Implement measures *to improve activity tolerance:*
	    1. perform actions *to promote rest and/or conserve energy:*
	      a. maintain activity restrictions as ordered
	      b. minimize environmental activity and noise
	      c. organize nursing care to allow for periods of uninterrupted rest
	      d. limit the number of visitors and their length of stay
	      e. assist client with self-care activities as needed
	      f. keep supplies and personal articles within easy reach
	      g. instruct client in energy-saving techniques (e.g. using shower chair when showering, sitting to brush teeth or comb hair)
	      h. implement measures to reduce fear and anxiety (see Nursing Diagnosis 6, action b)
	      i. implement measures to promote sleep (see Nursing Diagnosis 4, action c)
	      j. implement measures to relieve pain (see Nursing Diagnosis 2, action d)
	    2. perform actions to improve cardiac output (see Nursing Diagnosis 1, action c)
	    3. maintain oxygen therapy as ordered
	    4. increase client's activity gradually as allowed and tolerated.
	  c. Instruct client to:
	    1. report a decreased tolerance for activity
	    2. stop any activity that causes chest pain, shortness of breath, dizziness, or extreme fatigue or weakness.
	  d. Consult physician if signs and symptoms of activity intolerance persist or worsen.

■━━━

4. NURSING DIAGNOSIS: **Sleep pattern disturbance**

related to pain, frequent assessments and treatments, fear, and anxiety.

Desired Outcome	Nursing Actions and **Selected Purposes/Rationales**

4. The client will attain optimal amounts of sleep as evidenced by:
  a. statements of feeling well rested
  b. usual mental status
  c. absence of frequent yawning, dark circles under eyes, and hand tremors.
	4.a. Assess for signs and symptoms of a sleep pattern disturbance (e.g. statements of difficulty falling asleep, sleep interruptions, or not feeling well rested; irritability; lethargy; disorientation; frequent yawning; dark circles under eyes; slight hand tremors).
	  b. Determine the client's usual sleep habits.
	  c. Implement measures *to promote sleep:*
	    1. discourage long periods of sleep during the day unless signs and symptoms of sleep deprivation exist or daytime sleep is usual for client
	    2. perform actions to relieve pain (see Nursing Diagnosis 2, action d)

3. perform actions to reduce fear and anxiety (see Nursing Diagnosis 6, action b)
4. encourage participation in relaxing diversional activities during the evening
5. discourage intake of fluids high in caffeine (e.g. coffee, tea, colas), especially in the evening
6. offer client an evening snack that includes milk or cheese unless contraindicated (*the L-tryptophan in milk and cheese helps induce and maintain sleep*)
7. allow client to continue usual sleep practices (e.g. position; time; presleep routines such as reading, watching television, listening to music, and meditating) unless contraindicated
8. satisfy basic needs such as comfort and warmth before sleep
9. encourage client to urinate just before bedtime
10. reduce environmental distractions (e.g. close door to client's room; use night light rather than overhead light whenever possible; lower volume of paging system; keep staff conversations at a low level and away from client's room; close curtains between clients in a semi-private room or ward; keep beepers and alarms on low volume; provide client with "white noise" such as tape-recorded sounds of the ocean or rain; have earplugs available for client if needed)
11. administer prescribed sedative-hypnotics if indicated
12. perform actions *to reduce interruptions during sleep (80–100 minutes of uninterrupted sleep is usually needed to complete one sleep cycle)*:
    a. restrict visitors
    b. group care (e.g. medications, treatments, physical care, assessments) whenever possible.
d. Consult physician if signs and symptoms of sleep deprivation persist or worsen.

---

5. COLLABORATIVE DIAGNOSES:

Potential complications of myocardial infarction:

a. **cardiac dysrhythmias** related to impaired nodal function and/or altered myocardial conductivity associated with damage to the myocardium, hypoxia, sympathetic nervous system stimulation (a response to low cardiac output, pain, and anxiety), reperfusion of ischemic area, and possible electrolyte and acid-base imbalances;
b. **heart failure** related to impaired diastolic and systolic function of the heart associated with decreased compliance and contractility of the infarcted area;
c. **thromboembolism** related to:
    1. stasis of blood in the cardiac chambers associated with incomplete emptying
    2. formation of mural thrombi on the infarcted endocardium
    3. venous stasis associated with peripheral pooling of blood if activity restrictions are prolonged;
d. **rupture of a portion of the heart (e.g. ventricular free wall, interventricular septum, papillary muscle)** related to thinning and weakening of the necrotic area in the myocardium;
e. **pericarditis** related to an inflammatory response to epicardial necrosis;
f. **infarct extension or recurrence** related to insufficient myocardial blood supply to meet the myocardial oxygen requirements associated with decreased cardiac output or reocclusion of coronary artery(ies);
g. **cardiogenic shock** related to inability of damaged heart, intrinsic compensatory mechanisms, and treatment measures to maintain adequate tissue perfusion to vital organs (can occur as a result of extensive damage to the left ventricle, severe heart failure, severe or prolonged dysrhythmias, or rupture of the ventricle wall).

Desired Outcomes	Nursing Actions and *Selected Purposes/Rationales*

5.a. The client will maintain normal sinus rhythm as evidenced by:
1. regular apical pulse at 60–100 beats/minute
2. equal apical and radial pulse rates
3. absence of syncope and palpitations
4. ECG reading showing normal sinus rhythm.

5.a.1. Assess for and report signs and symptoms of cardiac dysrhythmias (e.g. irregular apical pulse; pulse rate below 60 or above 100 beats/minute; apical-radial pulse deficit; syncope; palpitations; abnormal rate, rhythm, or configurations on ECG).

2. Implement measures to improve cardiac output (see Nursing Diagnosis 1, action c) *in order to promote adequate myocardial tissue perfusion and oxygenation and reduce the risk of cardiac dysrhythmias.*

3. If cardiac dysrhythmias occur:
   a. initiate cardiac monitoring if not still being done
   b. administer antidysrhythmics (e.g. lidocaine, procainamide, bretylium, digoxin, metoprolol, atenolol, adenosine, diltiazem, verapamil, atropine) if ordered
   c. restrict client's activity based on his/her tolerance and severity of the dysrhythmia
   d. maintain oxygen therapy as ordered
   e. prepare client for electrophysiological studies (EPS) if planned *to diagnose the conduction problem or evaluate the effectiveness of antidysrhythmic agents*
   f. assess cardiovascular status frequently and report signs and symptoms of a further decrease in cardiac output and tissue perfusion
   g. prepare client for the following if planned:
      1. cardioversion
      2. insertion of a pacemaker or automatic implantable cardioverter defibrillator (AICD)
      3. electrode catheter ablation or surgical resection of irritable site
   h. have emergency cart readily available for defibrillation or cardiopulmonary resuscitation.

5.b. The client will not develop heart failure as evidenced by:
1. pulse 60–100 beats/minute
2. absence of an S_3 heart sound
3. usual mental status
4. clear, audible breath sounds
5. absence of or no increase in dyspnea and orthopnea
6. absence of cough
7. palpable peripheral pulses
8. increased strength and activity tolerance
9. skin warm and dry
10. urine output at least 30 ml/hour
11. stable weight
12. absence of edema; distended neck veins; and enlarged, tender liver.

5.b.1. Assess for and report signs and symptoms of heart failure:
   a. tachycardia
   b. presence of an S_3 heart sound
   c. increased restlessness or anxiousness, confusion, or other change in mental status
   d. crackles (rales)
   e. development of or increased shortness of breath
   f. dry, hacking cough or cough productive of frothy or blood-tinged sputum
   g. diminished or absent peripheral pulses
   h. increased weakness and fatigue
   i. cool, diaphoretic skin
   j. decreased urine output
   k. weight gain
   l. edema
   m. distended neck veins
   n. enlarged, tender liver.

2. Monitor chest x-ray results. Report findings of cardiomegaly, pleural effusion, or pulmonary edema.

3. Implement measures *to prevent heart failure:*
   a. perform actions to improve cardiac output (see Nursing Diagnosis 1, action c)
   b. perform actions to treat cardiac dysrhythmias if present (see action a.3 in this diagnosis) *because dysrhythmias contribute to the development of heart failure.*

4. If signs and symptoms of heart failure occur:
   a. continue with above actions
   b. administer the following medications if ordered:
      1. positive inotropic agents (e.g. dobutamine, dopamine, amrinone) *to increase myocardial contractility*
      2. vasodilators (e.g. nitroglycerin, captopril) *to decrease cardiac workload*

3. diuretics (usually not used initially unless pulmonary capillary wedge pressure is above 18 mm Hg *because volume expansion is often not a factor in acute heart failure*)
4. morphine sulfate *to reduce preload and anxiety* (used primarily in clients with pulmonary edema)

c. refer to Care Plan on Heart Failure for additional care measures.

5.c. The client will not develop a thromboembolism as evidenced by: 1. absence of pain, tenderness, swelling, and numbness in extremities 2. usual temperature and color of extremities 3. palpable and equal peripheral pulses 4. usual mental status 5. usual sensory and motor function 6. absence of sudden chest pain and dyspnea.	5.c.1. Assess for and report signs and symptoms of: a. deep vein thrombus (e.g. pain, tenderness, swelling, unusual warmth, and/or positive Homans' sign in extremity) b. arterial embolus (e.g. diminished or absent peripheral pulses; pallor, coolness, numbness, and/or pain in extremity) c. cerebral ischemia (e.g. decreased level of consciousness, alteration in usual sensory and motor function) d. pulmonary embolism (e.g. sudden chest pain, dyspnea, increased restlessness and apprehension).

2. Monitor echocardiogram results and report finding of a cardiac thrombus.
3. Implement measures *to prevent the development of thromboemboli:*
   a. perform actions *to reduce the risk of thrombus formation in the heart:*
      1. implement measures to improve cardiac output (see Nursing Diagnosis 1, action c)
      2. implement measures to treat dysrhythmias if present (see action a.3 in this diagnosis)
      3. implement measures to treat heart failure if it occurs (see action b.4 in this diagnosis)
   b. if client remains on bed rest or activity is significantly limited for longer than 48 hours, refer to Care Plan on Immobility, Collaborative Diagnosis 12, actions a.1.b and c and a.2.b and c (pp. 137–138) for measures to prevent and treat a deep vein thrombus and pulmonary embolism
   c. administer anticoagulants (e.g. warfarin, heparin) and antiplatelet agents (e.g. low-dose aspirin) if ordered.
4. If signs and symptoms of an arterial embolus occur:
   a. maintain client on bed rest with affected extremity in a level or slightly dependent position *to improve arterial blood flow*
   b. prepare client for diagnostic studies (e.g. Doppler or duplex ultrasound, arteriography) if planned
   c. prepare client for the following if planned:
      1. injection of a thrombolytic agent (e.g. streptokinase)
      2. embolectomy
   d. administer anticoagulants (e.g. continuous intravenous heparin, warfarin) as ordered
   e. provide emotional support to client and significant others.
5. If signs and symptoms of cerebral ischemia occur:
   a. maintain client on bed rest
   b. administer anticoagulants (e.g. continuous intravenous heparin, warfarin) as ordered
   c. provide emotional support to client and significant others
   d. refer to Care Plan on Cerebrovascular Accident for additional care measures if signs and symptoms persist.

5.d. The client will not experience rupture of any portion of the heart as evidenced by absence of signs of acute heart failure and/or cardiogenic shock (see outcomes b and g in this diagnosis for outcome criteria).	5.d.1. Assess for and report signs and symptoms of the following: a. papillary muscle rupture (e.g. holosystolic murmur, dyspnea, evidence of papillary muscle rupture on echocardiography or cardiac catheterization) b. ventricular septal defect (e.g. holosystolic murmur, parasternal thrill, finding of septal defect on echocardiography or cardiac catheterization) c. cardiac tamponade resulting from ventricular wall rupture (e.g. significant decrease in B/P, narrowed pulse pressure, pulsus paradoxus, distant or muffled heart sounds, jugular vein distention, increased central venous pressure [CVP]).

Desired Outcomes	Nursing Actions and *Selected Purposes/Rationales*

2. Assess for and immediately report signs and symptoms of acute heart failure and/or cardiogenic shock (see actions b.1 and 2 and g.1 in this diagnosis) that may occur as a result of rupture of a portion of the heart.
3. Implement measures to reduce cardiac workload (see Nursing Diagnosis 1, action c.2) *in order to reduce risk of rupture of the papillary muscle and ventricular free wall or septum.*
4. If signs and symptoms of rupture of a portion of the heart occur:
   a. maintain client on bed rest
   b. assist with pericardiocentesis if performed
   c. assist with measures to treat heart failure or cardiogenic shock (see actions b.4 and g.3 in this diagnosis)
   d. prepare client for surgical intervention (e.g. valve replacement, repair of ventricular septal defect) if planned
   e. provide emotional support to client and significant others.

5.e. The client will experience resolution of pericarditis if it develops as evidenced by:
   1. fewer reports of precordial pain
   2. absence of pericardial friction rub
   3. temperature declining toward normal
   4. WBC count and sedimentation rate declining toward normal range.

5.e.1. Assess for and report signs and symptoms of pericarditis:
   a. precordial pain that frequently radiates to shoulder, neck, back, and arm (usually left); is intensified during deep inspiration, movement, and coughing; and usually is relieved by sitting up and leaning forward
   b. pericardial friction rub (may be transient)
   c. persistent temperature elevation
   d. further increase in WBC count and sedimentation rate (both can be elevated as a result of the infarction).
2. If signs and symptoms of pericarditis occur:
   a. allay client's anxiety (client may believe that symptoms indicate recurrent MI)
   b. assist client to assume position of comfort (usually sitting up and leaning forward on overbed table)
   c. administer anti-inflammatory agents (e.g. aspirin) if ordered.

5.f. The client will not experience infarct extension or recurrence as evidenced by:
   1. no further episodes of persistent chest pain
   2. stable vital signs
   3. cardiac enzyme levels declining toward normal range
   4. improved ECG readings.

5.f.1. Assess for and report signs and symptoms of infarct extension or recurrence (e.g. recurrent episode of persistent chest pain; significant change in vital signs; further increase in cardiac enzymes; recurrent or further increase in ST segment elevation, T wave changes, and development of abnormal Q waves [if not already present] on ECG).
2. Implement measures to improve cardiac output (see Nursing Diagnosis 1, action c) *in order to reduce risk of infarct extension or recurrence.*
3. If client experiences signs and symptoms of infarct extension or recurrence, prepare him/her for coronary angiogram, thrombolytic therapy, or mechanical revascularization (e.g. PTCA, coronary artery bypass grafting [CABG]) if planned.

5.g. The client will not develop cardiogenic shock as evidenced by:
   1. stable or improved mental status
   2. systolic B/P greater than 80 mm Hg
   3. palpable peripheral pulses
   4. stable or improved skin temperature and color
   5. urine output at least 30 ml/hour
   6. pulmonary capillary wedge pressure (PCWP) between 15–18 mm Hg.

5.g.1. Assess for and immediately report signs and symptoms of cardiogenic shock:
   a. increased restlessness, lethargy, or confusion
   b. systolic B/P below 80 mm Hg
   c. rapid, weak pulse
   d. diminished or absent peripheral pulses
   e. increased coolness and duskiness or cyanosis of skin
   f. urine output less than 30 ml/hour
   g. PCWP greater than 18 mm Hg.
2. Implement measures *to prevent cardiogenic shock:*
   a. perform actions to improve cardiac output (see Nursing Diagnosis 1, action c)
   b. perform actions to treat cardiac dysrhythmias if present (see action a.3 in this diagnosis)
   c. perform actions to treat heart failure if it occurs (see action b.4 in this diagnosis)
   d. perform actions to treat rupture of any portion of the heart if it occurs (see action d.4 in this diagnosis).

3. If signs and symptoms of cardiogenic shock occur:
   a. continue with above actions
   b. maintain oxygen therapy as ordered
   c. prepare client for diagnostic studies (e.g. echocardiography, cardiac catheterization)
   d. administer the following if ordered:
      1. sympathomimetics (e.g. dopamine, dobutamine) *to increase cardiac output and maintain arterial pressure*
      2. phosphodiesterase inhibitors (e.g. amrinone) *to increase myocardial contractility and decrease systemic vascular resistance*
      3. vasodilators (e.g. nitroglycerin) *to reduce cardiac workload* (vasodilators are usually not given if the systolic B/P is less than 100 mm Hg)
      4. intravenous fluids (usually ordered if signs of hypoperfusion are present and the PCWP falls to 15 mm Hg or less)
   e. assist with intubation and insertion of hemodynamic monitoring device (e.g. Swan-Ganz catheter) and intra-aortic balloon pump (IABP) if indicated
   f. provide emotional support to client and significant others.

---

6. NURSING DIAGNOSIS:

Anxiety

related to severe pain; feeling of suffocation; possibility of severe disability or impending death; unfamiliar environment; and lack of understanding of diagnostic tests, the diagnosis, and treatment plan.

Desired Outcome	Nursing Actions and *Selected Purposes/Rationales*
6. The client will experience a reduction in anxiety as evidenced by: a. verbalization of feeling less anxious b. usual sleep pattern c. relaxed facial expression and body movements d. stable vital signs e. usual perceptual ability and interactions with others.	6.a. Assess client for signs and symptoms of anxiety (e.g. verbalization of feeling anxious, insomnia, tenseness, shakiness, restlessness, diaphoresis, tachycardia, facial pallor, self-focused behaviors). Validate perceptions carefully, remembering that some behaviors may result from hypoxia. b. Implement measures *to reduce fear and anxiety:* 　1. provide care in a calm, supportive, confident manner 　2. if client is having severe pain: 　　a. do not leave alone during period of acute distress 　　b. perform actions to relieve pain (see Nursing Diagnosis 2, action d) 　3. encourage significant others to project a caring, concerned attitude without obvious anxiousness 　4. once the period of acute distress has subsided: 　　a. orient client to hospital environment, equipment, and routines; include an explanation of cardiac monitoring devices 　　b. introduce client to staff who will be participating in care; if possible, maintain consistency in staff assigned to his/her care *to provide feelings of stability and comfort with the environment* 　　c. assure client that staff members are nearby; respond to call signal as soon as possible 　　d. keep cardiac monitor out of client's view and the sound turned as low as possible 　　e. encourage verbalization of fear and anxiety; provide feedback 　　f. explain all diagnostic tests 　　g. reinforce physician's explanation of invasive measures that are planned to improve coronary blood flow (e.g. streptokinase, tissue plasminogen activator [tPA], or anistreplase [APSAC, Eminase] infusion; percutaneous transluminal coronary angioplasty [PTCA]; intra-aortic balloon pump [IABP])

Desired Outcome	Nursing Actions and *Selected Purposes/Rationales*

      h. reinforce physician's explanations and clarify misconceptions client has about an MI, the treatment plan, and prognosis

      i. provide a calm, restful environment

      j. instruct client in relaxation techniques and encourage participation in diversional activities

      k. assist client to identify specific stressors and ways to cope with them

      l. provide information based on current needs of client at a level he/she can understand; encourage questions and clarification of information provided

      m. include significant others in orientation and teaching sessions and encourage their continued support of the client

      n. administer prescribed antianxiety agents if indicated.

   c. Consult physician if above actions fail to control fear and anxiety.

---

7. NURSING DIAGNOSIS:	**Grieving***

related to loss of normal function of the heart; possible changes in life style, occupation, and roles; and uncertainty of prognosis.

*This diagnostic label includes anticipatory grieving and grieving following the actual losses.

Desired Outcome	Nursing Actions and *Selected Purposes/Rationales*

7. The client will demonstrate beginning progression through the grieving process as evidenced by:
   a. verbalization of feelings about having had an MI
   b. usual sleep pattern
   c. participation in treatment plan and self-care activities
   d. utilization of available support systems
   e. verbalization of a plan for integrating prescribed follow-up care into life style.

7.a. Assess for signs and symptoms of grieving (e.g. change in eating habits, inability to concentrate, insomnia, anger, sadness, withdrawal from significant others, denial of having had an MI).

  b. Implement measures *to facilitate the grieving process:*
    1. assist the client to acknowledge the loss of normal heart function and the need to alter usual life style *so grief work can begin;* assess for factors that may hinder and facilitate acknowledgment
    2. discuss the grieving process and assist client to accept the phases of grieving as an expected response following an MI
    3. allow time for client to progress through the phases of grieving (phases vary among theorists but progress from shock and alarm to acceptance); be aware that not every phase is expressed by all individuals, that recurrence of phases is common, and that the grieving process may take months to years
    4. assist client to identify and utilize techniques that have helped him/her to cope in previous situations of loss
    5. perform actions *to promote trust* (e.g. answer questions honestly, provide requested information)
    6. provide an atmosphere of care and concern (e.g. provide privacy, be available and nonjudgmental, display empathy and respect) *so that client will feel free to express feelings*
    7. encourage the verbal expression of anger and sadness about having had an MI; recognize displacement of anger and assist client to see the actual cause of angry feelings and resentment
    8. encourage client to express feelings in whatever ways are comfortable (e.g. writing, drawing, conversation)
    9. support realistic hope regarding the prognosis
    10. support behaviors suggesting successful grief work (e.g. verbalizing feelings about loss of normal heart function, expressing sorrow, focusing on ways to adapt to changes)
    11. explain the phases of the grieving process to significant others; encourage their support and understanding

12. facilitate communication between the client and significant others; be aware that they may be in different phases of the grieving process
13. provide information regarding counseling services and support groups that might assist client in working through grief
14. when appropriate, assist client to meet spiritual needs (e.g. arrange for a visit from clergy).

c. Consult physician regarding referral for counseling if signs of dysfunctional grieving (e.g. persistent denial of losses, excessive anger or sadness, emotional lability) occur.

Discharge Teaching

■━━━━━━━━━━━━━━━━━━━━━━━━━━━━━━

8. NURSING DIAGNOSIS: **Knowledge deficit, Ineffective management of therapeutic regimen, or Altered health maintenance***

---

*The nurse should select the diagnostic label that is most appropriate for the client's discharge teaching needs.

Desired Outcomes	Nursing Actions and *Selected Purposes/Rationales*

8.a. The client will verbalize a basic understanding of a myocardial infarction.

8.b. The client will demonstrate accuracy in counting pulse.

8.c. The client will identify modifiable cardiovascular risk factors and ways to alter these factors.

8.d. The client will verbalize an understanding of the rationale for and components of a diet restricted in saturated fat and cholesterol.

8.a. Explain a myocardial infarction in terms the client can understand. Utilize appropriate teaching aids (e.g. pictures, videotapes, heart models). Inform client that it takes approximately 6–8 weeks for the heart to heal after a myocardial infarction.

8.b.1. Teach client how to count his/her pulse, being alert to the regularity of the rhythm.
2. Allow time for return demonstration and accuracy check.

8.c.1. Inform client that the following modifiable factors have been shown to contribute to cardiovascular disease:
   a. obesity
   b. elevated serum lipids
   c. lack of regular aerobic exercise
   d. cigarette smoking
   e. hypertension
   f. diabetes mellitus
   g. stressful life style.

2. Encourage client to discuss alcohol intake with health care provider. (The health care provider may advise the client to limit alcohol consumption because there is evidence that a daily alcohol intake exceeding 1 oz of ethanol [i.e. 2 oz of 100-proof whiskey, 8 oz of wine, 24 oz of beer] contributes to the development of hypertension and some forms of heart disease.)

3. Assist the client to identify ways he/she can make appropriate changes in life style to modify the above factors. Provide information about weight reduction plans; stress management classes; and cardiovascular fitness, smoking cessation, and alcohol rehabilitation programs. Initiate a referral if indicated.

8.d.1. Explain the rationale for restricting saturated fat and cholesterol intake.
2. Provide instructions on ways the client can reduce intake of saturated fat and cholesterol:
   a. reduce intake of red meat
   b. trim visible fat off meat and remove all skin from poultry
   c. use vegetable oil rather than coconut or palm oil in cooking and food preparation
   d. use cooking methods such as steaming, baking, broiling, poaching, microwaving, and grilling rather than frying
   e. restrict intake of eggs (recommendations about the number of whole eggs allowed per week vary depending on the client's lipid levels)

Desired Outcomes	Nursing Actions and *Selected Purposes/Rationales*

f. avoid commercial baked goods

g. avoid dairy products containing more than 1% fat.

8.e. The client will verbalize an understanding of medications ordered including rationale, food and drug interactions, side effects, schedule for taking, and importance of taking as prescribed.

8.e.1. Explain the rationale for, side effects of, and importance of taking the medications prescribed. Inform client of pertinent food and drug interactions.

2. If client is discharged on sublingual or buccal nitroglycerin, instruct to:

a. avoid drinking alcoholic beverages

b. have tablets readily available at all times

c. take a tablet before strenuous activity and in emotionally stressful situations

d. take one tablet when chest pain occurs and another every 5 minutes up to a total of 3 times if necessary; notify physician or obtain emergency medical assistance if pain persists

e. place tablet under tongue or in the buccal pouch and allow it to dissolve thoroughly before swallowing

f. store tablets in a tightly capped, dark-colored glass container away from heat and moisture

g. replace tablets every 6 months or sooner if they do not relieve discomfort

h. avoid rising to a standing position quickly after taking nitroglycerin in order to reduce dizziness associated with its vasodilatory effect

i. recognize that dizziness, flushing, and mild headache may occur after taking nitroglycerin

j. report fainting, persistent or severe headache, blurred vision, or dry mouth.

3. If nitroglycerin skin patches are prescribed:

a. provide instructions about correct application, skin care, need to rotate sites and remove old patches, and frequency of change; if physician prescribes the patch be left off for a certain length of time each day, explain that this helps prevent nitrate tolerance

b. caution client that activities that increase blood flow to the skin (e.g. hot bath or shower, sauna) can cause a sudden reduction in blood pressure

c. caution client about drinking alcoholic beverages

d. instruct client to remove skin patch if faintness, dizziness, or flushing occurs following application and to then notify health care provider

e. instruct client to report persistent redness or itching at the patch site.

4. If client is discharged on a beta-adrenergic blocking agent (e.g. metoprolol, atenolol), instruct to:

a. take the medication at the same time every day

b. check pulse before taking medication; consult physician before taking medication if pulse rate is unusually slow (it is expected that pulse will be lower than normal)

c. avoid skipping doses, altering the prescribed dose, trying to make up for missed doses, and discontinuing medication without first discussing it with health care provider

d. change from a lying to a sitting or standing position slowly if dizziness is a problem

e. limit intake of alcoholic beverages

f. monitor blood glucose on a regular basis if diabetic (beta blockers may affect blood sugar and mask symptoms of hypoglycemia)

g. wear or carry medical identification specifying the name of the medication being taken

h. report the following:

1. persistent lightheadedness or dizziness

2. significant weight gain, night cough, difficulty breathing, or swelling of feet or ankles (may be indicative of heart failure)

3. cold, painful toes or fingers

4. persistent fatigue or depression.

5. Instruct client to take lipid-lowering agents (e.g. lovastatin, gemfibrozil, pravastatin, simvastatin) and antiplatelet agents (e.g. aspirin) as prescribed.
6. Instruct client to consult physician before taking other prescription and nonprescription medications.
7. Instruct client to inform all health care providers of medications being taken.

8.f. The client will verbalize an understanding of activity restrictions and the rate at which activity can be progressed.	8.f.1. Reinforce physician's instructions about activity. Instruct client to: a. gradually increase activity tolerance by adhering to a regular exercise program (often begins with walking) b. take frequent rest periods for about 4–8 weeks after discharge c. avoid physical conditioning programs such as jogging and aerobic dancing until advised by physician d. avoid isometric exercise/activities (e.g. weight lifting, pushing, straining) e. avoid activity immediately after meals and in extreme heat or cold f. stop any activity that causes chest pain, shortness of breath, palpitations, dizziness, or extreme fatigue or weakness g. begin a cardiovascular fitness program when approved by physician. 2. Reinforce instructions regarding sexual activity: a. sexual activity with usual partner can be resumed after the prescribed length of time (many physicians consider a client ready to resume sexual activity when he/she is able to climb 2 flights of stairs briskly without dyspnea or angina) b. assume a comfortable and unstrenuous position for intercourse (e.g. side-lying, partner on top) c. a new sexual relationship can be started but may result in greater energy expenditure until it becomes a more familiar or usual experience d. take nitroglycerin before sexual activity in order to prevent angina e. avoid intercourse for at least 1–2 hours after a heavy meal or alcohol consumption f. avoid sexual activity when fatigued or stressed g. avoid hot or cold showers just before and after intercourse.
8.g. The client will state signs and symptoms to report to the health care provider.	8.g. Instruct the client to report: 1. chest, arm, neck, or jaw pain unrelieved by nitroglycerin 2. shortness of breath 3. significant weight gain or swelling of feet or ankles 4. irregular pulse or a significant unexpected change in the pulse rate 5. persistent impotence or decreased libido (can be a side effect of certain medications or result from anxiety, depression, or fatigue) 6. inability to tolerate prescribed activity.
8.h. The client will identify community resources that can assist with cardiac rehabilitation and adjustment to the effects of a myocardial infarction.	8.h.1. Provide information on community resources and support groups that can assist client with cardiac rehabilitation and adjustment to the effects of an MI (e.g. American Heart Association, "coronary clubs," counseling services). 2. Initiate a referral if indicated.
8.i. The client will verbalize an understanding of and a plan for adhering to recommended follow-up care including future appointments with health care provider.	8.i.1. Reinforce the importance of keeping follow-up appointments with health care provider and for exercise stress testing and laboratory studies to monitor serum lipid levels. 2. Implement measures to improve client compliance: a. include significant others in teaching sessions if possible b. encourage questions and allow time for reinforcement and clarification of information provided c. provide written instructions on future appointments with health care provider, dietary modifications, activity progression, medications prescribed, and signs and symptoms to report.

Bibliography

See pages 897–898 and 903.

⊒ PACEMAKER INSERTION

A pacemaker is a battery-powered device used to stimulate the heart electrically when the heart fails to initiate or conduct intrinsic electrical impulses at a rate that is sufficient to maintain adequate perfusion. Pacemaker insertion is indicated for treatment of symptomatic bradydysrhythmias (e.g. sinus bradycardia, second- and third-degree heart block, sick sinus syndrome) and on rare occasions, for treatment of tachydysrhythmias that have been unresponsive to other forms of therapy.

Pacemakers are either temporary or permanent. Temporary pacemakers are used to regulate the heart rate in emergency or short-term situations. In most instances, temporary pacing is done using external transcutaneous pacing electrodes or using temporary pacemaker electrodes that have been placed on the epicardium during thoracic surgery (e.g. heart surgery). Temporary pacemakers are attached to and regulated by an external power source. Permanent pacemakers are utilized for long-term management of certain dysrhythmias. There are a number of permanent pacemakers available. Their functional capabilities are described by a 3- or 5-letter code that specifies the chamber being paced, the chamber being sensed, mode of response (triggered or inhibited), programmability, and antitachycardia functions.

The components of a permanent pacemaker are the pulse generator (contains the battery and electric circuitry) and the pacemaker electrode catheter (lead or wire) that provides communication between the pulse generator and the electrode on the distal end of the catheter that lodges in the endocardium and delivers the electrical stimulus to the heart. The majority of pacemakers used now are dual-chambered pacemakers with electrodes in both the atrium and ventricle. Dual-chamber pacing allows for the physiological timing between atrial systole and ventricular systole to be maintained, which improves cardiac output. Present day pacemakers can also be programmed externally and the majority operate in a synchronous mode (a chamber of the heart is triggered to fire or is inhibited by the intrinsic activity of the heart) or a rate-responsive mode. The most frequently used rate-responsive systems have an activity sensor in the pulse generator that detects movement and then appropriately increases or decreases the pacing rate. Insertion of a permanent pacemaker is usually performed using local anesthesia. The pacemaker electrode catheter is inserted into the heart transvenously, usually via the subclavian or cephalic vein, and then attached to the pulse generator which is implanted in the subcutaneous tissue in the chest or abdomen. Most pulse generators are now powered by a lithium battery that has an average lifespan of 7–10 years.

This care plan focuses on the adult client with a symptomatic dysrhythmia hospitalized for probable transvenous insertion of a permanent pacemaker under local anesthesia. Preoperative goals of care are to maintain adequate cardiac output and assist the client to adjust psychologically to the idea of having a permanent pacemaker. Postoperatively, the goals of care are to prevent complications and educate the client regarding follow-up care.

DIAGNOSTIC TESTS

Electrocardiogram (ECG)
Electrophysiological studies (EPS)

DISCHARGE CRITERIA

Prior to discharge, the client will:

- have adequate cardiac output
- have no signs and symptoms of postoperative complications
- verbalize a basic understanding of the rationale for and function of a permanent pacemaker
- demonstrate knowledge of how to monitor pacemaker function
- verbalize an understanding of how to correctly perform range of motion exercises of arm and shoulder on the side of pacemaker insertion
- identify appropriate safety precautions associated with having a permanent pacemaker
- state signs and symptoms to report to the health care provider
- verbalize an understanding of and a plan for adhering to recommended follow-up care including future appointments with health care provider, medications prescribed, wound care, and activity restrictions.

NURSING/ COLLABORATIVE DIAGNOSES	**Preoperative**

Preoperative
1. Decreased cardiac output △ 387
2. Anxiety △ 388

Postoperative
1. Potential complications:
   a. pacemaker malfunction: failure to fire, capture, or sense
   b. cardiac tamponade
   c. pneumothorax
   d. undesirable stimulation of the heart and/or certain nerves and muscles △ 389

DISCHARGE TEACHING
2. Knowledge deficit, Ineffective management of therapeutic regimen, or Altered health maintenance △ 390

See Standardized Preoperative and Postoperative Care Plans for additional diagnoses.

PREOPERATIVE

Use in conjunction with the Standardized Preoperative Care Plan.

1. NURSING DIAGNOSIS:

Decreased cardiac output

related to abnormal heart rate and/or rhythm associated with a disorder in the initiation or conduction of intrinsic electrical impulses.

Desired Outcome	Nursing Actions and *Selected Purposes/Rationales*
1. The client will maintain adequate cardiac output as evidenced by: a. systolic B/P of at least 90 mm Hg b. palpable peripheral pulses c. no increase in number or duration of syncopal episodes d. no further decline in mental status e. absence of cyanosis f. urine output at least 30 ml/hour.	1.a. Assess client upon admission for baseline data regarding status of cardiac output. Expect that many of the following signs and symptoms of dysrhythmias and low cardiac output will be present: 1. B/P less than 110/70 mm Hg or below normal for client 2. irregular pulse 3. pulse rate less than 60 or greater than 100 beats/minute 4. fatigue and weakness 5. diminished peripheral pulses 6. dizziness, lightheadedness, syncope 7. restlessness, change in mental status 8. tachypnea, exertional dyspnea 9. cool, pale skin 10. capillary refill time greater than 3 seconds. b. Monitor ECG readings and report worsening of or additional dysrhythmias. c. Reassess cardiac status frequently and report the following signs and symptoms that may indicate the need for emergency pacemaker insertion: 1. systolic B/P below 90 mm Hg 2. absent peripheral pulses 3. prolonged or increased frequency of syncopal episodes 4. persistent decline in mental status 5. cyanosis 6. urine output less than 30 ml/hour. d. Implement measures *to maintain an adequate cardiac output before surgery:* 1. perform actions *to reduce cardiac workload:* a. maintain activity restrictions as ordered b. place client in a semi- to high Fowler's position

Desired Outcome	Nursing Actions and *Selected Purposes/Rationales*

	c. implement measures *to promote emotional rest* (e.g. reduce fear and anxiety)
	d. maintain oxygen therapy as ordered
	e. discourage smoking *(smoke has a cardiostimulatory effect, causes vasoconstriction, and reduces oxygen availability)*
	2. instruct client to avoid activities that create a Valsalva response (e.g. straining to have a bowel movement, holding breath while moving up in bed) *in order to reduce vagal stimulation and the subsequent slowing of heart rate and to prevent the sudden increase in cardiac workload that occurs with exhalation*
	3. administer the following if ordered:
	  a. medications *to treat tachydysrhythmias if present* (e.g. procainamide, disopyramide, quinidine, adenosine, diltiazem)
	  b. anticholinergic agents (e.g. atropine) or sympathomimetics (e.g. isoproterenol) *to increase heart rate if client has a bradydysrhythmia*
	4. notify physician if serum potassium level is abnormal *(abnormal potassium levels affect myocardial conductivity)*
	5. if client has heart block, consult physician before giving prescribed digitalis preparations *(digitalis preparations delay AV node conductivity)*
	6. assist with/maintain temporary pacing if ordered.

■

2. NURSING DIAGNOSIS: **Anxiety**

related to unfamiliar environment, lack of understanding of surgical procedure, anticipated postoperative discomfort, possibility of pacemaker malfunction, and possible changes in life style as a result of having a pacemaker.

Desired Outcome	Nursing Actions and *Selected Purposes/Rationales*

2. The client will experience a reduction in anxiety (see Standardized Preoperative Care Plan, Nursing Diagnosis 1 [pp. 96–97], for outcome criteria).	2.a. Refer to Standardized Preoperative Care Plan, Nursing Diagnosis 1 (pp. 96–97), for measures related to assessment and reduction of fear and anxiety.
	b. Implement additional measures *to reduce fear and anxiety:*
	  1. explain the rationale for and function of a pacemaker; utilize diagrams, pamphlets, and a pacemaker unit if available
	  2. explain that procedure will be performed using local anesthesia
	  3. if client is to receive an antimicrobial agent before surgery, explain that antimicrobial agents are routinely used before and for a short time after surgery to reduce the risk for infection
	  4. inform client that pacemakers are electrically safe and are not harmed during usual daily activities
	  5. inform client of the expected life span of the particular pacemaker to be implanted; explain that only the generator will need to be replaced when the battery gets weak
	  6. discuss the client's concerns regarding whether his/her occupation and hobbies can be continued safely with a pacemaker in place; if the occupation or interests involve contact sports or contact with high-voltage electrical equipment and large electromagnetic fields, instruct him/her to consult physician about the safety of continuing these activities.

POSTOPERATIVE

Use in conjunction with the Standardized Postoperative Care Plan.

1. COLLABORATIVE DIAGNOSES:

Potential complications of pacemaker insertion:

a. **pacemaker malfunction: failure to fire, capture, or sense** related to break in or faulty attachment of the pacemaker catheter to the generator, pulse generator malfunction, or improper placement or dislodgment of the pacemaker electrode(s);

b. **cardiac tamponade** related to perforation of the atria or ventricle by the pacemaker electrode catheter;

c. **pneumothorax** related to accumulation of air in the pleural space associated with accidental puncture of the pleura during subclavian insertion of the pacemaker electrode catheter;

d. **undesirable stimulation of the heart and/or certain nerves and muscles** related to the presence of a foreign body in the heart and the emission of electrical impulses from the pacemaker electrode to nearby muscles and nerves (e.g. diaphragm, intercostal muscles, phrenic nerve).

Desired Outcomes	Nursing Actions and *Selected Purposes/Rationales*

1.a. The client will experience normal pacemaker function as evidenced by:
  1. regular pulse at a rate equal to or greater than the preset level
  2. stable B/P
  3. absence of dizziness, syncope, and dyspnea
  4. ECG readings showing pacer spikes before the P wave and/or QRS complex when the pulse rate falls below the preset rate.
	1.a.1. Ascertain the method of pacing being used and the rate set by the physician in surgery. Use this information when assessing pacemaker function.
	  2. Assess for and report signs and symptoms of pacemaker malfunction:
	    a. apical pulse less than preset pacemaker rate
	    b. significant decrease in B/P
	    c. dizziness, lightheadedness, syncope
	    d. dyspnea
	    e. ECG readings showing any of the following:
	      1. absence of pacer spikes when heart rate falls below the preset level
	      2. pacer spikes present with normal P waves and QRS complexes
	      3. absence of P wave (if an atrial pacer) or QRS complex following a pacer spike
	      4. presence of premature beats.
	  3. Implement measures *to reduce the risk for pacemaker catheter breakage and dislodgment of the electrode(s) in order to prevent pacemaker malfunction:*
	    a. maintain activity restrictions as ordered
	    b. instruct client to limit movement of the arm and shoulder on the side of pacemaker insertion for the first 48 hours after surgery.
	  4. If signs and symptoms of pacemaker malfunction occur:
	    a. turn client to either side (preferably the left) *to help achieve placement of the electrode against the endocardium*
	    b. follow manufacturer's suggestions for problem solving (e.g. have a pacemaker magnet readily available to test function and convert pacemaker to asynchronous [fixed rate] mode if necessary, increase milliamperage of pacing threshold within prescribed or unit protocol limits until capture occurs)
	    c. prepare client for chest x-ray to check placement of the electrode catheter
	    d. prepare client for surgical repair or replacement of pacemaker if indicated
	    e. provide emotional support to client and significant others.

1.b. The client will not experience cardiac tamponade as evidenced by:	1.b.1. Assess for and report signs and symptoms of cardiac tamponade (e.g. significant decrease in B/P, narrowed pulse pressure, pulsus paradoxus, distant or muffled heart sounds, sense of fullness in chest, jugular vein distention).

Desired Outcomes	Nursing Actions and *Selected Purposes/Rationales*

1. stable vital signs
2. audible heart sounds
3. absence of jugular vein distention.
	2. Implement measures to prevent dislodgment of the electrode catheter (see action a.3 in this diagnosis) *in order to reduce the risk for perforation of the heart wall.*
	3. If signs and symptoms of cardiac tamponade occur:
	  a. prepare client for chest x-ray and echocardiogram
	  b. prepare client for repositioning or replacement of the electrode catheter, repair of perforation, and/or pericardiocentesis if planned
	  c. provide emotional support to client and significant others.

1.c. The client will have resolution of pneumothorax if it occurs as evidenced by:
1. audible breath sounds and a resonant percussion note over lungs
2. normal respiratory rate and pattern
3. usual mental status
4. blood gases returning to normal range.
	1.c.1. Assess for and immediately report signs and symptoms of pneumothorax (e.g. absent breath sounds with hyperresonant percussion note over involved area; rapid, shallow, and/or labored respirations; tachycardia; sudden onset of chest pain; restlessness; confusion).
	2. Monitor for and report the following:
	  a. abnormal blood gases
	  b. significant decrease in oximetry results
	  c. chest x-ray results showing lung collapse.
	3. If signs and symptoms of pneumothorax occur:
	  a. maintain client on bed rest in a semi- to high Fowler's position
	  b. maintain oxygen therapy as ordered
	  c. assess for and immediately report signs and symptoms of tension pneumothorax with mediastinal shift (e.g. severe dyspnea, increased restlessness and agitation, rapid and/or irregular heart rate, hypotension, neck vein distention, shift in trachea from midline)
	  d. prepare client for insertion of chest tube if indicated
	  e. provide emotional support to client and significant others.

1.d. The client will have resolution of ventricular irritability and undesired nerve and muscle stimulation as evidenced by:
1. absence of ventricular ectopic beats
2. absence of hiccoughs
3. absence of abdominal and intercostal muscle twitching.
	1.d.1. Assess for the following:
	  a. ventricular ectopic beats on ECG readings
	  b. hiccoughs
	  c. reports of abdominal or chest wall twitching.
	2. If the above signs and symptoms of ventricular irritability or undesired nerve or muscle stimulation persist:
	  a. consult physician
	  b. prepare client for the following procedures if planned:
	    1. chest x-ray to determine placement of the pacemaker electrode(s)
	    2. repositioning of the pacemaker electrode catheter.

Discharge Teaching

▪━━

2. NURSING DIAGNOSIS: **Knowledge deficit, Ineffective management of therapeutic regimen, or Altered health maintenance***

---

*The nurse should select the diagnostic label that is most appropriate for the client's discharge teaching needs.

Desired Outcomes	Nursing Actions and *Selected Purposes/Rationales*
2.a. The client will verbalize a basic understanding of the rationale for and function of a permanent pacemaker.	2.a. Reinforce preoperative teaching regarding the rationale for and basic function of a permanent pacemaker.
2.b. The client will demonstrate knowledge of how to monitor pacemaker function.	2.b.1. Inform client of pacemaker's set rate. 2. If appropriate, provide instructions about how to take pulse and monitor both the rate and regularity. (Many physicians prefer that their clients not monitor their own pulse because of the confusion between paced beats and spontaneous beats.)

3. If client is to monitor own pulse, instruct him/her to check resting pulse at least once a week or more frequently if experiencing prepacemaker symptoms.
4. Instruct client to have pulse generator function checked regularly per physician's instructions or if experiencing prepacemaker symptoms. Inform client that monitoring may be done at the physician's office or by a telephone monitoring device.

2.c. The client will verbalize an understanding of how to correctly perform range of motion exercises of arm and shoulder on the side of pacemaker insertion.

2.c.1. Teach client about range of motion exercises for arm and shoulder on the side of pacemaker insertion. Instruct client to start range of motion exercises 48–72 hours after the pacemaker implant and perform them at least 3 times/day. Caution client to do the exercises slowly and gently in order to prevent dislodgment of the pacemaker catheter.
2. Allow adequate time for questions and clarification of information provided.

2.d. The client will identify appropriate safety precautions associated with having a permanent pacemaker.

2.d. Instruct client to adhere to the following safety precautions:
1. avoid activities that may cause blunt trauma to the pulse generator (e.g. contact sports, firing rifle with butt end of a gun against affected shoulder)
2. avoid pressure on the insertion site and pulse generator (e.g. do not wear constrictive clothing or purse strap over the shoulder on operative side)
3. avoid close proximity with high-voltage electrical equipment and large electromagnetic fields
4. do not place any electrical device directly over pacemaker
5. move away from any electrical device if dizziness, lightheadedness, or decrease in pulse rate occurs
6. if planning to travel, obtain name of a physician and/or pacemaker clinic at point(s) of destination
7. alert airport personnel to pacemaker (the pacemaker may set off the security alarm) and request a seat away from the galley since most meals are heated in a large microwave oven
8. always wear a medical alert bracelet or tag and carry a pacemaker identification card; identification card should have insertion date, model and serial number of pacemaker, 3- to 5-letter function code, and rate setting.

2.e. The client will state signs and symptoms to report to the health care provider.

2.e.1. Refer to Standardized Postoperative Care Plan, Nursing Diagnosis 21, action c (p. 123), for signs and symptoms to report to the health care provider.
2. Instruct client to report these additional signs and symptoms:
a. increased irregularity of pulse or pulse rate lower than the pacemaker's preset rate (if self-monitoring is being done)
b. unexplained fatigue
c. lightheadedness, dizziness, fainting
d. shortness of breath
e. swelling of feet and ankles
f. chest pain
g. hiccoughing lasting more than 2 hours
h. redness, swelling, drainage, or increased soreness at implant site.

2.f. The client will verbalize an understanding of and a plan for adhering to recommended follow-up care including future appointments with health care provider, medications prescribed, wound care, and activity restrictions.

2.f.1. Refer to Standardized Postoperative Care Plan, Nursing Diagnosis 21 (pp. 123–124), for routine postoperative instructions and measures to improve client compliance.
2. Instruct client to progress activity as tolerated.
3. Instruct client to limit vigorous movement of arms and shoulders and avoid heavy lifting the first 6 weeks after surgery.

Bibliography

See pages 897–898 and 903.

UNIT TEN

NURSING CARE OF THE CLIENT WITH DISTURBANCES OF PERIPHERAL VASCULAR FUNCTION

ABDOMINAL AORTIC ANEURYSM REPAIR

An abdominal aortic aneurysm is an abnormal dilation of the wall of the abdominal aorta. The aneurysm usually develops in the segment of the vessel that is between the renal arteries and the iliac branches of the aorta. The most common cause of an abdominal aortic aneurysm is atherosclerosis. The plaque that forms on the wall of the artery causes degenerative changes in the medial layer of the vessel. These changes lead to loss of elasticity, weakening, and eventual dilation of the affected segment. Some other causes of abdominal aortic aneurysm include inflammation (arteritis), trauma, cystic medial necrosis, and infection.

Most abdominal aortic aneurysms are asymptomatic and are discovered during a routine physical examination (signs include palpation of a pulsatile mass in the abdomen and/or auscultation of a bruit over the abdominal aorta) or during a review of x-ray results of the abdomen or lower spine. The presence of symptoms such as mild to severe abdominal, lumbar, or flank pain and/or lower extremity arterial insufficiency is usually indicative of a large aneurysm that is exerting pressure on surrounding tissues or an aneurysm that is leaking. Surgical repair of an aneurysm is usually performed if the aneurysm is growing rapidly and/or reaches a size of 5–6 cm or larger or if the client experiences symptoms.

This care plan focuses on the adult client hospitalized for surgical repair of an abdominal aortic aneurysm. Preoperatively, goals of care are to reduce fear and anxiety and decrease the risk of aneurysm rupture. The goals of postoperative care are to maintain comfort, prevent complications, and educate the client regarding follow-up care.

DIAGNOSTIC TESTS

Abdominal x-ray
Abdominal ultrasound
Abdominal aortography
Computed tomography (CT)
Magnetic resonance imaging (MRI)

DISCHARGE CRITERIA

Prior to discharge, the client will:

- tolerate prescribed diet
- tolerate expected level of activity
- have surgical pain controlled
- have clear, audible breath sounds throughout lungs
- have evidence of normal healing of surgical wounds
- have no signs and symptoms of postoperative complications
- identify modifiable factors that increase the risk of vascular disease and ways to alter these factors
- state signs and symptoms to report to the health care provider
- verbalize an understanding of and a plan for adhering to recommended follow-up care including future appointments with health care provider, medications prescribed, activity level, and wound care.

NURSING/ COLLABORATIVE DIAGNOSES

Preoperative
1. Anxiety △   395
2. Potential complication: hypovolemic shock △   395

Postoperative
1. Altered fluid and electrolyte balance:
   a. third-spacing of fluid
   b. fluid volume excess or water intoxication
   c. fluid volume deficit
   d. hypokalemia, hypochloremia, and metabolic alkalosis △   397
2. Potential complications:
   a. hypovolemic shock
   b. lower extremity arterial embolization

  c. cardiac dysrhythmias
  d. bowel ischemia
  e. impaired renal function △ 398
 3. Sexual dysfunction △ 401

DISCHARGE TEACHING **4.** Knowledge deficit, Ineffective management of therapeutic regimen, or Altered health maintenance △ 401

See Standardized Preoperative and Postoperative Care Plans for additional diagnoses.

PREOPERATIVE

Use in conjunction with the Standardized Preoperative Care Plan.

1. NURSING DIAGNOSIS:

Anxiety

related to:
a. unfamiliar environment and separation from significant others;
b. lack of understanding of diagnostic tests, surgical procedure, and postoperative care;
c. anticipated loss of control associated with effects of anesthesia;
d. risk of disease if blood transfusions are necessary;
e. anticipated postoperative discomfort and potential change in sexual functioning;
f. possibility of death.

Desired Outcome	Nursing Actions and *Selected Purposes/Rationales*

1. The client will experience a reduction in anxiety (see Standardized Preoperative Care Plan, Nursing Diagnosis 1 [pp. 96–97], for outcome criteria).	1.a. Refer to Standardized Preoperative Care Plan, Nursing Diagnosis 1 (pp. 96–97), for measures related to the assessment and reduction of fear and anxiety.
	 b. Implement additional measures *to reduce fear and anxiety:*
	  1. orient client to critical care unit if appropriate
	  2. describe and explain the rationale for equipment and tubes that may be present postoperatively (e.g. cardiac monitor, ventilator, intravenous and intra-arterial lines, nasogastric tube, urinary catheter)
	  3. explain that B/P may be taken in both arms and thighs in order to better evaluate circulatory status
	  4. establish an alternative method of communicating (e.g. paper and pencil, magic slate) if client is expected to be on a ventilator postoperatively (mechanical ventilatory support is occasionally needed for 1–2 days following this major surgery)
	  5. reinforce physician's explanations and clarify misconceptions client has about effects of the surgery on sexual functioning (impotence can result from diminished blood flow in the mesenteric or internal iliac arteries during or after surgery and/or from nerve damage during surgery).

2. COLLABORATIVE DIAGNOSIS:

Potential complication of abdominal aortic aneurysm: hypovolemic shock related to excessive blood loss if the aneurysm ruptures.

Desired Outcome	Nursing Actions and *Selected Purposes/Rationales*

2. The client will not develop hypovolemic shock as evidenced by:
   a. usual mental status
   b. stable vital signs
   c. skin warm, dry, and usual color
   d. palpable peripheral pulses
   e. urine output at least 30 ml/hour.

2.a. Assess for and immediately report signs and symptoms of conditions that indicate impending aneurysm rupture:
   1. leaking aneurysm:
      a. increasing abdominal girth
      b. ecchymosis of flank area or perineum
      c. frank or occult gastrointestinal bleeding (*occurs if the aneurysm ruptures into the duodenum*)
      d. decreasing RBC, Hct, and Hb levels
      e. new or increased reports of lumbar, flank, abdominal, pelvic, or groin pain (*accumulation of blood in the peritoneum and/or retroperitoneal spaces causes irritation of and pressure on the tissues and nerves*)
      f. diminishing or absent peripheral pulses
      g. further decline in thigh B/P as compared with B/P in arm (thigh B/P is usually slightly lower than B/P in arm of a client with an abdominal aortic aneurysm)
   2. expanding aneurysm:
      a. new or increased reports of lumbar, flank, or groin pain (*results from pressure on lumbar nerves*)
      b. increased size of pulsating mass in abdomen
      c. increasing sense of abdominal and/or gastric fullness (*results from pressure on duodenum*)
      d. decreasing motor or sensory function of lower extremities (*results from pressure on lumbar and/or sacral nerves*).
   b. Assess for and report signs and symptoms of hypovolemic shock:
      1. restlessness, agitation, confusion, or other change in mental status
      2. significant decrease in B/P
      3. postural hypotension
      4. rapid, weak pulse
      5. rapid respirations
      6. cool, moist skin
      7. pallor, cyanosis
      8. diminished or absent peripheral pulses
      9. urine output less than 30 ml/hour.
   c. Implement measures *to decrease risk of aneurysm rupture:*
      1. instruct client to avoid elevating legs when in bed, using knee gatch, and crossing legs *in order to prevent restriction of blood flow to the lower extremities and subsequent increase in pressure on aneurysm site*
      2. perform actions *to prevent an increase in blood pressure:*
         a. limit client's activity as ordered
         b. instruct client to avoid activities that create a Valsalva response (e.g. straining to have a bowel movement, holding breath while moving up in bed, lifting heavy objects)
         c. implement measures to reduce fear and anxiety (see Preoperative Nursing Diagnosis 1)
      3. administer antihypertensives if ordered *to reduce pressure in the dilated vessel.*
   d. If signs and symptoms of hypovolemic shock occur:
      1. place client flat in bed unless contraindicated
      2. monitor vital signs frequently
      3. administer oxygen as ordered
      4. administer blood and/or volume expanders as ordered (these need to be used with caution *since increased vascular pressure can extend a tear at site of rupture*)
      5. prepare client for insertion of hemodynamic monitoring devices (e.g. central venous catheter, intra-arterial catheter) if indicated
      6. prepare client for emergency surgical repair of aneurysm if indicated
      7. provide emotional support to client and significant others.

POSTOPERATIVE **Use in conjunction with the Standardized Postoperative Care Plan.**

1. NURSING/COLLABORATIVE DIAGNOSIS:

Altered fluid and electrolyte balance:

a. **third-spacing of fluid** related to:
   1. increased capillary permeability in surgical area associated with the inflammation that occurs following extensive dissection of tissue during major abdominal surgery
   2. increased vascular hydrostatic pressure associated with fluid volume excess if present
   3. hypoalbuminemia associated with the escape of proteins from the vascular space into the peritoneum (a result of increased capillary permeability in the surgical area);

b. **fluid volume excess or water intoxication** related to:
   1. vigorous fluid replacement
   2. decreased water excretion associated with increased secretion of antidiuretic hormone (output of ADH is stimulated by trauma, pain, and anesthetic agents)
   3. reabsorption of third-space fluid (occurs about the 3rd postoperative day)
   4. fluid retention associated with renal insufficiency (can occur if there is inadequate blood flow to the kidneys during or after surgery);

c. **fluid volume deficit** related to restricted oral fluid intake before, during, and after surgery; blood loss; loss of fluid associated with nasogastric tube drainage; and inadequate fluid replacement;

d. **hypokalemia, hypochloremia, and metabolic alkalosis** related to loss of electrolytes and hydrochloric acid associated with nasogastric tube drainage.

Desired Outcomes	Nursing Actions and *Selected Purposes/Rationales*
1.a. The client will experience resolution of third-spacing as evidenced by: 1. absence of ascites 2. B/P and pulse within normal range for client and stable with position change.	1.a.1. Assess for and report signs and symptoms of third-spacing: a. ascites (e.g. increase in abdominal girth, dull percussion note over abdomen with finding of shifting dullness) b. evidence of vascular depletion (e.g. postural hypotension; weak, rapid pulse). 2. Monitor serum albumin levels. Report below-normal levels (*low serum albumin levels result in fluid shifting out of vascular space because albumin normally maintains plasma colloid osmotic pressure*). 3. Implement measures *to prevent further third-spacing and/or promote mobilization of fluid back into the vascular space:* a. perform actions to reduce fluid volume excess (see Standardized Postoperative Care Plan, Nursing Diagnosis 4, action b.3 [p. 105]) b. administer albumin infusions if ordered *to increase colloid osmotic pressure.* 4. Consult physician if signs and symptoms of third-spacing worsen or fail to resolve within expected length of time (reabsorption usually begins on 3rd postoperative day).
1.b. The client will not experience fluid volume excess or water intoxication (see Standardized Postoperative Care Plan, Nursing Diagnosis 4, outcome b [p. 105], for outcome criteria).	1.b. Refer to Standardized Postoperative Care Plan, Nursing Diagnosis 4, action b (p. 105), for measures related to assessment, prevention, and treatment of fluid volume excess and water intoxication.
1.c. The client will not experience fluid volume deficit, hypokalemia, hypochloremia, or metabolic alkalosis (see Standardized Postoperative Care Plan, Nursing Diagnosis 4, outcome a [p. 104], for outcome criteria).	1.c. Refer to Standardized Postoperative Care Plan, Nursing Diagnosis 4, action a (pp. 104–105), for measures related to assessment, prevention, and treatment of fluid volume deficit, hypokalemia, hypochloremia, and metabolic alkalosis.

2. COLLABORATIVE DIAGNOSES:

Potential complications of abdominal aortic aneurysm repair:

a. **hypovolemic shock** related to hypovolemia associated with blood loss during surgery, third-space fluid shift, nasogastric tube drainage, inadequate fluid replacement, and hemorrhage (can occur as a result of inadequate wound closure and/or stress on and subsequent leakage or rupture of anastomosis sites);

b. **lower extremity arterial embolization** related to dislodgment of necrotic debris or clot from surgical site;

c. **cardiac dysrhythmias** related to altered nodal function and myocardial conductivity associated with:
   1. myocardial hypoxia resulting from:
      a. altered respiratory function
      b. diminished myocardial blood flow that can result from pre-existing coronary artery disease, hypotension (can occur as a result of hypovolemia, vasodilation associated with rapid warming, and effects of some medications), and sympathetic nervous system-mediated vasoconstriction that results from pain, stress, and hypothermia)
   2. myocardial damage if a perioperative myocardial infarction has occurred
   3. hypokalemia if present;

d. **bowel ischemia** related to diminished blood supply to bowel associated with ligation of the inferior mesenteric artery during surgery, hypovolemia, and/or embolization;

e. **impaired renal function** related to insufficient blood flow to the kidneys associated with hypovolemia and prolonged aortic clamp time.

Desired Outcomes	Nursing Actions and *Selected Purposes/Rationales*
2.a. The client will not develop hypovolemic shock (see Standardized Postoperative Care Plan, Collaborative Diagnosis 19, outcome a [p. 120], for outcome criteria).	2.a.1. Assess for and report signs and symptoms of leakage at anastamosis sites: a. new or expanding hematoma at incision site and/or ecchymosis of flank or perineal area b. increased abdominal girth (can also occur with third-spacing) c. new or increased reports of lumbar, flank, abdominal, pelvic, or groin pain d. increasing feeling of abdominal and/or gastric fullness unrelated to oral intake e. diminishing or absent peripheral pulses f. decreased motor or sensory function in lower extremities g. decreasing B/P, increasing pulse h. decreasing RBC, Hct, and Hb values. 2. Assess for and report signs and symptoms of hypovolemic shock (see Standardized Postoperative Care Plan, Collaborative Diagnosis 19, action a.3 [p. 120]). 3. Implement measures *to prevent hypovolemic shock:* a. perform actions *to prevent or treat hypovolemia:* 1. implement measures to prevent further third-spacing and/or promote mobilization of fluid back into vascular space (see Postoperative Nursing Diagnosis 1, action a.3) 2. provide maximum fluid intake allowed (a fluid restriction may be ordered *to prevent fluid overload and subsequent pressure on the anastomosis sites*) 3. administer blood and/or volume expanders as ordered b. perform actions *to reduce stress on and subsequent separation of anastomosis sites:* 1. instruct client to avoid positions that compromise peripheral blood flow (e.g. elevating legs when in bed, use of knee gatch, crossing legs)

2. implement measures to reduce the accumulation of gastrointestinal gas and fluid and prevent nausea and vomiting (see Standardized Postoperative Care Plan, Nursing Diagnoses 7.A, action 3 and 7.B, action 2 [pp. 107–109])

3. implement measures to prevent or treat fluid volume excess and water intoxication (see Standardized Postoperative Care Plan, Nursing Diagnosis 4, action b.3 [p. 105])

4. instruct client to avoid activities that create a Valsalva response (e.g. straining to have a bowel movement, holding breath while moving up in bed)

5. instruct client to avoid vigorous coughing; consult physician about an order for an antitussive if indicated

6. administer antihypertensives if ordered *to reduce vascular pressure.*

4. If signs and symptoms of hypovolemic shock occur:
   a. place client flat in bed unless contraindicated
   b. monitor vital signs frequently
   c. administer oxygen as ordered
   d. administer blood products and/or volume expanders if ordered (these need to be used with caution if anastomosis site separation is suspected)
   e. prepare client for surgery if indicated
   f. provide emotional support to client and significant others.

2.b. The client will not experience lower extremity arterial embolization as evidenced by:
1. no reports of pain or diminished sensation in lower extremities
2. palpable peripheral pulses
3. usual temperature and color of extremities.

2.b.1. Assess for and report signs and symptoms of lower extremity arterial embolization:
   a. reports of pain (onset is often sudden and severe) and/or numbness in lower extremity(ies)
   b. diminishing or absent peripheral pulses (pulses can be absent for a short time after surgery *as a result of vasospasm and perioperative hypothermia*)
   c. cool, pale, or mottled extremities.

2. Implement measures *to reduce risk of embolization:*
   a. limit client's activity as ordered
   b. instruct client to avoid activities that create a Valsalva response (e.g. straining to have a bowel movement, holding breath while moving up in bed) *in order to prevent dislodgment of existing thrombi.*

3. If signs and symptoms of lower extremity arterial embolization occur:
   a. maintain client on bed rest
   b. prepare client for the following if planned:
      1. diagnostic studies (e.g. Doppler ultrasound, arteriography)
      2. embolectomy
   c. provide emotional support to client and significant others.

2.c. The client will maintain normal sinus rhythm as evidenced by:
1. regular apical pulse at 60–100 beats/minute
2. equal apical and radial pulse rates
3. absence of syncope and palpitations
4. ECG reading showing normal sinus rhythm.

2.c.1. Assess for and report signs and symptoms of cardiac dysrhythmias (e.g. irregular apical pulse; pulse rate below 60 or above 100 beats/minute; apical-radial pulse deficit; syncope; palpitations; abnormal rate, rhythm, or configurations on ECG).

2. Implement measures *to prevent cardiac dysrhythmias:*
   a. perform actions to maintain an adequate respiratory status (see Standardized Postoperative Care Plan, Nursing Diagnoses 2, action c and 3, action b [pp. 102–104]) *in order to maintain adequate myocardial tissue oxygenation*
   b. perform actions *to decrease stimulation of the sympathetic nervous system (sympathetic stimulation increases the heart rate and causes vasoconstriction, both of which increase cardiac workload and decrease oxygen availability to the myocardium):*
      1. implement measures to reduce pain and anxiety (see Standardized Postoperative Care Plan, Nursing Diagnoses 6, action e and 20, action b [pp. 107 and 122])
      2. implement measures *to keep client from getting cold* (e.g. maintain a comfortable room temperature, provide adequate clothing and blankets)

Desired Outcomes	Nursing Actions and *Selected Purposes/Rationales*
	c. perform actions to prevent or treat hypokalemia (see Standardized Postoperative Care Plan, Nursing Diagnosis 4, action a.3 [p. 104])
	d. perform actions *to prevent or treat hypotension:*
	1. consult physician before giving negative inotropic agents, diuretics, and vasodilating agents if systolic B/P is below 90–100 mm Hg
	2. perform actions to prevent hypovolemic shock (see action a.3 in this diagnosis) *in order to maintain an adequate vascular volume*
	3. administer narcotic (opioid) analgesics judiciously, being alert to the synergistic effect of the narcotic ordered and the anesthetic that was used during surgery
	4. gradually bring client's body temperature to normal if hypothermic (*rapid warming results in vasodilation*)
	5. administer sympathomimetics (e.g. norepinephrine, dopamine) if ordered.
	3. If cardiac dysrhythmias occur:
	a. continue with above actions
	b. administer antidysrhythmics as ordered
	c. restrict client's activity based on his/her tolerance and severity of the dysrhythmia
	d. maintain oxygen therapy as ordered
	e. assess cardiovascular status frequently and report signs and symptoms of inadequate tissue perfusion (e.g. decrease in B/P; cool, moist skin; cyanosis; diminished peripheral pulses; urine output less than 30 ml/hour; restlessness and agitation; shortness of breath)
	f. have emergency cart readily available for cardioversion, defibrillation, or cardiopulmonary resuscitation.

2.d. The client will not develop bowel ischemia as evidenced by:
 1. absence of blood in stools
 2. absence of diarrhea
 3. absence of or decrease in abdominal pain
 4. soft, nontender abdomen.
	2.d.1. Assess for and report signs and symptoms of bowel ischemia (e.g. blood in stools, diarrhea, reports of new or increasing abdominal pain, distended abdomen).
	 2. Implement measures to prevent hypovolemic shock and embolization (see actions a.3 and b.2 in this diagnosis) *in order to maintain adequate blood supply to the bowel.*
	 3. If signs and symptoms of bowel ischemia occur:
	   a. administer antimicrobials if ordered
	   b. prepare client for the following if planned:
	     1. colonoscopy
	     2. bowel resection (usually performed if client has extensive bowel tissue necrosis or gangrenous patches have developed)
	     3. embolectomy
	   c. provide emotional support to client and significant others.

2.e. The client will maintain adequate renal function as evidenced by:
 1. urine output at least 30 ml/hour
 2. BUN, serum creatinine, and creatinine clearance within normal range.
	2.e.1. Assess for and report signs and symptoms of impaired renal function (e.g. urine output less than 30 ml/hour, urine specific gravity fixed at or less than 1.010, elevated BUN and serum creatinine levels).
	 2. Collect a 24-hour urine specimen if ordered. Report decreased creatinine clearance.
	 3. Implement measures to prevent hypovolemic shock (see action a.3 in this diagnosis) *in order to maintain adequate renal blood flow.*
	 4. If signs and symptoms of impaired renal function occur:
	   a. continue with above actions
	   b. administer diuretics if ordered *to increase urine output*
	   c. assess for and report signs of acute renal failure (e.g. oliguria or anuria; weight gain; edema; elevated B/P; lethargy and confusion; increasing BUN and serum creatinine, phosphorus, and potassium levels)
	   d. refer to Care Plan on Renal Failure for additional care measures.

3. NURSING DIAGNOSIS:

Sexual dysfunction

related to:
a. decreased libido associated with operative site discomfort and fear of surgical site bleeding;
b. impotence associated with prolonged reduction in blood flow in the mesenteric or internal iliac arteries (can occur as a result of prolonged aortic clamp time during surgery, persistent hypovolemia, embolization, or graft occlusion) and/or nerve damage (can occur during surgery).

Desired Outcome	Nursing Actions and *Selected Purposes/Rationales*

3. The client will demonstrate beginning acceptance of changes in sexual functioning as evidenced by:
a. verbalization of a perception of self as sexually acceptable and adequate
b. statements reflecting beginning adjustment to the effects of surgery on sexual functioning
c. maintenance of relationship with significant other.
	3.a. Assess for signs and symptoms of sexual dysfunction (e.g. verbalization of sexual concerns, alteration in relationship with significant other, limitations imposed by the surgery).
	b. Provide accurate information about the effects of the surgery on sexual functioning. Encourage questions and clarify misconceptions.
	c. Implement measures *to promote optimal sexual functioning:*
	  1. facilitate communication between client and partner; focus on feelings the couple share and assist them to identify changes that may affect their sexual relationship
	  2. discuss ways to be creative in expressing sexuality (e.g. massage, fantasies, cuddling)
	  3. arrange for uninterrupted privacy during hospital stay if desired by the couple
	  4. if impotence is a problem:
	    a. encourage client to discuss it and various treatment options (e.g. vacuum erection aids, penile prosthesis) with physician
	    b. suggest alternative methods of sexual gratification if appropriate
	    c. discuss alternative methods of becoming a parent (e.g. adoption) if of concern to client
	  5. if client is concerned that operative site discomfort will interfere with usual sexual activity:
	    a. assure him/her that the discomfort is temporary and will diminish as incision heals
	    b. encourage alternatives to intercourse or use of positions that decrease pressure on the surgical site (e.g. side-lying)
	  6. reinforce the physician's instructions regarding when client can safely resume sexual activity; inform client that the incision and anastomosis sites should be secure when healing is complete
	  7. include partner in above discussions and encourage continued support of the client.
	d. Consult physician if counseling appears indicated.

Discharge Teaching

4. NURSING DIAGNOSIS:

Knowledge deficit, Ineffective management of therapeutic regimen, or Altered health maintenance*

*The nurse should select the diagnostic label that is most appropriate for the client's discharge teaching needs.

Desired Outcomes	Nursing Actions and *Selected Purposes/Rationales*
4.a. The client will identify modifiable factors that increase the risk of vascular disease and ways to alter these factors.	4.a.1. Inform the client of modifiable factors that have been shown to increase the risk of vascular disease: a. obesity b. elevated serum lipids c. lack of regular aerobic exercise d. cigarette smoking e. hypertension f. stressful life style. 2. Encourage client to discuss alcohol intake with health care provider. (The health care provider may advise the client to limit alcohol consumption because there is evidence that a daily alcohol intake exceeding 1 oz of ethanol [i.e. 2 oz of 100-proof whiskey, 8 oz of wine, 24 oz of beer] contributes to the development of hypertension and some forms of heart disease.) 3. Assist the client to identify ways he/she can make appropriate changes in life style. Provide information about stress management classes and weight loss, smoking cessation, cardiovascular fitness, and alcohol rehabilitation programs if appropriate. Initiate a referral if indicated. 4. Provide instructions on ways the client can reduce intake of saturated fat and cholesterol: a. reduce intake of red meat b. trim visible fat off meat and remove all skin from poultry c. use vegetable oil rather than coconut or palm oil in cooking and food preparation d. use cooking methods such as steaming, baking, broiling, poaching, microwaving, and grilling rather than frying e. restrict intake of eggs (recommendations about the number of whole eggs allowed per week vary depending on the client's lipid levels) f. avoid commercial baked goods g. avoid dairy products containing more than 1% fat. 5. Instruct client to take lipid-lowering agents (e.g. lovastatin, gemfibrozil, pravastatin) if prescribed.
4.b. The client will state signs and symptoms to report to the health care provider.	4.b.1. Refer to Standardized Postoperative Care Plan, Nursing Diagnosis 21, action c (p. 123), for signs and symptoms to report to the health care provider. 2. Instruct client to report these additional signs and symptoms: a. sudden or gradual increase in lower back, flank, groin, or abdominal pain b. chest pain c. coolness, pallor, or blueness of lower extremities d. increased weakness and fatigue e. decreased urine output f. dark brown, bloody, or persistent diarrhea g. increased bruising of incision site, flank area, or perineum h. impotence.
4.c. The client will verbalize an understanding of and a plan for adhering to recommended follow-up care including future appointments with health care provider, medications prescribed, activity level, and wound care.	4.c.1. Refer to Standardized Postoperative Care Plan, Nursing Diagnosis 21 (pp. 123–124), for routine postoperative instructions and measures to improve client compliance. 2. Reinforce the physician's instructions regarding: a. importance of scheduling adequate rest periods b. ways to prevent constipation and subsequent straining to have a bowel movement (e.g. drink at least 10 glasses of liquid/day unless contraindicated, increase intake of foods high in fiber, take stool softeners if necessary) c. the need to avoid sexual intercourse, isometric exercise/activity (e.g. lifting objects over 10 pounds, pushing heavy objects), and strenuous exercise for specified length of time (usually 6–12 weeks depending on the activity).

Bibliography

See pages 897–898 and 903.

◾ CAROTID ENDARTERECTOMY

Carotid endarterectomy is the surgical removal of atherosclerotic plaque from the intima of the carotid artery. The most common site of plaque formation in the carotid artery is the bifurcation. Access to this extracranial area is gained through an incision along the anterior sternocleidomastoid muscle. Surgery is performed to improve carotid artery blood flow and to reduce the risk of cerebral embolization and stroke.

This care plan focuses on the adult client hospitalized for a carotid endarterectomy. Preoperatively, the goals of care are to reduce fear and anxiety and maintain adequate cerebral tissue perfusion. Postoperative goals of care are to prevent complications and educate the client regarding follow-up care.

DIAGNOSTIC TESTS

Carotid ultrasound
Cerebral angiography
Oculoplethysmography (OPG)

DISCHARGE CRITERIA

Prior to discharge, the client will:

- have adequate cerebral blood flow
- have surgical pain controlled
- have evidence of normal wound healing
- identify ways to prevent or slow the progression of atherosclerosis
- identify ways to manage signs and symptoms resulting from cranial nerve damage if it has occurred
- state signs and symptoms to report to the health care provider
- verbalize an understanding of and a plan for adhering to recommended follow-up care including future appointments with health care provider, medications prescribed, activity level, and wound care.

NURSING/ COLLABORATIVE DIAGNOSES

Preoperative
1. Altered cerebral tissue perfusion △ 403
Postoperative
1. Potential complications:
   a. cerebral ischemia
   b. respiratory distress
   c. cranial nerve damage (particularly the facial, hypoglossal, glossopharyngeal, vagus, and/or accessory nerves) △ 404

DISCHARGE TEACHING
2. Knowledge deficit, Ineffective management of therapeutic regimen, or Altered health maintenance △ 407

See Standardized Preoperative and Postoperative Care Plans for additional diagnoses.

PREOPERATIVE

Use in conjunction with the Standardized Preoperative Care Plan.

---

1. NURSING DIAGNOSIS: **Altered cerebral tissue perfusion**

related to:

a. partial or complete occlusion of the carotid artery by atherosclerotic plaque and/or a thrombus;
b. a cerebral embolus associated with dislodgment of atherosclerotic plaque or a thrombus from the carotid artery.

Desired Outcome	Nursing Actions and *Selected Purposes/Rationales*
1. The client will maintain adequate cerebral tissue perfusion as evidenced by: a. mentally alert and oriented b. absence of dizziness, visual disturbances, and speech impairments c. normal motor and sensory function.	1.a. Assess for and report signs and symptoms of carotid artery occlusion and/or cerebral embolization (e.g. agitation, lethargy, confusion, dizziness, diplopia, ipsilateral blindness, homonymous hemianopsia, slurred speech, expressive aphasia, paresthesias, contralateral hemiparesis or hemiplegia). b. Implement measures *to maintain adequate cerebral tissue perfusion:* 1. administer anticoagulants (e.g. heparin, warfarin) or antiplatelet agents (e.g. low-dose aspirin, ticlopidine) if ordered *to prevent new or extended thrombus formation and further occlusion of the carotid artery* (these medications might be discontinued before surgery *to reduce the risk of intraoperative and postoperative hemorrhage*) 2. caution client to avoid activities that create a Valsalva response (e.g. straining to have a bowel movement, holding breath while moving up in bed) *in order to prevent dislodgment of existing thrombi* 3. perform actions *to prevent hypertension in order to reduce the risk of cerebral embolism:* a. implement measures *to reduce stress* (e.g. explain procedures, maintain calm environment) b. administer antihypertensives as ordered (these medications are sometimes discontinued before surgery *to reduce the risk of a critical drop in B/P during and immediately following surgery*). c. If signs and symptoms of altered cerebral tissue perfusion occur: 1. maintain client on bed rest with head of bed flat unless contraindicated 2. administer anticoagulants (e.g. continuous intravenous heparin, warfarin) if ordered 3. provide emotional support to client and significant others; be aware that the development of signs and symptoms usually necessitates postponement or cancellation of planned surgery 4. refer to Care Plan on Cerebrovascular Accident for additional care measures if signs and symptoms persist.

POSTOPERATIVE

Use in conjunction with the Standardized Postoperative Care Plan.

---

1. COLLABORATIVE DIAGNOSES:

Potential complications of carotid endarterectomy:

a. **cerebral ischemia** related to:
1. prolonged carotid artery clamp time during surgery and/or vasospasm associated with clamping and manipulation of cerebral vessels
2. hypovolemia associated with intraoperative and/or postoperative blood loss
3. compression of carotid vessels associated with edema and/or development of a hematoma in the operative area
4. hypotension associated with stimulation of the carotid sinus baroreceptors resulting from surgical manipulation and/or improved blood flow in the carotid artery following surgery
5. embolization during or after surgery and/or formation of a thrombus at surgical site;
b. **respiratory distress** related to airway obstruction associated with tracheal

compression (can occur as a result of hematoma formation and/or edema in the surgical area);

c. **cranial nerve damage (particularly the facial, hypoglossal, glossopharyngeal, vagus, and/or accessory nerves)** related to surgical trauma and/or compression of the nerves (can occur as a result of hematoma formation and/or edema).

Desired Outcomes	Nursing Actions and *Selected Purposes/Rationales*

1.a. The client will maintain adequate cerebral blood flow as evidenced by:
1. mentally alert and oriented
2. absence of dizziness, visual disturbances, and speech impairments
3. normal sensory and motor function.
	1.a.1. Assess for and report signs and symptoms of:
	  a. excessive operative site bleeding (e.g. new or expanding hematoma; continued bright red bleeding from incision or wound drain [a drain is sometimes in place for about 24 hours after surgery]; decreasing RBC, Hct, and Hb levels)
	  b. hypovolemic shock (see Standardized Postoperative Care Plan, Collaborative Diagnosis 19, action a.3 [p. 120])
	  c. cerebral ischemia:
	    1. agitation, irritability, lethargy, confusion
	    2. dizziness
	    3. visual disturbances (e.g. blurred or dimmed vision, diplopia, ipsilateral blindness, homonymous hemianopsia)
	    4. speech impairments (e.g. slurred speech, expressive aphasia)
	    5. paresthesias, paresis, paralysis.
	2. Implement measures *to prevent cerebral ischemia*:
	  a. perform actions to prevent or treat hypovolemic shock (see Standardized Postoperative Care Plan, Collaborative Diagnosis 19, actions a.4 and 5 [p. 120])
	  b. perform actions *to reduce pressure on carotid vessels*:
	    1. implement measures *to reduce operative site edema*:
	      a. keep head of bed elevated 30° unless contraindicated
	      b. apply ice pack to incisional area as ordered
	      c. administer corticosteroids if ordered
	    2. maintain patency of wound drain (e.g. keep tubing free of kinks, empty collection device as often as necessary) if present
	    3. instruct client to support head and neck with hands during position changes and to avoid turning head abruptly or hyperextending neck in order *to reduce stress on the suture line and prevent subsequent bleeding and hematoma formation*
	  c. caution client to avoid activities that create a Valsalva response (e.g. straining to have a bowel movement, holding breath while moving up in bed) *in order to prevent dislodgment of existing thrombi and reduce stress on and subsequent bleeding from the suture line*
	  d. administer the following medications if ordered *to maintain blood pressure within a safe range*:
	    1. antihypertensives *to prevent rupture of the operative vessel or reduce the risk of dislodgment of any existing thrombus* (hypertension may occur *as a result of the underlying disease process or damage to the carotid sinus baroreceptors during surgery*)
	    2. sympathomimetics (e.g. dopamine) *to treat hypotension resulting from carotid sinus baroreceptor stimulation*.
	3. If signs and symptoms of cerebral ischemia occur:
	  a. continue with above measures
	  b. maintain client on bed rest with head of bed flat unless contraindicated
	  c. prepare client for surgical removal of thrombus if planned
	  d. provide emotional support to client and significant others
	  e. refer to Care Plan on Cerebrovascular Accident for additional care measures if signs and symptoms persist.

Desired Outcomes	Nursing Actions and **Selected Purposes/Rationales**

1.b. The client will not experience respiratory distress as evidenced by:
  1. usual mental status
  2. unlabored respirations at 14–20/minute
  3. absence of stridor and sternocleidomastoid muscle retraction
  4. blood gases within normal range.

1.b.1. Assess for and report:
  a. increased edema or expanding hematoma in surgical area
  b. deviation of trachea from midline
  c. new or increased difficulty swallowing
  d. signs and symptoms of respiratory distress (e.g. restlessness, agitation, rapid and/or labored respirations, stridor, sternocleidomastoid muscle retraction)
  e. abnormal blood gases
  f. significant decrease in oximetry results.
  2. Have tracheostomy and suction equipment readily available.
  3. Implement measures *to prevent compression of the trachea and subsequent respiratory distress:*
  a. perform actions to prevent edema and hematoma formation in the operative area (see action a.2.b in this diagnosis)
  b. perform actions *to prevent excessive pressure in the operative vessel and subsequent bleeding and hematoma formation:*
    1. caution client to avoid activities that create a Valsalva response (e.g. straining to have a bowel movement, holding breath while moving up in bed)
    2. administer antihypertensives if ordered.
  4. If signs and symptoms of respiratory distress occur:
  a. place client in a high Fowler's position unless contraindicated
  b. loosen neck dressing if it appears tight
  c. administer oxygen as ordered
  d. assist with intubation or tracheostomy if indicated
  e. prepare client for evacuation of hematoma or surgical repair of the bleeding vessel if planned
  f. provide emotional support to client and significant others.

1.c. The client will experience beginning resolution of cranial nerve damage if it occurs as evidenced by:
  1. gradual return of facial symmetry and usual taste sensation
  2. increased ability to chew and swallow
  3. improved speech
  4. return of usual shoulder movements.

1.c.1. Assess for signs and symptoms of the following:
  a. facial nerve damage (e.g. facial ptosis on affected side, impaired sense of taste)
  b. vagus and glossopharyngeal nerve damage (e.g. loss of gag reflex, difficulty swallowing, hoarseness, inability to speak clearly, asymmetrical movement of soft palate when saying "ah")
  c. hypoglossal nerve damage (e.g. tongue biting when chewing, tongue deviation toward affected side, difficulty swallowing and speaking)
  d. accessory nerve damage (e.g. unilateral shoulder sag, difficulty raising shoulder against resistance).
  2. Implement measures to prevent compression of the cranial nerves at the operative site (see actions a.2.b and b.3.b in this diagnosis).
  3. If signs and symptoms of cranial nerve damage occur:
  a. if the facial, hypoglossal, vagus, and/or glossopharyngeal nerves are affected:
    1. withhold oral foods/fluids until gag reflex returns and client is better able to chew and swallow *in order to reduce the risk of aspiration;* provide parenteral nutrition or tube feeding if indicated
    2. when oral intake is allowed and tolerated:
      a. implement measures *to improve client's ability to chew and/or swallow:*
        1. place client in high Fowler's position for meals and snacks
        2. assist client to select foods that require little or no chewing and are easily swallowed (e.g. custard, eggs, canned fruits, mashed potatoes)
        3. avoid serving foods that are sticky (e.g. peanut butter, soft bread, honey)
        4. serve thick rather than thin fluids or add a thickening agent (e.g. "Thick-it," gelatin, baby cereal) to thin fluids
        5. moisten dry foods with gravy or sauces (e.g. catsup, sour cream, salad dressing)

     b. instruct client to add extra sweeteners or seasonings to foods/fluids if desired *in order to compensate for impaired sense of taste*

     3. implement measures *to facilitate communication* (e.g. maintain quiet environment; provide pad and pencil, magic slate, or word cards; listen carefully when client speaks)

     4. consult speech pathologist about additional ways to facilitate swallowing and communication

  b. if the accessory nerve is affected, instruct client in and assist with exercises *to prevent atrophy of trapezius and sternocleidomastoid muscles* (e.g. range of motion of affected shoulder, wall climbing with fingers, shoulder shrugs)

  c. provide emotional support to client and significant others; assure them that the nerve damage is usually not permanent but caution them that the symptoms may take months to resolve.

Discharge Teaching

■━━

2. NURSING DIAGNOSIS: **Knowledge deficit, Ineffective management of therapeutic regimen, or Altered health maintenance***

    *The nurse should select the diagnostic label that is most appropriate for the client's discharge teaching needs.

Desired Outcomes	Nursing Actions and *Selected Purposes/Rationales*

2.a. The client will identify ways to prevent or slow the progression of atherosclerosis.	2.a.1. Inform the client that certain modifiable factors such as elevated serum lipids and hypertension have been shown to increase the risk of atherosclerosis.
	2. Assist client to identify changes in life style that could reduce the risk for atherosclerosis (e.g. stress management, dietary modifications, physical exercise on a regular basis).
	3. Provide instructions on ways the client can reduce intake of saturated fat and cholesterol:
	  a. reduce intake of red meat
	  b. trim visible fat off meat and remove all skin from poultry
	  c. use vegetable oil rather than coconut or palm oil in cooking and food preparation
	  d. use cooking methods such as steaming, baking, broiling, poaching, microwaving, and grilling rather than frying
	  e. restrict intake of eggs (recommendations about the number of whole eggs allowed per week vary depending on the client's lipid levels)
	  f. avoid commercial baked goods
	  g. avoid dairy products containing more than 1% fat.
	4. Instruct client to take lipid-lowering agents (e.g. lovastatin, pravastatin, gemfibrozil) if prescribed.

2.b. The client will identify ways to manage signs and symptoms resulting from cranial nerve damage if it has occurred.	2.b.1. If signs and symptoms of hypoglossal, facial, vagus, and/or glossopharyngeal nerve damage are present:
	  a. reinforce techniques to improve swallowing and speaking
	  b. assist client in identifying foods that are nutritious and easy to chew and swallow; obtain a dietary consult if needed
	  c. instruct client to increase the amount of sweeteners and seasonings usually used and/or to try different seasonings in foods and beverages if sense of taste is altered.
	2. If signs and symptoms of accessory nerve damage are present, reinforce exercises that should be performed to maintain shoulder muscle tone and prevent contractures.
	3. Allow time for questions, clarification, and return demonstration.

Desired Outcomes	Nursing Actions and *Selected Purposes/Rationales*
2.c. The client will state signs and symptoms to report to the health care provider.	2.c.1. Refer to Standardized Postoperative Care Plan, Nursing Diagnosis 21, action c (p. 123), for signs and symptoms to report to the health care provider. 2. Instruct client to also report: a. increased swelling or purple discoloration at wound site b. new or increased difficulty chewing, swallowing, or speaking c. any loss of or change in vision d. dizziness e. numbness, tingling, or weakness of arm(s) or leg(s) f. increasing irritability g. lethargy, confusion h. failure of signs and symptoms of cranial nerve damage to resolve as expected; remind client that it can take months for reversible signs and symptoms to resolve.
2.d. The client will verbalize an understanding of and a plan for adhering to recommended follow-up care including future appointments with health care provider, medications prescribed, activity level, and wound care.	2.d.1. Refer to Standardized Postoperative Care Plan, Nursing Diagnosis 21 (pp. 123–124), for routine postoperative instructions and measures to improve client compliance. 2. Reinforce the physician's instructions regarding: a. ways to prevent constipation and subsequent straining to have a bowel movement (e.g. drink at least 10 glasses of liquid/day unless contraindicated, increase intake of foods high in fiber, take stool softeners if necessary) b. the need to avoid isometric exercise/activity (e.g. lifting objects over 10 pounds, pushing heavy objects) and strenuous exercise for specified length of time (usually 6–12 weeks depending on the activity).

Bibliography

See pages 897–898 and 904.

 # DEEP VEIN THROMBOSIS

Venous thrombosis occurs when a thrombus forms in a superficial or deep vein. This condition is often called thrombophlebitis because of the associated inflammation in the involved vessel wall. The predisposing factors for venous thrombus formation are venous stasis, trauma to the endothelium of the vein wall, and/or hypercoagulability. Conditions/factors associated with a high risk for venous thrombosis include surgery (especially orthopedic and abdominal surgery), immobility, age (over 40), heart failure, malignancy, fractures or other injuries of the pelvis or lower extremities, varicose veins, pregnancy, obesity, estrogen and oral contraceptive use, history of deep vein thrombosis, and inherited coagulation abnormalities.

Deep vein thrombosis usually develops in a lower extremity; however, the incidence of axillary-subclavian venous thrombosis is rising because of the increased use of central venous catheters. Clinical manifestations of deep vein thrombosis are often not distinctive and, in many cases, the client is asymptomatic. Signs and symptoms that may be present include pain, tenderness, swelling, unusual warmth, and/or positive Homans' sign in the involved extremity. The greatest danger associated with deep vein thrombosis is that the clot, or parts of it, will detach and cause embolic occlusion of a pulmonary vessel.

Persons with deep vein thrombosis are usually treated medically rather than surgically unless there is massive occlusion of a vessel and anticoagulation and thrombolytic therapy are contraindicated. With the increasing use of thrombolytic therapy, thrombectomies and embolectomies are rarely performed. Medical treatment varies depending on the location of the thrombus, the person's risk for bleeding and history of previous thrombus, and availability of serial duplex scanning or plethysmography. Anticoagulant therapy is not universally used to treat calf vein thrombosis because the incidence of pulmonary embolism is low if there is no proximal vein involvement. However, there is a risk of extension of calf vein thrombi into a proximal venous segment if untreated, and because of this risk, many persons with calf vein thrombosis are treated with anticoagulants. There is also some variation in the anticoagulant regimen in relation to the time that oral anticoagulants are initiated and the route and type of heparin ordered (e.g. continuous intravenous heparin, intermittent intravenous heparin, adjusted-dose subcutaneous heparin, low-molecular-weight heparin).

This care plan focuses on the adult client hospitalized **for treatment of deep vein thrombosis in a lower extremity.** The goals of care are to promote adequate peripheral circulation, prevent complications, reduce discomfort, and educate the client regarding follow-up care.

DIAGNOSTIC TESTS

Duplex ultrasound
Impedance plethysmography
Venography

DISCHARGE CRITERIA

Prior to discharge, the client will:

- have adequate tissue perfusion in affected extremity
- have no evidence of tissue irritation or breakdown
- have no signs and symptoms of complications
- identify ways to promote venous blood flow and reduce the risk of chronic venous insufficiency and recurrent thrombus formation
- verbalize an understanding of medications ordered including rationale, food and drug interactions, side effects, schedule for taking, and importance of taking as prescribed
- demonstrate the ability to correctly draw up and administer heparin subcutaneously if prescribed
- identify precautions necessary to prevent bleeding associated with anticoagulant therapy
- state signs and symptoms to report to the health care provider
- verbalize an understanding of and a plan for adhering to recommended follow-up care including future appointments with health care provider and activity level.

Use in conjunction with the Care Plan on Immobility.

NURSING/	1. Altered peripheral tissue perfusion △ 409
COLLABORATIVE	2. Pain: affected extremity △ 410
DIAGNOSES	3. Risk for impaired tissue integrity △ 411
	4. Potential complications:
	a. pulmonary embolism
	b. bleeding △ 411
DISCHARGE TEACHING	5. Knowledge deficit, Ineffective management of therapeutic regimen, or Altered health maintenance △ 413

See Care Plan on Immobility for additional diagnoses.

1. NURSING DIAGNOSIS:

Altered peripheral tissue perfusion

related to:
a. obstructed venous blood flow in affected extremity associated with the presence of a thrombus and inflammation of the vessel;
b. venous stasis associated with decreased mobility.

Desired Outcome	Nursing Actions and *Selected Purposes/Rationales*

1. The client will have improved venous blood flow in the affected extremity as evidenced by diminished pain, tenderness, swelling, and distended superficial blood vessels in extremity.	1.a. Assess for signs and symptoms of impaired venous blood flow in the affected extremity:
	   1. pain or tenderness in extremity
	   2. increase in circumference of extremity
	   3. distention of superficial blood vessels in extremity.
	  b. In the acute phase, implement measures *to treat deep vein thrombosis and improve venous blood flow:*
	   1. maintain activity restrictions as ordered (client is usually on bed rest for 5–7 days)
	   2. elevate affected leg or foot of bed as ordered
	   3. discourage positions that compromise venous blood flow (e.g. crossing legs, pillows under knees, sitting for long periods)
	   4. maintain a minimum fluid intake of 2500 ml/day (unless contraindicated) *to prevent increased blood viscosity*
	   5. administer anticoagulants (e.g. continuous intravenous heparin, warfarin) as ordered
	   6. prepare client for injection of a thrombolytic agent (e.g. streptokinase) if planned (thrombolytic therapy is reserved for treatment of ileofemoral and axillary-subclavian venous thromboses).
	  c. When ambulation is allowed, implement additional measures *to prevent venous stasis and promote adequate venous blood flow:*
	   1. consult physician about an order for antiembolism stockings; apply before client gets out of bed
	   2. instruct client to avoid prolonged sitting or standing.
	  d. Consult physician if signs and symptoms of impaired venous blood flow in affected extremity persist or worsen.

■━━━━━━━━━━━━━━━━━━━━━━━━━━━━━━━━━━━━━━

2. NURSING DIAGNOSIS: **Pain: affected extremity**

related to:
a. decreased tissue perfusion and swelling associated with obstructed venous blood flow;
b. inflammation of vein.

Desired Outcome	Nursing Actions and *Selected Purposes/Rationales*

2. The client will experience diminished pain in the affected extremity as evidenced by:
  a. verbalization of a decrease in pain
  b. relaxed facial expression and body positioning
  c. increased participation in activities when allowed.
	2.a. Assess for signs and symptoms of pain (e.g. verbalization of pain, grimacing, rubbing affected area, restlessness, reluctance to move).
	  b. Assess client's perception of the severity of pain using a pain intensity rating scale.
	  c. Assess client's pain pattern (e.g. location, quality, onset, duration, precipitating factors, aggravating factors, alleviating factors).
	  d. Implement measures *to reduce pain:*
	   1. perform actions to treat deep vein thrombosis and improve venous blood flow (see Nursing Diagnosis 1, actions b and c)
	   2. apply heat to affected area if ordered
	   3. perform actions *to protect the affected extremity from trauma, pressure, or excessive movement:*
	    a. avoid jarring the bed
	    b. use a bed cradle or footboard *to relieve pressure from bed linens*
	    c. support extremity during position changes
	    d. maintain activity restrictions as ordered
	    e. instruct client to move affected extremity slowly and cautiously
	   4. provide or assist with nonpharmacologic methods for pain relief

(e.g. position change, relaxation techniques, restful environment, diversional activities); caution client and significant others that the painful extremity should not be rubbed to relieve pain (*rubbing could dislodge the thrombus*)

    5. administer analgesics and anti-inflammatory agents if ordered.

  e. Consult physician if above measures fail to provide adequate pain relief.

---

3. NURSING DIAGNOSIS:

Risk for impaired tissue integrity

related to:

a. accumulation of waste products and decreased oxygen and nutrient supply to the skin and subcutaneous tissue associated with prolonged pressure on tissues as a result of decreased mobility;

b. damage to the skin and/or subcutaneous tissue associated with friction or shearing;

c. increased skin fragility in affected extremity associated with insufficient blood flow and edema.

Desired Outcome	Nursing Actions and *Selected Purposes/Rationales*

3. The client will maintain tissue integrity as evidenced by:
   a. absence of redness and irritation
   b. no skin breakdown.

3.a. Inspect the skin (especially bony prominences, dependent areas, and affected extremity) for pallor, redness, and breakdown.

  b. Refer to Care Plan on Immobility, Nursing Diagnosis 4, action b (pp. 129–130), for measures to prevent tissue breakdown.

  c. Implement measures *to prevent tissue breakdown in involved extremity:*

    1. perform actions to treat deep vein thrombosis and improve venous blood flow (see Nursing Diagnosis 1, actions b and c)

    2. perform actions *to protect affected extremity from trauma and/or excessive pressure:*

      a. use a bed cradle or footboard *to relieve pressure from bed linens*

      b. keep heel off bed by elevating extremity on foam block or pillows or using heel protector

      c. instruct and assist client to move affected extremity cautiously

      d. remove antiembolism stockings for 30–60 minutes at least twice daily

      e. use caution when applying heat to extremity.

  d. If tissue breakdown occurs:

    1. notify physician

    2. continue with above measures to prevent further irritation and breakdown

    3. perform care of involved area(s) as ordered or per standard hospital procedure

    4. implement measures to treat stasis ulcers (e.g. Unna boot, hydrocolloid dressings)

    5. assess client closely and report signs and symptoms of infection (e.g. elevated temperature; redness, heat, pain, and swelling around area of breakdown; unusual drainage from site).

---

4. COLLABORATIVE DIAGNOSES:

Potential complications:

a. **pulmonary embolism** related to dislodgment of thrombus;

b. **bleeding** related to prolonged coagulation time associated with anticoagulant therapy.

Desired Outcomes	Nursing Actions and *Selected Purposes/Rationales*

4.a. The client will not experience a pulmonary embolism as evidenced by:
1. absence of sudden chest pain
2. unlabored respirations at 14–20/minute
3. pulse 60–100 beats/minute
4. blood gases within normal range.

4.a.1. Assess for and report signs and symptoms of a pulmonary embolism (e.g. sudden chest pain, dyspnea, tachypnea, tachycardia, apprehension, low PaO_2).

2. Implement measures *to prevent a pulmonary embolism:*
   a. perform actions *to prevent dislodgment of thrombus:*
      1. maintain client on bed rest as ordered
      2. do not exercise or check for Homans' sign in affected extremity during acute phase of deep vein thrombosis
      3. never massage affected extremity and caution client not to allow significant others to massage extremity
      4. caution client to avoid activities that create a Valsalva response (e.g. straining to have a bowel movement, holding breath while moving up in bed)
   b. administer anticoagulants (e.g. continuous intravenous heparin, warfarin) as ordered
   c. prepare client for a vena caval interruption (e.g. insertion of an intracaval filtering device) if planned.

3. If signs and symptoms of a pulmonary embolism occur:
   a. maintain client on strict bed rest in a semi- to high Fowler's position
   b. maintain oxygen therapy as ordered
   c. prepare client for diagnostic tests (e.g. blood gases, ventilation-perfusion lung scan, pulmonary angiography)
   d. administer anticoagulants (e.g. continuous intravenous heparin, warfarin) as ordered
   e. prepare client for the following if planned:
      1. injection of a thrombolytic agent (streptokinase, urokinase, tissue plasminogen activator [tPA])
      2. vena caval interruption (e.g. insertion of an intracaval filtering device) *to prevent further pulmonary emboli*
      3. embolectomy (rarely performed)
   f. provide emotional support to client and significant others
   g. refer to Care Plan on Pulmonary Embolism for additional care measures.

4.b. The client will not experience unusual bleeding as evidenced by:
1. skin and mucous membranes free of petechiae, purpura, ecchymoses, and active bleeding
2. absence of unusual joint pain
3. no increase in abdominal girth
4. absence of frank and occult blood in stool, urine, and vomitus
5. usual menstrual flow
6. vital signs within normal range for client
7. stable Hct and Hb.

4.b.1. Assess client for and report signs and symptoms of unusual bleeding:
   a. petechiae, purpura, ecchymoses
   b. gingival bleeding
   c. prolonged bleeding from puncture sites
   d. epistaxis, hemoptysis
   e. unusual joint pain
   f. increase in abdominal girth
   g. frank or occult blood in stool, urine, or vomitus
   h. menorrhagia
   i. restlessness, confusion
   j. decreasing B/P and increased pulse rate
   k. decrease in Hct and Hb levels.

2. Monitor platelet count and coagulation test results (e.g. prothrombin time or International Normalized Ratio [INR], activated partial thromboplastin time, partial thromboplastin time). Report a low platelet count and coagulation test results that exceed the therapeutic range.

3. If platelet count is low, coagulation test results are abnormal, or Hct and Hb levels decrease, test all stool, urine, and vomitus for occult blood. Report positive results.

4. Implement measures *to prevent bleeding:*
   a. avoid giving injections whenever possible; consult physician about prescribing an alternative route for medications ordered to be given intramuscularly or subcutaneously

b. when giving injections or performing venous or arterial punctures, use the smallest gauge needle possible and apply gentle, prolonged pressure to the site after the needle is removed

c. caution client to avoid activities that increase the risk for trauma (e.g. shaving with a straight-edge razor, using stiff-bristle toothbrush or dental floss)

d. pad side rails if client is confused or restless

e. whenever possible, avoid intubations (e.g. nasogastric) and procedures that can cause injury to rectal mucosa (e.g. inserting a rectal suppository or tube, administering an enema)

f. perform actions *to reduce the risk for falls* (e.g. keep bed in low position with side rails up when client is in bed, avoid unnecessary clutter in room, instruct client to wear shoes with nonslip soles when ambulating)

g. instruct client to avoid blowing nose forcefully or straining to have a bowel movement; consult physician about an order for a decongestant and/or laxative if indicated.

5. If bleeding occurs and does not subside spontaneously:

a. apply firm, prolonged pressure to bleeding area(s) if possible

b. if epistaxis occurs, place client in a high Fowler's position and apply pressure and ice pack to nasal area

c. maintain oxygen therapy as ordered

d. perform gastric lavage as ordered *to control gastric bleeding*

e. administer protamine sulfate (antidote for heparin), vitamin K (e.g. phytonadione), and plasma or whole blood as ordered

f. assess for and report signs and symptoms of hypovolemic shock (e.g. restlessness; confusion; significant decrease in B/P; rapid, weak pulse; rapid respirations; cool, pale skin; urine output less than 30 ml/hour)

g. prepare client for surgical repair of bleeding vessels if indicated

h. provide emotional support to client and significant others.

Discharge Teaching

■

5. NURSING DIAGNOSIS:	**Knowledge deficit, Ineffective management of therapeutic regimen, or Altered health maintenance***

*The nurse should select the diagnostic label that is most appropriate for the client's discharge teaching needs.

Desired Outcomes	Nursing Actions and *Selected Purposes/Rationales*
5.a. The client will identify ways to promote venous blood flow and reduce the risk for chronic venous insufficiency and recurrent thrombus formation.	5.a.1. Provide the following instructions on ways to promote venous blood flow and reduce the risk for chronic venous insufficiency (can result from residual vein damage) and recurrent thrombus development: a. avoid wearing constrictive clothing (e.g. garters, girdles, narrow-banded knee-high hose) b. avoid sitting and standing in one position for long periods of time c. wear graduated compression stockings or support hose during the day d. avoid crossing legs and lying or sitting with pillows under knees e. engage in regular aerobic exercise (e.g. swimming, walking, bicycling) f. elevate legs periodically, especially when sitting g. dorsiflex feet regularly h. maintain an ideal body weight for age, height, and body frame. 2. Inform client that smoking and the use of estrogen or oral contraceptives can increase the risk for recurrent thrombus formation.

Desired Outcomes	Nursing Actions and *Selected Purposes/Rationales*

5.b. The client will verbalize an understanding of medications ordered including rationale, food and drug interactions, side effects, schedule for taking, and importance of taking as prescribed.	5.b.1. Explain the rationale for, side effects of, and importance of taking medications prescribed.
	    2. If client is discharged on warfarin (e.g. Coumadin), instruct to:
	      a. keep scheduled appointments for periodic blood studies to monitor coagulation times
	      b. take medication at the same time each day, do not stop taking medication abruptly, and do not attempt to make up for missed doses
	      c. avoid taking over-the-counter products containing aspirin and other nonsteroidal anti-inflammatory agents (these products enhance the action of warfarin)
	      d. avoid regular and/or excessive intake of alcohol (may alter responsiveness to warfarin)
	      e. avoid eating large amounts of foods high in vitamin K (e.g. green leafy vegetables)
	      f. report prolonged or excessive bleeding from skin, nose, or mouth; blood in urine, vomitus, sputum, or stool; prolonged or excessive menses; excessive bruising; severe headache; or sudden abdominal or back pain
	      g. inform physician immediately if pregnancy is suspected (warfarin crosses the placental barrier)
	      h. wear a medical alert bracelet or tag identifying self as being on anticoagulant therapy.
	    3. Instruct client to inform physician of any other prescription and nonprescription medications he/she is taking.
	    4. Instruct client to inform all health care providers of medications being taken.

5.c. The client will demonstrate the ability to correctly draw up and administer heparin subcutaneously if prescribed.	5.c.1. If client is to be discharged on subcutaneous heparin, provide instructions on subcutaneous injection technique. 2. Allow time for questions, practice, and return demonstration.

5.d. The client will identify precautions necessary to prevent bleeding associated with anticoagulant therapy.	5.d.1. Instruct client about ways to minimize risk of bleeding:
	      a. use an electric rather than straight-edge razor
	      b. floss and brush teeth gently
	      c. avoid putting sharp objects (e.g. toothpicks) in mouth
	      d. do not walk barefoot
	      e. cut nails carefully
	      f. avoid situations that could result in injury (e.g. contact sports)
	      g. avoid blowing nose forcefully
	      h. avoid straining to have a bowel movement.
	    2. Instruct client to control any bleeding by applying firm, prolonged pressure to the area if possible.

5.e. The client will state signs and symptoms to report to the health care provider.	5.e. Instruct client to report:
	    1. recurrent tenderness, pain, or swelling in extremity
	    2. sudden chest pain accompanied by shortness of breath
	    3. unusual bleeding (see action b.2.f in this diagnosis)
	    4. discoloration or itching of affected extremity (indicative of stasis dermatitis associated with chronic venous insufficiency)
	    5. skin breakdown on affected extremity.

5.f. The client will verbalize an understanding of and a plan for adhering to recommended follow-up care including future appointments with health care provider and activity level.	5.f.1. Reinforce importance of keeping follow-up appointments with health care provider.
	    2. Reinforce physician's instructions regarding activity limitations.
	    3. Implement measures to improve client compliance:
	      a. include significant others in teaching sessions if possible
	      b. encourage questions and allow time for reinforcement and clarification of information provided
	      c. provide written instructions regarding future appointments with health care provider, medications prescribed, activity restrictions, signs and symptoms to report, and future laboratory studies.

Bibliography

See pages 897–898 and 904.

⬓ FEMOROPOPLITEAL BYPASS

Lower extremity arterial bypass is performed to treat peripheral artery insufficiency that has not responded well to conservative management. The impaired blood flow can occur as a result of acute conditions (e.g. trauma, embolization) but most often is caused by atherosclerotic changes in the vessels. The femoropopliteal arterial segment is the most common site of occlusion in persons with lower extremity arterial disease. Signs and symptoms that usually indicate the need for surgical intervention include intermittent claudication that has become disabling, foot pain that is present at rest, and/or the presence of lower extremity ischemic ulcers.

Surgical treatment of the diseased femoropopliteal arterial segment can be accomplished by endarterectomy or removal of the segment and replacement with a synthetic graft, but the usual procedure is to bypass the segment using a synthetic or, more frequently, an autogenous vein graft. The saphenous vein is the preferred graft for femoropopliteal bypass because it is thick walled and has an adequate lumen diameter. Prior to grafting the saphenous vein proximal and distal to the occluded arterial segment, reversal of the vein or division of its valve cusps is done to allow unimpeded arterial blood flow.

This care plan focuses on the adult client with atherosclerotic occlusion of the femoropopliteal arterial segment who has been hospitalized for a femoropopliteal bypass. Preoperatively, goals of care are to reduce fear and anxiety, control pain, and maintain optimal tissue perfusion in the affected lower extremity. The goals of postoperative care are to maintain comfort, prevent complications, and educate the client regarding follow-up care.

DIAGNOSTIC TESTS

Duplex ultrasound
Plethysmography
Arteriography of affected lower extremity
Magnetic resonance imaging (MRI)
Segmental limb pressure measurements

DISCHARGE CRITERIA

Prior to discharge, the client will:

- have adequate circulation in the operative extremity
- have surgical pain controlled
- tolerate expected level of activity
- have evidence of normal wound healing
- have no signs and symptoms of postoperative complications
- identify ways to prevent or slow the progression of atherosclerosis
- identify ways to promote blood flow in the operative extremity
- state signs and symptoms to report to the health care provider
- verbalize an understanding of and a plan for adhering to recommended follow-up care including future appointments with health care provider, medications prescribed, activity level, and wound care.

NURSING/ COLLABORATIVE DIAGNOSES	**Preoperative**
	1. Altered peripheral tissue perfusion △ 416
	2. Pain: intermittent claudication and rest pain △ 416
	Postoperative
	1. Altered peripheral tissue perfusion △ 417
	2. Potential complications:
	a. graft occlusion
	b. compartment syndrome
	c. saphenous nerve damage △ 418
DISCHARGE TEACHING	3. Knowledge deficit, Ineffective management of therapeutic regimen, or Altered health maintenance △ 420

See Standardized Preoperative and Postoperative Care Plans for additional diagnoses.

PREOPERATIVE

Use in conjunction with the Standardized Preoperative Care Plan.

---

1. NURSING DIAGNOSIS:

Altered peripheral tissue perfusion

related to diminished blood flow in the affected lower extremity associated with atherosclerotic changes in the femoral and popliteal arteries.

Desired Outcome	Nursing Actions and *Selected Purposes/Rationales*
1. The client will not experience further reduction in arterial blood flow in the affected lower extremity as evidenced by: a. no increase in lower extremity pain b. no further decrease in peripheral pulses c. no increase in capillary refill time d. usual temperature and color of extremity.	1.a. Assess for signs and symptoms of a further reduction in arterial blood flow in the affected lower extremity: 1. intermittent claudication occurring with increased intensity and/or with less activity than previously 2. development of or increase in intensity of rest pain (this foot and toe pain that occurs when the client is in a horizontal position results from decreased blood flow to the skin and subcutaneous tissue; because it occurs in the absence of lower extremity muscle activity, it reflects a severe reduction in the femoropopliteal arterial blood flow) 3. diminishing peripheral pulses 4. increase in usual capillary refill time 5. increased coolness and numbness of foot and lower leg 6. increased pallor or blanching of foot and lower leg when extremity is elevated 7. more rapid appearance of rubor or cyanosis in foot and lower leg when extremity is in a dependent position. b. Implement measures *to prevent further reduction in and/or improve blood flow in the affected lower extremity:* 1. discourage positions that compromise blood flow in lower extremities (e.g. crossing legs, pillows under knees, use of knee gatch, elevating legs when in bed, sitting for long periods) 2. perform actions *to prevent vasoconstriction:* a. implement measures *to reduce stress* (e.g. maintain a calm environment, control pain, explain preoperative and postoperative care) b. discourage smoking c. implement measures *to keep client from getting cold* (e.g. maintain a comfortable room temperature; provide adequate clothing, warm socks, and blankets) 3. encourage short walks as tolerated 4. administer pentoxifylline (Trental) if ordered *to improve the flow of blood to the ischemic area.* c. Consult physician if signs and symptoms of further reduction in lower extremity tissue perfusion occur.

---

2. NURSING DIAGNOSIS:

Pain: intermittent claudication and rest pain

related to diminished arterial blood flow in the affected lower extremity (ischemia results in the release of anaerobic metabolites that irritate the nerve endings of the affected lower extremity).

Desired Outcome	Nursing Actions and *Selected Purposes/Rationales*

2. The client will experience diminished lower extremity pain as evidenced by:
a. verbalization of same
b. relaxed facial expression and body positioning.
	2.a. Assess for signs and symptoms of pain in the affected lower extremity:
	  1. intermittent claudication (e.g. verbalization of pain, aching, and/or cramping [usually in the calf muscle] during ambulation)
	  2. rest pain (e.g. awakening at night with reports of severe burning or aching in foot or toes)
	  3. grimacing, restlessness, reluctance to move, and/or rubbing lower leg or foot.
	b. Assess client's perception of the severity of pain using a pain intensity rating scale.
	c. Assess the client's pain pattern (e.g. location, quality, onset, duration, precipitating factors, aggravating factors, alleviating factors).
	d. Implement measures *to reduce pain in the affected extremity:*
	  1. perform actions to prevent further reduction in and/or improve blood flow in the affected lower extremity (see Preoperative Nursing Diagnosis 1, action b)
	  2. perform actions *to reduce fear and anxiety about the pain experience* (e.g. assure client that his/her need for pain relief is understood, plan methods for achieving pain control with client)
	  3. administer analgesics before activities and procedures that can cause pain and before pain becomes severe
	  4. perform actions *to reduce the number of episodes of intermittent claudication:*
	    a. encourage client to stop activity minutes before symptoms are usually experienced (intermittent claudication is predictable and the client is often aware of how far or how long he/she can ambulate before the discomfort begins or intensifies)
	    b. maintain client on bed rest if experiencing severe intermittent claudication (*limiting activity decreases muscle contractions in and subsequent ischemia of the affected lower extremity*)
	  5. if client is experiencing rest pain in the affected extremity, perform actions *to facilitate gravity flow of arterial blood to the ischemic area:*
	    a. allow client to sleep in a recliner with legs in a dependent position or, if in bed, to hang affected lower leg over the side of bed
	    b. instruct client to avoid horizontal positioning and elevation of affected extremity for prolonged periods
	  6. provide or assist with nonpharmacologic measures for relief of pain (e.g. progressive relaxation exercises; position change; diversional activities such as conversing, watching television, or reading)
	  7. administer analgesics if ordered.
	e. Consult physician if above measures fail to provide adequate pain relief.

POSTOPERATIVE

Use in conjunction with the Standardized Postoperative Care Plan.

---

1. NURSING DIAGNOSIS:

Altered peripheral tissue perfusion

related to diminished blood flow in the operative extremity associated with:
a. inflammation of the femoral and popliteal arteries at the sites of graft anastomosis;
b. pressure on vessels in the operative extremity resulting from edema that can occur as a result of decreased venous return and dissection around perivascular lymphatics;

c. venous stasis resulting from decreased mobility and decreased venous return if the saphenous vein was used for the bypass graft (can result in impaired venous return until collateral venous circulation improves);

d. hypovolemia resulting from blood loss during surgery and decreased fluid intake.

Desired Outcome	Nursing Actions and *Selected Purposes/Rationales*

1. The client will maintain adequate tissue perfusion in the operative extremity as evidenced by:
   a. resolution of leg and foot pain
   b. palpable peripheral pulses
   c. adequate Doppler flow readings in operative extremity
   d. absence of coolness, numbness, and cyanosis in foot and lower leg
   e. resolution of edema in operative extremity
   f. capillary refill time less than 3 seconds.

1.a. Assess for and report signs and symptoms of diminished tissue perfusion in operative extremity:
   1. pain unrelieved by prescribed analgesics
   2. diminished or absent pulses (the pulses may be difficult to palpate for 4–12 hours after surgery *because of vasospasm that can occur in the operative extremity*)
   3. diminished or absent Doppler flow readings over operative extremity
   4. coolness, numbness, or cyanosis of foot and lower leg
   5. increase in edema in the operative extremity
   6. capillary refill time greater than 3 seconds.

b. Implement measures *to promote adequate tissue perfusion in operative extremity:*
   1. avoid 90° flexion of the hip as much as possible (e.g. place client in high Fowler's position for meals only, limit length of time that client is in straight-back chair, provide recliner for client's use when sitting up)
   2. limit length of time that operative leg is in dependent position (e.g. allow client to sit up for meals only; encourage short, frequent walks rather than long walks)
   3. maintain knee in a neutral or slightly flexed position
   4. if lower extremity edema is present, elevate foot of bed 15° as ordered *to promote venous return without compromising arterial flow*
   5. place a bed cradle over lower extremities *to minimize pressure from bed linens*
   6. instruct client to perform active foot and leg exercises every 1–2 hours while awake
   7. perform actions *to prevent vasoconstriction:*
      a. implement measures *to reduce stress* (e.g. control pain, maintain a calm environment, explain postoperative care)
      b. discourage smoking
      c. implement measures *to keep client from getting cold* (e.g. maintain a comfortable room temperature; provide adequate clothing, warm socks, and blankets)
   8. maintain a minimum fluid intake of 2500 ml/day unless contraindicated; if oral intake is inadequate or contraindicated, maintain intravenous fluid therapy as ordered
   9. administer blood and blood products as ordered.

c. Consult physician if signs and symptoms of diminished tissue perfusion in the operative extremity persist or worsen.

---

2. COLLABORATIVE DIAGNOSES:

Potential complications of femoropopliteal bypass:

a. **graft occlusion** related to thrombus formation, kink in graft, or inadequate vessel diameter at sites of anastomosis;

b. **compartment syndrome** related to severe edema of the operative extremity (an infrequent, but serious complication that can occur as a result of surgical site inflammation, reperfusion of the ischemic muscles, or dissection around the perivascular lymphatics);

c. **saphenous nerve damage** related to:
   1. inadvertent or unavoidable dissection of the nerve during surgery
   2. trauma to the nerve during surgery.

Desired Outcomes	Nursing Actions and *Selected Purposes/Rationales*

2.a. The client will maintain a patent graft in the operative extremity as evidenced by:
1. no reports of sudden, severe toe or foot pain
2. palpable peripheral pulses
3. capillary refill time less than 3 seconds
4. absence of cyanosis, coolness, and diminishing sensation in the foot.
	2.a.1. Assess for and report signs and symptoms of graft occlusion in the operative extremity (e.g. sudden, severe pain in toes or foot; diminishing or absent peripheral pulses; capillary refill time greater than 3 seconds; cyanosis, coolness, or diminished sensation in the foot).
	    2. Implement measures *to prevent graft occlusion:*
	      a. avoid prolonged flexion of the knee on the operative extremity (e.g. limit sitting as ordered, do not place pillows under knees when in bed) *to prevent kinking of graft*
	      b. perform actions to promote adequate tissue perfusion in operative extremity (see Postoperative Nursing Diagnosis 1, action b) *in order to reduce the risk of thrombus formation.*
	    3. If signs and symptoms of graft occlusion occur:
	      a. maintain client on bed rest with operative leg in horizontal position
	      b. prepare client for surgical intervention (e.g. thrombectomy, straightening of graft, widening of lumen at site[s] of anastomosis) if planned
	      c. provide emotional support to client and significant others.

2.b. The client will not experience compartment syndrome in the operative extremity as evidenced by:
1. no complaints of increasing leg pain
2. no statements of new or increasing numbness and tingling in foot or leg or tightness and tenseness of thigh or calf muscle
3. ability to move leg and foot
4. no decrease in or absence of peripheral pulses
5. absence of cyanosis and coldness of leg and foot.
	2.b.1. Assess for and report signs and symptoms of compartment syndrome in the operative extremity:
	      a. complaints of increasing leg pain
	      b. statements of new or increasing numbness and tingling in foot or leg or tightness and tenseness of thigh or calf muscle
	      c. difficulty moving foot
	      d. diminishing or absent peripheral pulses
	      e. cyanotic, cold foot and leg.
	    2. Implement measures *to prevent an increase in edema in operative leg in order to reduce the risk of development of compartment syndrome:*
	      a. limit length of time that operative leg is in a dependent position (e.g. limit sitting and walking as ordered)
	      b. elevate operative extremity 15° if ordered
	      c. administer osmotic diuretics (e.g. mannitol) if ordered.
	    3. If signs and symptoms of compartment syndrome occur:
	      a. maintain client on bed rest
	      b. assess for and report brown discoloration of urine (*could indicate myoglobinuria resulting from the release of myoglobin from the damaged muscle cells; if an excessive amount of myoglobin is released, it can get trapped in the renal tubules and cause renal failure*)
	      c. prepare client for a fasciotomy if planned
	      d. provide emotional support to client and significant others.

2.c. The client will have resolution of or adapt to operative extremity saphenous nerve damage if it has occurred.	**2.c.1.** Assess for and report signs and symptoms of saphenous nerve damage (e.g. numbness, tingling, or hypersensitivity of the operative extremity).
	    2. If signs and symptoms of saphenous nerve damage are present:
	      a. adhere to and instruct client in the following safety precautions:
	        1. wear shoes or slippers whenever out of bed
	        2. do not apply heat or cold to the affected extremity
	        3. test temperature of bath water before use
	        4. protect operative extremity from trauma
	      b. reinforce information from physician regarding permanence of numbness, tingling, or hypersensitivity (these symptoms are permanent if the nerve was severed during surgery; if the nerve was just traumatized, the symptoms are temporary and expected to resolve within 1 year)
	      c. consult physician if signs and symptoms increase in severity.

Discharge Teaching

■━━━━━━━━━━━━━━━━━━━━━━━━━━

3. NURSING DIAGNOSIS: **Knowledge deficit, Ineffective management of therapeutic regimen, or Altered health maintenance***

---

*The nurse should select the diagnostic label that is most appropriate for the client's discharge teaching needs.

Desired Outcomes	Nursing Actions and *Selected Purposes/Rationales*

3.a. The client will identify ways to prevent or slow the progression of atherosclerosis.	3.a.1. Inform the client that certain modifiable factors such as elevated serum lipids and hypertension have been shown to increase the risk of atherosclerosis.
	2. Assist client to identify changes in life style that could reduce the risk for atherosclerosis (e.g. stress management, dietary modifications, physical exercise on a regular basis).
	3. Provide instructions on ways the client can reduce intake of saturated fat and cholesterol:
	  a. reduce intake of red meat
	  b. trim visible fat off meat and remove all skin from poultry
	  c. use vegetable oil rather than coconut or palm oil in cooking and food preparation
	  d. use cooking methods such as steaming, baking, broiling, poaching, microwaving, and grilling rather than frying
	  e. restrict intake of eggs (recommendations about the number of whole eggs allowed per week vary depending on the client's lipid levels)
	  f. avoid commercial baked goods
	  g. avoid dairy products containing more than 1% fat.
	4. Instruct client to take lipid-lowering agents (e.g. pravastatin, colestipol) if prescribed.

3.b. The client will identify ways to promote blood flow in the operative extremity.	3.b. Provide the following instructions about ways to promote blood flow in the operative extremity: 1. avoid wearing constrictive clothing (e.g. garters, girdles, narrow-banded knee-high stockings) 2. avoid positions that compromise blood flow (e.g. pillows under knees, crossing legs, sitting or standing for prolonged periods) 3. do active foot and leg exercises for 5 minutes every hour while awake 4. maintain a regular exercise program (walking and swimming are recommended) 5. stop smoking 6. drink at least 10 glasses of liquid/day unless contraindicated.

3.c. The client will state signs and symptoms to report to the health care provider.	3.c.1. Refer to Standardized Postoperative Care Plan, Nursing Diagnosis 21, action c (p. 123), for signs and symptoms to report to the health care provider.
	2. Instruct client to report these additional signs and symptoms:
	  a. sudden or gradual increase in operative leg or foot pain
	  b. increased swelling or purple discoloration at incision sites
	  c. pallor, coldness, or bluish color of the operative extremity
	  d. diminishing or sudden absence of peripheral pulses (client may be instructed to monitor his/her peripheral pulses)
	  e. significant increase in swelling of operative extremity (edema is expected to resolve gradually in 1–6 weeks)
	  f. difficulty moving foot on operative side
	  g. increasing numbness and/or tingling sensation of operative lower leg or foot.

3.d. The client will verbalize an understanding of and a plan for adhering to recommended follow-up care including future appointments with health care provider, medications prescribed, activity level, and wound care.

3.d.1. Refer to Standardized Postoperative Care Plan, Nursing Diagnosis 21 (pp. 123–124), for routine postoperative instructions and measures to improve client compliance.

2. Reinforce the physician's instructions regarding:
   a. importance of scheduling adequate rest periods
   b. need to avoid sitting or standing for long periods.

Bibliography

See pages 897–898 and 904.

UNIT ELEVEN

NURSING CARE OF THE CLIENT WITH DISTURBANCES OF RESPIRATORY FUNCTION

CANCER OF THE LUNG

Cancer of the lung, a malignant neoplasm involving lung tissue, is the leading cause of cancer-related deaths in the United States today. The rising incidence of cancer of the lung in both men and women is related to several factors, the chief of which is cigarette smoking. Other factors include environmental pollution; exposure to carcinogens such as asbestos, radioactive substances, arsenic, nickel, iron oxide, chromium, and chloromethyl ether; genetic factors; and lung scarring from previous inflammatory processes or chronic respiratory disease.

Cancer of the lung can occur as a primary tumor or as a metastasis from a site elsewhere in the body. The majority of primary lung neoplasms fall into one of 4 histological types. The types are small cell (oat cell) lung cancer (SCLC) and three non-small cell types of lung cancer (NSCLC), which include squamous cell (epidermoid) carcinoma, adenocarcinoma, and large cell cancer. These four types vary in relation to where they arise in the lung, responsiveness to the major modes of treatment, pattern of spread, clinical course, and prognosis. Squamous cell carcinoma and adenocarcinoma are the most common types. Squamous cell carcinoma is almost always associated with smoking, usually occurs as a central tumor, and produces early symptoms of local disease because of bronchial obstruction. It generally spreads by direct extension to surrounding tissue and has the best 5-year survival rate. Adenocarcinoma occurs most frequently in the periphery of the lungs, has a slow growth rate, tends to invade the pleura, typically does not produce symptoms until late in the course of the disease, and occurs more frequently in women and nonsmokers. Large cell tumors usually arise in the peripheral area of the lung, grow rapidly, and metastasize early. Small cell lung carcinoma tends to occur in the hilar or perihilar area, is usually a systemic disease at the time of diagnosis, is the type most frequently associated with paraneoplastic syndromes, and has a very poor prognosis.

The treatment selected depends on the tumor type(s), presence and extent of metastasis, and the client's health status. Surgery, with or without adjunctive chemotherapy or radiation therapy, is performed to resect the tumor if feasible. Unfortunately, surgery is usually not an option because the disease is often too advanced at the time of diagnosis. In these situations, chemotherapy or radiation therapy can be used alone or together in curative or palliative efforts.

The signs and symptoms of cancer of the lung are a result of a variety of factors including the actual presence of tumor in the lung; extension of the tumor into the thoracic cavity; extrathoracic metastasis of tumor; and systemic conditions that are not caused directly by the primary tumor, metastasis, or the treatment. The local manifestations can include dyspnea, cough or change in character of an established cough, change in amount and character of sputum produced (hemoptysis is often present), wheezing, and chest pain. If the tumor has extended into the thoracic cavity, signs and symptoms are those resulting from conditions such as pleural effusion, lung abscess formation, superior vena cava syndrome, and involvement of segments of the cervical and thoracic nerves. The signs and symptoms of metastasis vary depending on the area affected. Common sites of metastasis are the lymph nodes, liver, adrenal glands, brain, bones, and kidneys. Nonmetastatic systemic manifestations (referred to as paraneoplastic syndromes) include metabolic conditions such as Cushing's syndrome, syndrome of inappropriate antidiuretic hormone (SIADH), and hypercalcemia and neuromuscular conditions such as myasthenic (Lambert-Eaton) syndrome. These syndromes may predate x-ray evidence of lung cancer by many months.

This care plan focuses on care of the adult client with cancer of the lung hospitalized either for staging and initiation of treatment or for management of complications that have developed as a result of the disease process or its treatment. The goals of care are to reduce fear and anxiety, manage symptoms associated with the disease process and its treatment, and educate the client regarding follow-up care. If surgery is planned, this care plan should be used in conjunction with the Care Plan on Thoracic Surgery.

DIAGNOSTIC/STAGING TESTS*

Chest x-ray
Magnetic resonance imaging (MRI)
Computed tomography (CT)
Blood chemistry
Sputum cytology
Pulmonary function studies
Blood gases
Bronchoscopy
Biopsies (may include peripheral nodular lesions; lymph nodes such as scalene, mediastinal, and supraclavicular; pleura; bone marrow)
Thoracentesis
Radionuclide bone, brain, and liver scans
Pulmonary angiography

*Tests will vary according to the histological type of the tumor and the client's symptoms.

DISCHARGE CRITERIA

Prior to discharge, the client will:

- have an adequate respiratory status
- have no signs and symptoms of complications
- have an adequate or improving nutritional status
- have pain controlled
- tolerate expected level of activity
- identify ways to improve oxygenation status and maximize pulmonary health
- demonstrate proper chest physiotherapy techniques and the ability to use the equipment recommended to maximize pulmonary health
- identify ways to minimize the risk of infection
- verbalize ways to improve appetite and nutritional status
- verbalize ways to manage chronic syndrome of inappropriate antidiuretic hormone (SIADH) if present
- state signs and symptoms to report to the health care provider
- share thoughts and feelings about the diagnosis of lung cancer, the prognosis, and the effects of the disease process and its treatment on self-concept, life style, and roles
- identify community resources that can assist with home management and adjustment to the diagnosis and the effects of treatment
- verbalize an understanding of and a plan for adhering to recommended follow-up care including future appointments with health care provider, medications prescribed, activity level, and plans for subsequent treatment.

Use in conjunction with the Care Plans on Chemotherapy and External Radiation Therapy if appropriate.

NURSING/ COLLABORATIVE DIAGNOSES

1. Anxiety △   426
2. Impaired respiratory function:
   a. ineffective breathing pattern
   b. ineffective airway clearance
   c. impaired gas exchange △   426
3. Altered nutrition: less than body requirements △   428
4. Pain:
   a. tissue and skeletal pain
   b. chest pain
   c. pain within the irradiated area
   d. pharyngeal and esophageal pain
   e. oral pain △   429
5. Impaired verbal communication △   430
6. Activity intolerance △   430
7. Self-care deficit △   431
8. Sleep pattern disturbance △   432
9. Altered thought processes △   432
10. Risk for infection △   433
11. Risk for trauma: falls △   433
12. Potential complications:
    a. atelectasis
    b. lung abscess
    c. pleural effusion
    d. superior vena cava syndrome (SVCS)
    e. spinal cord compression
    f. syndrome of inappropriate antidiuretic hormone (SIADH)
    g. hypercalcemia
    h. Cushing's syndrome △   434
13. Self-concept disturbance △   438
14. Ineffective individual coping △   438
15. Grieving △   439

DISCHARGE TEACHING	**16.** Knowledge deficit, Ineffective management of therapeutic regimen, or Altered health maintenance △ 439

See Care Plans on Chemotherapy and External Radiation Therapy for additional diagnoses.

---

1. NURSING DIAGNOSIS: **Anxiety**

related to current signs and symptoms; lack of understanding of the diagnosis, diagnostic tests, and treatment plan; unfamiliar environment; financial concerns; anticipated effects of cancer and its treatment on body functioning and usual life style and roles; and probability of premature death.

Desired Outcome	Nursing Actions and *Selected Purposes/Rationales*

1. The client will experience a reduction in anxiety as evidenced by:
  a. verbalization of feeling less anxious
  b. usual sleep pattern
  c. relaxed facial expression and body movements
  d. stable vital signs
  e. usual perceptual ability and interactions with others.
	1.a. Assess client on admission for:
	  1. fears, misconceptions, and level of understanding about lung cancer, tests to stage the disease, and possible treatment modes
	  2. perception of anticipated results of diagnostic tests and planned treatment
	  3. significance of the diagnosis of lung cancer to client
	  4. availability of an adequate support system
	  5. past experiences with cancer and its treatment
	  6. signs and symptoms of anxiety (e.g. verbalization of feeling anxious, insomnia, tenseness, shakiness, restlessness, diaphoresis, tachycardia, elevated blood pressure, facial pallor, self-focused behaviors).
	 b. Refer to Nursing Diagnosis 1, action b (pp. 174 and 202–203), in Care Plans on Chemotherapy and External Radiation Therapy for measures to reduce fear and anxiety associated with the diagnosis and planned treatment.
	 c. Implement additional measures *to reduce fear and anxiety:*
	  1. explain all diagnostic tests performed to stage lung cancer
	  2. perform actions to reduce pain (see Nursing Diagnosis 4)
	  3. perform actions to improve respiratory status (see Nursing Diagnosis 2, action d) *in order to reduce dyspnea*
	  4. inform client that the amount of blood in sputum does not necessarily correlate with severity of the disease; provide an opaque, covered container for sputum collection *to reduce anxiety associated with hemoptysis*
	  5. perform actions to assist client to cope with the diagnosis and its implications (see Nursing Diagnosis 14).
	 d. Consult physician if above actions fail to control fear and anxiety.

---

2. NURSING DIAGNOSIS: **Impaired respiratory function:***

a. **ineffective breathing pattern** related to:
  1. increased rate and decreased depth of respirations associated with fear and anxiety

---

*This diagnostic label includes the following nursing diagnoses: ineffective breathing pattern, ineffective airway clearance, and impaired gas exchange.

2. decreased rate and depth of respirations associated with the depressant effect of some medications (e.g. narcotic [opioid] analgesics)
3. diminished lung/chest wall expansion associated with compression of lung tissue by the tumor, weakness, fatigue, reluctance to breathe deeply because of pain, pleural effusion if present, and paralysis of diaphragm on involved side (can occur if the tumor has invaded the phrenic nerve);

b. **ineffective airway clearance** related to:
1. excessive mucus production associated with inflammation of lung tissue resulting from the disease process
2. stasis of secretions associated with:
    a. difficulty coughing up secretions resulting from the depressant effect of some medications (e.g. narcotic [opioid] analgesics), pain, weakness, fatigue, and presence of tenacious secretions (can occur if fluid intake is inadequate)
    b. impaired ciliary function resulting from the disease process
    c. decreased mobility
3. invasion of and/or pressure on airways by tumor;

c. **impaired gas exchange** related to decrease in effective lung surface associated with replacement of lung tissue by neoplastic cells, accumulation of secretions, and/or atelectasis.

Desired Outcome	Nursing Actions and *Selected Purposes/Rationales*

2. The client will experience adequate respiratory function as evidenced by:
a. normal rate and depth of respirations
b. decreased dyspnea
c. usual or improved breath sounds
d. usual mental status
e. usual skin color
f. blood gases within normal range.
	2.a. Assess for and report signs and symptoms of impaired respiratory function:
	  1. rapid, shallow, or slow respirations
	  2. dyspnea, orthopnea
	  3. use of accessory muscles when breathing
	  4. adventitious breath sounds (e.g. crackles [rales], wheezes)
	  5. diminished or absent breath sounds
	  6. cough
	  7. restlessness, irritability
	  8. confusion, somnolence
	  9. central cyanosis (a late sign).
	b. Monitor for and report the following:
	  1. abnormal blood gases
	  2. significant decrease in oximetry results
	  3. significant changes in chest x-ray results.
	c. Assist with pulmonary function studies (e.g. tidal volume, vital capacity, inspiratory force) if done to evaluate respiratory status and effectiveness of treatment measures.
	d. Implement measures *to improve respiratory status:*
	  1. place client in a semi- to high Fowler's position unless contraindicated; position overbed table so client can lean on it if desired
	  2. perform actions to reduce fear and anxiety (see Nursing Diagnosis 1, actions b and c)
	  3. perform actions to reduce pain (see Nursing Diagnosis 4)
	  4. perform actions to increase strength and activity tolerance (see Nursing Diagnosis 6, action b) *in order to increase client's willingness and ability to move, cough, deep breathe, and use incentive spirometer*
	  5. instruct client to breathe slowly if hyperventilating
	  6. maintain oxygen therapy as ordered
	  7. assist client to turn at least every 2 hours while in bed
	  8. instruct client to deep breathe or use incentive spirometer every 1–2 hours
	  9. assist with positive airway pressure techniques (e.g. IPPB, continuous positive airway pressure [CPAP], biphasic positive airway pressure [BiPAP], expiratory positive airway pressure [EPAP]) if ordered

Desired Outcome	Nursing Actions and *Selected Purposes/Rationales*

10. instruct client in and assist with diaphragmatic breathing if appropriate (may be necessary if the tumor has invaded the phrenic nerve)
11. perform actions *to facilitate removal of pulmonary secretions:*
    a. instruct and assist client to cough or "huff" every 1–2 hours
    b. implement measures *to thin tenacious secretions and reduce drying of the respiratory mucous membrane:*
        1. maintain a fluid intake of 2500 ml/day unless contraindicated
        2. humidify inspired air as ordered
    c. assist with administration of mucolytics and diluent or hydrating agents via nebulizer if ordered
    d. assist with or perform postural drainage therapy (PDT) if ordered
    e. perform suctioning if needed
12. instruct client to avoid intake of gas-forming foods (e.g. beans, cauliflower, cabbage, onions), carbonated beverages, and large meals *in order to prevent gastric distention and subsequent pressure on the diaphragm*
13. discourage smoking (*smoke increases mucus production, impairs ciliary function, decreases oxygen availability, and can cause inflammation and damage to the bronchial walls*)
14. maintain activity restrictions if ordered; increase activity as allowed and tolerated
15. administer central nervous system depressants judiciously; hold medication and consult physician if respiratory rate is less than 12/minute
16. administer the following medications if ordered:
    a. bronchodilators (e.g. methylxanthines, beta-adrenergic agonists)
    b. corticosteroids (*may be given to decrease airway inflammation and thereby improve bronchial airflow*)
17. assist with thoracentesis if performed *to remove excessive pleural fluid and improve lung expansion*
18. prepare client for treatment of the malignancy (e.g. radiation therapy, chemotherapy, surgical resection of tumor) if planned *to reduce the tumor mass.*
    e. Consult physician if signs and symptoms of impaired respiratory function persist or worsen.

---

3. NURSING DIAGNOSIS:

Altered nutrition: less than body requirements

related to:
a. decreased oral intake associated with:
   1. oral, pharyngeal, or esophageal pain (can be a side effect of cytotoxic drugs and/or radiation therapy)
   2. difficulty swallowing resulting from narrowing of the esophagus (can occur if the tumor has invaded or is compressing the esophagus)
   3. anorexia resulting from factors such as depression, fear, anxiety, fatigue, discomfort, dyspnea, early satiety, and altered sense of taste (often reported by persons with cancer);
b. loss of nutrients associated with vomiting resulting from administration of cytotoxic agents;
c. impaired utilization of nutrients associated with:
   1. accelerated and inefficient metabolism of proteins, carbohydrates, and fats resulting from the disease process
   2. decreased absorption of nutrients resulting from loss of intestinal absorptive surface if mucositis has developed as a result of the administration of cytotoxic agents;
d. utilization of available nutrients by the malignant cells rather than the host.

Desired Outcome	Nursing Actions and *Selected Purposes/Rationales*
3. The client will have or attain an adequate nutritional status (see Care Plan on Chemotherapy, Nursing Diagnosis 2 [p. 175], for outcome criteria).	3.a. Refer to Care Plan on Chemotherapy, Nursing Diagnosis 2 (pp. 175–176), for measures related to assessment and maintenance or promotion of an adequate nutritional status. b. Place client in a high Fowler's position for meals and provide supplemental oxygen therapy during meals if indicated *to help relieve dyspnea.*

■—————————————————————————————

4. NURSING DIAGNOSIS:　**Pain:**

    a. **tissue and skeletal pain** related to pressure from the tumor and enlarged lymph nodes, nerve involvement, and metastasis to the bone or other organs if it has occurred;

    b. **chest pain** related to:
      1. irritation of the parietal pleura associated with extension of the primary tumor or pleural effusion (if present)
      2. muscle strain associated with excessive coughing
      3. extension of the primary tumor into the chest wall;

    c. **pain within the irradiated area** related to inflammation and exposure of nerve endings associated with moist desquamation if it occurs;

    d. **pharyngeal and esophageal pain** related to inflammation and/or ulceration of the mucosa associated with the effects of radiation to upper chest and/or administration of cytotoxic drugs;

    e. **oral pain** related to mucositis associated with the effects of cytotoxic drugs on the rapidly dividing cells of the oral mucosa.

Desired Outcome	Nursing Actions and *Selected Purposes/Rationales*

4. The client will experience diminished pain (see Care Plan on External Radiation Therapy, Nursing Diagnosis 4 [pp. 205–206], for outcome criteria).	4.a. Refer to Care Plan on External Radiation Therapy, Nursing Diagnosis 4 (pp. 205–206), for measures related to assessment and management of pain.
	b. Implement additional measures *to reduce pain:*
	  1. perform actions *to reduce tissue and/or skeletal pain:*
	    a. move client carefully; obtain adequate assistance when needed
	    b. when turning client, logroll and support all extremities
	    c. utilize smooth motions when moving client; avoid pushing or pulling on body parts
	    d. caution client to avoid sudden twisting and turning
	    e. provide a firm mattress or place a bed board under mattress for added support
	    f. administer anti-inflammatory agents if ordered
	    g. prepare client for radiation therapy to painful skeletal areas if planned *to shrink metastatic tumor and reduce pressure on the bone*
	  2. perform actions *to reduce chest pain:*
	    a. instruct and assist client to splint chest with hands or pillow when deep breathing, coughing, or changing position
	    b. implement measures to treat pleural effusion if present (see Collaborative Diagnosis 12, action c.3)
	    c. implement measures to control excessive coughing (see Nursing Diagnosis 6, action b.1.h)
	    d. assist with an intercostal nerve block if performed *for intractable pain.*

5. NURSING DIAGNOSIS: **Impaired verbal communication**

related to pressure on the recurrent laryngeal nerve (can occur if the tumor invades the mediastinum).

Desired Outcome	Nursing Actions and *Selected Purposes/Rationales*

5. The client will successfully communicate needs and desires.	5.a. Assess client for impaired verbal communication (e.g. hoarseness, difficulty speaking).
	b. Implement measures *to facilitate communication:*
	  1. maintain a patient, calm approach; listen attentively and allow ample time for communication
	  2. maintain a quiet environment *so that client does not have to speak loudly*
	  3. ask questions that require short answers or nod of head if client is having difficulty speaking and/or is fatigued
	  4. provide materials such as magic slate, pad and pencil, and/or word cards if appropriate; try to ensure that placement of intravenous line does not interfere with client's use of these communication aids
	  5. answer call signal in person rather than using intercommunication system.
	c. Inform significant others and health care personnel of techniques being used to facilitate client's ability to communicate.
	d. Consult physician if client experiences increasing impairment of verbal communication.

6. NURSING DIAGNOSIS: **Activity intolerance**

related to:
a. tissue hypoxia associated with impaired gas exchange;
b. possible loss of muscle mass, tone, and strength associated with inadequate nutritional status and decreased physical activity;
c. difficulty resting and sleeping associated with discomfort, fear, anxiety, grief, and unfamiliar environment;
d. increased energy expenditure associated with strenuous breathing efforts, persistent coughing, and an increase in the metabolic rate resulting from continuous, active tumor growth.

Desired Outcome	Nursing Actions and *Selected Purposes/Rationales*

6. The client will demonstrate an increased tolerance for activity as evidenced by:
a. verbalization of feeling less fatigued and weak
b. ability to perform activities of daily living without increased dyspnea, chest pain, diaphoresis, dizziness, and a significant change in vital signs.
	6.a. Assess for signs and symptoms of activity intolerance:
	  1. statements of fatigue or weakness
	  2. exertional dyspnea, chest pain, diaphoresis, or dizziness
	  3. abnormal heart rate response to activity (e.g. increase in rate of 20 beats/minute above resting rate, rate not returning to preactivity level within 3 minutes after stopping activity, change from regular to irregular rate)
	  4. decreased systolic B/P or a significant increase (10–15 mm Hg) in diastolic pressure with activity.
	b. Implement measures *to improve activity tolerance:*
	  1. perform actions *to promote rest and/or conserve energy:*
	    a. maintain activity restrictions as ordered

   b. minimize environmental activity and noise
   c. organize nursing care to allow for periods of uninterrupted rest
   d. limit the number of visitors and their length of stay
   e. assist client with self-care activities as needed
   f. keep supplies and personal articles within easy reach
   g. instruct client in energy-saving techniques (e.g. using shower chair when showering, sitting to brush teeth or comb hair)
   h. implement measures *to control excessive coughing:*
      1. instruct client to avoid intake of extremely hot or cold foods/fluids (*these can stimulate cough*)
      2. protect client from exposure to irritants such as flowers, smoke, and powder
      3. encourage client not to smoke (*smoke irritates the respiratory tract*)
      4. administer prescribed antitussives if indicated
   i. implement measures to promote sleep (see Nursing Diagnosis 8)
   j. implement measures to reduce pain (see Nursing Diagnosis 4)
   2. discourage smoking and excessive intake of beverages high in caffeine such as coffee, tea, and colas (*nicotine and caffeine increase cardiac workload and myocardial oxygen utilization, thereby decreasing oxygen availability*)
   3. perform actions to improve respiratory status (see Nursing Diagnosis 2, action d) *in order to help relieve dyspnea and improve tissue oxygenation*
   4. if oxygen therapy is necessary during activity, keep portable oxygen equipment readily available for client's use
   5. perform actions to promote an adequate nutritional status (see Nursing Diagnosis 3)
   6. increase client's activity gradually as allowed and tolerated.
   c. Instruct client to:
      1. report a decreased tolerance for activity
      2. stop any activity that causes chest pain, increased shortness of breath, dizziness, or extreme fatigue or weakness.
   d. Consult physician if signs and symptoms of activity intolerance persist or worsen.

---

7. NURSING DIAGNOSIS: **Self-care deficit**

related to:
a. altered thought processes if present;
b. activity limitations imposed by dyspnea, weakness, fatigue, and discomfort associated with the disease process, diagnostic tests, and/or the side effects of radiation therapy or treatment with cytotoxic drugs.

Desired Outcome	Nursing Actions and *Selected Purposes/Rationales*
7. The client will perform self-care activities within physical limitations.	7.a. Refer to Care Plan on Chemotherapy, Nursing Diagnosis 8 (p. 181), for measures related to planning for and meeting client's self-care needs. b. Implement measures to increase strength and improve activity tolerance (see Nursing Diagnosis 6, action b) *in order to further facilitate client's ability to perform self-care.*

8. NURSING DIAGNOSIS: **Sleep pattern disturbance**

related to:
a. fear, anxiety, and grief;
b. decreased activity, unfamiliar environment, and frequent assessments and treatments;
c. excessive coughing and inability to assume usual sleep position associated with orthopnea;
d. discomfort associated with the disease process and side effects of treatment.

Desired Outcome	Nursing Actions and *Selected Purposes/Rationales*

8. The client will attain optimal amounts of sleep (see Care Plan on Chemotherapy, Nursing Diagnosis 10 [p. 182], for outcome criteria).	8.a. Refer to Care Plan on Chemotherapy, Nursing Diagnosis 10 (pp. 182–183), for measures related to assessment and promotion of sleep.
	 b. Implement additional measures *to promote sleep:*
	  1. perform actions to reduce fear and anxiety (see Nursing Diagnosis 1, actions b and c)
	  2. perform actions to improve respiratory status (see Nursing Diagnosis 2, action d) *in order to relieve orthopnea*
	  3. perform actions to reduce pain (see Nursing Diagnosis 4)
	  4. perform actions to control excessive coughing (see Nursing Diagnosis 6, action b.1.h)
	  5. if client has orthopnea, assist him/her to assume a position *that facilitates breathing* (e.g. head of bed elevated with arms supported on pillows, resting forward on overbed table with good pillow support, sitting in chair)
	  6. maintain oxygen therapy during sleep.

9. NURSING DIAGNOSIS: **Altered thought processes***

related to:
a. cerebral hypoxia associated with impaired gas exchange;
b. central nervous system depressant effect of hypercalcemia if present;
c. damage to cerebral tissue (can occur if lung cancer has metastasized to the brain or if client is experiencing certain paraneoplastic neurological conditions).

*The diagnostic label of acute or chronic confusion may be more appropriate depending on the client's symptoms.

Desired Outcome	Nursing Actions and *Selected Purposes/Rationales*

9. The client will experience an improvement in thought processes as evidenced by:
a. improved verbal response time
b. improved memory
c. longer attention span
d. improved level of orientation.
	9.a. Assess client for altered thought processes (e.g. slowed verbal responses, impaired memory, shortened attention span, confusion).
	 b. Ascertain from significant others client's usual level of cognitive functioning.
	 c. Implement measures *to maintain optimal thought processes:*
	  1. perform actions to improve respiratory status (see Nursing Diagnosis 2, action d) *in order to reduce cerebral hypoxia*
	  2. perform actions to prevent or treat hypercalcemia (see Collaborative Diagnosis 12, action g.2)

3. prepare client for radiation therapy treatment of brain metastasis if planned
4. administer corticosteroids (e.g. dexamethasone) if ordered *to reduce cerebral edema and/or nerve inflammation if brain metastasis has occurred or a paraneoplastic neurological condition is present.*

d. If client shows evidence of altered thought processes:
1. reorient client to person, place, and time as necessary
2. address client by name
3. place familiar objects, clock, and calendar within client's view
4. approach client in a slow, calm, manner; allow adequate time for communication
5. repeat instructions as necessary using clear, simple language and short sentences
6. maintain a consistent and fairly structured routine and write out a schedule of activities for client to refer to if desired
7. have client perform only one activity at a time and allow adequate time for performance of activities
8. encourage client to make lists of planned activities, questions, and concerns
9. encourage significant others to be supportive of client; instruct them in methods of dealing with client's altered thought processes
10. discuss physiological basis for altered thought processes with client and significant others; inform them that cognitive and emotional functioning usually improve if treatment of the underlying cause is effective
11. consult physician if altered thought processes persist or worsen.

---

10. NURSING DIAGNOSIS: **Risk for infection**

related to:
a. stasis of pulmonary secretions associated with airway obstruction, poor cough effort, and decreased activity;
b. lowered natural resistance associated with an inadequate nutritional status, stress, and immunosuppressive effects of certain drugs (e.g. cytotoxic agents, corticosteroids);
c. break in skin integrity associated with radiation-induced desquamation if it has occurred;
d. break in mucosal surfaces associated with effects of cytotoxic drugs.

Desired Outcome	Nursing Actions and *Selected Purposes/Rationales*
10. The client will remain free of infection (see Care Plan on Chemotherapy, Nursing Diagnosis 11 [pp. 183–184], for outcome criteria).	10.a. Refer to Care Plan on Chemotherapy, Nursing Diagnosis 11 (pp. 183–185), for measures related to assessment and prevention of infection. b. Implement measures to facilitate removal of pulmonary secretions (see Nursing Diagnosis 2, action d.11) *in order to prevent pneumonia.*

---

11. NURSING DIAGNOSIS: **Risk for trauma: falls**

related to:
a. confusion and lethargy associated with impaired gas exchange, hypercalcemia if present, and brain metastasis (if it has occurred);

b. weakness associated with nutritional and sleep deficits, impaired gas exchange, hypercalcemia, side effect of radiation therapy and/or chemotherapy, and/or presence of paraneoplastic conditions such as myasthenic syndrome.

Desired Outcome	Nursing Actions and *Selected Purposes/Rationales*

11. The client will not experience falls.	11.a. Implement measures *to prevent falls:*
	   1. keep bed in low position with side rails up when client is in bed
	   2. keep needed items within easy reach
	   3. encourage client to request assistance whenever needed; have call signal within easy reach
	   4. use lap belt when client is in chair if indicated
	   5. instruct client to wear well-fitting slippers/shoes with nonslip soles and low heels when ambulating
	   6. keep floor free of clutter and wipe up spills promptly
	   7. carefully position tubings and equipment so that they will not interfere with ambulation
	   8. accompany client during ambulation utilizing a transfer safety belt if he/she is weak or dizzy
	   9. provide ambulatory aids (e.g. walker, cane) if client is weak or unsteady on feet
	  10. instruct client to ambulate in well-lit areas and to utilize handrails if needed
	  11. do not rush client; allow adequate time for ambulation to the bathroom and in hallway
	  12. make sure that shower has a nonslip bottom surface and that shower chair, secure bath mat, call signal, grab bars, and adequate lighting are present
	  13. administer central nervous system depressants judiciously
	  14. perform actions to prevent or treat hypercalcemia (see Collaborative Diagnosis 12, action g.2) *in order to help maintain mental alertness and normal neuromuscular function*
	  15. perform actions to improve respiratory status (see Nursing Diagnosis 2, action d) *in order to facilitate gas exchange and reduce cerebral hypoxia*
	  16. perform actions *to treat brain metastasis and/or paraneoplastic neurological conditions* (e.g. prepare client for radiation therapy treatments, administer corticosteroids if ordered) if present
	  17. perform actions to increase strength and improve activity tolerance (see Nursing Diagnosis 6, action b)
	  18. if client is confused or irrational:
	    a. reorient frequently to surroundings and necessity of adhering to safety precautions
	    b. provide appropriate level of supervision
	    c. consult physician about the temporary use of a bed alarm or jacket or wrist restraints if necessary
	    d. administer prescribed antianxiety and antipsychotic medications if indicated.
	b. Include client and significant others in planning and implementing measures to prevent falls.
	c. If client falls, initiate first aid if appropriate and notify physician.

---

12. COLLABORATIVE DIAGNOSES:

Potential complications of lung cancer:

a. **atelectasis** related to:
  1. stasis of secretions in the alveoli and bronchioles associated with poor cough effort, decreased activity, and obstruction by primary tumor

2. shallow respirations associated with restricted lung expansion resulting from fatigue, weakness, chest pain, presence of primary tumor, and/or pleural effusion if present

3. obstructed airflow associated with tumor involvement of major airways;

b. **lung abscess** related to necrosis of tissue within and around tumor;

c. **pleural effusion** related to:
   1. increased capillary permeability associated with inflammation resulting from presence of malignant cells in the pleura
   2. increased capillary hydrostatic pressure in the visceral pleura associated with obstruction of the pulmonary veins by the tumor
   3. impaired absorption of pleural fluid into the pleural lymphatic channels associated with lymph node obstruction resulting from the presence of a tumor
   4. increased colloid osmotic pressure in the pleural space associated with the presence of necrotic malignant cells;

d. **superior vena cava syndrome (SVCS)** related to obstruction of the superior vena cava associated with extrinsic pressure by the tumor or enlarged paratracheal lymph nodes, intraluminal thrombosis, or invasion of the vein wall by tumor cells (occurs most frequently with a superior mediastinal mass);

e. **spinal cord compression** related to metastasis to the vertebrae and/or epidural space;

f. **syndrome of inappropriate antidiuretic hormone (SIADH)** related to:
   1. ectopic production and secretion of antidiuretic hormone (ADH) by tumor cells (occurs most frequently with SCLC)
   2. administration of some antineoplastic agents found to be associated with the occurrence of SIADH (e.g. cisplatin, cyclophosphamide, vincristine)
   3. stimulation of ADH output associated with pain and stress;

g. **hypercalcemia** related to:
   1. increased bone resorption associated with the release of substances such as parathyroid hormone-related protein (PTHrP) by tumor cells (particularly with squamous cell carcinoma), bone metastasis if present, decreased mobility, and side effect of some cytotoxic agents
   2. increased renal tubular reabsorption of calcium associated with the release of substances such as parathyroid hormone-related protein (PTHrP) by tumor cells (particularly with squamous cell carcinoma);

h. **Cushing's syndrome** related to ectopic adrenocorticotropic hormone (ACTH) production by tumor cells and/or metastatic lesions of the adrenal glands.

Desired Outcomes	Nursing Actions and *Selected Purposes/Rationales*

12.a. The client will not develop atelectasis or will experience resolution of atelectasis if it occurs as evidenced by:
1. usual or improved breath sounds
2. resonant percussion note over lungs
3. no increase in dyspnea
4. pulse rate within normal range for client
5. afebrile status.
	12.a.1. Assess for and report signs and symptoms of atelectasis (e.g. diminished or absent breath sounds, dull percussion note over affected area, increased respiratory rate, increased dyspnea, tachycardia, elevated temperature).
	2. Monitor chest x-ray results. Report findings of atelectasis.
	3. Implement measures to improve respiratory status (see Nursing Diagnosis 2, action d) *in order to reduce the risk of or help resolve atelectasis.*
	4. If signs and symptoms of atelectasis occur:
	  a. increase frequency of turning, coughing or "huffing," deep breathing, and use of incentive spirometer
	  b. increase activity as allowed and tolerated
	  c. consult physician if signs and symptoms of atelectasis persist or worsen.

12.b. The client will have resolution of a lung abscess if it occurs as evidenced by: 1. absence of chills and fever	12.b.1. Assess for and report signs and symptoms of a lung abscess (e.g. chills; fever; increased respiratory rate; diminished or absent breath sounds and dull percussion note over affected area; cough productive of purulent, foul-smelling sputum; increased chest pain). 2. Monitor chest x-ray, computed tomography, and lung scan results. Report findings of lung abscess.

Desired Outcomes | Nursing Actions and **Selected Purposes/Rationales**

2. improved breath sounds and resonant percussion note over affected area
3. cough productive of clear mucus only
4. decreased chest pain.

3. If signs and symptoms of a lung abscess occur:
   a. prepare client for surgical drainage of abscess if planned
   b. administer antimicrobials if ordered.

12.c. The client will experience resolution of pleural effusion if it occurs as evidenced by:
1. decreased dyspnea
2. symmetrical chest movement
3. improved breath sounds and resonant percussion note over affected area
4. decreased chest pain.

12.c.1. Assess for and report signs and symptoms of pleural effusion (e.g. increased dyspnea; decreased chest excursion on affected side; diminished or absent breath sounds and dull percussion note over affected area; increase in chest pain).
2. Monitor chest x-ray and computed tomography results. Report findings of pleural effusion.
3. If signs and symptoms of pleural effusion occur:
   a. prepare client for and assist with procedures to remove excess fluid from the pleural space (e.g. thoracentesis with or without insertion of chest tube, insertion of a pleuroperitoneal shunt)
   b. prepare client for the following if planned *to prevent recurrence of the pleural effusion:*
      1. radiation therapy and/or chemotherapy *to treat the underlying malignancy*
      2. procedures to obliterate the pleural space (e.g. pleurodesis, pleurectomy).

12.d. The client will experience a reduction in signs and symptoms of SVCS if it occurs as evidenced by:
1. decreased dyspnea
2. decreased edema and erythema of face, neck, and upper trunk
3. decreased chest pain
4. absence of hoarseness, headache, and vertigo.

12.d.1. Assess for and report signs and symptoms of SVCS (e.g. increased dyspnea; edema and/or erythema of face, neck, or upper trunk; distended neck veins; increased chest pain; hoarseness; headache; vertigo). Symptoms usually become more pronounced if client bends forward or lies flat.
2. If signs and symptoms of SVCS occur:
   a. prepare client for chest x-ray, computed tomography, and/or venography if planned
   b. maintain client on bed rest with head of bed elevated
   c. prepare client for the following if planned:
      1. radiation therapy and/or chemotherapy *to shrink the obstructing tumor*
      2. surgery such as superior vena cava bypass if SVCS is caused by thrombosis or if symptoms are severe and have not been controlled by radiation therapy and/or chemotherapy
   d. administer the following medications if ordered:
      1. corticosteroids (e.g. dexamethasone) *to decrease edema at the site of obstruction of superior vena cava*
      2. diuretics *to reduce edema,* particularly if client is experiencing respiratory distress (diuretics provide only temporary relief and are used cautiously *because they can further decrease venous return*)
      3. thrombolytic agents (e.g. urokinase, streptokinase) if etiology is intraluminal thrombosis.

12.e. The client will experience a reduction in signs and symptoms of spinal cord compression if it occurs as evidenced by:
1. decreased back pain
2. improved motor and sensory function
3. improved bowel and bladder control.

12.e.1. Assess for and report signs and symptoms of spinal cord compression (e.g. back pain that may or may not radiate and is not relieved by lying down, progressive weakness, sensory deficits, loss of bowel and bladder control). Signs and symptoms manifested depend on which segment of the spinal cord is involved and extent of compression.
2. If signs and symptoms of spinal cord compression occur:
   a. prepare client for the following if planned:
      1. diagnostic tests (e.g. computed tomography, magnetic resonance imaging)
      2. radiation therapy *to reduce the size of the metastatic tumor*
      3. surgical decompression and spine stabilization if neurological deterioration is rapid and relief is not achieved with radiation to affected area
   b. administer the following medications if ordered:
      1. corticosteroids (e.g. dexamethasone) *to reduce edema at the site of metastasis*

2. analgesics *to reduce pain*
c. assist client with activities of daily living as needed
d. provide emotional support to client and significant others
e. refer to Care Plan on Spinal Cord Injury for additional care measures.

12.f. The client will experience resolution of SIADH if it develops as evidenced by:	12.f.1. Assess for and report signs and symptoms of SIADH:

12.f.1. Assess for and report signs and symptoms of SIADH:
a. sudden weight gain
b. intake greater than output
c. lethargy, confusion
d. reports of persistent headache
e. muscle weakness
f. fingerprint edema over sternum (indicative of cellular edema)
g. abdominal cramping, nausea, vomiting
h. seizures
i. elevated urine sodium and osmolality levels
j. low serum sodium and osmolality levels.

12.f. The client will experience resolution of SIADH if it develops as evidenced by:
1. decline in weight toward normal
2. balanced intake and output
3. usual mental status
4. absence of headache, muscle weakness, cellular edema, abdominal cramping, nausea, vomiting, and seizure activity
5. serum and urine sodium and osmolality levels within normal limits.

2. If signs and symptoms of SIADH occur:
a. maintain fluid restrictions if ordered (usually 500–1000 ml/day) *to prevent further fluid retention*
b. implement measures *to prevent further ADH stimulation:*
   1. perform actions to reduce pain (see Nursing Diagnosis 4)
   2. perform actions to reduce fear and anxiety (see Nursing Diagnosis 1, actions b and c)
c. encourage intake of foods/fluids high in sodium (e.g. cured meats, processed cheese, canned soups, catsup, dill pickles, tomato juice, canned vegetables, bouillon)
d. initiate seizure precautions
e. administer the following if ordered:
   1. diuretics (usually furosemide) *to promote water excretion*
   2. intravenous infusions of a hypertonic saline solution *to treat hyponatremia*
   3. demeclocycline *to promote water excretion* (*inhibits effect of ADH at the renal tubular level*)
f. prepare client for treatment of the underlying malignancy if planned.

12.g. The client will maintain a safe serum calcium level as evidenced by:
1. usual mental status
2. usual muscle strength and tone and reflex responses
3. absence of nausea, vomiting, and anorexia
4. regular pulse at 60–100 beats/minute
5. serum calcium within normal range.

12.g.1. Assess for and report signs and symptoms of hypercalcemia (e.g. change in mental status, muscle weakness, depressed reflexes, nausea, vomiting, anorexia, constipation, polyuria, cardiac dysrhythmias, elevated serum calcium level).

2. Implement measures *to prevent or treat hypercalcemia:*
a. prepare client for treatment of underlying malignancy
b. consult physician prior to administering calcium-containing antacids (e.g. Tums, Titralac), vitamin D preparations, or thiazide diuretics (*these can all increase serum calcium levels*)
c. encourage mobility as tolerated (*weight-bearing reduces calcium loss from the bones*)
d. maintain a minimum fluid intake of 2500 ml/day unless contraindicated (*hydrating the client lowers serum calcium by dilution*)
e. administer the following if ordered:
   1. saline infusions *to increase urinary calcium excretion*
   2. calcitonin *to inhibit bone resorption and increase renal clearance of calcium*
   3. loop diuretics (e.g. furosemide) *to increase renal excretion of calcium*
   4. medications such as gallium nitrate, etidronate, pamidronate, or plicamycin *to inhibit bone resorption.*
3. Consult physician if serum calcium levels remain above a safe level.

12.h. The client will experience a reduction in signs and symptoms associated with Cushing's syndrome if it occurs as evidenced by:

12.h.1. Assess for and report signs and symptoms of Cushing's syndrome (e.g. muscle weakness, edema, mild hypertension, psychosis, hyperglycemia, decreased serum potassium, high serum ACTH and cortisol levels, increased urinary cortisol and 17-hydroxycorticosteroid levels, increased pH and CO_2 content).

Desired Outcomes	Nursing Actions and *Selected Purposes/Rationales*
1. increased muscle strength 2. resolution of edema 3. usual mental status 4. serum glucose, potassium, ACTH, and cortisol levels within normal range 5. normal urinary cortisol and 17-hydroxycorticosteroid levels 6. blood gases within normal range for client.	2. If signs and symptoms of Cushing's syndrome occur: a. ensure that precautions are taken to prevent infection (*the increased cortisol level lowers the client's natural resistance to infection*) b. administer the following if ordered: 1. medications such as metyrapone, aminoglutethimide, or ketoconazole *to inhibit adrenal cortisol synthesis* 2. potassium supplements *to treat hypokalemia* c. prepare client for treatment of the malignancy if planned (e.g. radiation therapy, chemotherapy, bilateral adrenalectomy).

---

13. NURSING DIAGNOSIS: **Self-concept disturbance***

related to:
a. change in appearance (e.g. excessive weight loss, hair loss associated with chemotherapy, skin changes associated with radiation therapy, gynecomastia associated with ectopic hormone production by tumor cells);
b. temporary or permanent infertility associated with hormonal imbalance resulting from ectopic hormone production by tumor cells and/or cytotoxic drug therapy;
c. changes in sexual functioning associated with weakness, fatigue, dyspnea, pain, and anxiety;
d. increased dependence on others to meet self-care needs;
e. anticipated changes in life style and roles associated with effects of the disease process and its treatment.

---

*This diagnostic label includes the nursing diagnoses of body image disturbance, self-esteem disturbance, and altered role performance.

Desired Outcome	Nursing Actions and *Selected Purposes/Rationales*
13. The client will demonstrate beginning adaptation to changes in appearance, body functioning, life style, and roles (see Care Plan on Chemotherapy, Nursing Diagnosis 13 [p. 191], for outcome criteria).	13. Refer to Care Plan on Chemotherapy, Nursing Diagnosis 13 (pp. 191–192), for measures related to assessment and promotion of a positive self-concept.

---

14. NURSING DIAGNOSIS: **Ineffective individual coping**

related to:
a. persistent discomfort associated with the disease process and the side effects of chemotherapy and/or radiation therapy;
b. guilt associated with the diagnosis of lung cancer if a personal habit such as smoking was the major cause;
c. fear, anxiety, fatigue, feeling of powerlessness, and uncertainty of the effectiveness of treatment.

Desired Outcome	Nursing Actions and *Selected Purposes/Rationales*
14. The client will demonstrate effective coping skills (see Care Plan on Chemotherapy, Nursing Diagnosis 14 [p. 193]), for outcome criteria).	14.a. Refer to Care Plan on Chemotherapy, Nursing Diagnosis 14 (p. 193), for measures related to assessment and management of ineffective coping. b. Assist the client to work through feelings of guilt about factors that contributed to the development of lung cancer (e.g. smoking, occupation).

15. NURSING DIAGNOSIS: **Grieving***

related to:
a. loss of normal function of the lung;
b. changes in body image and usual life style and roles associated with the disease process and its treatment;
c. diagnosis of cancer with probability of premature death.

*This diagnostic label includes anticipatory grieving and grieving following the actual losses.

Desired Outcome	Nursing Actions and *Selected Purposes/Rationales*
15. The client will demonstrate beginning progression through the grieving process (see Care Plan on Chemotherapy, Nursing Diagnosis 15 [p. 194], for outcome criteria).	15. Refer to Care Plan on Chemotherapy, Nursing Diagnosis 15 (p. 194), for measures related to assessment and facilitation of grieving.

Discharge Teaching

16. NURSING DIAGNOSIS: **Knowledge deficit, Ineffective management of therapeutic regimen, or Altered health maintenance***

*The nurse should select the diagnostic label that is most appropriate for the client's discharge teaching needs.

Desired Outcomes	Nursing Actions and *Selected Purposes/Rationales*
16.a. The client will identify ways to improve oxygenation status and maximize pulmonary health.	16.a. Instruct client in ways to improve oxygenation status and maximize pulmonary health: 1. schedule adequate rest periods 2. avoid exposure to respiratory irritants such as smoke, dust, perfume, aerosol sprays, paint fumes, and solvents whenever possible 3. stop smoking 4. wear a mask or scarf over nose and mouth if exposure to high levels of irritants such as smoke, fumes, and dust is unavoidable 5. avoid high altitudes; if air travel is required, consult physician about the need for supplemental oxygen 6. continue with prescribed chest physiotherapy (e.g. breathing exercises, postural drainage therapy)

Desired Outcomes	Nursing Actions and *Selected Purposes/Rationales*

7. take medications such as bronchodilators and mucolytics as prescribed
8. minimize risk of respiratory tract infections:
   a. avoid contact with persons who have respiratory tract infections
   b. avoid crowds and poorly ventilated areas
   c. maintain good oral hygiene
   d. cleanse all respiratory care equipment properly
   e. drink at least 10 glasses of liquid/day unless contraindicated.

16.b. The client will demonstrate proper chest physiotherapy techniques and the ability to use the equipment recommended to maximize pulmonary health.

16.b.1. Reinforce instructions about proper breathing techniques (e.g. pursed-lip breathing, diaphragmatic breathing) and postural drainage therapy (PDT may be indicated if large amounts of mucus continue to be produced).
2. Reinforce instructions about use of respiratory equipment (e.g. oxygen, incentive spirometer, metered-dose inhalers).
3. Allow time for questions, clarification, and return demonstration.

16.c. The client will identify ways to minimize the risk of infection.

16.c. Refer to Care Plan on Chemotherapy, Nursing Diagnosis 17, action a (p. 196), for instructions related to preventing infection.

16.d. The client will verbalize ways to improve appetite and nutritional status.

16.d. Refer to Care Plan on Chemotherapy, Nursing Diagnosis 17, action e (p. 197), for instructions related to improving appetite and maintaining an adequate nutritional status.

16.e. The client will verbalize ways to manage chronic SIADH if present.

16.e. If appropriate, provide the following instructions related to management of chronic SIADH:
1. continue fluid restriction (usually 1 quart/day) if recommended by physician
2. take medications (e.g. furosemide, demeclocycline) as prescribed
3. increase intake of foods/fluids high in sodium (e.g. tomato juice, cured meats, processed cheese, canned vegetables and soups, catsup, dill pickles, bouillon)
4. report new or intensified signs and symptoms of SIADH (e.g. sudden weight gain, decrease in urine output, drowsiness, confusion, weakness, headache, nausea, vomiting, abdominal cramping, seizures).

16.f. The client will state signs and symptoms to report to the health care provider.

16.f.1. Instruct client to report the following:
a. drainage from and/or persistent redness of biopsy site(s)
b. signs and symptoms of hypercalcemia (e.g. nausea, vomiting, increased urination, muscle weakness, confusion)
c. persistent fever
d. development of or increased difficulty swallowing
e. excessive weight loss
f. increasing fatigue, weakness, or shortness of breath
g. swollen, painful joints (may indicate the development of hypertrophic pulmonary osteoarthropathy [a paraneoplastic condition])
h. swelling of upper body
i. persistent headache
j. development or worsening of a cough especially if productive of purulent, green, foul-smelling, or blood-tinged sputum
k. muscle weakness, numbness or tingling in extremities, or uncoordinated movements (may indicate development of a paraneoplastic neuromuscular syndrome)
l. signs and symptoms of Pancoast's syndrome (e.g. pain in shoulder and arm) and Horner's syndrome (e.g. very small pupil, drooping of eyelid, and loss of sweating on one side of face); these two syndromes usually occur together, are a result of extension of the primary tumor into the lower cervical and upper thoracic nerves, and occur most frequently with squamous cell carcinoma
m. irritability, drowsiness, or confusion
n. signs and symptoms of SIADH (see action e.4 in this diagnosis)
o. excessive depression or difficulty coping with the diagnosis.

2. If appropriate, refer to the Care Plan on Chemotherapy, Nursing Diagnosis 17, action l (p. 199) and/or the Care Plan on External Radiation Therapy, Nursing Diagnosis 16, action j (p. 226), for additional signs and symptoms client should report if receiving chemotherapy and/or radiation therapy.

16.g. The client will identify community resources that can assist with home management and adjustment to the diagnosis and the effects of treatment.

16.g.1. Provide information about and encourage utilization of community resources that can assist client and significant others with home management and adjustment to the diagnosis of lung cancer and effects of prescribed treatment (e.g. American Cancer Society, counselors, social service agencies, home health agencies, I Can Cope, Meals on Wheels, local support groups, Hospice).

2. Initiate a referral if indicated.

16.h. The client will verbalize an understanding of and a plan for adhering to recommended follow-up care including future appointments with health care provider, medications prescribed, activity level, and plans for subsequent treatment.

16.h.1. Reinforce physician's explanation of planned radiation therapy and/or chemotherapy schedule if appropriate. Stress importance of strictly following the prescribed protocol for the treatments and keeping all appointments for follow-up examinations and laboratory work.

2. Explain rationale for, side effects of, and importance of taking medications prescribed. Inform client of pertinent food and drug interactions.

3. Emphasize need for planned rest periods and adjusting activity according to tolerance.

4. Implement measures to improve client compliance:
   a. include significant others in teaching sessions if possible
   b. encourage questions and allow time for reinforcement and clarification of information provided
   c. provide written instructions regarding scheduled appointments with health care provider and for chemotherapy, radiation therapy, and laboratory work; medications prescribed; and signs and symptoms to report.

Bibliography

See pp. 897–898 and 904.

CHRONIC OBSTRUCTIVE PULMONARY DISEASE

Chronic obstructive pulmonary disease (COPD) is a term used to describe a process characterized by lower airway obstruction and a reduction in airflow on expiration. Other terms sometimes used to describe this condition are chronic obstructive lung disease (COLD), chronic airflow limitation (CAL), and chronic obstructive airways syndrome. Signs and symptoms usually include dyspnea, cough, and sputum production that worsen over time and during periodic exacerbations. The two major diseases that comprise COPD are chronic bronchitis and emphysema. Chronic bronchitis is characterized by a cough that persists at least 3 months of the year for 2 consecutive years and an excessive production of mucus in the bronchi due to inflammation of the bronchioles and hypertrophy and hyperplasia of the mucous glands. In contrast, emphysema is characterized by dyspnea and a mild cough. The impaired airflow that occurs with emphysema is related to loss of lung elasticity and narrowed bronchioles. Both chronic bronchitis and emphysema are usually present to some degree in the person with COPD, although one of the two conditions usually predominates.

Causative factors of COPD include chronic irritation of the lungs by cigarette smoke, exposure to air pollution and chemical irritants, and recurrent respiratory tract infections. In a small percentage of cases of emphysema, the destruction of lung tissue by proteolytic enzymes is a result of a genetic deficiency of homozygous alpha$_1$-protease inhibitor.

This care plan focuses on care of the adult client with COPD who is hospitalized during an acute exacerbation. Goals of care are to improve respiratory function, prevent complications, and educate the client regarding ways to manage existing symptoms and slow the progression of the disease process.

DIAGNOSTIC TESTS

Chest x-ray
Pulmonary function studies
Arterial blood gases
Oximetry

DISCHARGE CRITERIA

Prior to discharge, the client will:

- have improved respiratory function
- tolerate expected level of activity
- have no signs and symptoms of complications
- identify ways to prevent or minimize further respiratory problems
- demonstrate proper chest physiotherapy and use of respiratory equipment
- verbalize an understanding of medications ordered including rationale, food and drug interactions, side effects, methods of administering, and importance of taking as prescribed
- identify appropriate safety measures related to COPD and its treatment
- state signs and symptoms to report to the health care provider
- share feelings and thoughts about the effects of COPD on life style and roles
- identify community resources that can assist with home management and adjustment to changes resulting from COPD
- verbalize an understanding of and a plan for adhering to recommended follow-up care including future appointments with health care provider and graded exercise program.

NURSING/ COLLABORATIVE DIAGNOSES	1. Impaired respiratory function:
	  a. ineffective breathing pattern
	  b. ineffective airway clearance
	  c. impaired gas exchange △ 442
	2. Altered nutrition: less than body requirements △ 444
	3. Activity intolerance △ 445
	4. Self-care deficit △ 446
	5. Sleep pattern disturbance △ 447
	6. Risk for infection: pneumonia △ 448
	7. Potential complications:
	  a. right-sided heart failure (cor pulmonale)
	  b. respiratory failure △ 449
	8. Anxiety △ 450
	9. Self-concept disturbance △ 451
	10. Powerlessness △ 452
	11. Ineffective management of therapeutic regimen △ 453

DISCHARGE TEACHING	12. Knowledge deficit or Altered health maintenance △ 454

1. NURSING DIAGNOSIS:

Impaired respiratory function:*

a. **ineffective breathing pattern** related to:
  1. increased rate and decreased depth of respirations associated with fear and anxiety
  2. diminished lung/chest wall expansion associated with weakness, fatigue, and presence of a flattened diaphragm (a result of prolonged hyperinflation of the lungs);

---

*This diagnostic label includes the following nursing diagnoses: ineffective breathing pattern, ineffective airway clearance, and impaired gas exchange.

 b. **ineffective airway clearance** related to:
  1. narrowing of the bronchioles associated with:
   a. production of excessive mucus
   b. inflammation and hyperplasia of the bronchial walls (especially with chronic bronchitis)
   c. bronchospasm resulting from irritation of the bronchioles by excessive mucus
  2. collapse of the alveoli associated with destruction of lung tissue (occurs primarily with emphysema)
  3. stasis of secretions associated with:
   a. difficulty coughing up secretions resulting from fatigue and weakness and presence of tenacious secretions if fluid intake is inadequate
   b. impaired ciliary function resulting from loss of ciliated epithelium (occurs with inflammation and destruction and fibrosis of bronchial walls)
   c. decreased mobility;
 c. **impaired gas exchange** related to narrowing or obstruction of the small airways and a decrease in effective lung surface (occurs as a result of collapse, destruction, and fibrosis of alveolar walls).

Desired Outcome	Nursing Actions and *Selected Purposes/Rationales*

1. The client will experience adequate respiratory function as evidenced by:
 a. usual rate and depth of respirations
 b. decreased dyspnea
 c. usual or improved breath sounds
 d. usual mental status
 e. usual skin color
 f. blood gases within normal range for client.
	1.a. Assess for signs and symptoms of impaired respiratory function:
	  1. shallow, rapid respirations
	  2. dyspnea, orthopnea
	  3. use of accessory muscles when breathing
	  4. adventitious breath sounds (e.g. rhonchi)
	  5. diminished or absent breath sounds
	  6. cough
	  7. restlessness, irritability
	  8. confusion, somnolence
	  9. central cyanosis (a late sign).
	 b. Monitor for and report significant abnormalities of blood gas values, oximetry results, and chest x-ray reports.
	 c. Assist with pulmonary function studies. Report results that worsen or do not improve after treatment begins.
	 d. Implement measures *to improve respiratory status:*
	  1. perform actions to increase strength and improve activity tolerance (see Nursing Diagnosis 3, action b) *in order to increase client's willingness and ability to move, cough, deep breathe, and use incentive spirometer*
	  2. perform actions to reduce fear and anxiety (see Nursing Diagnosis 8, action b)
	  3. place client in a semi- to high Fowler's position; position overbed table so client can lean on it if desired
	  4. maintain oxygen therapy as ordered (question any order for high oxygen concentration *since many persons with COPD are dependent on hypoxemia as the stimulus to breathe*)
	  5. assist client to turn from side to side every 2 hours while in bed
	  6. instruct client in and assist with diaphragmatic and pursed-lip breathing techniques
	  7. instruct client to deep breathe or use incentive spirometer every 1–2 hours
	  8. perform actions *to facilitate removal of pulmonary secretions:*
	   a. instruct and assist client to cough or ''huff'' every 1–2 hours
	   b. implement measures *to thin tenacious secretions and reduce dryness of the respiratory mucous membrane:*
	    1. maintain a fluid intake of at least 2500 ml/day unless contraindicated
	    2. humidify inspired air as ordered
	   c. assist with administration of mucolytics and diluent or hydrating agents via nebulizer if ordered

Desired Outcome	Nursing Actions and *Selected Purposes/Rationales*

    d. assist with or perform postural drainage therapy (PDT) if ordered
    e. perform suctioning if needed
    f. administer prescribed expectorants if indicated
  9. instruct client to avoid intake of large meals, gas-forming foods (e.g. beans, cauliflower, cabbage, onions), and carbonated beverages *in order to prevent gastric distention and increased pressure on the diaphragm*
  10. discourage smoking (*smoke increases mucus production, impairs ciliary function, decreases oxygen availability, and can cause inflammation and damage to the bronchial walls*)
  11. maintain activity restrictions if ordered; increase activity as allowed and tolerated
  12. avoid use of central nervous system depressants (*these further depress respiratory status*)
  13. administer the following medications if ordered:
    a. bronchodilators:
      1. methylxanthines (e.g. theophylline)
      2. beta-adrenergic agonists (e.g. metaproterenol, albuterol, terbutaline)
      3. anticholinergics (e.g. ipratropium)
    b. corticosteroids (e.g. prednisone, methylprednisolone) which may be given *to decrease airway inflammation and thereby improve bronchial air flow.*
  e. Consult physician if signs and symptoms of impaired respiratory function persist or worsen.

---

2. NURSING DIAGNOSIS: **Altered nutrition: less than body requirements**

related to:
a. decreased oral intake associated with:
  1. dyspnea, weakness, fatigue, and depression
  2. nausea (can occur in response to noxious stimuli such as sight of expectorated sputum)
  3. early satiety resulting from compression of the stomach by flattened diaphragm;
b. increased metabolic needs associated with increased energy expenditure resulting from strenuous breathing efforts and persistent coughing.

Desired Outcome	Nursing Actions and *Selected Purposes/Rationales*

2. The client will maintain an adequate nutritional status as evidenced by:
a. weight within normal range for client's age, height, and body frame
b. normal BUN and serum albumin, transferrin, and lymphocyte levels
c. usual strength and activity tolerance
d. healthy oral mucous membrane.

2.a. Assess for and report signs and symptoms of malnutrition:
  1. weight below normal for client's age, height, and body frame
  2. abnormal BUN and low serum albumin, transferrin, and lymphocyte levels
  3. increased weakness and fatigue
  4. sore, inflamed oral mucous membrane
  5. pale conjunctiva.
b. Monitor percentage of meals and snacks client consumes. Report a pattern of inadequate intake.
c. Implement measures *to maintain an adequate nutritional status:*
  1. perform actions *to improve oral intake:*
    a. implement measures to improve respiratory status (see Nursing Diagnosis 1, action d) *in order to help relieve dyspnea*
    b. implement measures to facilitate client's psychological adjustment to COPD (see Nursing Diagnoses 9, actions c–t and 10, actions c–l) *in order to reduce depression*
    c. schedule treatments that assist in mobilizing mucus (e.g. aerosol

treatments, postural drainage therapy) at least 1 hour before or after meals *to prevent nausea*

   d. increase activity as allowed and tolerated (*activity usually promotes a sense of well-being and improves appetite*)

   e. obtain a dietary consult if necessary to assist client in selecting foods/fluids that meet nutritional needs, are appealing, and adhere to personal and cultural preferences

   f. encourage a rest period before meals *to minimize fatigue*

   g. eliminate noxious sights and odors from the environment; provide client with an opaque, covered container for expectorated sputum; empty container frequently and remove it from the table during mealtime if it is not needed (*noxious stimuli can cause nausea*)

   h. maintain a clean environment and a relaxed, pleasant atmosphere

   i. provide oral hygiene before meals and after respiratory treatments

   j. if client is quite dyspneic, assist him/her to select foods that require little or no chewing

   k. serve frequent, small meals rather than large ones if client is weak, fatigues easily, or has a poor appetite

   l. place client in a high Fowler's position for meals and provide supplemental oxygen therapy during meals if indicated *to help relieve dyspnea*

   m. allow adequate time for meals; reheat foods/fluids if necessary

   n. limit fluid intake with meals (unless the fluid has high nutritional value) *to reduce early satiety and subsequent decreased food intake*

  2. ensure that meals are well balanced and high in essential nutrients; offer dietary supplements if indicated

  3. administer vitamins and minerals if ordered.

  d. Perform a calorie count if ordered. Report information to dietitian and physician.

  e. Consult physician about an alternative method of providing nutrition (e.g. parenteral nutrition, tube feedings) if client does not consume enough food or fluids to meet nutritional needs.

---

3. NURSING DIAGNOSIS:

Activity intolerance

related to:

  a. tissue hypoxia associated with impaired gas exchange;

  b. inadequate nutritional status;

  c. difficulty resting and sleeping associated with dyspnea, excessive coughing, fear, anxiety, frequent assessments and treatments, and side effects of medication therapy (e.g. some bronchodilators);

  d. increased energy expenditure associated with strenuous breathing efforts and persistent coughing.

Desired Outcome	Nursing Actions and *Selected Purposes/Rationales*

3. The client will demonstrate an increased tolerance for activity as evidenced by:
  a. verbalization of feeling less fatigued and weak
  b. ability to perform activities of daily living without increased dyspnea, chest pain, diaphoresis, dizziness, and a significant change in vital signs.
	3.a. Assess for signs and symptoms of activity intolerance:
	  1. statements of fatigue or weakness
	  2. exertional dyspnea, chest pain, diaphoresis, or dizziness
	  3. abnormal heart rate response to activity (e.g. increase in rate of 20 beats/minute above resting rate, rate not returning to preactivity level within 3 minutes after stopping activity, change from regular to irregular rate)
	  4. decreased systolic B/P or a significant increase (10–15 mm Hg) in diastolic pressure with activity.
	b. Implement measures *to improve activity tolerance:*
	  1. perform actions *to promote rest and/or conserve energy:*
	    a. maintain activity restrictions as ordered
	    b. minimize environmental activity and noise

Desired Outcome	Nursing Actions and *Selected Purposes/Rationales*

c. organize nursing care to allow for periods of uninterrupted rest

d. limit the number of visitors and their length of stay

e. assist client with self-care activities as needed

f. keep supplies and personal articles within easy reach

g. instruct client in energy-saving techniques (e.g. using shower chair when showering, sitting to brush teeth or comb hair)

h. implement measures to reduce fear and anxiety (see Nursing Diagnosis 8, action b)

i. implement measures to promote sleep (see Nursing Diagnosis 5, action c)

j. implement measures *to control cough:*
1. instruct client to avoid intake of very hot or cold foods/fluids (*these can stimulate cough*)
2. protect client from exposure to irritants such as flowers, smoke, and powder
3. administer prescribed antitussives if indicated *to suppress cough* (when cough is productive, antitussives should be used only when coughing is excessive and interfering significantly with the client's ability to rest and sleep)

2. discourage smoking and excessive intake of beverages high in caffeine such as coffee, tea, and colas (*nicotine and caffeine increase cardiac workload and myocardial oxygen utilization, thereby decreasing oxygen availability*)

3. perform actions to improve respiratory status (see Nursing Diagnosis 1, action d) *in order to improve tissue oxygenation and help relieve dyspnea*

4. perform actions to maintain an adequate nutritional status (see Nursing Diagnosis 2, action c)

5. reinforce use of controlled breathing techniques (e.g. inhaling through nose and exhaling slowly through pursed lips) during activity

6. if oxygen therapy is necessary during activity, keep portable oxygen equipment readily available for client's use

7. increase client's activity gradually as allowed and tolerated.

c. Instruct client to:
1. report a decreased tolerance for activity
2. stop any activity that causes chest pain, increased shortness of breath, dizziness, or extreme fatigue or weakness.

d. Consult physician if signs and symptoms of activity intolerance persist or worsen.

---

4. NURSING DIAGNOSIS: **Self-care deficit**

related to weakness, fatigue, and dyspnea.

Desired Outcome	Nursing Actions and *Selected Purposes/Rationales*
4. The client will demonstrate increased participation in self-care activities within physical limitations.	4.a. With client, develop a realistic plan for meeting daily physical needs. b. Implement measures *to facilitate client's ability to perform self-care activities:* 1. schedule care at a time when client is most likely to be able to participate: a. a couple of hours after arising (*bronchial secretions and inflammation are greater immediately upon awakening because of client's inactivity through the night*) b. after rest periods c. not immediately after meals or treatments

2. keep needed objects within easy reach
3. perform actions to increase strength and improve activity tolerance (see Nursing Diagnosis 3, action b)
4. perform actions to improve respiratory status (see Nursing Diagnosis 1, action d) *in order to reduce dyspnea*
5. consult occupational therapist about assistive devices available (e.g. long-handled hairbrush and shoehorn); reinforce use of these devices if indicated
6. allow adequate time for accomplishment of self-care activities.

c. Encourage maximum independence within limitations imposed by dyspnea, weakness, and fatigue. Provide positive feedback for all efforts and accomplishments of self-care.
d. Assist client with activities he/she is unable to perform independently.
e. Inform significant others of client's abilities to perform own care. Explain the importance of encouraging and allowing client to maintain an optimal level of independence.

---

5. NURSING DIAGNOSIS:

Sleep pattern disturbance

related to fear, anxiety, unfamiliar environment, excessive coughing, frequent assessments and treatments, side effects of medications (e.g. some bronchodilators), and inability to assume usual sleep position associated with orthopnea.

Desired Outcome	Nursing Actions and *Selected Purposes/Rationales*

5. The client will attain optimal amounts of sleep as evidenced by:
a. statements of feeling well rested
b. usual mental status
c. absence of frequent yawning, dark circles under eyes, and hand tremors.
	5.a. Assess for signs and symptoms of a sleep pattern disturbance (e.g. statements of difficulty falling asleep, sleep interruptions, or not feeling well rested; irritability; lethargy; disorientation; frequent yawning; dark circles under eyes; slight hand tremors).
	b. Determine the client's usual sleep habits.
	c. Implement measures *to promote sleep:*
	  1. discourage long periods of sleep during the day unless signs and symptoms of sleep deprivation exist or daytime sleep is usual for client
	  2. perform actions to reduce fear and anxiety (see Nursing Diagnosis 8, action b)
	  3. perform actions to improve respiratory status (see Nursing Diagnosis 1, action d) *in order to relieve orthopnea*
	  4. encourage participation in relaxing diversional activities during the evening
	  5. discourage intake of fluids high in caffeine (e.g. coffee, tea, colas), especially in the evening
	  6. offer client an evening snack that includes cheese unless contraindicated (*the L-tryptophan in cheese helps induce and maintain sleep*)
	  7. allow client to continue usual sleep practices (e.g. position; time; presleep routines such as reading, watching television, listening to music, and meditating) unless contraindicated
	  8. satisfy basic needs such as comfort and warmth before sleep
	  9. encourage client to urinate just before bedtime
	  10. perform actions to control cough (see Nursing Diagnosis 3, action b.1.j)
	  11. assist client to assume a position *that facilitates breathing* (e.g. head of bed elevated with arms supported on pillows, resting forward on overbed table with good pillow support, sitting in a chair)

Desired Outcome	Nursing Actions and *Selected Purposes/Rationales*

12. maintain oxygen therapy during sleep
13. reduce environmental distractions (e.g. close door to client's room, use night light rather than overhead light whenever possible, lower volume of paging system, keep staff conversations at a low level and away from client's room, close curtains between clients in a semi-private room or ward, keep beepers and alarms on low volume, have earplugs available for client if needed)
14. administer prescribed sedative-hypnotics if indicated (use these medications with caution *because of their respiratory depressant effect*)
15. perform actions *to reduce interruptions during sleep (80–100 minutes of uninterrupted sleep is usually needed to complete one sleep cycle)*:
    a. restrict visitors
    b. group care (e.g. medications, treatments, physical care, assessments) whenever possible.
d. Consult physician if signs and symptoms of sleep deprivation persist or worsen.

---

6. NURSING DIAGNOSIS: **Risk for infection: pneumonia**

related to stasis of secretions in the lungs (secretions provide a good medium for bacterial growth).

Desired Outcome	Nursing Actions and *Selected Purposes/Rationales*

6. The client will not develop pneumonia as evidenced by:
   a. usual breath sounds and percussion note over lungs
   b. absence of tachypnea
   c. cough productive of clear mucus only
   d. afebrile status
   e. absence of pleuritic pain
   f. WBC count within normal range
   g. blood gases returning to normal range for client
   h. negative sputum culture.

6.a. Assess for and report signs and symptoms of pneumonia:
   1. abnormal breath sounds (e.g. crackles [rales], pleural friction rub, bronchial breath sounds, diminished or absent breath sounds)
   2. dull percussion note over affected lung area
   3. increase in respiratory rate
   4. cough productive of purulent, green, or rust-colored sputum
   5. chills and fever
   6. pleuritic pain
   7. elevated WBC count.
b. Monitor oximetry and blood gas results. Report values that have worsened.
c. Obtain sputum specimen for culture if ordered. Report abnormal results.
d. Monitor chest x-ray results. Report findings indicative of pneumonia.
e. Implement measures *to prevent pneumonia*:
   1. perform actions to improve respiratory status (see Nursing Diagnosis 1, action d)
   2. protect client from persons with respiratory tract infections
   3. encourage and assist client to perform frequent oral hygiene *in order to reduce the colonization of bacteria in the oropharynx and subsequent aspiration of these microorganisms*
   4. replace or cleanse equipment used for respiratory care as often as needed.
f. If signs and symptoms of pneumonia occur:
   1. continue with above measures
   2. administer antimicrobials if ordered
   3. refer to Care Plan on Pneumonia for additional care measures.

7. COLLABORATIVE DIAGNOSES:

Potential complications of COPD:

a. **right-sided heart failure (cor pulmonale)** related to increased cardiac workload associated with:
   1. pulmonary hypertension resulting from pulmonary vasoconstriction that occurs in response to hypoxia
   2. compensatory response to the decreased pulmonary blood flow that occurs when there is loss of large portions of the pulmonary vascular bed (can result from destruction and fibrosis of lung tissue);

b. **respiratory failure** related to severe ventilation-perfusion imbalance associated with end-stage COPD, acute exacerbation of COPD, and/or presence of conditions that further compromise respiratory status (e.g. pneumonia, abdominal or thoracic surgery, pneumothorax).

Desired Outcomes	Nursing Actions and *Selected Purposes/Rationales*

7.a. The client will not develop right-sided heart failure as evidenced by:
   1. pulse 60–100 beats/minute
   2. no increase in intensity of S_2 heart sound or development of summation gallop
   3. usual mental status
   4. no increase in dyspnea, weakness, and fatigue
   5. adequate urine output
   6. stable weight
   7. absence of edema; distended neck veins; and enlarged, tender liver.

7.a.1. Assess for and report signs and symptoms of right-sided heart failure:
   a. increase in pulse rate
   b. development of a loud S_2 heart sound and/or summation gallop
   c. restlessness, anxiousness, confusion
   d. increased dyspnea, weakness, and/or fatigue
   e. decreased urine output
   f. weight gain
   g. edema
   h. distended neck veins
   i. enlarged, tender liver.
   2. Monitor chest x-ray results. Report findings of cardiomegaly.
   3. Implement measures to improve respiratory status (see Nursing Diagnosis 1, action d) *in order to reduce cardiac workload and the subsequent risk for right-sided heart failure.*
   4. If signs and symptoms of right-sided heart failure occur:
   a. maintain oxygen therapy as ordered
   b. maintain fluid and sodium restrictions if ordered
   c. maintain client on strict bed rest in a semi- to high Fowler's position
   d. administer medications that may be ordered *to reduce vascular congestion and/or cardiac workload* (e.g. diuretics, cardiotonics, vasodilators)
   e. refer to Care Plan on Heart Failure for additional care measures.

7.b. The client will not experience respiratory failure as evidenced by:
   1. usual skin color
   2. usual mental status
   3. PaO_2 above 50 mm Hg and $PaCO_2$ below 50 mm Hg.

7.b.1. Assess for and report signs and symptoms of severe respiratory distress (e.g. increased sternocleidomastoid and intercostal muscle retraction, cyanotic skin color, drowsiness, confusion).
   2. Monitor blood gas and oximetry results. Report values that have worsened.
   3. Implement measures *to prevent respiratory failure:*
   a. perform actions to improve respiratory status (see Nursing Diagnosis 1, action d)
   b. perform actions to prevent and treat pneumonia (see Nursing Diagnosis 6, actions e and f) *in order to prevent a further compromise in respiratory status.*
   4. If signs and symptoms of respiratory failure occur:
   a. continue with above actions
   b. assist with intubation, mechanical ventilatory support, and transfer to intensive care unit if indicated
   c. if life-saving measures are not indicated, refer to Care Plan on Terminal Care for additional nursing actions
   d. provide emotional support to client and significant others.

8. NURSING DIAGNOSIS:

Anxiety

related to dyspnea and feeling of suffocation, unfamiliar environment, financial concerns, prognosis, and feeling of lack of control over progression of the disease.

Desired Outcome	Nursing Actions and *Selected Purposes/Rationales*

8. The client will experience a reduction in anxiety as evidenced by:
a. verbalization of feeling less anxious
b. usual sleep pattern
c. relaxed facial expression and body movements
d. stable vital signs
e. usual perceptual ability and interactions with others.
	8.a. Assess client for signs and symptoms of anxiety (e.g. verbalization of feeling anxious, insomnia, tenseness, shakiness, restlessness, diaphoresis, elevated blood pressure, tachycardia, facial pallor, self-focused behaviors). Validate perceptions carefully, remembering that some behavior may result from tissue hypoxia.
	b. Implement measures *to reduce fear and anxiety:*
	  1. maintain a calm, supportive, confident manner when interacting with client
	  2. do not leave client alone during period of acute respiratory distress
	  3. perform actions to improve respiratory status (see Nursing Diagnosis 1, action d) *in order to reduce dyspnea*
	  4. perform actions *to decrease client's feeling of suffocation:*
	    a. open curtains and doors
	    b. approach client from the side rather than face-on (*close face-on contact may make client feel closed in*)
	    c. limit number of visitors in room at any one time
	    d. remove unnecessary equipment from room
	    e. administer oxygen via nasal cannula rather than mask if possible
	  5. encourage significant others to project a caring, concerned attitude without obvious anxiousness
	  6. once the period of acute respiratory distress has subsided:
	    a. orient client to hospital environment, equipment, and routines
	    b. introduce client to staff who will be participating in care; if possible, maintain consistency in staff assigned to his/her care *to provide feelings of stability and comfort with the environment*
	    c. assure client that staff members are nearby; respond to call signal as soon as possible
	    d. provide a calm, restful environment
	    e. encourage verbalization of fear and anxiety; provide feedback
	    f. reinforce physician's explanations and clarify misconceptions the client has about COPD, the treatment plan, and prognosis
	    g. explain all diagnostic tests
	    h. instruct client in relaxation techniques and encourage participation in diversional activities
	    i. assist client to identify specific stressors and ways to cope with them
	    j. provide information based on current needs of client at a level he/she can understand; encourage questions and clarification of information provided
	    k. perform actions to reduce client's feeling of powerlessness (see Nursing Diagnosis 10, actions c–l)
	    l. initiate financial and/or social service referrals if indicated
	    m. include significant others in orientation and teaching sessions and encourage their continued support of the client
	    n. administer prescribed antianxiety agents if indicated.
	c. Consult physician if above actions fail to control fear and anxiety.

9. NURSING DIAGNOSIS:

Self-concept disturbance*

related to:
a. change in appearance (e.g. ''barrel'' chest, clubbing of fingers, retraction of tissues around the neck and supraclavicular spaces);
b. dependence on others to meet self-care needs;
c. possible alteration in sexual functioning (may result from dyspnea, weakness, fatigue, and persistent cough);
d. stigma associated with chronic illness;
e. possible changes in life style and roles.

---

*This diagnostic label includes the nursing diagnoses of body image disturbance, self-esteem disturbance, and altered role performance.

Desired Outcome	Nursing Actions and *Selected Purposes/Rationales*
9. The client will demonstrate beginning adaptation to changes in appearance, body functioning, level of independence, life style, and roles as evidenced by: a. verbalization of feelings of self-worth b. maintenance of relationships with significant others c. active participation in activities of daily living d. verbalization of a plan for adapting life style to changes resulting from the effects of COPD.	9.a. Assess for signs and symptoms of a self-concept disturbance (e.g. verbalization of negative feelings about self, withdrawal from significant others, lack of participation in activities of daily living, lack of plan for adapting to necessary changes in life style). b. Determine the meaning of changes in appearance, body functioning, life style, and roles to the client by encouraging verbalization of feelings and by noting nonverbal responses to changes experienced. c. Be aware that client will grieve the progressive loss of respiratory function. Provide support during the grieving process. d. Discuss with client realistic expectations of improvements in body functioning and ability to resume usual activities. e. Implement measures *to assist client to increase self-esteem* (e.g. limit negative self-assessment, encourage positive comments about self, assist to identify strengths, give positive feedback about accomplishments and behaviors that are indicative of high self-esteem). f. Assist client to identify and utilize coping techniques that have been helpful in the past. g. If client is self-conscious about appearance, suggest clothing styles that make physical changes less apparent (e.g. loose-fitting shirts, shirts with high collars). h. Assist client with usual grooming and makeup habits if necessary. i. Reinforce measures that can help client improve his/her activity tolerance (e.g. resting prior to activity, maintaining a good nutritional status, sitting rather than standing when performing tasks, adhering to a graded exercise program, taking medications as prescribed, using portable oxygen as prescribed). j. If appropriate, discuss with client ways in which he/she can reduce dyspnea during sexual activity (e.g. obtain adequate rest and use inhaled bronchodilators before sexual activity, use oxygen before and during sexual activity, assume positions such as side-lying that reduce energy expenditure). k. Consult occupational therapist if indicated about a home evaluation before discharge to identify assistive devices and environmental modifications that could help the client to be more independent in his/her living situation. l. Encourage significant others to allow client to do as much as he/she is able *so that independence can be re-established and/or self-esteem redeveloped.* m. Implement measures to reduce client's feelings of powerlessness (see Nursing Diagnosis 10, actions c–l). n. Support behaviors suggesting positive adaptation to changes that have occurred (e.g. compliance with treatment plan, verbalization of feelings of self-worth, maintenance of relationships with significant others).

Desired Outcome	Nursing Actions and *Selected Purposes/Rationales*
	o. Assist client's and significant others' adjustment by listening, facilitating communication, and providing information.
	p. Assist client and significant others to have similar expectations and understanding of future life style and to identify ways that personal and family goals can be adjusted rather than abandoned.
	q. Encourage visits and support from significant others.
	r. Encourage client to pursue usual roles and interests and to continue involvement in social activities. If previous roles, interests, and hobbies cannot be pursued, encourage development of new ones.
	s. Provide information about and encourage utilization of community agencies and support groups (e.g. vocational rehabilitation; family, individual, and/or financial counseling).
	t. Consult physician about psychological counseling if client desires or seems unwilling or unable to adapt to changes resulting from COPD.

■━━━

10. NURSING DIAGNOSIS: **Powerlessness**

related to physical limitations; disease progression despite efforts to comply with treatment plan; dependence on others to meet self-care needs; and alterations in roles, life style, and future plans.

Desired Outcome	Nursing Actions and *Selected Purposes/Rationales*
10. The client will demonstrate increased feelings of control over his/her situation as evidenced by: a. verbalization of same b. active participation in planning of care c. participation in self-care activities within physical limitations.	10.a. Assess for behaviors that may indicate feelings of powerlessness (e.g. verbalization of lack of control over self-care or current situation, anger, irritability, passivity, lack of participation in care planning or self-care). b. Obtain information from client and significant others regarding client's usual response to situations in which he/she has had limited control (e.g. loss of job, financial stress). c. Evaluate client's perceptions of current situation, strengths, weaknesses, expectations, and parts of current situation that are under his/her control. Correct misinformation and inaccurate perceptions and encourage discussion of feelings about areas in which there is a perceived lack of control. d. Assist client to establish realistic short- and long-term goals. e. Reinforce physician's explanations about COPD and the importance of adhering to the treatment plan as a way to slow disease progression and prevent or delay the development of complications. Clarify misconceptions. f. Support realistic hope about the client's ability to slow the progression of COPD and adapt to changes that have occurred as a result of it. g. Remind client of the right to ask questions about current condition and the prescribed treatment plan. h. Support client's efforts to increase knowledge of and control over condition. Provide relevant pamphlets and audiovisual materials. i. Include client in the planning of care, encourage maximum participation in the treatment plan, and allow choices whenever possible *to promote a sense of control.* j. Inform client of scheduled procedures and tests *so that he/she knows what to expect, which promotes a sense of control.* k. Encourage client to be as active as possible in making decisions about his/her living situation. l. Encourage client's participation in self-help groups if indicated.

11. NURSING DIAGNOSIS: **Ineffective management of therapeutic regimen**

related to:
a. lack of understanding of the implications of not following the prescribed treatment plan;
b. feeling of lack of control over disease progression;
c. difficulty modifying personal habits (e.g. smoking) and integrating necessary treatments into life style;
d. insufficient financial resources.

Desired Outcome	Nursing Actions and *Selected Purposes/Rationales*
11. The client will demonstrate the probability of effective management of the therapeutic regimen as evidenced by: a. willingness to learn about and participate in treatments and care b. statements reflecting ways to modify personal habits and integrate treatments into life style c. statements reflecting an understanding of the implications of not following the prescribed treatment plan.	11.a. Assess for indications that the client may be unable to effectively manage the therapeutic regimen: 1. statements reflecting inability to manage care at home 2. failure to adhere to treatment plan while in hospital (e.g. refusing to use proper breathing techniques, refusing medications) 3. statements reflecting a lack of understanding of factors that may cause further progression of COPD 4. statements reflecting an unwillingness or inability to modify personal habits and integrate necessary treatments into life style 5. statement reflecting view that COPD is curable or that the situation is hopeless and efforts to comply with the treatment plan are useless. b. Implement measures *to promote effective management of the therapeutic regimen:* 1. explain COPD in terms the client can understand; stress the fact that COPD is a chronic condition and adherence to the treatment program is necessary in order to delay and/or prevent complications; caution client that some complications may occur despite strict adherence to treatment plan 2. encourage questions and clarify misconceptions client has about COPD and its effects 3. encourage client to participate in treatment plan (e.g. postural drainage therapy, breathing exercises) 4. provide instruction regarding respiratory care (e.g. use of nebulizers and metered-dose devices, pursed-lip and diaphragmatic breathing techniques); allow time for return demonstration; determine areas of difficulty and misunderstanding and reinforce teaching as necessary 5. perform actions to promote a positive self-concept and reduce feelings of powerlessness (see Nursing Diagnoses 9, actions c–t and 10, actions c–l) *in order to promote a sense of self-reliance and control over the effects of COPD* 6. initiate and reinforce the discharge teaching outlined in Nursing Diagnosis 12 *in order to promote a sense of control over disease progression* 7. provide client with written instructions about chest physiotherapy, ways to prevent further respiratory problems, prescribed medications, signs and symptoms to report, and future appointments with health care provider 8. assist client to identify ways treatments can be incorporated into life style; focus on modifications of life style rather than complete change 9. encourage client to discuss concerns regarding cost of hospitalization, medications, oxygen equipment, and follow-up care; obtain a social service consult to assist with financial planning and to obtain financial aid if indicated 10. provide information about and encourage utilization of community resources that can assist client to make necessary life-style changes (e.g. American Lung Association; pulmonary rehabilitation groups; counseling, vocational, and social services; smoking cessation programs)

Desired Outcome | Nursing Actions and **Selected Purposes/Rationales**

11. reinforce behaviors suggesting future compliance with prescribed treatments (e.g. statements reflecting plans for integrating treatments into life style, active participation in treatment plan, changes in personal habits)
12. include significant others in explanations and teaching sessions and encourage their support; reinforce the need for client to assume responsibility for managing as much of care as possible.
   c. Consult physician about referrals to community health agencies if continued instruction, support, or supervision is needed.

Discharge Teaching

■ ───────────────────────────────────────

12. NURSING DIAGNOSIS: **Knowledge deficit or Altered health maintenance***

*The nurse should select the diagnostic label that is most appropriate for the client's discharge teaching needs.

Desired Outcomes | Nursing Actions and **Selected Purposes/Rationales**

12.a. The client will identify ways to prevent or minimize further respiratory problems.

12.a.1. Instruct client in ways to prevent or minimize further respiratory problems:
   a. maintain overall general good health:
      1. eat a well-balanced diet
      2. schedule adequate rest periods to avoid undue fatigue
      3. adhere to prescribed graded exercise program
   b. stop smoking
   c. avoid exposure to respiratory irritants such as smoke, dust, some perfumes, aerosol sprays, paint fumes, and solvents
   d. remain indoors when air pollution levels and/or pollen counts are high and/or outdoor temperatures are extremely hot or cold
   e. wear a mask or scarf over nose and mouth if exposure to high levels of irritants such as smoke, fumes, and dust is unavoidable
   f. avoid high altitudes; if air travel is required, consult physician about the need for supplemental oxygen
   g. adhere to chest physiotherapy (e.g. breathing exercises, postural drainage therapy) as ordered
   h. take medications such as bronchodilators and mucolytics as prescribed
   i. decrease the risk of respiratory tract infections:
      1. avoid contact with persons who have respiratory tract infections
      2. avoid crowds and poorly ventilated areas
      3. receive immunizations against influenza and pneumococcal pneumonia
      4. take antimicrobials as prescribed (many physicians instruct clients to begin antimicrobial therapy if sputum color becomes yellow or green)
      5. cleanse all respiratory care equipment properly
      6. drink at least 10 glasses of liquid/day.
   2. Assist client in identifying ways he/she can make appropriate changes in personal habits and life style to reduce modifiable risk factors.

12.b. The client will demonstrate proper chest physiotherapy and use of respiratory equipment.

12.b.1. Reinforce instructions about proper breathing techniques (e.g. pursed-lip breathing, diaphragmatic breathing) and postural drainage therapy (PDT may be indicated if large amounts of mucus continue to be produced).
   2. Reinforce instructions about use of respiratory equipment (e.g. oxygen, incentive spirometer).

12.c. The client will verbalize an understanding of medications ordered including rationale, food and drug interactions, side effects, methods of administering, and importance of taking as prescribed.

3. Allow time for questions, clarification, and return demonstration.

12.c.1. Explain the rationale for, side effects of, and importance of taking medications prescribed.

2. Inform client of pertinent food and drug interactions.

3. Instruct in proper use of nebulizers and metered-dose inhalers (MDI) if prescribed. Allow time for client to practice the techniques.

4. If client is discharged on theophylline, instruct to:
   a. take it with food to minimize nausea, vomiting, and epigastric pain
   b. take it on a regular basis as ordered to maintain therapeutic blood levels
   c. report signs and symptoms that could indicate overdose (e.g. persistent nausea, vomiting, dizziness, insomnia, rapid pulse, muscle twitching, seizures)
   d. have blood theophylline levels evaluated periodically.

5. Reinforce the need to consult physician before taking additional prescription and nonprescription medications.

12.d. The client will identify appropriate safety measures related to COPD and its treatment.

12.d. Instruct client regarding the following safety measures:
   1. do not smoke when using oxygen therapy
   2. do not set oxygen flow rate at a level higher than prescribed by physician
   3. do not allow any source of spark or flame within 10 feet of the oxygen source
   4. ensure that all electrical equipment in the area of the oxygen source is grounded
   5. always wear a medical alert identification bracelet or tag to ensure that proper medications and appropriate oxygen flow rate are administered in emergency situations
   6. notify health care providers of having COPD and current therapy.

12.e. The client will state signs and symptoms to report to the health care provider.

12.e. Instruct client to report:
   1. changes in sputum characteristics (e.g. increase in volume or consistency, yellow or green color)
   2. sputum that does not return to usual color after 3 days of antimicrobial therapy
   3. cough that becomes worse
   4. increased fatigue, weakness, and shortness of breath
   5. increased need for medications and/or oxygen therapy
   6. elevated temperature
   7. drowsiness, confusion
   8. chest pain
   9. persistent weight loss or sudden weight gain
   10. swelling in ankles and/or feet
   11. signs and symptoms of theophylline overdose (see action c.4.c in this diagnosis).

12.f. The client will identify community resources that can assist with home management and adjustment to changes resulting from COPD.

12.f.1. Provide information regarding community resources that can assist client and significant others with home management and adjustment to changes resulting from COPD (e.g. American Lung Association; respiratory equipment companies; pulmonary rehabilitation groups; counseling, vocational, and social services; Meals on Wheels; transportation services; home health agencies).

2. Initiate a referral if indicated.

12.g. The client will verbalize an understanding of and a plan for adhering to recommended follow-up care including future appointments with health care provider and graded exercise program.

12.g.1. Reinforce importance of lifelong follow-up care.

2. Reinforce physician's instructions about a graded exercise program (e.g. walking for 20 minutes 3 times a week, stationary bicycling).

3. Implement measures to promote effective management of the therapeutic regimen (see Nursing Diagnosis 11, action b).

Bibliography

See pages 897–898 and 904.

▣ PNEUMONIA

Pneumonia is an acute inflammation of lung tissue. There are many causes including exposure to pathogenic organisms (e.g. bacteria, viruses, fungi, mycoplasmas) or inhalation of environmental irritants such as toxic chemicals, gases, and dust. Pneumonia may also result from aspiration of oropharyngeal secretions, food, fluid, or vomitus.

Pneumonia is usually classified according to the causative organism, anatomic site, and/or etiological factor. It may also be classified as community-acquired, hospital-acquired (nosocomial), or atypical. The types differ in relation to the mechanism of lung invasion (i.e. inhalation, aspiration, vascular system, direct extension), incubation period, signs and symptoms experienced by the client, complications that can result, and mortality rate.

The majority of persons hospitalized with pneumonia have bacterial pneumonia. The most common type of community-acquired bacterial pneumonia is pneumococcal pneumonia which occurs most often in the winter and usually follows an upper respiratory infection. It usually has an abrupt onset marked by a sudden, shaking chill; fever; cough; and pleuritic chest pain. The elderly client may not exhibit the classic signs and symptoms and often presents with weakness, fatigue, a poor appetite, and a change in mental status. Persons at greatest risk for development of pneumococcal pneumonia are those who have impaired pulmonary defense mechanisms (e.g. the immunosuppressed, the very young or old, persons with chronic pulmonary disease or alcoholism, those with neurological deficits that result in a decreased level of consciousness or swallowing impairments, smokers).

This care plan focuses on the adult client hospitalized with signs and symptoms of pneumococcal pneumonia. Goals of care are to improve respiratory function, relieve discomfort, prevent complications, and educate the client regarding follow-up care.

DIAGNOSTIC TESTS

Chest x-ray
White blood cell count and differential
Serological studies (e.g. cold agglutinins)
Sputum studies for Gram's stain, culture, and sensitivity
Pleural fluid examination and analysis
Blood cultures
Oximetry
Blood gases

DISCHARGE CRITERIA

Prior to discharge, the client will:

- have improved respiratory function
- tolerate expected level of activity
- have no signs and symptoms of complications
- identify ways to maintain respiratory health
- state signs and symptoms to report to the health care provider
- verbalize an understanding of and a plan for adhering to recommended follow-up care including future appointments with health care provider, medications prescribed, and activity limitations.

NURSING/ COLLABORATIVE DIAGNOSES

1. Impaired respiratory function
   a. ineffective breathing pattern
   b. ineffective airway clearance
   c. impaired gas exchange △   457
2. Risk for fluid volume deficit △   458
3. Altered nutrition: less than body requirements △   459
4. Pain: chest △   459
5A. Altered comfort: chills and excessive diaphoresis △   460
5B. Altered comfort: nausea △   460
6. Hyperthermia △   461
7. Activity intolerance △   461
8. Sleep pattern disturbance △   463

9. Risk for infection: extrapulmonary (e.g. bacteremia, pericarditis, meningitis, septic arthritis) and/or superinfection (e.g. candidiasis) △   464
10. Potential complications:
  a. pleural effusion
  b. atelectasis △   465

DISCHARGE TEACHING   **11.** Knowledge deficit, Ineffective management of therapeutic regimen, or Altered health maintenance △   465

---

1. NURSING DIAGNOSIS: **Impaired respiratory function:***

a. **ineffective breathing pattern** related to:
  1. diminished lung/chest wall expansion associated with weakness, fatigue, chest pain, and pleural effusion if present
  2. increased rate and decreased depth of respirations associated with the increase in metabolic rate that occurs with an infectious process;
b. **ineffective airway clearance** related to:
  1. increased production of secretions associated with the inflammatory process
  2. stasis of secretions associated with decreased activity, poor cough effort resulting from fatigue and chest pain, and impaired ciliary function (results from the increased viscosity and volume of mucus with the infectious process);
c. **impaired gas exchange** related to a decrease in effective lung surface associated with the accumulation of secretions and consolidation of lung tissue.

---

*This diagnostic label includes the following nursing diagnoses: ineffective breathing pattern, ineffective airway clearance, and impaired gas exchange.

Desired Outcome	Nursing Actions and *Selected Purposes/Rationales*

1. The client will experience adequate respiratory function as evidenced by:
a. normal rate and depth of respirations
b. decreased dyspnea
c. improved breath sounds
d. usual mental status
e. usual skin color
f. blood gases within normal range.
	1.a. Assess for and report signs and symptoms of impaired respiratory function:
	  1. rapid, shallow respirations
	  2. dyspnea, orthopnea
	  3. use of accessory muscles when breathing
	  4. abnormal breath sounds (e.g. diminished, bronchial, crackles [rales], wheezes)
	  5. cough (usually a productive cough of rust-colored, purulent, or blood-tinged sputum)
	  6. restlessness, irritability
	  7. confusion, somnolence
	  8. central cyanosis (a late sign).
	b. Monitor for and report the following:
	  1. abnormal blood gases
	  2. significant decrease in oximetry results
	  3. abnormal chest x-ray results.
	c. Implement measures *to improve respiratory status:*
	  1. maintain client on bed rest as ordered during the acute phase *to reduce oxygen needs*
	  2. place client in a semi- to high Fowler's position unless contraindicated; position with pillows *to prevent slumping*
	  3. instruct client to breathe slowly if hyperventilating
	  4. assist client to turn from side to side at least every 2 hours while in bed
	  5. instruct client to deep breathe or use incentive spirometer every 1–2 hours

Desired Outcome	Nursing Actions and *Selected Purposes/Rationales*
	6. assist with positive airway pressure techniques (e.g. IPPB, continuous positive airway pressure [CPAP], biphasic positive airway pressure [BiPAP], expiratory positive airway pressure [EPAP]) if ordered
	7. perform actions *to facilitate removal of pulmonary secretions:*
	a. instruct and assist client to cough or "huff" every 1–2 hours
	b. implement measures *to thin tenacious secretions and reduce dryness of the respiratory mucous membrane:*
	1. maintain a fluid intake of at least 2500 ml/day unless contraindicated
	2. humidify inspired air as ordered
	c. assist with administration of mucolytics and diluent or hydrating agents via nebulizer if ordered
	d. assist with or perform postural drainage therapy (PDT) if ordered
	e. perform suctioning if ordered
	f. administer expectorants if ordered
	8. perform actions to reduce chest pain (see Nursing Diagnosis 4, action d)
	9. maintain oxygen therapy as ordered
	10. discourage smoking (*smoke increases mucus production, impairs ciliary function, decreases oxygen availability, and can cause inflammation and damage to the bronchial walls*)
	11. perform actions to increase strength and activity tolerance (see Nursing Diagnosis 7, action b) *in order to increase client's willingness and ability to move, cough, deep breathe, and use incentive spirometer*
	12. administer central nervous system depressants judiciously; hold medication and consult physician if respiratory rate is less than 12/minute
	13. administer the following medications if ordered:
	a. bronchodilators (e.g. theophylline)
	b. antimicrobials.
	d. Consult physician if signs and symptoms of impaired respiratory function persist or worsen.

■━━━

2. NURSING DIAGNOSIS: **Risk for fluid volume deficit**

related to decreased oral intake and excessive fluid loss (occurs with profuse diaphoresis and hyperventilation if present).

Desired Outcome	Nursing Actions and *Selected Purposes/Rationales*

2. The client will not experience a fluid volume deficit as evidenced by:
  a. normal skin turgor
  b. moist mucous membranes
  c. stable weight
  d. B/P and pulse within normal range for client and stable with position change
  e. hand vein filling time less than 3–5 seconds
  f. usual mental status
  g. BUN and Hct within normal range
	2.a. Assess for and report signs and symptoms of fluid volume deficit:
	  1. decreased skin turgor
	  2. dry mucous membranes, thirst
	  3. sudden weight loss of 2% or greater
	  4. postural hypotension and/or low B/P
	  5. weak, rapid pulse
	  6. delayed hand vein filling time (longer than 3–5 seconds)
	  7. change in mental status
	  8. elevated BUN and Hct
	  9. decreased urine output with increased specific gravity (reflects an actual rather than potential fluid volume deficit).
	  b. Implement measures *to prevent fluid volume deficit:*
	  1. perform actions to improve oral intake (see Nursing Diagnosis 3, action c.1)
	  2. perform actions to reduce fever (see Nursing Diagnosis 6, action b)

h. balanced intake and output
i. urine specific gravity within normal range.

in order to reduce fluid loss resulting from the diaphoresis and hyperventilation that may accompany an increase in temperature
3. maintain a fluid intake of at least 2500 ml/day unless contraindicated; if oral intake is inadequate or contraindicated, maintain intravenous therapy as ordered.

---

3. NURSING DIAGNOSIS:

Altered nutrition: less than body requirements

related to:
a. decreased oral intake associated with weakness, fatigue, excessive coughing, the foul odor and taste of sputum and some aerosol treatments, nausea, and dyspnea;
b. increased nutritional needs associated with the increase in metabolic rate that occurs with an infectious process.

Desired Outcome	Nursing Actions and *Selected Purposes/Rationales*

3. The client will maintain an adequate nutritional status as evidenced by:
a. weight within normal range for client's age, height, and body frame
b. normal BUN and serum albumin, Hct, Hb, and transferrin levels
c. usual strength and activity tolerance
d. healthy oral mucous membrane.

3.a. Assess for and report signs and symptoms of malnutrition:
  1. weight below normal for client's age, height, and body frame
  2. abnormal BUN and low serum albumin, Hct, Hb, and transferrin levels
  3. increased weakness and fatigue
  4. sore, inflamed oral mucous membrane
  5. pale conjunctiva.
b. Monitor percentage of meals and snacks client consumes. Report a pattern of inadequate intake.
c. Implement measures *to maintain an adequate nutritional status:*
  1. perform actions *to improve oral intake:*
    a. implement measures to prevent or treat nausea (see Nursing Diagnosis 5.B, action 2)
    b. schedule respiratory therapy 1 hour before or after meals if possible
    c. increase activity as allowed and tolerated (*activity usually promotes a sense of well-being and stimulates appetite*)
    d. obtain a dietary consult if necessary to assist client in selecting foods/fluids that meet nutritional needs, are appealing, and adhere to personal and cultural preferences whenever possible
    e. encourage a rest period before meals *to minimize fatigue*
    f. maintain a clean environment and a relaxed, pleasant atmosphere
    g. assist with oral hygiene before meals and after respiratory therapy
    h. place client in a high Fowler's position for meals and provide supplemental oxygen therapy during meals if indicated *to help relieve dyspnea*
    i. serve frequent, small meals rather than large ones if client is weak, fatigues easily, or has a poor appetite
    j. allow adequate time for meals; reheat foods/fluids if necessary
  2. ensure that meals are well balanced and high in essential nutrients; offer dietary supplements if indicated
  3. administer vitamins and minerals if ordered.
d. Perform a calorie count if ordered. Report information to dietitian and physician.
e. Consult physician about an alternative method of providing nutrition (e.g. parenteral nutrition, tube feedings) if client does not consume enough food or fluids to meet nutritional needs.

---

4. NURSING DIAGNOSIS:

Pain: chest

related to:
a. irritation of the parietal pleura associated with the inflammatory process;
b. muscle strain associated with excessive coughing.

Desired Outcome	Nursing Actions and *Selected Purposes/Rationales*

4. The client will experience diminished chest pain as evidenced by:
  a. verbalization of a decrease in or absence of pain
  b. relaxed facial expression and body positioning
  c. increased participation in activities.
	4.a. Assess for signs and symptoms of pain (e.g. verbalization of pain, grimacing, reluctance to move, restlessness, guarding of affected side of chest).
	  b. Assess client's perception of the severity of pain using a pain intensity rating scale.
	  c. Assess the client's pain pattern (e.g. location, quality, onset, duration, precipitating factors, aggravating factors, alleviating factors).
	  d. Implement measures *to reduce chest pain:*
	    1. perform actions *to reduce fear and anxiety about the pain experience* (e.g. assure client that his/her need for pain relief is understood)
	    2. administer analgesics prior to any painful procedures (e.g. transtracheal sputum aspiration)
	    3. instruct and assist client to splint chest with hands or pillow when deep breathing, coughing, or changing position
	    4. provide or assist with nonpharmacologic methods for pain relief (e.g. position change, relaxation techniques, restful environment, diversional activities)
	    5. perform actions to decrease excessive coughing (see Nursing Diagnosis 7, action b.1.j)
	    6. administer analgesics if ordered.
	  e. Consult physician if above actions fail to provide adequate relief of chest pain.

5.A. NURSING DIAGNOSIS: **Altered comfort: chills and excessive diaphoresis**

related to persistent fever associated with the infectious process.

Desired Outcome	Nursing Actions and *Selected Purposes/Rationales*

5.A. The client will not experience discomfort associated with chills and excessive diaphoresis as evidenced by:
  1. verbalization of comfort
  2. ability to rest.
	5.A.1. Assess client for chills and excessive diaphoresis.
	  2. Implement measures to reduce fever (see Nursing Diagnosis 6, action b).
	  3. Implement measures *to promote comfort if client is having chills:*
	    a. maintain a room temperature that is comfortable for client
	    b. protect client from drafts
	    c. provide extra blankets and clothing as needed
	    d. provide warm liquids to drink.
	  4. Implement measures *to promote comfort if excessive diaphoresis is present:*
	    a. change linen and clothing whenever damp
	    b. bathe client and sponge his/her face as needed.
	  5. Consult physician if client continues to have chills and excessive diaphoresis.

5.B. NURSING DIAGNOSIS: **Altered comfort: nausea**

related to stimulation of the vomiting center associated with noxious stimuli (e.g. the foul taste of sputum and some aerosol treatments, sight of sputum).

Desired Outcome	Nursing Actions and **Selected Purposes/Rationales**

5.B. The client will verbalize relief of nausea.	5.B.1. Assess client for nausea.
	2. Implement measures *to prevent or treat nausea:*
	  a. encourage client to take deep, slow breaths when nauseated
	  b. eliminate noxious sights and odors from the environment; provide client with an opaque, covered container for expectorated sputum; empty container frequently and remove it from the table during mealtime if it is not needed (*noxious stimuli can cause stimulation of the vomiting center*)
	  c. provide oral hygiene after chest physical therapy and aerosol treatments and before meals
	  d. schedule treatments that assist in mobilizing mucus (e.g. aerosol treatments, postural drainage) at least 1 hour before or after meals
	  e. provide small, frequent meals; instruct client to ingest foods and fluids slowly
	  f. avoid serving foods with an overpowering aroma; remove lids from hot foods before entering room
	  g. encourage client to eat dry foods (e.g. toast, crackers) and avoid drinking liquids with meals if nauseated
	  h. administer antiemetics if ordered.
	3. Consult physician if above measures fail to control nausea.

---

6. NURSING DIAGNOSIS:

Hyperthermia

related to stimulation of the thermoregulatory center in the hypothalamus by endogenous pyrogens that are released in an infectious process.

Desired Outcome	Nursing Actions and **Selected Purposes/Rationales**

6. The client will experience resolution of hyperthermia as evidenced by:
  a. skin usual temperature and color
  b. pulse rate between 60–100 beats/minute
  c. respirations 14–20/minute
  d. normal body temperature.
	6.a. Assess for signs and symptoms of hyperthermia (e.g. warm, flushed skin; tachycardia; tachypnea; elevated temperature).
	  b. Implement measures *to reduce fever:*
	    1. perform actions *to resolve the infectious process:*
	      a. implement measures to facilitate removal of pulmonary secretions (see Nursing Diagnosis 1, action c.7)
	      b. implement measures to promote rest and/or conserve energy (see Nursing Diagnosis 7, action b.1)
	      c. implement measures to maintain an adequate nutritional status (see Nursing Diagnosis 3, action c)
	      d. administer antimicrobials as ordered
	    2. administer tepid sponge bath and/or apply cool cloths to groin and axillae
	    3. apply cooling blanket if ordered
	    4. utilize a room fan *to provide cool circulating air*
	    5. administer antipyretics if ordered.
	  c. Consult physician if temperature remains elevated.

---

7. NURSING DIAGNOSIS:

Activity intolerance

related to:
a. tissue hypoxia associated with impaired gas exchange;

    b. difficulty resting and sleeping associated with excessive coughing, dyspnea, discomfort, unfamiliar environment, anxiety, and frequent assessments and treatments;

    c. inadequate nutritional status;

    d. increased energy expenditure associated with persistent coughing and the increased metabolic rate that is present in an infectious process.

Desired Outcome	Nursing Actions and *Selected Purposes/Rationales*

7. The client will demonstrate an increased tolerance for activity as evidenced by:
  a. verbalization of feeling less fatigued and weak
  b. ability to perform activities of daily living without dizziness; increased dyspnea, chest pain, and diaphoresis; and a significant change in vital signs.
	7.a. Assess for signs and symptoms of activity intolerance:
	  1. statements of fatigue or weakness
	  2. exertional dyspnea, chest pain, diaphoresis, or dizziness
	  3. abnormal heart rate response to activity (e.g. increase in rate of 20 beats/minute above resting rate, rate not returning to preactivity level within 3 minutes after stopping activity, change from regular to irregular rate)
	  4. decreased systolic B/P or a significant increase (10–15 mm Hg) in diastolic pressure with activity.
	 b. Implement measures *to improve activity tolerance:*
	  1. perform actions *to promote rest and/or conserve energy:*
	    a. maintain activity restrictions as ordered
	    b. minimize environmental activity and noise
	    c. organize nursing care to allow for periods of uninterrupted rest
	    d. limit the number of visitors and their length of stay
	    e. assist client with self-care activities as needed
	    f. keep supplies and personal articles within easy reach
	    g. instruct client in energy-saving techniques (e.g. using shower chair when showering, sitting to brush teeth or comb hair)
	    h. implement measures to promote sleep (see Nursing Diagnosis 8, action c)
	    i. implement measures to reduce discomfort (see Nursing Diagnoses 4, action d; 5.A, actions 3 and 4; and 5.B, action 2)
	    j. implement measures *to decrease excessive coughing:*
	      1. protect client from exposure to irritants such as smoke, flowers, and powder
	      2. instruct client to avoid intake of extremely hot or cold foods/fluids (*these can stimulate cough*)
	      3. administer prescribed antitussives if indicated (when cough is productive, antitussives should be used only when coughing is excessive and interfering significantly with the client's ability to rest and sleep)
	  2. perform actions to reduce fever and resolve the infectious process (see Nursing Diagnosis 6, action b) *in order to lower the metabolic rate*
	  3. discourage smoking and excessive intake of beverages high in caffeine such as coffee, tea, and colas (*nicotine and caffeine increase cardiac workload and myocardial oxygen utilization, thereby decreasing oxygen availability*)
	  4. perform actions to improve respiratory status (see Nursing Diagnosis 1, action c) *in order to relieve dyspnea and improve tissue oxygenation*
	  5. if oxygen therapy is necessary during activity, keep portable oxygen equipment readily available for client's use
	  6. perform actions to maintain an adequate nutritional status (see Nursing Diagnosis 3, action c)
	  7. increase client's activity gradually as allowed and tolerated.
	 c. Instruct client to:
	  1. report a decreased tolerance for activity
	  2. stop any activity that causes increased chest pain, increased shortness of breath, dizziness, or extreme fatigue or weakness.
	 d. Consult physician if signs and symptoms of activity intolerance persist or worsen.

8. NURSING DIAGNOSIS:

Sleep pattern disturbance

related to unfamiliar environment, discomfort, excessive coughing, anxiety, inability to assume usual sleep position because of dyspnea, and frequent assessments and treatments.

Desired Outcome	Nursing Actions and *Selected Purposes/Rationales*

8. The client will attain optimal amounts of sleep as evidenced by:
a. statements of feeling well rested
b. usual mental status
c. absence of frequent yawning, dark circles under eyes, and hand tremors.
	8.a. Assess for signs and symptoms of a sleep pattern disturbance (e.g. statements of difficulty falling asleep, sleep interruptions, or not feeling well rested; irritability; lethargy; disorientation; frequent yawning; dark circles under eyes; slight hand tremors).
	b. Determine the client's usual sleep habits.
	c. Implement measures *to promote sleep:*
	  1. discourage long periods of sleep during the day unless signs and symptoms of sleep deprivation exist or daytime sleep is usual for client
	  2. perform actions to reduce discomfort (see Nursing Diagnoses 4, action d; 5.A, actions 3 and 4; and 5.B, action 2)
	  3. perform actions to reduce excessive coughing (see Nursing Diagnosis 7, action b.1.j)
	  4. encourage participation in relaxing diversional activities during the evening
	  5. discourage intake of fluids high in caffeine (e.g. coffee, tea, colas), especially in the evening
	  6. perform actions to reduce anxiety (e.g. explain treatments; assure client that difficulty breathing should subside with treatment; provide care in a calm, confident manner).
	  7. allow client to continue usual sleep practices (e.g. time; presleep routines such as reading, watching television, listening to music, and meditating) unless contraindicated
	  8. satisfy basic needs such as comfort and warmth before sleep
	  9. have client empty bladder just before bedtime
	  10. reduce environmental distractions (e.g. close door to client's room; use night light rather than overhead light whenever possible; lower volume of paging system; keep staff conversations at a low level and away from client's room; close curtains between clients in a semi-private room or ward; keep beepers and alarms on low volume; have earplugs available for client if needed)
	  11. if client has orthopnea, assist him/her to assume a position *that facilitates breathing* (e.g. head of bed elevated with arms supported on pillows, resting forward on overbed table with good pillow support, sitting in a chair)
	  12. maintain oxygen therapy during sleep
	  13. administer prescribed sedative-hypnotics if indicated
	  14. perform actions *to reduce interruptions during sleep* (*80–100 minutes of uninterrupted sleep is usually needed to complete one sleep cycle*):
	    a. restrict visitors
	    b. group care (e.g. medications, treatments, physical care, assessments) whenever possible.
	d. Consult physician if signs and symptoms of sleep deprivation persist or worsen.

9. NURSING DIAGNOSIS: **Risk for infection: extrapulmonary (e.g. bacteremia, pericarditis, meningitis, septic arthritis) and/or superinfection (e.g. candidiasis)**
related to:
a. spread of pneumococcus via the blood stream associated with inadequate host defenses;
b. resistance of pneumococcus to antimicrobial agents;
c. interruption in the balance of usual endogenous microbial flora associated with the administration of antimicrobial agents.

Desired Outcome	Nursing Actions and *Selected Purposes/Rationales*
9. The client will not develop an extrapulmonary infection or a superinfection as evidenced by: a. gradual return of vital signs to normal b. usual mental status c. absence of pericardial friction rub and precordial pain d. absence of joint pain and swelling e. absence of unusual drainage from any body cavity f. absence of white patches and ulcerations in mouth g. absence of stiff neck and headache h. WBC and differential counts returning toward normal range for client.	9.a. Assess for and report signs and symptoms of an extrapulmonary infection or a superinfection: 1. increase in temperature and pulse above previous levels 2. change in mental status 3. pericardial friction rub, precordial pain 4. swollen, red, painful joints 5. unusual color, amount, and odor of vaginal drainage; perineal itching; white patches or ulcerated areas in the mouth (*fungal infections are common superinfections with antimicrobial therapy*) 6. stiff neck, headache 7. increase in WBC count above previous levels and/or significant change in differential. b. Implement measures *to prevent an extrapulmonary infection and/or a superinfection:* 1. perform actions to resolve the infectious process (see Nursing Diagnosis 6, action b.1) 2. use good handwashing technique and encourage client to do the same 3. maintain sterile technique during all invasive procedures (e.g. urinary catheterizations, venous and arterial punctures, injections) 4. rotate intravenous insertion sites according to hospital policy 5. protect client from others with infection 6. anchor catheters/tubings (e.g. urinary, intravenous) securely *in order to reduce trauma to the tissues and the risk for introduction of pathogens associated with in-and-out movement of the tubing* 7. change equipment, tubings, and solutions used for treatments such as intravenous infusions and respiratory care according to hospital policy 8. maintain a closed system for drains (e.g. urinary catheters) and intravenous infusions whenever possible 9. instruct and assist client to perform good perineal care at least every shift and after each bowel movement 10. reinforce importance of frequent oral hygiene. c. If signs and symptoms of an extrapulmonary infection or a superinfection occur: 1. continue with above measures 2. prepare client for and/or assist with diagnostic tests (e.g. lumbar puncture, cultures, joint aspiration) if planned 3. implement appropriate comfort measures for symptoms experienced 4. implement measures *to ensure client safety* (e.g. raise side rails, assist client with ambulation) if changes in mental status are present 5. administer antimicrobials as ordered.

10. COLLABORATIVE DIAGNOSES:

Potential complications of pneumonia:

a. **pleural effusion** related to an increase in pulmonary capillary permeability associated with the inflammatory process;
b. **atelectasis** related to shallow respirations, stasis of secretions in the alveoli and bronchioles, and decreased surfactant production (results from inadequate deep breathing and changes in regional blood flow in the lungs that can occur when mobility is decreased).

Desired Outcomes	Nursing Actions and *Selected Purposes/Rationales*

10.a. The client will not develop pleural effusion as evidenced by:
1. no increase in chest pain
2. unlabored respirations at 14–20/minute
3. symmetrical chest excursion
4. improved breath sounds and percussion note throughout lung fields.
	10.a.1. Assess for and report signs and symptoms of pleural effusion:
	  a. increase in chest pain
	  b. increased dyspnea
	  c. decreased chest excursion on affected side
	  d. dull percussion note and diminished or absent breath sounds over affected area.
	2. Monitor chest x-ray, ultrasound, and computed tomography results. Report findings of pleural effusion.
	3. Implement measures to resolve the infectious process (see Nursing Diagnosis 6, action b.1) *in order to reduce the risk for the development of pleural effusion.*
	4. If signs and symptoms of pleural effusion occur:
	  a. continue with actions to improve respiratory status (see Nursing Diagnosis 1, action c)
	  b. prepare client for a thoracentesis and/or insertion of chest tube if planned.

10.b. The client will not develop atelectasis as evidenced by:
1. improved breath sounds and percussion note over lungs
2. unlabored respirations at 14–20/minute
3. no increase in dyspnea, pulse rate, or temperature.
	10.b.1. Assess for and report signs and symptoms of atelectasis (e.g. diminished or absent breath sounds; dull percussion note over affected area; further increase in respiratory rate, dyspnea, and temperature).
	2. Monitor chest x-ray results. Report findings of atelectasis.
	3. Implement measures to improve respiratory status (see Nursing Diagnosis 1, action c) *in order to reduce the risk of atelectasis.*
	4. If signs and symptoms of atelectasis occur:
	  a. increase frequency of turning, coughing or "huffing," deep breathing, and use of incentive spirometer
	  b. increase activity as allowed and tolerated
	  c. consult physician if signs and symptoms of atelectasis persist or worsen.

Discharge Teaching

11. NURSING DIAGNOSIS:

Knowledge deficit, Ineffective management of therapeutic regimen, or Altered health maintenance*

*The nurse should select the diagnostic label that is most appropriate for the client's discharge teaching needs.

Desired Outcomes	Nursing Actions and *Selected Purposes/Rationales*
11.a. The client will identify ways to maintain respiratory health.	11.a. Instruct client in ways to maintain respiratory health: 1. consume a well-balanced diet 2. drink at least 10 glasses of liquid/day unless contraindicated

Desired Outcome	Nursing Actions and *Selected Purposes/Rationales*
	3. maintain a balanced program of rest and exercise
	4. avoid crowds during flu and cold season
	5. avoid contact with persons who have respiratory infections
	6. consult physician about vaccinations available if at high risk for recurrent pneumonia
	7. continue coughing and deep breathing exercises for at least 6–8 weeks after discharge and during any period of decreased physical activity or respiratory infection
	8. maintain good oral hygiene in order to reduce the number of organisms in the oropharynx
	9. avoid excessive alcohol intake and stop smoking to prevent depression of pulmonary antimicrobial defenses
	10. avoid exposure to respiratory irritants (e.g. smoke and other environmental pollutants).
11.b. The client will state signs and symptoms to report to the health care provider.	11.b. Instruct client to report the following signs and symptoms:
	1. persistent or recurrent temperature elevation
	2. chills
	3. difficulty breathing
	4. restlessness, irritability, drowsiness, or confusion
	5. persistent or increased chest pain
	6. persistent weight loss
	7. persistent fatigue
	8. persistent cough
	9. unusual color, amount, and odor of vaginal secretions
	10. white patches or ulcerated areas in the mouth
	11. stiff neck and headache
	12. swollen, red, painful joints.
11.c. The client will verbalize an understanding of and a plan for adhering to recommended follow-up care including future appointments with health care provider, medications prescribed, and activity limitations.	11.c.1. Reinforce the importance of keeping follow-up appointments with health care provider.
	2. Explain the rationale for, side effects of, and importance of taking medications prescribed (e.g. antimicrobials). Inform client of pertinent food and drug interactions.
	3. Implement measures to improve client compliance:
	a. include significant others in all discharge teaching sessions if possible
	b. encourage questions and allow time for reinforcement and clarification of information provided
	c. provide written instructions regarding scheduled appointments with health care provider, medications prescribed, fluid requirements, respiratory care, and signs and symptoms to report.

Bibliography

See pages 897–898 and 904.

PNEUMOTHORAX

Pneumothorax occurs when air accumulates in the pleural space and causes extensive lung tissue recoil and complete alveolar collapse in one or more lobes. It is classified as open or closed. An open pneumothorax can result when a surgical or traumatic opening of the chest wall or diaphragm allows air to enter the pleural space. It can also occur as a complication of a diagnostic or therapeutic procedure (e.g. thoracentesis, subclavian venipuncture). A closed pneumothorax occurs when air enters the pleural space through a tear or weakening in an internal respiratory structure (e.g. pleural lining, bronchus, alveoli). Spontaneous pneumothorax, a type of closed pneumothorax, is most commonly caused by the rupture of a bleb on the visceral pleural lining. A primary spontaneous pneumothorax occurs in the absence of obvious respiratory disease. The persons at greatest risk for this condition are men who are tall, 20–40 years of age, smokers, and have a family history of spontaneous pneumothorax. A less common type of closed pneumothorax is a secondary spontaneous pneumothorax. This can occur as a complication of a variety of pulmonary diseases such as chronic obstructive pulmonary disease, cystic fibrosis, malignancy, and tuberculosis.

Clinical manifestations of a pneumothorax vary with the degree of lung collapse. Common signs and symptoms include sudden onset of unilateral sharp chest pain, tachypnea, dyspnea, anxiety, absent or diminished breath sounds, and tachycardia. When the pneumothorax is symptomatic and involves greater than 15% of the lung tissue, it is usually managed with thoracostomy and placement of a chest tube in the intrapleural space. The tube is connected to suction through a closed water-seal drainage system or, less frequently, to a flutter (Heimlich) valve to evacuate the intrapleural air, re-establish negative intrapleural pressure, and re-expand the lung. Following lung re-expansion, pleurodesis (the obliteration of the pleural space by instillation of an irritant such as doxycycline or bleomycin through the chest tube into the pleural space) is a treatment option for a person who has had a primary spontaneous pneumothorax. Pleurodesis results in only minor changes in lung function as long as adherence of the pleural linings occurs after the lung is reinflated. A secondary or a recurrent primary spontaneous pneumothorax can be treated by surgically resecting or closing areas that contain multiple blebs.

This care plan focuses on the adult client hospitalized for diagnosis and treatment of a primary spontaneous pneumothorax. Goals of care are to promote an adequate respiratory status, relieve pain, prevent complications, reduce fear and anxiety, and educate the client regarding follow-up care.

DIAGNOSTIC TESTS

Chest x-ray
Blood gas analysis
Oximetry

DISCHARGE CRITERIA

Prior to discharge, the client will:

- experience re-expansion of affected lung
- have adequate respiratory function
- identify safety measures related to care of chest tube insertion site and flutter valve (if present)
- identify ways to reduce the risk of recurrent spontaneous pneumothorax
- state signs and symptoms to report to the health care provider
- verbalize an understanding of and plan for adhering to recommended follow-up care including future appointments with health care provider and activity restrictions.

1. NURSING DIAGNOSIS:

Ineffective breathing pattern

related to:
a. increased rate and decreased depth of respirations associated with fear and anxiety;
b. decreased rate and depth of respirations associated with the depressant effect of some medications (e.g. narcotic [opioid] analgesics);
c. diminished lung/chest wall expansion associated with:

1. reluctance to breathe deeply resulting from chest pain and fear of dislodging chest tube or experiencing another pneumothorax
2. collapse of lung tissue.

Desired Outcome	Nursing Actions and *Selected Purposes/Rationales*

1. The client will experience an effective breathing pattern as evidenced by:
  a. normal rate and depth of respirations
  b. decreased dyspnea
  c. symmetrical chest excursion
  d. blood gases within normal range.
	1.a. Assess for signs and symptoms of an ineffective breathing pattern (e.g. shallow respirations, tachypnea, dyspnea, asymmetrical chest excursion, use of accessory muscles when breathing).
	  b. Monitor for and report the following:
	    1. abnormal blood gases
	    2. significant decrease in oximetry results.
	  c. Implement measures *to improve breathing pattern:*
	    1. perform actions to reduce chest pain (see Nursing Diagnosis 3, action d)
	    2. perform actions to reduce fear and anxiety (see Nursing Diagnosis 5, action b)
	    3. place client in a semi- to high Fowler's position unless contraindicated
	    4. assist client to turn from side to side at least every 2 hours while in bed
	    5. instruct client to deep breathe or use incentive spirometer every 1–2 hours
	    6. assure client that deep breathing and turning should not dislodge the chest tube or increase the risk of a recurrent pneumothorax
	    7. instruct client to breathe slowly if hyperventilating
	    8. increase activity as allowed and tolerated
	    9. administer central nervous system depressants judiciously; hold medication and consult physician if respiratory rate is less than 12/minute.
	  d. Consult physician if ineffective breathing pattern continues.

■

2. NURSING DIAGNOSIS: Impaired gas exchange

related to loss of effective lung surface associated with lung collapse.

Desired Outcome	Nursing Actions and *Selected Purposes/Rationales*

2. The client will experience adequate O_2/CO_2 exchange as evidenced by:
  a. usual mental status
  b. unlabored respirations at 14–20/minute
  c. blood gases within normal range.
	2.a. Assess for and report signs and symptoms of impaired gas exchange:
	    1. restlessness, irritability
	    2. confusion, somnolence
	    3. tachypnea, dyspnea
	    4. decreased PaO_2 and/or increased $PaCO_2$.
	  b. Monitor for and report a significant decrease in oximetry results.
	  c. Implement measures *to improve gas exchange:*
	    1. perform actions *to promote lung re-expansion:*
	      a. prepare client for and assist with insertion of chest tube (the tube is then connected to a drainage system [with or without suction] or, less commonly, to a flutter valve)
	      b. following chest tube insertion, implement measures *to maintain patency and integrity of chest drainage system:*
	        1. maintain fluid level in water seal and suction chambers as ordered
	        2. maintain occlusive dressing over chest tube insertion site
	        3. tape all connections securely
	        4. tape the tubing close to insertion site to the chest wall *in order to reduce the risk of inadvertent removal of the tube*
	        5. position tubing *to promote optimum drainage* (e.g. coil excess

tubing on bed rather than allowing it to hang down below the collection device, keep tubing free of kinks)
6. drain fluid that accumulates in tubing into the collection chamber; milk chest tube only if ordered
7. keep drainage collection device below level of client's chest at all times
  c. perform actions *to facilitate the escape of air from the pleural space* (e.g. maintain suction as ordered; ensure that the air vent is open on the drainage collection device if system is to water seal only; if a flutter valve is present, ensure that there is no fluid in the valve and that the distal end is open)
2. perform actions to improve breathing pattern (see Nursing Diagnosis 1, action c)
3. maintain oxygen therapy as ordered
4. discourage smoking (*smoke decreases oxygen availability*)
5. maintain activity restrictions as ordered; increase activity gradually as allowed and tolerated
6. following lung re-expansion, assist with pleurodesis if planned (*may be done to reduce the risk of a recurrent spontaneous pneumothorax*).
  d. Consult physician if signs and symptoms of impaired gas exchange persist or worsen.

---

3. NURSING DIAGNOSIS: **Pain: chest**

related to:
a. irritation of the parietal pleura associated with:
   1. stretching of the pleura resulting from air in the pleural space
   2. inflammatory process if pleurodesis is performed;
b. tissue irritation associated with insertion and presence of chest tube.

Desired Outcome	Nursing Actions and *Selected Purposes/Rationales*
3. The client will experience diminished chest pain as evidenced by: a. verbalization of a decrease in or absence of pain b. relaxed facial expression and body positioning c. improved breathing pattern d. increased participation in activities e. stable vital signs.	3.a. Assess for signs and symptoms of chest pain (e.g. verbalization of pain, grimacing, rubbing chest, guarding of affected side of chest, reluctance to move, shallow respirations, restlessness, increased B/P, tachycardia). b. Assess client's perception of the severity of pain using a pain intensity rating scale. c. Assess the client's pain pattern (e.g. location, quality, onset, duration, precipitating factors, aggravating factors, alleviating factors). d. Implement measures *to reduce chest pain:* 1. perform actions to reduce fear and anxiety (see Nursing Diagnosis 5, action b) *in order to promote relaxation and subsequently increase the client's threshold and tolerance for pain* 2. administer analgesics before activities and procedures that can cause pain and before pain becomes severe 3. instruct and assist client to splint chest with hands or pillow when deep breathing, coughing, and changing position 4. provide or assist with nonpharmacologic methods for pain relief (e.g. position change; progressive relaxation exercises; restful environment; diversional activities such as watching television, reading, or conversing) 5. securely anchor chest tube *to limit its movement and resulting tissue irritation* 6. administer analgesics as ordered 7. assist with intercostal nerve block if performed. e. Consult physician if the above measures fail to provide adequate pain relief.

4. COLLABORATIVE DIAGNOSIS:

Potential complication of pneumothorax: tension pneumothorax with mediastinal shift

related to a significant increase in intrapleural pressure associated with inability of air to leave pleural space during expiration (can occur as a result of chest tube or flutter valve malfunction).

Desired Outcome	Nursing Actions and *Selected Purposes/Rationales*
4. The client will not develop tension pneumothorax with mediastinal shift as evidenced by: a. no sudden increase in dyspnea b. vital signs within normal range for client c. usual mental status d. absence of neck vein distention e. trachea in midline position f. usual skin color g. blood gases returning toward normal h. chest x-ray showing re-expansion of lung on affected side.	4.a. Assess for and immediately report signs and symptoms of: 1. malfunction of chest drainage system (e.g. respiratory distress, lack of fluctuation in the water seal chamber without evidence of lung re-expansion, excessive bubbling in water seal chamber, significant increase in subcutaneous emphysema) 2. malfunction of the flutter valve if present (e.g. respiratory distress, presence of fluid at the proximal end of the valve, abrupt cessation of air flow from the distal end of the valve during exhalation) 3. extended pneumothorax (e.g. extended area of absent breath sounds with hyperresonant percussion note, increased dyspnea, chest x-ray showing an increase in size of pneumothorax) 4. tension pneumothorax (e.g. severe dyspnea, rapid and/or irregular heart rate, hypotension, restlessness and agitation, neck vein distention, shift in trachea from midline). b. Monitor blood gases. Report values that have worsened. c. Monitor chest x-ray results. Report findings of mediastinal shifting. d. Implement measures to promote lung re-expansion (see Nursing Diagnosis 2, action c.1) *in order to reduce the risk of tension pneumothorax with mediastinal shift.* e. If signs and symptoms of tension pneumothorax with mediastinal shift occur: 1. maintain client on bed rest in a semi- to high Fowler's position 2. maintain oxygen therapy as ordered 3. assist with clearing of existing chest tube or flutter valve, insertion of new tube, and/or needle aspiration of air from the pleural space *to reduce intrapleural pressure* 4. provide emotional support to client and significant others.

5. NURSING DIAGNOSIS:

Anxiety

related to difficulty breathing; chest pain; unfamiliar environment; lack of understanding of diagnostic tests, diagnosis, and treatment measures; and possibility of recurrence of pneumothorax.

Desired Outcome	Nursing Actions and *Selected Purposes/Rationales*
5. The client will experience a reduction in anxiety as evidenced by: a. verbalization of feeling less anxious b. usual sleep pattern	5.a. Assess client for signs and symptoms of anxiety (e.g. verbalization of feeling anxious, insomnia, tenseness, shakiness, restlessness, diaphoresis, tachycardia, elevated blood pressure, facial pallor, self-focused behaviors). Validate perceptions carefully, remembering that some behaviors may be the result of tissue hypoxia and respiratory distress. b. Implement measures *to reduce fear and anxiety:*

c. relaxed facial expression and body movements
d. stable vital signs
e. usual perceptual ability and interactions with others.

1. orient client to hospital environment, equipment, and routines
2. introduce client to staff who will be participating in care; if possible, maintain consistency in staff assigned to his/her care *to provide feelings of stability and comfort with the environment*
3. assure client that staff members are nearby; respond to call signal as soon as possible
4. maintain a calm, supportive, confident manner when interacting with client
5. encourage verbalization of fear and anxiety; provide feedback
6. reinforce physician's explanations and clarify misconceptions the client has about the pneumothorax, treatment plan, and possible recurrence
7. explain all diagnostic tests
8. perform actions to reduce chest pain (see Nursing Diagnosis 3, action d)
9. perform actions to improve gas exchange (see Nursing Diagnosis 2, action c) *in order to relieve respiratory distress*
10. provide a calm, restful environment
11. instruct client in relaxation techniques and encourage participation in diversional activities once the period of acute pain and respiratory distress has subsided
12. assist client to identify specific stressors and ways to cope with them
13. provide information based on current needs of client and significant others at a level he/she can understand; encourage questions and clarification of information provided
14. encourage significant others to project a caring, concerned attitude without obvious anxiousness
15. include significant others in orientation and teaching sessions and encourage their continued support of the client
16. administer prescribed antianxiety agents if indicated.

c. Consult physician if above actions fail to control fear and anxiety.

Discharge Teaching

███───────────────────────────────────────

6. **NURSING DIAGNOSIS:**   **Knowledge deficit, Ineffective management of therapeutic regimen, or Altered health maintenance***

*The nurse should select the diagnostic label that is most appropriate for the individual client's teaching needs.

Desired Outcomes	Nursing Actions and *Selected Purposes/Rationales*
6.a. The client will identify safety measures related to care of chest tube insertion site and flutter valve (if present).	6.a.1. If chest tube was removed before discharge, explain the importance of maintaining an occlusive dressing over the insertion site until instructed by physician to remove it.

6.a.2. If client is discharged with a flutter valve in place, reinforce the following safety measures:
   a. maintain an occlusive dressing around the insertion site
   b. ensure that the connection between the chest tube and flutter valve is taped securely and that it is anchored to the chest wall using tape
   c. maintain patency of the flutter valve (e.g. avoid occluding the distal end of the flutter valve, contact physician if fluid collects in the valve, avoid activities such as swimming and bathing [the valve should not be submerged in water]).

3. Allow time for questions and clarification of information provided.

Desired Outcomes	Nursing Actions and *Selected Purposes/Rationales*
6.b. The client will identify ways to reduce the risk of recurrent spontaneous pneumothorax.	6.b.1. Caution client to avoid activities that involve experiencing marked changes in atmospheric pressure (e.g. scuba diving, flying in unpressurized aircraft, mountain climbing). 2. Encourage client to stop smoking.
6.c. The client will state signs and symptoms to report to the health care provider.	6.c. Instruct client to report the following signs and symptoms: 1. difficulty breathing 2. chest pain 3. elevated temperature 4. chills 5. increased redness and warmth at chest tube insertion site 6. purulent drainage from chest tube insertion site or flutter valve.

6.d. The client will verbalize an understanding of and plan for adhering to recommended follow-up care including future appointments with health care provider and activity restrictions.	6.d.1. Reinforce importance of keeping follow-up appointments with health care provider.
	2. Instruct client to avoid excessive physical exertion and lifting objects over 10 pounds until permitted by physician.
	3. Reinforce physician's explanation about the possibility of recurrent spontaneous pneumothorax (occurs in approximately 30–50% of clients after initial episode). Assist client to develop a plan for obtaining emergency assistance if spontaneous pneumothorax recurs.
	4. Encourage client to continue with deep breathing exercises and use of incentive spirometer for time period recommended by physician.
	5. Implement measures to improve client compliance:
	  a. include significant others in teaching sessions if possible
	  b. encourage questions and allow time for reinforcement and clarification of information provided
	  c. provide written instructions about precautions related to chest tube insertion site and flutter valve (if present), signs and symptoms to report, future appointments with health care provider, and activity restrictions.

Bibliography

See pages 897–898 and 905.

PULMONARY EMBOLISM

Pulmonary embolism is the partial or complete occlusion of one of the pulmonary arteries or its branches by an embolus. The most common source of the embolus is a thrombus that originates in a deep vein of the lower extremities. Less frequently, the embolus results from a thrombus that originates in the right side of the heart or the upper extremities or from a nonthrombic source such as air, fat, amniotic fluid, tumor cells, and foreign material (e.g. broken intravenous catheter, talc [often used to 'cut' drugs injected by intravenous drug abusers]).

The clinical manifestations of pulmonary embolism are varied and nonspecific. The extensiveness of the signs and symptoms depends on the size and number of emboli, size of the vessel that is occluded, extent of vessel occlusion, and presence of pre-existing cardiac or pulmonary disease. The classic signs and symptoms of a moderate-size pulmonary embolism are sudden onset of dyspnea, tachypnea, tachycardia, and a feeling of apprehension or impending doom. The person may also experience chest pain and syncope.

Medical treatment varies depending on the source of the embolus and its effect on cardiopulmonary function. When the source is a thrombus, treatment usually consists of bed rest and initiation of intravenous anticoagulant therapy. A thrombolytic agent might be administered if the thromboembolus is occluding a large vessel and/or cardiopulmonary status is severely compromised. Anticoagulant therapy (subcutaneous and/or oral) often continues for 3–6 months following discharge. If thrombolytic agents and anticoagulant therapy are contraindicated or unsuccessful or the source of the embolus is nonthrombic, surgical removal of the embolus may be indicated.

This care plan focuses on the adult client hospitalized for treatment of pulmonary embolism resulting from a deep vein thrombus. The goals of care are to promote adequate respiratory function, prevent complications, reduce fear and anxiety, and educate the client regarding follow-up care.

DIAGNOSTIC TESTS

Lung scan (ventilation-perfusion [V/Q] scan or perfusion scan)
Pulmonary angiography
Arterial blood gases
Chest x-ray

DISCHARGE CRITERIA

Prior to discharge, the client will:

- have adequate respiratory function
- have no reports of chest pain
- have no signs and symptoms of complications
- identify ways to reduce the risk of recurrent thrombus formation and pulmonary embolism
- verbalize an understanding of medications ordered including rationale, food and drug interactions, side effects, schedule for taking, and importance of taking as prescribed
- demonstrate the ability to correctly draw up and administer heparin subcutaneously if prescribed
- identify ways to prevent bleeding associated with anticoagulant therapy
- state signs and symptoms to report to the health care provider
- verbalize an understanding of and a plan for adhering to recommended follow-up care including future appointments with health care provider and activity level.

Use in conjunction with the Care Plan on Immobility.

NURSING/ COLLABORATIVE DIAGNOSES

1. Ineffective breathing pattern △ 473
2. Impaired gas exchange △ 474
3. Pain: chest △ 475
4. Potential complications:
   a. right-sided heart failure
   b. extended or recurrent pulmonary embolism
   c. atelectasis
   d. bleeding △ 476
5. Anxiety △ 478

DISCHARGE TEACHING

6. Knowledge deficit, Ineffective management of therapeutic regimen, or Altered health maintenance △ 478

See Care Plan on Immobility for additional diagnoses.

---

1. NURSING DIAGNOSIS:

Ineffective breathing pattern

related to:
a. increased rate and decreased depth of respirations associated with fear, anxiety, and stimulant effects of hypoxia;

b. decreased rate and depth of respirations associated with depressant effect of some medications (e.g. narcotic [opioid] analgesics);
c. diminished lung/chest wall expansion associated with reluctance to breathe deeply because of pain if present.

Desired Outcome	Nursing Actions and *Selected Purposes/Rationales*

1. The client will maintain an effective breathing pattern as evidenced by:
a. normal rate and depth of respirations
b. absence of dyspnea
c. blood gases within normal range.
	1.a. Assess for signs and symptoms of an ineffective breathing pattern (e.g. rapid, shallow respirations; dyspnea; use of accessory muscles when breathing).
	b. Monitor for and report the following:
	  1. abnormal blood gases
	  2. significant decrease in oximetry results.
	c. Implement measures *to improve breathing pattern:*
	  1. perform actions to reduce pain (see Nursing Diagnosis 3, action d)
	  2. perform actions to reduce fear and anxiety (see Nursing Diagnosis 5)
	  3. perform actions to improve gas exchange (see Nursing Diagnosis 2, action c) *in order to reduce hypoxia and subsequent stimulation of the respiratory center*
	  4. place client in a semi- to high Fowler's position unless contraindicated
	  5. instruct client to breathe slowly if hyperventilating
	  6. instruct client to deep breathe or use incentive spirometer every 1–2 hours
	  7. administer central nervous system depressants judiciously; hold medication and consult physician if respiratory rate is less than 12/minute
	  8. increase activity when allowed.
	d. Consult physician if ineffective breathing pattern persists or worsens.

■───

2. NURSING DIAGNOSIS: **Impaired gas exchange**

related to:
a. decreased pulmonary perfusion associated with partial or complete occlusion of pulmonary arterial blood flow by the embolus and vasoconstriction resulting from the release of vasoactive mediators (e.g. serotonin, prostaglandin, thromboxane) from the platelets that coat the embolus;
b. decreased bronchial airflow associated with bronchoconstriction resulting from:
  1. the release of mediators such as serotonin, prostaglandin, and thromboxane from the platelets that coat the embolus
  2. a compensatory response to an increase in the amount of dead space in the underperfused lung area (the compensatory bronchoconstriction also affects airways in perfused lung areas);
c. alveolar collapse associated with atelectasis if it occurs.

Desired Outcome	Nursing Actions and *Selected Purposes/Rationales*

2. The client will experience adequate O_2/CO_2 exchange as evidenced by:
a. usual mental status
	2.a. Assess for and report signs and symptoms of impaired gas exchange:
	  1. restlessness, irritability
	  2. confusion, somnolence
	  3. tachypnea, dyspnea.

b. unlabored respirations at 14–20/minute
c. blood gases within normal range.

b. Monitor for and report the following:
   1. abnormal blood gases
   2. significant decrease in oximetry results.
c. Implement measures *to improve gas exchange:*
   1. maintain client on bed rest *to reduce oxygen demand during acute respiratory distress*; increase activity gradually as allowed and tolerated
   2. maintain oxygen therapy as ordered
   3. perform actions to improve breathing pattern (see Nursing Diagnosis 1, action c)
   4. discourage smoking (*smoke decreases oxygen availability and can cause further vasoconstriction as well as inflammation of the bronchial walls*)
   5. perform actions *to improve pulmonary blood flow:*
      a. administer anticoagulants (e.g. continuous intravenous heparin, warfarin) if ordered
      b. prepare client for the following if planned:
         1. injection of a thrombolytic agent (e.g. streptokinase, urokinase, tissue plasminogen activator [tPA])
         2. embolectomy.
d. Consult physician if signs and symptoms of impaired gas exchange persist or worsen.

---

3. NURSING DIAGNOSIS: **Pain: chest**

related to:
a. decreased pulmonary tissue perfusion associated with obstructed pulmonary blood flow;
b. inflammation of the parietal pleura associated with tissue damage if infarction occurs.

Desired Outcome	Nursing Actions and *Selected Purposes/Rationales*

3. The client will experience diminished chest pain as evidenced by:
  a. verbalization of a decrease in pain
  b. relaxed facial expression and body positioning
  c. increased participation in activities when allowed
  d. pulse and B/P within normal range for client.
	3.a. Assess for signs and symptoms of pain (e.g. verbalization of pain, grimacing, rubbing chest, reluctance to move, shallow respirations, restlessness, increased B/P, tachycardia).
	  b. Assess client's perception of the severity of pain using a pain intensity rating scale.
	  c. Assess the client's pain pattern (e.g. location, quality, onset, duration, precipitating factors, aggravating factors, alleviating factors).
	  d. Implement measures *to reduce pain:*
	    1. perform actions to reduce fear and anxiety (see Nursing Diagnosis 5) *in order to promote relaxation and subsequently increase the client's threshold and tolerance for pain*
	    2. perform actions to improve gas exchange (see Nursing Diagnosis 2, action c) *in order to reduce tissue hypoxia in the involved lung area*
	    3. instruct and assist client to splint chest with hands or pillow when deep breathing, coughing, and changing position
	    4. provide or assist with nonpharmacologic methods for pain relief (e.g. position change, relaxation techniques, restful environment, diversional activities)
	    5. administer analgesics if ordered.
	  e. Consult physician if above actions fail to provide adequate pain relief.

4. COLLABORATIVE DIAGNOSES:

Potential complications:

a. **right-sided heart failure** related to increased cardiac workload associated with:
   1. pulmonary hypertension (can result from pulmonary vasoconstriction that occurs in response to hypoxia and the release of vasoactive mediators)
   2. compensatory response to the decreased pulmonary blood flow that occurs when there is obstruction of multiple vessels and/or of large vessels of the pulmonary vascular bed;
b. **extended or recurrent pulmonary embolism** related to inadequate response to treatment and/or continued presence of predisposing conditions;
c. **atelectasis** related to:
   1. shallow respirations associated with chest pain, fear, and anxiety
   2. stasis of secretions in the alveoli and bronchioles associated with bronchoconstriction and decreased mobility during time that activity is restricted
   3. decreased surfactant production associated with reduced pulmonary blood flow and inadequate deep breathing;
d. **bleeding** related to prolonged coagulation time associated with anticoagulant therapy.

Desired Outcomes	Nursing Actions and *Selected Purposes/Rationales*

4.a. The client will not develop right-sided heart failure as evidenced by:
1. pulse 60–100 beats/minute
2. no increase in intensity of S_2 heart sound or development of summation gallop
3. usual mental status
4. no increase in dyspnea
5. usual strength and activity tolerance
6. adequate urine output
7. stable weight
8. absence of edema and distended neck veins.
	4.a.1. Assess for and report signs and symptoms of right-sided heart failure:
	  a. further increase in pulse
	  b. development of a loud S_2 heart sound and/or summation gallop
	  c. restlessness, anxiousness, confusion
	  d. increased dyspnea
	  e. weakness and fatigue
	  f. decreased urine output
	  g. weight gain
	  h. edema
	  i. distended neck veins.
	  2. Monitor chest x-ray results. Report findings of cardiomegaly.
	  3. Implement measures to improve pulmonary blood flow (see Nursing Diagnosis 2, action c.5) *in order to reduce cardiac workload and the subsequent risk for right-sided heart failure.*
	  4. If signs and symptoms of right-sided heart failure occur:
	    a. maintain oxygen therapy as ordered
	    b. maintain client on strict bed rest in a semi- to high Fowler's position
	    c. maintain fluid and sodium restrictions if ordered
	    d. administer medications that may be ordered *to reduce vascular congestion and/or cardiac workload* (e.g. diuretics, cardiotonics, vasodilators)
	    e. refer to Care Plan on Heart Failure for additional care measures.

4.b. The client will not experience extension or recurrence of a pulmonary embolism as evidenced by:
1. absence of or diminishing chest pain
2. absence of or decrease in dyspnea
3. pulse 60–100 beats/minute
4. blood gases returning toward normal.
	4.b.1. Assess for and report signs and symptoms of extended or recurrent pulmonary embolism (e.g. development of, persistent, or increased chest pain, dyspnea, tachypnea, or tachycardia; declining Pao_2).
	  2. Administer heparin and/or assist with administration of thrombolytic agents (e.g. urokinase, tissue plasminogen activator [tPA], streptokinase) if ordered *to prevent extension of the embolism.*
	  3. Implement measures *to prevent recurrence of a pulmonary embolism:*
	    a. perform actions to prevent and treat a deep vein thrombus (see Care Plan on Immobility, Collaborative Diagnosis 12, actions a.1.b and c [p. 137])
	    b. perform actions *to prevent dislodgment of thrombus:*
	      1. maintain client on bed rest as ordered
	      2. do not exercise, check for Homans' sign in, or massage any extremity known to have a thrombus

3. caution client to avoid activities that create a Valsalva response (e.g. straining to have a bowel movement, holding breath while moving up in bed)

c. prepare client for a vena caval interruption (e.g. insertion of an intracaval filtering device) if planned.

4. If signs and symptoms of extended or recurrent pulmonary embolism occur:

a. continue with above actions

b. maintain client on strict bed rest in a semi- to high Fowler's position

c. maintain oxygen therapy as ordered

d. prepare client for diagnostic tests (e.g. ventilation-perfusion lung scan, blood gases, pulmonary angiography) if indicated

e. prepare client for surgical intervention (e.g. embolectomy) if planned

f. assess for and report signs and symptoms of pulmonary infarction (e.g. hemoptysis, fever, increased WBC count)

g. provide emotional support to client and significant others.

4.c. The client will not develop atelectasis (see Care Plan on Immobility, Collaborative Diagnosis 12, outcome b [p. 138], for outcome criteria).

4.c.1. Refer to Care Plan on Immobility, Collaborative Diagnosis 12, action b (p. 138), for measures related to assessment, prevention, and treatment of atelectasis.

2. Implement measures to improve breathing pattern and gas exchange (see Nursing Diagnoses 1, action c and 2, action c) *in order to further reduce the risk for atelectasis.*

4.d. The client will not experience unusual bleeding as evidenced by:

1. skin and mucous membranes free of petechiae, purpura, ecchymoses, and active bleeding

2. absence of unusual joint pain

3. no increase in abdominal girth

4. absence of frank and occult blood in stool, urine, and vomitus

5. usual menstrual flow

6. vital signs within normal range for client

7. stable Hct and Hb.

4.d.1. Assess client for and report signs and symptoms of unusual bleeding:

a. petechiae, purpura, ecchymoses

b. gingival bleeding

c. prolonged bleeding from puncture sites

d. epistaxis, hemoptysis

e. unusual joint pain

f. increase in abdominal girth

g. frank or occult blood in stool, urine, or vomitus

h. menorrhagia

i. restlessness, confusion

j. decreasing B/P and increased pulse rate

k. decrease in Hct and Hb levels.

2. Monitor platelet count and coagulation test results (e.g. prothrombin time or International Normalized Ratio [INR], activated partial thromboplastin time). Report a low platelet count and coagulation test results that exceed the therapeutic range.

3. If platelet count is low, coagulation test results are abnormal, or Hct and Hb levels decrease, test all stools, urine, and vomitus for occult blood. Report positive results.

4. Implement measures *to prevent bleeding:*

a. avoid giving injections whenever possible; consult physician about prescribing an alternative route for medications ordered to be given intramuscularly or subcutaneously

b. when giving injections or performing venous or arterial punctures, use the smallest gauge needle possible and apply gentle, prolonged pressure to the site after the needle is removed

c. caution client to avoid activities that increase the risk for trauma (e.g. shaving with a straight-edge razor, using stiff-bristle toothbrush or dental floss)

d. whenever possible, avoid intubations (e.g. nasogastric) and procedures that can cause injury to the rectal mucosa (e.g. taking temperature rectally, inserting a rectal suppository, administering an enema)

e. perform actions *to reduce the risk for falls* (e.g. keep bed in low position with side rails up when client is in bed, avoid unnecessary clutter in room, instruct client to wear slippers/shoes with nonslip soles when ambulating)

f. pad side rails if client is confused or restless

g. instruct client to avoid blowing nose forcefully or straining to have a bowel movement; consult physician about an order for a decongestant and/or laxative if indicated.

Desired Outcomes	Nursing Actions and *Selected Purposes/Rationales*

	5. If bleeding occurs and does not subside spontaneously:
	   a. apply firm, prolonged pressure to bleeding area(s) if possible
	   b. if epistaxis occurs, place client in a high Fowler's position and apply pressure and ice pack to nasal area
	   c. maintain oxygen therapy as ordered
	   d. perform gastric lavage as ordered *to control gastric bleeding*
	   e. administer protamine sulfate (antidote for heparin), vitamin K (e.g. phytonadione), and plasma or whole blood as ordered
	   f. assess for and report signs and symptoms of hypovolemic shock (e.g. restlessness; confusion; significant decrease in B/P; rapid, weak pulse; rapid respirations; cool, pale skin; urine output less than 30 ml/hour)
	   g. prepare client for surgical repair of bleeding vessels if indicated
	   h. provide emotional support to client and significant others.

5. NURSING DIAGNOSIS: **Anxiety**

related to dyspnea; chest pain; lack of understanding of diagnostic tests, diagnosis, and treatments; unfamiliar environment; possibility of recurrent embolism; and threat of death.

Desired Outcome	Nursing Actions and *Selected Purposes/Rationales*

5. The client will experience a reduction in anxiety (see Care Plan on Immobility, Nursing Diagnosis 13 [p. 140], for outcome criteria).	5.a. Refer to Care Plan on Immobility, Nursing Diagnosis 13 (p. 140), for measures related to assessment and reduction of fear and anxiety.
	  b. Implement additional measures *to reduce fear and anxiety:*
	   1. do not leave client alone during period of acute respiratory distress
	   2. perform actions to improve gas exchange (see Nursing Diagnosis 2, action c) *in order to relieve dyspnea*
	   3. perform actions to reduce chest pain (see Nursing Diagnosis 3, action d)
	   4. explain all diagnostic tests
	   5. reassure client that extreme apprehension or "sense of doom" is a common symptom of pulmonary embolism and will diminish as condition stabilizes.

Discharge Teaching

6. NURSING DIAGNOSIS: **Knowledge deficit, Ineffective management of therapeutic regimen, or Altered health maintenance***

*The nurse should select the diagnostic label that is most appropriate for the individual client's teaching needs.

Desired Outcomes	Nursing Actions and *Selected Purposes/Rationales*

6.a. The client will identify ways to reduce the risk of recurrent thrombus formation and pulmonary embolism.	6.a.1. Provide the following instructions on ways to promote venous blood flow and reduce the risk of thrombus recurrence:
	   a. avoid wearing constrictive clothing (e.g. garters, girdles, narrow-banded knee-high hose)
	   b. avoid sitting and standing in one position for long periods of time
	   c. wear graduated compression stockings or support hose during the day
	   d. avoid crossing legs and lying or sitting with pillows under knees
	   e. engage in regular aerobic exercise (e.g. swimming, walking, cycling)

f. elevate legs periodically, especially when sitting

g. dorsiflex feet regularly

h. maintain an ideal body weight for age, height, and body frame.

2. Inform client that smoking and the use of estrogen or oral contraceptives can increase the risk for recurrent thrombus formation.

3. Instruct client to avoid trauma to or massage of any area of suspected thrombus formation in order to decrease risk of pulmonary embolism.

4. Provide information regarding exercise programs and support groups that can assist the client to stop smoking and/or lose weight.

6.b. The client will verbalize an understanding of medications ordered including rationale, food and drug interactions, side effects, schedule for taking, and importance of taking as prescribed.

6.b.1. Explain the rationale for, side effects of, and importance of taking medications prescribed.

2. If client is discharged on warfarin (e.g. Coumadin), instruct to:

a. keep scheduled appointments for periodic blood studies to monitor coagulation times

b. take medication at the same time each day, do not stop taking medication abruptly, and do not attempt to make up for missed doses

c. avoid taking over-the-counter products containing aspirin and other nonsteroidal anti-inflammatory agents (these products enhance the action of warfarin)

d. avoid regular and/or excessive intake of alcohol (may alter responsiveness to warfarin)

e. avoid eating large amounts of foods high in vitamin K (e.g. green leafy vegetables)

f. report prolonged or excessive bleeding from skin, nose, or mouth; blood in urine, vomitus, sputum, or stool; prolonged or excessive menses; excessive bruising; severe headache; or sudden abdominal or back pain

g. inform physician immediately if pregnancy is suspected (warfarin crosses the placental barrier)

h. wear a medical alert identification bracelet or tag identifying self as being on anticoagulant therapy.

3. Instruct client to inform physician of any other prescription and nonprescription medications he/she is taking.

4. Instruct client to inform all health care providers of medications being taken.

6.c. The client will demonstrate the ability to correctly draw up and administer heparin subcutaneously if prescribed.

6.c.1. If client is to be discharged on subcutaneous heparin, provide instructions about subcutaneous injection technique.

2. Allow time for questions, practice, and return demonstration.

6.d. The client will identify ways to prevent bleeding associated with anticoagulant therapy.

6.d.1. Instruct client about ways to minimize the risk of bleeding while on anticoagulant therapy:

a. use an electric rather than straight-edge razor

b. floss and brush teeth gently

c. avoid putting sharp objects (e.g. toothpicks) in mouth

d. do not walk barefoot

e. cut nails carefully

f. avoid situations that could result in injury (e.g. contact sports)

g. do not blow nose forcefully

h. avoid straining to have a bowel movement.

2. Instruct client to control any bleeding by applying firm, prolonged pressure to the area if possible.

6.e. The client will state signs and symptoms to report to the health care provider.

6.e. Stress the importance of reporting the following signs and symptoms:

1. tenderness, swelling, or pain in extremity

2. sudden chest pain

3. new or increased shortness of breath

4. extreme anxiousness or restlessness

5. cough productive of blood-tinged sputum

6. unusual bleeding (see action b.2.f in this diagnosis)

7. fever.

6.f. The client will verbalize an understanding of and a

6.f.1. Reinforce the importance of keeping follow-up appointments with health care provider.

Desired Outcomes	Nursing Actions and *Selected Purposes/Rationales*

plan for adhering to recommended follow-up care including future appointments with health care provider and activity level.	2. Reinforce the physician's instructions regarding activity limitations.
	3. Implement measures to improve client compliance:
	  a. include significant others in teaching sessions if possible
	  b. encourage questions and allow time for reinforcement and clarification of information provided
	  c. provide written instructions regarding future appointments with health care provider, medications prescribed, activity restrictions, signs and symptoms to report, and future laboratory studies.

Bibliography

See pages 897–898 and 905.

 # THORACIC SURGERY

Thoracic surgery is a term used to encompass a variety of procedures that involve entry into the thoracic cavity for access to the lungs, heart, aorta, or esophagus. Types of thoracic surgery commonly performed to treat pulmonary disorders include pneumonectomy, lobectomy, segmental resection, and wedge resection. These procedures may be performed to treat benign or malignant tumors, confined areas of bronchiectasis or tuberculosis, lung trauma, lung abscesses, blebs, and bullae. Although advances in endoscopic and laser technology allow for the removal of small peripheral tumors or defects through an intercostally inserted endoscope, an open thoracic approach is still required for extensive tissue removal.

This care plan focuses on the adult client hospitalized for thoracic surgery to remove a portion or all of a lung. Preoperative goals of care are to reduce fear and anxiety and assist the client to maintain an optimal respiratory status. The goals of postoperative care are to prevent and detect complications, maintain comfort, and educate the client regarding follow-up care. The care plan will need to be individualized according to the client's diagnosis, extensiveness of the surgery, prognosis, and plans for subsequent treatment.

DIAGNOSTIC TESTS

Pulmonary function studies
Chest x-ray
Computed tomography (CT)
Bronchoscopy with or without biopsy
Ventilation-perfusion scan
Blood gases
Electrocardiogram (ECG)

DISCHARGE CRITERIA

Prior to discharge, the client will:

- have optimal respiratory function
- have evidence of normal healing of surgical wound
- have surgical pain controlled
- have no signs and symptoms of postoperative complications
- demonstrate the ability to perform prescribed arm and shoulder exercises
- state signs and symptoms to report to the health care provider
- identify community resources that can assist with home management and adjustment to the diagnosis, effects of surgery, and adjuvant treatment if planned
- verbalize an understanding of and a plan for adhering to recommended follow-up care including future appointments with health care provider, medications prescribed, activity level, pain management, wound care, and subsequent treatment of the underlying disorder.

NURSING/ COLLABORATIVE DIAGNOSES	**Preoperative**
	1. Anxiety △ 481
	2. Ineffective airway clearance △ 482
	3. Impaired gas exchange △ 482
	Postoperative
	1. Impaired respiratory function:
	a. ineffective breathing pattern
	b. ineffective airway clearance
	c. impaired gas exchange △ 483
	2. Potential complications:
	a. extended pneumothorax
	b. hemothorax
	c. mediastinal shift
	d. cardiac dysrhythmias
	e. acute pulmonary edema
	f. bronchopleural fistula
	g. restricted arm and shoulder movement △ 484
	3. Grieving △ 488
DISCHARGE TEACHING	**4.** Knowledge deficit, Ineffective management of therapeutic regimen, or Altered health maintenance △ 489

See Standardized Preoperative and Postoperative Care Plans for additional diagnoses.

PREOPERATIVE

Use in conjunction with the Standardized Preoperative Care Plan.

■

1. NURSING DIAGNOSIS: **Anxiety**

related to:
a. lack of understanding of diagnostic tests, diagnosis, surgical procedure, and postoperative management;
b. unfamiliar environment and financial concerns;
c. anticipated loss of control associated with effects of anesthesia;
d. potential embarrassment or loss of dignity associated with body exposure;
e. anticipated pain and/or difficulty breathing;
f. possible changes in usual life style (e.g. activity limitations, cessation of smoking).

Desired Outcome	Nursing Actions and *Selected Purposes/Rationales*
1. The client will experience a reduction in anxiety (see Standardized Preoperative Care Plan, Nursing Diagnosis 1 [pp. 96–97], for outcome criteria).	1.a. Refer to Standardized Preoperative Care Plan, Nursing Diagnosis 1 (pp. 96–97), for measures related to assessment and reduction of fear and anxiety.
	b. Implement additional measures *to reduce fear and anxiety:*
	1. reinforce physician's explanations about anticipated effect of loss of lung tissue on activity tolerance
	2. provide instruction about the purpose of chest drainage system that will be present after partial removal of a lung (chest tubes are rarely inserted if a pneumonectomy is performed)
	3. assure client that he/she will receive supplemental oxygen following surgery if needed.

2. NURSING DIAGNOSIS: **Ineffective airway clearance**

related to difficulty coughing up secretions associated with:
a. excessive or tenacious pulmonary secretions resulting from the underlying disease process;
b. weakness and pain (may occur as a result of underlying disease process).

Desired Outcome	Nursing Actions and *Selected Purposes/Rationales*

2. The client will experience effective airway clearance as evidenced by:
a. usual breath sounds
b. usual rate and depth of respirations
c. absence of dyspnea
d. absence of cyanosis.
	2.a. Assess for signs and symptoms of ineffective airway clearance (e.g. abnormal breath sounds; rapid, shallow respirations; dyspnea; development of or increase in cough; cyanosis).
	b. Implement measures *to promote effective airway clearance:*
	  1. instruct and assist client to turn, cough or "huff," and deep breathe every 1–2 hours
	  2. perform actions *to facilitate removal of pulmonary secretions:*
	    a. implement measures *to thin tenacious secretions and reduce drying of the respiratory mucous membrane:*
	      1. maintain a fluid intake of at least 2500 ml/day unless contraindicated
	      2. humidify inspired air as ordered
	    b. assist with administration of mucolytics and diluent or hydrating agents via nebulizer as ordered
	    c. assist with or perform postural drainage therapy (PDT) if ordered
	    d. perform suctioning if ordered
	    e. administer expectorants if ordered
	  3. increase activity as allowed and tolerated
	  4. administer bronchodilators (e.g. theophylline) if ordered *to improve bronchial airflow.*
	c. Consult physician if signs and symptoms of ineffective airway clearance persist or worsen.

3. NURSING DIAGNOSIS: **Impaired gas exchange**

related to loss of effective lung surface associated with the underlying disease process.

Desired Outcome	Nursing Actions and *Selected Purposes/Rationales*

3. The client will experience adequate O_2/CO_2 exchange as evidenced by:
a. usual mental status
b. unlabored respirations at 14–20/minute
c. blood gases within normal range for client.
	3.a. Assess for and report signs and symptoms of impaired gas exchange:
	  1. restlessness, irritability
	  2. confusion, somnolence
	  3. tachypnea, dyspnea
	  4. decreased PaO_2 and/or increased $PaCO_2$.
	b. Monitor for and report a decrease in oximetry results.
	c. Implement measures *to improve gas exchange:*
	  1. perform actions to promote effective airway clearance (see Preoperative Nursing Diagnosis 2, action b)
	  2. place client in a semi- to high Fowler's position unless contraindicated; position overbed table so client can rest on it if desired
	  3. maintain oxygen therapy as ordered

4. discourage smoking (*smoke increases mucus production, impairs ciliary function, decreases oxygen availability, and can cause inflammation and damage to the bronchial walls*)
5. administer central nervous system depressants judiciously; hold medication and consult physician if respiratory rate is less than 12/minute.

d. Consult physician if signs and symptoms of impaired gas exchange persist or worsen.

POSTOPERATIVE

Use in conjunction with the Standardized Postoperative Care Plan.

---

1. NURSING DIAGNOSIS:

Impaired respiratory function:*

a. **ineffective breathing pattern** related to:
  1. increased rate and decreased depth of respirations associated with fear and anxiety
  2. decreased rate and depth of respirations associated with the depressant effect of anesthesia and some medications (e.g. narcotic [opioid] analgesics, central-acting muscle relaxants)
  3. diminished lung/chest wall expansion associated with:
     a. reluctance to breathe deeply resulting from incisional pain and fear of dislodging chest tube(s) if in place
     b. positioning, weakness, fatigue, and elevation of the diaphragm (can occur if abdominal distention is present or if the phrenic nerve was injured during surgery);
b. **ineffective airway clearance** related to:
  1. occlusion of the pharynx associated with relaxation of the tongue resulting from effect of anesthesia and some medications (e.g. narcotic [opioid] analgesics, central-acting muscle relaxants)
  2. stasis of secretions associated with:
     a. decreased activity
     b. depressed ciliary function resulting from effects of anesthesia
     c. difficulty coughing up secretions resulting from the depressant effect of anesthesia and some medications (e.g. narcotic [opioid] analgesics, central-acting muscle relaxants), pain, weakness, fatigue, and presence of tenacious secretions (can occur as a result of fluid volume deficit)
  3. increased secretions associated with irritation of the respiratory tract (can result from inhalation anesthetics, endotracheal intubation, and surgically induced lung tissue injury and inflammation);
c. **impaired gas exchange** related to the decrease in alveolar surface and pulmonary vasculature associated with the extensive removal of lung tissue.

---

*This diagnostic label includes the following nursing diagnoses: ineffective breathing pattern, ineffective airway clearance, and impaired gas exchange.

Desired Outcome	Nursing Actions and *Selected Purposes/Rationales*
1. The client will experience adequate respiratory function as evidenced by: a. improved rate and depth of respirations b. absence of or decrease in dyspnea	1.a. Assess for and report signs and symptoms of impaired respiratory function: 1. rapid, shallow, or slow respirations 2. dyspnea, orthopnea 3. use of accessory muscles when breathing 4. adventitious breath sounds (e.g. crackles [rales], rhonchi) 5. diminished or absent breath sounds over remaining lung tissue

Desired Outcome	Nursing Actions and *Selected Purposes/Rationales*

c. normal breath sounds over remaining lung tissue
d. usual mental status
e. usual skin color
f. blood gases returning toward normal range.

    6. development of or increase in cough
    7. restlessness, irritability
    8. confusion, somnolence
    9. central cyanosis (a late sign).
  b. Monitor for and report significant changes in blood gases and oximetry and chest x-ray results.
  c. Implement measures *to improve respiratory status:*
    1. perform actions to improve breathing pattern and promote effective airway clearance (see Standardized Postoperative Care Plan, Nursing Diagnoses 2, action c and 3, action b [pp. 102–104])
    2. perform actions to reduce pain (see Standardized Postoperative Care Plan, Nursing Diagnosis 6, action e [p. 107])
    3. perform actions to maintain patency and integrity of chest drainage system (see Postoperative Collaborative Diagnosis 2, action a.4.a) *in order to promote re-expansion of residual lung tissue*
    4. if chest tube(s) present, assure client that deep breathing and coughing will not dislodge the tube(s)
    5. position client as ordered (e.g. on back or on operative side after pneumonectomy, on back or either side following removal of a portion of the lung) *to allow full expansion of remaining lung tissue*
    6. when positioning client on his/her side, use a 30–45° "tip" position (rather than complete lateral positioning) *to minimize lateral compression of lung tissue*
    7. keep head of bed elevated *to facilitate lung expansion and promote drainage of fluid and residual air via chest tube(s)*
    8. maintain oxygen therapy as ordered
    9. administer bronchodilators (e.g. theophylline) if ordered.
  d. Consult physician if signs and symptoms of impaired respiratory function persist or worsen.

---

2. COLLABORATIVE DIAGNOSES:

Potential complications of thoracic surgery:

a. **extended pneumothorax** related to an increase in intrapleural pressure associated with accumulation of air in pleural space (can occur if the chest drainage system malfunctions and/or air leaks into the pleural space through the incision);

b. **hemothorax** related to intraoperative or postoperative bleeding and/or malfunction of the chest drainage system;

c. **mediastinal shift** related to:
  1. a significant increase in intrapleural pressure on the operative side following a lobectomy associated with an accumulation of fluid and air in the pleural space
  2. excessive negative pressure on the operative side following pneumonectomy associated with inadequate serous fluid accumulation in the empty thoracic space (the position of the mediastinum is maintained by accumulation of serous fluid in the empty thoracic space);

d. **cardiac dysrhythmias** related to altered nodal function and myocardial conductivity associated primarily with myocardial hypoxia (may result from impaired gas exchange, diminished myocardial blood flow that can occur with hypovolemia and sympathetic nervous system-mediated vasoconstriction in the immediate postoperative period, and/or mediastinal shifting if present);

e. **acute pulmonary edema** related to:
  1. increased pulmonary capillary permeability associated with hypoxia
  2. increased hydrostatic pressure in the remaining pulmonary vessels associated with reduced size of the pulmonary vasculature bed and decreased effectiveness of lymphatic drainage resulting from removal of pulmonary tissue (especially if pneumonectomy was performed);

f. **bronchopleural fistula** related to:
  1. inadequate bronchial closure and healing following a partial or complete

resection of the lung (most often associated with preoperative radiation and/or residual cancer at the bronchial stump)

    2. presence of empyema in residual lung tissue (can occur following removal of a portion of the lung);

g. **restricted arm and shoulder movement** related to decreased activity of the arm and shoulder on the operative side associated with pain and adhesion formation between incised muscles.

Desired Outcomes	Nursing Actions and *Selected Purposes/Rationales*

2.a. The client will experience normal lung re-expansion as evidenced by:
  1. audible breath sounds and resonant percussion note over remaining lung tissue by 3rd–4th postoperative day
  2. unlabored respirations at 14–20/minute
  3. blood gases returning toward normal
  4. chest x-ray showing lung re-expansion.

2.a.1. Assess for and immediately report signs and symptoms of:
  a. malfunction of chest drainage system (e.g. respiratory distress, lack of fluctuation in water seal chamber without evidence of lung re-expansion, excessive bubbling in water seal chamber, significant increase in subcutaneous emphysema)
  b. extended pneumothorax (e.g. extended area of absent breath sounds with hyperresonant percussion note; rapid, shallow, and/or labored respirations; increased chest pain; restlessness; confusion).

2. Monitor blood gases. Report values that have worsened.

3. Monitor chest x-ray results. Report findings of delayed lung re-expansion or further lung collapse.

4. Implement measures *to promote lung re-expansion and prevent extended pneumothorax*:
  a. perform actions *to maintain patency and integrity of chest drainage system if present*:
    1. maintain fluid level in the water seal and suction chambers as ordered
    2. maintain occlusive dressing over chest tube insertion site(s)
    3. tape all connections securely
    4. tape the tubing close to insertion site to the chest wall *to reduce the risk of inadvertent removal of the tube*
    5. position tubing *to promote optimum drainage* (e.g. coil excess tubing on bed rather than allowing it to hang down below the collection device, keep tubing free of kinks)
    6. drain fluid that accumulates in tubing into the collection chamber; milk chest tube(s) only if ordered
    7. keep drainage collection device below level of client's chest at all times
  b. perform actions *to facilitate the escape of air from the pleural space* (e.g. maintain suction as ordered, ensure that the air vent is open on the drainage collection device if system is to water seal only)
  c. perform actions to improve respiratory status (see Postoperative Nursing Diagnosis 1, action c).

5. If signs and symptoms of extended pneumothorax occur:
  a. maintain client on bed rest in a semi- to high Fowler's position
  b. maintain oxygen therapy as ordered
  c. assess for and immediately report signs and symptoms of mediastinal shift (see action c.1 in this diagnosis)
  d. assist with clearing of existing chest tube(s) and/or insertion of a new tube.

2.b. The client will not develop hemothorax as evidenced by:
  1. audible breath sounds and resonant percussion note over remaining lung tissue by 3rd–4th postoperative day
  2. unlabored respirations at 14–20/minute

2.b.1. Assess for and immediately report signs and symptoms of:
  a. thoracic bleeding (e.g. unexpected increase in the amount of bloody drainage from chest tube(s), increase in bloody drainage on dressing, further decrease in Hct and Hb)
  b. hemothorax (e.g. diminished or absent breath sounds with dull percussion note over affected area, dyspnea).

2. Monitor blood gases. Report values that have worsened.

3. Implement measures to maintain patency and integrity of chest drainage system (see action a.4.a in this diagnosis) *in order to reduce risk of hemothorax.*

Desired Outcomes	Nursing Actions and *Selected Purposes/Rationales*

3. blood gases returning toward normal range.

4. If signs and symptoms of hemothorax occur:
   a. maintain client on bed rest in a semi- to high Fowler's position
   b. maintain oxygen therapy as ordered
   c. assess for and report signs and symptoms of a mediastinal shift (see action c.1 in this diagnosis)
   d. assess for and report signs and symptoms of shock (e.g. hypotension; increased pulse and respirations; urine output less than 30 ml/hour; cool, moist skin; restlessness; confusion)
   e. administer blood products and/or volume expanders if ordered
   f. assist with clearing of existing chest tube(s), thoracentesis, or insertion of chest tube if not already present
   g. prepare client for surgical intervention to ligate bleeding vessels if indicated.

2.c. The client will not develop a mediastinal shift as evidenced by:
1. absence of or no sudden increase in dyspnea
2. vital signs within normal range for client
3. usual mental status
4. trachea in midline position
5. absence of neck vein distention
6. blood gases returning toward normal range.

2.c.1. Assess for and immediately report signs and symptoms of mediastinal shift (e.g. severe dyspnea, rapid and/or irregular pulse rate, hypotension, restlessness and agitation, shift in trachea from midline, neck vein distention).
2. Monitor blood gases and report values that have worsened.
3. Implement measures *to reduce risk of mediastinal shift:*
   a. keep chest tube clamped if one is in place after a pneumonectomy (*serous fluid accumulation is essential to maintain proper pressure gradient on operative side*)
   b. position client as ordered (e.g. on back or on operative side after pneumonectomy)
   c. perform actions to prevent and treat pneumothorax and hemothorax (see actions a.4 and 5 and b.3 and 4 in this diagnosis).
4. If signs and symptoms of mediastinal shift occur:
   a. maintain client on bed rest in a semi- to high Fowler's position
   b. maintain oxygen therapy as ordered
   c. if chest tube(s) malfunctioning or not present, assist with clearing of existing tube(s), thoracentesis, or insertion of new tube(s) if indicated
   d. provide emotional support to client and significant others.

2.d. The client will maintain normal sinus rhythm as evidenced by:
1. regular apical pulse at 60–100 beats/minute
2. equal apical and radial pulse rates
3. absence of syncope and palpitations
4. ECG reading showing normal sinus rhythm.

2.d.1. Assess for and report signs and symptoms of cardiac dysrhythmias (e.g. irregular apical pulse; pulse rate below 60 or above 100 beats/minute; apical-radial pulse deficit; syncope; palpitations; abnormal rate, rhythm, or configurations on ECG).
2. Implement measures *to prevent cardiac dysrhythmias:*
   a. perform actions to improve respiratory status (see Postoperative Nursing Diagnosis 1, action c) *in order to maintain adequate myocardial tissue oxygenation*
   b. perform actions to reduce pain and fear and anxiety (see Standardized Postoperative Care Plan, Nursing Diagnoses 6, action e and 20, action b [pp. 107 and 122]) *in order to decrease stimulation of the sympathetic nervous system (sympathetic stimulation increases the heart rate and causes vasoconstriction, both of which increase cardiac workload and decrease oxygen availability to the myocardium)*
   c. perform actions to prevent or treat mediastinal shift (see actions c.3 and 4 in this diagnosis).
3. If cardiac dysrhythmias occur:
   a. continue with above actions
   b. administer antidysrhythmics (e.g. digoxin) as ordered
   c. restrict client's activity based on his/her tolerance and severity of the dysrhythmia
   d. maintain oxygen therapy as ordered
   e. assess cardiovascular status frequently and report signs and symptoms of inadequate tissue perfusion (e.g. decrease in B/P; cool, moist skin; cyanosis; diminished peripheral pulses; urine output less than 30 ml/hour; restlessness and agitation; increased shortness of breath)

f. have emergency cart readily available for cardioversion, defibrillation, or cardiopulmonary resuscitation.

2.e. The client will not develop pulmonary edema as evidenced by:

1. unlabored respirations at 14–20/minute
2. pulse 60–100 beats/minute
3. clear breath sounds and resonant percussion note over unoperative area
4. absence of productive, persistent cough
5. usual skin color
6. blood gases returning toward normal range.

2.e.1. Assess for and report signs and symptoms of pulmonary edema (e.g. severe dyspnea, tachycardia, adventitious breath sounds, dull percussion note over remaining lung tissue, persistent cough productive of frothy and/or blood-tinged sputum, cyanosis).

2. Monitor for and report the following:
   a. decrease in PaO_2 or increase in $PaCO_2$
   b. significant decrease in oximetry results.

3. Monitor chest x-ray results. Report findings of pulmonary edema.

4. Implement measures *to prevent hypoxia and reduce the risk of pulmonary edema:*
   a. perform actions to improve respiratory status (see Postoperative Nursing Diagnosis 1, action c)
   b. perform actions to maintain patency and integrity of chest drainage system if present (see action a.4.a in this diagnosis) *in order to promote lung re-expansion.*

5. If signs and symptoms of pulmonary edema occur:
   a. continue with above measures
   b. administer the following medications if ordered:
      1. bronchodilators (e.g. theophylline) *to increase bronchial airflow*
      2. agents *to reduce pulmonary vascular congestion* (e.g. diuretics, morphine sulfate).

2.f. The client will experience resolution of a bronchopleural fistula if it occurs as evidenced by:

1. afebrile status
2. cough productive of clear mucus only
3. absence of continuous bubbling in water seal chamber of chest drainage system
4. unlabored respirations at 14–20/minute
5. WBC and differential counts returning toward normal.

2.f.1. Assess for and report signs and symptoms of a bronchopleural fistula (e.g. fever, cough productive of serosanguinous or purulent sputum, continuous bubbling in water seal chamber of chest drainage system, increasing subcutaneous emphysema around incision and neck, respiratory distress).

2. Monitor for and report the following:
   a. persistent elevation of WBC count and significant change in differential
   b. chest x-ray results showing probable bronchopleural fistula.

3. If signs and symptoms of a bronchopleural fistula occur:
   a. turn client to operative side if he/she has had a pneumonectomy until thoracotomy drainage can be established (*this will reduce the risk for aspiration of pleural fluid into the remaining lung*)
   b. have tracheostomy tray readily available (*severe subcutaneous emphysema in the neck can compress the trachea and obstruct the airway*)
   c. prepare client for the following if planned:
      1. chest tube insertion
      2. thoracentesis
      3. surgical repair of bronchial stump
   d. provide emotional support to client and significant others.

2.g. The client will maintain normal arm and shoulder function as evidenced by ability to move arm and shoulder on operative side through usual range of motion.

2.g.1. Assess for and report signs and symptoms of restricted arm and shoulder movement on operative side (e.g. inability to move arm and shoulder through usual range of motion, inability to use arm in activities of daily living).

2. Implement measures *to prevent restriction of arm and shoulder movement on operative side:*
   a. instruct client in and assist with arm and shoulder exercises as ordered
   b. perform actions to reduce pain (see Standardized Postoperative Care Plan, Nursing Diagnosis 6, action e [p. 107]) *in order to increase client's ability and willingness to move arm and shoulder*
   c. encourage client to use arm on operative side to perform self-care activities
   d. place frequently used articles and bed stand on operative side *so that client will be encouraged to reach with affected arm*
   e. anchor pull rope at foot of bed; encourage client to use arm on operative side to pull self to sitting position.

Desired Outcomes	Nursing Actions and *Selected Purposes/Rationales*

3. If signs and symptoms of restricted arm and shoulder movement occur:
   a. continue with above actions
   b. assist with planned physical therapy program.

---

3. NURSING DIAGNOSIS: **Grieving***

related to loss of all or part of a lung and anticipated changes in usual life style as a result of diminished lung capacity.

*This diagnostic label includes anticipatory grieving and grieving following the actual losses.

Desired Outcome	Nursing Actions and *Selected Purposes/Rationales*

3. The client will demonstrate beginning progression through the grieving process as evidenced by:
   a. verbalization of feelings about the loss of all or part of a lung and its anticipated effects on life style
   b. usual sleep pattern
   c. participation in treatment plan and self-care activities
   d. utilization of available support systems
   e. verbalization of ways to modify current life style to compensate for altered lung capacity.

3.a. Assess for signs and symptoms of grieving (e.g. change in eating habits, inability to concentrate, insomnia, anger, sadness, withdrawal from significant others, denial of loss).

   b. Implement measures *to facilitate the grieving process:*
   1. assist client to acknowledge the changes resulting from loss of lung function *so grief work can begin*; assess for factors that may hinder and facilitate acknowledgment
   2. discuss the grieving process and assist client to accept the phases of grieving as an expected response to the actual and/or anticipated loss
   3. allow time for client to progress through the phases of grieving (phases vary among theorists but progress from shock and alarm to acceptance); be aware that not every phase is expressed by all individuals, that recurrence of phases is common, and that the grieving process may take months to years
   4. provide an atmosphere of care and concern (e.g. provide privacy, be available and nonjudgmental, display empathy and respect) *so client will feel free to express feelings*
   5. perform actions *to promote trust* (e.g. answer questions honestly, provide requested information)
   6. encourage the verbal expression of anger and sadness about the loss of the lung; recognize displacement of anger and assist client to see the actual cause of angry feelings and resentment
   7. encourage client to express feelings in whatever ways are comfortable (e.g. writing, drawing, conversation)
   8. assist client to identify and utilize techniques that have helped him/her to cope in previous situations of loss
   9. support realistic hope about client's ability to resume usual activities
   10. support behaviors suggesting successful grief work (e.g. verbalizing feelings about the loss of a lung, expressing sorrow, focusing on ways to adapt to altered lung capacity)
   11. explain the phases of the grieving process to significant others; encourage their support and understanding
   12. facilitate communication between client and significant others
   13. provide information regarding counseling services and support groups that might assist client in working through grief
   14. when appropriate, assist client to meet spiritual needs (e.g. arrange for visit from clergy).

   c. Consult physician regarding referral for counseling if signs of dysfunctional grieving (e.g. persistent denial of loss, excessive anger or sadness, emotional lability) occur.

Discharge Teaching

4. NURSING DIAGNOSIS:	**Knowledge deficit, Ineffective management of therapeutic regimen, or Altered health maintenance***

**The nurse should select the diagnostic label that is most appropriate for the client's teaching needs.

Desired Outcomes	Nursing Actions and *Selected Purposes/Rationales*
4.a. The client will demonstrate the ability to perform prescribed arm and shoulder exercises.	4.a.1. Instruct client regarding importance of exercising the arm and shoulder on operative side. Emphasize that the exercises should be performed at least 5 times/day for several weeks. 2. Demonstrate appropriate arm and shoulder exercises (e.g. shoulder shrugs, arm circles). 3. Allow time for questions, clarification, and return demonstration.
4.b. The client will state signs and symptoms to report to the health care provider.	4.b.1. Refer to Standardized Postoperative Care Plan, Nursing Diagnosis 21, action c (p. 123), for signs and symptoms to report to the health care provider. 2. Instruct the client to report these additional signs and symptoms: a. increased discomfort in or decreased ability to move arm and shoulder on operative side b. increased shortness of breath c. persistent cough.
4.c. The client will identify community resources that can assist with home management and adjustment to the diagnosis, effects of surgery, and adjuvant treatment if planned.	4.c.1. Provide information about community resources that can assist the client and significant others with home management and adjustment to the diagnosis, effects of surgery, and adjuvant treatment if planned (e.g. American Lung Association, American Cancer Society, smoking cessation program, Meals on Wheels, counselors, support groups, home health agencies). 2. Initiate a referral if indicated.
4.d. The client will verbalize an understanding of and a plan for adhering to recommended follow-up care including future appointments with health care provider, medications prescribed, activity level, pain management, wound care, and subsequent treatment of the underlying disorder.	4.d.1. Refer to Standardized Postoperative Care Plan, Nursing Diagnosis 21 (pp. 123–124), for routine postoperative instructions and measures to improve client compliance. 2. Reinforce physician's instructions about activity level: a. gauge activity according to tolerance and ensure adequate rest periods b. stop any activity that causes excessive fatigue, dyspnea, or chest pain c. avoid lifting heavy objects until complete healing of chest muscles has occurred. 3. Inform client that numbness and discomfort in the operative area can persist for several weeks but are usually temporary. 4. Clarify plans for subsequent treatment of underlying disorder (e.g. chemotherapy, radiation therapy) if appropriate.

Bibliography

See pages 897–898 and 905.

UNIT TWELVE

NURSING CARE OF THE CLIENT WITH DISTURBANCES OF THE KIDNEY AND URINARY TRACT

BLADDER NECK SUSPENSION (VESICOURETHRAL SUSPENSION)

A bladder neck suspension is a surgical procedure performed to restore the bladder neck and proximal urethra to their normal anatomical position. It is performed to correct urinary stress incontinence associated with excessive mobility of the urethra and/or lowering of the position of the bladder neck (vesicourethral segment) resulting from pelvic floor weakness. The surgery is indicated when conservative measures for treating stress incontinence (e.g. pelvic floor exercises, biofeedback, estrogen therapy, alpha-adrenergic agonists) have failed to produce significant improvement.

A number of techniques can be utilized to suspend the vesicourethral junction in a physiological position. They all involve placement of sutures in the periurethral and/or vaginal fascia and anchoring those sutures to the underside of the pubic symphysis. The surgery can be accomplished by an abdominal approach (e.g. Marshall-Marchetti-Krantz, Burch) or a vaginal approach in com-bination with suprapubic endoscopy (e.g. Stamey, Raz). A "no incision" approach done by suprapubic endoscopy (e.g. Gittes) can be performed on persons who are unable to tolerate a general or spinal anesthetic. The approach selected depends on the physiological condition of the client, the type of incontinence, previous procedures, the presence of associated pelvic floor abnormalities (e.g. enterocele, uterine prolapse, cystocele, rectocele), and the need for additional abdominal surgery.

This care plan focuses on the adult client hospitalized for a bladder neck suspension. Preoperative goals of care are to reduce fear and anxiety and prepare the client for the surgical experience. Postoperatively, goals of care are to maintain comfort, prevent complications, and educate the client regarding follow-up care. If repair of a cystocele and/or rectocele is planned concurrently, use this care plan in conjunction with the Care Plan on Colporrhaphy.

DIAGNOSTIC TESTS

Cystoscopy
Lateral cystogram
Cystometrogram
Urethral pressure profile
Voiding cystourethrogram
Videourodynamic studies

DISCHARGE CRITERIA

Prior to discharge, the client will:

- have evidence of normal healing of surgical wound(s)
- have clear, audible breath sounds throughout lungs
- have adequate urine output
- have no evidence of wound or urinary tract infection
- have no signs and symptoms of postoperative complications
- demonstrate care of suprapubic catheter if present
- demonstrate the ability to measure residual urine
- state signs and symptoms to report to the health care provider
- verbalize an understanding of and a plan for adhering to recommended follow-up care including future appointments with health care provider, medications prescribed, activity restrictions, and measures to prevent constipation.

NURSING/ COLLABORATIVE DIAGNOSES	**Postoperative**	
	1. Urinary retention △ 493	
	2. Constipation △ 493	
	3. Risk for infection:	
	a. urinary tract infection	
	b. wound infection △ 494	
	4. Potential complication: bladder, urethral, or ureteral injury △ 494	
DISCHARGE TEACHING	5. Knowledge deficit, Ineffective management of therapeutic regimen, or Altered health maintenance △ 495	

See Standardized Preoperative and Postoperative Care Plans for additional diagnoses.

PREOPERATIVE   Refer to the Standardized Preoperative Care Plan.

POSTOPERATIVE   Use in conjunction with the Standardized Postoperative Care Plan.

---

1. NURSING DIAGNOSIS: **Urinary retention**

related to:
a. obstruction of the urethral and/or suprapubic catheters if present;
b. impaired urination following removal of the catheter(s) associated with:
   1. edema of the bladder neck and urethra resulting from surgical trauma
   2. increased tone of the urinary sphincters resulting from sympathetic nervous system stimulation (can result from pain, fear, and anxiety)
   3. decreased perception of bladder fullness resulting from the depressant effect of some medications (e.g. narcotic [opioid] analgesics)
   4. relaxation of the bladder muscle resulting from the depressant effect of some medications (e.g. narcotic [opioid] analgesics) and stimulation of the sympathetic nervous system (can result from pain, fear, and anxiety).

Desired Outcome	Nursing Actions and *Selected Purposes/Rationales*

1. The client will not experience urinary retention as evidenced by:
a. no reports of bladder fullness and suprapubic discomfort
b. absence of bladder distention
c. balanced intake and output within 48 hours after surgery
d. voiding adequate amounts at expected intervals after removal of the catheter(s).
	1.a. Assess for and report the following:
	  1. urinary retention when suprapubic and/or urethral catheters are present (e.g. reports of bladder fullness or suprapubic discomfort, bladder distention, absence of fluid in urinary drainage tubing, output that continues to be less than intake 48 hours after surgery)
	  2. urinary retention following catheter removal (e.g. reports of bladder fullness or suprapubic discomfort, bladder distention, output that continues to be less than intake 48 hours after surgery, frequent voiding of small amounts [25–60 ml] of urine).
	 b. Implement measures *to prevent urinary retention:*
	  1. perform actions *to maintain patency of urinary catheter(s):*
	    a. keep drainage tubing free of kinks
	    b. keep collection container below level of bladder
	    c. tape catheter tubing securely (suprapubic catheter tubing to abdomen, urethral catheter tubing to thigh) *in order to prevent inadvertent removal*
	    d. irrigate catheter if ordered
	  2. after urethral catheter is removed, open suprapubic catheter as scheduled or if client is unable to void voluntarily
	  3. when both urethral and suprapubic catheters have been removed, refer to Standardized Postoperative Care Plan, Nursing Diagnosis 13, actions d and e (pp. 113–114), for measures related to prevention and treatment of urinary retention.

---

2. NURSING DIAGNOSIS: **Constipation**

related to:
a. decreased gastrointestinal motility associated with manipulation of the bowel (if an abdominal approach was used), decreased activity, and the depressant effect of the anesthetic and narcotic (opioid) analgesics;
b. decreased intake of fluids and foods high in fiber;
c. reluctance to defecate associated with fear of pain and possible disruption of sutures.

Desired Outcome	Nursing Actions and *Selected Purposes/Rationales*
2. The client will not experience constipation (see Standardized Postoperative Care Plan, Nursing Diagnosis 14 [p. 114], for outcome criteria).	2.a. Refer to Standardized Postoperative Care Plan, Nursing Diagnosis 14 (pp. 114–115), for measures related to assessment and prevention of constipation. b. Implement additional measures *to prevent constipation:* 1. consult physician about an order for a stool softener if one has not been ordered 2. instruct client to request an analgesic prior to attempting to defecate *in order to ease the surgical site pain associated with the increased intra-abdominal and perineal pressure that occur with defecation.*

---

3. NURSING DIAGNOSIS: **Risk for infection:**

a. **urinary tract infection** related to:
 1. increased growth and colonization of microorganisms associated with urinary stasis
 2. introduction of pathogens associated with the presence of urethral and/or suprapubic catheters and performance of intermittent catheterizations if done to determine residual urine volume;

b. **wound infection** related to:
 1. wound contamination associated with introduction of pathogens during or following surgery (particularly high risk with a vaginal approach because of the proximity of the incision to the perianal area)
 2. decreased resistance to infection (can result if blood flow to wound area is diminished or client has an inadequate nutritional status).

Desired Outcomes	Nursing Actions and *Selected Purposes/Rationales*
3.a. The client will remain free of urinary tract infection (see Standardized Postoperative Care Plan, Nursing Diagnosis 16, outcome c [p. 117], for outcome criteria).	3.a.1. Refer to Standardized Postoperative Care Plan, Nursing Diagnosis 16, action c (p. 117), for measures related to assessment, prevention, and treatment of urinary tract infection. 2. Implement measures to prevent urinary retention (see Postoperative Nursing Diagnosis 1, action b) *in order to further reduce the risk of urinary stasis and subsequent urinary tract infection.*
3.b. The client will remain free of wound infection (see Standardized Postoperative Care Plan, Nursing Diagnosis 16, outcome b [pp. 116–117], for outcome criteria).	3.b.1. Refer to Standardized Postoperative Care Plan, Nursing Diagnosis 16, action b (pp. 116–117), for measures related to assessment, prevention, and management of postoperative wound infection. 2. Implement additional measures *to reduce the risk for wound infection if a vaginal incision is present:* a. instruct client to wipe from front to back following urination and defecation b. assist client with perineal care every shift and after each bowel movement.

---

4. COLLABORATIVE DIAGNOSIS: **Potential complication of bladder neck suspension surgery: bladder, urethral, or ureteral injury**

related to accidental tear or ligation during the surgical procedure.

Desired Outcome	Nursing Actions and *Selected Purposes/Rationales*

4. The client will experience healing of bladder, urethral, or ureteral injury if it occurs as evidenced by:
  a. gradual resolution of hematuria and backache
  b. urine output greater than 200 ml within 6–8 hours after surgery.
	4.a. Assess for and report signs and symptoms of bladder, urethral, or ureteral injury (e.g. persistent or increasing hematuria or backache, urine output less than 200 ml in first 6–8 hours after surgery).
	  b. If signs and symptoms of bladder, urethral, or ureteral injury are present:
	    1. continue to monitor output carefully
	    2. prepare client for surgical repair if indicated
	    3. provide emotional support to client and significant others.

Discharge Teaching

■

5. NURSING DIAGNOSIS: **Knowledge deficit, Ineffective management of therapeutic regimen, or Altered health maintenance***

       *The nurse should select the diagnostic label that is most appropriate for the client's discharge teaching needs.

Desired Outcomes	Nursing Actions and *Selected Purposes/Rationales*

5.a. The client will demonstrate care of suprapubic catheter if present.	5.a.1. Provide the following instructions about care of suprapubic catheter if client is discharged with one in place:
	    a. tape catheter securely to abdomen
	    b. keep drainage tubing free of kinks
	    c. keep collection bag below level of bladder.
	    2. Allow time for questions, clarification, and return demonstration.

5.b. The client will demonstrate the ability to measure residual urine.	5.b.1. Provide the following instructions about how to measure residual urine (the client who needs to measure residual urine and does not have a suprapubic catheter will need to be instructed on how to perform self-catheterization):
	    a. unclamp the suprapubic catheter after urinating or at prescribed intervals (usually every 4 hours if unable to urinate)
	    b. leave the suprapubic catheter unclamped for 10 minutes, reclamp the catheter, and then empty the bag and measure the amount of urine
	    c. measure and record the amount of urine voided and the amount of residual urine.
	    2. Instruct client to contact physician's office once the residual urine amounts are consistently less than 100 ml for 2 consecutive days (most physicians want the suprapubic catheter to be removed at this point).
	    3. Allow time for questions, clarification, and return demonstration.

5.c. The client will state signs and symptoms to report to the health care provider.	5.c.1. Refer to Standardized Postoperative Care Plan, Nursing Diagnosis 21, action c (p. 123), for signs and symptoms to report to the health care provider.
	    2. Instruct client to report these additional signs and symptoms:
	    a. stress incontinence
	    b. unusual and continuous abdominal or pelvic pain
	    c. temperature above 38° C (100.5° F)
	    d. persistent bright red vaginal bleeding or clots
	    e. persistent inability to void voluntarily
	    f. persistent residual urine amounts in excess of 100 ml.

Desired Outcomes	Nursing Actions and **Selected Purposes/Rationales**

5.d. The client will verbalize an understanding of and a plan for adhering to recommended follow-up care including future appointments with health care provider, medications prescribed, activity restrictions, and measures to prevent constipation.	5.d.1. Refer to Standardized Postoperative Care Plan, Nursing Diagnosis 21 (pp. 123–124), for routine postoperative instructions and measures to improve client compliance.
	
	2. Instruct client to avoid lifting objects over 15 pounds until healing is complete (about 6 weeks).
	
	3. If client has a vaginal incision, instruct her to:
	  a. perform good perineal hygiene, particularly after defecation
	  b. avoid inserting anything into vagina (e.g. tampons, douches) or having sexual intercourse until advised by physician (usually for 6 weeks).
	
	4. Reinforce measures to prevent constipation:
	  a. drink 8–10 glasses of water a day unless contraindicated
	  b. eat foods that are high in fiber (e.g. fresh fruits and vegetables, whole grain cereals)
	  c. take 1–2 stool softeners (e.g. Dialose) a day.
	
	5. Instruct client to contact physician's office or follow physician's instructions regarding the appropriate measures to take if there is a two-day span without a bowel movement (at this point, the physician will often recommend that client self-administer a small-volume enema [e.g. Fleet] or laxative suppository [e.g. Dulcolax]).

Bibliography

See pages 897–898 and 905.

CHRONIC RENAL FAILURE

Chronic renal failure (CRF) is a progressive, irreversible loss of kidney function that usually develops gradually over many years. The leading causes of CRF are diabetes mellitus, hypertension, and glomerulonephritis. Other causes include pyelonephritis/interstitial nephritis, obstruction of the urinary tract by conditions such as benign prostatic hypertrophy, and hereditary conditions such as polycystic kidney disease. Chronic renal failure can also develop following acute renal failure that has resulted in irreversible renal damage.

Creatinine clearance is the measurement that is used to determine the effectiveness of renal function. As renal failure progresses, creatinine clearance results decline, reflecting a decrease in the glomular filtration rate (GFR) and the percent of functioning nephrons. The severity of CRF can be classified by the proportion of renal function that has been lost and is often divided into three stages. In the first stage, diminished renal reserve, the GFR can be as low as 30% of normal, but the renal dysfunction usually goes undiagnosed because homeostatic mechanisms are able to maintain fluid balance and keep serum electrolytes, urea nitrogen, and creatinine within normal ranges.

Renal insufficiency, the second stage, begins when the GFR is about 25% of normal. In this stage, creatinine clearance continues to decline and azotemia (the retention of nitrogenous substances in the blood) begins. The blood urea nitrogen (BUN) and serum creatinine are elevated in this stage but they are not high enough to cause symptoms that are problematic for the client. During this stage, the client progresses from a nonoliguric phase, in which the kidneys are unable to concentrate the urine, to a state of oliguria. When this occurs, symptoms become evident and result mainly from a decreased ability of the kidneys to excrete fluid and electrolytes.

The third stage of CRF is uremia or end-stage renal disease (ESRD). It occurs when the GFR is less than 10% of normal and nitrogenous substances (e.g. urea, creatinine, phenols) accumulate to levels high enough to cause toxic effects on other body systems. Typical signs and symptoms of ESRD can include lethargy, irritability, extreme fatigue and weakness, pruritus, nausea and vomiting, muscle cramping, and stomatitis. Fluid, electrolyte, and acid-base imbalances also worsen and, in this stage, dialysis or kidney transplantation is necessary for survival.

This care plan focuses on the adult client with renal insufficiency who has progressed from the nonoliguric to the oliguric phase and is hospitalized for treatment and further evaluation of renal function. The goals of care are to reduce fear and anxiety; control fluid, electrolyte, and acid-base imbalances; prevent complications; and educate the client regarding follow-up care.

DIAGNOSTIC TESTS

Urine studies (e.g. creatinine clearance, osmolality, specific gravity, electrolytes, protein)
Blood studies (e.g. BUN, creatinine, CBC, electrolytes, CO_2 content, protein, osmolality)
Computed tomography of the kidneys (nephrotomography)
Renal ultrasonography (nephrosonography)
Intravenous pyelogram (IVP)
X-ray of the kidneys, ureters, and bladder (KUB)
Renal angiography
Renal biopsy

DISCHARGE CRITERIA

Prior to discharge, the client will:

- not have signs or symptoms of uremic syndrome
- have blood pressure within a safe range
- have fluid, electrolyte, and acid-base balance stabilized within a safe range
- tolerate expected level of activity
- have no evidence of infection
- have an adequate nutritional status
- verbalize a basic understanding of CRF
- identify ways to slow the progression of kidney damage
- verbalize an understanding of fluid restrictions and dietary modifications
- demonstrate the ability to accurately weigh self, measure fluid intake and output, and monitor own blood pressure
- identify ways to reduce the risk of infection
- identify ways to manage signs and symptoms that often occur as a result of CRF
- share feelings and concerns about the effects of CRF on life style and roles
- state signs and symptoms to report to the health care provider
- identify community resources that can assist with adjustment to changes resulting from CRF
- verbalize an understanding of and a plan for adhering to recommended follow-up care including future appointments with health care provider and medications prescribed.

NURSING/ COLLABORATIVE DIAGNOSES

1. Altered fluid and electrolyte balance:
   a. fluid volume excess
   b. hyponatremia
   c. hypernatremia
   d. hyperkalemia
   e. hypocalcemia
   f. hyperphosphatemia
   g. hypermagnesemia
   h. metabolic acidosis △ 498
2. Altered nutrition: less than body requirements △ 501
3. Altered oral mucous membrane: dryness △ 502
4. Activity intolerance △ 502
5. Constipation △ 503
6. Risk for infection △ 504
7. Potential complications:
   a. uremic syndrome
   b. hypertension △ 505
8. Anxiety △ 506
9. Grieving △ 507
10. Ineffective management of therapeutic regimen △ 508

DISCHARGE TEACHING

11. Knowledge deficit or Altered health maintenance △ 509

1. NURSING/COLLABORATIVE DIAGNOSIS:

Altered fluid and electrolyte balance:

a. **fluid volume excess** related to retention of sodium and water associated with:
   1. decrease in number of functioning nephrons and subsequent decreased GFR
   2. activation of the renin-angiotensin-aldosterone mechanism resulting from decreased renal blood flow (can occur as a result of the underlying disease process);

b. **hyponatremia** related to excessive fluid intake in relation to output (causes a relative hyponatremia), restricted dietary intake of sodium, and loss of sodium associated with diuretic therapy;

c. **hypernatremia** related to:
   1. decreased ability of the kidneys to excrete sodium
   2. increased aldosterone output associated with activation of the renin-angiotensin-aldosterone mechanism if decreased renal blood flow has occurred as a result of the underlying disease process
   3. dietary sodium intake in excess of prescribed restrictions;

d. **hyperkalemia** related to:
   1. decreased ability of the kidneys to excrete potassium
   2. increased cellular release of potassium associated with progressive renal tissue damage and metabolic acidosis
   3. dietary potassium intake in excess of prescribed restrictions
   4. use of potassium-sparing diuretics or salt substitutes containing potassium;

e. **hypocalcemia** related to:
   1. decreased absorption of calcium associated with inability of the kidneys to activate vitamin D (the active metabolite of vitamin D is needed to stimulate calcium absorption from the small intestine)
   2. hyperphosphatemia (causes a reciprocal drop in calcium);

f. **hyperphosphatemia** related to decreased ability of the kidneys to excrete phosphorus, excessive intake of dietary phosphorus, and hypocalcemia (an inverse relationship exists between phosphorus and calcium);

g. **hypermagnesemia** related to:
   1. decreased ability of the kidneys to excrete magnesium
   2. excessive intake of magnesium-containing antacids;

h. **metabolic acidosis** related to:
   1. decreased ability of the kidneys to excrete hydrogen ions and reabsorb bicarbonate
   2. hyperkalemia (the body attempts to compensate for high serum potassium levels by shifting hydrogen ions into the vascular space in exchange for potassium ions).

Desired Outcomes	Nursing Actions and *Selected Purposes/Rationales*
1.a. The client will experience resolution of fluid volume excess as evidenced by: 1. decline in weight toward client's normal 2. B/P within normal range for client 3. absence of an S_3 heart sound 4. normal pulse volume 5. balanced intake and output 6. usual mental status 7. normal breath sounds 8. absence of dyspnea,	1.a.1. Assess for and report signs and symptoms of fluid volume excess: a. weight gain of 2% or greater over a short period b. elevated B/P (B/P may not be elevated if fluid has shifted out of vascular space) c. presence of an S_3 heart sound d. bounding pulse e. intake greater than output f. change in mental status g. crackles (rales) and diminished or absent breath sounds h. dyspnea, orthopnea i. peripheral edema j. distended neck veins k. delayed hand vein emptying time (longer than 3–5 seconds) l. elevated CVP (use internal jugular vein pulsation method to estimate CVP if monitoring device not present).

orthopnea, peripheral edema, and distended neck veins
9. hand vein emptying time less than 3–5 seconds
10. CVP within normal range.

1.b. The client will maintain a safe serum sodium level as evidenced by:
1. absence of nausea, vomiting, abdominal cramps, and thirst
2. moist mucous membranes
3. usual mental status
4. usual muscle strength
5. absence of seizure activity
6. serum sodium within a safe range for client.

1.c. The client will maintain a safe serum potassium level as evidenced by:
1. regular pulse at 60–100 beats/minute
2. absence of paresthesias
3. usual muscle tone and strength
4. absence of diarrhea and intestinal colic
5. normal ECG reading
6. serum potassium within a safe range for client.

2. Monitor chest x-ray results. Report findings of pulmonary vascular congestion, pleural effusion, or pulmonary edema.
3. Implement measures *to reduce fluid volume excess:*
   a. maintain fluid restrictions as ordered (intake allowed is usually 400–700 ml plus the amount of urine output in the previous 24 hours)
   b. restrict sodium intake as ordered
   c. administer the following medications if ordered:
      1. diuretics *to increase excretion of water*
      2. arterial vasodilators *to improve renal blood flow* (*reduced renal perfusion stimulates the renin-angiotensin-aldosterone mechanism*).
4. Consult physician if signs and symptoms of fluid volume excess persist or worsen.

1.b.1. Assess for and report signs and symptoms of:
   a. hyponatremia (e.g. nausea, vomiting, abdominal cramps, lethargy, confusion, weakness, seizures)
   b. hypernatremia (e.g. thirst; dry, sticky mucous membranes; restlessness; lethargy; weakness; elevated temperature; seizures).
2. Monitor serum sodium results. Report values that are not within a safe range for client.
3. Implement measures *to prevent or treat hyponatremia:*
   a. maintain fluid restrictions as ordered *to prevent dilutional hyponatremia*
   b. increase dietary allotment of sodium if ordered
   c. administer loop diuretics (e.g. furosemide) if ordered *to treat dilutional hyponatremia* (*loop diuretics induce a fairly isotonic diuresis so that water loss can occur without further hyponatremia*).
4. Implement measures *to prevent or treat hypernatremia:*
   a. maintain maximum fluid intake allowed
   b. maintain dietary sodium restrictions if ordered
   c. administer thiazide diuretics if ordered.
5. Consult physician if unsafe serum sodium levels persist.

1.c.1. Assess for and report signs and symptoms of hyperkalemia (e.g. slow or irregular pulse; paresthesias; muscle weakness and flaccidity; diarrhea and intestinal colic; ECG reading showing peaked T wave, prolonged PR interval, and/or widened QRS; elevated serum potassium level).
2. Implement measures *to prevent or treat hyperkalemia:*
   a. maintain dietary restrictions of potassium as ordered
   b. instruct client to consult physician or dietitian about which salt substitute can safely be used (*most salt substitutes contain potassium*)
   c. perform actions *to reduce the cellular release of potassium:*
      1. implement measures *to spare body proteins and prevent excessive tissue breakdown:*
         a. encourage client to consume the amount of dietary protein allotted
         b. provide allotted amount of carbohydrates (*spares the protein by providing a quick energy source*)
         c. perform actions to prevent infection (see Nursing Diagnosis 6, action c) *in order to prevent an increase in metabolic rate and subsequent increase in protein catabolism*
      2. implement measures to prevent or treat metabolic acidosis (see action g.2 in this diagnosis)
   d. if signs and symptoms of hyperkalemia are present, consult physician before administering prescribed potassium supplements and other medications that can increase potassium levels (e.g. potassium penicillin G, potassium-sparing diuretics)
   e. if transfusions are necessary:
      1. request fresh blood (*the potassium content of blood stored longer than 48–72 hours is higher than that of fresh blood*)

Desired Outcomes	Nursing Actions and *Selected Purposes/Rationales*
	2. follow recommended precautions *to prevent damage to cells* (e.g. fill drip chamber above filter top, use 18 gauge needle)
	f. administer the following medications if ordered:
	1. loop diuretics (e.g. ethacrynic acid, furosemide) *to increase renal excretion of potassium*
	2. cation-exchange resins (e.g. sodium polystyrene sulfonate [Kayexalate]) *to increase potassium excretion via the intestines* (*act by exchanging sodium for potassium*)
	3. intravenous insulin and hypertonic glucose solutions *to enhance transport of potassium back into cells.*
	3. If signs and symptoms of hyperkalemia persist or worsen:
	a. consult physician
	b. have intravenous calcium preparation (e.g. calcium gluconate) readily available (*may be ordered to counteract the effect of a high potassium level on the heart*).

1.d. The client will maintain a safe serum calcium level as evidenced by:
  1. usual mental status
  2. negative Chvostek's and Trousseau's signs
  3. absence of numbness and tingling in fingers, toes, and circumoral area; hyperreflexia; tetany; and seizure activity
  4. serum calcium within a safe range for client.
	1.d.1. Assess for and report signs and symptoms of hypocalcemia (e.g. anxiousness; irritability; positive Chvostek's and Trousseau's signs; numbness or tingling of fingers, toes, or circumoral area; hyperactive reflexes; tetany; seizures; serum calcium level that is lower than normal for client).
	  2. Implement measures *to prevent or treat hypocalcemia:*
	    a. provide sources of calcium (e.g. milk, milk products) in diet unless contraindicated
	    b. administer activated vitamin D (e.g. calcitriol, calcifediol) and calcium supplements if ordered
	    c. avoid rapid transfusion of citrated blood (*the citrate that is added to blood to prevent clotting binds calcium; the liver normally removes citrate unless it is infused too rapidly*)
	    d. perform actions to prevent or treat hyperphosphatemia (see action e.2 in this diagnosis)
	    e. avoid rapid or aggressive treatment of acidosis (*rapidly reversing acidosis can result in decreased ionization of calcium*).
	  3. If signs and symptoms of hypocalcemia occur:
	    a. institute seizure precautions
	    b. administer calcium preparations (e.g. calcium gluconate, calcium carbonate) as ordered.

1.e. The client will maintain a safe serum phosphorus level as evidenced by:
  1. absence of paresthesias, tetany, and seizure activity
  2. serum phosphorus within a safe range for client.
	1.e.1. Assess for and report signs and symptoms of hyperphosphatemia (e.g. paresthesias, tetany, seizures, higher than normal serum phosphorus level for client).
	  2. Implement measures *to prevent or treat hyperphosphatemia:*
	    a. restrict dietary intake of phosphorus if ordered by limiting foods/fluids such as organ meats, poultry, milk, milk products, eggs, and legumes
	    b. administer phosphate-binding medications such as aluminum hydroxide (e.g. Amphojel), aluminum carbonate (e.g. Basaljel), and calcium carbonate (e.g. Tums) if ordered.
	  3. Consult physician if signs and symptoms of hyperphosphatemia persist or worsen.

1.f. The client will maintain a safe serum magnesium level as evidenced by:
  1. absence of flushing, nausea, vomiting, and muscle weakness
  2. usual mental status
  3. vital signs within normal range for client
  4. serum magnesium within a safe range for client.
	1.f.1. Assess for and report signs and symptoms of hypermagnesemia (e.g. flushed, warm skin; nausea; vomiting; muscle weakness; drowsiness; lethargy; hypotension; bradypnea; bradycardia; higher than normal serum magnesium level for client).
	  2. Implement measures *to prevent or treat hypermagnesemia:*
	    a. avoid giving laxatives and antacids that contain magnesium (e.g. Milk of Magnesia, Gelusil, Mylanta, Maalox)
	    b. maintain dietary restrictions of magnesium if ordered by limiting intake of foods/fluids such as nuts, whole-grain breads and cereals, and legumes.
	  3. Consult physician if signs and symptoms of hypermagnesemia persist or worsen.

1.g. The client will not experience metabolic acidosis as evidenced by:
1. usual mental status
2. unlabored respirations at 14–20/minute
3. absence of headache, nausea, vomiting, and cardiac dysrhythmias
4. blood gases within a safe range for client
5. anion gap within normal range.

1.g.1. Assess for and report signs and symptoms of metabolic acidosis (e.g. drowsiness; disorientation; stupor; rapid, deep respirations; headache; nausea; vomiting; cardiac dysrhythmias; lower than usual pH and CO_2 content; increased anion gap).
2. Implement measures *to prevent or treat metabolic acidosis:*
   a. perform actions to prevent or treat hyperkalemia (see action c.2 in this diagnosis)
   b. administer sodium bicarbonate if ordered (usually reserved for treatment of severe acidosis [pH less than 7.1–7.2]).
3. Consult physician if signs and symptoms of acidosis persist or worsen.

---

2. NURSING DIAGNOSIS:

Altered nutrition: less than body requirements

related to decreased oral intake associated with:
a. dislike of prescribed diet;
b. prescribed dietary modifications (especially protein restrictions that are necessary in order to control the serum levels of nitrogenous substances).

Desired Outcome	Nursing Actions and *Selected Purposes/Rationales*

2. The client will maintain an adequate nutritional status as evidenced by:
a. weight within normal range for client's age, height, and body frame
b. serum albumin, Hct, Hb, transferrin, and lymphocyte levels within normal range
c. usual or improved strength and activity tolerance
d. healthy oral mucous membrane.

2.a. Assess for and report signs and symptoms of malnutrition:
1. weight below normal for client's age, height, and body frame
2. low serum albumin, Hct, Hb, transferrin, and lymphocyte levels (some of these values may be abnormal as a result of decreased renal function)
3. weakness and fatigue (may also be a reflection of decreasing renal function)
4. sore, inflamed oral mucous membrane
5. pale conjunctiva.
b. Monitor percentage of meals and snacks client consumes. Report a pattern of inadequate intake.
c. Implement measures *to maintain an adequate nutritional status:*
1. perform actions *to improve oral intake:*
   a. increase activity as tolerated (*activity usually promotes a sense of well-being and improves appetite*)
   b. obtain a dietary consult if necessary to assist client in selecting foods/fluids that meet nutritional needs, are appealing, and adhere to personal and cultural preferences as well as the prescribed dietary modifications
   c. encourage a rest period before meals *to minimize fatigue*
   d. maintain a clean environment and a relaxed, pleasant atmosphere
   e. provide oral hygiene before meals
   f. serve frequent, small meals rather than large ones if client is weak, fatigues easily, and/or has a poor appetite
   g. allow adequate time for meals; reheat foods/fluids if necessary
2. encourage client to eat the maximum amount of protein allowed; instruct him/her to satisfy protein requirements with foods/fluids that are complete proteins and contain essential amino acids (e.g. eggs, milk, meat, poultry) if client's serum phosphorus level is not too high
3. offer dietary supplements if indicated
4. administer vitamins and minerals if ordered.

Desired Outcome	Nursing Actions and *Selected Purposes/Rationales*
	d. Perform a calorie count if ordered. Report information to dietitian and physician.
	e. Consult physician if client does not consume enough food or fluids to meet nutritional needs.

---

3. NURSING DIAGNOSIS: **Altered oral mucous membrane: dryness**

related to prescribed fluid restriction.

Desired Outcome	Nursing Actions and *Selected Purposes/Rationales*
3. The client will maintain a moist, intact oral mucous membrane.	3.a. Assess client for dryness of the oral mucosa.
	b. Implement measures *to relieve dryness of the oral mucous membrane:*
	1. maintain the maximum fluid intake allowed; encourage client to space fluid intake evenly throughout the hours he/she is awake
	2. instruct and assist client to perform oral hygiene as often as needed
	3. instruct client to avoid use of products that contain lemon and glycerin and mouthwashes containing alcohol (*these products have a drying and irritating effect on the oral mucous membrane*)
	4. encourage client to rinse mouth frequently with water
	5. encourage client to lubricate lips frequently
	6. encourage client to breathe through nose rather than mouth
	7. encourage client not to smoke (*smoking irritates and dries the mucosa*)
	8. provide hard candy for client to suck on unless contraindicated *in order to stimulate salivation.*
	c. Consult physician if dryness worsens and/or cracking or breakdown of oral mucous membrane occurs.

---

4. NURSING DIAGNOSIS: **Activity intolerance**

related to:
a. inadequate tissue oxygenation associated with anemia resulting from:
   1. decreased secretion of erythropoietin as a result of impaired renal function (erythropoietin stimulates the bone marrow to produce RBCs)
   2. shortened survival time of RBCs (as renal failure progresses, the nitrogenous substances in the blood increase and cause increased hemolysis of RBCs);
b. inadequate nutritional status.

Desired Outcome	Nursing Actions and *Selected Purposes/Rationales*
4. The client will demonstrate an increased tolerance for activity as evidenced by:	4.a. Assess for signs and symptoms of activity intolerance:
a. verbalization of feeling less fatigued and weak	1. statements of fatigue or weakness
b. ability to perform activities of daily living without exertional dyspnea, chest pain,	2. exertional dyspnea, chest pain, diaphoresis, or dizziness
	3. abnormal heart rate response to activity (e.g. increase in rate of 20 beats/minute above resting rate, rate not returning to preactivity level within 3 minutes after stopping activity, change from regular to irregular rate)
	4. decreased systolic B/P or a significant increase (10–15 mm Hg) in diastolic pressure with activity.

diaphoresis, dizziness, and a significant change in vital signs.

b. Implement measures *to improve activity tolerance:*
   1. perform actions *to promote rest and/or conserve energy:*
      a. maintain activity restrictions if ordered
      b. minimize environmental activity and noise
      c. organize nursing care to allow for periods of uninterrupted rest
      d. limit the number of visitors and their length of stay
      e. assist client with self-care activities as needed
      f. keep supplies and personal articles within easy reach
      g. instruct client in energy-saving techniques (e.g. using shower chair when showering, sitting to brush teeth or comb hair)
   2. perform actions to reduce the levels of serum nitrogenous substances (see Collaborative Diagnosis 7, action a.4) *in order to reduce the rate of RBC hemolysis*
   3. perform actions to maintain an adequate nutritional status (see Nursing Diagnosis 2, action c)
   4. administer hematopoietic agents (e.g. epoetin alfa) and/or androgens (e.g. testosterone propionate, fluoxymesterone) if ordered *to stimulate RBC production*
   5. increase client's activity gradually as tolerated.
c. Instruct client to:
   1. report a decreased tolerance for activity
   2. stop any activity that causes chest pain, shortness of breath, dizziness, or extreme fatigue or weakness.
d. Consult physician if signs and symptoms of activity intolerance persist or worsen.

---

5. NURSING DIAGNOSIS:

Constipation

related to:
a. decreased intake of fluids and foods high in fiber associated with prescribed restrictions;
b. decreased gastrointestinal motility associated with decreased activity and effect of antacids containing aluminum or calcium (may be given to prevent or treat hyperphosphatemia).

Desired Outcome	Nursing Actions and *Selected Purposes/Rationales*

5. The client will not experience constipation as evidenced by:
a. usual frequency of bowel movements
b. passage of soft, formed stool
c. absence of abdominal distention and pain, rectal fullness or pressure, and straining during defecation.
	5.a. Ascertain client's usual bowel elimination habits.
	b. Assess for signs and symptoms of constipation (e.g. decrease in frequency of bowel movements; passage of hard, formed stools; anorexia; abdominal distention and pain; feeling of fullness or pressure in rectum; straining during defecation).
	c. Assess bowel sounds. Report diminishing sounds.
	d. Implement measures *to prevent constipation:*
	  1. increase activity as tolerated
	  2. encourage client to consume the allotted amount of fluid
	  3. encourage client to defecate whenever the urge is felt
	  4. assist client to bathroom or bedside commode for bowel movements unless contraindicated
	  5. encourage client to relax, provide privacy, and have call signal within reach during attempts to defecate (*measures to promote relaxation enable client to relax the levator ani muscle and external anal sphincter, which facilitates evacuation of stool*)
	  6. encourage client to establish a regular time for defecation, preferably an hour after a meal
	  7. encourage client to drink hot liquids upon arising in the morning *in order to stimulate peristalsis*

Desired Outcome	Nursing Actions and *Selected Purposes/Rationales*

8. encourage client to increase intake of bran (bran is recommended *because it is a good source of fiber and is low in phosphorus*)
9. consult physician about alternating antacids that are constipating (e.g. Amphojel, Rolaids, Tums) with those that have a laxative effect (e.g. Milk of Magnesia, Gelusil, Mylanta, Maalox) if client's magnesium level is not too high.

   e. Consult physician if signs and symptoms of constipation persist.

---

6. NURSING DIAGNOSIS: **Risk for infection**

related to:
a. lowered natural resistance associated with:
   1. a depressed immune response resulting from the effects of increasing levels of serum nitrogenous substances
   2. inadequate nutritional status;
b. stasis of respiratory secretions and urinary stasis if mobility is decreased.

Desired Outcome	Nursing Actions and *Selected Purposes/Rationales*

6. The client will remain free of infection as evidenced by:
  a. absence of fever and chills
  b. pulse within normal limits
  c. normal breath sounds
  d. usual mental status
  e. cough productive of clear mucus only
  f. voiding clear urine without reports of frequency, urgency, and burning
  g. absence of heat, pain, redness, swelling, and unusual drainage in any area
  h. no reports of increased weakness and fatigue
  i. WBC and differential counts within normal range
  j. negative results of cultured specimens.

6.a. Assess for and report signs and symptoms of infection (be aware that some signs and symptoms vary depending on the site of infection, the causative organism, and the age and immune status of the client):
   1. elevated temperature
   2. chills
   3. increased pulse
   4. abnormal breath sounds
   5. malaise, lethargy, acute confusion
   6. loss of appetite
   7. cough productive of purulent, green, or rust-colored sputum
   8. cloudy, foul-smelling urine
   9. reports of frequency, urgency, or burning when urinating
   10. presence of WBCs, bacteria, and/or nitrites in urine
   11. heat, pain, redness, swelling, or unusual drainage in any area
   12. reports of increased weakness or fatigue
   13. elevated WBC count and/or significant change in differential.
  b. Obtain specimens (e.g. urine, vaginal drainage, sputum, blood) for culture as ordered. Report positive results.
  c. Implement measures *to prevent infection:*
   1. perform actions to reduce the levels of serum nitrogenous substances (see Collaborative Diagnosis 7, action a.4)
   2. maintain the maximum fluid intake allowed
   3. use good handwashing technique and encourage client to do the same
   4. use sterile technique during all invasive procedures (e.g. urinary catheterizations, venous and arterial punctures, injections)
   5. anchor catheters/tubings (e.g. urinary, intravenous) securely *in order to reduce trauma to the tissues and the risk for introduction of pathogens associated with the in-and-out movement of the tubing*
   6. rotate intravenous sites according to hospital policy
   7. change equipment, tubings, and solutions used for treatments such as intravenous infusions and respiratory care according to hospital policy
   8. maintain a closed system for drains (e.g. urinary catheter) and intravenous infusions whenever possible
   9. protect client from others who have an infection and instruct him/her to continue this after discharge
   10. perform actions to maintain an adequate nutritional status (see Nursing Diagnosis 2, action c)

11. perform actions to reduce stress (see Nursing Diagnosis 8, action b) *in order to prevent excessive secretion of cortisol* (*cortisol inhibits the immune response*)
12. reinforce importance of good oral hygiene
13. perform actions *to prevent stasis of respiratory secretions* (e.g. instruct and assist client to turn, cough, and deep breathe; increase activity as tolerated)
14. perform actions to prevent urinary retention (e.g. instruct client to urinate when the urge is first felt, promote relaxation during voiding attempts) *in order to prevent urinary stasis*
15. instruct and assist client to perform good perineal care routinely and after each bowel movement.

---

7. COLLABORATIVE DIAGNOSES:

Potential complications of chronic renal failure:

a. **uremic syndrome** related to accumulation of serum nitrogenous substances (e.g. creatinine, urea, phenols) associated with extensive loss of renal function (signs and symptoms usually occur when GFR falls to less than 10% of normal);
b. **hypertension** related to:
   1. fluid volume excess associated with the decreased GFR
   2. peripheral vasoconstriction associated with increased stimulation of the renin-angiotensin mechanism (possibly in response to diminished renal blood flow).

Desired Outcomes	Nursing Actions and *Selected Purposes/Rationales*

7.a. The client will not experience uremic syndrome as evidenced by:
1. pulse regular at 60–100 beats/minute
2. usual mental status
3. usual skin color
4. improved strength and activity tolerance
5. no reports of nausea, insomnia, itching, muscle cramping, joint pain, paresthesias, and taste alterations
6. intact oral mucous membrane
7. absence of vomiting, unusual bleeding, pericarditis, asterixis, and seizure activity.
	7.a.1. Assess for signs and symptoms of uremic syndrome:
	  a. cardiac dysrhythmias
	  b. difficulty concentrating, lethargy, confusion, or hallucinations
	  c. sallow or grayish-bronze skin color
	  d. increased weakness or fatigue
	  e. reports of nausea, insomnia, itching, muscle cramps, joint pain, paresthesias, restless feeling in legs during periods of inactivity, or metallic or bitter taste in mouth
	  f. stomatitis
	  g. vomiting
	  h. unusual bleeding (e.g. ecchymoses; prolonged bleeding from puncture sites; gingival bleeding; frank or occult blood in stool, urine, or vomitus)
	  i. pericarditis (e.g. precordial pain that frequently radiates to shoulder, neck, back, and arm [usually left]; pericardial friction rub; elevated temperature)
	  j. asterixis, seizures.
	2. Monitor BUN and serum creatinine results. Report levels that increase.
	3. Collect a 24-hour urine specimen if ordered. Report creatinine clearance levels that decrease.
	4. Implement measures *to reduce the levels of serum nitrogenous substances in order to prevent uremic syndrome:*
	  a. perform actions to maintain an adequate nutritional status (see Nursing Diagnosis 2, action c) *in order to reduce catabolism of body proteins*
	  b. maintain dietary protein restrictions
	  c. perform actions to prevent infection (see Nursing Diagnosis 6, action c) *in order to prevent an increase in metabolic rate and subsequent cellular catabolism*

Desired Outcomes	Nursing Actions and *Selected Purposes/Rationales*

    d. perform actions *to prevent further renal damage:*
      1. implement measures as ordered to control disease conditions such as diabetes that have caused or contributed to CRF
      2. consult the physician before administering medications that are known to be nephrotoxic (e.g. gentamicin, streptomycin, naproxen, ibuprofen).
  5. If signs and symptoms of uremic syndrome occur:
    a. consult physician
    b. continue with above measures
    c. prepare client for dialysis if planned
    d. maintain a safe environment for client (e.g. side rails up while in bed, assistance with ambulation as needed, constant supervision if indicated, seizure precautions)
    e. perform actions *to treat cardiac dysrhythmias if present* (e.g. administer antidysrhythmics as ordered, restrict activity if indicated)
    f. perform actions *to control nausea and vomiting if present* (e.g. administer antiemetics as ordered; provide small, frequent meals; instruct client to ingest foods/fluids slowly)
    g. perform actions *to reduce pruritus if present* (e.g. use tepid water and mild soap for bathing, apply emollient creams or ointments frequently, administer antihistamines if ordered)
    h. perform actions *to control muscle cramps if they occur* (e.g. instruct client to push feet against footboard when leg cramps occur, apply warm packs to affected areas)
    i. perform actions *to reduce the severity of stomatitis if present* (e.g. instruct client to avoid substances such as extremely hot, spicy, or acidic foods/fluids; assist with frequent oral hygiene; apply oral protective pastes as ordered)
    j. perform actions *to prevent bleeding* (e.g. apply gentle, prolonged pressure after injections and venous and arterial punctures; instruct client to use an electric rather than a straight-edge razor and to use a soft-bristle toothbrush for oral hygiene)
    k. perform actions *to control bleeding if it occurs* (e.g. apply firm, prolonged pressure to bleeding area if possible; administer clotting factors, vitamin K, or hemostatic agent if ordered)
    l. perform actions *to treat pericarditis if present* (e.g. maintain activity restrictions as ordered, administer an anti-inflammatory agent and analgesics if ordered)
    m. provide emotional support to client and significant others.

7.b. The client will not experience hypertension as evidenced by:
  1. B/P within a safe range for client
  2. no reports of headache and dizziness.

7.b.1. Assess for and report signs and symptoms of hypertension (e.g. B/P greater than client's usual level [a B/P of 140–159/90–99 is usually classified as mild hypertension], headache, dizziness).
  2. Implement measures *to prevent or control hypertension:*
    a. perform actions to reduce fluid volume excess and prevent or treat hypernatremia (see Nursing Diagnosis 1, actions a.3 and b.4)
    b. perform actions to reduce fear and anxiety (see Nursing Diagnosis 8, action b)
    c. administer antihypertensives (e.g. nifedipine, enalapril).
  3. If hypertension persists or worsens:
    a. consult physician
    b. continue with above actions
    c. refer to Care Plan on Hypertension for additional care measures.

■━━

8. NURSING DIAGNOSIS: **Anxiety**

related to lack of understanding of diagnosis, diagnostic tests, and treatment plan; uncertainty regarding extensiveness of disease progression; prognosis; financial concerns; unfamiliar environment; and the effects of CRF on life style and roles.

Desired Outcome	Nursing Actions and *Selected Purposes/Rationales*

8. The client will experience a reduction in anxiety as evidenced by:
  a. verbalization of feeling less anxious
  b. usual sleep pattern
  c. relaxed facial expression and body movements
  d. stable vital signs
  e. usual perceptual ability and interactions with others.
	8.a. Assess client for signs and symptoms of anxiety (e.g. verbalization of feeling anxious, insomnia, tenseness, shakiness, restlessness, diaphoresis, tachycardia, elevated blood pressure, facial pallor, self-focused behaviors). Validate perceptions carefully, remembering that some behavior may result from fluid and electrolyte imbalances.
	  b. Implement measures *to reduce fear and anxiety:*
	    1. orient client to hospital environment, equipment, and routines
	    2. introduce client to staff who will be participating in care; if possible, maintain consistency in staff assigned to his/her care *to provide feelings of stability and comfort with the environment*
	    3. assure client that staff members are nearby; respond to call signal as soon as possible
	    4. maintain a calm, supportive, confident manner when interacting with client
	    5. encourage verbalization of fear and anxiety; provide feedback
	    6. reinforce physician's explanations and clarify misconceptions the client has about CRF, diagnostic tests, the treatment plan, and prognosis
	    7. explain all diagnostic tests performed to assess the level of renal function
	    8. provide a calm, restful environment
	    9. instruct client in relaxation techniques and encourage participation in diversional activities
	    10. initiate financial and/or social service referrals if indicated
	    11. assist client to identify specific stressors and ways to cope with them
	    12. provide information based on current needs of client at a level he/she can understand; encourage questions and clarification of information provided
	    13. encourage significant others to project a caring, concerned attitude without obvious anxiousness
	    14. include significant others in orientation and teaching sessions and encourage their continued support of the client
	    15. administer prescribed antianxiety agents if indicated.
	  c. Consult physician if above measures fail to control fear and anxiety.

---

9. NURSING DIAGNOSIS:

Grieving*

related to progressive loss of kidney function and the effects of this on life style and roles.

---

*This diagnostic label includes anticipatory grieving and grieving following the actual losses.

Desired Outcome	Nursing Actions and *Selected Purposes/Rationales*

9. The client will demonstrate beginning progression through the grieving process as evidenced by:
  a. verbalization of feelings about having chronic renal failure
  b. usual sleep pattern
  c. participation in treatment
	9.a. Assess for signs and symptoms of grieving (e.g. change in eating habits, inability to concentrate, insomnia, anger, sadness, withdrawal from significant others, denial of progressive loss of kidney function).
	  b. Implement measures *to facilitate the grieving process:*
	    1. assist client to acknowledge the progressive loss of kidney function *so grief work can begin*; assess for factors that may hinder and facilitate acknowledgment
	    2. discuss the grieving process and assist client to accept the phases of grieving as an expected response to an actual and/or anticipated loss;

Desired Outcome	Nursing Actions and *Selected Purposes/Rationales*
plan and self-care activities d. utilization of available support systems e. verbalization of a plan for integrating prescribed follow-up care into life style.	support the realization that grief may recur because of the chronic, progressive nature of the disease 3. allow time for client to progress through the phases of grieving (phases vary among theorists but progress from shock and alarm to acceptance); be aware that not every phase is expressed by all individuals, that recurrence of phases is common, and that the grieving process will probably continue in varying degrees throughout life because of the progressive nature of chronic renal failure 4. provide an atmosphere of care and concern (e.g. provide privacy, be available and nonjudgmental, display empathy and respect) *so that client will feel free to express feelings* 5. perform actions *to promote trust* (e.g. answer questions honestly, provide requested information) 6. encourage the verbal expression of anger and sadness about the loss experienced; recognize displacement of anger and assist client to see the actual cause of angry feelings and resentment; establish limits on abusive behavior if demonstrated 7. encourage client to express feelings in whatever ways are comfortable (e.g. writing, drawing, conversation) 8. assist client to identify and utilize techniques that have helped him/her to cope in previous situations of loss 9. support realistic hope about the effect that adherence to the treatment plan has on prognosis 10. support behaviors suggesting successful grief work (e.g. verbalizing feelings about loss, focusing on ways to adapt to progressive loss of kidney function) 11. explain the phases of the grieving process to significant others; encourage their support and understanding 12. facilitate communication between the client and significant others; be aware that they may be in different phases of the grieving process 13. provide information regarding counseling services and support groups that might assist client in working through grief 14. when appropriate, assist client to meet spiritual needs (e.g. arrange for visit from clergy). c. Consult physician regarding referral for counseling if signs of dysfunctional grieving (e.g. persistent denial of loss, excessive anger or sadness, emotional lability) occur.

■───

10. NURSING DIAGNOSIS: **Ineffective management of therapeutic regimen**

related to lack of understanding of the implications of not following the prescribed treatment plan, difficulty integrating necessary treatments into life style, and lack of financial resources.

Desired Outcome	Nursing Actions and *Selected Purposes/Rationales*
10. The client will demonstrate the probability of effective management of the therapeutic regimen as evidenced by: a. willingness to learn about and participate in treatments and care b. statements reflecting ways to modify personal	10.a. Assess for indications that the client may be unable to effectively manage the therapeutic regimen: 1. statements reflecting inability to manage care at home 2. failure to adhere to treatment plan while in the hospital (e.g. not adhering to dietary modifications and fluid restrictions, refusing medications) 3. statements reflecting a lack of understanding of factors that will cause further renal damage 4. statements reflecting an unwillingness or inability to modify personal habits and integrate necessary treatments into life style

habits and integrate prescribed care into life style

c. statements reflecting an understanding of the implications of not following the prescribed treatment plan.

5. statements reflecting view that kidney damage will reverse itself or that the situation is hopeless and efforts to comply with prescribed care are useless.

b. Implement measures *to promote effective management of the therapeutic regimen:*

1. explain renal failure in terms client can understand; stress the fact that it is a chronic disease and that adherence to treatment plan is necessary in order to delay and/or prevent complications

2. initiate and reinforce discharge teaching outlined in Nursing Diagnosis 11 *in order to promote a sense of control and self-reliance*

3. encourage client to participate in prescribed care (e.g. monitoring intake and output, calculating allowed fluid intake, selecting foods and fluids within dietary restrictions)

4. assist client to identify ways treatments can be incorporated into life style; focus on modifications of life style rather than complete change

5. obtain a dietary consult to assist client in planning a dietary program based on prescribed modifications and client's likes, dislikes, cultural preferences, and daily routines

6. encourage questions and clarify misconceptions the client has about CRF and its effects

7. perform actions to facilitate the grieving process (see Nursing Diagnosis 9, action b)

8. provide client with verbal and written instructions about future appointments with health care provider, ways to prevent further kidney damage, dietary modifications, fluid restrictions, medications, and signs and symptoms to report; determine areas of difficulty and misunderstanding and reinforce teaching as necessary

9. encourage client to discuss concerns about the cost of medications and follow-up medical care; obtain a social service consult to assist with financial planning and to obtain financial aid if indicated

10. provide information about and encourage utilization of community resources that can assist client to make necessary life-style changes (e.g. local chapter of the American Kidney Association, vocational rehabilitation, counseling services)

11. reinforce behaviors suggesting future compliance with the therapeutic regimen (e.g. statements reflecting plans for integrating care into life style, active participation in treatment plan, changes in personal habits)

12. include significant others in explanations and teaching sessions and encourage their support; reinforce the need for client to assume responsibility for managing as much of care as possible.

c. Consult physician regarding referrals to community health agencies if continued instruction, support, or supervision is needed.

Discharge Teaching

■

11. NURSING DIAGNOSIS:	**Knowledge deficit or Altered health maintenance***

*The nurse should select the diagnostic label that is most appropriate for the client's discharge teaching needs.

Desired Outcomes	Nursing Actions and *Selected Purposes/Rationales*
11.a. The client will verbalize a basic understanding of CRF.	11.a. Explain renal failure in terms that client can understand. Utilize appropriate teaching aids (e.g. pictures, videotapes, kidney models).

Desired Outcomes	Nursing Actions and *Selected Purposes/Rationales*

11.b. The client will identify ways to slow the progression of kidney damage.	11.b.1. Provide instructions regarding ways to slow the progression of kidney damage:
	  a. control hypertension by adhering to dietary modifications and taking medications as prescribed
	  b. reduce the risk of urinary tract infection by:
	    1. cleaning perianal area thoroughly after each bowel movement
	    2. consuming the maximum amount of fluids allowed
	    3. wiping from front to back after urination and defecation (if female)
	  c. reduce the risk of nephrotoxic reactions by:
	    1. consulting the physician before:
	      a. taking any additional prescription and nonprescription drugs
	      b. receiving any vaccines
	      c. resuming any occupation or hobby involving exposure to chemicals or fumes
	    2. avoiding contact with products such as antifreeze, pesticides, carbon tetrachloride, mercuric chloride, lead, arsenic, and creosote.
	  2. With client and significant others, discuss ways in which above health care measures can be incorporated into life style.

11.c. The client will verbalize an understanding of fluid restrictions and dietary modifications.	11.c.1. Reinforce the importance of adhering to prescribed fluid restrictions and dietary modifications.
	  2. Reinforce physician's instructions about specific fluid restrictions and dietary modifications.
	  3. Reinforce dietitian's instructions on how to calculate and measure dietary allotments. Have client develop sample menus.
	  4. If client is on a protein- and sodium-restricted diet, inform him/her that numerous salt-free and protein-free products are available. Provide names of local stores that carry these products.
	  5. If client is on fluid restrictions, instruct to:
	    a. take oral medications with soft foods (e.g. applesauce, pudding) rather than liquids
	    b. reduce thirst by:
	      1. sucking on hard candy, popsicles, or ice cubes made with favorite juices (caution client that the fluid volume of the popsicles and ice cubes must be considered as oral fluid intake)
	      2. spacing fluids evenly throughout the hours he/she is awake
	    c. set out the 24-hour allotment of liquids in the morning in order to visualize the amount allowed for the day.

11.d. The client will demonstrate the ability to accurately weigh self, measure fluid intake and output, and monitor own blood pressure.	11.d.1. If client needs to monitor weight, instruct him/her to weigh at the same time, on the same scale, and with similar amounts of clothing on.
	  2. Demonstrate how to measure and record fluid intake and urinary output if indicated. Stress that any substance that is liquid at room temperature is counted as fluid intake.
	  3. If client needs to monitor blood pressure, provide instructions on how to take, read, and record it.
	  4. Allow time for questions, clarification, practice, and return demonstration. Instruct client to take record of weights, fluid intake and urinary output, and B/P readings to appointments with health care provider.

11.e. The client will identify ways to reduce the risk of infection.	11.e. Instruct client in ways to reduce the risk of infection:
	  1. avoid contact with persons who have an infection
	  2. avoid crowds during the flu or cold season
	  3. decrease or stop smoking
	  4. drink allotted amounts of liquids
	  5. maintain good personal hygiene
	  6. maintain a good nutritional status
	  7. maintain an adequate balance between activity and rest
	  8. take antimicrobials as prescribed before scheduled dental work, invasive diagnostic procedures, or surgery.

11.f. The client will identify ways to manage signs and symptoms that often occur as a result of CFR.

11.f. Provide instructions regarding ways to manage the following signs and symptoms that often occur as a result of CRF:
1. weakness and fatigue:
   a. schedule frequent rest periods throughout the day
   b. maintain a good nutritional status
2. dry mouth:
   a. space fluid allotments evenly throughout waking hours
   b. perform oral hygiene frequently
3. decreased libido (can occur as a result of weakness and fatigue, depression, and side effects of some medications):
   a. schedule rest periods before and after sexual activity
   b. explore creative ways of expressing sexuality (e.g. massage, fantasies, cuddling).

11.g. The client will state signs and symptoms to report to the health care provider.

11.g. Instruct client to report the following:
1. weight gain of more than 0.5 kg (1 pound)/day or a continued weight loss
2. persistent nausea or vomiting
3. increasing fatigue or weakness
4. difficulty concentrating and making decisions
5. confusion
6. persistent or severe headache
7. palpitations or chest pain
8. blood in stools, urine, or vomitus; persistent bleeding from nose, mouth, or any cut; prolonged or excessive menses; excessive bruising; or sudden abdominal or back pain
9. fever or chills
10. numbness or tingling in extremities, persistent restless feeling in legs during periods of inactivity
11. change in skin color (bronze, yellow-gray)
12. impotence, infertility, or amenorrhea (could indicate hormonal imbalances caused by increasing serum levels of nitrogenous substances)
13. increasing blood pressure (if B/P is monitored at home)
14. swelling of feet, ankles, or hands
15. diarrhea or constipation (either can occur as a side effect of some antacid therapy; physicians generally recommend alternating antacids containing magnesium with those containing aluminum or calcium to prevent these bowel problems)
16. fainting or persistent dizziness or lightheadedness
17. persistent itching
18. oral pain or breakdown of oral mucous membrane
19. shortness of breath
20. muscle cramping
21. twitching or seizures
22. joint or bone pain (could indicate osteodystrophy resulting from effects of hypocalcemia and hyperphosphatemia).

11.h. The client will identify community resources that can assist with adjustment to changes resulting from CRF.

11.h.1. Provide information about community resources that can assist the client and significant others to adjust to changes resulting from chronic renal failure (e.g. local chapter of the American Kidney Association, vocational rehabilitation, social services, counseling services).
2. Initiate a referral if indicated.

11.i. The client will verbalize an understanding of and a plan for adhering to recommended follow-up care including future appointments with health care provider and medications prescribed.

11.i.1. Reinforce the importance of keeping follow-up appointments with health care provider.
2. Explain the rationale for, side effects of, and importance of taking prescribed medications (e.g. antihypertensives, antacids, vitamins, electrolyte supplements, diuretics, hematopoietic agents). Inform client of pertinent food and drug interactions.
3. Reinforce the importance of consulting the physician before taking any prescription and nonprescription drugs because some drugs are nephrotoxic (e.g. ibuprofen, cimetidine, neomycin, naproxen, gentamicin) and can hasten the progression of CRF, some drugs such as aspirin and digoxin are excreted by the kidneys and can rapidly build to toxic levels in the body (usual dosages may need to be reduced or a

Desired Outcomes	Nursing Actions and *Selected Purposes/Rationales*

different medication taken), and some drugs contain ingredients that could affect electrolyte balance and elevate blood pressure (e.g. many cold remedies).

4. Refer to Nursing Diagnosis 10, action b, for measures to promote the client's ability to effectively manage the therapeutic regimen.

Bibliography

See pages 897–898 and 905.

 # CYSTECTOMY WITH URINARY DIVERSION

Cystectomy is the removal of the bladder and is accompanied by a procedure to divert urinary flow. It may be performed to treat a malignancy of the bladder, congenital bladder anomalies, neurogenic bladder, and irreparable bladder trauma. A cystectomy may also be performed to prevent further deterioration of renal function associated with chronic bladder infection. In some cases, the surgery includes removal of just the bladder (simple cystectomy) but when there is an invasive malignancy, a more radical procedure is performed. In men, a radical cystectomy usually includes removal of the bladder, prostate, seminal vesicles, a portion of the vas deferens, and some or all of the pelvic lymph nodes. In women, a radical cystectomy usually includes removal of the bladder, urethra, uterus, fallopian tubes, ovaries, a portion of the anterior vaginal wall, and some or all of the pelvic lymph nodes.

There are several ways to accomplish urinary diversion. The most common surgical method is the conventional conduit. In this procedure, the ureters are implanted in one end of a resected segment of intestine and the other end of the intestinal segment is brought through the abdominal wall to create a stoma. Because no valves are incorporated into the construction of the conventional conduit, drops of urine usually flow from the stoma every few seconds, resulting in the client's need to wear a urinary collection appliance at all times.

The second most common surgical method to accomplish urinary diversion is the continent internal reservoir (e.g. Kock pouch, Indiana pouch). In this method, the ureters are implanted in one end of a resected portion of intestine that has been remodeled to create a reservoir. A segment of the other end of the reservoir is used to create the stoma that is brought out through the abdominal wall. The reflux of urine from the reservoir back through the ureters and the uncontrolled flow of urine from the reservoir through the stoma is prevented by the surgical positioning of the ureters, reservoir, and stoma or by the use of one-way valves at these sites. After healing occurs, a catheter is inserted into the stoma at regularly scheduled intervals (usually every 4–6 hours once the reservoir stretches to its full capacity) to drain the reservoir. If the system functions properly, the client does not need to wear a urinary collection appliance over the stoma.

Another method of urinary diversion is the direct implantation of the ureters into the abdominal wall (cutaneous ureterostomy). Because of the high rate of stenosis of ureteral stomas, this method is usually reserved for clients who cannot tolerate lengthy surgery and/or have a short life expectancy.

The type of urinary diversion selected depends on many factors including the client's preference, age, body build, ability to learn about and participate in care of the urinary diversion, prognosis, and ability to tolerate lengthy surgery; the integrity of the client's ureters, kidneys, and intestinal tract; the advice of the enterostomal therapist nurse; and the expertise of the surgeon.

This care plan focuses on the adult client hospitalized for a cystectomy with urinary diversion by means of a conventional conduit. Some additional nursing interventions are also included for the client with a continent internal reservoir. The goals of preoperative care are to reduce fear and anxiety and prepare the client for the change in body image and function. Postoperatively, goals of care are to maintain peristomal skin integrity, prevent complications, facilitate psychological adjustment to the changes experienced, and educate the client regarding management of the urinary diversion and follow-up care.

DIAGNOSTIC TESTS

Intravenous pyelogram (IVP)
Ultrasonography
Computed tomography (CT)
Urinalysis
Cystoscopy (with or without biopsy)
Cystography
Urodynamic studies

DISCHARGE CRITERIA

Prior to discharge, the client will:

- maintain an adequate urine output via the urinary diversion
- have surgical pain controlled
- have evidence of normal healing of surgical wound
- have a medium pink to red, moist stoma and intact peristomal skin
- have no signs and symptoms of postoperative complications
- verbalize a basic understanding of the anatomical changes that have occurred as a result of the surgery
- demonstrate the ability to change the urostomy appliance and maintain stomal and peristomal skin integrity
- demonstrate the ability to properly clean reusable urostomy equipment
- demonstrate the ability to drain and irrigate a continent internal reservoir if present
- identify ways to control odor of the urostomy drainage and appliance
- identify ways to prevent urinary tract infection
- state signs and symptoms to report to the health care provider
- share thoughts and feelings about altered urinary elimination and its effect on body image and life style
- identify appropriate community resources that can assist with home management and adjustment to changes resulting from the urinary diversion
- verbalize an understanding of and a plan for adhering to recommended follow-up care including future appointments with health care provider, wound care, activity level, and medications prescribed.

NURSING/ COLLABORATIVE DIAGNOSES

Preoperative
1. Anxiety △   514
2. Knowledge deficit △   514

Postoperative
1. Actual/Risk for impaired tissue integrity △   516
2. Risk for infection: urinary tract △   518
3. Potential complications:
   a. stomal changes:
      1. prolapse
      2. excessive bleeding
      3. necrosis
   b. urinary obstruction
   c. peritonitis △   519
4. Sexual dysfunction △   521
5. Self-concept disturbance △   522
6. Ineffective individual coping △   524
7. Grieving △   525

DISCHARGE TEACHING
8. Knowledge deficit, Ineffective management of therapeutic regimen, or Altered health maintenance △   526

See Standardized Preoperative and Postoperative Care Plans for additional diagnoses.

PREOPERATIVE

Use in conjunction with the Standardized Preoperative Care Plan.

---

1. NURSING DIAGNOSIS: **Anxiety**

related to:
a. unfamiliar environment and separation from significant others;
b. lack of understanding of diagnostic tests, planned surgical procedure, and care that will be required for the urinary diversion;
c. anticipated loss of control associated with effects of anesthesia;
d. anticipated discomfort, surgical findings, changes in appearance and body functioning, and effects of urinary diversion on future life style and roles;
e. financial concerns associated with hospitalization;
f. ability to independently care for urinary diversion following discharge.

Desired Outcome	Nursing Actions and *Selected Purposes/Rationales*

1. The client will experience a reduction in anxiety (see Standardized Preoperative Care Plan, Nursing Diagnosis 1 [pp. 96–97], for outcome criteria).	1.a. Refer to Standardized Preoperative Care Plan, Nursing Diagnosis 1 (pp. 96–97), for measures related to assessment and reduction of fear and anxiety.
	 b. Implement additional measures *to reduce fear and anxiety:*
	  1. provide client with information about preoperative routines, the surgical procedure, general postoperative care, the function and appearance of the stoma, and management of the urinary diversion (see Preoperative Nursing Diagnosis 2) *so he/she will know what to expect*
	  2. explain that every attempt will be made to place the stoma in an area that he/she can easily see and reach and where the appliance will lie flat, adhere well to the skin, and allow the client freedom of movement (the tentative stoma site is mapped out preoperatively by the physician and/or enterostomal therapist)
	  3. inform client that instructions about the management of the urinary diversion will be repeated as often as necessary prior to discharge and that there will be resources available to provide assistance/supervision following discharge
	  4. assure client that stoma has no pain receptors and will not be painful when touched
	  5. explain that current urostomy collection devices are odorproof and available in sizes to fit various body contours
	  6. if acceptable to client, arrange for a visit with a person of similar age and same sex who has successfully adapted to a urinary diversion
	  7. assure client that the urinary diversion need not dramatically alter life style (only contact sports are contraindicated).

Client Teaching

---

2. NURSING DIAGNOSIS: **Knowledge deficit**

regarding hospital routines associated with surgery, physical preparation for the cystectomy with urinary diversion, the surgical procedure, sensations that normally occur following surgery and anesthesia, expected appearance and function of the urostomy, and postoperative care and management of the urinary diversion.

Desired Outcomes	Nursing Actions and *Selected Purposes/Rationales*

2.a. The client will verbalize an understanding of the surgical procedure, preoperative care, and postoperative sensations and care.

2.a.1. Refer to Standardized Preoperative Care Plan, Nursing Diagnosis 4, actions a.1–4 (pp. 99–100), for information to include in preoperative teaching.

    2. Provide additional information about specific preoperative care and postoperative sensations and care for clients having a cystectomy with urinary diversion:

      a. explain the preoperative bowel preparation (e.g. low-residue or clear liquid diet, cleansing enemas, laxatives, antimicrobial therapy); reinforce the fact that bowel preparation is necessary since a portion of the bowel will be used to create the urinary diversion

      b. if a conventional conduit is the planned method of urinary diversion, explain that ureteral stents (small, firm catheters) may be inserted in surgery to maintain patency of the ureters (the stents will extend from the stoma and are removed once surgical site edema subsides [usually about 5–10 days after surgery])

      c. if a continent internal reservoir is the planned method of urinary diversion, inform the client that:

        1. ureteral stents or a catheter will be inserted in surgery and will extend from the stoma and drain continually into an external collection device; stress that this is a temporary measure (usually for 10–14 days) to keep the ureters patent (if stents are present) while surgical site edema subsides and to keep the reservoir from becoming distended while the suture lines are healing

        2. the reservoir will need to be irrigated regularly in the early postoperative period to remove mucus that accumulates in the reservoir (the bowel used to construct the reservoir initially secretes quite a bit of mucus)

        3. following removal of the ureteral stents or catheter, a catheter will be inserted into the stoma at regularly scheduled intervals to drain the reservoir and an external collection device will not be needed.

    3. Allow time for questions and clarification of information provided.

2.b. The client will demonstrate the ability to perform activities designed to prevent postoperative complications.

2.b. Refer to Standardized Preoperative Care Plan, Nursing Diagnosis 4, action b (p. 100), for instructions on ways to prevent postoperative complications.

2.c. The client will verbalize an understanding of the appearance of the stoma and management of the urinary diversion.

2.c.1. Arrange for a visit with enterostomal therapist if available.

    2. Reinforce basic information provided by physician and/or enterostomal therapist regarding:

      a. expected location of stoma

      b. expected appearance of stoma postoperatively (red, initially edematous)

      c. expected drainage (slight bleeding of stoma, some blood in urine for 24–48 hours, mucus in urine [occurs because the urinary diversion is constructed using a section of bowel and the bowel mucosa normally secretes mucus])

      d. management of urinary diversion (e.g. peristomal skin care, odor control, use of various types of appliances, irrigation and drainage of an internal reservoir)

      e. urostomy products that client will be using in the immediate postoperative period.

    3. Provide visual aids and allow client to handle appliances he/she will be using in the immediate postoperative period.

    4. Encourage client to try wearing an appliance partially filled with water in order to experience how it feels and to validate whether planned stoma site will be adequate for successful adhesion of appliance.

    5. Allow time for questions and clarification of information provided.

POSTOPERATIVE

Use in conjunction with the Standardized Postoperative Care Plan.

---

1. NURSING DIAGNOSIS: **Actual/Risk for impaired tissue integrity**

related to:

a. disruption of tissue associated with the surgical procedure;

b. delayed wound healing associated with factors such as decreased nutritional status, inadequate blood supply to wound area, and preoperative radiation therapy (may have been done if the underlying disease process is a malignancy);

c. irritation of skin around suture lines and wound drains associated with contact with wound drainage, pressure from tubes, and use of tape;

d. irritation of peristomal area associated with:

1. chemical irritation resulting from prolonged contact with urine; soap residue and perspiration under the appliance; and allergic reaction to tape, adhesives, and/or other substances used to secure the appliance to the skin

2. mechanical irritation resulting from frequent and/or improper removal of tape, adhesives, and/or other substances used to secure the appliance to the skin; and aggressive cleansing of peristomal area.

Desired Outcomes	Nursing Actions and *Selected Purposes/Rationales*
1.a. The client will experience normal healing of surgical wounds (see Standardized Postoperative Care Plan, Nursing Diagnosis 9, outcome a [pp. 109–110], for outcome criteria).	1.a. Refer to Standardized Postoperative Care Plan, Nursing Diagnosis 9, action a (pp. 109–110), for measures related to assessment and promotion of wound healing.
1.b. The client will maintain integrity of the peristomal skin and skin in contact with wound drainage, tape, and tubings as evidenced by: 1. absence of redness and irritation 2. no skin breakdown.	1.b.1. Inspect skin areas that are in contact with wound drainage, tape, and tubings for signs of irritation and breakdown.

2. Assess for signs and symptoms of peristomal irritation or breakdown (e.g. redness, inflammation, and/or excoriation of peristomal skin; reports of itching and burning under the appliance; inability to keep appliance on).

3. Refer to Standardized Postoperative Care Plan, Nursing Diagnosis 9, actions b.2 and 3 (pp. 110–111), for measures to prevent and treat tissue irritation and breakdown in areas in contact with wound drainage, tape, and tubings.

4. Implement measures *to prevent peristomal irritation and breakdown:*

a. patch test all products that will come in contact with the skin (e.g. adhesives, solvents, sealants, barriers) before initial use; do not use products that cause redness, itching, or burning

b. change appliance only when necessary (e.g. as ordered, if appliance is leaking, if client reports burning or itching of the peristomal skin, when the stoma size changes); appliance is typically changed every 3 days in the early postoperative period and then should be able to remain in place for 5–7 days

c. use a 2-piece appliance (skin barrier and pouch) in the initial postoperative period *so that the pouch can be removed to assess the stoma without having to remove the adhesive from the skin*

d. remove hair from peristomal skin using an electric razor *to help achieve an adequate appliance seal and to reduce irritation when the appliance is removed*

e. perform actions *to reduce peristomal irritation during removal of appliance:*

    1. place drops of warm water or solvent where the appliance adheres to the skin *in order to facilitate removal*; allow time for adhesive to loosen before removing appliance from the skin

    2. remove appliance gently and in direction of hair growth; hold skin adjacent to the skin barrier taut and push down on skin slightly *to facilitate separation*

f. perform actions *to prevent urine from coming in contact with the skin when changing appliance:*

    1. change appliance when the urostomy is least active (in the morning before drinking liquids or when fluid intake has been reduced for a few hours)

    2. place a wick (rolled gauze pad, tampon) on the stoma opening when the appliance is off

g. cleanse peristomal skin thoroughly with mild soap and water, rinse completely, and pat dry; use tepid rather than hot water *to prevent burns*

h. apply skin sealant before application of skin barrier *to protect skin from irritating effect of the adhesive*

i. use a skin barrier composed of synthetic material (e.g. Stomahesive); avoid the use of a hydrophilic barrier (e.g. karaya) *because it will dissolve when in contact with urine*

j. perform actions *to prevent urine from contacting the skin when appliance is on:*

    1. measure diameter of stoma and cut skin barrier and pouch openings no more than 0.3 cm (⅛ inch) larger than stoma (it may be necessary to create a pattern to use for cutting the openings if stoma has an irregular shape)

    2. instruct and assist client to remeasure the stoma size frequently during first 6 weeks after surgery and to alter size of skin barrier and pouch openings as stomal edema decreases

    3. implement measures *to achieve an adequate appliance seal:*

       a. avoid use of ointments or lotions on peristomal skin (*these can interfere with adequate adhesive bonding*)

       b. follow manufacturer's instructions carefully when applying products such as skin sealant and barrier and the pouch

       c. use ostomy paste (e.g. Stomahesive paste) to fill in irregularities around stoma site (e.g. body folds, scars) before applying skin barrier

       d. apply firm pressure and remove wrinkles and air pockets when applying skin barrier and pouch; place client in a supine position *to increase tautness of skin surface during application*

    4. use a pouch with an antireflux valve

    5. empty pouch when it is about 1/3 full (*the weight of pouch could cause the appliance to separate from the skin*)

    6. position pouch so gravity flow facilitates drainage away from stoma and peristomal skin

    7. close valve or clamp tightly after emptying pouch *to prevent leakage*

k. if a belted appliance is used, fasten the belt so that 2 fingers can easily slip between belt and skin *to prevent excessive pressure on the skin*

l. instruct and assist client to check appliance periodically to ensure that clamp or valve is not placing pressure on the skin.

5. If signs and symptoms of peristomal irritation and breakdown occur:

a. avoid use of any product that may have caused the peristomal irritation or breakdown

b. cleanse area gently with warm water

c. perform skin care according to enterostomal therapist's or physician's order or hospital procedure (usual care may include exposing affected area to air for 20–30 minutes when appliance is changed; covering all irritated skin with a properly fitted, hypoallergenic, solid skin barrier; avoiding appliance changes unless there are signs of leakage; and applying an antifungal agent or corticosteroid preparation to affected area)

Desired Outcomes	Nursing Actions and *Selected Purposes/Rationales*

d. consult physician and/or enterostomal therapist if:
   1. condition of peristomal skin does not improve within 48 hours
   2. signs and symptoms of infection (e.g. elevated temperature; redness, heat, pain, and swelling around area of breakdown; unusual drainage or odor from site) are present.

---

2. NURSING DIAGNOSIS: **Risk for infection: urinary tract**

related to:
a. increased growth and colonization of microorganisms associated with stasis of urine resulting from:
   1. obstruction of urine flow (can occur as a result of edema of the stoma or ureteral junctions, excessive collection of mucus in the stoma, malfunction of ureteral stents if present, or blockage of stomal catheter [catheter is usually present for 7–10 days postoperatively if client has an internal reservoir and does not have ureteral stents])
   2. incomplete or infrequent emptying of the internal reservoir (if present) following removal of the stomal catheter or ureteral stents;
b. introduction of pathogens into the urinary tract associated with:
   1. reflux of urine from the collection device into the stoma, ureteral stents, or stomal catheter
   2. reflux of urine from the conduit or internal reservoir into the ureters or kidney
   3. presence of stomal catheter or ureteral stents
   4. incorrect or inadequate cleansing of reusable urostomy appliances or peristomal skin
   5. intermittent catheterization and irrigation of the internal reservoir (if present).

Desired Outcome	Nursing Actions and *Selected Purposes/Rationales*

2. The client will remain free of urinary tract infection as evidenced by:
   a. no increase in sediment in urine
   b. no unusual color or odor of urine
   c. absence of chills and fever
   d. absence of bacteria, nitrites, and WBCs in urine
   e. negative urine culture.

2.a. Assess for and report signs and symptoms of urinary tract infection (e.g. increased sediment in urine; bloody or cloudy, foul-smelling urine; chills; elevated temperature).
   b. Monitor urinalysis and report presence of bacteria, nitrites, and/or WBCs.
   c. Obtain a urine specimen for culture and sensitivity if ordered. Report abnormal results.
   d. Test pH of urine if ordered. Consult physician if the pH is greater than 6.5.
   e. Implement measures *to prevent urinary tract infection:*
      1. perform actions *to prevent reflux and/or stasis of urine:*
         a. implement measures to prevent urinary obstruction (see Postoperative Collaborative Diagnosis 3, action b.2)
         b. use a pouch with an antireflux valve
         c. instruct and assist client to empty pouch when it is 1/3 full *in order to prevent reflux and reduce risk of bacterial growth resulting from stasis of urine in pouch*
         d. instruct and assist client to change to a bedside collection system before lying down for an extended period
         e. if client has an internal reservoir, instruct and assist him/her to empty it as often as necessary (frequency depends on the reservoir capacity and the client's fluid intake) *to reduce the risk for urinary stasis*
         f. increase activity as tolerated
      2. maintain sterile technique during catheterization and irrigation of the internal reservoir (if present)
      3. cleanse peristomal skin thoroughly each time appliance is changed
      4. maintain fluid intake of at least 2500 ml/day (unless contraindicated) *to*

promote urine formation (*if client has a conventional conduit, this increases the amount of urine that passes through the conduit and subsequently flushes pathogens out of the conduit*)

5. ensure that any reusable urostomy appliances are cleansed thoroughly, rinsed, and allowed to dry completely between applications
6. if client's urine is too alkaline (pH greater than 6.5):
   a. encourage client to increase intake of foods/fluids that will make urine more acidic (e.g. cranberry juice, prune juice, plums, poultry, fish, whole grains)
   b. instruct client to avoid excessive intake of milk, citrus fruits, and carbonated beverages (*these tend to alkalinize urine*)
   c. administer medications such as ascorbic acid if ordered.
   f. If signs and symptoms of urinary tract infection occur:
   1. continue with above actions
   2. administer antimicrobial agents if ordered.

---

3. COLLABORATIVE DIAGNOSES:

Potential complications of cystectomy with urinary diversion:

a. **stomal changes:**
   1. **prolapse** related to pressure around the stoma, poor tissue turgor, and loss of integrity of suture line
   2. **excessive bleeding** related to irritation associated with aggressive cleansing of stoma and/or improper fit or application of appliance
   3. **necrosis** related to intraoperative and/or postoperative interruption of blood supply to the stoma;
b. **urinary obstruction** related to:
   1. loss of patency of stomal catheter or ureteral stents if present
   2. edema of stoma and/or ureters associated with surgical trauma
   3. collection of mucus at stoma and/or ureteral openings;
c. **peritonitis** related to:
   1. leakage of urine and/or intestinal contents into the peritoneum associated with loss of integrity of the sutures at sites of surgical anastomoses
   2. leakage of urine into and/or exposure of the peritoneum associated with retraction of peristomal skin from stoma (mucocutaneous separation) resulting from slippage of the sutures or impaired healing of surgical site
   3. accumulation of wound drainage in the peritoneum
   4. wound infection.

Desired Outcomes	Nursing Actions and *Selected Purposes/Rationales*

3.a. The client will maintain integrity of the stoma as evidenced by:
1. medium pink to red coloring of stoma
2. expected stomal height
3. absence of excessive bleeding and increasing edema of the stoma.

3.a.1. Assess for and report signs and symptoms of impaired stomal integrity (e.g. pale, dark red, or blue-black color of stoma; increased stomal height; increased stomal edema or bleeding). Use only clear appliances during immediate postoperative period *to allow easy visibility of stoma.*
2. Implement measures *to maintain integrity of stoma:*
   a. perform actions *to maintain adequate stomal circulation:*
      1. ensure that the openings of the skin barrier and pouch are not too small and that the stoma is centered in the openings *in order to prevent pressure on and around the stoma*
      2. instruct client to avoid wearing clothing that puts pressure on the stoma
   b. apply appliance securely *to prevent it from slipping and irritating or shearing the stoma*
   c. always cleanse stoma gently using a soft cloth, gauze, or tissue.
3. If signs and symptoms of impaired stomal integrity occur:
   a. perform stomal care as ordered
   b. prepare client for surgical revision of stoma if indicated
   c. provide emotional support to client and significant others.

Desired Outcomes	Nursing Actions and *Selected Purposes/Rationales*

3.b. The client will not experience urinary obstruction as evidenced by:
   1. balanced intake and output beginning 48 hours postoperatively
   2. gradual resolution of abdominal tenderness and distention
   3. expected volume of drainage from abdominal incision and drain.

3.b.1. Assess for and report signs and symptoms of ureteral or stomal obstruction (e.g. significant decrease in urinary output from stoma, ureteral stents, or stomal catheter; increasing abdominal tenderness and distention; increase in drainage from abdominal incision or drain).
   2. Implement measures *to prevent urinary obstruction:*
      a. encourage a fluid intake of 2500 ml/day unless contraindicated *to keep urine dilute and maintain adequate urine flow (mucus is not as likely to congeal in dilute urine and an adequate urine flow helps flush mucus through the conduit and stoma)*
      b. flush ureteral stents or irrigate stomal catheter if ordered (*mucus can accumulate in and subsequently obstruct the stents or catheter*)
      c. if client has an internal reservoir, irrigate the reservoir as ordered *to remove mucus (excessive mucus can obstruct the ureteral openings)*
      d. change the appliance carefully *in order to avoid dislodgment of the ureteral stents or stomal catheter if present.*
   3. If signs and symptoms of urinary obstruction occur:
      a. prepare client for dilation of the stoma, surgical revision of stoma or sites of ureteral anastomoses, and/or insertion of ureteral stents
      b. provide emotional support to client and significant others.

3.c. The client will not develop peritonitis as evidenced by:
   1. gradual resolution of abdominal pain
   2. soft, nondistended abdomen
   3. temperature declining toward normal
   4. stable vital signs
   5. absence of nausea and vomiting
   6. gradual return of normal bowel sounds
   7. WBC count declining toward normal.

3.c.1. Assess for and report signs and symptoms of peritonitis (e.g. increase in severity of abdominal pain; rebound tenderness; distended, rigid abdomen; increase in temperature; tachycardia; tachypnea; hypotension; nausea; vomiting; failure of bowel sounds to return to normal).
   2. Monitor WBC counts. Report levels that increase or fail to decline toward normal.
   3. Implement measures *to prevent peritonitis:*
      a. perform actions to prevent and treat wound infection (see Standardized Postoperative Care Plan, Nursing Diagnosis 16, actions b.4 and 5 [pp. 116–117])
      b. perform actions *to maintain patency of wound drain if present:*
         1. keep tubing free of kinks
         2. empty collection device as often as necessary
         3. maintain suction as ordered
      c. perform actions *to prevent inadvertent removal of wound drain if present:*
         1. use caution when changing dressings surrounding drain
         2. provide extension tubing if necessary *to enable client to move without placing tension on the drain*
         3. instruct client not to pull on drain and drainage tubing
      d. perform actions *to prevent distention of the conduit or internal reservoir (distention can cause strain on the suture lines and subsequent leakage of urine into the peritoneal cavity):*
         1. implement measures to prevent urinary obstruction (see action b.2 in this diagnosis)
         2. assist client with intermittent catheterization of the internal reservoir (if present) at scheduled intervals and when he/she feels increased abdominal pressure
      e. do not reposition ureteral stents or stomal catheter if present *because repositioning them could disrupt the suture lines*
      f. if separation of stoma from peristomal skin occurs:
         1. perform wound care as ordered *to facilitate the formation of granulation tissue in retracted area*
         2. prepare client for surgical reconstruction of the stoma if planned.
   4. If signs and symptoms of peritonitis occur:
      a. withhold oral intake as ordered
      b. place client on bed rest in a semi-Fowler's position *to assist in pooling or localizing gastrointestinal contents and urine in the pelvis rather than under the diaphragm*
      c. prepare client for diagnostic tests (e.g. abdominal x-ray, peritoneal aspiration, computed tomography, ultrasonography) if planned

    d. insert a nasogastric tube and maintain suction as ordered

    e. administer antimicrobials if ordered

    f. administer intravenous fluids and/or blood volume expanders if ordered *to prevent or treat shock* (*can result from the increased capillary permeability that occurs with inflammation and the subsequent escape of protein, fluid, and electrolytes from the vascular space into the peritoneal cavity*)

    g. prepare client for surgical intervention (e.g. drainage and irrigation of peritoneum, repair of sites of anastomoses) if indicated

    h. provide emotional support to client and significant others.

---

4. NURSING DIAGNOSIS:

Sexual dysfunction

related to:

a. decreased libido associated with feelings of loss of femininity/masculinity and sexual attractiveness, fear of offensive odor or leakage of urine from the stoma (if client has an internal reservoir) or urostomy appliance, fear of rejection by partner, discomfort resulting from surgical incision, and depression;

b. impotence (can occur as a result of nerve damage during a radical cystectomy);

c. decreased potential for orgasm in the female client associated with clitoral injury (can occur with radical cystectomy);

d. dyspareunia associated with narrowing and shortening of the vaginal canal resulting from removal of a portion of the anterior vaginal wall if a radical cystectomy was performed.

Desired Outcome	Nursing Actions and *Selected Purposes/Rationales*

4. The client will demonstrate beginning acceptance of changes in sexual functioning as evidenced by:
  a. verbalization of a perception of self as sexually acceptable and adequate
  b. statements reflecting beginning adjustment to the effects of the urinary diversion on sexuality
  c. maintenance of relationship with significant other.
	4.a. Assess for signs and symptoms of sexual dysfunction (e.g. verbalization of sexual concerns or inability to achieve sexual satisfaction, alteration in relationship with significant other, limitations imposed by nerve damage and structural changes incurred during surgery).
	  b. Provide accurate information about effects of the surgery and urinary diversion on sexual functioning. Encourage questions and clarify misconceptions.
	  c. Implement measures *to promote optimal sexual functioning:*
	    1. facilitate communication between client and partner; focus on the feelings the couple share and assist them to identify changes that may affect their sexual relationship
	    2. perform actions to facilitate psychological adjustment to the changes that have occurred (see Postoperative Nursing Diagnoses 5, actions d–r; 6, action c; and 7, action b)
	    3. instruct client in ways *to reduce risk of leakage of urine during sexual activity:*
	      a. empty the pouch or drain internal reservoir (if present) before sexual activity
	      b. secure appliance seal with tape for added security
	    4. if client is concerned about odor, instruct him/her to:
	      a. shower or bathe before sexual activity
	      b. use an odorproof pouch or pouch deodorant
	      c. use cologne or perfume if desired
	      d. keep room well ventilated
	    5. if appropriate, involve partner in urostomy care *to facilitate partner's adjustment to the changes in client's appearance and body functioning and subsequently decrease the possibility of partner's rejection of client*

Desired Outcome	Nursing Actions and *Selected Purposes/Rationales*

6. if client is concerned about the presence of the stoma and appliance, discuss the possibility of:
   a. using opaque or patterned pouches or decorative pouch covers
   b. wearing underwear with the crotch removed (for females), boxer shorts (for males), or a cummerbund or stretch tube top around abdomen during sexual activity
7. arrange for uninterrupted privacy during hospital stay if desired by the couple
8. if client is concerned that operative site discomfort will interfere with usual sexual activity:
   a. assure him/her that discomfort is temporary and will diminish as the incision heals
   b. encourage alternatives to intercourse or use of positions that decrease pressure on surgical site (e.g. side-lying)
9. if impotence is a problem:
   a. encourage client to discuss it and various treatment options (e.g. vacuum erection aids, penile prosthesis) with physician
   b. suggest alternative methods of sexual gratification if appropriate
   c. discuss alternative methods of becoming a parent (e.g. artificial insemination, adoption) if of concern to client
10. discuss ways to be creative in expressing sexuality (e.g. massage, fantasies, cuddling)
11. if appropriate, discuss with female client the need for vaginal dilatation after healing has occurred *to prevent further contraction and shortening of the vaginal canal*
12. encourage client to obtain written information regarding sexual activity from the United Ostomy Association and from manufacturers of urostomy appliances
13. include partner in above discussion and encourage continued support of the client.
   d. Consult physician if counseling appears indicated.

---

5. **NURSING DIAGNOSIS:**   **Self-concept disturbance***

related to:
a. loss of ability to urinate normally;
b. dependence (usually temporary) on others for assistance with urostomy management;
c. loss of control of urinary elimination if client has a conventional conduit;
d. change in appearance associated with the presence of a stoma and urostomy appliance;
e. changes in usual sexual functioning;
f. embarrassment associated with odor of urostomy drainage and appliance;
g. sterility associated with:
   1. loss of ejaculatory function in the male client resulting from removal of the prostate and seminal vesicles if a radical cystectomy was performed
   2. removal of the ovaries, uterus, and fallopian tubes in the female client if a radical cystectomy was performed.

---

*This diagnostic label includes the nursing diagnoses of body image disturbance, self-esteem disturbance, and altered role performance.

Desired Outcome	Nursing Actions and *Selected Purposes/Rationales*

5. The client will demonstrate beginning adaptation to changes in appearance, body

5.a. Assess for signs and symptoms of a self-concept disturbance (e.g. verbalization of negative feelings about self, withdrawal from significant others, lack of participation in activities of daily living, refusal to look at

functioning, and life style as evidenced by:

a. verbalization of feelings of self-worth
b. maintenance of relationships with significant others
c. active participation in activities of daily living
d. verbalization of a beginning plan for integrating changes in appearance and body functioning into life style.

or touch stoma, lack of plan for adapting to necessary changes in life style).

b. Determine the meaning of changes in appearance, body functioning, and life style to the client by encouraging verbalization of feelings and by noting nonverbal responses to the changes experienced.

c. Implement measures to facilitate the grieving process (see Postoperative Nursing Diagnosis 7, action b).

d. Discuss with client improvements in body functioning and appearance that can realistically be expected.

e. Implement measures *to assist client to increase self-esteem* (e.g. limit negative self-assessment, encourage positive comments about self, assist to identify strengths, give positive feedback about accomplishments and behaviors that are indicative of high self-esteem).

f. Reinforce actions to assist client to cope with effects of the urinary diversion (see Postoperative Nursing Diagnosis 6, action c).

g. Implement measures to promote optimal sexual functioning (see Postoperative Nursing Diagnosis 4, action c).

h. Instruct and assist client in ways *to decrease odor of urostomy drainage and appliance:*
   1. use odorproof pouches and change appliance regularly
   2. use disposable appliances or clean reusable items thoroughly
   3. empty appliance regularly
   4. perform actions to achieve an adequate appliance seal (see Postoperative Nursing Diagnosis 1, action b.4.j.3)
   5. drain the internal reservoir (if present) at scheduled intervals and when it feels full to reduce the possibility of urine leakage from stoma
   6. increase intake of foods/fluids that are known to help reduce odor of urine (e.g. cranberry juice, yogurt, buttermilk) unless contraindicated
   7. avoid foods that cause urine to have a strong odor (e.g. asparagus, cabbage)
   8. use room or pouch deodorizers
   9. change bed linens and clothing as soon as they become soiled.

i. Assure client that once the edema and discomfort associated with the surgery have resolved, he/she will be able to dress as before with minor, if any, modifications.

j. Show client and significant others some of the attractive urostomy products that are available (e.g. opaque or patterned pouches, pouch covers).

k. Assist client with usual grooming and makeup habits if necessary.

l. Promote activities that require client to confront the body changes that have occurred (e.g. active participation in urostomy care). Be aware that the integration of the change in body image does not usually occur until 2–6 months after the actual physical change has occurred.

m. Demonstrate acceptance of client using techniques such as touch and frequent visits. Encourage significant others to do the same.

n. Support behaviors suggesting positive adaptation to changes that have occurred (e.g. willingness to care for urostomy, compliance with the treatment plan, verbalization of feelings of self-worth, maintenance of relationships with significant others).

o. Encourage significant others to allow client to do what he/she is able *so that independence can be re-established and/or self-esteem redeveloped.*

p. Assist client's and significant others' adjustment by listening, facilitating communication, and providing information.

q. Encourage visits and support from significant others.

r. Encourage client to pursue usual roles and interests and to continue involvement in social activities.

s. Consult physician about psychological counseling if client desires or seems unwilling or unable to adapt to changes resulting from the urinary diversion.

6. NURSING DIAGNOSIS: **Ineffective individual coping**

related to:
a. fear, anxiety, and depression associated with the diagnosis, prognosis, loss of control over urinary elimination (especially with a conventional conduit), and possibility of rejection by others;
b. difficulty performing urostomy care and incorporating the care into life style;
c. need for lifelong medical supervision.

Desired Outcome	Nursing Actions and *Selected Purposes/Rationales*

6. The client will demonstrate effective coping as evidenced by:
a. verbalization of ability to cope with the urinary diversion and its effects
b. utilization of appropriate problem-solving techniques
c. willingness to participate in treatment plan and meet basic needs
d. absence of destructive behavior toward self and others
e. appropriate use of defense mechanisms
f. utilization of available support systems.
	6.a. Assess for and report signs and symptoms of ineffective individual coping (e.g. verbalization of inability to cope; inability to ask for help, problem solve, or meet basic needs; insomnia; withdrawal; reluctance to participate in treatment plan; destructive behavior toward self or others; inappropriate use of defense mechanisms; inability to meet role expectations).
	b. Assess client's perception of current situation.
	c. Implement measures *to promote effective coping:*
	  1. allow time for client to begin to adjust to the urinary diversion
	  2. assist client to recognize and manage inappropriate denial if it is present
	  3. if acceptable to client, arrange for a visit with an ostomate of similar age and same sex who has successfully adjusted to a urinary diversion
	  4. perform actions to reduce fear and anxiety (see Standardized Postoperative Care Plan, Nursing Diagnosis 20, action b [p. 122])
	  5. encourage verbalization about current situation
	  6. assist client to identify personal strengths and resources that can be utilized to facilitate coping with the current situation
	  7. demonstrate acceptance of client but set limits on inappropriate behavior
	  8. create an atmosphere of trust and support
	  9. maintain consistency of approaches and explanations
	  10. do not overload client with information irrelevant to present stage of urostomy management unless client is questioning or expressing an interest
	  11. encourage participation in urostomy care as soon as possible
	  12. use products that client is expected to use when discharged
	  13. ensure adequate time for and privacy during urostomy care
	  14. include client in planning of care, encourage maximum participation in urostomy care, and allow choices when possible *to enable him/her to maintain a sense of control*
	  15. instruct client in effective problem-solving techniques (e.g. accurate identification of stressors, determination of various options to solve problem)
	  16. assist client to maintain usual daily routines whenever possible
	  17. discuss with significant others the fear of rejection client may be experiencing and encourage their support
	  18. instruct client to have extra urostomy products readily available at all times
	  19. administer antianxiety and/or antidepressant agents if ordered
	  20. assist client to identify and utilize available support systems; provide information about available community resources that can assist client and significant others in coping with effects of urinary diversion and the underlying disease process (e.g. United Ostomy Association, American Cancer Society, counseling services, local ostomy support groups, community health agencies)
	  21. encourage the client to share with significant others the kind of

support that would be most beneficial (e.g. listening, inspiring hope, providing reassurance and accurate information)

22. support behaviors indicative of effective coping (e.g. participation in urostomy care, verbalization of ability to cope, utilization of effective problem-solving strategies).

d. Consult physician about psychological counseling if appropriate. Initiate a referral if necessary.

---

7. NURSING DIAGNOSIS:	**Grieving***

related to loss of the ability to urinate normally, change in appearance, and possible effects of the surgery on sexual functioning.

*This diagnostic label includes anticipatory grieving and grieving following the actual losses.

Desired Outcome	Nursing Actions and *Selected Purposes/Rationales*

7. The client will demonstrate beginning progression through the grieving process as evidenced by:
   a. verbalization of feelings about the urinary diversion and its effects
   b. usual sleep pattern
   c. participation in treatment plan and self-care activities
   d. utilization of available support systems
   e. verbalization of a plan for integrating urostomy care into life style.

7.a. Assess for signs and symptoms of grieving (e.g. change in eating habits, inability to concentrate, insomnia, anger, sadness, withdrawal from significant others, denial of loss).

b. Implement measures *to facilitate the grieving process:*

1. assist client to acknowledge the losses *so grief work can begin*; assess for factors that may hinder and facilitate acknowledgment
2. discuss the grieving process and assist client to accept the phases of grieving as an expected response to actual and anticipated losses
3. allow time for client to progress through the phases of grieving (phases vary among theorists but progress from shock and alarm to acceptance); be aware that not every phase is expressed by all individuals, that recurrence of phases is common, and that the grieving process may take months to years
4. provide an atmosphere of care and concern (e.g. provide privacy, be available and nonjudgmental, display empathy and respect) *so client will feel free to express feelings*
5. perform actions *to promote trust* (e.g. answer questions honestly, provide requested information)
6. encourage the verbal expression of anger and sadness about the losses experienced; recognize displacement of anger and assist client to see the actual cause of angry feelings and resentment
7. encourage client to express feelings in whatever ways are comfortable (e.g. writing, drawing, conversation)
8. perform actions to promote effective coping (see Postoperative Nursing Diagnosis 6, action c)
9. support realistic hope about the effects of the surgery on his/her life (e.g. increased comfort, improved urinary elimination, treatment of underlying disease process)
10. support behaviors suggesting successful grief work (e.g. verbalizing feelings about the urinary diversion, focusing on ways to adapt to losses, learning to care for urostomy)
11. explain the phases of the grieving process to significant others; encourage their support and understanding
12. facilitate communication between the client and significant others; be aware that they may be in different phases of the grieving process
13. provide information regarding counseling services and support groups that might assist client in working through grief
14. when appropriate, assist client to meet spiritual needs (e.g. arrange for visit from clergy).

Desired Outcome	Nursing Actions and *Selected Purposes/Rationales*
	c. Consult physician about referral for counseling if signs of dysfunctional grieving (e.g. persistent denial of losses, excessive anger or sadness, emotional lability) occur.

Discharge Teaching

■──

8. NURSING DIAGNOSIS: **Knowledge deficit, Ineffective management of therapeutic regimen, or Altered health maintenance***

> *The nurse should select the diagnostic label that is most appropriate for the client's discharge teaching needs.

Desired Outcomes	Nursing Actions and *Selected Purposes/Rationales*
8.a. The client will verbalize a basic understanding of the anatomical changes that have occurred as a result of the surgery.	8.a. Reinforce teaching about the anatomical changes that have occurred as a result of the cystectomy and urinary diversion. Use appropriate teaching aids (e.g. pictures, videotapes, anatomical models).
8.b. The client will demonstrate the ability to change the urostomy appliance and maintain stomal and peristomal skin integrity.	8.b.1. Reinforce teaching regarding application of the appliance, prevention of peristomal skin irritation and breakdown, and maintenance of stomal integrity (see Postoperative Nursing Diagnosis 1, actions b.4 and 5 and Collaborative Diagnosis 3, action a.2, for appropriate measures).
	2. Instruct and assist client to establish a routine for emptying the pouch and changing the appliance. Support client's efforts to maintain integrity of stoma and peristomal skin and keep the pouch from overfilling but discourage excessive emptying of the pouch and changing appliance more often than necessary.
	3. Inform client that despite good urostomy care, urine crystals (a result of continued exposure to alkaline urine over time) and encrustations (from mucus accumulation) can form on the stoma and peristomal skin. Explain that if client notices crystals or encrustations, he/she should:
	a. cleanse the stoma and peristomal skin with a solution of white vinegar and water (usually 1:1) each time appliance is changed
	b. replace reusable appliances from which crystals or encrustations cannot be completely removed
	c. consult physician or enterostomal therapist about additional care measures.
	4. Instruct client to follow special precautions for products used (e.g. inert, moldable skin barriers must be kept in airtight container; skin sealants should be used only on healthy peristomal skin because they can further irritate reddened and excoriated skin).
	5. Allow time for questions, clarification, practice, and return demonstration of emptying the pouch, changing the appliance, and performing appropriate stoma and peristomal skin care.
8.c. The client will demonstrate the ability to properly clean reusable urostomy equipment.	8.c.1. Discuss recommended method of cleaning reusable urostomy equipment based on manufacturer's recommendations.
	2. Demonstrate appropriate appliance cleansing. Emphasize importance of:
	a. washing and rinsing appliance thoroughly upon removal
	b. soaking pouch according to manufacturer's instructions
	c. allowing appliance to dry thoroughly before reusing
	d. storing appliance according to manufacturer's instructions (e.g. apply powder or cornstarch to inside of pouch; keep items in a clean, dry place).
	3. Allow time for questions, clarification, and return demonstration.

8.d. The client will demonstrate the ability to drain and irrigate a continent internal reservoir if present.

8.d.1. Demonstrate the correct method of inserting a catheter through the stoma to drain or irrigate the internal reservoir.

2. Reinforce physician's instructions about the frequency of draining the reservoir (initially the reservoir may need to be emptied every 2–3 hours but, as the incisions heal and the reservoir stretches, the client should be able to extend this to every 4–6 hours during the day and once during the night).

3. Demonstrate correct technique for irrigating an internal reservoir. Caution client to use only the prescribed amount of irrigant in order to avoid overdistending and damaging the reservoir. Inform client that the irrigation is done to remove mucus that is secreted by the bowel segment used to construct the reservoir, that this mucus production decreases over time, and that irrigations will be needed less frequently or not at all as time goes by.

4. Allow time for questions, clarification, practice, and return demonstration of drainage and irrigation of an internal reservoir.

8.e. The client will identify ways to control odor of the urostomy drainage and appliance.

8.e. Provide instructions on ways to control odor of urostomy drainage and appliance:

1. drink at least 10 glasses of liquid/day unless contraindicated; increase volume of liquid if urine appears concentrated

2. avoid foods that cause urine to have a strong odor (e.g. asparagus, cabbage)

3. increase intake of foods/fluids that reduce urine odor (e.g. cranberry juice, yogurt, buttermilk) unless contraindicated

4. place a small amount of deodorizer in bottom of pouch

5. change appliance at appropriate intervals

6. cleanse reusable appliances thoroughly

7. use odorproof pouch and empty it regularly.

8.f. The client will identify ways to prevent urinary tract infection.

8.f. Provide instructions on ways to prevent urinary tract infection:

1. drink at least 10 glasses of liquid/day unless contraindicated

2. prevent reflux of urine by:
   a. emptying pouch when it is 1/3 full
   b. attaching a bedside collection system when lying down for an extended period
   c. using a pouch with an antireflux valve

3. maintain urine acidity by:
   a. increasing intake of foods/fluids that acidify the urine (e.g. cranberry juice, prune juice, plums, poultry, fish, whole grains)
   b. avoiding excessive intake of milk, carbonated beverages, and citrus fruit
   c. taking medications such as ascorbic acid as prescribed

4. clean reusable appliances thoroughly (see action c.2 in this diagnosis).

8.g. The client will state signs and symptoms to report to the health care provider.

8.g.1. Refer to Standardized Postoperative Care Plan, Nursing Diagnosis 21, action c (p. 123), for signs and symptoms to report to the health care provider.

2. Instruct client to also report:
   a. dark red, blue-black, or pale stoma
   b. absence of or reduction in urinary output despite an adequate fluid intake
   c. excessive bleeding of stoma or bloody drainage from stoma
   d. excessive mucus drainage from urinary meatus (some drainage should be expected for several weeks postoperatively)
   e. change in contour of stoma (use diagrams and descriptive terms so client does not confuse decreasing stomal size due to resolving edema with actual stomal retraction)
   f. persistent skin irritation or breakdown of peristomal skin
   g. persistent presence of urine crystals or encrustations on stoma or peristomal skin
   h. persistent leakage of urostomy appliance
   i. persistent leakage of urine from stoma (if client has a continent internal reservoir)
   j. difficulty draining or irrigating an internal reservoir if present

Desired Outcomes	Nursing Actions and *Selected Purposes/Rationales*

	k. signs and symptoms of urinary tract infection (e.g. fever; chills; bloody or cloudy, foul-smelling urine; increased sediment in urine)
	   l. signs and symptoms of renal calculi (e.g. dull, aching or severe, colicky flank pain; blood in urine; nausea; vomiting); stone formation, a late complication of a urinary diversion, may result from persistent urinary stasis, urinary tract infection, or inadequate fluid intake
	  m. difficulty adjusting to change in appearance, urostomy care, or altered urinary elimination.

8.h. The client will identify appropriate community resources that can assist with home management and adjustment to changes resulting from the urinary diversion.	8.h.1. Provide information about community resources that can assist the client and significant others with home management and adjustment to changes resulting from urinary diversion (e.g. local ostomy support groups; American Cancer Society; community health agencies; enterostomal therapist; home health agencies; financial, individual, and family counseling services). 2. Initiate a referral if indicated.

8.i. The client will verbalize an understanding of and a plan for adhering to recommended follow-up care including future appointments with health care provider, wound care, activity level, and medications prescribed.	8.i.1. Refer to Standardized Postoperative Care Plan, Nursing Diagnosis 21 (pp. 123–124), for routine postoperative instructions and measures to improve client compliance.
	   2. Reinforce the physician's instructions regarding activity limitations:
	     a. avoid lifting heavy objects until permitted by physician
	     b. avoid participating in contact sports.
	   3. Explain the rationale for, side effects of, and importance of taking medications prescribed (e.g. antimicrobials, ascorbic acid). Inform client of pertinent food and drug interactions.
	   4. Provide client with a list of urostomy products he/she is using (include product name, size, and number) and where these supplies can be obtained.

Bibliography

See pages 897–898 and 905.

NEPHRECTOMY

Nephrectomy is the surgical removal of the kidney. Conditions that are commonly treated by nephrectomy include renal carcinoma, massive traumatic injury to the kidney, polycystic kidney disease (especially if the kidney is bleeding or severely infected), calculi, renal tuberculosis, pyelonephritis, glomerulonephritis, and renal sclerosis resulting from hypertension. The kidney may also be removed for the purpose of donation.

The surgical approach used to perform a nephrectomy depends on the extensiveness of the planned surgery; the client's age, body build, and physiological status; the underlying pathology; and prior surgical incisions. A common approach utilized for a simple nephrectomy is the subcostal flank approach. Other approaches (e.g. thoracoabdominal, transabdominal, dorsolumbar) may be necessary when greater visualization, improved access, or a more radical procedure is necessary.

This care plan focuses on the adult client hospitalized for a simple unilateral nephrectomy. Preoperatively, the goals of care are to reduce fear and anxiety and prepare the client for the surgical experience. Postoperative goals of care are to maintain comfort, prevent complications, and educate the client regarding follow-up care. The care plan will need to be individualized according to the client's diagnosis, prognosis, and plans for subsequent treatment.

DIAGNOSTIC TESTS

Intravenous pyelogram (IVP)
Magnetic resonance imaging (MRI)
Ultrasonography
Computed tomography (CT)

Radionuclide renal scan
Renal angiography
X-ray of kidneys, ureters, and bladder (KUB)
Blood chemistry
Urinalysis
Creatinine clearance

DISCHARGE CRITERIA

Prior to discharge, the client will:

- have evidence of normal healing of surgical wound
- have adequate functioning of the remaining kidney
- have clear, audible breath sounds throughout lungs
- have no signs and symptoms of postoperative complications
- verbalize ways to maintain health of the remaining kidney
- state signs and symptoms to report to the health care provider
- share thoughts and feelings about the loss of the kidney
- verbalize an understanding of and a plan for adhering to recommended follow-up care including future appointments with health care provider, medications prescribed, activity level, wound care, and plans for subsequent treatment of the underlying disorder.

NURSING/ COLLABORATIVE DIAGNOSES

Preoperative
1. Anxiety △ 529
Postoperative
1. Ineffective breathing pattern △ 530
2. Potential complications:
   a. hypovolemic shock
   b. paralytic ileus
   c. pneumothorax △ 530

DISCHARGE TEACHING

3. Knowledge deficit, Ineffective management of therapeutic regimen, or Altered health maintenance △ 532

See Standardized Preoperative and Postoperative Care Plans for additional diagnoses.

PREOPERATIVE

Use in conjunction with the Standardized Preoperative Care Plan.

1. NURSING DIAGNOSIS:

Anxiety

related to:
a. unfamiliar environment and separation from significant others;
b. anticipated loss of control associated with effects of anesthesia;
c. lack of understanding of diagnostic tests and planned surgical procedure;
d. financial concerns associated with hospitalization;
e. anticipated discomfort, surgical findings, and change in body functioning as a result of loss of a kidney.

Desired Outcome	Nursing Actions and *Selected Purposes/Rationales*

1. The client will experience a reduction in anxiety (see Standardized Preoperative Care Plan, Nursing Diagnosis 1 [pp. 96–97], for outcome criteria).	1.a. Refer to Standardized Preoperative Care Plan, Nursing Diagnosis 1 (pp. 96–97), for measures related to assessment and reduction of fear and anxiety.
	b. Implement additional measures *to reduce fear and anxiety:*
	  1. reinforce physician's explanation that normal kidney function can be maintained by a single healthy kidney
	  2. begin teaching the client about ways to maintain the health of the kidney that will remain; assure him/her that this information will be reviewed again in detail prior to discharge.

POSTOPERATIVE

Use in conjunction with the Standardized Postoperative Care Plan.

---

1. NURSING DIAGNOSIS:

Ineffective breathing pattern

related to:
a. increased rate and decreased depth of respirations associated with fear and anxiety;
b. decreased rate and depth of respirations associated with the depressant effect of anesthesia and some medications (e.g. narcotic [opioid] analgesics);
c. diminished lung/chest wall expansion associated with:
  1. reluctance to breathe deeply resulting from incisional pain and fear of dislodging chest tube if present (a chest tube is usually inserted following a thoracoabdominal approach)
  2. positioning, weakness, fatigue, and elevation of the diaphragm (can occur if abdominal distention is present).

Desired Outcome	Nursing Actions and *Selected Purposes/Rationales*

1. The client will maintain an effective breathing pattern (see Standardized Postoperative Care Plan, Nursing Diagnosis 2 [p. 102], for outcome criteria).	1.a. Refer to Standardized Postoperative Care Plan, Nursing Diagnosis 2 (pp. 102–103), for measures related to assessment and management of an ineffective breathing pattern.
	b. Implement additional measures *to improve breathing pattern:*
	  1. assure client that deep breathing will not dislodge chest tube if present
	  2. provide pillow support between lower costal margin and iliac crest when client is lying on operative side *in order to decrease strain on flank incision and subsequently increase ease of deep breathing.*

---

2. COLLABORATIVE DIAGNOSES:

Potential complications of nephrectomy:

a. **hypovolemic shock** related to hypovolemia associated with excessive blood loss during surgery (the renal area is highly vascular), inadequate fluid replacement, and hemorrhage (can occur if there is excessive stress on the newly ligated operative site vessels);
b. **paralytic ileus** related to manipulation of the bowel during surgery, effect of anesthesia and some medications (e.g. central nervous system depressants) on bowel motility, and hypovolemia if it occurs (can cause decreased blood supply to the intestine);
c. **pneumothorax** related to an accumulation of air in the pleural space associated with surgical opening of the pleura (occurs most frequently with the thoracoabdominal approach) and/or malfunction of chest tube if present.

Desired Outcomes	Nursing Actions and *Selected Purposes/Rationales*

2.a. The client will not develop hypovolemic shock (see Standardized Postoperative Care Plan, Collaborative Diagnosis 19, outcome a [p. 120], for outcome criteria).

2.a.1. Refer to Standardized Postoperative Care Plan, Collaborative Diagnosis 19, action a (p. 120), for measures related to assessment, prevention, and treatment of hypovolemic shock.
   2. Implement additional measures *to prevent hypovolemic shock:*
      a. perform actions *to reduce stress on the surgical wound in order to reduce the risk for hemorrhage:*
         1. instruct client to splint incisional area with hands or pillow when turning and coughing
         2. implement measures to prevent nausea and vomiting (see Standardized Postoperative Care Plan, Nursing Diagnosis 7.B, action 2 [pp. 108–109]).
      b. prepare client for surgery (e.g. ligation of bleeding vessels) if indicated.

2.b. The client will have resolution of a paralytic ileus if it occurs (see Standardized Postoperative Care Plan, Collaborative Diagnosis 19, outcome d [p. 121], for outcome criteria).

2.b. Refer to Standardized Postoperative Care Plan, Collaborative Diagnosis 19, action d (p. 121), for measures related to assessment and management of a paralytic ileus.

2.c. The client will experience normal lung re-expansion if pneumothorax occurs as evidenced by:
   1. audible breath sounds and resonant percussion note by the 3rd–4th postoperative day
   2. unlabored respirations at 14–20/minute
   3. blood gases returning toward normal
   4. chest x-ray showing lung re-expansion.

2.c.1. Assess for and immediately report signs and symptoms of:
      a. malfunction of the chest drainage system (e.g. respiratory distress, lack of fluctuation in water seal chamber without evidence of lung re-expansion, excessive bubbling in water seal chamber, significant increase in subcutaneous emphysema)
      b. further lung collapse (e.g. extended area of absent breath sounds with hyperresonant percussion note; rapid, shallow, and/or labored respirations; tachycardia; increased chest pain; restlessness; confusion).
   2. Monitor for and report the following:
      a. blood gas results that have worsened
      b. significant decrease in oximetry results
      c. chest x-ray results showing delayed lung re-expansion or further lung collapse.
   3. Implement measures *to promote lung re-expansion and prevent further lung collapse:*
      a. perform actions *to maintain patency and integrity of chest drainage system:*
         1. maintain fluid levels in the water seal and suction chambers as ordered
         2. maintain occlusive dressing over chest tube insertion site
         3. tape all connections securely
         4. tape the tubing close to insertion site to the chest wall *to reduce the risk of inadvertent removal of the tube*
         5. position tubing *to promote optimum drainage* (e.g. coil excess tubing on bed rather than allowing it to hang down below the collection device, keep tubing free of kinks)
         6. drain fluid that accumulates in tubing into the collection chamber; milk chest tube only if ordered
         7. keep drainage collection device below level of client's chest at all times
      b. implement measures *to facilitate the escape of air from the pleural space* (e.g. maintain suction as ordered, ensure that the air vent is open on the drainage collection device if system is to water seal only)
      c. perform actions to improve breathing pattern (see Postoperative Nursing Diagnosis 1) and facilitate airway clearance (see Standardized Postoperative Care Plan, Nursing Diagnosis 3, action b [pp. 103–104]).
   4. If signs and symptoms of further lung collapse occur:

Desired Outcomes	Nursing Actions and **Selected Purposes/Rationales**
	a. maintain client on bed rest in a semi- to high Fowler's position
	b. maintain oxygen therapy as ordered
	c. assess for and immediately report signs and symptoms of tension pneumothorax with mediastinal shift (e.g. severe dyspnea, increased restlessness and agitation, rapid and/or irregular pulse rate, hypotension, neck vein distention, shift in trachea from midline)
	d. assist with clearing of existing chest tube and/or insertion of a new tube.

Discharge Teaching

■━━

3. NURSING DIAGNOSIS: **Knowledge deficit, Ineffective management of therapeutic regimen, or Altered health maintenance***

_____

*The nurse should select the diagnostic label that is most appropriate for the client's discharge teaching needs.

Desired Outcomes	Nursing Actions and **Selected Purposes/Rationales**

3.a. The client will verbalize ways to maintain health of the remaining kidney.	3.a. Instruct client regarding ways to maintain health of the remaining kidney:
	1. adhere to precautions to prevent a urinary tract infection:
	  a. perform actions to prevent urinary stasis:
	    1. drink at least 10 glasses of liquid/day unless contraindicated
	    2. urinate whenever the urge is felt
	    3. avoid long periods of inactivity (if unable to maintain a program of moderate activity, be sure to change positions frequently)
	  b. wipe from front to back after urinating and defecating (if female)
	  c. keep perineal area clean and dry
	2. immediately report signs and symptoms of a urinary tract infection (e.g. chills; fever; urgency, frequency, or burning on urination; cloudy, foul-smelling urine)
	3. notify physician if a cold or other infection persists for more than 2–3 days or if unable to maintain an adequate fluid intake
	4. inform other health care providers about the nephrectomy so that prophylactic antimicrobials may be initiated before dental work and invasive procedures such as cystoscopy and minor surgeries
	5. avoid activities that might cause trauma to the remaining kidney (e.g. contact sports, horseback riding)
	6. consult physician before taking any prescription and nonprescription medications that could damage the remaining kidney (e.g. ibuprofen, cimetidine, naproxen, neomycin, gentamicin)
	7. if nephrectomy was performed because of renal calculi, reinforce physician's instructions about diet, drug therapy, and daily fluid requirements to prevent formation of stones in the remaining kidney
	8. if surgery was necessary because of renal hypertension, reinforce the physician's instructions about methods of controlling B/P (e.g. dietary modifications, medications, stress management).

3.b. The client will state signs and symptoms to report to the health care provider.	3.b.1. Refer to Standardized Postoperative Care Plan, Nursing Diagnosis 21, action c (p. 123), for signs and symptoms to report to the health care provider.
	2. Instruct client to report these additional signs and symptoms:
	  a. unexplained weight gain
	  b. decreased urine output
	  c. flank pain on the unoperative side
	  d. blood in the urine.

3.c. The client will verbalize an understanding of and a plan for adhering to recommended follow-up care including future appointments with health care provider, medications prescribed, activity level, wound care, and plans for subsequent treatment of the underlying disorder.

3.c.1. Refer to Standardized Postoperative Care Plan, Nursing Diagnosis 21, (pp. 123–124), for routine postoperative instructions and measures to improve client compliance.

2. Reinforce physician's instructions regarding activity:
   a. gauge activity according to tolerance and allow adequate rest periods
   b. avoid lifting objects over 7–10 pounds, pushing heavy objects, and exercising strenuously for specified length of time (usually 6–12 weeks).

3. Clarify plans for subsequent treatment of the underlying disorder (e.g. chemotherapy, radiation therapy) if appropriate.

Bibliography

See pages 897–898 and 905–906.

UNIT THIRTEEN

NURSING CARE OF THE CLIENT WITH DISTURBANCES OF HEMATOPOIETIC AND LYMPHATIC FUNCTION

HUMAN IMMUNODEFICIENCY VIRUS (HIV) INFECTION AND ACQUIRED IMMUNE DEFICIENCY SYNDROME (AIDS)

Acquired immune deficiency syndrome (AIDS) is an infectious disease of the immune system and is considered to be the last phase of the clinical spectrum of infection by the human immunodeficiency virus (HIV). HIV is a retrovirus that affects the cells in the body that have a CD4 molecule (a glycoprotein) on their surface. The virus can infect several types of human cells including lymphocytes, monocytes, macrophages, glial cells, bone marrow progenitors, and the gut epithelium. The CD4+ T lymphocytes (also called T_4 or T-helper lymphocytes) have the greatest number of CD4 receptors and are consequently the major target of HIV. These lymphocytes are ultimately destroyed by HIV, which results in severely impaired cell-mediated immunity in the host. Humoral immune function is also impaired because the B cells are unable to respond appropriately to the presence of a new antigen without the help of normal CD4+ T lymphocytes. The effect of HIV on the macrophage as well as the effect of the altered CD4+ T lymphocyte function on macrophage activity further depresses immune system function.

HIV has been isolated from all body fluids but at this point, transmission has been associated only with blood, semen, vaginal secretions, and breast milk. The known routes of transmission are by intimate sexual contact, mucous membrane or percutaneous exposure to infected blood or blood products, and perinatal transmission from mother to child.

Infection with HIV tends to follow a particular course, with the clinical expression being attributed to either the effects of the virus itself or the consequences of CD4+ T lymphocyte depletion. The initial event in the course of the disease is acute (primary) HIV infection ("acute retroviral syndrome"), which occurs about the time of seroconversion (usually within 3–12 weeks after exposure to HIV). The person experiences mononucleosis or flu-like symptoms (e.g. fever, headache, myalgias, lymphadenopathy, rash) that may persist for a week or longer. Following resolution of these initial symptoms, the HIV-infected person enters an asymptomatic or latent phase that often lasts as long as 10–12 years, de-pending on the rate of viral replication and the rapidity of CD4+ T lymphocyte destruction. The next phase of HIV infection is manifested by the development of various nonspecific symptoms such as chronically enlarged lymph nodes (persistent generalized lymphadenopathy [PGL]), persistent localized viral or fungal infections, unexplained fever and weight loss, fatigue, night sweats, peripheral neuropathy, and persistent diarrhea. AIDS is the last phase of HIV infection. In addition to the symptoms experienced in the previous phase, AIDS is heralded by immune suppression (serologically defined as a CD4+ T lymphocyte count less than 200/µL) and the presence of a condition that meets the criteria for definition of an AIDS case as specified by the Centers for Disease Control and Prevention (CDC). These AIDS-indicator conditions include HIV-related encephalopathy, wasting syndrome, opportunistic infections (e.g. *Pneumocystis carinii* pneumonia [PCP], candidiasis, *Mycobacterium* tuberculosis, *Mycobacterium-avium* complex [MAC], cryptococcosis, cytomegalovirus disease, *Toxoplasma* encephalitis, coccidioidomycosis), and AIDS-related cancers (e.g. Kaposi's sarcoma, non-Hodgkin's lymphoma, invasive cervical cancer).

At this time, there is no cure for HIV infection or the subsequent immunodeficiency. Treatment is aimed primarily at controlling replication of HIV and preventing and controlling the potentially fatal opportunistic diseases. The antiretroviral agents used to control replication of HIV in the host include the reverse transcriptase inhibitors such as zidovudine (ZDV, Retrovir, AZT), zalcitabine (dideoxycytidine [ddC, Hivid]), didanosine (ddI, Videx), stavudine (d4T, Zerit), and lamivudine (3TC, Epivir) and the protease inhibitors (e.g. saquinavir, ritonavir, indinavir).

This care plan focuses on the adult client with HIV infection hospitalized for treatment of a probable opportunistic infection. The goals of care are to assist with measures to treat the infection and reduce the risk for additional infection, maintain fluid balance and an adequate nutritional status, maintain comfort, reduce fear and anxiety, assist the client to cope with the diagnosis, and educate him/her regarding follow-up care.

DIAGNOSTIC TESTS

Tests to Diagnose HIV Infection
Antibody tests (e.g. enzyme-linked immunosorbent assay [ELISA], western blot assay, immunofluorescence assay [IFA], radioimmunoprecipitation assay [RIPA])
P24-antigen assay
Polymerase chain reaction (PCR)
Viral cultures
Immune function tests (e.g. absolute CD4+ T lymphocyte count, percentage of CD4+ T lymphocytes, CD4/CD8 ratio, beta-2 microglobulin, serum neopterin)

Tests to Diagnose HIV and AIDS-Related Conditions
Complete blood count (CBC) and differential
Anergy testing (if in an area where tuberculosis is prevalent)
Tuberculin skin testing (PPD)

Specimen (e.g. blood, urine, sputum, cerebrospinal fluid, stool, drainage) testing for infectious agents (e.g. Gram's stain, acid-fast stains, acid-Schiff stain, stool cultures, antibody titers)

Neurological studies (e.g. MRI, CT scan, EMG)

Biopsies (e.g. mucocutaneous lesions, lung, brain, cervix)

Tests for sexually transmitted diseases (e.g. antigen and antibody tests for hepatitis B, VDRL or RPR for syphilis)

Chest x-ray

Pulmonary function tests

GI studies (e.g. barium swallow, endoscopy, colonoscopy)

Cervicovaginal cytology (Pap smear)

DISCHARGE CRITERIA

Prior to discharge, the client will:

- have an adequate respiratory status
- have an adequate or improved nutritional status
- be able to perform activities of daily living without undue fatigue or dyspnea
- demonstrate evidence that opportunistic infection is resolving
- be effectively managing the signs and symptoms of neurological dysfunction
- have discomfort at a manageable level
- show evidence that skin and oral mucous membranes are intact or healing appropriately
- have fewer episodes of diarrhea
- identify ways to prevent the spread of HIV
- identify ways to decrease the risk for developing opportunistic infections
- state signs and symptoms to report to the health care provider
- share feelings about change in self-concept and the social isolation that may result from the diagnosis
- identify resources that can assist in adjustment to changes resulting from the diagnosis of AIDS
- verbalize an understanding of and a plan for adhering to recommended follow-up care including regular laboratory studies, future appointments with health care providers, and medications prescribed.

NURSING/ COLLABORATIVE DIAGNOSES

1. Impaired respiratory function:
   a. ineffective breathing pattern
   b. ineffective airway clearance
   c. impaired gas exchange △ 538
2. Altered fluid and electrolyte balance:
   a. fluid volume deficit
   b. hypokalemia
   c. hyponatremia △ 539
3. Altered nutrition: less than body requirements △ 540
4. Pain:
   a. oral, pharyngeal, and/or esophageal pain
   b. abdominal pain
   c. neuropathic pain (e.g. painful paresthesias)
   d. headache
   e. chest pain
   f. skin and local tissue pain △ 542
5A. Altered comfort: chills and excessive diaphoresis △ 543
5B. Altered comfort: pruritus △ 543
6. Hyperthermia △ 544
7. Altered oral mucous membrane △ 545
8. Actual/Risk for impaired tissue integrity △ 546
9. Fatigue △ 547
10. Self-care deficit △ 548
11. Diarrhea △ 549

1. NURSING DIAGNOSIS:

Impaired respiratory function:*

a. **ineffective breathing pattern** related to:
   1. diminished lung/chest wall expansion associated with weakness, fatigue, and chest pain if present
   2. increased rate and decreased depth of respirations associated with anxiety and the increase in metabolic rate that occurs with infection;
b. **ineffective airway clearance** related to:
   1. increased production of secretions associated with some opportunistic infections of the lungs
   2. stasis of secretions associated with decreased activity and poor cough effort resulting from fatigue and pain;
c. **impaired gas exchange** related to a decrease in effective lung surface associated with:
   1. the presence of infiltrates and/or cavities in the lung tissue resulting from opportunistic infection of the lungs (e.g. *Pneumocystis carinii* pneumonia, pneumococcal pneumonia, *Mycobacterium* tuberculosis, histoplasmosis)
   2. compression and/or replacement of lung tissue if an AIDS-related cancer such as Kaposi's sarcoma or non-Hodgkin's lymphoma is present.

---

*This diagnostic label includes the following nursing diagnoses: ineffective breathing pattern, ineffective airway clearance, and impaired gas exchange.

Desired Outcome	Nursing Actions and *Selected Purposes/Rationales*

1. The client will experience adequate respiratory function as evidenced by:
a. normal rate and depth of respirations
b. decreased dyspnea
c. improved breath sounds
d. usual mental status
e. usual skin color
f. blood gases within normal range.
	1.a. Assess for and report signs and symptoms of impaired respiratory function:
	  1. rapid, shallow respirations
	  2. dyspnea, orthopnea
	  3. use of accessory muscles when breathing
	  4. abnormal breath sounds (e.g. diminished, bronchial, crackles [rales], wheezes)
	  5. cough (can be productive or dry and nonproductive depending on the opportunistic disease present)
	  6. restlessness, irritability
	  7. confusion, somnolence
	  8. central cyanosis (a late sign).

    b. Monitor for and report the following:
       1. abnormal blood gases
       2. significant decrease in oximetry results
       3. abnormal chest x-ray results.
    c. Implement measures *to improve respiratory status:*
       1. maintain activity restrictions as ordered *to reduce oxygen needs*
       2. place client in a semi- to high Fowler's position unless contraindicated; position with pillows *to prevent slumping*
       3. instruct client to breathe slowly if hyperventilating
       4. assist client to turn from side to side at least every 2 hours while in bed
       5. instruct client to deep breathe or use incentive spirometer every 1–2 hours
       6. assist with positive airway pressure techniques (e.g. IPPB, continuous positive airway pressure [CPAP], biphasic positive airway pressure [BiPAP], expiratory positive airway pressure [EPAP]) if ordered
       7. perform actions *to facilitate removal of pulmonary secretions:*
         a. instruct and assist client to cough or "huff" every 1–2 hours
         b. implement measures *to thin tenacious secretions and reduce dryness of the respiratory mucous membrane:*
           1. maintain a fluid intake of at least 2500 ml/day unless contraindicated
           2. humidify inspired air as ordered
         c. assist with administration of mucolytics and diluent or hydrating agents via nebulizer if ordered
         d. assist with or perform postural drainage therapy (PDT) if ordered
         e. perform suctioning if ordered
         f. administer expectorants if ordered
       8. perform actions to reduce pain and fatigue (see Nursing Diagnoses 4, action e and 9, action c) *in order to promote a more effective cough and increased activity*
       9. maintain oxygen therapy as ordered
      10. discourage smoking (*smoke increases mucus production, impairs ciliary function, decreases oxygen availability, and can cause inflammation and damage to the bronchial walls*)
      11. administer central nervous system depressants judiciously; hold medication and consult physician if respiratory rate is less than 12/ minute
      12. administer the following medications if ordered:
         a. bronchodilators (e.g. theophylline, albuterol)
         b. antimicrobials (e.g. trimethoprim-sulfamethoxazole [TMP/SMZ], amphotericin B, fluconazole, penicillin, ampicillin, antituberculosis regimen [isoniazid + rifampin + pyrazinamide + ethambutol or streptomycin])
         c. corticosteroids *to decrease pulmonary inflammation* (usually reserved for moderate to severe cases of *Pneumocystis carinii* pneumonia *because of the risk for further immunosuppression*).
    d. Consult physician if signs and symptoms of impaired respiratory function persist or worsen.

2. NURSING/COLLABORATIVE DIAGNOSES:

Altered fluid and electrolyte balance:
    a. **fluid volume deficit** related to:
       1. excessive loss of fluid associated with diarrhea, diaphoresis, and vomiting if present
       2. decreased oral intake associated with anorexia, weakness, nausea, and oropharyngeal pain;
    b. **hypokalemia** related to:

1. excessive loss of potassium associated with diarrhea, vomiting if present, and renal potassium wasting that can be induced by some antimicrobials (e.g. amphotericin B, sodium penicillin)
2. decreased oral intake;

c. **hyponatremia** related to:
1. excessive loss of sodium associated with diarrhea, profuse diaphoresis, and vomiting if present
2. fluid replacement with hypotonic solutions
3. water retention associated with increased ADH output resulting from opportunistic disease involvement of the lungs or central nervous system.

Desired Outcome	Nursing Actions and *Selected Purposes/Rationales*
2. The client will maintain fluid and electrolyte balance as evidenced by: a. normal skin turgor b. moist mucous membranes c. stable weight d. B/P and pulse within normal range for client and stable with position change e. hand vein filling time less than 3–5 seconds f. usual mental status g. balanced intake and output h. usual muscle strength i. soft, nondistended abdomen with normal bowel sounds j. absence of nausea, vomiting, abdominal cramps, and seizure activity k. BUN, Hct, and serum potassium and sodium within normal range.	2.a. Assess for and report signs and symptoms of: 1. fluid volume deficit: a. decreased skin turgor, dry mucous membranes, thirst b. sudden weight loss of 2% or greater c. postural hypotension and/or low B/P d. weak, rapid pulse e. delayed hand vein filling time (longer than 3–5 seconds) f. change in mental status g. decreased urine output (reflects an actual rather than potential fluid volume deficit) h. increased BUN and Hct (may not be increased if nutritional status is inadequate) 2. hypokalemia (e.g. cardiac dysrhythmias, postural hypotension, muscle weakness, nausea and vomiting, abdominal distention, hypoactive or absent bowel sounds, low serum potassium level) 3. hyponatremia (e.g. nausea, vomiting, abdominal cramps, lethargy, confusion, weakness, seizures, low serum sodium level). b. Implement measures *to prevent or treat fluid and electrolyte imbalances:* 1. perform actions to control diarrhea (see Nursing Diagnosis 11, action e) 2. perform actions to improve oral intake (see Nursing Diagnosis 3, action c.1) 3. perform actions to reduce fever (see Nursing Diagnosis 6, action b) 4. administer antiemetics if ordered *to control vomiting* 5. maintain a fluid intake of at least 2500 ml/day unless contraindicated 6. administer fluid and electrolyte replacements (e.g. oral solution containing water, sugar, baking soda, and salt; intravenous isotonic saline or lactated Ringer's; potassium supplements) if ordered 7. encourage intake of foods/fluids high in potassium (e.g. bananas, orange juice, potatoes, raisins, apricots, cantaloupe, tomato juice) and sodium (e.g. processed cheese, canned soups, canned vegetables, bouillon, tomato juice). c. Consult physician if signs and symptoms of fluid and electrolyte imbalances persist or worsen.

3. NURSING DIAGNOSIS:

Altered nutrition: less than body requirements

related to:
a. decreased oral intake associated with:
1. anorexia resulting from malaise, fatigue, fear, anxiety, pain, depression, and increased levels of certain cytokines that depress appetite (e.g. tumor necrosis factor [TNF])
2. nausea, dyspnea, and cognitive impairment if present
3. oral pain and/or dysphagia resulting from opportunistic lesions in the mouth, pharynx, and esophagus;

b. increased nutritional needs associated with:
  1. the increased metabolic rate that occurs with infection
  2. accelerated muscle breakdown resulting from increased levels of certain cytokines (e.g. TNF);
c. decreased absorption of nutrients if HIV and/or opportunistic infection involve the intestine;
d. loss of nutrients associated with persistent diarrhea and vomiting if present.

Desired Outcome	Nursing Actions and *Selected Purposes/Rationales*

3. The client will maintain an adequate nutritional status as evidenced by:
  a. weight within or returning toward normal range for client's age, height, and body frame
  b. normal BUN and serum albumin, Hct, Hb, and transferrin levels
  c. skinfold thickness and mid-arm circumference (MAC) within normal range
  d. usual strength and activity tolerance
  e. healthy oral mucous membrane.

3.a. Assess for and report signs and symptoms of malnutrition:
  1. weight below normal for client's age, height, and body frame
  2. abnormal BUN and low serum albumin, Hct, Hb, and transferrin levels
  3. skinfold thickness and mid-arm circumference (MAC) less than normal
  4. weakness and fatigue
  5. sore, inflamed oral mucous membrane
  6. pale conjunctiva.
b. Monitor percentage of meals and snacks client consumes. Report a pattern of inadequate intake.
c. Implement measures *to maintain an adequate nutritional status:*
  1. perform actions *to improve oral intake:*
    a. implement measures to maintain or regain integrity of the oral mucous membrane (see Nursing Diagnosis 7, action d)
    b. implement measures to reduce fear and anxiety (see Nursing Diagnosis 17, action b) and assist client to adjust psychologically to the diagnosis of AIDS (see Nursing Diagnoses 18, action c; 19, actions c–n; and 20, action b)
    c. perform actions *to reduce nausea* (e.g. administer prescribed antiemetics, encourage client to eat dry foods when nauseated, avoid serving foods with an overpowering aroma) if present
    d. perform actions to reduce pain (see Nursing Diagnosis 4, action e)
    e. increase activity as tolerated (*activity usually promotes a sense of well-being and improves appetite*)
    f. obtain a dietary consult if necessary to assist client in selecting foods/fluids that meet nutritional needs, are appealing, and adhere to personal and cultural preferences
    g. if client is having difficulty swallowing, assist him/her to select foods that are easily chewed and swallowed (e.g. eggs, custard, canned fruit) and avoid serving foods that are sticky (e.g. peanut butter, soft bread)
    h. encourage a rest period before meals *to minimize fatigue*
    i. maintain a clean environment and a relaxed, pleasant atmosphere
    j. provide oral hygiene before meals
    k. serve frequent, small meals rather than large ones if client is weak, fatigues easily, and/or has a poor appetite
    l. if client is dyspneic, place in a high Fowler's position for meals and provide supplemental oxygen therapy during meals
    m. if client's sense of taste is altered, suggest adding extra sweeteners and flavorings/seasonings to foods
    n. encourage significant others to bring in client's favorite foods and eat with him/her *to make eating more of a familiar social experience*
    o. assist client with meals if indicated
    p. allow adequate time for meals; reheat foods/fluids as necessary
  2. perform actions to control diarrhea (see Nursing Diagnosis 11, action e)
  3. ensure that meals are well balanced and high in essential nutrients; offer high-protein, high-calorie dietary supplements (e.g. Advera) if indicated

Desired Outcome	Nursing Actions and *Selected Purposes/Rationales*

4. administer the following if ordered:
   a. vitamins and minerals
   b. appetite stimulants (e.g. megestrol acetate, dronabinol)
   c. oxandrolone *to increase muscle mass* (*it also acts as an appetite stimulant*).
   d. Perform a calorie count if ordered. Report information to dietitian and physician.
   e. Consult physician about an alternative method of providing nutrition (e.g. parenteral nutrition, tube feedings) if client does not consume enough foods or fluids to meet nutritional needs.

---

4. NURSING DIAGNOSIS: **Pain:**

a. **oral, pharyngeal, and/or esophageal pain** related to the presence of aphthous ulcers in the mouth and/or infections involving the oropharyngeal and esophageal mucosa (e.g. candidiasis, herpes simplex);
b. **abdominal pain** related to nonspecific gastritis and opportunistic infection or neoplasm involvement of the intestine;
c. **neuropathic pain (e.g. painful paresthesias)** related to the possible direct effect of HIV on the nervous system and the side effects of some medications (e.g. didanosine, zalcitabine, isoniazid);
d. **headache** related to cranial inflammation/pressure associated with an opportunistic infection involving the sinuses or brain or the presence of a cerebral neoplasm;
e. **chest pain** related to:
   1. inflammation of the parietal pleura associated with an opportunistic infection of the lungs
   2. muscle strain associated with excessive coughing if present;
f. **skin and local tissue pain** related to:
   1. skin lesions associated with opportunistic infection and/or Kaposi's sarcoma
   2. pressure in subcutaneous tissues associated with lymphedema
   3. skin breakdown in perianal area associated with diarrhea.

Desired Outcome	Nursing Actions and *Selected Purposes/Rationales*

4. The client will experience diminished pain as evidenced by:
   a. verbalization of a decrease in or absence of pain
   b. relaxed facial expression and body positioning
   c. increased participation in activities
   d. stable vital signs.

4.a. Assess for signs and symptoms of pain (e.g. verbalization of pain, grimacing, reluctance to move or breathe deeply, rubbing head, reluctance to eat, restlessness, diaphoresis, facial pallor, increased blood pressure, tachycardia).
b. Assess client's perception of the severity of pain using a pain intensity rating scale.
c. Assess the client's pain pattern (e.g. location, quality, onset, duration, precipitating factors, aggravating factors, alleviating factors).
d. Ask the client to describe previous pain experiences and methods used to manage pain effectively.
e. Implement measures *to reduce pain:*
   1. perform actions *to reduce fear and anxiety about the pain experience* (e.g. assure client that his/her need for pain relief is understood, plan methods for achieving pain control with client)
   2. perform actions to reduce fear and anxiety (see Nursing Diagnosis 17, action b) *in order to promote relaxation and subsequently increase the client's threshold and tolerance for pain*
   3. administer analgesics before activities and procedures that can cause pain and before pain becomes severe
   4. perform actions to reduce fatigue (see Nursing Diagnosis 9, action c) *in order to increase the client's threshold and tolerance for pain*

   5. provide or assist with nonpharmacologic methods for pain relief (e.g. position change; progressive relaxation exercises; guided imagery; restful environment; diversional activities such as watching television, reading, or conversing)
   6. plan methods for achieving pain control with client *in order to assist him/her to maintain a sense of control over the pain experience*
   7. administer the following if ordered:
      a. nonopioid (nonnarcotic) analgesics such as salicylates and other nonsteroidal anti-inflammatory agents (acetaminophen should be avoided if the client is taking zidovudine *because it may increase the toxicity of zidovudine*)
      b. opioid (narcotic) analgesics
      c. tricyclic antidepressants (e.g. amitriptyline) and/or anticonvulsants (e.g. carbamazepine) *to treat painful neuropathies*
      d. topical anesthetic/analgesic ointments (e.g. capsaicin) *to treat skin and superficial neuropathic pain*
      e. oral anesthetic and/or protective agents (e.g. sucralfate, viscous xylocaine mixed with diphenhydramine elixir and a magnesium or aluminum antacid)
      f. corticosteroids (*may be utilized to relieve pain associated with some CNS lesions and sinusitis*)
      g. antimicrobials and/or antineoplastic agents (*may be given to treat HIV infection and/or opportunistic disease[s] causing the pain*).
   f. Consult physician about an order for patient-controlled analgesia (PCA) if adequate relief cannot be achieved with the above measures.

5.A. NURSING DIAGNOSIS: **Altered comfort: chills and excessive diaphoresis**

related to persistent or recurrent fever associated with HIV and opportunistic infections.

Desired Outcome	Nursing Actions and *Selected Purposes/Rationales*

5.A. The client will not experience discomfort associated with chills and diaphoresis as evidenced by:
1. verbalization of comfort
2. ability to rest.
	5.A.1. Assess client for chills and excessive diaphoresis.
	   2. Implement measures to reduce fever (see Nursing Diagnosis 6, action b) *in order to decrease chills and excessive diaphoresis.*
	   3. Implement measures *to promote comfort if client is having chills:*
	   a. maintain a room temperature that is comfortable for client
	   b. protect client from drafts
	   c. provide extra blankets and clothing as needed
	   d. provide warm liquids to drink.
	   4. Implement measures *to promote comfort if excessive diaphoresis is present:*
	   a. change linen and clothing whenever damp
	   b. bathe client and sponge his/her face as needed.
	   5. Consult physician if client continues to have chills and excessive diaphoresis.

5.B. NURSING DIAGNOSIS: **Altered comfort: pruritus**

related to:
1. dry skin associated with fluid volume deficit (can occur as a result of decreased oral intake, excessive diaphoresis, and/or persistent diarrhea);

2. pruritic folliculitis (e.g. staphylococcal folliculitis, eosinophilic folliculitis);
3. dermatological disorders such as seborrheic dermatitis, photodermatitis, and psoriasis;
4. a side effect of some antimicrobials (e.g. trimethoprim-sulfamethoxazole);
5. vulvovaginal candidiasis.

Desired Outcome	Nursing Actions and *Selected Purposes/Rationales*
5.B. The client will experience relief of pruritus as evidenced by: 1. verbalization of same 2. no scratching or rubbing of skin.	5.B.1. Assess for the following: 　a. reports of itchiness 　b. persistent scratching or rubbing of skin. 2. Instruct client in and/or implement measures *to reduce pruritus:* 　a. apply cool, moist compresses to pruritic areas 　b. perform actions *to reduce skin dryness:* 　　1. use tepid water and mild soaps for bathing 　　2. apply oil-based agents to skin immediately after bathing when skin is hydrated unless contraindicated 　　3. apply emollient creams or ointments frequently 　　4. encourage a fluid intake of 2500 ml/day unless contraindicated 　　5. utilize a room humidifier *to maintain moisture in the air* 　c. add emollients, cornstarch, or baking soda to bath water unless contraindicated 　d. pat skin dry after bathing, making sure to dry thoroughly 　e. encourage participation in diversional activity 　f. utilize relaxation techniques 　g. utilize cutaneous stimulation techniques (e.g. pressure, massage, vibration, stroking with a soft brush) at sites of itching or acupressure points 　h. encourage client to wear loose, cotton garments 　i. administer the following if ordered: 　　1. antihistamines 　　2. topical corticosteroids (e.g. triamcinolone, hydrocortisone, desonide) 　　3. systemic antimicrobial agents *to treat pruritic folliculitis* (e.g. dicloxacillin, itraconazole) 　　4. topical antifungal agents *to treat vulvovaginal candidiasis* (e.g. miconazole, clotrimazole) 　　5. topical antifungal agents *to treat seborrheic dermatitis* (e.g. ketoconazole, clotrimazole). 3. Consult physician if above measures fail to reduce pruritus or if the skin becomes excoriated.

6. NURSING DIAGNOSIS:

Hyperthermia

related to stimulation of the thermoregulatory center in the hypothalamus by endogenous pyrogens that are released in an infectious process.

Desired Outcome	Nursing Actions and *Selected Purposes/Rationales*
6. The client will experience resolution of hyperthermia as evidenced by:	6.a. Assess for signs and symptoms of hyperthermia (e.g. warm, flushed skin; tachycardia; tachypnea; elevated temperature). 　b. Implement measures *to reduce fever:*

a. skin usual temperature
   and color
b. pulse rate between 60–100
   beats/minute
c. respirations 14–20/minute
d. normal body temperature.

1. perform actions *to resolve the infectious process:*
   a. implement measures to promote rest (see Nursing Diagnosis 9,
      action c.1)
   b. implement measures to maintain an adequate nutritional status (see
      Nursing Diagnosis 3, action c)
   c. implement measures to facilitate removal of pulmonary secretions
      (see Nursing Diagnosis 1, action c.7) if a respiratory infection is
      present
   d. administer antimicrobials as ordered
2. administer tepid sponge bath and/or apply cool cloths to groin and
   axillae if indicated
3. use a room fan *to provide cool circulating air*
4. apply cooling blanket if ordered
5. administer antipyretics if ordered.
c. Consult physician if temperature remains higher than 38.5° C.

---

7. NURSING DIAGNOSIS:

Altered oral mucous membrane

related to:
a. malnutrition and fluid volume deficit;
b. infections such as *Candida albicans,* herpes simplex, oral hairy leukoplakia,
   and bacterial gingivitis/periodontitis;
c. Kaposi's sarcoma or lymphoma in the oral cavity.

Desired Outcome	Nursing Actions and *Selected Purposes/Rationales*
7. The client will have a healthy oral cavity as evidenced by: a. absence of inflammation b. pink, moist, intact mucosa c. absence of lesions d. absence of halitosis e. no report of oral dryness and pain f. ability to swallow without discomfort.	7.a. Assess client for and report signs and symptoms of altered oral mucous membrane (e.g. inflamed and/or ulcerated oral mucosa; corrugated, white thickenings, particularly on sides of tongue; groups of vesicles; removable white plaques; reddened and retracted gingivae; red or purple macules, papules, or nodules; halitosis; reports of oral dryness and pain; dysphagia). b. Culture oral lesions as ordered. Report positive results. c. Prepare client for and assist with biopsy of oral lesions if planned. Report positive results. d. Implement measures *to maintain or regain integrity of oral mucous membrane:* 　1. reinforce importance of and assist client with oral hygiene after meals and snacks; avoid use of products that contain lemon and glycerin and mouthwashes containing alcohol (*these products have a drying and irritating effect on the oral mucous membrane*) 　2. have client rinse mouth frequently with warm saline; baking soda and water; or a solution of salt, baking soda, and water 　3. use a soft-bristle brush, sponge-tipped applicator, or low-pressure power spray for oral hygiene 　4. lubricate client's lips frequently 　5. encourage client to breathe through nose rather than mouth *in order to reduce mouth dryness* 　6. encourage a fluid intake of at least 2500 ml/day unless contraindicated 　7. perform actions to maintain an adequate nutritional status (see Nursing Diagnosis 3, action c) 　8. encourage client not to smoke (*smoking irritates and dries the mucosa*) 　9. assist client with selection of soft, bland foods 　10. instruct client to avoid foods/fluids that are extremely hot 　11. administer antifungal agents (e.g. clotrimazole troches, nystatin suspension, fluconazole, ketoconazole) and antiviral agents (e.g. acyclovir, foscarnet) if ordered

Desired Outcome	Nursing Actions and *Selected Purposes/Rationales*

	12. if periodontal disease is present, administer the following if ordered:
	  a. oral antiseptic rinses (e.g. chlorhexidine gluconate [Peridex])
	  b. antimicrobial agents (e.g. metronidazole, augmentin, clindamycin)
	13. if Kaposi's sarcoma or lymphoma lesions are present in the oral cavity, prepare client for radiation therapy, chemotherapy, and/or excision of lesion(s) if planned
	14. if aphthous ulcers are present, administer topical corticosteroid preparations (e.g. fluocinonide [Lidex] ointment mixed with Orabase, Decadron elixir) if ordered
	15. if stomatitis is not controlled:
	  a. increase frequency of oral hygiene
	  b. if client has dentures, remove and replace only for meals.
	e. Consult physician if signs and symptoms of altered oral mucous membrane persist or worsen.

■───────────────────────────

8. NURSING DIAGNOSIS:

Actual/Risk for impaired tissue integrity

related to:
a. presence of cutaneous infections such as folliculitis, herpes zoster or simplex, bullous impetigo, bacillary angiomatosis, molluscum contagiosum, and/or abscesses;
b. presence of certain skin disorders (e.g. seborrheic dermatitis, photodermatitis, psoriasis);
c. skin lesions associated with Kaposi's sarcoma if present;
d. excessive scratching associated with pruritus;
e. increased skin fragility associated with dryness and malnutrition;
f. persistent contact with irritants associated with diarrhea;
g. damage to the skin and/or subcutaneous tissue associated with prolonged pressure on tissues, friction, or shearing if mobility is decreased.

Desired Outcome	Nursing Actions and *Selected Purposes/Rationales*

8. The client will maintain and/or regain tissue integrity as evidenced by:
a. absence of redness and irritation
b. no skin breakdown.
	8.a. Assess the client for the presence of cutaneous lesions (e.g. vesicles, papules, macules, plaques, scaling patches, nodules).
	b. Assess bony prominences, perineum, and dependent and pruritic areas for pallor, redness, and breakdown.
	c. Implement measures *to treat existing cutaneous conditions:*
	  1. administer systemic antimicrobial agents (e.g. dicloxacillin, erythromycin, doxycycline, acyclovir) if ordered *to treat cutaneous infections*
	  2. apply topical corticosteroids if ordered *to treat inflammatory skin conditions*
	  3. cleanse infected lesions with antiseptic solution (e.g. chlorhexidine) if ordered
	  4. assist with and/or prepare client for treatments such as chemotherapy, radiation therapy, and surgical excision if ordered *to treat Kaposi's sarcoma.*
	d. Implement measures *to prevent additional tissue breakdown:*
	  1. assist client to turn at least every 2 hours
	  2. position client properly; use pressure-reducing or pressure-relieving devices (e.g. pillows, gel or foam cushions, alternating pressure mattress, air-fluidized bed) if indicated
	  3. gently massage around reddened areas at least every 2 hours
	  4. apply a thin layer of powder or cornstarch to bottom sheet or skin and to opposing skin surfaces (e.g. axillae, beneath breasts) if indicated *to absorb moisture and/or reduce friction*
	  5. lift and move client carefully using a turn sheet and adequate assistance
	  6. limit length of time client is in semi-Fowler's position to 30 minutes (*in this position, client tends to slide down in bed, which can cause skin surface abrasion and shearing*)

    7. instruct client to shift weight at least every 30 minutes
    8. keep skin clean and dry
    9. keep bed linens dry and wrinkle-free
  10. increase activity as allowed and tolerated
  11. perform actions to maintain an adequate nutritional status (see Nursing Diagnosis 3, action c)
  12. perform actions to prevent skin dryness (see Nursing Diagnosis 5.B, action 2.b)
  13. perform actions *to prevent skin irritation resulting from diarrhea:*
    a. implement measures to reduce diarrhea (see Nursing Diagnosis 11, action e)
    b. assist client to thoroughly cleanse and dry perineal area with soft tissue or cloth after each bowel movement; apply a protective ointment or cream
    c. apply a fecal incontinence pouch if diarrhea is severe
    d. provide incontinence pads if needed to absorb moisture; do not allow skin to come in contact with plastic portion of pads
  14. perform actions *to prevent skin irritation resulting from scratching:*
    a. implement measures to relieve pruritus (see Nursing Diagnosis 5.B, action 2)
    b. keep nails trimmed and/or apply mittens if necessary
    c. instruct client to apply firm pressure to pruritic areas rather than scratching.
  e. If tissue breakdown occurs or existing breakdown progresses:
    1. notify physician
    2. continue with measures identified in actions c and d in this diagnosis to prevent further tissue irritation and breakdown
    3. perform care of involved areas as ordered or per standard hospital procedure.

---

9. NURSING DIAGNOSIS:

Fatigue

related to:
a. difficulty resting and sleeping;
b. increased energy utilization associated with the elevated metabolic rate that is present in infection;
c. malnutrition;
d. tissue hypoxia associated with:
  1. impaired alveolar gas exchange if respiratory infection is present
  2. anemia resulting from:
    a. bone marrow involvement by HIV, other infections, and/or AIDS-related neoplasms
    b. treatment with medications that can cause bone marrow depression (e.g. zidovudine, antineoplastic agents, trimethoprim-sulfamethoxazole);
e. overwhelming emotional demands associated with the diagnosis of AIDS.

Desired Outcome	Nursing Actions and *Selected Purposes/Rationales*

9. The client will experience a reduction in fatigue as evidenced by:
a. verbalization of feelings of increased energy
b. ability to perform usual activities of daily living
	9.a. Assess for signs and symptoms of fatigue (e.g. verbalization of unremitting, overwhelming lack of energy and inability to maintain usual routines; lack of interest in surroundings; decreased ability to concentrate; increased emotional lability).
	  b. Assess client's perception of the severity of fatigue using a fatigue rating scale.
	  c. Implement measures *to increase strength and reduce fatigue:*

Desired Outcome	Nursing Actions and **Selected Purposes/Rationales**

c. increased interest in surroundings and ability to concentrate
 	
d. decreased emotional lability.
	1. perform actions *to promote rest and/or conserve energy:*
	   a. maintain activity restrictions if ordered
	   b. minimize environmental activity and noise
	   c. organize nursing care to allow for periods of uninterrupted rest
	   d. limit the number of visitors and their length of stay
	   e. assist client with self-care activities as needed
	   f. keep supplies and personal articles within easy reach
	   g. instruct client in energy-saving techniques (e.g. using shower chair when showering, sitting to brush teeth or comb hair)
	   h. implement measures to reduce fear and anxiety (see Nursing Diagnosis 17, action b) and assist the client to adjust psychologically to the diagnosis of AIDS (see Nursing Diagnoses 18, action c; 19, actions c–n; and 20, action b)
	   i. implement measures to reduce discomfort (see Nursing Diagnoses 4, action e; 5.A, actions 3 and 4; and 5.B, action 2)
	   j. implement measures to promote sleep (see Nursing Diagnosis 13, action c)
	2. perform actions to resolve the infectious process (see Nursing Diagnosis 6, action b.1)
	3. perform actions to maintain an adequate nutritional status (see Nursing Diagnosis 3, action c)
	4. perform actions to improve respiratory status (see Nursing Diagnosis 1, action c)
	5. discourage smoking and excessive intake of beverages high in caffeine such as coffee, tea, and colas (*nicotine and caffeine increase cardiac workload and myocardial oxygen utilization, thereby decreasing oxygen availability*)
	6. administer the following if ordered:
	   a. packed red blood cells
	   b. recombinant human erythropoietin (e.g. epoetin alfa) *to stimulate RBC production*
	7. increase client's activity gradually as allowed and tolerated.
	d. Consult physician if signs and symptoms of fatigue worsen.

---

10. NURSING DIAGNOSIS: **Self-care deficit**

related to:
a. cognitive and/or motor impairments if present (can result from the direct effect of HIV on the nervous system or opportunistic disease involvement of the central nervous system);
b. fatigue, weakness, and dyspnea;
c. depression;
d. visual impairment if present (can result from cytomegalovirus retinitis).

Desired Outcome	Nursing Actions and **Selected Purposes/Rationales**

10. The client will demonstrate increased participation in self-care activities within physical limitations.	10.a. With client, develop a realistic plan for meeting daily physical needs.
	   b. Implement measures *to facilitate client's ability to perform self-care activities:*
	     1. perform actions to increase strength and reduce fatigue (see Nursing Diagnosis 9, action c)
	     2. schedule care at a time when client is most likely to be able to participate (e.g. after rest periods, not immediately after meals or treatments)
	     3. keep needed objects within easy reach
	     4. consult occupational therapist about assistive devices available (e.g. long-handled hairbrush, broad-handled utensils)

5. if client has a visual impairment, orient to surroundings and location of items needed for self-care
6. if oxygen therapy is needed during activity, keep portable oxygen equipment readily available for client's use
7. allow adequate time for accomplishment of self-care activities
8. perform actions to facilitate adjustment to the diagnosis of AIDS (see Nursing Diagnoses 18, action c; 19, actions c–n; and 20, action b).

c. Encourage maximum independence within physical limitations and prescribed activity restrictions. Provide positive feedback for all efforts and accomplishments of self-care.

d. Assist the client with activities he/she is unable to perform independently.

e. Inform significant others of client's abilities to perform own care. Explain the importance of encouraging and allowing client to maintain an optimal level of independence within prescribed activity restrictions and his/her activity tolerance level and cognitive and motor abilities.

---

11. NURSING DIAGNOSIS:

Diarrhea

related to a direct effect of HIV on the intestine or opportunistic disease involvement of the intestine (e.g. *Mycobacterium avium-intracellulare*, *Cryptosporidium*, *Salmonella*, cytomegalovirus, *Isospora belli*, *Clostridium difficile*, *Entamoeba histolytica*, *Giardia*, Kaposi's sarcoma).

Desired Outcome	Nursing Actions and *Selected Purposes/Rationales*
11. The client will have fewer bowel movements and more formed stool.	11.a. Ascertain client's usual bowel elimination habits.

b. Assess for signs and symptoms of diarrhea (e.g. frequent, loose stools; urgency; abdominal pain and cramping; hyperactive bowel sounds).

c. Obtain stool specimens for culture and/or examination for ova and parasites. Report positive results.

d. Prepare client for endoscopy if planned *to examine intestinal mucosa, obtain specimens for culture, and/or perform biopsies.*

e. Implement measures *to control diarrhea:*
   1. perform actions *to rest the bowel:*
      a. restrict oral intake if ordered
      b. when oral intake is allowed:
         1. gradually progress from fluids to small meals
         2. instruct client to avoid foods/fluids that may stimulate or irritate the inflamed bowel:
            a. those high in fiber (e.g. whole-grain cereals, raw fruits and vegetables)
            b. those that are spicy or extremely hot or cold
            c. those high in lactose (e.g. milk, milk products)
      c. implement measures to reduce fear and anxiety (see Nursing Diagnosis 17, action b)
      d. encourage client to rest
      e. discourage smoking (*nicotine has a stimulant effect on the gastrointestinal tract*)
   2. encourage client to drink pectin-containing juices (e.g. apple, pear)
   3. administer the following medications if ordered:
      a. opiate or opiate derivatives (e.g. paregoric, loperamide, diphenoxylate hydrochloride) *to decrease gastrointestinal motility*
      b. bulk-forming agents (e.g. methylcellulose, psyllium hydrophilic mucilloid) *to absorb water in the bowel, which results in a more formed stool*

Desired Outcome	Nursing Actions and *Selected Purposes/Rationales*

c. adsorbents (e.g. kaolin, pectin, attapulgite [Kaopectate], bismuth subsalicylate [Pepto-Bismol])

d. octreotide acetate (Sandostatin) *to suppress the output of motilin and subsequently reduce gastrointestinal activity*

e. antimicrobial agents (e.g. ganciclovir, foscarnet, ampicillin, ciprofloxacin, amoxicillin, metronidazole, azithromycin, paromomycin, trimethoprim-sulfamethoxazole, zidovudine, zalcitabine, saquinavir) *to treat the infectious process*

    4. assist with measures to treat intestinal neoplasms (e.g. chemotherapy, radiation therapy) if planned.

f. Consult physician if diarrhea persists or worsens.

---

12. NURSING DIAGNOSIS: **Altered thought processes***

related to:

a. HIV encephalopathy (AIDS dementia complex) associated with the direct effect of HIV on the central nervous system;

b. opportunistic infections and/or neoplasms involving the central nervous system (e.g. toxoplasmic encephalitis, cryptococcal meningitis, progressive multifocal leukoencephalopathy, herpes or cytomegalovirus [CMV] encephalitis, primary central nervous system lymphoma);

c. fluid and electrolyte imbalances and hypoxemia if present;

d. depression and severe anxiety.

---

*The diagnostic label of acute or chronic confusion may be more appropriate depending on the client's symptoms.

Desired Outcome	Nursing Actions and *Selected Purposes/Rationales*

12. The client will experience improvement in thought processes as evidenced by:
    a. improved verbal response time
    b. longer attention span
    c. improved memory
    d. improved reasoning ability and judgment
    e. decreased apathy
    f. decreased agitation
    g. absence of hallucinations.

12.a. Assess client for altered thought processes (e.g. slowed verbal responses, decreased ability to concentrate, impaired memory, poor reasoning ability or judgment, apathy, agitation, hallucinations).

b. Ascertain from significant others client's usual level of cognitive and emotional functioning.

c. Prepare client for diagnostic studies that may be done to determine the cause of altered thought processes (e.g. computed tomography [CT] or magnetic resonance imaging [MRI] of the brain, toxoplasma and cryptococcal serology studies, cerebrospinal fluid analysis, brain biopsy, neuropsychological tests).

d. Implement measures *to improve client's thought processes:*

    1. perform actions to improve tissue oxygenation (see Nursing Diagnoses 1, action c and 9, action c.6)

    2. perform actions to prevent or treat fluid and electrolyte imbalances (see Nursing Diagnosis 2, action b)

    3. administer the following medications if ordered:

        a. antimicrobials (e.g. clindamycin, pyrimethamine, sulfadiazine, amphotericin B, flucytosine, fluconazole, acyclovir, ganciclovir, foscarnet, zidovudine, zalcitabine, saquinavir) *to treat infectious processes*

        b. cytotoxic agents *to treat neoplastic conditions affecting nervous system*

        c. antipsychotic agents (e.g. haloperidol, perphenazine, chlorpromazine) *to reduce restlessness, agitation, or hallucinations*

  d. central nervous system stimulants (e.g. dextroamphetamine sulfate) *to reduce apathy and withdrawn behavior.*
  e. If client shows evidence of altered thought processes:
   1. reorient client to person, place, and time as necessary
   2. address client by name
   3. place familiar objects, clock, and calendar within client's view
   4. approach client in a slow, calm manner; allow adequate time for communication
   5. repeat instructions as necessary using clear, simple language and short sentences
   6. keep environmental stimuli to a minimum
   7. maintain a consistent and fairly structured routine and write out schedule of activities for client to refer to if desired
   8. have client perform only one activity at a time and allow adequate time for performance of activities
   9. encourage client to make lists of planned activities, questions, and concerns
   10. assist client to problem solve if necessary
   11. maintain realistic expectations of client's ability to learn, comprehend, and remember information provided; provide client with a written copy of instructions
   12. if client is experiencing hallucinations, allow significant others to remain with client *in order to provide constant reassurance*
   13. encourage significant others to be supportive of client; instruct them in methods of dealing with client's altered thought processes
   14. discuss physiological basis for altered thought processes with client and significant others; inform them that cognitive and emotional functioning may improve with drug therapy
   15. consult physician if altered thought processes persist or worsen.

---

13. NURSING DIAGNOSIS: **Sleep pattern disturbance**

related to fear, anxiety, depression, frequent assessments and treatments, pain, diarrhea, pruritus, chills, night sweats, coughing and dyspnea (may occur if respiratory infection is present), unfamiliar environment, and effect of some medications (e.g. zidovudine).

Desired Outcome	Nursing Actions and *Selected Purposes/Rationales*

13. The client will attain optimal amounts of sleep as evidenced by:
a. statements of feeling well rested
b. usual mental status
c. absence of frequent yawning, dark circles under eyes, and hand tremors.
	13.a. Assess for signs and symptoms of a sleep pattern disturbance (e.g. statements of difficulty falling asleep, sleep interruptions, or not feeling well rested; irritability; lethargy; disorientation; frequent yawning; dark circles under eyes; slight hand tremors).
	  b. Determine the client's usual sleep habits.
	  c. Implement measures *to promote sleep:*
	   1. discourage long periods of sleep during the day unless signs and symptoms of sleep deprivation exist or daytime sleep is usual for client
	   2. perform actions to reduce fear and anxiety (see Nursing Diagnosis 17, action b) and assist the client to adjust psychologically to the diagnosis of AIDS (see Nursing Diagnoses 18, action c; 19, actions c–n; and 20, action b)
	   3. perform actions to reduce discomfort associated with chills and excessive diaphoresis and pruritus (see Nursing Diagnoses 5.A, actions 3 and 4 and 5.B, action 2)

Desired Outcome	Nursing Actions and *Selected Purposes/Rationales*

4. perform actions to reduce pain (see Nursing Diagnosis 4, action e)
5. perform actions to control diarrhea (see Nursing Diagnosis 11, action e)
6. encourage participation in relaxing diversional activities during the evening
7. discourage intake of fluids high in caffeine (e.g. coffee, tea, colas), especially in the evening
8. allow client to continue usual sleep practices (e.g. position; time; presleep routines such as reading, watching television, listening to music, and meditating) unless contraindicated
9. satisfy basic needs such as comfort and warmth before sleep
10. encourage client to urinate just before bedtime
11. reduce environmental distractions (e.g. close door to client's room; use night light rather than overhead light whenever possible; lower volume of paging system; keep staff conversations at a low level and away from client's room; close curtains between clients in a semi-private room or ward; provide client with "white noise" such as fan, soft music, or tape-recorded sounds of ocean or rain; have sleep mask and earplugs available for client if needed)
12. ensure good room ventilation
13. if client has orthopnea:
    a. assist him/her to assume a position *that facilitates breathing* (e.g. head of bed elevated with arms supported on pillows, resting forward on overbed table with good pillow support, sitting in a chair)
    b. maintain oxygen therapy during sleep
14. if client has a persistent cough, perform actions *to control coughing:*
    a. instruct client to avoid intake of very hot or cold foods/fluids (*these can stimulate cough*)
    b. protect client from irritants such as flowers, smoke, and powder
    c. encourage client not to smoke (*smoking irritates the respiratory tract*)
    d. humidify inspired air as ordered
    e. administer antitussives if ordered
15. administer prescribed sedative-hypnotics if indicated
16. perform actions *to reduce interruptions during sleep* (*80–100 minutes of uninterrupted sleep is usually needed to complete one sleep cycle*):
    a. restrict visitors
    b. group care (e.g. medications, treatments, physical care, assessments) whenever possible.
    d. Consult physician if signs and symptoms of sleep deprivation persist or worsen.

---

14. NURSING DIAGNOSIS:

Risk for infection: opportunistic

related to:
a. decreased resistance to infection associated with:
   1. cellular and humoral immune deficiencies present in HIV infection
   2. inadequate nutritional status
   3. depletion of immune mechanisms resulting from presenting infection and treatment with antimicrobial agents;
b. stasis of respiratory secretions and/or urinary stasis if mobility is decreased;
c. break in integrity of skin associated with frequent venipunctures or placement of a central venous catheter (e.g. Groshong);
d. impaired integrity of skin or mucous membranes if present.

Desired Outcome	Nursing Actions and *Selected Purposes/Rationales*

14. The client will remain free of additional opportunistic infection(s) as evidenced by:
 a. return of temperature toward client's normal range
 b. decrease in episodes of chills and diaphoresis
 c. pulse returning toward normal range
 d. normal or improved breath sounds
 e. absence or resolution of dyspnea
 f. stable or improved mental status
 g. voiding clear urine without reports of frequency, urgency, and burning
 h. absence or resolution of painful, pruritic skin lesions
 i. stable or gradual increase in body weight
 j. no reports of increased weakness and fatigue
 k. absence of visual disturbances
 l. absence or resolution of heat, pain, redness, swelling, and unusual drainage in any area
 m. absence or resolution of oral mucous membrane irritation and ulceration
 n. ability to swallow without difficulty
 o. WBC and differential counts returning toward normal range
 p. negative results of cultured specimens.

14.a. Assess for and report signs and symptoms of additional opportunistic infection (be alert to subtle changes in client since the signs of infection may be minimal as a result of immunosuppression; also be aware that some signs and symptoms vary depending on the site of infection, the causative organism, and the age of the client):
 1. increase in temperature above client's usual level
 2. increase in episodes of chills and diaphoresis
 3. increased pulse
 4. development or worsening of abnormal breath sounds
 5. development or worsening of dyspnea
 6. development or worsening of cough
 7. decline in mental status
 8. cloudy, foul-smelling urine
 9. reports of frequency, urgency, or burning when urinating
 10. presence of WBCs, bacteria, and/or nitrites in urine
 11. vesicular lesions particularly on face, lips, and perianal area
 12. new or increased reports of pain in and/or itching of skin lesions and surrounding tissue
 13. further increase in weight loss, fatigue, or weakness
 14. visual disturbances
 15. new or increased heat, pain, redness, swelling, or unusual drainage in any area
 16. new or increased irritation or ulceration of oral mucous membrane
 17. development of or increased dysphagia
 18. significant change in WBC count and/or differential.
 b. Obtain specimens (e.g. urine, vaginal drainage, stool, sputum, blood, drainage from lesions) for culture as ordered. Report positive results.
 c. Implement measures *to prevent further infection:*
 1. administer the following medications if ordered:
 a. antiretroviral agents (e.g. zidovudine, didanosine, zalcitabine, stavudine, lamivudine, saquinavir, ritonavir) *to reduce the rate of replication of HIV*
 b. immunomodulating agents (e.g. interferon alfa, colony stimulating factors such as filgrastim and sargramostim) *to stimulate production/enhance activity of the white blood cells*
 c. antimicrobial agents *to treat current infection or prevent additional opportunistic infection (e.g. TMP/SMZ to prevent Pneumocystis carinii pneumonia once the CD4+ T lymphocyte count falls below 200 μL)*
 2. maintain a fluid intake of at least 2500 ml/day unless contraindicated
 3. use good handwashing technique and encourage client to do the same
 4. protect client from others with infection
 5. perform actions to maintain an adequate nutritional status (see Nursing Diagnosis 3, action c)
 6. perform actions identified in this care plan to reduce stressors such as discomfort, dyspnea, fear and anxiety, and feelings of powerlessness *in order to prevent excessive secretion of cortisol (cortisol inhibits the immune response)*
 7. perform actions to maintain or regain integrity of oral mucous membrane (see Nursing Diagnosis 7, action d)
 8. maintain sterile technique during all invasive procedures (e.g. urinary catheterization, venous and arterial punctures, injections)
 9. rotate intravenous insertion sites according to hospital policy
 10. anchor catheters/tubings (e.g. urinary, intravenous, wound) securely *in order to reduce trauma to the tissues and the risk for introduction of pathogens associated with the in-and-out movement of the tubing*

Desired Outcome	Nursing Actions and **Selected Purposes/Rationales**
	11. change equipment, tubings, and solutions used for treatments such as intravenous infusions, respiratory care, irrigations, and enteral feedings according to hospital policy
	12. maintain a closed system for drains (e.g. wound, urinary catheter) and intravenous infusions whenever possible
	13. encourage a low-microbe diet (e.g. cooked foods, scrupulously cleaned fruits and vegetables)
	14. perform actions *to prevent stasis of respiratory secretions* (e.g. assist client to turn, cough, and deep breathe; increase activity as allowed and tolerated)
	15. perform actions to prevent or treat skin breakdown (see Nursing Diagnosis 8, actions c–e)
	16. perform actions to prevent urinary retention (e.g. instruct client to urinate when the urge is first felt, promote relaxation during voiding attempts) *in order to prevent urinary stasis*
	17. instruct and assist client to perform good perineal care routinely and after each bowel movement
	18. if client has open lesions, perform actions *to prevent wound infection* (e.g. maintain sterile technique during wound care, instruct client to avoid touching wounds)
	19. if client has a central venous catheter, instruct and assist him/her with proper care of the exit site.

■━━

15. NURSING DIAGNOSIS:

Risk for trauma:

a. **falls** related to:
  1. weakness and fatigue
  2. decline in cognitive, behavioral, and/or motor function associated with the direct effect of HIV on the brain and spinal cord (e.g. AIDS dementia complex, vacuolar myelopathy) and/or opportunistic infection or neoplastic involvement of the central nervous system
  3. visual impairment if present (may result from cytomegalovirus retinitis);
b. **burns** related to diminished sensation associated with peripheral neuropathy if present (appears to be a result of the direct attack of HIV on the myelin and can also occur as a side effect of some antiretroviral agents).

Desired Outcome	Nursing Actions and **Selected Purposes/Rationales**

15. The client will not experience falls or burns.	15.a. Implement measures *to reduce the risk for trauma:*
	1. perform actions *to prevent falls:*
	  a. keep bed in low position with side rails up when client is in bed
	  b. keep needed items within easy reach
	  c. encourage client to request assistance whenever needed; have call signal within easy reach
	  d. use lap belt when client is in chair if indicated
	  e. instruct client to wear well-fitting slippers/shoes with nonslip soles and low heels when ambulating
	  f. keep floor free of clutter and wipe up spills promptly
	  g. accompany client during ambulation utilizing a transfer safety belt if he/she is weak or dizzy
	  h. provide ambulatory aids (e.g. walker, cane) if client is weak or unsteady on feet
	  i. reinforce instructions from physical therapist regarding correct transfer and ambulation techniques
	  j. instruct client to ambulate in well-lit areas and to use handrails if needed

    k. if vision is impaired, orient client to surroundings and identify obstacles during ambulation

    l. do not rush client; allow adequate time for ambulation to the bathroom and in hallway

    m. make sure that shower has a nonslip bottom surface and that shower chair, secure bath mat, call signal, grab bars, and adequate lighting are present

    n. perform actions to improve strength and reduce fatigue (see Nursing Diagnosis 9, action c)

    o. administer central nervous system depressants judiciously

    p. if client is confused or irrational:

        1. reorient frequently to surroundings and necessity of adhering to safety precautions

        2. provide appropriate level of supervision

        3. consult physician about the temporary use of a bed alarm or jacket or wrist restraints if necessary

        4. administer prescribed antianxiety and antipsychotic medications if indicated

  2. perform actions *to prevent burns:*

    a. let hot foods and fluids cool slightly before serving

    b. supervise client while smoking if indicated

    c. assess temperature of bath water and direct heat application devices (e.g. K-pad, warm compresses, hot water bottle) before and during use

  3. administer medications (e.g. antimicrobials, antineoplastic agents) as ordered *to treat the underlying disease condition and subsequently improve mental status and motor and sensory function.*

 b. Include client and significant others in planning and implementing measures to prevent trauma.

 c. If injury does occur, initiate first aid if appropriate and notify physician.

---

16. NURSING DIAGNOSIS:	**Altered sexuality patterns**

related to:

a. rejection by desired partner associated with his/her fear of contracting AIDS;

b. need to disclose to new partner(s) the diagnosis of AIDS;

c. decreased sexual desire associated with fatigue, weakness, anxiety, depression, and fear of transmitting or contracting disease.

Desired Outcome	Nursing Actions and *Selected Purposes/Rationales*

16. The client will demonstrate beginning adjustment to the effects of AIDS on sexuality patterns as evidenced by:
  a. verbalization of same
  b. verbalization of a perception of self as sexually adequate and acceptable.
	16.a. Assess for signs and symptoms of altered sexuality patterns (e.g. verbalization of sexual concerns, reports of changes in sexual activities or behaviors).
	  b. Determine the client's perception of desired sexuality, usual pattern of sexual expression, recent changes in sexuality patterns, and attitude and concerns about the impact of AIDS on sexuality.
	  c. Implement measures *to promote an optimal sexuality pattern:*
	    1. facilitate communication between client and partner; focus on the feelings they share and assist them to identify factors that may affect their sexual relationship
	    2. provide accurate information about the transmission of HIV during intimate contact; encourage questions, clarify misconceptions and fears, and encourage client and significant other to keep current on information about how HIV is spread

Desired Outcome	Nursing Actions and ***Selected Purposes/Rationales***
	3. discuss ways to be creative in expressing sexuality (e.g. massage, fantasies, cuddling)
	4. discuss various options for meeting sexual needs (e.g. masturbation, safer sexual activity with partner that takes into consideration the type[s] of opportunistic infection present)
	5. arrange for uninterrupted privacy during hospital stay if desired by couple
	6. instruct client to allow for adequate rest periods before sexual activity
	7. perform actions to reduce fear and anxiety (see Nursing Diagnosis 17, action b) and facilitate adjustment to the diagnosis of AIDS (see Nursing Diagnoses 18, action c; 19, actions c–n; and 20, action b)
	8. provide information about support groups and professional counselors that can assist client in adjusting to the effects of AIDS on sexuality
	9. include partner in above discussions and encourage continued support of the client.
	d. Consult physician if counseling appears indicated.

---

17. NURSING DIAGNOSIS: **Anxiety**

related to:
a. lack of understanding about HIV infection and AIDS, current symptoms, diagnostic tests, and treatment;
b. financial concerns;
c. diagnosis of a disabling and fatal disease;
d. stigma associated with having AIDS and possible changes in relationships with others if the diagnosis is disclosed;
e. possibility of having transmitted HIV infection to others and the need to inform them.

Desired Outcome	Nursing Actions and ***Selected Purposes/Rationales***

17. The client will experience a reduction in anxiety as evidenced by:
a. verbalization of feeling less anxious
b. usual sleep pattern
c. relaxed facial expression and body movements
d. stable vital signs
e. usual perceptual ability and interactions with others.
	17.a. Assess client for signs and symptoms of anxiety (e.g. verbalization of feeling anxious, insomnia, tenseness, shakiness, restlessness, diaphoresis, tachycardia, elevated blood pressure, facial pallor, self-focused behaviors).
	b. Implement measures *to reduce fear and anxiety:*
	  1. orient client to hospital environment, equipment, and routines
	  2. introduce client to staff who will be participating in care; if possible, maintain consistency in staff assigned to his/her care *to provide feelings of stability and comfort with the environment*
	  3. assure client that staff members are nearby; respond to call signal as soon as possible
	  4. maintain a calm, supportive, confident manner when interacting with client
	  5. encourage verbalization of fear and anxiety; provide feedback
	  6. explain all tests that may be performed to diagnose HIV infection, current immune status, and HIV/AIDS-related conditions
	  7. reinforce physician's explanation about HIV infection including mode of transmission, effects on immune system, and prognosis; encourage questions and clarify misconceptions
	  8. provide a calm, restful environment
	  9. instruct client in relaxation techniques and encourage participation in diversional activities
	  10. perform actions to assist client to cope with the diagnosis and its implications (see Nursing Diagnosis 18, action c)
	  11. initiate financial and/or social service referrals if indicated

12. provide information based on current needs of client at a level he/she can understand; encourage questions and clarification of information provided
13. encourage significant others to project a caring, concerned attitude without obvious anxiousness
14. include significant others in orientation and teaching sessions and encourage their continued support of the client
15. administer prescribed antianxiety agents if indicated.
    c. Consult physician if above actions fail to control fear and anxiety.

---

18. NURSING DIAGNOSIS:　　**Ineffective individual coping**

related to:
a. depression, fear, and anxiety associated with the diagnosis of AIDS and poor prognosis;
b. need for permanent change in life style associated with impaired immune system functioning and potential for disease transmission to others;
c. uncertainty of disease course and feelings of powerlessness over course of disease;
d. need for disclosure of diagnosis with possibility of subsequent rejection and/or distancing by others and loss of employment and health benefits;
e. guilt associated with past behavior (if it was a factor in contracting HIV) and/or possibility of having transmitted HIV to others;
f. lack of personal resources to deal with disability and premature death associated with youth (a significant number of clients are in their twenties or thirties and are not developmentally prepared to acknowledge and cope with disability and their own mortality);
g. multiple losses (e.g. death of close friends with AIDS; loss of normal body functioning, family support, financial security, and/or usual life style and roles);
h. chronic symptoms (e.g. pain, diarrhea, fatigue) if present.

Desired Outcome	Nursing Actions and *Selected Purposes/Rationales*
18. The client will demonstrate effective coping as evidenced by: a. verbalization of ability to cope with the diagnosis and its implications b. utilization of appropriate problem-solving techniques c. willingness to participate in treatment plan and meet basic needs d. absence of destructive behavior toward self and others e. appropriate use of defense mechanisms f. utilization of available support systems.	18.a. Assess for and report signs and symptoms of ineffective individual coping (e.g. verbalization of inability to cope; inability to ask for help, problem solve, or meet basic needs; insomnia; withdrawal; reluctance to participate in treatment plan; destructive behavior toward self or others; inappropriate use of defense mechanisms; inability to meet role expectations). b. Assess client's perception of current situation. c. Implement measures *to promote effective coping:* 　1. allow time for client to begin to adjust to the diagnosis and its implications, planned treatment, and anticipated changes in life style and roles 　2. assist client to recognize and manage inappropriate denial if it is present 　3. perform actions to reduce fear and anxiety, reduce feelings of powerlessness, and facilitate grieving (see Nursing Diagnoses 17, action b; 19, actions c–n; and 20, action b) 　4. perform actions to reduce pain (see Nursing Diagnosis 4, action e), control diarrhea (see Nursing Diagnosis 11, action e), and reduce fatigue (see Nursing Diagnosis 9, action c) 　5. encourage verbalization about current situation 　6. assist client to identify personal strengths and resources that can be utilized to facilitate coping with the current situation

Desired Outcome	Nursing Actions and *Selected* **Purposes/Rationales**
	7. demonstrate acceptance of client but set limits on inappropriate behavior
	8. create an atmosphere of trust and support
	9. if acceptable to client, arrange for a visit from another individual who is successfully living with AIDS
	10. include client in planning care, encourage maximum participation in treatment plan, and allow choices when possible *to enable him/her to maintain a sense of control*
	11. instruct client in effective problem-solving techniques (e.g. accurate identification of stressors, determination of various options to solve problem)
	12. assist client to maintain usual daily routines whenever possible
	13. assist client to identify priorities and attainable goals as he/she starts to plan for necessary life-style and role changes
	14. assist client and significant others to identify ways that personal and family goals can be adjusted rather than abandoned
	15. discuss ways to maintain optimal health; focus on methods of altering rather than changing life style
	16. assist client through methods such as role playing to prepare for negative reactions from others because of diagnosis of AIDS
	17. administer antianxiety and/or antidepressant agents if ordered
	18. assist client to identify and utilize available support systems; provide information about resources and support groups that can assist client and significant others in coping with effects of AIDS (e.g. American Foundation for AIDS Research, National AIDS Clearinghouse, National Association of People with AIDS, CDC National AIDS Hotline, Project Inform, hospice programs, drug abuse programs)
	19. when appropriate, assist client to meet spiritual needs (e.g. arrange for a visit from clergy)
	20. encourage continued emotional support from significant others
	21. encourage client to share with significant others the kind of support that would be most beneficial (e.g. listening, inspiring hope, providing reassurance and accurate information)
	22. support behaviors indicative of effective coping (e.g. participation in treatment plan, verbalization of the ability to cope with diagnosis of AIDS, utilization of effective problem-solving strategies).
	d. Consult physician about psychological counseling if appropriate. Initiate a referral if necessary.

---

19. NURSING DIAGNOSIS: **Powerlessness**

related to:
a. the disabling and terminal nature of AIDS;
b. increasing dependence on others to meet basic needs;
c. changes in roles, relationships, and future plans.

Desired Outcome	Nursing Actions and *Selected* **Purposes/Rationales**
19. The client will demonstrate increased feelings of control over his/her situation as evidenced by:	19.a. Assess client for behaviors that may indicate feelings of powerlessness (e.g. verbalization of lack of control over current situation, anger, irritability, passivity, lack of participation in care planning or self-care).
	b. Obtain information from client and significant others regarding client's

a. verbalization of same
b. active participation in planning of care
c. participation in self-care activities within physical limitations.

usual response to situations in which he/she has had limited control (e.g. loss of job, financial stress).

c. Evaluate client's perception of current situation, strengths, weaknesses, expectations, and parts of current situation which are under his/her control. Correct misinformation and inaccurate perceptions and encourage discussion of feelings about areas in which there is a perceived lack of control.

d. Assist client to establish realistic short- and long-term goals.

e. Reinforce physician's explanation about AIDS and the treatment plan. Clarify misconceptions.

f. Implement measures to promote effective coping (see Nursing Diagnosis 18, action c) *in order to promote an increased sense of control over situation.*

g. Support realistic hope about the possibility of future independence and effectiveness of drugs in controlling conditions that can result from an impaired immune system.

h. Remind client of the right to ask questions about current condition, prognosis, and treatment regimen.

i. Inform client of resources available to assist with the execution of advance directives.

j. Support client's efforts to increase knowledge of and control over condition. Provide relevant pamphlets, audiovisual materials, and information about resources and support groups for persons with HIV infection.

k. Inform client of scheduled procedures and tests *so that he/she knows what to expect, which promotes a sense of control.*

l. Consult occupational therapist (if indicated) about assistive devices and environmental modifications that would allow client more independence in performing activities of daily living.

m. Encourage significant others to allow client to do as much as he/she is able *so that a feeling of independence can be maintained.*

n. Encourage client's participation in support groups if indicated.

---

20. NURSING DIAGNOSIS: **Grieving***

related to:
a. diagnosis of an incurable illness with an uncertain course and a high probability of premature death;
b. changes in body functioning, appearance, life style, and roles associated with the disease process.

---

*This diagnostic label includes anticipatory grieving and grieving following the actual losses.

Desired Outcome	Nursing Actions and *Selected Purposes/Rationales*

20. The client will demonstrate beginning progression through the grieving process as evidenced by:
a. verbalization of feelings about AIDS and its implications
b. usual sleep pattern
	20.a. Assess for signs and symptoms of grieving (e.g. change in eating habits, inability to concentrate, insomnia, anger, sadness, withdrawal from significant others, denial of loss).
	b. Implement measures *to facilitate the grieving process:*
	  1. assist client to acknowledge the losses resulting from the diagnosis of AIDS *so grief work can begin;* assess for factors that may hinder and facilitate acknowledgment
	  2. discuss the grieving process and assist client to accept the phases

Desired Outcome	Nursing Actions and *Selected Purposes/Rationales*
c. participation in treatment plan and self-care activities d. utilization of available support systems e. verbalization of a plan for integrating prescribed follow-up care into life style.	of grieving as an expected response to actual and/or anticipated losses 3. allow time for client to progress through the phases of grieving (phases vary among theorists but progress from shock and alarm to acceptance); be aware that not every phase is expressed by all individuals, that recurrence of phases is common, and that the grieving process may take months to years 4. provide an atmosphere of care and concern (e.g. provide privacy, be available and nonjudgmental, display empathy and respect) *so that client will feel free to express feelings* 5. perform actions *to promote trust* (e.g. answer questions honestly, provide requested information) 6. encourage the verbal expression of anger and sadness about the diagnosis of AIDS; recognize displacement of anger and assist client to see actual cause of angry feelings and resentment; establish limits on abusive behavior if demonstrated 7. encourage client to express feelings in whatever ways are comfortable (e.g. writing, drawing, conversation) 8. perform actions to promote effective coping (see Nursing Diagnosis 18, action c) 9. support realistic hope by providing accurate information about research currently being done on HIV infection and the possibility of more effective treatment 10. support behaviors suggesting successful grief work (e.g. verbalizing feelings about the diagnosis of AIDS and changes in body functioning, learning needed skills, developing or renewing relationships, focusing on ways to adapt to losses) 11. explain the phases of the grieving process to significant others; encourage their support, understanding, and presence 12. facilitate communication between the client and significant others; be aware that they may be in different phases of the grieving process 13. provide information regarding counseling services and support groups that might assist client in working through grief. c. Consult physician about referral for counseling if signs of dysfunctional grieving (e.g. persistent denial of losses, excessive anger or sadness, emotional lability) occur.

■

21. NURSING DIAGNOSIS: **Social isolation**

related to:
a. fear of associating with others because of possibility of contracting an infection;
b. stigma and discrimination associated with the diagnosis of AIDS and others' fear of contracting HIV;
c. precautions necessary to prevent spread of HIV;
d. anger towards others responsible for disease transmission to him/her.

Desired Outcome	Nursing Actions and *Selected Purposes/Rationales*
21. The client will experience a decreased sense of isolation as evidenced by: a. maintenance of relationships with significant others	21.a. Ascertain client's usual degree of social interaction. b. Assess for indications of social isolation (e.g. absence of supportive significant others; uncommunicative; withdrawn; expression of feelings of rejection, being different from others, or aloneness imposed by others; hostility; sad, dull affect). c. Implement measures *to decrease social isolation:*

b. verbalization of decreasing feelings of aloneness and rejection.

1. assist client to identify reasons for feeling isolated and alone; aid him/her in developing a plan of action to reduce these feelings
2. reinforce physician's explanation about the immune deficiency; assure client that continued social contact with healthy people will not cause disease or infection
3. provide information to client and significant others about how HIV is known to be transmitted; assure them that HIV does not spread through ordinary physical contact
4. demonstrate acceptance of client using techniques such as touch and frequent visits
5. encourage significant others to visit
6. encourage client to maintain telephone contact with significant others
7. schedule time each day to sit and talk with client
8. assist client to identify a few persons he/she feels comfortable with and encourage interactions with them
9. encourage client to allow friends and family to share their feelings and fears *in order to reduce the possibility of their distancing from client*
10. make items such as telephone, TV, radio, greeting cards, and newspapers accessible to client
11. have significant others bring client's favorite objects from home and place in room.

---

22. NURSING DIAGNOSIS: **Altered family processes**

related to:
a. diagnosis of terminal, communicable disease in family member;
b. fear of disclosure of diagnosis with subsequent rejection of family unit;
c. change in family roles and structure associated with progressive disability and eventual death of family member;
d. financial burden associated with extended illness and progressive disability of client;
e. fear of contracting disease from client;
f. decisions made by client and his/her partner about such issues as treatment plan, life support, and disposition of property that may be in conflict with the client's family of origin;
g. anticipatory grief.

Desired Outcome	Nursing Actions and *Selected Purposes/Rationales*

22. The family members* will demonstrate beginning adjustment to diagnosis of AIDS in client and changes in functioning of family member and family roles and structure as evidenced by:
a. meeting client's needs
b. verbalization of ways to adapt to required role and life-style changes
c. active participation in decision making and client's care
	22.a. Assess for signs and symptoms of altered family processes (e.g. inability to meet client's needs, statements of not being able to accept client's diagnosis or make necessary role and life-style changes, inability to make decisions, inability or refusal to participate in client's care, negative family interactions).
	b. Identify components of the family and their patterns of communication and role expectations.
	c. Implement measures *to facilitate family members' adjustment to client's diagnosis, changes in his/her functioning within the family system, and altered family roles and structure:*
	  1. encourage and assist family members to verbalize feelings about client's diagnosis and its effect on their life style and family structure; actively listen to each family member and maintain a nonjudgmental attitude about feelings shared
	  2. reinforce physician's explanation about AIDS, how HIV is transmitted, and planned treatment program

---

*The term "family members" is being used here to include client's significant others.

Desired Outcome	Nursing Actions and *Selected Purposes/Rationales*
d. positive interactions with one another	3. assist family to gain a realistic perspective of client's situation, conveying as much hope as appropriate
	4. provide privacy *so that family members and client can share their feelings with one another*; stress the importance of and facilitate the use of good communication techniques
	5. assist family members to progress through their own grieving process; explain that they may encounter times when they need to focus on meeting their own rather than the client's needs
	6. emphasize the need for family members to obtain adequate rest and nutrition and to identify and utilize stress management techniques *so that they are better able to emotionally and physically deal with the changes that are being experienced, physical care of the client, and reactions of others when diagnosis is known*
	7. encourage and assist family members to identify coping strategies for dealing with the client's diagnosis and its effect on the family
	8. assist family to identify realistic goals and ways of reaching these goals
	9. include family members in decision making about client's care; convey appreciation for their input and continued support of the client
	10. encourage and allow family members to participate in client's care as appropriate
	11. assist family members to identify resources that can assist them in coping with their feelings and meeting their immediate and long-term needs (e.g. counseling and social services; pastoral care; service, church, and AIDS support groups); initiate a referral if indicated.
	d. Consult physician if family members continue to demonstrate difficulty adjusting to client's diagnosis and change in client's functioning and family structure.

Discharge Teaching

■──

23. NURSING DIAGNOSIS: **Knowledge deficit, Ineffective management of therapeutic regimen, or Altered health maintenance***

──────────────

*The nurse should select the diagnostic label that is most appropriate for the client's discharge teaching needs.

Desired Outcomes	Nursing Actions and *Selected Purposes/Rationales*
23.a. The client will identify ways to prevent the spread of HIV.	23.a. Instruct client in ways to prevent spread of HIV to others:
	1. if a spill of blood or other body fluids occurs, cleanse area with hot, soapy water or a household detergent and then disinfect with a solution of 1 part bleach to 10 parts water
	2. dispose of mop and sponge water used to clean up body fluid spills in the toilet
	3. do not share eating utensils, toothbrushes, razors, enema equipment, or sexual devices
	4. if sexually active with a partner:
	a. avoid multiple sexual partners
	b. be honest with desired partner about HIV infection
	c. modify techniques so that both partners are protected from contact with body fluids
	d. avoid unsafe sexual practices (e.g. sharing sex toys; allowing ejaculate to come in contact with broken skin or mucous membranes; intercourse without a condom; any activity that could

cause tears in lining of vagina, rectum, or penis; mouth contact with penis, vagina, or anal area)

e. avoid vaginal intercourse during menstruation (the contact with blood increases the risk of HIV transmission)

f. use the following guidelines in relation to condom use:
1. always use a condom during anal, vaginal, and oral penetration (condom should be applied prior to time a body orifice is entered because HIV is found in preseminal fluid)
2. use only latex condoms (HIV can penetrate other types of materials)
3. use only condoms with a receptacle tip to reduce the risk of spillage of semen; if that type is unavailable, create a receptacle for ejaculate by pinching tip of condom as it is rolled on erect penis
4. lubricate outside of condom and area to be penetrated to minimize possibility of condom breakage; use a water-based lubricant such as K-Y jelly or a spermicidal compound containing nonoxynol-9 (nonoxynol-9 is known to have some antiviral activity)
5. avoid lubricants made of mineral oil or petroleum distillates such as Vaseline or baby oil (these products weaken latex)
6. hold condom at base of penis during withdrawal and use caution during removal of condom to prevent spillage of semen (penis should be withdrawn and condom removed before the penis has totally relaxed)
7. dispose of condom immediately after use (a new one should be used for subsequent sexual activity)
8. store condoms in a cool place to prevent them from drying out and breaking during use
9. do not use a condom if the expiration date on the package has passed, the package looks worn or punctured, or if the condom looks brittle or discolored or is sticky

5. avoid getting pregnant but if pregnancy occurs, consult health care provider about antiretroviral therapy (e.g. zidovudine) to reduce the risk of perinatal transmission of HIV to infant
6. do not breast feed infant
7. do not donate blood, sperm, or body organs
8. if an intravenous drug user:
   a. get involved in a drug treatment program
   b. do not share drug paraphernalia with others
   c. discard disposable needles and syringes after one use or clean them with household bleach and rinse thoroughly with water.

23.b. The client will identify ways to decrease the risk for developing opportunistic infections.

23.b. Instruct client in ways to decrease risk for developing an opportunistic infection:
1. cleanse kitchen and bathroom surfaces regularly with a disinfectant to prevent growth of pathogens
2. use a 1:10 solution of household bleach and water for cleaning and/or disinfecting areas soiled with blood or other body fluids
3. wear gloves when gardening and when in contact with human or pet excreta (e.g. cleaning litter boxes, bird cages, and aquariums)
4. avoid exposure to body fluids during sexual activity and use latex condoms during sexual intercourse
5. avoid oral-anal sex
6. avoid touching mucous membranes while handling raw meat, seafood, or poultry and wash hands and kitchen surfaces with hot, soapy water after contact with these foods
7. prior to eating fruits and vegetables, wash them well
8. do not eat raw or undercooked poultry, meat, or seafood; anything containing raw eggs or unpasteurized milk; or anything that has passed its expiration date
9. consult health care provider about receiving immunizations (e.g. pneumococcal vaccine, influenza vaccine, hepatitis B vaccine)

Desired Outcomes	Nursing Actions and *Selected Purposes/Rationales*
	10. avoid swimming in lakes, rivers, and public pools
	11. if traveling to a developing country, consult health care provider about recommended immunizations and health care practices (e.g. drinking only bottled water, avoiding raw fruits and vegetables and unpasteurized dairy products)
	12. if a community "boil water" advisory is issued, boil water for a full minute
	13. do not share eating utensils, towels, washcloths, toothbrushes, razors, enema equipment, or sexual devices
	14. keep living quarters well ventilated and change furnace filters regularly to reduce exposure to airborne disease
	15. avoid contact with persons who have an infection and those who have been recently vaccinated
	16. maintain an adequate balance between activity and rest
	17. inform all health care providers of HIV infection so that drugs that further suppress the immune system (e.g. corticosteroids, immunosuppressants) will not be prescribed unnecessarily
	18. maintain an optimal nutritional status
	19. drink at least 10 glasses of liquid/day unless contraindicated.
23.c. The client will state signs and symptoms to report to the health care provider.	23.c. Stress importance of notifying the health care provider if the following signs and symptoms occur or if these existing signs and symptoms worsen: 1. persistent fever or chills 2. night sweats 3. persistent headache 4. swollen glands 5. painful, itchy skin lesions 6. reddish-purple patches or nodules on any body area 7. ulcerations or white patches in the mouth 8. difficulty swallowing 9. persistent diarrhea 10. perianal or vulvovaginal itching and/or pain 11. frequency, urgency, or burning on urination 12. cloudy, foul-smelling urine 13. dry cough or a cough productive of purulent, green, or rust-colored sputum 14. progressive shortness of breath 15. increasing weakness, fatigue, or weight loss 16. change in vision 17. loss of strength and coordination in extremity(ies) 18. numbness, tingling, or pain in extremity(ies) 19. inability to maintain an adequate fluid intake.
23.d. The client will identify resources that can assist in adjustment to changes resulting from the diagnosis of AIDS.	23.d.1. Provide information to client and significant others about resources that can assist in adjustment to the diagnosis of AIDS (e.g. American Foundation for AIDS Research, National Association of People with AIDS, hospice programs, community support groups, CDC National AIDS Hotline, Project Inform, counselors). 2. Initiate a referral if indicated.

23.e. The client will verbalize an understanding of and a plan for adhering to recommended follow-up care including regular laboratory studies, future appointments with health care providers, and medications prescribed.	23.e.1. Reinforce the importance of keeping scheduled follow-up appointments for laboratory studies and with health care providers.
	2. Explain the rationale for, side effects of, and importance of taking medications prescribed. Inform client of pertinent food and drug interactions.
	3. If trimethoprim-sulfamethoxazole is prescribed prophylactically to prevent PCP, provide the following instructions:
	  a. take the medication with a large glass of water at least 1 hour before or 2 hours after a meal
	  b. drink at least 10 glasses of liquid/day unless contraindicated
	  c. report development of a rash, nausea and vomiting, fever, or yellowing of skin.
	4. If client is discharged on zidovudine (e.g. ZDV, Retrovir, AZT), instruct him/her to:

    a. follow schedule of drug administration carefully

    b. avoid taking other medications unless approved by physician

    c. report the following:

       1. nausea that persists for longer than 6 weeks or frequent episodes of vomiting

       2. increased weakness and fatigue or shortness of breath upon exertion (anemia is a common adverse effect)

       3. sore throat, fever, or wound that does not heal (infection can result from the bone marrow depressant effects)

       4. muscle pain, persistent headache, or severe upper abdominal pain.

5. If client is discharged on didanosine, instruct to:

    a. take pills 1 hour before or 2–3 hours after eating

    b. take 2 pills at a time and thoroughly chew them or dissolve them in water in order to ensure release of buffering agent in the pills

    c. avoid intake of alcohol because of the increased risk of pancreatitis with this drug

    d. report upper abdominal pain; nausea; vomiting; persistent or severe diarrhea; or pain, numbness, or tingling in extremities.

6. Stress the importance of taking hematopoietic agents (e.g. epoetin alfa [Epogen], granulocyte colony-stimulating factor [filgrastim]) as prescribed.

7. Implement measures to improve client compliance:

    a. include significant others in discharge teaching sessions if possible

    b. encourage questions and allow time for reinforcement and clarification of information provided

    c. provide written instructions regarding scheduled appointments with health care providers and laboratory, medications prescribed, signs and symptoms to report, and ways to prevent infection.

Bibliography

See pages 897–898 and 906.

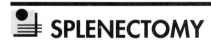

SPLENECTOMY

Splenectomy is the surgical removal of the spleen. The most common indication for the surgery is rupture of the spleen. Causes of rupture include penetrating or blunt trauma to the spleen, operative trauma to the spleen during surgery on nearby organs, and damage to the spleen as a result of disease (e.g. mononucleosis, tuberculosis of the spleen). A splenectomy may also be indicated if the spleen is removing excessive quantities of platelets, erythrocytes, or leukocytes from the circulation (hypersplenism). Conditions associated with hypersplenism include leukemia, idiopathic thrombocytopenic purpura, Felty's syndrome, thalassemia major, lymphoma, and hereditary spherocytosis. Additionally, splenectomy may be performed to treat splenic aneurysm, cysts, and neoplasm. When feasible, a partial splenectomy or splenic autotransplantation (transplantation of splenic fragments into other areas of the abdomen) is performed so that some of the spleen's immunological function is maintained.

This care plan focuses on the adult client hospitalized with a suspected splenic rupture resulting from trauma. Preoperatively, goals of care are to prevent hypovolemic shock and prepare the client for surgery. Postoperative goals of care are to maintain comfort, prevent complications, and educate the client regarding follow-up care.

DIAGNOSTIC TESTS

Computed tomography (CT)
Ultrasonography
Abdominal x-ray
Magnetic resonance imaging (MRI)
Complete blood count (CBC)

DISCHARGE CRITERIA

Prior to discharge, the client will:

- have surgical pain controlled
- have no signs and symptoms of infection
- have no signs and symptoms of postoperative complications
- identify appropriate safety measures to follow because of increased risk for infection
- state signs and symptoms to report to the health care provider
- verbalize an understanding of and a plan for adhering to recommended follow-up care including future appointments with health care provider, medications prescribed, wound care, and activity level.

NURSING/ COLLABORATIVE DIAGNOSES	**Preoperative**
	 1. Potential complication: hypovolemic shock △ 566
	 Postoperative
	 1. Risk for infection △ 567
	 2. Potential complications:
	   a. pancreatitis
	   b. subphrenic abscess
	   c. thromboembolism
	   d. postsplenectomy sepsis △ 568

DISCHARGE TEACHING	3. Knowledge deficit, Ineffective management of therapeutic regimen, or Altered health maintenance △ 570

See Standardized Preoperative and Postoperative Care Plans for additional diagnoses.

PREOPERATIVE

Use in conjunction with the Standardized Preoperative Care Plan.

---

1. COLLABORATIVE DIAGNOSIS:

Potential complication of ruptured spleen: hypovolemic shock

related to excessive blood loss associated with trauma to the spleen (the spleen is a highly vascular organ).

Desired Outcome	Nursing Actions and *Selected Purposes/Rationales*
1. The client will not develop hypovolemic shock as evidenced by:	1.a. Assess for and report: 1. signs and symptoms of splenic rupture (e.g. left upper abdominal pain and tenderness, generalized abdominal pain, pain in left shoulder

a. usual mental status
b. stable vital signs
c. skin warm, dry, and usual color
d. palpable peripheral pulses
e. urine output at least 30 ml/hour.

[a referred pain that results from irritation of the diaphragm by blood in the abdominal cavity and is known as Kehr's sign])
2. decreasing RBC, Hct, and Hb levels
3. signs and symptoms of hypovolemic shock:
   a. restlessness, agitation, confusion, or other change in mental status
   b. significant decrease in B/P
   c. postural hypotension
   d. rapid, weak pulse
   e. rapid respirations
   f. cool, moist skin
   g. pallor, cyanosis
   h. diminished or absent peripheral pulses
   i. urine output less than 30 ml/hour.
b. Administer blood products and/or volume expanders if ordered *to prevent hypovolemic shock.*
c. If signs and symptoms of hypovolemic shock occur:
   1. continue to administer blood products and/or volume expanders as ordered
   2. place client flat in bed with legs elevated unless contraindicated
   3. monitor vital signs frequently
   4. administer oxygen as ordered
   5. prepare client for splenectomy (surgery may need to be performed before scheduled time)
   6. provide emotional support to client and significant others.

POSTOPERATIVE

Use in conjunction with the Standardized Postoperative Care Plan.

---

1. NURSING DIAGNOSIS:

Risk for infection

related to decreased resistance to infection associated with removal of the spleen (the macrophages and lymphocytes in the spleen are responsible for phagocytizing infectious organisms and producing antibodies).

Desired Outcome	Nursing Actions and *Selected Purposes/Rationales*

1. The client will remain free of infection as evidenced by:
a. absence of fever and chills
b. pulse within normal limits
c. normal breath sounds
d. usual mental status
e. cough productive of clear mucus only
f. voiding clear urine without reports of frequency, urgency, and burning
g. absence of heat, redness, swelling, and unusual pain and drainage in any area
	1.a. Assess for and report signs and symptoms of infection (be aware that some signs and symptoms vary depending on the site of infection, the causative organism, and the age and immune status of the client):
	  1. elevated temperature
	  2. chills
	  3. increased pulse
	  4. abnormal breath sounds
	  5. malaise, lethargy, acute confusion
	  6. cough productive of purulent, green, or rust-colored sputum
	  7. cloudy, foul-smelling urine
	  8. reports of frequency, urgency, or burning when urinating
	  9. presence of WBCs, bacteria, and/or nitrites in urine
	  10. heat, redness, swelling, or unusual pain or drainage in any area
	  11. WBC count that continues to increase and/or a significant change in differential.
	b. Obtain specimens (e.g. wound drainage, urine, vaginal drainage, sputum, blood) for culture as ordered. Report positive results.

Desired Outcome	Nursing Actions and **Selected Purposes/Rationales**
h. no further increase in WBC count or significant change in differential i. negative results of cultured specimens.	c. Implement measures *to prevent infection:* 1. maintain a fluid intake of at least 2500 ml/day unless contraindicated 2. use good handwashing technique and encourage client to do the same 3. use sterile technique (surgical asepsis) during all invasive procedures (e.g. urinary catheterizations, venous and arterial punctures, injections, wound care) 4. anchor catheters/tubings (e.g. urinary, intravenous, wound drainage) securely *in order to reduce trauma to the tissues and the risk for introduction of pathogens associated with the in-and-out movement of the tubing* 5. rotate intravenous insertion sites according to hospital policy 6. change equipment, tubings, and solutions used for treatments such as intravenous infusions, respiratory care, and irrigations according to hospital policy 7. maintain a closed system for drains (e.g. wound, urinary catheter) and intravenous infusions whenever possible 8. protect client from others with infection and instruct him/her to continue this after discharge 9. perform actions to maintain an adequate nutritional status (see Standardized Postoperative Care Plan, Nursing Diagnosis 5, action d [p. 106]) 10. reinforce importance of good oral hygiene 11. perform actions *to prevent stasis of respiratory secretions* (e.g. assist client to turn, cough, and deep breathe; increase activity as allowed and tolerated) 12. perform actions to prevent urinary retention (e.g. instruct client to urinate when the urge is first felt, promote relaxation during voiding attempts, administer bethanechol as ordered) *in order to prevent urinary stasis* 13. instruct and assist client to perform good perineal care routinely and after each bowel movement 14. perform actions *to prevent wound infection* (e.g. maintain aseptic technique during wound care, instruct client to avoid touching wound, maintain patency of wound drain) 15. administer immunizations (e.g. influenza vaccine, pneumococcal vaccine) if ordered (whenever possible, immunizations are given before the splenectomy *so that immunity has already begun to develop at the time of surgery*) 16. administer prophylactic antimicrobials if ordered.

■━━━━━━━━━━━━━━━━━━━━━━━━━━━━━━━━━━━━━━━

2. COLLABORATIVE DIAGNOSES:

Potential complications of splenectomy:

a. **pancreatitis** related to trauma to the pancreas during surgery;

b. **subphrenic abscess** related to suppuration in the surgical area and decreased resistance to infection;

c. **thromboembolism** related to:
1. hypercoagulability associated with:
   a. increase in the number of circulating erythrocytes (contributes to hemoconcentration and increased blood viscosity) and platelets resulting from the spleen no longer being available to destroy the cells that are old or damaged and to store blood (usually stores 150–300 ml of blood including about 30% of the platelet mass)
   b. increased release of tissue thromboplastin into the blood (occurs as a result of trauma from the injury and surgery)
2. venous stasis associated with decreased activity, increased blood viscosity, and abdominal distention (the distended intestine can put pressure on the abdominal vessels)
3. trauma to vein walls during surgery;

d. **postsplenectomy sepsis** related to development of a fulminant infection associated with diminished immune system function following splenectomy.

Desired Outcomes	Nursing Actions and *Selected Purposes/Rationales*
2.a. The client will experience resolution of pancreatitis if it occurs as evidenced by: 1. gradual resolution of abdominal pain 2. temperature declining toward normal 3. stable B/P and pulse 4. serum amylase and lipase levels decreasing toward normal 5. renal amylase/creatinine clearance ratio returning toward normal 6. WBC count decreasing toward normal.	2.a.1. Assess for and report signs and symptoms of pancreatitis (e.g. extension of abdominal pain to back, increased midepigastric or left upper quadrant pain, increase in temperature, hypotension, tachycardia, elevated serum amylase and lipase levels). 2. Collect a timed (usually 2-hour) urine specimen if ordered. Report an elevated renal amylase/creatinine clearance ratio. 3. Monitor WBC counts. Report levels that increase or fail to decrease toward normal. 4. If signs and symptoms of pancreatitis occur: a. assist client to assume position of greatest comfort (e.g. side-lying or sitting with trunk and knees flexed) b. maintain food and fluid restrictions as ordered c. insert nasogastric tube and maintain suction as ordered (*removal of gastric secretions reduces pancreatic stimulation*) d. administer the following medications if ordered: 1. analgesics 2. antacids and/or histamine₂ receptor antagonists (e.g. famotidine, ranitidine, cimetidine) *to decrease the acidity of gastric contents and thereby reduce stimulation of the pancreas* (*when acidic gastric contents enter the duodenum and jejunum, secretin is released; secretin stimulates pancreatic secretion*) e. refer to Care Plan on Pancreatitis for additional care measures.
2.b. The client will experience resolution of a subphrenic abscess if it develops as evidenced by: 1. decrease in abdominal pain 2. temperature declining toward normal 3. WBC count decreasing toward normal.	2.b.1. Assess for and report signs and symptoms of a subphrenic abscess (e.g. increased, persistent abdominal pain; increase in temperature and pulse rate). 2. Monitor WBC count and report levels that increase or fail to decrease toward normal. 3. If signs and symptoms of subphrenic abscess occur: a. administer antimicrobials if ordered b. prepare client for surgical intervention (e.g. incision and drainage of abscess) if planned c. assess for and report signs and symptoms of peritonitis (e.g. distended, rigid abdomen; increased severity of abdominal pain; rebound tenderness; continued diminished or absent bowel sounds; nausea; vomiting; further increase in temperature; tachycardia, tachypnea; hypotension).
2.c. The client will not experience signs and symptoms of a deep vein thrombus or pulmonary embolism (see Standardized Postoperative Care Plan, Collaborative Diagnosis 19, outcomes c.1 and 2 [pp. 120–121], for outcome criteria).	2.c.1. Refer to Standardized Postoperative Nursing Care Plan, Collaborative Diagnosis 19, actions c.1 and 2 (pp. 120–121), for measures related to assessment, prevention, and treatment of a deep vein thrombus and pulmonary embolism. 2. Assess for and report increasing abdominal distention and pain (*may indicate portal vein or mesenteric venous thrombus*).
2.d. The client will not experience postsplenectomy sepsis as evidenced by: 1. absence of nausea, vomiting, and headache 2. usual mental status 3. stable vital signs.	2.d.1. Assess for and report signs and symptoms of postsplenectomy sepsis (e.g. nausea, vomiting, headache, confusion, hypotension, tachycardia, tachypnea). Be aware that client's condition can rapidly progress to shock, coma, and death following the onset of symptoms. 2. Implement measures *to reduce the risk for postsplenectomy sepsis:* a. perform actions to prevent infection (see Postoperative Nursing Diagnosis 1, action c) b. assess for and immediately report signs and symptoms of infection (see Postoperative Nursing Diagnosis 1, action a) *so that orders for treatment can be obtained and initiated promptly* (*a mild infection can develop into sepsis within hours*).

Desired Outcomes   Nursing Actions and *Selected Purposes/Rationales*

3. If signs and symptoms of postsplenectomy sepsis occur:
   a. maintain intravenous fluid therapy as ordered
   b. monitor vital signs frequently
   c. obtain specimens (e.g. urine, wound drainage, blood, sputum) for culture as ordered
   d. administer antimicrobials as ordered
   e. prepare client for transfer to critical care unit and insertion of hemodynamic monitoring devices (e.g. central venous catheter, intraarterial catheter) if planned
   f. provide emotional support to client and significant others.

Discharge Teaching

◼━━

3. NURSING DIAGNOSIS: **Knowledge deficit, Ineffective management of therapeutic regimen, or Altered health maintenance***

────────────

*The nurse should select the diagnostic label that is most appropriate for the client's discharge teaching needs.

Desired Outcomes   Nursing Actions and *Selected Purposes/Rationales*

3.a. The client will identify appropriate safety measures to follow because of increased risk for infection.

3.a.1. Explain to client that he/she is more prone to infection because the rest of the immune system cannot completely compensate for the loss of the spleen.
   2. Instruct client to:
      a. continue to adhere to measures to prevent infection (see Standardized Postoperative Care Plan, Nursing Diagnosis 21, action a [p. 123])
      b. consult health care provider about receiving vaccinations periodically to reduce the risk of pneumonia and influenza
      c. inform all health care providers of being asplenic so that prophylactic antimicrobials can be started before any dental work, invasive diagnostic procedure, or surgery is performed
      d. carry an identification card and wear a medical alert identification bracelet or tag identifying self as being asplenic and at increased risk for infection.

3.b. The client will state signs and symptoms to report to the health care provider.

3.b.1. Refer to Standardized Postoperative Care Plan, Nursing Diagnosis 21, action c (p. 123), for signs and symptoms to report to the health care provider.
   2. Instruct client to report these additional signs and symptoms:
      a. nausea, vomiting, headache, and/or confusion (could indicate postsplenectomy sepsis)
      b. any febrile illness
      c. any minor infection.

3.c. The client will verbalize an understanding of and a plan for adhering to recommended follow-up care including future appointments with health care provider, medications prescribed, wound care, and activity level.

3.c. Refer to Standardized Postoperative Care Plan, Nursing Diagnosis 21 (pp. 123–124), for routine postoperative instructions and measures to improve client compliance.

Bibliography

See pages 897–898 and 906.

UNIT FOURTEEN

NURSING CARE OF THE CLIENT WITH DISTURBANCES OF THE GASTROINTESTINAL TRACT

APPENDECTOMY

An appendectomy is the surgical removal of the appendix (a small cylindrical blind tube that extends from the inferior part of the cecum just below the ileocecal valve). It is performed to treat appendicitis, which most frequently occurs as a result of obstruction of the lumen of the appendix by a fecalith, a foreign body, an appendiceal calculus, a tumor, hyperplasia of submucosal lymphatic tissue, or retained barium following contrast radiography. Inflammation of the appendix with subsequent lumen obstruction may also occur concurrently with acute infections. Obstruction of the appendix leads to increased luminal pressure, vascular congestion, bacterial invasion, and ultimately, necrosis and perforation of the appendix.

An appendectomy is done via laparotomy or laparoscopy. A laparoscopic appendectomy offers the advantage of shorter hospitalization and decreased morbidity and mortality but is contraindicated in persons with extensive intraperitoneal adhesions or other intestinal problems that would impede mobilization and dissection of the appendix.

This care plan focuses on the adult client with suspected appendicitis who is hospitalized for a possible appendectomy. Preoperative goals of care are to reduce fear and anxiety, control discomfort, and prevent perforation of the appendix. The goals of postoperative care are to maintain comfort, prevent complications, and educate the client regarding follow-up care.

DIAGNOSTIC TESTS

White blood cell (WBC) count and differential
Ultrasonography
Computed tomography (CT)
Abdominal x-ray

DISCHARGE CRITERIA

Prior to discharge, the client will:

- have evidence of normal healing of surgical wound
- have clear, audible breath sounds
- tolerate prescribed diet
- have surgical pain controlled
- have no signs and symptoms of postoperative complications
- state signs and symptoms to report to the health care provider
- verbalize an understanding of and a plan for adhering to recommended follow-up care including future appointments with health care provider, medications prescribed, activity level, and wound care.

NURSING/ COLLABORATIVE DIAGNOSES	**Preoperative**
	1. Pain: abdominal (particularly in the periumbilical area or right lower quadrant) △ 573
	2. Altered comfort: nausea and vomiting △ 573
	3. Hyperthermia △ 574
	4. Potential complications:
	  a. abscess formation
	  b. peritonitis △ 574
	Postoperative
	1. Potential complications:
	  a. abscess formation
	  b. peritonitis △ 575

DISCHARGE TEACHING	2. Knowledge deficit, Ineffective management of therapeutic regimen, or Altered health maintenance △ 576

See Standardized Preoperative and Postoperative Care Plans for additional diagnoses.

PREOPERATIVE

Use in conjunction with the Standardized Preoperative Care Plan.

---

1. NURSING DIAGNOSIS:

Pain: abdominal (particularly in the periumbilical area or right lower quadrant)

related to:
a. stretching of the appendix associated with obstruction and inflammation of the appendix;
b. irritation of the peritoneum (occurs with transmural involvement of the appendix and subsequent contact of the inflamed serosal surface of the appendix with the peritoneum).

Desired Outcome	Nursing Actions and *Selected Purposes/Rationales*

1. The client will experience diminished abdominal pain as evidenced by:
a. verbalization of a decrease in pain
b. relaxed facial expression and body positioning
c. stable vital signs.
	1.a. Assess for signs and symptoms of pain (e.g. verbalization of pain, grimacing, reluctance to move, guarding or rubbing of abdomen, restlessness, diaphoresis, facial pallor, increased B/P, tachycardia).
	b. Assess client's perception of the severity of pain using a pain intensity rating scale.
	c. Assess the client's pain pattern (e.g. location, quality, onset, duration, precipitating factors, aggravating factors, alleviating factors); note that a finding of pain in the right lower quadrant elicited by palpation of the left lower quadrant (Rovsing's sign) and/or localized tenderness over McBurney's point are diagnostic indicators of appendicitis.
	d. Ask the client to describe previous pain experiences and methods used to manage pain effectively.
	e. Implement measures *to reduce pain*:
	  1. perform actions *to reduce fear and anxiety about the pain experience* (e.g. assure client that his/her need for pain relief is understood, plan methods for achieving pain control with client)
	  2. perform actions to reduce fear and anxiety (see Standardized Preoperative Care Plan, Nursing Diagnosis 1, action c [p. 97]) *in order to promote relaxation and subsequently increase the client's threshold and tolerance for pain*
	  3. assist client to assume a comfortable position (e.g. side-lying with right knee flexed)
	  4. administer analgesics if ordered (analgesics may be held until the diagnosis is established).
	f. Consult physician if above measures fail to provide adequate pain relief.

---

2. NURSING DIAGNOSIS:

Altered comfort: nausea and vomiting

related to stimulation of the vomiting center associated with:
a. stimulation of the visceral afferent pathways resulting from inflammation of the appendix;
b. stimulation of the cerebral cortex resulting from pain and stress.

Desired Outcome	Nursing Actions and *Selected Purposes/Rationales*

2. The client will experience relief of nausea and vomiting as evidenced by:
  a. verbalization of relief of nausea
  b. absence of vomiting.
	2.a. Assess client for nausea and vomiting.
	  b. Implement measures *to reduce nausea and vomiting:*
	    1. perform actions to reduce abdominal pain (see Preoperative Nursing Diagnosis 1, action e)
	    2. perform actions to reduce fear and anxiety (see Standardized Preoperative Care Plan, Nursing Diagnosis 1, action c [p. 97])
	    3. eliminate noxious sights and odors from the environment (*noxious stimuli can cause stimulation of the vomiting center*)
	    4. encourage client to take deep, slow breaths when nauseated
	    5. encourage client to change positions slowly (*rapid movement can result in stimulation of the chemoreceptor trigger zone and subsequent excitation of the vomiting center*)
	    6. provide oral hygiene after each emesis
	    7. restrict oral intake if indicated
	    8. administer antiemetics if ordered.
	  c. If above measures fail to control nausea and vomiting:
	    1. consult physician
	    2. be prepared to insert a nasogastric tube and maintain suction as ordered.

3. NURSING DIAGNOSIS:

Hyperthermia

related to stimulation of the thermoregulatory center in the hypothalamus by endogenous pyrogens that are released in an infectious process.

Desired Outcome	Nursing Actions and *Selected Purposes/Rationales*

3. The client will have hyperthermia adequately controlled as evidenced by:
  a. skin usual temperature and color
  b. pulse rate between 60–100 beats/minute
  c. respirations 14–20/minute
  d. temperature declining toward normal.
	3.a. Assess for signs and symptoms of hyperthermia (e.g. warm, flushed skin; tachycardia; tachypnea; elevated temperature).
	  b. Administer the following medications if ordered *to help reduce fever:*
	    a. antipyretics
	    b. antimicrobials *to resolve the infectious process.*
	  c. Consult physician if temperature remains higher than 38° C.

4. COLLABORATIVE DIAGNOSES:

Potential complications of appendicitis:

a. **abscess formation** related to perforation of the appendix into a localized, contained area;

b. **peritonitis** related to release of intestinal contents into the peritoneal cavity associated with perforation of the appendix or leakage of a periappendiceal abscess.

Desired Outcomes	Nursing Actions and *Selected Purposes/Rationales*

4.a. The client will not have formation of an abscess as evidenced by:
1. temperature stable and less than 38° C
2. no increase in abdominal pain or tenderness
3. no palpable mass in abdomen
4. no further increase in WBC count.
	4.a.1. Assess for and report signs and symptoms of abscess formation (e.g. further increase in temperature or temperature above 38° C, increase in abdominal pain and localized tenderness, presence of a palpable mass in abdomen).
	2. Monitor WBC counts. Report increasing levels or WBC count greater than 15,000/mm³).
	3. Implement measures *to reduce the risk for perforation of the appendix and subsequent abscess formation:*
	  a. perform actions *to prevent a further increase in intraluminal pressure:*
	    1. withhold oral intake if ordered
	    2. insert a nasogastric tube and maintain suction if ordered
	    3. do not administer an enema
	  b. avoid use of laxatives (*may cause excessive peristalsis*)
	  c. do not apply heat to abdomen (*may speed up the suppurative process and precipitate perforation*).
	4. If signs and symptoms of abscess formation occur:
	  a. prepare client for diagnostic studies (e.g. computed tomography, ultrasonography) if planned
	  b. administer antimicrobials as ordered
	  c. prepare client for surgery or percutaneous drainage of abscess.

4.b. The client will not develop peritonitis as evidenced by:
1. temperature stable and less than 38° C
2. soft, nondistended abdomen
3. no increase in abdominal pain and tenderness, nausea, and vomiting
4. normal bowel sounds
5. stable vital signs
6. no further increase in WBC count.
	4.b.1. Assess for and report signs and symptoms of peritonitis (e.g. further increase in temperature or temperature above 38° C; distended, rigid abdomen; increase in severity of abdominal pain; rebound tenderness; increased nausea and vomiting; diminished or absent bowel sounds; tachycardia; tachypnea; hypotension).
	2. Monitor WBC counts. Report increasing levels or a WBC count greater than 15,000/mm³.
	3. Implement measures to reduce the risk for perforation of the appendix (see action a.3 in this diagnosis) *in order to prevent peritonitis.*
	4. If signs and symptoms of peritonitis occur:
	  a. withhold oral intake as ordered
	  b. place client on bed rest in a semi-Fowler's position *to assist in pooling or localizing gastrointestinal contents in the pelvis rather than under the diaphragm*
	  c. prepare client for diagnostic tests (e.g. abdominal x-ray, computed tomography, ultrasonography) if planned
	  d. insert nasogastric or intestinal tube and maintain suction as ordered
	  e. administer antimicrobials as ordered
	  f. administer intravenous fluids and/or blood volume expanders if ordered *to prevent or treat shock (can result from the increased capillary permeability that occurs with inflammation and the subsequent escape of protein, fluid, and electrolytes from the vascular space into the peritoneal cavity)*
	  g. prepare client for surgery (e.g. appendectomy with drainage and irrigation of peritoneum) if planned
	  h. provide emotional support to client and significant others.

POSTOPERATIVE

Use in conjunction with the Standardized Postoperative Care Plan.

---

1. COLLABORATIVE DIAGNOSES:

Potential complications of appendectomy:

  a. **abscess formation** related to suppuration in the inflamed or infected area (more likely to occur following resection of a perforated appendix);

  b. **peritonitis** related to entrance of pathogens/irritants into peritoneal cavity associated with wound infection, leakage from an abscess, and/or release of intestinal contents into the peritoneal cavity resulting from preoperative or intraoperative perforation of the appendix and leakage of suture lines postoperatively.

Desired Outcomes	Nursing Actions and *Selected Purposes/Rationales*

1.a. The client will not develop or will have resolution of an abscess if it occurs as evidenced by:
1. temperature declining toward normal
2. absence of chills
3. gradual resolution of abdominal pain
4. WBC count declining toward normal.
	1.a.1. Assess for and report signs and symptoms of abscess formation (e.g. increase in temperature, chills, increased or more constant abdominal pain, presence of a palpable mass in abdomen, further increase in WBC count).
	  2. Implement measures to maintain patency and prevent inadvertent removal of wound drain if present (see actions b.3.b and c in this diagnosis) *in order to reduce the risk for abscess formation.*
	  3. If signs and symptoms of abscess formation occur:
	    a. prepare client for diagnostic tests (e.g. computed tomography, ultrasonography) if planned
	    b. administer antimicrobials as ordered
	    c. prepare client for surgical drainage of the abscess if planned
	    d. provide emotional support to client and significant others.

1.b. The client will not develop or will have resolution of peritonitis if it occurs as evidenced by:
1. gradual resolution of abdominal pain
2. soft, nondistended abdomen
3. temperature declining toward normal
4. stable vital signs
5. gradual return of normal bowel sounds
6. WBC count declining toward normal.
	1.b.1. Refer to Preoperative Collaborative Diagnosis 4, actions b.1 and 4 for measures related to assessment and treatment of peritonitis.
	  2. Monitor WBC counts. Report levels that increase or fail to decline toward normal.
	  3. Implement measures *to prevent peritonitis:*
	    a. perform actions to treat an abscess if it occurs (see action a.3 in this diagnosis)
	    b. perform actions *to maintain patency of wound drain if present in order to prevent increased pressure on the suture line:*
	      1. keep tubing free of kinks
	      2. empty collection device as often as necessary
	      3. maintain suction as ordered
	    c. perform actions *to prevent inadvertent removal of wound drain if present:*
	      1. use caution when changing dressings surrounding drain
	      2. provide extension tubing if necessary *to enable client to move without placing tension on the drain*
	      3. instruct client not to pull on drain and drainage tubing
	    d. maintain sterile technique during dressing changes and wound care
	    e. keep abdominal dressing clean and dry
	    f. administer antimicrobials if ordered.

Discharge Teaching

■━━━━━━━━━━━━━━━━━━━━━━━━━━━━━━━━━━━

2. NURSING DIAGNOSIS: **Knowledge deficit, Ineffective management of therapeutic regimen, or Altered health maintenance***

---

*The nurse should select the diagnostic label that is most appropriate for the client's discharge teaching needs.

Desired Outcomes	Nursing Actions and *Selected Purposes/Rationales*
2.a. The client will state signs and symptoms to report to the health care provider.	2.a. Refer to Standardized Postoperative Care Plan, Nursing Diagnosis 21, action c (p. 123), for signs and symptoms to report to the health care provider.

2.b. The client will verbalize an understanding of and a plan for adhering to recommended follow-up care including future appointments with health care provider, medications prescribed, activity level, and wound care.

2.b. Refer to Standardized Postoperative Care Plan, Nursing Diagnosis 21 (pp. 123–124), for routine postoperative instructions and measures to improve client compliance.

Bibliography

See pages 897–898 and 906.

BOWEL DIVERSION: ILEOSTOMY

An ileostomy is the diversion of the ileum from the abdominal cavity through an opening created in the abdominal wall. It may be performed following abdominal trauma or to treat conditions such as familial polyposis, intestinal cancer, and, most commonly, inflammatory bowel disease that is refractory to conservative management. An ileostomy can be temporary or permanent.

A temporary ileostomy is usually created to allow the bowel to heal following traumatic abdominal injury or to permit healing of a newly constructed ileoanal reservoir (pouch). The ileoanal reservoir is a treatment option for some persons with inflammatory bowel disease or familial polyposis. In the initial surgery, the diseased portion of the intestine is removed, a temporary ileostomy is performed, and a reservoir is created in the rectal area using a portion of the ileum. After 2–4 months, the ileostomy is closed and intestinal continuity is established between the remaining intestine and the ileoanal reservoir.

There are 2 types of permanent ileostomies. The conventional (Brooke) ileostomy is the most common one. It is created by bringing a portion of the terminal ileum through the abdominal wall, usually in the right lower quadrant. The ileostomy drains intermittently but, because it cannot be regulated, a collection device needs to be worn over the stoma at all times. Another type of permanent ileostomy is the continent ileostomy. In this procedure, the terminal ileum is used to construct an intra-abdominal reservoir (Kock pouch). Initially, the reservoir drains via a catheter that is placed through the stoma and a surgically constructed one-way valve. After the surgical area heals, the catheter is removed and the reservoir only needs to be drained periodically. If the system functions properly, the client does not need to wear a collection device over the stoma. The type of permanent ileostomy constructed depends on the client's age, underlying disease process, and preference and expertise of the surgeon. A proctocolectomy (removal of the colon, rectum, and anus) is often done at the same time as a permanent ileostomy to treat the disease process or to prevent future bowel changes that could occur. If a proctocolectomy is not performed, the rectal stump is sutured across the top; the rectum stays intact and secretes mucus that is expelled via the anus.

This care plan focuses on the adult client with inflammatory bowel disease hospitalized for bowel diversion with creation of a permanent ileostomy. Preoperatively, goals of care are to reduce fear and anxiety and begin to prepare the client for the changes in body image and function. The postoperative goals of care are to maintain fluid and electrolyte balance and an adequate nutritional status, maintain integrity of the peristomal and perianal skin, prevent complications, facilitate psychological adjustment to the ileostomy, and educate the client regarding follow-up care.

DIAGNOSTIC TESTS

Refer to Care Plan on Inflammatory Bowel Disease.

DISCHARGE CRITERIA

Prior to discharge, the client will:

- have surgical pain controlled
- have evidence of normal healing of the surgical wound
- have a medium pink to red, moist stoma and intact peristomal and perianal skin

- have no evidence of fluid and electrolyte imbalances
- maintain an adequate nutritional status
- have no signs and symptoms of postoperative complications
- verbalize a basic understanding of the anatomical changes that have occurred as a result of the bowel diversion
- identify ways to maintain fluid and electrolyte balance
- verbalize ways to maintain an optimal nutritional status
- identify methods of controlling odor and sound associated with ileostomy drainage and gas
- demonstrate the ability to change the pouch system, maintain integrity of the peristomal and perianal skin, and maintain adequate stomal circulation and integrity
- demonstrate the ability to properly use, clean, and store ostomy products
- demonstrate the ability to drain and irrigate a continent ileostomy if present
- identify ways to prevent and treat blockage of the stoma
- state signs and symptoms to report to the health care provider
- share thoughts and feelings about the effect of altered bowel function on self-concept and life style
- identify appropriate community resources that can assist with home management and adjustment to changes resulting from the bowel diversion
- verbalize an understanding of and a plan for adhering to recommended follow-up care including future appointments with health care provider, wound care, activity level, and medications prescribed.

NURSING/ COLLABORATIVE DIAGNOSES	**Preoperative**
	1. Anxiety △ 579
	2. Knowledge deficit △ 579
	Postoperative
	1. Altered fluid and electrolyte balance:
	   a. fluid volume deficit
	   b. hypokalemia, hypomagnesemia, and hypochloremia
	   c. metabolic alkalosis
	   d. metabolic acidosis △ 581
	2. Altered nutrition: less than body requirements △ 582
	3. Actual/Risk for impaired tissue integrity △ 582
	4. Potential complications:
	   a. peritonitis
	   b. stomal changes:
	      1. necrosis
	      2. excessive bleeding
	      3. prolapse
	   c. stomal obstruction △ 585
	5. Altered sexuality patterns △ 588
	6. Self-concept disturbance △ 589
	7. Ineffective individual coping △ 590
	8. Grieving △ 591

DISCHARGE TEACHING	9. Knowledge deficit, Ineffective management of therapeutic regimen, or Altered health maintenance △ 592

See Care Plan on Inflammatory Bowel Disease and the Standardized Preoperative and Postoperative Care Plans for additional diagnoses.

PREOPERATIVE

Use in conjunction with the Care Plan on Inflammatory Bowel Disease and the Standardized Preoperative Care Plan.

---

1. NURSING DIAGNOSIS: **Anxiety**

related to:
a. unfamiliar environment and separation from significant others;
b. anticipated loss of control associated with effects of anesthesia;
c. lack of understanding of diagnostic tests, planned surgical procedure, and care that will be required for the ileostomy;
d. financial concerns associated with hospitalization;
e. anticipated discomfort, surgical findings, changes in appearance and body functioning, and effects of ileostomy on future life style;
f. ability to independently perform ileostomy care following discharge.

Desired Outcome	Nursing Actions and *Selected Purposes/Rationales*
1. The client will experience a reduction in anxiety (see Standardized Preoperative Care Plan, Nursing Diagnosis 1 [pp. 96–97], for outcome criteria).	1.a. Refer to Standardized Preoperative Care Plan, Nursing Diagnosis 1 (pp. 96–97), for measures related to assessment and reduction of fear and anxiety. b. Implement additional measures *to reduce fear and anxiety:* 1. provide client with information about preoperative routines, the surgical procedure, general postoperative care, the function and appearance of the stoma, and management of the ileostomy (see Preoperative Nursing Diagnosis 2) *so he/she will know what to expect* 2. explain that every attempt will be made to place the stoma in an area that he/she can easily see and reach and where the appliance will lie flat, adhere well to the skin, and allow the client freedom of movement (the tentative stoma site is mapped out preoperatively by the physician and/or enterostomal therapist) 3. inform client that instructions about the management of the ileostomy will be repeated as often as necessary prior to discharge and that there will be resources available to provide assistance/supervision following discharge 4. assure client that the stoma has no pain receptors and will not be painful when touched 5. stress that effluent (intestinal drainage from the stoma) usually has a weakly acidic or sweet odor that is not unpleasant 6. assure client that ileostomy pouches are odorproof and available in sizes that fit various body contours 7. emphasize the positive effects of the surgery on future life style (the discomfort and frequent diarrhea associated with inflammatory bowel disease and the side effects of medications such as corticosteroids usually have had a disruptive effect on many aspects of the client's life) 8. if acceptable to client, arrange for a visit with a person of similar age and same sex who has successfully adjusted to an ileostomy.

Client Teaching

---

2. NURSING DIAGNOSIS: **Knowledge deficit**

regarding the surgical procedure, hospital routines associated with the surgery, physical preparation for the bowel diversion, sensations that normally occur following surgery and anesthesia, expected appearance and function of the ileostomy, and postoperative care and management of the ileostomy.

Desired Outcomes	Nursing Actions and *Selected Purposes/Rationales*

2.a. The client will verbalize an understanding of the surgical procedure, preoperative care, and postoperative sensations and care.

2.a.1. Refer to Standardized Preoperative Care Plan, Nursing Diagnosis 4, actions a.1–4 (pp. 99–100), for information to include in preoperative teaching.

 2. Provide additional information regarding specific preoperative care and postoperative sensations and care for clients having a bowel diversion with ileostomy:

 a. explain the preoperative bowel preparation (e.g. low-residue or clear liquid diet, cleansing enemas, laxatives, antimicrobial therapy)

 b. if proctocolectomy is planned, inform client that:

 1. a perineal wound drain will be present after surgery

 2. occasional feelings of pressure in the perineal area are expected after surgery and that these will subside as edema decreases

 c. if a continent ileostomy is planned, inform client that:

 1. a catheter will be inserted into the reservoir during surgery and will extend from the stoma and drain into an external collection device; stress that this is a temporary measure (usually for 3–4 weeks) to keep the reservoir from becoming distended while the suture lines are healing

 2. the reservoir will need to be irrigated periodically (especially in the early postoperative period) to remove mucus that accumulates in the reservoir (the bowel used to construct the reservoir initially secretes quite a bit of mucus)

 3. following removal of the stomal catheter, a catheter will be inserted into the stoma at regularly scheduled intervals for a short time (usually 10–15 minutes) to drain the reservoir and an external collection device will not be needed.

 3. Allow time for questions and clarification of information provided.

2.b. The client will demonstrate the ability to perform activities designed to prevent postoperative complications.

2.b. Refer to Standardized Preoperative Care Plan, Nursing Diagnosis 4, action b (p. 100), for instructions on ways to prevent postoperative complications.

2.c. The client will verbalize an understanding of the appearance, function, and management of the ileostomy.

2.c.1. Arrange for a visit with an enterostomal therapist if available.

 2. Reinforce information provided by physician and/or enterostomal therapist about the appearance and function of the ileostomy:

 a. the stoma will be medium pink to red in color and moist (similar in appearance to healthy oral mucous membrane)

 b. the stoma will shrink in size as edema resolves during the first 6 weeks after surgery (final stoma height is usually 1.5–2.5 cm [about ½–1 inch] from the skin surface)

 c. slight bleeding of the stoma is expected when it is wiped with tissue

 d. for the first day or two after surgery, the stoma will drain a small amount of clear to white, blood-tinged fluid containing some mucus; after a few days, the color of the drainage will change to green and then to light to medium brown as the diet progresses

 e. when the ileostomy begins to function (usually 2–3 days after surgery), the drainage will be watery and high-volume (up to 1–2 liters/day) but within a couple of weeks the amount will begin to decrease (expected amount of output after 2–3 months is 500–800 ml/day) and develop a thicker, paste-like consistency.

 3. Provide basic information about peristomal skin care, ways to control intestinal gas and odor of the effluent, irrigation and drainage of the reservoir if a continent ileostomy is planned, and use of various types of ileostomy products.

 4. Provide visual aids and allow client to handle ileostomy products he/she will be using in the immediate postoperative period. Provide a pouch clamp so that client can practice putting it on and taking it off of an empty pouch.

5. Encourage client to try wearing a pouch system partially filled with water in order to experience how it feels and to validate if planned stoma site will be adequate for successful adhesion of the pouch.
6. Allow time for questions and clarification of information provided.

POSTOPERATIVE

Use in conjunction with the Standardized Postoperative Care Plan.

---

1. NURSING/COLLABORATIVE DIAGNOSIS:

Altered fluid and electrolyte balance:

a. **fluid volume deficit** related to restricted oral fluid intake before, during, and after surgery; blood loss; loss of fluid associated with vomiting, nasogastric tube drainage, and/or high-volume ileostomy output; and inadequate fluid replacement;

b. **hypokalemia, hypomagnesemia, and hypochloremia** related to loss of electrolytes associated with vomiting, nasogastric tube drainage, decreased oral intake, and/or high-volume ileostomy output;

c. **metabolic alkalosis** related to loss of hydrochloric acid associated with vomiting and nasogastric tube drainage;

d. **metabolic acidosis** related to loss of bicarbonate ions associated with high-volume ileostomy output (effluent contains bicarbonate ions that would normally be absorbed throughout the large intestine).

Desired Outcome	Nursing Actions and *Selected Purposes/Rationales*

1. The client will not experience fluid volume deficit, hypokalemia, hypochloremia, hypomagnesemia, and acid-base imbalance as evidenced by:
a. normal skin turgor
b. moist mucous membranes
c. stable weight
d. B/P and pulse within normal range for client and stable with position change
e. hand vein filling time less than 3–5 seconds
f. balanced intake and output within 48 hours after surgery
g. urine specific gravity within normal range
h. return of peristalsis within expected time
i. usual mental status
j. absence of cardiac dysrhythmias, twitching, muscle weakness,
	1.a. Assess for and report:
	  1. signs and symptoms of fluid volume deficit, hypokalemia, hypochloremia, and metabolic alkalosis (see Standardized Postoperative Care Plan, Nursing Diagnosis 4, action a.1 [p. 104])
	  2. signs and symptoms of hypomagnesemia (e.g. anxiousness, irritability, cardiac dysrhythmias, tremors, positive Chvostek's and Trousseau's signs, seizures)
	  3. signs and symptoms of metabolic acidosis (e.g. drowsiness; disorientation; stupor; rapid, deep respirations; headache; nausea; vomiting; cardiac dysrhythmias)
	  4. elevated BUN and abnormal serum electrolyte and blood gas values.
	b. Monitor for and report excessive ileostomy output (after bowel activity returns, expected output may be as high as 2000 ml/day and then in 10–14 days it should begin to gradually decrease to 500–800 ml/day within 2–3 months).
	c. Refer to Standardized Postoperative Care Plan, Nursing Diagnosis 4, action a.3 (p. 104), for measures to prevent or treat fluid volume deficit, hypokalemia, hypochloremia, and metabolic alkalosis.
	d. Implement additional measures *to prevent or treat fluid volume deficit and electrolyte imbalances:*
	  1. administer additional electrolyte replacements (e.g. magnesium sulfate, sodium bicarbonate) if ordered
	  2. as diet advances, perform actions *to prevent or control excessive ileostomy output:*
	    a. instruct client to avoid excessive intake of foods/fluids that may cause diarrhea (e.g. raw fruits and vegetables, spicy or extremely hot or cold items, coffee)

Desired Outcome	Nursing Actions and *Selected Purposes/Rationales*

paresthesias, dizziness, headache, nausea, and vomiting
k. negative Chvostek's and Trousseau's signs
l. BUN, serum electrolytes, and blood gases within normal range.

b. encourage intake of bulk-forming foods (e.g. applesauce, bananas, boiled rice)
c. administer antidiarrheal agents (e.g. loperamide, diphenoxylate hydrochloride) if ordered.
e. Consult physician if signs and symptoms of fluid volume deficit and electrolyte imbalances persist or worsen.

---

2. NURSING DIAGNOSIS:

Altered nutrition: less than body requirements

related to:
a. decreased oral intake associated with prescribed dietary modifications; pain; weakness; fatigue; nausea; and fear of excessive ileostomy output, gas, and/or odor;
b. inadequate nutritional replacement therapy;
c. loss of nutrients associated with vomiting and excessive ileostomy output;
d. decreased absorption of nutrients associated with loss of absorptive surface of the bowel resulting from surgical removal of a large amount of the intestines;
e. increased nutritional needs associated with the increased metabolic rate that occurs during wound healing.

Desired Outcome	Nursing Actions and *Selected Purposes/Rationales*

2. The client will maintain an adequate nutritional status (see Standardized Postoperative Care Plan, Nursing Diagnosis 5 [pp. 105–106], for outcome criteria).

2.a. Refer to Standardized Postoperative Care Plan, Nursing Diagnosis 5 (pp. 105–106), for measures related to assessment and maintenance of an adequate nutritional status.
  b. Implement additional measures *to maintain an adequate nutritional status:*
   1. perform actions to prevent or control excessive ileostomy output (see Postoperative Nursing Diagnosis 1, action d.2)
   2. reinforce methods of reducing gas and odor of effluent (see Postoperative Nursing Diagnosis 6, actions g and h) *so that this concern does not cause client to limit oral intake*
   3. instruct client to chew food thoroughly *in order to enhance digestion and subsequent absorption of nutrients.*

---

3. NURSING DIAGNOSIS:

Actual/Risk for impaired tissue integrity

related to:
a. disruption of tissue associated with the surgical procedure;
b. delayed wound healing associated with factors such as decreased nutritional status and inadequate blood supply to wound area;
c. irritation of skin associated with:
   1. contact with wound drainage, ileostomy output (effluent is rich in proteolytic enzymes), soap residue and perspiration under the pouch, and/or mucous drainage from the anus (occurs if rectum was left intact)
   2. frequent and/or improper removal of tape and adhesives or other substances used to secure pouch to the skin
   3. aggressive cleansing of peristomal area

4. sensitivity to tape, pouch material, and/or substances used to secure pouch to the skin (e.g. adhesive disk, skin barrier, adhesive spray)
5. pressure from tubes, appliance belt, and/or pouch drainage valve or clamp.

Desired Outcomes	Nursing Actions and *Selected Purposes/Rationales*

3.a. The client will experience normal healing of surgical wounds (see Standardized Postoperative Care Plan, Nursing Diagnosis 9, outcome a [pp. 109–110], for outcome criteria).

3.b. The client will maintain integrity of peristomal and perianal skin and skin in contact with wound drainage, tape, and tubings as evidenced by:
1. absence of redness and irritation
2. no skin breakdown.

3.a. Refer to Standardized Postoperative Care Plan, Nursing Diagnosis 9, action a (pp. 109–110), for measures related to assessment and promotion of wound healing.

3.b.1. Inspect skin areas that are in contact with wound drainage, tape, and tubings for signs of irritation and breakdown.
   2. Assess for signs and symptoms of:
      a. peristomal irritation or breakdown (e.g. redness, inflammation, and/or excoriation of peristomal skin; reports of itching or burning under the pouch seal; inability to keep pouch on)
      b. perianal irritation or breakdown (e.g. redness, inflammation, and/or excoriation of perianal skin; reports of itching or burning in perianal area).
   3. Refer to Standardized Postoperative Care Plan, Nursing Diagnosis 9, actions b.2 and 3 (pp. 109–110), for measures to prevent and treat irritation and breakdown in areas in contact with wound drainage, tape, and tubings.
   4. Implement measures *to prevent peristomal irritation and breakdown:*
      a. remove hair from peristomal skin using an electric razor *to help achieve an adequate pouch seal and to reduce irritation when the pouch system is removed*
      b. patch test all products that will come in contact with the skin (e.g. sealant, barrier, adhesive, solvent) before initial use; do not use products that cause redness, rash, itching, or burning
      c. change entire pouch system only when necessary (e.g. as ordered, if pouch seal is leaking, if client reports burning or itching of the peristomal skin, when the stoma size changes); pouch system is usually changed every 3 days in the early postoperative period and then should be able to remain in place for 5–7 days
      d. use a 2-piece pouch system (e.g. faceplate and pouch, wafer with flange and pouch) during the initial postoperative period *so that pouch can be removed to assess the stoma without having to remove the adhesive from the skin*
      e. perform actions *to reduce peristomal irritation during removal of the pouch system:*
         1. place drops of warm water or solvent where the pouch system adheres to the skin *in order to facilitate removal;* allow time for adhesive to loosen before removing pouch system from the skin
         2. remove pouch system gently and in direction of hair growth; hold skin adjacent to faceplate taut and push down on skin slightly *to facilitate separation*
      f. perform actions *to prevent effluent from coming in contact with the skin when changing the pouch system or pouch:*
         1. change the pouch or pouch system when the ileostomy is least active (e.g. upon awakening in the morning, before meals, 2–4 hours after eating, before retiring at night)
         2. place a wick (rolled gauze pad, tampon) on the stoma opening when the pouch system or pouch is off

Desired Outcomes   Nursing Actions and *Selected Purposes/Rationales*

    g. cleanse peristomal skin thoroughly with mild soap and water, rinse completely, and pat dry; use tepid rather than hot water *to prevent burns*

    h. apply skin sealant to the clean, dry peristomal skin before applying the skin barrier *in order to protect skin from the irritating effect of the adhesive*

    i. always use a skin barrier (e.g. Stomahesive) *to protect skin from the proteolytic enzymes that are in the effluent*

    j. perform actions *to prevent effluent from contacting the skin when the pouch system is on:*
        1. measure the diameter of the stoma; cut skin barrier the same size as stoma and select a pouch with an opening that is not more than 0.3 cm (1/8 inch) larger than the stoma (it may be necessary to create a pattern to use for cutting barrier and pouch openings if stoma has an irregular shape and cannot be measured using appliance manufacturer's standard measuring guide)
        2. instruct and assist client to remeasure the stoma frequently during the first 6 weeks after surgery and to alter size of skin barrier and pouch openings as stomal edema decreases
        3. implement measures *to achieve an adequate pouch seal:*
            a. avoid use of ointments or lotions on peristomal skin (*these can interfere with adequate adhesive bonding*)
            b. follow manufacturer's instructions carefully when applying skin products and pouch system
            c. use products such as ostomy paste (e.g. Stomahesive paste) to fill in irregularities around stoma site (e.g. body folds, scars) before applying pouch system
            d. apply firm pressure and remove air pockets when applying pouch system; place client in a supine position *to increase tautness of skin surface during application*
        4. empty pouch when it is 1/3 full of effluent or inflated with gas (*a heavy or inflated pouch can cause the pouch system to separate from the skin*)
        5. position pouch so gravity flow facilitates drainage away from stoma and peristomal skin
        6. rinse out bottom of drainable pouch after emptying it and then close pouch securely *to prevent leakage*
        7. use a drainable pouch, 2-piece pouch system, and/or pouch with release valve if gas is a problem; never puncture or cut the pouch to release gas *because effluent can seep out of the opening*

    k. if a belted pouch system is used, fasten the belt so that 2 fingers can slip easily between belt and skin *to prevent excessive pressure on skin*

    l. instruct and assist client to check pouch periodically to ensure that clamp or valve is not placing pressure on the skin.

  5. Implement measures *to prevent perianal irritation and breakdown:*
    a. keep perianal area clean and dry
    b. instruct client to perform perineal exercises (e.g. relaxing and tightening perineal and gluteal muscles) regularly *to increase anal sphincter tone and reduce the risk of mucus leakage*
    c. place absorbent pads in client's underwear if needed and change pads when they become damp
    d. apply petroleum-based ointment to perianal area as ordered *to protect skin.*

  6. If signs and symptoms of peristomal or perianal skin irritation or breakdown occur:
    a. cleanse areas gently with warm water
    b. avoid use of any product that may have caused the irritation or breakdown
    c. perform skin care according to physician's order, enterostomal therapist's instructions, or hospital procedure (usual care may include exposing affected area to air for 20–30 minutes; covering all irritated

skin with a properly fitted, hypoallergenic, solid skin barrier; avoiding pouch system changes unless there are signs of leakage; and applying an antifungal agent or corticosteroid preparation to affected area)

    d. consult physician and/or enterostomal therapist if:

       1. areas of irritation or breakdown do not improve within 48 hours

       2. signs and symptoms of infection (e.g. elevated temperature; redness, heat, pain, and swelling around area of breakdown; unusual drainage or odor from site) are present.

---

4. COLLABORATIVE DIAGNOSES:

Potential complications of bowel diversion surgery:

a. **peritonitis** related to:

  1. wound infection (a client with inflammatory bowel disease often has a decreased resistance to infection as a result of long-term preoperative corticosteroid use and decreased nutritional status)

  2. leakage of intestinal contents into the peritoneum during surgery and/or postoperatively associated with loss of integrity of the sutures at sites of anastomoses or separation of the peristomal skin from the stoma (retraction of the stoma can occur as a result of slippage of sutures, impaired healing of surgical site, or shrinkage of the supporting tissues)

  3. accumulation of wound drainage in the peritoneum;

b. **stomal changes:**

  1. **necrosis** related to intraoperative and/or postoperative interruption of blood supply to the stoma

  2. **excessive bleeding** related to irritation associated with aggressive cleansing of stoma and/or improper fit or application of pouch system

  3. **prolapse** related to loss of integrity of the sutures or pressure around the stoma;

c. **stomal obstruction** related to stomal edema and/or blockage of stoma.

Desired Outcomes	Nursing Actions and *Selected Purposes/Rationales*

4.a. The client will not develop peritonitis as evidenced by:
1. gradual resolution of abdominal pain
2. soft, nondistended abdomen
3. temperature declining toward normal
4. stable vital signs
5. absence of nausea and vomiting
6. gradual return of normal bowel sounds
7. WBC count decreasing toward normal.
	4.a.1. Assess for and report signs and symptoms of peritonitis (e.g. increase in severity of abdominal pain; generalized abdominal pain; rebound tenderness; distended, rigid abdomen; increase in temperature; tachycardia; tachypnea; hypotension; nausea; vomiting; continued absent or diminished bowel sounds).
	  2. Monitor WBC counts. Report levels that increase or fail to decline toward normal.
	  3. Implement measures *to prevent peritonitis:*
	    a. perform actions to prevent and treat wound infection (see Standardized Postoperative Care Plan, Nursing Diagnosis 16, actions b.4 and 5 [pp. 116–117])
	    b. perform actions *to maintain patency of wound drain if present:*
	      1. keep tubing free of kinks
	      2. empty collection device as often as necessary
	      3. maintain suction as ordered
	    c. perform actions *to prevent inadvertent removal of wound drain if present:*
	      1. use caution when changing dressings surrounding drain
	      2. provide extension tubing if necessary *to enable client to move without placing tension on drain*
	      3. instruct client not to pull on drain and drainage tubing
	    d. perform actions *to prevent distention of the internal reservoir (if client has a continent ileostomy) or of the remaining segment of*

Desired Outcomes | Nursing Actions and **Selected Purposes/Rationales**

ileum (*distention can cause strain on the suture lines and subsequent leakage of intestinal contents into the peritoneal cavity*):

1. implement measures to prevent stomal obstruction (see action c.2 in this diagnosis)
2. instruct client to avoid activities such as drinking carbonated beverages, chewing gum, smoking, and eating gas-producing foods (e.g. cabbage, onions, beans, cucumbers) *in order to prevent the accumulation of air and gas in the remaining intestine or internal reservoir*
3. use only the prescribed amount of irrigating solution (usually 20–30 ml) when irrigating the stoma or internal reservoir
4. maintain patency of stomal catheter if present (e.g. keep stomal catheter and drainage bag below level of reservoir *to promote gravity drainage,* keep catheter free of kinks, irrigate catheter as ordered)
5. change pouch system carefully *in order to avoid dislodgment of the stomal catheter* (*if present*)
6. if client has a continent ileostomy and the stomal catheter is removed prior to discharge, assist him/her with drainage of the internal reservoir at scheduled intervals and when he/she feels increased abdominal pressure

e. do not reposition the stomal catheter if present (*repositioning could disrupt the suture line*)

f. if the peristomal skin separates from the stoma:
1. perform wound care as ordered *to facilitate the formation of granulation tissue in the affected area*
2. prepare client for surgical reconstruction of the stoma if planned

g. administer antimicrobials if ordered.

4. If signs and symptoms of peritonitis occur:
a. withhold oral intake as ordered
b. place client on bed rest in a semi-Fowler's position *to assist in pooling or localizing gastrointestinal contents in the pelvis rather than under the diaphragm*
c. prepare client for diagnostic tests (e.g. abdominal x-ray, computed tomography, ultrasonography) if planned
d. insert a nasogastric tube and maintain suction as ordered
e. administer antimicrobials if ordered
f. administer intravenous fluids and/or blood volume expanders if ordered *to prevent or treat shock* (*can result from the increased capillary permeability that occurs with inflammation and the subsequent escape of protein, fluid, and electrolytes from the vascular space into the peritoneal cavity*)
g. prepare client for surgical intervention (e.g. drainage and irrigation of peritoneum, repair of site of anastomosis) if planned
h. provide emotional support to client and significant others.

4.b. The client will maintain adequate stomal circulation and integrity as evidenced by:
1. medium pink to red stomal coloring
2. expected stomal height
3. absence of excessive bleeding and increasing edema of the stoma.

4.b.1. Assess for and report signs and symptoms of impaired stomal circulation and/or integrity (e.g. pale, dark red, blue-black, or purple color of stoma; increased height of stoma; increased stomal edema or bleeding). Use only clear pouches and a 2-piece pouch system during the immediate postoperative period *to allow easy visibility of stoma.*

2. Implement measures *to maintain adequate stomal circulation and integrity:*
a. ensure that openings of the skin barrier and pouch system are not too small and that the stoma is carefully centered in the openings *in order to prevent pressure on and around the stoma*
b. apply pouch system securely *to prevent it from slipping and irritating or shearing stoma*

c. always cleanse stoma gently using a soft cloth, gauze, or tissue
d. instruct client to avoid wearing clothing that puts pressure on the stoma.
3. If signs and symptoms of impaired stomal circulation and/or integrity occur:
   a. perform stomal care as ordered
   b. prepare client for surgical revision of stoma if planned
   c. provide emotional support to client and significant others.

4.c. The client will not develop stomal obstruction as evidenced by:
1. expected amount and consistency of ileostomy output
2. no reports of abdominal cramping, nausea, or increased feeling of fullness
3. absence of vomiting.

4.c.1. Assess for and report signs and symptoms of stomal obstruction:
   a. less than expected amount of ileostomy output (after return of peristalsis, output may be as high as 2000 ml/day and will gradually decrease to about 500–800 ml/day)
   b. change in effluent consistency from a thicker consistency to a thin, watery liquid (postoperatively, effluent gradually becomes thicker; a return to thin, watery consistency may indicate blockage of stoma)
   c. reports of abdominal cramping, nausea, or increased feeling of fullness
   d. vomiting.
2. Implement measures *to prevent stomal obstruction:*
   a. irrigate stoma if ordered *to remove excessive mucus that could block stoma*
   b. maintain a fluid intake of 2500 ml/day unless contraindicated *to keep effluent from becoming too thick*
   c. administer oral medications crushed and mixed in water or in liquid or chewable form (*undigested pills can block stoma*)
   d. when oral intake is allowed, perform actions *to prevent blockage of stoma by food:*
      1. encourage client to eat small, frequent meals rather than 3 large ones
      2. instruct client to chew food thoroughly
      3. instruct client to avoid or eat only small amounts of foods that are high in fiber (*fibrous foods absorb water in the intestinal tract*) and/or are hard to digest (e.g. popcorn, coconut, raw vegetables, fruits with seeds, bean sprouts, bamboo shoots, whole kernel corn, potato skins, bran, nuts, fruit skins).
3. If stomal edema seems to be obstructing the stoma, consult physician about gently inserting a catheter through the stoma into the ileal segment *to drain effluent until edema decreases.*
4. If food particles or mucus seem to be obstructing the stoma, implement measures *to promote the flow of effluent through the stoma:*
   a. perform actions *to relax the abdominal muscle that surrounds the stoma* (e.g. administer analgesic if ordered, apply warm compress to the abdomen unless contraindicated, encourage participation in relaxing activities such as reading and listening to music)
   b. perform actions *to break up or shift food or mucus:*
      1. encourage fluid intake unless contraindicated
      2. instruct and assist client to assume a knee-chest position
      3. gently massage peristomal area unless contraindicated
      4. assist with or gently perform digital dilation of stoma if ordered
      5. irrigate the ileostomy if ordered.
5. If signs and symptoms of stomal obstruction persist:
   a. withhold oral intake as ordered
   b. maintain intravenous therapy as ordered *to prevent fluid volume deficit and increased viscosity of effluent*
   c. insert a nasogastric tube and maintain suction as ordered
   d. prepare client for surgical intervention to remove obstruction if indicated
   e. provide emotional support to client and significant others.

5. NURSING DIAGNOSIS: **Altered sexuality patterns**

related to feelings of loss of femininity/masculinity and sexual attractiveness, fear of offensive odor or leakage of effluent from the stoma (if client has an internal reservoir) or the pouch, fear of rejection by partner, discomfort associated with surgical incision, and depression.

Desired Outcome	Nursing Actions and *Selected Purposes/Rationales*

5. The client will demonstrate beginning adjustment to effects of the ileostomy on sexuality as evidenced by:
a. verbalization of a perception of self as sexually acceptable and adequate
b. statements reflecting ways to adjust to effects of ileostomy on sexual functioning.
	5.a. Assess for signs and symptoms of altered sexuality patterns (e.g. verbalization of sexual concerns, reports of anticipated changes in sexual activities or behaviors).
	b. Determine client's perception of desired sexuality and usual pattern of sexual expression.
	c. Implement measures *to promote an optimal sexuality pattern:*
	  1. facilitate communication between client and partner; focus on feelings the couple share and assist them to identify changes which may affect their sexual relationship
	  2. perform actions to facilitate psychological adjustment to the changes that have occurred (see Postoperative Nursing Diagnoses 6, actions d–u; 7, action c; and 8, action b)
	  3. instruct client in ways *to reduce risk for leakage of effluent during sexual activity:*
	    a. empty pouch or drain internal reservoir (if present) before sexual activity
	    b. secure pouch seal with tape for added security
	  4. if client is concerned about odor, instruct to:
	    a. shower or bathe before sexual activity
	    b. use an odorproof pouch or a pouch deodorizer
	    c. use cologne or perfume if desired
	    d. keep room well ventilated
	  5. if client is concerned about the presence of the stoma and pouch system, discuss the possibility of:
	    a. using opaque or patterned pouches or decorative pouch covers
	    b. wearing underwear with the crotch removed (for females), boxer shorts (for males), or stretch tube top or cummerbund around abdomen during sexual activity
	  6. if client is concerned that operative site discomfort will interfere with usual sexual activity:
	    a. assure him/her that discomfort is temporary and will diminish as the incision heals
	    b. encourage use of positions that decrease pressure on surgical site (e.g. side-lying) until the incision heals
	  7. discuss ways to be creative in expressing sexuality (e.g. massage, fantasies, cuddling)
	  8. if appropriate, involve partner in ileostomy care *to facilitate partner's adjustment to the changes in client's appearance and body functioning and subsequently decrease the possibility of partner's rejection of client*
	  9. arrange for uninterrupted privacy during hospital stay if desired by the couple
	  10. encourage client to obtain written information regarding sexual activity and sexuality from the United Ostomy Association and from manufacturers of ostomy products
	  11. include partner in above discussions and encourage continued support of the client.
	d. Consult physician if counseling appears indicated.

6. NURSING DIAGNOSIS: **Self-concept disturbance***

related to:
a. change in appearance associated with presence of stoma and pouch system;
b. embarrassment associated with sound and odor resulting from gas and effluent;
c. dependence (usually temporary) on others for assistance with ileostomy management;
d. loss of control over bowel elimination if client has conventional ileostomy;
e. possibility of impotence if nerve damage occurred during a proctocolectomy (use of nerve-sparing surgical techniques has greatly reduced the occurrence of nerve damage and subsequent impotence).

---

*This diagnostic label includes the nursing diagnoses of body image disturbance, self-esteem disturbance, and altered role performance.

Desired Outcome	Nursing Actions and *Selected Purposes/Rationales*

6. The client will demonstrate beginning adaptation to changes in appearance and body functioning as evidenced by:
a. verbalization of feelings of self-worth
b. maintenance of relationships with significant others
c. active participation in activities of daily living
d. verbalization of a beginning plan for integrating changes in appearance and body functioning into life style.
	6.a. Assess for signs and symptoms of a self-concept disturbance (e.g. verbalization of negative feelings about self, withdrawal from significant others, lack of participation in activities of daily living, refusal to look at or touch stoma, lack of plan for adapting to necessary changes in life style).
	b. Determine the meaning of changes in appearance and body functioning to the client by encouraging verbalization of feelings and by noting nonverbal responses to the changes experienced.
	c. Implement measures to facilitate the grieving process (see Postoperative Nursing Diagnosis 8, action b).
	d. Implement measures *to assist client to increase self-esteem* (e.g. limit negative self-assessment, encourage positive comments about self, assist to identify strengths, give positive feedback about accomplishments and behaviors that are indicative of high self-esteem).
	e. Reinforce actions to assist client to cope with the effects of the ileostomy (see Postoperative Nursing Diagnosis 7, action c).
	f. Implement measures to promote an optimal sexuality pattern (see Postoperative Nursing Diagnosis 5, action c).
	g. Instruct client in ways *to reduce gas formation:*
	  1. avoid activities that can cause air swallowing (e.g. chewing gum, smoking)
	  2. limit intake of carbonated beverages and gas-producing foods (e.g. cabbage, onions, beans, radishes, cucumbers).
	h. Instruct client in and assist with measures *to reduce odor of ileostomy drainage and/or gas:*
	  1. use odorproof pouches, a pouch deodorizer, and/or a pouch with a deodorizing flatus filter
	  2. empty pouch regularly; rinse inside of pouch and clean off any effluent before closing pouch
	  3. drain the reservoir of continent ileostomy at scheduled intervals and when it feels full to reduce possibility of leakage from stoma
	  4. use a disposable pouch and change it regularly or clean reusable pouch thoroughly
	  5. empty or change pouch in a well-ventilated area; use room deodorizers if desired
	  6. perform actions to achieve an adequate pouch seal (see Postoperative Nursing Diagnosis 3, action b.4.j.3)
	  7. limit intake of foods that cause effluent to have a strong odor (e.g. onions, fish, eggs, strong cheeses, asparagus)
	  8. increase intake of foods/fluids that control odor (e.g. spinach, parsley, yogurt, buttermilk)
	  9. change bed linens and clothing promptly if they become soiled.

Desired Outcome	Nursing Actions and *Selected Purposes/Rationales*
	i. Inform client that the pouch and clothing muffle sounds of bowel activity.

j. Assure client that once the stomal edema and surgical discomfort have resolved, he/she will be able to dress as before with minor, if any, modifications.

k. Show client and significant others some of the attractive ileostomy products that are available (e.g. opaque or patterned pouches, pouch covers).

l. Assist client with usual grooming and makeup habits if necessary.

m. If nerve damage that could result in impotence is believed to have occurred during a proctocolectomy:
1. encourage client to discuss impotence and various treatment options (e.g. vacuum erection aids, penile prosthesis) with physician
2. suggest alternative methods of sexual gratification if appropriate
3. discuss alternative methods of becoming a parent (e.g. artificial insemination, adoption) if of concern to client.

n. Promote activities that require client to confront the body changes that have occurred (e.g. active participation in ileostomy care). Be aware that integration of the change in body image does not usually occur until 2–6 months after the actual physical change has occurred.

o. Demonstrate acceptance of client using techniques such as touch and frequent visits. Encourage significant others to do the same.

p. Support behaviors suggesting positive adaptation to changes that have occurred (e.g. willingness to care for ileostomy, compliance with treatment plan, verbalization of feelings of self-worth, maintenance of relationships with significant others).

q. Encourage significant others to allow client to do what he/she is able *so that independence can be re-established and/or self-esteem redeveloped.*

r. Assist client's and significant others' adjustment by listening, facilitating communication, and providing information.

s. Encourage visits and support from significant others.

t. Encourage client to pursue usual roles and interests and to continue involvement in social activities.

u. Provide information about and encourage utilization of community agencies and support groups (e.g. ostomy groups; sexual, family, individual, and/or financial counseling).

v. Consult physician about psychological counseling if client desires or seems unwilling or unable to adapt to changes resulting from the bowel diversion.

---

7. NURSING DIAGNOSIS: **Ineffective individual coping**

related to:
a. fear, anxiety, and depression associated with loss of control over bowel elimination (especially with a conventional ileostomy) and possibility of rejection by others;
b. difficulty performing ileostomy care and incorporating the care into life style;
c. need for lifelong medical supervision.

Desired Outcome	Nursing Actions and *Selected Purposes/Rationales*
7. The client will demonstrate effective coping as evidenced by: a. verbalization of ability to cope with the ileostomy	7.a. Assess for and report signs and symptoms of ineffective individual coping (e.g. verbalization of inability to cope; inability to ask for help, problem solve, or meet basic needs; insomnia; withdrawal; reluctance to participate in treatment plan; destructive behavior toward self or others; inappropriate use of defense mechanisms; inability to meet role expectations).

b. utilization of appropriate problem-solving techniques

c. willingness to participate in treatment plan and meet basic needs

d. absence of destructive behavior toward self and others

e. appropriate use of defense mechanisms

f. utilization of available support systems.

b. Assess client's perception of current situation.

c. Implement measures *to promote effective coping*:

1. allow time for client to begin to adjust to the ileostomy; if frequent diarrhea and cramping had limited client's activities before surgery, stress positive effects ileostomy will have on life style

2. assist client to recognize and manage inappropriate denial if it is present

3. if acceptable to client, arrange for a visit from a person of similar age and same sex who has successfully adjusted to an ileostomy

4. perform actions to reduce fear and anxiety (see Standardized Postoperative Care Plan, Nursing Diagnosis 20, action b [p. 122])

5. encourage verbalization about current situation

6. assist client to identify personal strengths and resources that can be utilized to facilitate coping with the current situation

7. demonstrate acceptance of client but set limits on inappropriate behavior

8. create an atmosphere of trust and support

9. maintain consistency of approaches and explanations

10. do not overload client with information irrelevant to present stage of ileostomy management unless client is questioning or expressing an interest

11. encourage participation in ileostomy care as soon as possible

12. use products that client will be using when discharged

13. ensure adequate time for and privacy during ileostomy care

14. include client in planning of care, encourage maximum participation in ileostomy care, and allow choices when possible *to enable him/her to maintain a sense of control*

15. instruct client in effective problem-solving techniques (e.g. accurate identification of stressors, determination of various options to solve problem)

16. assist client to maintain usual daily routines whenever possible

17. assist client through methods such as role playing to prepare for negative reactions from others because of ileostomy

18. instruct client to have extra ileostomy products readily available at all times

19. administer antianxiety and/or antidepressant agents if ordered

20. assist client to identify and use available support systems; provide information about available community resources that can assist client and significant others in coping with effects of the ileostomy (e.g. stress management classes, local ostomy support groups, United Ostomy Association, counseling services)

21. discuss with significant others the fear of rejection client may be experiencing and encourage their continued support

22. encourage client to share with significant others the kind of support that would be most beneficial (e.g. listening, inspiring hope, providing reassurance and accurate information)

23. support behaviors indicative of effective coping (e.g. participation in ileostomy care, verbalization of ability to cope, utilization of effective problem-solving strategies).

d. Consult physician about psychological counseling if appropriate. Initiate a referral if necessary.

---

8. **NURSING DIAGNOSIS:**   **Grieving***

related to loss of usual manner of bowel elimination and changes associated with the surgical procedure and presence of the ileostomy.

---

*This diagnostic label includes anticipatory grieving and grieving following the actual losses.

Desired Outcome	Nursing Actions and *Selected Purposes/Rationales*

8. The client will demonstrate beginning progression through the grieving process as evidenced by:
a. verbalization of feelings about the ileostomy
b. usual sleep pattern
c. participation in treatment plan and self-care activities
d. utilization of available support systems
e. verbalization of a plan for integrating ileostomy care into life style.
	8.a. Assess for signs and symptoms of grieving (e.g. change in eating habits, inability to concentrate, insomnia, anger, sadness, withdrawal from significant others, denial of loss).
	b. Implement measures *to facilitate the grieving process:*
	  1. assist client to acknowledge losses *so grief work can begin*; assess for factors that may hinder and facilitate acknowledgment
	  2. discuss the grieving process and assist client to accept the phases of grieving as an expected response to actual and/or anticipated losses
	  3. allow time for client to progress through the phases of grieving (phases vary among theorists but progress from shock and alarm to acceptance); be aware that not every phase is expressed by all individuals, that recurrence of phases is common, and that the grieving process may take months to years
	  4. provide an atmosphere of care and concern (e.g. provide privacy, be available and nonjudgmental, display empathy and respect) *so client will feel free to express feelings*
	  5. perform actions *to promote trust* (e.g. answer questions honestly, provide requested information)
	  6. encourage the verbal expression of anger and sadness about the losses experienced; recognize displacement of anger and assist client to see the actual cause of angry feelings and resentment
	  7. encourage client to express feelings in whatever ways are comfortable (e.g. writing, drawing, conversation)
	  8. perform actions to promote effective coping (see Postoperative Nursing Diagnosis 7, action c)
	  9. support realistic hope about effects of the bowel diversion on his/her life (e.g. increased comfort, treatment of the underlying disease process)
	  10. support behaviors suggesting successful grief work (e.g. verbalizing feelings about ileostomy, focusing on ways to adapt to changes in bowel elimination and presence of stoma, learning ileostomy care)
	  11. explain the phases of the grieving process to significant others; encourage their support and understanding
	  12. facilitate communication between the client and significant others; be aware that they may be in different phases of the grieving process
	  13. provide information regarding counseling services and support groups that might assist client in working through grief
	  14. when appropriate, assist client to meet spiritual needs (e.g. arrange for a visit from clergy).
	c. Consult physician regarding referral for counseling if signs of dysfunctional grieving (e.g. persistent denial of losses, excessive anger or sadness, emotional lability) occur.

Discharge Teaching

■━━━

9. NURSING DIAGNOSIS: **Knowledge deficit, Ineffective management of therapeutic regimen, or Altered health maintenance***

---

*The nurse should select the diagnostic label that is most appropriate for the client's discharge teaching needs.

Desired Outcomes	Nursing Actions and *Selected Purposes/Rationales*
9.a. The client will verbalize a basic understanding of the anatomical changes that have occurred as a result of the bowel diversion.	9.a. Reinforce teaching regarding the anatomical changes that have occurred as a result of the bowel diversion. Use appropriate teaching aids (e.g. pictures, videotapes, anatomical models).

9.b. The client will identify ways to maintain fluid and electrolyte balance.	9.b. Provide the following instructions on ways to maintain fluid and electrolyte balance:
	1. instruct client to drink at least 10 glasses of liquid/day unless contraindicated and to increase fluid intake during hot weather, during and following intense physical activity, when perspiring profusely, and during episodes of diarrhea
	2. instruct client to perform the following actions to prevent excessive ileostomy output:
	  a. avoid excessive intake of foods/liquids that may cause diarrhea (e.g. raw fruits and vegetables, extremely hot or cold beverages, spicy foods, coffee)
	  b. do not take laxatives or excessive amounts of magnesium-containing antacids (e.g. Milk of Magnesia, Mylanta, Maalox)
	  c. take antidiarrheal agents (e.g. loperamide, diphenoxylate hydrochloride) as prescribed
	3. if ileostomy output increases or becomes more watery, instruct client to:
	  a. increase intake of bulk-forming foods (e.g. applesauce, bananas, boiled rice)
	  b. increase intake of foods/liquids such as fruit juices, Gatorade, potatoes, tea, bananas, and bouillon to maintain electrolyte balance
	  c. drink a mixture of baking soda and water ($\frac{1}{4}$–$\frac{1}{2}$ teaspoon baking soda and 1 cup of water) if prescribed by physician to maintain acid-base balance.

9.c. The client will verbalize ways to maintain an optimal nutritional status.	9.c. Provide instructions regarding ways to maintain an optimal nutritional status: 1. reinforce ways to prevent excessive ileostomy output (see action b.2 in this diagnosis) 2. stress the need to chew food thoroughly in order to enhance digestion and subsequent absorption of nutrients 3. stress the importance of taking vitamins and minerals as prescribed.
9.d. The client will identify methods of controlling odor and sound associated with ileostomy drainage and gas.	9.d.1. Reinforce instructions regarding ways to reduce gas formation and odor associated with ileostomy drainage and gas (see Postoperative Nursing Diagnosis 6, actions g and h). 2. Inform client that the ostomy pouch and clothing will muffle the sounds from the ileostomy.
9.e. The client will demonstrate the ability to change the pouch system, maintain integrity of the peristomal and perianal skin, and maintain adequate stomal circulation and integrity.	9.e.1. Reinforce teaching regarding application of the pouch system, prevention of peristomal and perianal skin irritation and breakdown, and maintenance of adequate stomal circulation and integrity (see Postoperative Nursing Diagnosis 3, actions b.4 and 5 and Collaborative Diagnosis 4, action b.2, for appropriate measures). 2. Support client's efforts to decrease odor of effluent and gas but discourage excessive changing and emptying of pouch or pouch system. 3. Instruct and assist client to establish a routine for emptying and changing pouch or emptying continent ileostomy in order to reduce risk of leakage of effluent. 4. Instruct client to follow special precautions for products used (e.g. inert, moldable skin barriers must be kept in airtight container; skin sealants should be used only on healthy peristomal skin because they can further irritate reddened and excoriated skin).

Desired Outcomes	Nursing Actions and *Selected Purposes/Rationales*
	5. Allow time for questions, clarification, practice, and return demonstration of emptying the pouch, changing the pouch system, and performing appropriate stoma and skin care.
9.f. The client will demonstrate the ability to properly use, clean, and store ostomy products.	9.f.1. Instruct client regarding proper use of ostomy products he/she will be using after discharge.
	2. Demonstrate appropriate pouch system cleansing. Emphasize importance of:
	a. rinsing inside of pouch each time it is emptied
	b. soaking reusable pouch according to manufacturer's instructions and allowing it to dry thoroughly before reusing.
	3. Instruct client to avoid reusing disposable products and to discard a reusable pouch if it retains an odor after thorough cleansing or if it becomes brittle.
	4. Discuss recommended methods of storing ostomy products based on manufacturer's recommendations.
	5. Allow time for questions, clarification, and return demonstration.
9.g. The client will demonstrate the ability to drain and irrigate a continent ileostomy if present.	9.g.1. Explain the gradual and progressive clamping routine if catheter will still be in the stoma of a continent ileostomy at time of discharge.
	2. If the stomal catheter has been removed, demonstrate the correct method of and explain the schedule for stomal catheter insertion (initially the reservoir will need to be drained for 10–15 minutes every 3–4 hours but after about 6 months it may need emptying only 2–3 times/day).
	3. Demonstrate the correct technique for irrigating a continent ileostomy. Caution client to use only the prescribed amount of irrigant (usually 20–30 ml) in order to avoid overdistending and damaging the internal reservoir.
	4. Allow time for questions, clarification, and return demonstration of clamping, draining, and irrigating techniques.
9.h. The client will identify ways to prevent and treat blockage of the stoma.	9.h.1. Instruct client in ways to prevent blockage of the stoma:
	a. drink at least 10 glasses of liquid/day unless contraindicated
	b. irrigate stoma routinely if instructed to do so by physician
	c. chew food thoroughly
	d. avoid or eat only small amounts of foods that are high in fiber and/or hard to digest (e.g. popcorn, coconut, raw vegetables, bean sprouts, bamboo shoots, whole kernel corn, potato skins, fruit with seeds, nuts, fruit skins).
	2. Instruct client to do the following if stoma is blocked:
	a. apply a warm compress to abdomen
	b. participate in relaxing activities (e.g. warm bath, reading)
	c. attempt to break-up or shift blockage (e.g. assume a knee-chest position, gently massage peristomal area, irrigate the stoma or gently perform digital dilation of the stoma if prescribed).
	3. Demonstrate techniques such as massage of abdomen, irrigation of stoma, and digital dilation of stoma if appropriate.
	4. Allow time for questions, clarification, and return demonstration.
9.i. The client will state signs and symptoms to report to the health care provider.	9.i.1. Refer to Standardized Postoperative Care Plan, Nursing Diagnosis 21, action c (p. 123), for signs and symptoms to report to the health care provider.
	2. Instruct client to also report:
	a. dark red, blue-black, purple, or pale stoma
	b. change in color, consistency, or odor of effluent that is not readily identified as a response to food or fluid intake
	c. absence of or persistent increase in ileostomy output
	d. change in contour or height of stoma (use diagrams and descriptive terms so client does not confuse decreasing stoma size due to resolving edema with actual stomal retraction)
	e. excessive bleeding of stoma or bloody drainage from stoma
	f. difficulty accomplishing ileostomy care

g. persistent skin irritation

h. skin breakdown

i. persistent thirst, dry mucous membranes, or decreased urine output (may indicate fluid volume deficit)

j. signs and symptoms of low potassium (e.g. irregular pulse, muscle weakness and cramping, nausea, vomiting)

k. signs and symptoms of low sodium (e.g. headache, abdominal cramps, fatigue, irritability)

l. thin, watery ileostomy output; absence of ileostomy output; unusual foul odor of gas; abdominal distention; and/or nausea and vomiting that does not resolve within 2 hours of implementing measures to relieve stomal blockage

m. persistent leakage of pouch system

n. persistent leakage of effluent from stoma (if client has a continent ileostomy)

o. difficulty draining or irrigating an internal reservoir if present

p. fever; pain or cramping in reservoir area; pain when draining the reservoir; and/or watery, high-volume ileostomy output (these signs and symptoms can indicate inflammation of the internal reservoir [pouchitis], which is a long-term complication that can develop in the client with a continent ileostomy)

q. difficulty adjusting to changes in appearance and body functioning.

9.j. The client will identify appropriate community resources that can assist with home management and adjustment to changes resulting from the bowel diversion.

9.j.1. Provide information about community resources that can assist the client and significant others with home management and adjustment to changes resulting from bowel diversion (e.g. local ostomy support groups; community health agencies; enterostomal therapist; home health agencies; financial, individual, and family counseling services).

2. Initiate a referral if appropriate.

9.k. The client will verbalize an understanding of and a plan for adhering to recommended follow-up care including future appointments with health care provider, wound care, activity level, and medications prescribed.

9.k.1. Refer to Standardized Postoperative Care Plan, Nursing Diagnosis 21 (pp. 123–124), for routine postoperative instructions and measures to improve client compliance.

2. Reinforce physician's instructions regarding activity limitations:

a. avoid lifting objects over 10 pounds for at least 6 weeks

b. avoid participating in contact sports.

3. Provide client with a list of ostomy products he/she is using (include product name, size, and number) and where these supplies can be obtained.

4. Explain the rationale for, side effects of, and importance of taking medications prescribed (e.g. electrolyte supplements, vitamins, antimicrobials). Inform client of pertinent food and drug interactions.

5. Stress the fact that oral medications should be crushed or in liquid, chewable, uncoated, or sugar-coated form rather than enteric-coated tablets or timed-release spansules so absorption can take place before the medication is excreted.

Bibliography

See pages 897–898 and 906–907.

GASTRECTOMY

Gastrectomy is the surgical removal of all or part of the stomach. A total gastrectomy involves removal of the entire stomach and anastomosis of the esophagus to the jejunum (esophagojejunostomy). It may be indicated for treatment of advanced stomach cancer or Zollinger-Ellison syndrome that is not controlled by more conservative measures but, because it is so difficult to maintain an adequate nutritional status postoperatively, a total gastrectomy is performed infrequently. The more common type of gastrectomy performed is a partial gastrectomy. This less extensive surgery is most often done to treat peptic ulcer disease that continues to be symptomatic despite conservative management or to treat complications that develop as a result of the disease (e.g. perforation, gastric outlet obstruction, hemorrhage). A partial gastrectomy may also be performed to resect ulcerated lesions that are believed to be precancerous.

A partial gastrectomy usually involves excision of 40–75% of the distal stomach including the antrum (which contains the gastrin-secreting cells) and a portion of the body of the stomach that contains much of the parietal cell mass. Gastrointestinal continuity is re-established by anastomosis of the remaining stomach to the duodenum (gastroduodenostomy or Billroth I) or jejunum (gastrojejunostomy or Billroth II). In the latter procedure, the duodenal stump is left intact so that bile and pancreatic secretions can enter the jejunum. The decreased output of gastric secretions that results from a partial gastrectomy can be enhanced by a vagotomy, which is often performed concurrently to further reduce stimulation of gastric secretions. A truncal vagotomy (resection of the vagal nerve trunks at the level of the esophageal hiatus) is more effective than a selective (partial) vagotomy in reducing gastric secretions; however, the denervation also greatly suppresses gastric motility and impairs normal functioning of the pancreas, gallbladder, and small intestine so it is not performed as often as a selective vagotomy.

This care plan focuses on the adult client with intractable peptic ulcer disease who is hospitalized for a partial gastrectomy. Preoperatively, the goals of care are to reduce fear and anxiety and prepare the client for the postoperative period. Postoperative goals of care are to maintain comfort, assist the client to maintain an adequate nutritional status, prevent complications, and educate the client regarding follow-up care.

DIAGNOSTIC TESTS

Refer to Care Plan on Peptic Ulcer.

DISCHARGE CRITERIA

Prior to discharge, the client will:
- have surgical pain controlled
- have evidence of normal healing of the surgical wound
- have clear, audible breath sounds throughout lungs
- have no signs and symptoms of postoperative complications
- tolerate prescribed diet
- identify ways to prevent recurrence of peptic ulcers
- verbalize an understanding of ways to maintain an adequate nutritional status
- identify ways to control postvagotomy diarrhea if it occurs
- identify ways to manage dumping syndrome if it occurs
- state signs and symptoms to report to the health care provider
- verbalize an understanding of and a plan for adhering to recommended follow-up care including future appointments with health care provider, medications prescribed, activity level, and wound care.

NURSING/ COLLABORATIVE DIAGNOSES

Postoperative
1. Ineffective breathing pattern △   597
2. Altered nutrition: less than body requirements △   597
3. Diarrhea △   598
4. Potential complications:
   a. hypovolemic shock
   b. peritonitis
   c. afferent loop syndrome
   d. early dumping syndrome
   e. late dumping syndrome (postprandial hypoglycemia) △   599

DISCHARGE TEACHING   **5.** Knowledge deficit, Ineffective management of therapeutic regimen, or Altered health maintenance △   601

See Care Plan on Peptic Ulcer and the Standardized Preoperative and Postoperative Care Plans for additional diagnoses.

PREOPERATIVE

Refer to the Care Plan on Peptic Ulcer and the Standardized Preoperative Care Plan.

POSTOPERATIVE

Use in conjunction with the Standardized Postoperative Care Plan.

---

1. NURSING DIAGNOSIS:

Ineffective breathing pattern

related to:
a. increased rate and decreased depth of respirations associated with fear and anxiety;
b. decreased rate and depth of respirations associated with the depressant effect of anesthesia and some medications (e.g. narcotic [opioid] analgesics);
c. diminished lung/chest wall expansion associated with positioning, weakness, fatigue, abdominal distention, and reluctance to breathe deeply because of a high abdominal incision.

Desired Outcome	Nursing Actions and *Selected Purposes/Rationales*

1. The client will maintain an effective breathing pattern (see Standardized Postoperative Care Plan, Nursing Diagnosis 2 [p. 102], for outcome criteria).	1.a. Refer to Standardized Postoperative Care Plan, Nursing Diagnosis 2 (pp. 102–103), for measures related to assessment and management of an ineffective breathing pattern.
	  b. Implement additional measures *to improve breathing pattern:*
	    1. instruct client to bend knees while coughing and deep breathing *in order to relieve tension on abdominal muscles and incision*
	    2. instruct and assist client to splint incision with hands or pillow when coughing and deep breathing.

---

2. NURSING DIAGNOSIS:

Altered nutrition: less than body requirements

related to:
a. decreased oral intake associated with prescribed dietary modifications, pain, weakness, fatigue, nausea, feeling of fullness (can occur as a result of abdominal distention), fear of experiencing dumping syndrome (especially with a gastrojejunostomy) or diarrhea (following a truncal vagotomy), and early satiety resulting from reduced stomach size;
b. decreased absorption of nutrients associated with impaired digestion resulting from:
  1. decreased gastric acid secretion (occurs with vagotomy and removal of gastrin-secreting cells and parietal cells)
  2. rapid entry of food into small intestine (a result of reduced stomach size and removal of pylorus)

3. decreased stimulation and secretion of pancreatic juice and bile associated with:
   a. reduction in hydrochloric acid and gastrin secretion (these gastric secretions stimulate pancreatic enzyme secretion and gallbladder contraction)
   b. absence of food moving through the duodenum following gastrojejunostomy (the presence of food in the duodenum causes the release of cholecystokinin, which stimulates gallbladder contraction and pancreatic enzyme secretion);
   c. decreased absorption of iron associated with bypassing the duodenum if a gastrojejunostomy was performed;
   d. inadequate nutritional replacement therapy;
   e. loss of nutrients associated with diarrhea if present;
   f. increased nutritional needs associated with the increased metabolic rate that occurs during wound healing.

Desired Outcome	Nursing Actions and *Selected Purposes/Rationales*

2. The client will maintain an adequate nutritional status (see Standardized Postoperative Care Plan, Nursing Diagnosis 5 [pp. 105–106], for outcome criteria).	2.a. Refer to Standardized Postoperative Care Plan, Nursing Diagnosis 5 (pp. 105–106), for measures related to assessment and maintenance of an adequate nutritional status.
	b. Implement additional measures *to maintain an adequate nutritional status when oral intake is allowed:*
	  1. provide small, frequent meals if client is weak, fatigues easily, has a poor appetite, and/or experiences early satiety
	  2. instruct client to chew food thoroughly (*small food particles are more easily and completely digested*)
	  3. perform actions to prevent or control postvagotomy diarrhea (see Postoperative Nursing Diagnosis 3, action b) and dumping syndrome (see Postoperative Collaborative Diagnosis 4, actions d.2 and 3) *in order to reduce the client's fear of precipitating these conditions and to promote increased absorption of nutrients*
	  4. administer the following if ordered:
	    a. vitamins and minerals (may be ordered in liquid or chewable form *to facilitate absorption*)
	    b. pancreatic enzymes (e.g. pancreatin, pancrelipase) and/or bile salts *to facilitate digestion.*

---

3. NURSING DIAGNOSIS: **Diarrhea***

related to rapid passage of foods/fluids through the small intestine associated with loss of nervous system regulation of bowel activity.

---

*Referred to as "postvagotomy diarrhea" and is more likely to occur if a truncal rather than selective vagotomy was performed.

Desired Outcome	Nursing Actions and *Selected Purposes/Rationales*

3. The client will not experience or will have diminished postvagotomy diarrhea as evidenced by:
a. passage of formed stool
b. no reports of urgency or abdominal cramping.
	3.a. Assess for and report signs and symptoms of postvagotomy diarrhea (e.g. watery stools, urgency, and abdominal cramping usually occurring within 1–2 hours after eating).
	b. When oral intake is allowed, implement measures *to prevent or control postvagotomy diarrhea:*
	  1. advance diet gradually
	  2. encourage client to eat small rather than large meals

3. instruct client to drink fluids between rather than with meals
4. administer antidiarrheal agents (e.g. kaolin/pectin compounds, loperamide, diphenoxylate hydrochloride) if ordered.

c. Consult physician if postvagotomy diarrhea persists.

---

4. COLLABORATIVE DIAGNOSES:

Potential complications of gastrectomy:

a. **hypovolemic shock** related to hypovolemia associated with excessive blood loss during surgery (many major arteries and veins supply and surround the stomach), inadequate fluid replacement, and postoperative hemorrhage (can occur if there is excessive stress on the newly ligated operative site vessels);

b. **peritonitis** related to:
  1. wound infection
  2. leakage of upper gastrointestinal contents into the peritoneal cavity associated with loss of integrity of the suture line at the duodenal stump (with gastrojejunostomy) or the site of anastomosis;

c. **afferent loop syndrome** related to partial obstruction of the remaining portion of the duodenum associated with factors such as edema or presence of a kink in the efferent jejunal limb after gastrojejunostomy;

d. **early dumping syndrome** related to rapid emptying of hypertonic food into the jejunum especially after a gastrojejunostomy (the bolus of food is hypertonic and attracts fluid from the vascular space; this distends the bowel lumen and increases intestinal peristalsis and motility);

e. **late dumping syndrome (postprandial hypoglycemia)** related to rapid emptying of food/fluid high in carbohydrates into the jejunum especially after a gastrojejunostomy (this results in increased absorption of glucose into the blood causing increased release of insulin and subsequent hypoglycemia).

Desired Outcomes	Nursing Actions and *Selected Purposes/Rationales*

4.a. The client will not develop hypovolemic shock (see Standardized Postoperative Care Plan, Collaborative Diagnosis 19, outcome a [p. 120], for outcome criteria).	4.a.1. Refer to Standardized Postoperative Care Plan, Collaborative Diagnosis 19, action a (p. 120), for measures related to assessment, prevention, and treatment of hypovolemic shock.
	2. Implement additional measures *to prevent hypovolemic shock:*
	  a. perform actions to prevent stress on the newly ligated vessels (see action b.3.d in this diagnosis)
	  b. prepare client for surgery (e.g. ligation of bleeding vessels) if indicated.

4.b. The client will not develop peritonitis as evidenced by:
1. gradual resolution of abdominal pain
2. soft, nondistended abdomen
3. temperature declining toward normal
4. stable vital signs
5. absence of nausea and vomiting
6. gradual return of normal bowel sounds
7. WBC count declining toward normal.
	4.b.1. Assess for and report:
	  a. bile in wound drain (*indicates leakage from suture lines*)
	  b. hiccoughs (can occur as a result of distention of remaining stomach; distention increases pressure on the suture lines)
	  c. signs and symptoms of peritonitis (e.g. increase in severity of abdominal pain; generalized abdominal pain; rebound tenderness; distended, rigid abdomen; increase in temperature; tachycardia; tachypnea; hypotension; nausea; vomiting; continued diminished or absent bowel sounds).
	2. Monitor WBC counts. Report levels that increase or fail to decline toward normal.
	3. Implement measures *to prevent peritonitis:*
	  a. perform actions to prevent and treat wound infection (see Standardized Postoperative Care Plan, Nursing Diagnosis 16, actions b.4 and 5 [pp. 116–117])
	  b. perform actions *to maintain patency of wound drain if present:*
	    1. keep tubing free of kinks
	    2. empty collection device as often as necessary
	    3. maintain suction as ordered

Desired Outcomes	Nursing Actions and *Selected Purposes/Rationales*

    c. perform actions *to prevent inadvertent removal of wound drain if
        present:*
        1. use caution when changing dressings surrounding drain
        2. provide extension tubing if necessary *to enable client to move
            without placing tension on the drain*
        3. instruct client not to pull on drain and drainage tubing
    d. perform actions *to prevent stress on and subsequent leakage from the
        suture line at site of anastomosis:*
        1. do not change position of the nasogastric tube unless ordered (*the
            tube is positioned during surgery and moving it can traumatize the
            suture line*)
        2. implement measures to prevent nausea and vomiting (see
            Standardized Postoperative Care Plan, Nursing Diagnosis 7.B,
            action 2 [pp. 108–109])
        3. implement measures *to prevent distention of the remaining portion
            of the stomach:*
            a. irrigate nasogastric tube only if ordered and with no more than
                prescribed amount of solution
            b. perform actions to reduce the accumulation of gastrointestinal
                gas and fluid (see Standardized Postoperative Care Plan,
                Nursing Diagnosis 7.A, action 3 [pp. 107–108])
            c. when oral intake is allowed, progress diet slowly and instruct
                client to avoid drinking fluids with meals
    e. perform actions to treat afferent loop syndrome if it occurs (see action
        c.2 in this diagnosis) *in order to prevent distention of the duodenal
        stump and subsequently reduce the risk of disruption of the duodenal
        stump sutures following gastrojejunostomy.*
4. If signs and symptoms of peritonitis occur:
    a. withhold oral intake as ordered
    b. place client on bed rest in a semi-Fowler's position *to assist in
        pooling or localizing gastrointestinal contents in the pelvis rather
        than under the diaphragm*
    c. prepare client for diagnostic tests (e.g. abdominal x-ray, computed
        tomography, ultrasound) if planned
    d. assist physician with insertion of a nasogastric tube and maintain
        suction as ordered
    e. administer antimicrobials as ordered
    f. administer intravenous fluids and/or blood volume expanders if
        ordered *to prevent or treat shock (can result from the increased
        capillary permeability that occurs with inflammation and the
        subsequent escape of protein, fluid, and electrolytes from the vascular
        space into the peritoneal cavity)*
    g. prepare client for surgical intervention (e.g. repair of anastomosis) if
        planned
    h. provide emotional support to client and significant others.

4.c. The client will have
      resolution of afferent loop
      syndrome if it occurs as
      evidenced by:
      1. no reports of intense
          nausea or epigastric
          fullness and pain after
          eating
      2. no episodes of vomiting
          bile after eating.

4.c.1. Assess for and report signs and symptoms of afferent loop syndrome (e.g.
        reports of intense nausea and/or epigastric fullness and pain after eating,
        forceful vomiting of large amounts of bile after eating). Signs and
        symptoms usually occur 20–90 minutes after eating.
    2. If signs and symptoms of afferent loop syndrome occur:
        a. restrict oral intake as ordered
        b. prepare client for diagnostic tests (e.g. ultrasound, computed
            tomography) if planned
        c. assist physician with insertion of a nasogastric tube and maintain
            suction as ordered
        d. administer antimicrobials as ordered (*infection can develop as a
            result of stasis of secretions in the afferent loop*)
        e. prepare client for surgical intervention if obstruction is caused by
            kinking of the efferent jejunal limb.

4.d. The client will not experience dumping syndrome after eating as evidenced by:
1. no reports of abdominal cramping
2. normal bowel sounds
3. skin dry and usual color
4. absence of palpitations, weakness, dizziness, and diarrhea
5. usual mental status.

4.d.1. Assess for signs and symptoms of:
a. early dumping syndrome (e.g. reports of abdominal cramping, hyperactive bowel sounds, diaphoresis, flushing, palpitations, weakness, dizziness, and/or diarrhea within 30 minutes after meals)
b. late dumping syndrome (e.g. anxiety, palpitations, dizziness, weakness, diaphoresis, inability to concentrate, decreased coordination, and/or confusion occurring 1–3 hours after meals).
2. Implement measures *to prevent dumping syndrome:*
a. instruct client to avoid intake of simple carbohydrates (e.g. jelly, cake, pie, pudding, candy) *because they are hypertonic and tend to rapidly draw fluid into the intestine and because they are rapidly absorbed into the blood leading to increased insulin release and subsequent hypoglycemia*
b. encourage intake of foods containing moderate to high amounts of fat and protein (*these foods leave the stomach more slowly and are less hypertonic*)
c. instruct client in ways *to delay gastric emptying:*
1. eat small, dry meals
2. eat meals slowly
3. drink fluids between rather than with meals; avoid fluids for at least 1 hour before and after meals
4. eat in a semi-recumbent position, then lie down for at least 30 minutes after each meal unless contraindicated.
3. If signs and symptoms of dumping syndrome occur:
a. provide client with a rapid-acting carbohydrate (e.g. hard candy, sugar-containing soft drink) or glucose tablets *to treat the hypoglycemia that characterizes late dumping syndrome*
b. review dietary management and revise as necessary (e.g. reduce size of meals, reduce sugar intake)
c. administer anticholinergics (e.g. propantheline) 30 minutes before meals if ordered *to delay gastric emptying.*

Discharge Teaching

5. NURSING DIAGNOSIS: **Knowledge deficit, Ineffective management of therapeutic regimen, or Altered health maintenance***

*The nurse should select the diagnostic label that is most appropriate for the client's discharge teaching needs.

Desired Outcomes

Nursing Actions and *Selected Purposes/Rationales*

5.a. The client will identify ways to prevent recurrence of peptic ulcers.

5.a.1. Instruct the client in ways to prevent peptic ulcer recurrence:
a. drink decaffeinated or caffeine-free tea and colas rather than those containing caffeine
b. avoid drinking coffee and alcohol or drink these beverages only in small amounts immediately following a meal
c. avoid intake of any foods and fluids that cause gastric distress
d. eat regularly scheduled meals and snacks (recommended frequency and amount will vary depending on the size of the remaining stomach); do not skip meals
e. eat slowly and chew food thoroughly
f. maintain a calm, relaxed atmosphere at mealtime and whenever possible
g. stop smoking
h. maintain a balance of physical activity and rest
i. avoid stressful situations

Desired Outcomes	Nursing Actions and *Selected Purposes/Rationales*
	j. avoid ingestion of medications such as aspirin, aspirin-containing products, and ibuprofen; if it is necessary to take these or other ulcerogenic medications (e.g. corticosteroids, indomethacin), take them with food whenever possible
	k. take medications (e.g. antacids, histamine$_2$ receptor antagonists, cholestyramine [may be indicated if client is experiencing reflux of bile into the stomach]) as prescribed.
	2. Obtain a dietary consult if client needs assistance in planning meals that incorporate recommended dietary modifications.
	3. Provide information on community resources that can assist the client in making life-style changes (e.g. stress management classes, smoking cessation programs, counseling services). Initiate a referral if indicated.
5.b. The client will verbalize an understanding of ways to maintain an adequate nutritional status.	**5.b.1.** Instruct client regarding ways to maintain an adequate nutritional status: a. eat regularly scheduled meals and snacks (recommended frequency and amount will vary depending on the size of the remaining stomach); do not skip meals b. eat slowly and chew food thoroughly to enhance digestion and absorption of nutrients c. continue with actions to prevent or control postvagotomy diarrhea and dumping syndrome (see actions c.3 and 4 and d.3–5 in this diagnosis); contact health care provider if these conditions are not controlled since they can result in excessive loss of nutrients d. take vitamin and mineral supplements as prescribed (usually prescribed in liquid or chewable form to ensure maximum absorption) e. take pancreatic enzymes (e.g. pancreatin, pancrelipase) and/or bile salts as prescribed (may be prescribed to facilitate digestion of food).
	2. Instruct client to adhere to scheduled follow-up blood studies to determine need for vitamin B$_{12}$ injections (pernicious anemia can develop years after the surgery as a result of decreased secretion of the intrinsic factor resulting from surgical removal of the gastrin-secreting and parietal cells).
5.c. The client will identify ways to control postvagotomy diarrhea if it occurs.	**5.c.1.** Inform client that episodes of diarrhea may occur if a truncal vagotomy was performed.
	2. Explain that postvagotomy diarrhea can be mild or explosive, usually occurs within 1–2 hours after eating, is episodic (can occur 2–3 times a week for 1–3 days), and is unpredictable (episodes may last 1–2 months and then not recur for weeks or months). Emphasize that if this condition occurs, it usually resolves within a year.
	3. Instruct client that eating small rather than large meals and drinking liquids between rather than with meals may help prevent postvagotomy diarrhea.
	4. Provide teaching regarding antidiarrheal medications recommended or prescribed by physician.
5.d. The client will identify ways to manage dumping syndrome if it occurs.	**5.d.1.** Reinforce physician's explanation regarding the factors that cause dumping syndrome. Emphasize that if this condition occurs, it usually resolves within 6–12 months.
	2. Instruct client to be alert for signs and symptoms of: a. early dumping syndrome (e.g. abdominal cramping, weakness, flushing, palpitations, dizziness, and/or diarrhea within 30 minutes after eating) b. late dumping syndrome (e.g. anxiety, palpitations, dizziness, weakness, sweating, inability to concentrate, and/or decreased coordination 1–3 hours after meals).
	3. Reinforce teaching regarding ways to prevent dumping syndrome (see Postoperative Collaborative Diagnosis 4, action d.2).
	4. Provide teaching regarding medications prescribed to prevent dumping syndrome (small doses of an anticholinergic agent may need to be taken 30 minutes before meals if symptoms cannot be prevented with above actions).
	5. Instruct client to drink fluids with high sugar content (e.g. sugar-

containing soft drinks), eat candy that contains sugar or graham crackers, or take glucose tablets unless contraindicated if signs and symptoms of late dumping syndrome occur.

5.e. The client will state signs and symptoms to report to the health care provider.	5.e.1. Refer to Standardized Postoperative Care Plan, Nursing Diagnosis 21, action c (p. 123), for signs and symptoms to report to the health care provider.

      2. Instruct client to also report:

        a. persistent nausea and/or vomiting

        b. persistent, increasing, or recurrent abdominal or epigastric discomfort

        c. abdominal distention or rigidity

        d. bloody, coffee-ground, or green-yellow vomitus

        e. foul-smelling, greasy stools that float (indicative of impaired absorption of dietary fat)

        f. persistent diarrhea

        g. persistent or increasing fatigue and weakness

        h. persistent weight loss

        i. signs and symptoms of dumping syndrome (see action d.2 in this diagnosis) that are not controlled using recommended measures

        j. epigastric burning or aching that gets worse after eating and/or frequent vomiting or eructation of bile and food particles (these signs and symptoms are indicative of alkaline reflux gastritis, which can develop when alkaline pancreatic secretions and bile reflux into the remaining portion of the stomach).

5.f. The client will verbalize an understanding of and a plan for adhering to recommended follow-up care including future appointments with health care provider, medications prescribed, activity level, and wound care.	5.f. Refer to Standardized Postoperative Care Plan, Nursing Diagnosis 21 (pp. 123–124), for routine postoperative instructions and measures to improve client compliance.

Bibliography

See pages 897–898 and 907.

GASTRIC REDUCTION

Gastric reduction is a type of bariatric surgery (surgery performed to control obesity) that is accomplished by vertical-banded gastroplasty or, less frequently, by gastric bypass. Both of these methods involve reducing the capacity of the stomach to 30–50 ml by partitioning off a small portion of the stomach distal to the gastroesophageal junction to form a gastric pouch. A narrow outlet is then created for the gastric pouch so that it does not empty quickly. As a result of the decreased gastric capacity and delayed pouch emptying, it is expected that the client will experience early satiety and subsequently decrease his/her oral intake and lose weight.

The most frequently performed method of gastric reduction is vertical-banded gastroplasty. In this method, the gastric pouch is formed on the lesser curvature side of the stomach by the placement of 2 adjacent rows of vertical staple lines. The narrow channel created between the pouch and remaining stomach is reinforced with a ring of mesh or plastic to reduce the risk of channel widening. Food/fluid then pass from the pouch, through the channel, into the remaining stomach, and through the intestinal tract. Gastric bypass also incorporates gastric partitioning but, in this method of gastric reduction, the gastric pouch is created by the placement of horizontal rows of staples or by actual surgical transection of the stomach. A gastrojejunostomy (Roux-en-Y) is then performed so that foods/fluids pass from the gastric pouch directly into the jejunum. The opening created between the pouch and the jejunal loop is about 1 cm in diameter.

Clients are carefully screened physically and psychologically and must meet certain criteria before undergoing gastric reduction surgery. The criteria usually include massive obesity for at least 5 years, inability to reduce weight using other forms of treatment, weight that is at least 100 pounds or 100% or more over ideal body weight, and obesity that results from a caloric intake greater than the body's needs rather than an underlying metabolic disorder. The client must also be emotionally stable, have no major illness, and have access to adequate follow-up medical care.

This care plan focuses on the adult client hospitalized for gastric reduction surgery. Preoperative goals of care are to reduce fear and anxiety, prepare the client for the surgery and the postoperative period, and assist him/her to maintain a positive self-concept. Postoperatively, the goals of care are to maintain adequate nutrition, maintain comfort, prevent complications, assist the client to develop strategies that will help ensure compliance with dietary modifications, and educate the client regarding follow-up care.

DISCHARGE CRITERIA

Prior to discharge, the client will:

- have evidence of normal healing of surgical wounds
- have clear, audible breath sounds throughout lungs
- tolerate prescribed diet
- have no signs and symptoms of postoperative complications
- identify ways to prevent excessive stretching of the gastric pouch
- verbalize an understanding of ways to maintain an adequate nutritional status
- identify ways to reduce the risk of consuming excessive amounts of food, fluid, and calories
- demonstrate the ability to accurately calculate and measure the allotted amounts of food and fluid
- state signs and symptoms to report to the health care provider
- identify community resources that can assist in the adjustment to prescribed dietary modifications and future changes in body image
- verbalize an understanding of and a plan for adhering to recommended follow-up care including future appointments with health care provider, activity level, medications prescribed, and wound care.

NURSING/ COLLABORATIVE DIAGNOSES	**Preoperative**
	 1. Self-concept disturbance △ 604
	 Postoperative
	 1. Ineffective breathing pattern △ 605
	 2. Altered nutrition: less than body requirements △ 606
	 3. Actual/Risk for impaired tissue integrity △ 607
	 4. Potential complications:
	    a. overdistention of the gastric pouch
	    b. peritonitis
	    c. thromboembolism
	    d. atelectasis △ 608
	 5. Ineffective management of therapeutic regimen △ 610

DISCHARGE TEACHING	**6.** Knowledge deficit or Altered health maintenance △ 611

See Standardized Preoperative and Postoperative Care Plans for additional diagnoses.

PREOPERATIVE

Use in conjunction with the Standardized Preoperative Care Plan.

1. NURSING DIAGNOSIS:

Self-concept disturbance*

related to obesity and the inability to lose weight by more conventional methods.

---

*This diagnostic label includes the nursing diagnoses of body image disturbance and self-esteem disturbance.

Desired Outcome	Nursing Actions and *Selected Purposes/Rationales*

1. The client will demonstrate a positive self-concept as evidenced by:
  a. verbalization of feelings of self-worth
  b. positive statements regarding anticipated effects of surgical procedure
  c. maintenance of relationships with significant others
  d. active participation in preoperative care and self-care.
	1.a. Assess for signs and symptoms of a self-concept disturbance (e.g. verbalization of negative feelings about self, withdrawal from significant others, lack of participation in preoperative care or self-care).
	  b. Determine the meaning of obesity and anticipated effects of the gastric reduction to the client by encouraging verbalization of feelings and by noting nonverbal responses.
	  c. Implement measures *to assist client to increase self-esteem* (e.g. limit negative self-assessment, encourage positive comments about self, assist to identify strengths, give positive feedback about accomplishments, provide positive feedback about decision to have the surgery and lose weight).
	  d. Implement measures *to reduce client's embarrassment about obesity:*
	    1. obtain information from physician regarding client's height and weight so that oversized equipment and supplies (e.g. bed, chair, commode, blood pressure cuff, gowns, bathrobe) can be obtained before client is admitted
	    2. remove unnecessary furniture and equipment from room so client can move around easily
	    3. provide privacy when weighing client
	    4. transfer client to and from operating room in own hospital bed rather than attempting to use a regular-sized stretcher.
	  e. Allow client to wear own clothes rather than hospital gown before and after surgery if desired.
	  f. Assure client that he/she will be assisted with usual grooming and makeup habits after surgery if necessary.
	  g. Demonstrate acceptance of client using techniques such as touch and frequent visits.
	  h. Arrange for a visit from an individual who has achieved weight loss after gastric reduction surgery if client desires.
	  i. If client is expressing concerns about the amount of excess skin that will be present after the majority of weight loss occurs (usually after 1–1½ years), provide information about various clothing styles that may be most flattering (e.g. long-sleeved shirts or blouses) and reconstructive surgery that is available to remove excess skin from abdomen, breasts, upper arms, and thighs.
	  j. Consult physician if client has unrealistic expectations of postoperative weight loss and dietary management.

POSTOPERATIVE

Use in conjunction with the Standardized Postoperative Care Plan.

---

1. NURSING DIAGNOSIS:

Ineffective breathing pattern

related to:
a. increased rate and decreased depth of respirations associated with fear and anxiety;
b. decreased rate and depth of respirations associated with the depressant effect of anesthesia (effect lasts longer in the obese client because adipose tissue more readily absorbs and stores anesthetic agents) and some medications (e.g. narcotic [opioid] analgesics);
c. diminished lung/chest wall expansion associated with:
  1. limited diaphragmatic excursion resulting from large amounts of abdominal adipose tissue, abdominal distention, and reluctance to breathe deeply because of a high abdominal incision
  2. decreased activity (lung expansion is restricted by the bed surface when client is lying in bed)
  3. increased weight of the chest wall of an obese client (especially in women with pendulous breasts).

Desired Outcome	Nursing Actions and *Selected Purposes/Rationales*
1. The client will maintain an effective breathing pattern (see Standardized Postoperative Care Plan, Nursing Diagnosis 2 [p. 102], for outcome criteria).	1.a. Refer to Standardized Postoperative Care Plan, Nursing Diagnosis 2 (pp. 102–103), for measures related to assessment and improvement of breathing pattern. b. Implement additional measures *to improve breathing pattern:* 1. position client with head of bed elevated at least 30° at all times 2. instruct and assist client to use overhead trapeze and turn at least every 2 hours 3. add extensions to tubings if necessary *to enable client to turn and move without fear of dislodging tubes* 4. instruct client to bend knees while coughing and deep breathing *in order to relieve tension on abdominal muscles and incision* 5. instruct and assist client to splint incision with hands or pillow when coughing and deep breathing 6. assist with ambulation the evening of surgery and at least 4 times/day as ordered.

■

2. NURSING DIAGNOSIS:　**Altered nutrition: less than body requirements**

related to:
a. decreased oral intake associated with nausea, pain, weakness, fatigue, prescribed dietary modifications, and early satiety resulting from small pouch size;
b. inadequate nutritional replacement therapy;
c. increased nutritional needs associated with the increased metabolic rate that occurs during wound healing.

Desired Outcome	Nursing Actions and *Selected Purposes/Rationales*
2. The client will maintain an adequate nutritional status as evidenced by: a. normal BUN and serum albumin, Hct, Hb, transferrin, and lymphocyte levels b. usual strength and activity tolerance c. healthy oral mucous membrane.	2.a. Assess for and report signs and symptoms of malnutrition: 1. abnormal BUN and low serum albumin, Hct, Hb, transferrin, and lymphocyte levels (decreased Hct and Hb may also result from surgical blood loss) 2. weakness and fatigue 3. sore, inflamed oral mucous membrane 4. pale conjunctiva. b. Assess for return of bowel function every 2–4 hours. Notify physician when client has normal bowel sounds and is expelling flatus *so that jejunostomy tube feedings and/or oral intake can be started as soon as possible.* c. When oral intake is allowed, monitor client's intake. Report if the prescribed amounts or types of fluids are not consumed. d. Implement measures *to maintain an adequate nutritional status:* 1. maintain jejunostomy tube feeding if ordered 2. when oral intake is allowed: 　a. perform actions to reduce pain (see Standardized Postoperative Care Plan, Nursing Diagnosis 6, action e [p. 107]) 　b. administer antiemetics and/or gastrointestinal stimulants (e.g. metoclopramide) if ordered *to control nausea* 　c. maintain a clean environment and a relaxed, pleasant atmosphere 　d. provide oral hygiene before offering fluids 　e. provide high-protein liquid nourishment as part of fluid allotment as soon as allowed (client is usually allowed to drink dilute liquid protein supplements 4–5 days after surgery)

      f. reinforce the importance of consuming fluids at scheduled frequency and consuming more nutritious fluids and foods as soon as allowed (client is usually allowed to progress from fluids to solids after 6–8 weeks)

    3. administer vitamins and minerals if ordered.

  e. Consult physician if client is unable to tolerate or adhere to prescribed diet.

---

3. NURSING DIAGNOSIS: **Actual/Risk for impaired tissue integrity**

related to:

a. disruption of tissue associated with the surgical procedure;

b. delayed wound healing associated with factors such as decreased nutritional status and inadequate blood supply to wound area;

c. irritation of skin associated with contact with wound drainage, pressure from tubes, and use of tape;

d. difficulty keeping deep skin fold areas dry;

e. damage to the skin and/or subcutaneous tissue associated with:
    1. friction or shearing when moving in bed
    2. pressure on tissues as a result of excessive body weight and decreased activity.

Desired Outcomes	Nursing Actions and *Selected Purposes/Rationales*
3.a. The client will experience normal healing of surgical wounds (see Standardized Postoperative Care Plan, Nursing Diagnosis 9, outcome a [pp. 109–110], for outcome criteria).	3.a.1. Refer to Standardized Postoperative Care Plan, Nursing Diagnosis 9, action a (pp. 109–110), for measures related to assessment and promotion of wound healing. 2. Implement measures to maintain an adequate nutritional status (see Postoperative Nursing Diagnosis 2, action d) *in order to further promote wound healing.*

3.b. The client will maintain tissue integrity as evidenced by:
1. absence of redness and irritation
2. no skin breakdown.
	3.b.1. Inspect the following sites for pallor, redness, and breakdown:
	   a. skin folds of abdomen and groin and under breasts
	   b. skin areas in contact with wound drainage, tape, and tubings
	   c. back, coccyx, and buttocks
	   d. elbows and heels.
	  2. Refer to Standardized Postoperative Care Plan, Nursing Diagnosis 9, action b.2 (pp. 110–111), for measures to prevent tissue irritation and breakdown in areas in contact with wound drainage, tape, and tubings.
	  3. Implement additional measures *to reduce the risk for tissue breakdown:*
	   a. assist client to turn at least every 2 hours when in bed
	   b. assist client to position self properly; use pressure-reducing or pressure-relieving devices (e.g. pillows, gel or foam cushions, alternating pressure mattress, air-fluidized bed) if indicated
	   c. assist client with ambulation as ordered and as frequently as tolerated
	   d. gently massage heels, elbows, and around reddened areas at least every 2 hours
	   e. apply a thin layer of powder or cornstarch to bottom sheet or skin and to opposing skin surfaces (e.g. axillae, beneath breasts, abdominal folds) if indicated *to absorb moisture and/or reduce friction*
	   f. instruct and assist client to use overhead trapeze to lift self off the bed when moving
	   g. instruct and assist client to shift weight at least every 30 minutes
	   h. keep skin clean and dry
	   i. keep bed linens dry and wrinkle-free
	   j. perform actions *to reduce irritation resulting from friction and pressure on elbows and heels:*

Desired Outcomes	Nursing Actions and *Selected Purposes/Rationales*

       1. encourage client to use overhead trapeze to move self rather than pushing with heels and elbows

       2. provide elbow and heel protectors if indicated.

    4. If tissue breakdown occurs:

      a. notify physician

      b. continue with above measures to prevent further irritation and breakdown

      c. perform care of involved areas as ordered or per standard hospital procedure

      d. assess client closely and report signs and symptoms of infection (e.g. elevated temperature; heat, pain, and swelling around area of breakdown; unusual drainage from site).

---

4. COLLABORATIVE DIAGNOSES:

Potential complications of gastric reduction surgery:

a. **overdistention of the gastric pouch** related to:
   1. accumulation of gas and fluid in the pouch associated with:
     a. decreased peristalsis and/or impaired functioning of nasogastric or gastrostomy tube
     b. obstruction of the pouch outlet (the channel between the pouch and distal stomach if gastroplasty performed or the opening between the pouch and jejunal loop if gastric bypass performed) resulting from edema and/or ingestion of medications or thick fluids that are not able to pass through pouch outlet
   2. excessive oral intake;

b. **peritonitis** related to:
   1. wound infection
   2. leakage of gastric contents into the peritoneum associated with disruption of the staple line (if gastroplasty performed) or proximal anastomosis (if gastric bypass performed);

c. **thromboembolism** related to:
   1. venous stasis associated with decreased activity, increased blood viscosity (can result from fluid volume deficit), and pressure on abdominal vessels from excessive adipose tissue and abdominal distention
   2. hypercoagulability associated with increased release of thromboplastin into the blood (occurs as a result of surgical trauma) and hemoconcentration and increased blood viscosity (can occur as a result of fluid volume deficit)
   3. trauma to vein walls during surgery;

d. **atelectasis** related to shallow respirations and stasis of secretions in the alveoli and bronchioles.

Desired Outcomes	Nursing Actions and *Selected Purposes/Rationales*

4.a. The client will not experience overdistention of the gastric pouch as evidenced by:
1. decreased reports of epigastric fullness
2. absence of nausea and vomiting.

4.a.1. Assess for and report signs and symptoms of overdistention of the gastric pouch (e.g. increasing reports of epigastric fullness, nausea, vomiting).

    2. Implement measures *to prevent overdistention of the gastric pouch:*

     a. maintain patency of nasogastric or gastric tube *to reduce gas and fluid accumulation during period of decreased peristalsis*; irrigate the tube only if ordered and with no more than prescribed amount of solution

     b. encourage and assist client with frequent position changes and ambulation as soon as allowed and tolerated (*activity stimulates peristalsis*)

     c. instruct the client to avoid activities such as chewing gum and smoking *in order to reduce air swallowing*

     d. do not change position of nasogastric or gastric tube unless ordered (*the tube is usually positioned at the pouch outlet to help prevent obstruction of the opening into the distal stomach [if gastroplasty performed] or jejunal loop [if gastric bypass performed]*)

    e. when oral intake is allowed:

      1. adhere strictly to prescribed oral intake schedule (clients usually begin with hourly liquid feedings of 30 ml and, over at least 6 weeks, progress to 5 or 6 small [1–2 ounce] liquid meals/day with 1–2 ounces of water allowed periodically between meals)

      2. provide client with allotted amounts of fluids at the proper times; discard skipped "meals" *so client does not ingest feedings too close together*

      3. instruct client to adhere to the liquid or blenderized diet as ordered (*oral intake that is too thick can block the pouch outlet, which may be narrower in the early postoperative period because of edema*)

      4. administer oral medication in liquid or chewable form or crushed thoroughly *to prevent blockage of the pouch outlet*

    f. encourage client to eructate whenever the urge is felt

    g. encourage use of nonnarcotic analgesics once severe pain has subsided (*narcotic [opioid] analgesics depress gastrointestinal motility*).

  3. If signs and symptoms of overdistention occur:

    a. withhold all oral intake as ordered

    b. prepare client for upper abdominal x-rays to check placement of nasogastric or gastric tube if present

    c. assist physician with adjustment or reinsertion of the nasogastric or gastric tube if indicated.

4.b. The client will not develop peritonitis as evidenced by:

1. gradual resolution of abdominal pain
2. soft, nondistended abdomen
3. temperature declining toward normal
4. stable vital signs
5. absence of nausea and vomiting
6. gradual return of normal bowel sounds
7. WBC count declining toward normal.

4.b.1. Assess for and report signs and symptoms of peritonitis (e.g. increase in severity of abdominal pain; generalized abdominal pain; rebound tenderness; distended, rigid abdomen; increase in temperature; tachycardia; tachypnea; hypotension; nausea; vomiting; continued diminished or absent bowel sounds).

  2. Monitor WBC counts. Report levels that increase or fail to decline toward normal.

  3. Implement measures *to prevent peritonitis*:

    a. perform actions to prevent and treat wound infection (see Standardized Postoperative Care Plan, Nursing Diagnosis 16, actions b.4 and 5 [pp. 116–117])

    b. perform actions *to maintain patency of wound drain(s) if present*:

      1. keep tubing free of kinks

      2. empty collection device(s) as often as necessary

      3. maintain suction as ordered

    c. perform actions *to prevent inadvertent removal of wound drain(s) if present*:

      1. use caution when changing dressings surrounding drain(s)

      2. provide extension tubing if necessary *to enable client to move without placing tension on the drain(s)*

      3. instruct client not to pull on drain(s) and drainage tubing(s)

    d. perform actions *to prevent stress on and subsequent leakage of gastric contents from the staple line or site of proximal anastomosis*:

      1. implement measures to prevent overdistention of the gastric pouch (see action a.2 in this diagnosis)

      2. implement measures to prevent nausea and vomiting (e.g. maintain patency of nasogastric or gastric tube, eliminate noxious sights and odors from the environment, instruct client to change positions slowly, administer antiemetics and/or gastrointestinal stimulants as ordered)

      3. do not adjust position of nasogastric or gastric tube unless ordered (*adjustment may cause disruption of staples or perforation at site of proximal anastomosis*).

  4. If signs and symptoms of peritonitis occur:

    a. withhold oral intake and jejunostomy tube feeding as ordered

Desired Outcomes	Nursing Actions and *Selected Purposes/Rationales*
	b. place client on bed rest in a semi-Fowler's position *to assist in pooling or localizing gastric contents in the pelvis rather than under the diaphragm*
	c. prepare client for diagnostic tests (e.g. abdominal x-ray, computed tomography, ultrasound) if planned
	d. assist physician with insertion of a nasogastric or gastric tube and maintain suction as ordered
	e. administer antimicrobials as ordered
	f. administer intravenous fluids and/or blood volume expanders if ordered *to prevent or treat shock (can result from the increased capillary permeability that occurs with inflammation and the subsequent escape of protein, fluid, and electrolytes from the vascular space into the peritoneal cavity)*
	g. prepare client for surgical intervention (e.g. repair of perforation) if planned
	h. provide emotional support to client and significant others.
4.c. The client will not develop a deep vein thrombus and pulmonary embolism (see Standardized Postoperative Care Plan, Collaborative Diagnosis 19, outcomes c.1 and 2 [pp. 120–121], for outcome criteria).	4.c. Refer to Standardized Postoperative Care Plan, Collaborative Diagnosis 19, actions c.1 and 2 (pp. 120–121), for measures related to assessment, prevention, and treatment of a deep vein thrombus and pulmonary embolism.
4.d. The client will not develop atelectasis (see Standardized Postoperative Care Plan, Collaborative Diagnosis 19, outcome b [p. 120], for outcome criteria).	4.d.1. Refer to Standardized Postoperative Care Plan, Collaborative Diagnosis 19, action b (p. 120), for measures related to assessment, prevention, and treatment of atelectasis. 2. Implement additional measures to improve breathing pattern (see Postoperative Nursing Diagnosis 1) *in order to further reduce the risk of atelectasis.*

---

5. NURSING DIAGNOSIS:

Ineffective management of therapeutic regimen

related to lack of understanding of the implications of not following the prescribed treatment plan and difficulty integrating prescribed dietary modifications into life style.

Desired Outcome	Nursing Actions and *Selected Purposes/Rationales*
5. The client will demonstrate the probability of effective management of the therapeutic regimen as evidenced by: a. willingness to learn about and participate in treatments and care b. statements reflecting ways to integrate prescribed dietary plan and exercise program into life style c. statements reflecting an understanding of the implications of not following the prescribed treatment plan.	5.a. Assess for indications that the client may be unable to effectively manage the therapeutic regimen: 1. failure to adhere to treatment plan while in hospital (e.g. not adhering to dietary modifications and fluid restrictions, refusing to increase activity) 2. statements reflecting a lack of understanding of dietary modifications and factors that will cause stretching of the gastric pouch 3. verbalization of an inability to integrate necessary dietary modifications and exercise program into life style 4. statements reflecting the belief that the surgical procedure will result in continued weight loss even without adherence to the prescribed dietary modifications or that he/she will return to preoperative weight despite adherence to dietary modifications. b. Implement measures *to promote effective management of the therapeutic regimen:* 1. explain the surgical procedure and importance of dietary modifications and a balanced exercise program in terms the client can

understand; emphasize that adherence to the treatment program is necessary if an optimal weight is to be attained

2. inform the client that prescribed food and fluid modifications are not as strict after the surgical area has healed (usually 6–8 weeks)

3. stress the positive effects of compliance with dietary modifications and exercise program (e.g. weight loss resulting in change in appearance; decreased risk of development of conditions such as diabetes mellitus, cardiovascular disease, respiratory problems, and arthritis)

4. assist client to identify ways dietary modifications and exercise program can be incorporated into life style; focus on modifications of life style rather than complete change (e.g. schedule meetings after rather than during lunch, meet friends at a park rather than a restaurant)

5. provide a dietary consult to assist client in planning a dietary program based on prescribed modifications and client's personal and cultural preferences and daily routines

6. encourage activities other than eating to cope with stress (e.g. exercise)

7. initiate and reinforce the discharge teaching outlined in Postoperative Nursing Diagnosis 6 *in order to promote a sense of control*

8. encourage questions and allow time for reinforcement and clarification of information provided

9. provide written instructions about future appointments with health care provider, dietary modifications, and signs and symptoms to report

10. provide information about and encourage utilization of community resources that can assist client to make necessary life-style changes (e.g. weight reduction groups, counseling services, support groups of persons who have had the same or similar surgery, stress management classes)

11. reinforce behaviors suggesting future compliance with the therapeutic regimen (e.g. statements reflecting plans for integrating dietary modifications into life style, active participation in planning dietary program)

12. include significant others in explanations and teaching sessions and encourage their support; reinforce the need for client to assume responsibility for managing as much of care as possible.

c. Consult physician regarding referrals to community agencies and/or support groups if continued instruction, support, or supervision is needed.

Discharge Teaching

∎━━━

6. NURSING DIAGNOSIS: **Knowledge deficit or Altered health maintenance***

*The nurse should select the diagnostic label that is most appropriate for the client's discharge teaching needs.

Desired Outcomes	Nursing Actions and *Selected Purposes/Rationales*

6.a. The client will identify ways to prevent excessive stretching of the gastric pouch.	6.a. Instruct client in ways to prevent excessive stretching of the gastric pouch:
	1. decrease risk of blockage of the gastric outlet by:
	  a. limiting oral intake to liquids and blenderized foods for about 6–8 weeks after surgery as prescribed
	  b. taking all prescription and nonprescription medications in liquid or chewable form or crushing them thoroughly
	  c. chewing foods thoroughly
	2. do not exceed prescribed volume of food/fluid intake

Desired Outcomes	Nursing Actions and *Selected Purposes/Rationales*
	3. do not make up for skipped meals while on an hourly drinking/eating schedule 4. eat and drink slowly 5. avoid intake of carbonated beverages for 6–8 weeks after surgery and limit intake of these beverages after that time 6. when solid foods are allowed, consume fluids between rather than with meals.

6.b. The client will verbalize an understanding of ways to maintain an adequate nutritional status.	6.b.1. Instruct client regarding ways to maintain an adequate nutritional status:
	  a. do not skip meals
	  b. consume foods/fluids from each food group daily as diet advances
	  c. consume adequate amounts of protein (e.g. blenderized drinks containing peanut butter, pureed meats and fish, creamed cottage cheese) as diet advances
	  d. take vitamin and mineral supplements as prescribed.
	  2. Obtain dietary consult if indicated to assist client in planning meals.

6.c. The client will identify ways to reduce the risk of consuming excessive amounts of food, fluid, and calories.	6.c. Instruct client in ways to reduce the risk of consuming excessive amounts of food, fluid, and calories:
	  1. limit food/fluid intake to prescribed volume
	  2. prepare foods ahead of time, freeze in 1-ounce portions using plastic ice cube trays or plastic bags, and then reheat only allowed amounts at mealtime
	  3. have jars of prepared strained baby food products rather than high-calorie puddings and snacks on hand
	  4. have only low-calorie drinks available (other than the required high-protein supplements)
	  5. decrease the risk of hunger by adhering to a schedule of 5 or 6 meals/day as diet advances (each meal will usually consist of 2–4 tablespoons of food)
	  6. serve food on a small plate (this provides an illusion that meals are larger than they really are)
	  7. eat and drink very slowly (use techniques such as putting fork down between bites of food and putting glass down between sips of fluid)
	  8. if going out to dinner, order an appetizer and have it served with everyone else's entree
	  9. avoid excessive intake of high-calorie foods/fluids (it is possible to maintain or gain weight if only high-calorie substances are consumed).

6.d. The client will demonstrate the ability to accurately calculate and measure the allotted amounts of food and fluid.	6.d.1. Demonstrate ways to measure foods/fluids accurately using measuring spoons and a cup with 1-ounce markings. 2. Allow time for questions, clarification, and return demonstration.

6.e. The client will state signs and symptoms to report to the health care provider.	6.e.1. Refer to Standardized Postoperative Care Plan, Nursing Diagnosis 21, action c (p. 123), for signs and symptoms to report to the health care provider.
	  2. Instruct client to also report:
	    a. nausea and vomiting after consuming prescribed amount of foods/fluids
	    b. inability to adhere to dietary modifications
	    c. weight gain
	    d. inability to lose weight or excessive weight loss (expected weight loss is usually about 10 pounds/month for the 1st year or 30% of preoperative body weight by the end of the 1st year)
	    e. abdominal cramping, flushing, palpitations, weakness, and/or dizziness within 30 minutes after eating (indicative of dumping syndrome, which sometimes occurs when a client who has had a gastric bypass begins to eat solid food; if dumping syndrome does occur, symptoms are usually mild and self-limiting or easily controlled with minor dietary modifications).

6.f. The client will identify community resources that	6.f.1. Provide information about community resources that can assist the client with adjustment to prescribed dietary modifications and future changes

can assist in the adjustment to prescribed dietary modifications and future changes in body image.

6.g. The client will verbalize an understanding of and a plan for adhering to recommended follow-up care including future appointments with health care provider, activity level, medications prescribed, and wound care.

in body image (e.g. weight reduction groups, counseling services, support groups of persons who have had the same or similar surgery).

2. Initiate a referral if indicated.

6.g.1. Refer to Standardized Postoperative Care Plan, Nursing Diagnosis 21 (pp. 123–124), for routine postoperative instructions.

2. Reinforce the physician's instructions regarding need to adhere to a schedule of moderate exercise (clients are usually instructed to begin a walking program and should be walking 1–2 miles/day by the 4th week after discharge).

3. Refer to Postoperative Nursing Diagnosis 5, action b, for measures to promote the client's ability to effectively manage the therapeutic regimen.

Bibliography

See pages 897–898 and 907.

INFLAMMATORY BOWEL DISEASE: ULCERATIVE COLITIS AND CROHN'S DISEASE

Crohn's disease and ulcerative colitis are idiopathic chronic inflammatory bowel diseases, which are often jointly referred to as inflammatory bowel disease (IBD). These disorders have similarities but can usually be differentiated by clinical, radiological, and pathologic findings. The classic clinical manifestations of inflammatory bowel disease include diarrhea, abdominal pain and cramping, and fever. The severity and pattern of signs and symptoms depend on the portion(s) of the bowel affected and depth of bowel wall involvement. Ulcerative colitis primarily involves the mucosa of the bowel wall, extending to the submucosa only in severe cases. It typically starts in the rectum and sigmoid colon and progresses in a continuous pattern through the colon. It rarely involves the small intestine. Crohn's disease can occur anywhere in the gastrointestinal tract. The most frequent sites of involvement are the terminal ileum and right colon. The entire thickness of the bowel wall is involved and it has a segmental, discontinuous pattern of progression.

Clients with either condition may experience a number of the same complications; however, those with ulcerative colitis have a higher incidence of rectal bleeding, whereas clients with Crohn's disease have a higher incidence of perianal involvement and fistula formation. Some clients also experience extraintestinal manifestations such as liver and biliary involvement; kidney stones; arthritis; and skin, eye, and oral lesions. Clients with inflammatory bowel disease may require hospitalization during periods of exacerbation or if complications are suspected.

This care plan focuses on the adult client with severe abdominal pain and diarrhea who is hospitalized for medical management of inflammatory bowel disease. The goals of care are to increase comfort, rest the bowel, maintain adequate nutrition and hydration, prevent complications, and educate the client regarding effective home management of the disease.

DIAGNOSTIC TESTS

Sigmoidoscopy/proctosigmoidoscopy
Colonoscopy (may be contraindicated during acute illness)
Abdominal x-rays
Air-contrast or double-contrast (barium followed by air) radiography of the colon (may be contraindicated during acute illness)
Computed tomography (CT)
Barium contrast x-ray of upper gastrointestinal tract (small bowel follow-through)
Mucosal biopsies
Stool examination
Complete blood count (CBC)
Erythrocyte sedimentation rate (ESR)
Serum albumin, total protein, and electrolyte levels

DISCHARGE CRITERIA

Prior to discharge, the client will:

- have decreased abdominal pain
- have fewer episodes of diarrhea
- tolerate prescribed diet and have an improved nutritional status
- be free of signs and symptoms of complications
- identify ways to reduce the incidence of disease exacerbation
- verbalize ways to maintain an optimal nutritional status
- state ways to prevent perianal skin breakdown
- verbalize an understanding of medications ordered including rationale, food and drug interactions, side effects, schedule for taking, and importance of taking as prescribed
- state signs and symptoms to report to the health care provider
- identify resources that can assist in the adjustment to changes resulting from inflammatory bowel disease and its treatment
- share feelings and thoughts about the effects of inflammatory bowel disease on life style and self-concept
- verbalize an understanding of and a plan for adhering to recommended follow-up care including future appointments with health care provider and activity level.

**NURSING/
COLLABORATIVE
DIAGNOSES**

1. Altered fluid and electrolyte balance:
   a. fluid volume deficit, hypokalemia, hypochloremia, hypomagnesemia, and hypocalcemia
   b. metabolic acidosis △   615
2. Altered nutrition: less than body requirements △   616
3. Pain:
   a. abdominal pain and cramping
   b. joint pain
   c. perianal pain △   617
4. Risk for impaired tissue integrity △   618
5. Hyperthermia △   619
6. Activity intolerance △   620
7. Diarrhea △   621
8. Sleep pattern disturbance △   622
9. Risk for infection △   622
10. Potential complications:
    a. renal calculi
    b. perirectal, rectovaginal, enterovesical, and enteroenteric abscesses and fistulas
    c. toxic megacolon
    d. bowel obstruction
    e. peritonitis
    f. thromboembolism △   624
11. Anxiety △   627
12. Self-concept disturbance △   628
13. Ineffective individual coping △   629

DISCHARGE TEACHING

14. Knowledge deficit, Ineffective management of therapeutic regimen, or Altered health maintenance △   630

1. NURSING/COLLABORATIVE DIAGNOSIS:

Altered fluid and electrolyte balance:

a. **fluid volume deficit, hypokalemia, hypochloremia, hypomagnesemia, and hypocalcemia** related to:
  1. prolonged inadequate oral intake associated with pain, fatigue, prescribed dietary restrictions, and fear of precipitating an attack of abdominal cramping and diarrhea
  2. impaired absorption of fluid and electrolytes associated with inflammation, ulceration, and scarring of the intestine
  3. excessive loss of fluid and electrolytes associated with persistent diarrhea (loss of potassium can also occur as a result of treatment with corticosteroids);

b. **metabolic acidosis** related to excessive loss of bicarbonate associated with persistent diarrhea.

Desired Outcome	Nursing Actions and *Selected Purposes/Rationales*
1. The client will maintain fluid and electrolyte balance as evidenced by: a. normal skin turgor b. moist mucous membranes c. stable weight d. B/P and pulse within normal range for client and stable with position change e. hand vein filling time less than 3–5 seconds f. usual mental status g. balanced intake and output h. urine specific gravity within normal range i. soft, nondistended abdomen with active bowel sounds j. absence of cardiac dysrhythmias, muscle weakness, paresthesias, twitching, spasms, and dizziness k. absence of headache, nausea, and vomiting l. negative Chvostek's and Trousseau's signs m. serum electrolytes and blood gases within normal range.	1.a. Assess for and report signs and symptoms of: 1. fluid volume deficit: a. decreased skin turgor, dry mucous membranes, thirst b. sudden weight loss of 2% or greater c. postural hypotension and/or low B/P d. weak, rapid pulse e. delayed hand vein filling time (longer than 3–5 seconds) f. change in mental status g. decreased urine output with increased specific gravity (reflects an actual rather than potential fluid volume deficit) h. significant increase in BUN and Hct above previous levels 2. hypokalemia (e.g. cardiac dysrhythmias, postural hypotension, muscle weakness, nausea and vomiting, abdominal distention, hypoactive or absent bowel sounds) 3. hypochloremia (e.g. dizziness, irritability, paresthesias, muscle twitching or spasms) 4. hypomagnesemia and/or hypocalcemia (e.g. anxiousness; irritability; cardiac dysrhythmias; positive Chvostek's and Trousseaus's signs; numbness or tingling of fingers, toes, or circumoral area; hyperactive reflexes; tetany; seizures) 5. metabolic acidosis (e.g. drowsiness; disorientation; stupor; rapid, deep respirations; headache; nausea and vomiting; cardiac dysrhythmias). b. Monitor serum electrolyte and blood gas results. Report abnormal values. c. Implement measures *to prevent or treat fluid and electrolyte imbalances:* 1. perform actions to control diarrhea (see Nursing Diagnosis 7, action c) 2. maintain a fluid intake of at least 2500 ml/day unless contraindicated; if oral intake is inadequate or contraindicated, maintain intravenous therapy as ordered 3. when oral intake is allowed: a. perform actions to improve oral intake (see Nursing Diagnosis 2, action c.4.c) b. assist client to select foods/fluids within the prescribed dietary regimen that would replenish electrolytes (be aware that many foods/fluids high in potassium and magnesium are contraindicated on a low-residue diet): 1. foods/fluids high in potassium (e.g. bananas, apricots, potatoes, cantaloupe) 2. foods/fluids high in sodium (e.g. canned soups and vegetables, bouillon) 3. foods/fluids high in magnesium (e.g. seafood)

Desired Outcome	Nursing Actions and *Selected Purposes/Rationales*

4. administer the following if ordered:
    a. electrolyte replacements (e.g. potassium chloride, magnesium sulfate, calcium gluconate, calcium carbonate, sodium chloride, sodium bicarbonate)
    b. vitamin D preparations *to increase intestinal absorption of calcium.*
d. If signs and symptoms of hypomagnesemia or hypocalcemia occur, institute seizure precautions.
e. Consult physician if signs and symptoms of fluid and electrolyte imbalances persist or worsen.

---

2. NURSING DIAGNOSIS: **Altered nutrition: less than body requirements**

related to:
a. decreased oral intake associated with pain, fatigue, prescribed dietary restrictions, and the knowledge that eating often precipitates abdominal cramping and diarrhea;
b. decreased absorption of nutrients associated with inflammation, ulceration, and scarring of the bowel;
c. loss of nutrients associated with diarrhea and protein exudation from the inflamed bowel;
d. impaired folate absorption associated with treatment with sulfasalazine;
e. increased metabolism of nutrients associated with the increased metabolic rate that may be present during periods of exacerbation.

Desired Outcome	Nursing Actions and *Selected Purposes/Rationales*

2. The client will have an improved nutritional status as evidenced by:
  a. weight approaching a normal range for client's age, height, and body frame
  b. improved BUN and serum albumin, Hct, Hb, folate, transferrin, and lymphocyte levels
  c. increased strength and activity tolerance
  d. healthy oral mucous membrane.

2.a. Assess for signs and symptoms of malnutrition:
    1. weight below normal for client's age, height, and body frame
    2. abnormal BUN and low serum albumin, Hct, Hb, folate, transferrin, and lymphocyte levels
    3. weakness and fatigue
    4. sore, inflamed oral mucous membrane
    5. pale conjunctiva.
b. When oral intake is allowed, monitor the percentage of meals and snacks client consumes. Report a pattern of inadequate intake.
c. Implement measures *to improve nutritional status:*
    1. administer total parenteral nutrition if ordered
    2. perform actions to reduce inflammation and hypermotility of the bowel (see Nursing Diagnosis 7, action c) *in order to reduce episodes of diarrhea and increase absorption of nutrients*
    3. maintain activity restrictions as ordered (usually bed rest with bedside commode or bathroom privileges) *to reduce caloric requirements*
    4. when food or fluid is allowed:
      a. provide elemental formulas (e.g. Vivonex, Criticare HN) if ordered (these formulas are high in calories and nutrients, free of lactose and fiber, and absorbed in the proximal small bowel)
      b. progress diet as tolerated (usual progression is from elemental formulas to a low-residue, high-calorie, high-protein diet)
      c. perform actions *to improve oral intake:*
        1. implement measures to reduce pain (see Nursing Diagnosis 3, action e)
        2. encourage a rest period before meals *to minimize fatigue*
        3. maintain a clean environment and a relaxed, pleasant atmosphere
        4. provide oral hygiene before meals
        5. implement measures *to improve the palatability of elemental formulas* (e.g. offer a variety of flavors, serve chilled)

      6. obtain a dietary consult if necessary to assist client in selecting foods/fluids that are appealing and adhere to personal and cultural preferences as well as the prescribed dietary modifications

      7. serve frequent, small meals rather than large ones if client is weak, fatigues easily, or has a poor appetite

      8. allow adequate time for meals; reheat foods/fluids if necessary

   5. administer the following if ordered:

      a. iron preparations (oral iron preparations may not be effective during an acute attack *because they may be poorly absorbed from the inflamed bowel*)

      b. vitamin preparations (e.g. fat-soluble vitamins, vitamin B_{12}, folic acid)

      c. medium-chain triglycerides (MCT) *to provide an absorbable source of fatty acids* (*MCT are absorbed more proximally and do not require bile salts for absorption*).

   d. Perform a calorie count if ordered. Report information to dietitian and physician.

   e. Consult physician if nutritional status continues to decline.

---

3. NURSING DIAGNOSIS:　　**Pain:**

   a. **abdominal pain and cramping** related to:
     1. inflammation and ulceration of the bowel
     2. interference with the flow of intestinal contents associated with narrowing of the intestinal lumen as a result of inflammation and hypertrophy and fibrosis of the bowel wall if present;
   b. **joint pain** related to extraintestinal involvement of the joints (peripheral arthritis, ankylosing spondylitis, and sacroiliitis are the most common joint disorders that occur);
   c. **perianal pain** related to irritation and breakdown of skin in the perianal area associated with persistent diarrhea and/or the presence of an anorectal abscess or fistula.

Desired Outcome	Nursing Actions and *Selected Purposes/Rationales*

3. The client will experience diminished pain as evidenced by:
  a. verbalization of same
  b. relaxed facial expression and body positioning
  c. increased participation in activities
  d. stable vital signs.
	3.a. Assess for signs and symptoms of pain (e.g. verbalization of pain; grimacing; reluctance to move; rubbing abdomen, back, or joints; restlessness; diaphoresis; facial pallor; increased B/P; tachycardia).
	  b. Assess client's perception of the severity of pain using a pain intensity rating scale.
	  c. Assess the client's pain pattern (e.g. location, quality, onset, duration, precipitating factors, aggravating factors, alleviating factors).
	  d. Ask the client to describe previous pain experiences and methods used to manage pain effectively.
	  e. Implement measures *to reduce pain*:
	    1. perform actions *to reduce fear and anxiety about the pain experience* (e.g. assure client that his/her need for pain relief is understood, plan methods for achieving pain control with client)
	    2. perform actions to reduce fear and anxiety (see Nursing Diagnosis 11, action b) *in order to promote relaxation and subsequently increase the client's threshold and tolerance for pain*
	    3. administer analgesics before activities and procedures that can cause pain and before pain becomes severe

Desired Outcome	Nursing Actions and **Selected Purposes/Rationales**
	4. perform actions to promote rest (e.g. minimize environmental activity and noise, limit number of visitors and their length of stay) *in order to reduce fatigue and subsequently increase the client's threshold and tolerance for pain*
	5. perform actions to reduce inflammation and hypermotility of the bowel (see Nursing Diagnosis 7, action c) *in order to reduce abdominal pain and cramping*
	6. consult physician regarding measures *to help relieve joint pain if present* (e.g. application of brace/splint to affected joint, application of heat to affected joint)
	7. perform actions *to relieve perianal pain if present:*
	a. implement measures to control diarrhea (see Nursing Diagnosis 7, action c)
	b. clean perianal area with medicated wipes such as Tucks after each bowel movement
	c. apply protective ointment or cream to perianal area after each bowel movement
	d. consult physician about order for sitz baths
	e. apply anesthetic preparation (e.g. Nupercainal, Tronolane) to perianal area or into rectum if ordered
	f. administer corticosteroid foam or enema or mesalamine suppository or enema if ordered
	8. provide or assist with nonpharmacologic measures for pain relief (e.g. position change; relaxation exercises; restful environment; diversional activities such as watching television, reading, or conversing)
	9. administer the following medications if ordered:
	a. analgesics (narcotic [opioid] analgesics must be administered judiciously *because they slow gastrointestinal motility and can cause toxic megacolon*)
	b. anticholinergic agents (e.g. propantheline bromide, dicyclomine hydrochloride) *to reduce abdominal cramping* (these agents must also be given with caution *because they slow gastrointestinal motility and can cause toxic megacolon*).
	f. Consult physician if above measures fail to provide adequate pain relief.

---

4. NURSING DIAGNOSIS: **Risk for impaired tissue integrity**

related to:
a. damage to the skin and/or subcutaneous tissue associated with prolonged pressure on the tissues, friction, and shearing that can occur when mobility is decreased;
b. frequent contact with irritants associated with persistent diarrhea;
c. increased fragility of skin associated with malnutrition and dryness of skin (may result from fluid volume deficit).

Desired Outcome	Nursing Actions and **Selected Purposes/Rationales**

4. The client will maintain tissue integrity as evidenced by:
  a. absence of redness and irritation
  b. no skin breakdown.
	4.a. Inspect the skin (especially bony prominences, dependent areas, and perianal area) for pallor, redness, and breakdown.
	  b. Implement measures *to prevent tissue breakdown:*
	    1. instruct and/or assist client to turn at least every 2 hours
	    2. position client properly; use pressure-reducing or pressure-relieving devices (e.g. pillows, gel or foam cushions, alternating pressure mattress, air-fluidized bed) if indicated

3. gently massage around reddened areas at least every 2 hours
4. apply a thin layer of powder or cornstarch to bottom sheet or skin and opposing skin surfaces if indicated *to absorb moisture and/or reduce friction*
5. encourage client to limit length of time he/she is in semi-Fowler's position to 30 minutes (*in this position, client tends to slide down in bed, which can cause skin surface abrasion and shearing*)
6. instruct or assist client to shift weight at least every 30 minutes
7. keep skin clean and dry
8. keep bed linens dry and wrinkle-free
9. increase activity as allowed and tolerated
10. perform actions to improve nutritional status (see Nursing Diagnosis 2, action c)
11. perform actions *to prevent drying of the skin:*
    a. encourage a fluid intake of 2500 ml/day unless contraindicated
    b. provide a mild soap for bathing
    c. apply moisturizing lotion and/or emollient to skin at least once a day
12. perform actions *to prevent skin irritation resulting from diarrhea:*
    a. implement measures to control diarrhea (see Nursing Diagnosis 7, action c)
    b. assist client to gently cleanse and dry perianal area with a soft tissue or cloth after each bowel movement; apply a protective ointment or cream
    c. provide incontinence pads if needed to absorb moisture; do not allow skin to come in contact with plastic portion of the pads.
c. If tissue breakdown occurs:
  1. notify physician
  2. continue with above measures to prevent further irritation and breakdown
  3. perform care of involved areas as ordered or per standard hospital procedure
  4. assess client closely and report signs and symptoms of infection (e.g. elevated temperature; redness, heat, pain, and swelling around area of breakdown; unusual drainage from site).

---

5. NURSING DIAGNOSIS: **Hyperthermia**

related to stimulation of the thermoregulatory center in the hypothalamus by endogenous pyrogens that are released in an inflammatory process.

Desired Outcome	Nursing Actions and *Selected Purposes/Rationales*

5. The client will experience resolution of hyperthermia as evidenced by:
a. skin usual temperature and color
b. pulse rate between 60–100 beats/minute
c. respirations 14–20/minute
d. normal body temperature.
	5.a. Assess for signs and symptoms of hyperthermia (e.g. warm, flushed skin; tachycardia; tachypnea; elevated temperature).
	b. Implement measures *to reduce fever:*
	  1. perform actions to reduce inflammation and hypermotility of the bowel (see Nursing Diagnosis 7, action c)
	  2. administer antipyretics if ordered.
	c. Consult physician if temperature remains higher than 38° C.

6. NURSING DIAGNOSIS: **Activity intolerance**

related to:
a. inadequate nutritional status;
b. difficulty resting and sleeping associated with pain, frequent need to defecate, fear, and anxiety;
c. tissue hypoxia associated with anemia resulting from:
   1. blood loss from the ulcerated bowel
   2. decreased oral intake and impaired absorption of iron, vitamin B_{12}, and folate;
d. increased energy expenditure associated with the increased metabolic rate that may be present during period of exacerbation.

Desired Outcome	Nursing Actions and *Selected Purposes/Rationales*

6. The client will demonstrate an increased tolerance for activity as evidenced by:
a. verbalization of feeling less fatigued and weak
b. ability to perform activities of daily living without exertional dyspnea, chest pain, diaphoresis, dizziness, and a significant change in vital signs.
	6.a. Assess for signs and symptoms of activity intolerance:
	   1. statements of fatigue or weakness
	   2. exertional dyspnea, chest pain, diaphoresis, or dizziness
	   3. abnormal heart rate response to activity (e.g. increase in rate of 20 beats/minute above resting rate, rate not returning to preactivity level within 3 minutes after stopping activity, change from regular to irregular rate)
	   4. decreased systolic B/P or a significant increase (10–15 mm Hg) in diastolic pressure with activity.
	  b. Implement measures *to improve activity tolerance:*
	   1. perform actions *to promote rest and/or conserve energy:*
	     a. maintain activity restrictions as ordered
	     b. minimize environmental activity and noise
	     c. organize nursing care to allow for periods of uninterrupted rest
	     d. limit the number of visitors and their length of stay
	     e. assist client with self-care activities as needed
	     f. keep supplies and personal articles within easy reach
	     g. instruct client in energy-saving techniques (e.g. using shower chair when showering, sitting to brush teeth or comb hair)
	     h. implement measures to reduce fear and anxiety (see Nursing Diagnosis 11, action b)
	     i. implement measures to promote sleep (see Nursing Diagnosis 8, action c)
	     j. implement measures to reduce pain (see Nursing Diagnosis 3, action e)
	   2. perform actions to reduce inflammation and hypermotility of the bowel (see Nursing Diagnosis 7, action c) *in order to reduce excess energy demands associated with inflammation, improve absorption of nutrients, reduce pain, and increase client's ability to rest and sleep*
	   3. perform actions to improve nutritional status (see Nursing Diagnosis 2, action c)
	   4. administer packed red blood cells if ordered
	   5. increase client's activity gradually as allowed and tolerated.
	  c. Instruct client to:
	   1. report a decreased tolerance for activity
	   2. stop any activity that causes chest pain, shortness of breath, dizziness, or extreme fatigue or weakness.
	  d. Consult physician if signs and symptoms of activity intolerance persist or worsen.

7. NURSING DIAGNOSIS: **Diarrhea**

related to increased peristalsis and disorders of intestinal secretion and absorption associated with damage to the intestinal mucosa.

Desired Outcome	Nursing Actions and *Selected Purposes/Rationales*

7. The client will have fewer bowel movements and more formed stool.	7.a. Ascertain client's usual bowel elimination habits.
	  b. Assess for signs and symptoms of diarrhea (e.g. frequent, loose stools; urgency; abdominal pain and cramping; hyperactive bowel sounds).
	  c. Implement measures *to reduce inflammation and hypermotility of the bowel in order to control diarrhea:*
	  1. perform actions *to rest the bowel:*
	  a. restrict oral intake if ordered (usually NPO during acute stage)
	  b. maintain activity restrictions as ordered (may initially be limited to bed rest with bedside commode or bathroom privileges)
	  c. implement measures *to reduce stress* (e.g. explain procedures, provide for consistency in staff assigned, perform actions to reduce pain)
	  d. discourage smoking (*nicotine has a stimulant effect on the gastrointestinal tract*)
	  e. when oral intake is allowed:
	  1. progress diet as ordered (diet usually progresses from elemental formulas [these formulas are absorbed in the proximal small bowel and thereby minimize stimulation of the bowel] to a low-residue diet)
	  2. instruct client to avoid foods/fluids that may be poorly digested or can act as irritants to the inflamed bowel:
	  a. milk and milk products (*clients with Crohn's disease may have an intolerance to lactose-rich foods because of a deficiency of lactase*)
	  b. those high in fat (e.g. butter, cream, whole milk, ice cream, fried foods, gravies)
	  c. those high in fiber or residue (e.g. whole-grain cereals, nuts, raw fruits and vegetables)
	  d. those high in caffeine (e.g. coffee, tea, colas)
	  e. spicy foods
	  f. extremely hot or cold foods/fluids
	  3. instruct client to add new foods one at a time
	  4. provide small, frequent meals rather than 3 large ones
	  2. administer the following medications if ordered:
	  a. corticosteroids or ACTH *to reduce inflammation of the bowel*
	  b. sulfasalazine or a nonsulfa-aminosalicylate (e.g. olsalazine, controlled-release mesalamine) *to reduce inflammation of the bowel*
	  c. antidiarrheal agents (e.g. loperamide) or anticholinergic agents (e.g. propantheline bromide, dicyclomine hydrochloride) *to slow intestinal motility* (both agents must be used cautiously in severe disease *because of the risk for toxic megacolon*)
	  d. bulk-forming agents (e.g. methylcellulose, psyllium hydrophilic mucilloid) *to absorb water in the bowel, which results in a more formed stool*
	  e. cholestyramine *to bind bile salts* (might be prescribed if it is likely that diarrhea is related to decreased absorption of bile salts by the ileum)
	  f. immunosuppressive agents such as azathioprine, mercaptopurine, or cyclosporine (used to reduce intestinal symptoms in cases that are persistent and severe; the effectiveness and action of these agents are still undetermined).
	  d. Consult physician if diarrhea persists.

8. NURSING DIAGNOSIS: **Sleep pattern disturbance**

related to frequent need to defecate, pain, fear, and anxiety.

Desired Outcome	Nursing Actions and *Selected Purposes/Rationales*

8. The client will attain optimal amounts of sleep as evidenced by:
a. statements of feeling well rested
b. usual mental status
c. absence of frequent yawning, dark circles under eyes, and hand tremors.
	8.a. Assess for signs and symptoms of a sleep pattern disturbance (e.g. statements of difficulty falling asleep, sleep interruptions, or not feeling well rested; irritability; lethargy; disorientation; frequent yawning; dark circles under eyes; slight hand tremors).
	b. Determine the client's usual sleep habits.
	c. Implement measures *to promote sleep:*
	  1. discourage long periods of sleep during the day unless signs and symptoms of sleep deprivation exist or daytime sleep is usual for client
	  2. perform actions to reduce fear and anxiety (see Nursing Diagnosis 11, action b)
	  3. perform actions to reduce pain (see Nursing Diagnosis 3, action e)
	  4. perform actions to reduce inflammation and hypermotility of the bowel (see Nursing Diagnosis 7, action c) *in order to reduce abdominal pain and cramping and the frequency of bowel movements*
	  5. encourage participation in relaxing diversional activities during the evening
	  6. discourage intake of fluids high in caffeine (e.g. coffee, tea, colas), especially in the evening
	  7. allow client to continue usual sleep practices (e.g. position; time; presleep routines such as reading, watching television, listening to music, and meditating) unless contraindicated
	  8. satisfy basic needs such as comfort and warmth before sleep
	  9. encourage client to urinate just before bedtime
	  10. reduce environmental distractions (e.g. close door to client's room; use night light rather than overhead light whenever possible; lower volume of paging system; keep staff conversations at a low level and away from client's room; close curtains between clients in a semi-private room or ward; provide client with "white noise" such as fan, soft music, or tape-recorded sounds of the ocean or rain; have earplugs available for client if needed)
	  11. administer prescribed sedative-hypnotics if indicated
	  12. perform actions *to reduce interruptions during sleep (80–100 minutes of uninterrupted sleep is usually needed to complete one sleep cycle):*
	    a. restrict visitors
	    b. group care (e.g. medications, treatments, physical care, assessments) whenever possible.
	d. Consult physician if signs and symptoms of sleep deprivation persist or worsen.

9. NURSING DIAGNOSIS: **Risk for infection**

related to:
a. ulcerations in the bowel wall;
b. lowered resistance to infection associated with malnutrition and treatment with corticosteroids and/or immunosuppressives;
c. stasis of respiratory secretions and urine associated with decreased mobility if activity restrictions are prescribed.

Desired Outcome	Nursing Actions and *Selected Purposes/Rationales*

9. The client will remain free of infection as evidenced by:
a. temperature declining toward normal
b. absence of chills
c. pulse within normal limits
d. normal breath sounds
e. usual mental status
f. cough productive of clear mucus only
g. voiding clear urine without reports of frequency, urgency, and burning
h. no increase in episodes of diarrhea and abdominal cramping and pain
i. absence of heat, pain, redness, swelling, and unusual drainage in any area
j. no reports of increased weakness and fatigue
k. WBC and differential counts returning toward normal
l. negative results of cultured specimens.
	9.a. Assess for and report signs and symptoms of infection (be aware that some signs and symptoms vary depending on the site of infection, the causative organism, and the age and immune status of the client):
	  1. significant increase in temperature (an elevated temperature may be present due to the bowel inflammation)
	  2. chills
	  3. increased pulse
	  4. abnormal breath sounds
	  5. lethargy, acute confusion
	  6. cough productive of purulent, green, or rust-colored sputum
	  7. cloudy, foul-smelling urine
	  8. reports of frequency, urgency, or burning when urinating
	  9. reports of increased weakness or fatigue
	  10. presence of WBCs, bacteria, and/or nitrites in urine
	  11. increase in episodes of diarrhea and abdominal cramping and pain
	  12. heat, pain, redness, swelling, or unusual drainage in any area
	  13. increase in WBC count above previous levels (WBC count will usually be elevated as a result of bowel inflammation) and/or significant change in differential.
	b. Obtain specimens (e.g. urine, vaginal drainage, stool, sputum, blood) for culture as ordered. Report positive results.
	c. Implement measures *to prevent infection:*
	  1. maintain a fluid intake of at least 2500 ml/day unless contraindicated
	  2. use good handwashing technique and encourage client to do the same
	  3. use sterile technique during all invasive procedures (e.g. urinary catheterizations, venous and arterial punctures, injections)
	  4. protect client from others with infection
	  5. rotate intravenous insertion sites according to hospital policy
	  6. anchor catheter/tubings (e.g. urinary, intravenous) securely *in order to reduce trauma to the tissues and the risk for introduction of pathogens associated with the in-and-out movement of the tubing*
	  7. change equipment, tubings, and solutions used for treatments such as intravenous infusions and enteral feedings according to hospital policy
	  8. maintain a closed system on drains (e.g. urinary catheter) and intravenous infusions whenever possible
	  9. perform actions to improve nutritional status (see Nursing Diagnosis 2, action c)
	  10. reinforce importance of good oral hygiene
	  11. perform actions *to reduce stress* (e.g. explain procedures, provide for consistency in staff assigned, perform actions to reduce pain) *in order to prevent excessive secretion of cortisol (cortisol inhibits the immune system)*
	  12. perform actions *to prevent stasis of respiratory secretions* (e.g. instruct client to turn, cough, and deep breathe; increase activity as allowed and tolerated)
	  13. perform actions to prevent tissue breakdown (see Nursing Diagnosis 4, action b)
	  14. perform actions to prevent urinary retention (e.g. instruct client to urinate when the urge is first felt, promote relaxation during voiding attempts) *in order to prevent urinary stasis*
	  15. instruct and assist client to perform good perineal care routinely and after each bowel movement
	  16. perform actions to reduce inflammation of the bowel (see Nursing Diagnosis 7, action c) *in order to prevent further ulceration of the bowel and subsequently reduce the risk for intestinal infection*
	  17. administer antimicrobials if ordered (antimicrobials are generally given only if surgery is planned or if the client has severe colitis and is at high risk for infection; however, metronidazole is currently being prescribed by many practitioners for the relief of symptoms in clients with Crohn's disease).

10. COLLABORATIVE DIAGNOSES:

Potential complications of inflammatory bowel disease:

a. **renal calculi** related to crystalline deposits in the urine associated with:
   1. increased serum oxalate (dietary oxalate normally binds with calcium in the intestine and is excreted in the stool; in clients with IBD, calcium is bound with the poorly absorbed fat and oxalate becomes available for absorption)
   2. stasis of urine resulting from decreased activity
   3. decreased flushing of solutes from the urinary tract if urine formation is reduced as a result of fluid volume deficit
   4. treatment with sulfasalazine;
b. **perirectal, rectovaginal, enterovesical, and enteroenteric abscesses and fistulas** related to extension of a mucosal fissure or ulcer through the intestinal wall;
c. **toxic megacolon** related to loss of colonic muscle tone associated with the effects of widespread inflammation in the bowel, use of some medications (e.g. opiates, anticholinergics), and hypokalemia;
d. **bowel obstruction** related to narrowing of the intestinal lumen associated with inflammation and scar tissue formation in the bowel;
e. **peritonitis** related to perforation of the bowel or leakage from an abscess or fistula;
f. **thromboembolism** related to:
   1. hypercoagulability associated with increased levels of certain clotting factors, thrombocytosis (a frequent manifestation of acute inflammation), and increased blood viscosity (may result from fluid volume deficit)
   2. venous stasis associated with decreased mobility and increased blood viscosity if fluid intake is inadequate.

Desired Outcomes	Nursing Actions and *Selected Purposes/Rationales*

10.a. The client will not develop renal calculi as evidenced by:
  1. absence of flank pain, hematuria, nausea, and vomiting
  2. clear urine without calculi.

10.a.1. Assess for and report signs and symptoms of renal calculi (e.g. dull, aching or severe, colicky flank pain; hematuria; nausea; vomiting).
   2. Implement measures *to prevent renal calculi:*
     a. perform actions *to prevent urinary stasis:*
        1. assist client to change positions at least every 2 hours
        2. progress activity as allowed and tolerated
        3. implement measures *to facilitate voiding* (e.g. provide privacy, allow client to assume normal voiding position unless contraindicated, pour warm water over perineum)
        4. instruct client to void whenever the urge is felt
        5. maintain patency of urinary catheter if present
     b. maintain a minimum fluid intake of 2500 ml/day unless contraindicated
     c. perform actions *to decrease absorption of oxalate from the intestine:*
        1. encourage client to decrease intake of foods/fluids high in oxalate (e.g. tea, chocolate, spinach, rhubarb)
        2. encourage client to adhere to a low-fat diet (*this reduces the amount of fat available to bind calcium, thereby freeing calcium to bind with oxalate*)
     d. administer the following medications if ordered:
        1. anion-exchange resins (e.g. cholestyramine) *to bind oxalate and decrease its absorption from the bowel*
        2. calcium preparations (e.g. calcium carbonate, calcium gluconate) *to bind oxalate and decrease its absorption from the bowel*
        3. citrate preparations *to increase solubility of minerals in the urine.*
   3. If signs and symptoms of renal calculi occur:
     a. strain all urine and save any calculi for analysis; report finding to physician
     b. maintain a minimum fluid intake of 2500 ml/day unless contraindicated

c. administer analgesics as ordered

d. prepare client for removal of calculi (e.g. extracorporeal shock wave lithotripsy [ESWL], percutaneous ultrasonic lithotripsy, pyelolithotomy) if planned.

10.b. The client will have resolution of any abscesses and fistulas that develop as evidenced by:

1. temperature declining toward normal
2. resolution of abdominal pain
3. absence of perianal redness and swelling
4. no unusual vaginal drainage
5. clear, yellow urine
6. WBC count declining toward normal.

10.b.1. Assess for and report signs and symptoms of abscess and/or fistula formation (e.g. further increase in temperature, increased or more constant abdominal pain, perianal redness and swelling, foul vaginal discharge or passage of stool from vagina, dysuria, fecaluria, further increase in WBC count).

2. Implement measures to reduce inflammation of the bowel (see Nursing Diagnosis 7, action c) *in order to promote healing of the intestinal mucosa and subsequently decrease the risk for development of abscesses and fistulas and promote healing of any that exist.*

3. If signs and symptoms of abscesses or fistulas occur:
   a. prepare client for diagnostic studies (e.g. computed tomography, ultrasonography, barium enema)
   b. administer antimicrobials (e.g. metronidazole) as ordered
   c. if cutaneous fistula is present, perform wound care as ordered
   d. prepare client for surgical intervention (e.g. incision and drainage of abscess, resection of involved area) if planned
   e. provide emotional support to client and significant others.

10.c. The client will not develop toxic megacolon as evidenced by:

1. absence of abdominal distention
2. gradual resolution of abdominal pain
3. active bowel sounds
4. gradual resolution of diarrhea
5. temperature and WBC count declining toward normal.

10.c.1. Assess for and report signs and symptoms of toxic megacolon:
   a. abdominal distention and increased abdominal pain and tenderness
   b. hypoactive or absent bowel sounds with tympanic percussion note over abdomen
   c. sudden decrease in episodes of diarrhea
   d. fever (usually greater than 38.6° C) and tachycardia
   e. increase in WBC count.

2. Monitor abdominal x-ray results. Report findings of colonic dilation.

3. Implement measures *to prevent development of toxic megacolon:*
   a. perform actions to reduce inflammation of the bowel (see Nursing Diagnosis 7, action c)
   b. administer opiates, opiate derivatives, and anticholinergics judiciously (*all decrease intestinal motility*)
   c. perform actions to prevent or treat hypokalemia (see Nursing Diagnosis 1, action c).

4. If signs and symptoms of toxic megacolon occur:
   a. withhold oral intake as ordered
   b. consult physician about discontinuing any opiates, opiate derivatives, and anticholinergics ordered
   c. insert nasogastric tube and maintain suction as ordered
   d. administer the following if ordered:
      1. intravenous fluids *to maintain adequate vascular volume (third-space fluid shifting occurs as a result of increased capillary permeability associated with the inflammation and increased intraluminal pressure that are present with toxic megacolon)*
      2. corticosteroids *to reduce intestinal inflammation*
      3. antimicrobials (e.g. metronidazole) *to prevent infection (the risk of perforation is increased when toxic megacolon develops)*
   e. prepare client for surgical intervention (e.g. colectomy) if planned
   f. provide emotional support to client and significant others.

10.d. The client will not develop a bowel obstruction as evidenced by:

1. absence of vomiting and abdominal distention
2. gradual return of normal bowel sounds.

10.d.1. Assess for and report signs and symptoms of a bowel obstruction:
   a. vomiting
   b. abdominal distention
   c. change in bowel sounds (bowel sounds can be high-pitched and more hyperactive if the bowel is partially obstructed or they can be absent once there is complete obstruction).

2. Monitor abdominal x-ray results. Report findings of partial or complete bowel obstruction.

3. Implement measures to reduce inflammation of the bowel (see Nursing Diagnosis 7, action c) *in order to reduce intestinal narrowing and scar tissue formation.*

Desired Outcomes	Nursing Actions and *Selected Purposes/Rationales*

4. If signs and symptoms of a bowel obstruction occur:
   a. withhold oral intake as ordered
   b. insert nasogastric or intestinal tube and maintain suction as ordered
   c. administer intravenous fluids if ordered *to maintain an adequate vascular volume (dehydration occurs with prolonged vomiting and third-spacing occurs due to the increased capillary permeability that results from increased intraluminal pressure in a bowel obstruction)*
   d. prepare client for endoscopic balloon dilatation of strictures or surgical intervention (e.g. stricturoplasty, bowel resection) if planned
   e. provide emotional support to client and significant others.

10.e. The client will not develop peritonitis as evidenced by:
1. temperature declining toward normal
2. soft, nondistended abdomen
3. gradual resolution of abdominal pain
4. gradual return of normal bowel sounds
5. absence of nausea and vomiting
6. stable vital signs
7. WBC count declining toward normal.

10.e.1. Assess for and report signs and symptoms of peritonitis (e.g. further increase in temperature; distended, rigid abdomen; increased abdominal pain; rebound tenderness; diminished or absent bowel sounds; nausea; vomiting; tachycardia; tachypnea; hypotension).
2. Monitor WBC counts. Report levels that increase or fail to decline toward normal.
3. Implement measures to prevent and treat abscesses, fistulas, toxic megacolon, and/or bowel obstruction (see actions b.2 and 3, c.3 and 4, and d.3 and 4 in this diagnosis) *in order to reduce the risk for peritonitis.*
4. If signs and symptoms of peritonitis occur:
   a. withhold oral intake as ordered
   b. place client on bed rest in a semi-Fowler's position *to assist in pooling or localizing intestinal contents in the pelvis rather than under the diaphragm*
   c. prepare client for diagnostic tests (e.g. abdominal x-ray, computed tomography, ultrasonography) if planned
   d. insert nasogastric or intestinal tube and maintain suction as ordered
   e. administer antimicrobials (e.g. metronidazole) as ordered
   f. administer intravenous fluids and/or blood volume expanders if ordered *to prevent or treat shock (can result from the increased capillary permeability that occurs with inflammation and the subsequent escape of protein, fluid, and electrolytes from the vascular space into the peritoneal cavity)*
   g. prepare client for surgical intervention (e.g. repair of perforation, bowel resection) if planned
   h. provide emotional support to client and significant others.

10.f.1. The client will not develop a deep vein thrombus as evidenced by:
a. absence of pain, tenderness, swelling, and distended superficial vessels in extremities
b. usual temperature of extremities
c. negative Homans' sign.

10.f.1.a. Assess for and report signs and symptoms of a deep vein thrombus:
1. pain or tenderness in extremity
2. increase in circumference of extremity
3. distention of superficial vessels in extremity
4. unusual warmth of extremity
5. positive Homans' sign (not always a reliable indicator).
b. Implement measures *to prevent thrombus formation:*
1. encourage client to perform active foot and leg exercises every 1–2 hours while awake
2. instruct client to avoid positions that compromise blood flow (e.g. pillows under knees, crossing legs, sitting for long periods)
3. consult physician about an order for antiembolism stockings
4. maintain a minimum fluid intake of 2500 ml/day unless contraindicated *to prevent increased blood viscosity*
5. administer anticoagulants (e.g. low- or adjusted-dose heparin, low-molecular-weight heparin) if ordered
6. progress activity as allowed.
c. If signs and symptoms of a deep vein thrombus occur:
1. maintain client on bed rest until activity orders are received
2. elevate foot of bed 15–20° above heart level if ordered
3. discourage positions that compromise blood flow (e.g. pillows under knees, crossing legs, sitting for long periods)
4. prepare client for diagnostic studies (e.g. venography, duplex ultrasound, impedance plethysmography) if indicated

5. administer anticoagulants (e.g. heparin, warfarin) as ordered
6. refer to Care Plan on Deep Vein Thrombosis for additional care measures.

10.f.2. The client will not experience a pulmonary embolism as evidenced by:
a. absence of sudden chest pain
b. unlabored respirations at 14–20/minute
c. pulse 60–100 beats/ minute
d. blood gases within normal range.

10.f.2.a. Assess for and report signs and symptoms of pulmonary embolism (e.g. sudden chest pain, dyspnea, tachypnea, tachycardia, apprehension, low PaO$_2$).
b. Implement measures *to prevent a pulmonary embolism:*
1. perform actions to prevent and treat a deep vein thrombus (see actions f.1.b and c in this diagnosis)
2. do not exercise, check for Homans' sign in, or massage any extremity known to have a thrombus
3. caution client to avoid activities that create a Valsalva response (e.g. straining to have a bowel movement, holding breath while moving up in bed) *in order to prevent dislodgment of existing thrombi.*
c. If signs and symptoms of a pulmonary embolism occur:
1. maintain client on strict bed rest in a semi- to high Fowler's position
2. maintain oxygen therapy as ordered
3. prepare client for diagnostic tests (e.g. blood gases, ventilation-perfusion lung scan, pulmonary angiography)
4. administer anticoagulants (e.g. continuous intravenous heparin, warfarin) as ordered
5. prepare client for a vena caval interruption (e.g. insertion of an intracaval filtering device) if planned *to prevent further pulmonary emboli*
6. provide emotional support to client and significant others
7. refer to Care Plan on Pulmonary Embolism for additional care measures.

---

11. NURSING DIAGNOSIS: **Anxiety**

related to pain; persistent diarrhea; lack of understanding of diagnosis, diagnostic tests, and treatments; unfamiliar environment; uncertain prognosis; and possibility of surgery if current symptoms cannot be controlled.

Desired Outcome	Nursing Actions and *Selected Purposes/Rationales*

11. The client will experience a reduction in anxiety as evidenced by:
a. verbalization of feeling less anxious
b. usual sleep pattern
c. relaxed facial expression and body movements
d. stable vital signs
e. usual perceptual ability and interactions with others.

11.a. Assess client for signs and symptoms of anxiety (e.g. verbalization of feeling anxious, insomnia, tenseness, shakiness, restlessness, diaphoresis, tachycardia, elevated blood pressure, facial pallor, self-focused behaviors).
b. Implement measures *to reduce fear and anxiety:*
1. orient client to hospital environment, equipment, and routines
2. introduce client to staff who will be participating in care; if possible, maintain consistency in staff assigned to his/her care *to provide feelings of stability and comfort with the environment*
3. assure client that staff members are nearby; respond to call signal as soon as possible
4. maintain a calm, supportive, confident manner when interacting with client
5. encourage verbalization of fear and anxiety; provide feedback
6. explain all diagnostic tests
7. reinforce physician's explanations and clarify misconceptions the client has about inflammatory bowel disease, the treatment plan, and prognosis

Desired Outcome	Nursing Actions and *Selected Purposes/Rationales*
	8. perform actions to reduce pain (see Nursing Diagnosis 3, action e) 9. perform actions to reduce inflammation and hypermotility of the bowel (see Nursing Diagnosis 7, action c) *in order to reduce episodes of diarrhea* 10. provide a calm, restful environment 11. instruct client in relaxation techniques and encourage participation in diversional activities 12. assist client to cope with the diagnosis and its implications (see Nursing Diagnosis 13, action c) 13. provide information based on current needs of the client at a level he/she can understand; encourage questions and clarification of information provided 14. encourage significant others to project a caring, concerned attitude without obvious anxiousness 15. include significant others in orientation and teaching sessions and encourage their continued support of the client 16. if surgical intervention is indicated, begin preoperative teaching 17. administer prescribed antianxiety agents if indicated. c. Consult physician if above actions fail to control fear and anxiety.

■━━

12. NURSING DIAGNOSIS: **Self-concept disturbance***

related to:
a. dependence on others to meet self-care needs;
b. embarrassment associated with diarrhea;
c. changes in sexual functioning associated with pain, fatigue, and weakness;
d. changes in life style imposed by inflammatory bowel disease and its treatment.

---

*This diagnostic label includes the nursing diagnoses of body image disturbance, self-esteem disturbance, and altered role performance.

Desired Outcome	Nursing Actions and *Selected Purposes/Rationales*

12. The client will demonstrate beginning adaptation to changes in body functioning, life style, and roles as evidenced by:
a. verbalization of feelings of self-worth and sexual adequacy
b. maintenance of relationships with significant others
c. active participation in activities of daily living
d. verbalization of a beginning plan for adapting life style to changes resulting from inflammatory bowel disease.
	12.a. Assess for signs and symptoms of a self-concept disturbance (e.g. verbalization of negative feelings about self, withdrawal from significant others, lack of participation in activities of daily living, lack of a plan for adapting to necessary changes in life style).
	  b. Determine the meaning of changes in body functioning, life style, and roles to the client by encouraging verbalization of feelings and by noting nonverbal responses to changes experienced.
	  c. Discuss with client improvements in bowel function, comfort, and energy levels that can realistically be expected.
	  d. Implement measures *to assist client to increase self-esteem* (e.g. limit negative self-assessment, encourage positive comments about self, assist to identify strengths, give positive feedback about accomplishments and behaviors that are indicative of high self-esteem).
	  e. Implement measures to assist client to cope with the effects of inflammatory bowel disease (see Nursing Diagnosis 13, action c).
	  f. Implement measures *to reduce embarrassment associated with diarrhea:*
	    1. provide a private room if possible
	    2. keep bedside commode or bedpan within easy reach
	    3. use room deodorizers and empty bedpan or commode as soon as possible after each bowel movement *to reduce odor.*
	  g. Encourage client to discuss concerns about sexual functioning. Offer suggestions to assist client to regain optimal level of sexual functioning (e.g. rest before sexual activity).

h. Support behaviors suggesting positive adaptation to changes that have occurred (e.g. compliance with treatment plan, verbalization of feelings of self-worth, maintenance of relationships with significant others).
i. Encourage significant others to allow client to do what he/she is able *so that independence can be re-established and/or self-esteem redeveloped.*
j. Assist client's and significant others' adjustment by listening, facilitating communication, and providing information.
k. Assist client and significant others to have similar expectations of future life style and to identify ways that personal and family goals can be adjusted rather than abandoned.
l. Encourage visits and support from significant others.
m. Encourage client to pursue usual roles and interests and to continue involvement in social activities. If previous roles, interests, and hobbies cannot be pursued, encourage development of new ones.
n. Provide information about and encourage utilization of community resources (e.g. support groups; sexual, family, and individual counseling).
o. Consult physician about psychological counseling if client desires or seems unwilling or unable to adapt to changes resulting from inflammatory bowel disease.

---

13. NURSING DIAGNOSIS: **Ineffective individual coping**

related to:
a. chronicity of condition and effect of inflammatory bowel disease on life style;
b. pain;
c. fear of eventual need for an ileal diversion;
d. feeling of powerlessness.

Desired Outcome	Nursing Actions and *Selected Purposes/Rationales*

13. The client will demonstrate effective coping as evidenced by:
a. verbalization of ability to cope with inflammatory bowel disease and its effects
b. utilization of appropriate problem-solving techniques
c. willingness to participate in treatment plan and meet basic needs
d. absence of destructive behavior toward self and others
e. appropriate use of defense mechanisms
f. utilization of available support systems.
	13.a. Assess for and report signs and symptoms of ineffective individual coping (e.g. verbalization of inability to cope; inability to ask for help, problem solve, or meet basic needs; insomnia; withdrawal; reluctance to participate in treatment plan; destructive behavior toward self or others; inappropriate use of defense mechanisms; inability to meet role expectations).
	b. Assess client's perception of current situation.
	c. Implement measures *to promote effective coping:*
	  1. assist client to recognize and manage inappropriate denial if it is present
	  2. perform actions to reduce fear and anxiety (see Nursing Diagnosis 11, action b)
	  3. perform actions to reduce pain (see Nursing Diagnosis 3, action e)
	  4. encourage verbalization about current situation and ways comparable situations have been handled in the past
	  5. assist client to identify personal strengths and resources that can be used to facilitate coping with the current situation
	  6. demonstrate acceptance of client but set limits on inappropriate behavior
	  7. create an atmosphere of trust and support
	  8. if acceptable to client, arrange for a visit with another individual who has successfully adjusted to inflammatory bowel disease
	  9. provide consistency in caregivers when possible; inform client if there will be a change in caregivers *so he/she will not interpret the change as rejection*

Desired Outcome	Nursing Actions and *Selected Purposes/Rationales*
	10. include client in planning of care, encourage maximum participation in treatment plan, and allow choices when possible *to enable him/her to maintain a sense of control*
	11. instruct client in effective problem-solving techniques (e.g. accurate identification of stressors, determination of various options to solve problem)
	12. assist client to maintain usual daily routines whenever possible
	13. assist client to identify priorities and attainable goals as he/she starts to plan for necessary life-style and role changes
	14. assist client to prepare for negative reactions from others because of diarrhea and odor of flatus
	15. assist client to identify and utilize available support systems; provide information regarding available community resources that can assist client and significant others in coping with inflammatory bowel disease (e.g. support groups, counseling services, Crohn's and Colitis Foundation of America)
	16. administer antianxiety and/or antidepressant agents if ordered
	17. encourage continued emotional support from significant others; reinforce the importance of maintaining a calm, nonstressful atmosphere during visits
	18. encourage client to share with significant others the kind of support that would be the most beneficial (e.g. listening, inspiring hope, providing reassurance and accurate information)
	19. support behaviors indicative of effective coping (e.g. increased participation in self-care activities and treatment plan, verbalization of ways to adapt to necessary changes in life style).
	d. Consult physician about psychological counseling if appropriate. Initiate a referral if necessary.

Discharge Teaching

■━━

14. NURSING DIAGNOSIS: **Knowledge deficit, Ineffective management of therapeutic regimen, or Altered health maintenance***

————————

*The nurse should select the diagnostic label that is most appropriate for the client's discharge teaching needs.

Desired Outcomes	Nursing Actions and *Selected Purposes/Rationales*
14.a. The client will identify ways to reduce the incidence of disease exacerbation.	14.a.1. Reinforce the importance of adhering to the prescribed treatment regimen in order to reduce the incidence of disease exacerbation.
	2. Instruct the client regarding ways to reduce bowel irritation:
	a. reduce intake of or avoid foods/fluids likely to be poorly digested or that may irritate the bowel (e.g. raw fruits and vegetables, whole-grain cereals, gravy, fried foods, spicy foods, milk and milk products, caffeine-containing beverages, extremely hot drinks, iced drinks)
	b. avoid use of laxatives
	c. avoid smoking and alcohol intake.
	3. Explain that stress can precipitate periods of exacerbation. Provide information about stress management classes and counseling services that may assist client to manage stress.
14.b. The client will verbalize ways to maintain an optimal nutritional status.	14.b. Provide instructions regarding ways to maintain an optimal nutritional status:
	1. reinforce instructions regarding prescribed diet (a low-residue, high-calorie, high-protein diet is often recommended)

2. inform client that eating small, frequent meals rather than 3 large meals may help achieve the recommended high-calorie intake
3. reinforce the benefits of eating when rested and in a relaxed atmosphere
4. stress the importance of taking vitamins and minerals as prescribed.

14.c. The client will state ways to prevent perianal skin breakdown.

14.c. Provide the following instructions about ways to prevent perianal skin breakdown:
1. use soft toilet tissue for wiping after each bowel movement
2. cleanse perianal area with a mild soap and warm water after each bowel movement; dry thoroughly
3. apply a protective ointment or cream to perianal area after skin has been cleansed.

14.d. The client will verbalize an understanding of medications ordered including rationale, food and drug interactions, side effects, schedule for taking, and importance of taking as prescribed.

14.d.1. Explain rationale for, side effects of, and importance of taking medications prescribed. Inform client of pertinent food and drug interactions.
2. If client is discharged on sulfasalazine, instruct to:
   a. drink at least 10 glasses of liquid/day to reduce risk of kidney stone formation
   b. expect that urine might be an orange-yellow color
   c. take medication with food or after meals to reduce gastric irritation
   d. report a sore throat or mouth, fever, unusual fatigue, continuous headache or aching joint(s), unusual bruising or bleeding, nausea, vomiting, or rash
   e. notify health care provider if unable to impregnate partner (sulfasalazine can cause a reduction in sperm count or a change in sperm morphology)
   f. keep scheduled appointments for blood and urine studies.
3. If client is discharged on a corticosteroid preparation, instruct to:
   a. take medication exactly as prescribed
   b. adjust dosage only if prescribed by physician
   c. notify physician if unable to tolerate oral medication
   d. gradually taper off medication as directed; do not discontinue medication suddenly or of own accord
   e. take with food or antacids to reduce gastric irritation
   f. eat smaller, more frequent meals if gastric irritation occurs
   g. expect that certain effects such as facial rounding, slight weight gain and swelling, increased appetite, and slight mood changes may occur
   h. report undesirable effects of corticosteroid therapy such as marked swelling in extremities, significant weight gain, extreme emotional and behavioral changes, extreme weakness, tarry stools, bloody or coffee-ground vomitus, frequent or persistent headaches, insomnia, and lack of menses
   i. avoid contact with persons who have an infection because corticosteroids lower resistance to infection.
4. If client is to administer corticosteroid enemas or rectal foam or mesalamine enemas or rectal suppositories at home, instruct in technique, schedule (it is usually recommended that these products be administered at bedtime), and length of time he/she should retain the solution or suppository. Allow time for questions, clarification, and return demonstration.
5. Instruct client to inform physician before taking other prescription and nonprescription medications.
6. Instruct client to inform all health care providers of medications being taken.

14.e. The client will state signs and symptoms to report to the health care provider.

14.e. Instruct client to report the following signs and symptoms:
1. recurrent episodes of diarrhea and abdominal pain and cramping
2. increasing abdominal distention
3. persistent vomiting
4. unusual rectal or vaginal drainage
5. burning on urination or brownish, foul-smelling urine

Desired Outcomes	Nursing Actions and **Selected Purposes/Rationales**
	6. pain, swelling, or open sores in perianal area
	7. continued weight loss
	8. constipation
	9. yellowing of skin, flank pain, change in vision, eye pain, or joint pain or swelling (can indicate extraintestinal involvement).
14.f. The client will identify resources that can assist in the adjustment to changes resulting from inflammatory bowel disease and its treatment.	14.f.1. Provide information about resources that can assist the client and significant others in adjusting to inflammatory bowel disease and its effects (e.g. local support groups, Crohn's and Colitis Foundation of America, counseling services, stress management classes).
	2. Initiate a referral if indicated.
14.g. The client will verbalize an understanding of and a plan for adhering to recommended follow-up care including future appointments with health care provider and activity level.	14.g.1. Reinforce importance of keeping follow-up appointments with health care provider.
	2. Reinforce importance of frequent rest periods throughout the day.
	3. Implement measures to improve client compliance:
	a. include significant others in teaching sessions if possible
	b. encourage questions and allow time for reinforcement and clarification of information provided
	c. provide written instructions on future appointments with health care provider, medications prescribed, signs and symptoms to report, and future laboratory studies.

Bibliography

See pages 897–898 and 907.

MANDIBULAR (JAW) FRACTURE WITH INTERMAXILLARY FIXATION

Fracture of the mandible (lower jaw) is one of the most common fractures and is usually the result of blunt trauma to the jaw. The goal of treatment for a mandibular fracture is to correct deformity and restore functional dental occlusion. This is accomplished by closed reduction and 4–6 weeks of intermaxillary fixation (maxillary-mandibular fixation [MMF]) or by open reduction and internal fixation, which is sometimes followed by a shorter period (1–2 weeks) of intermaxillary fixation. Intermaxillary fixation involves attaching wires or arch bars along the upper and lower teeth and connecting these with cross wires or orthodontic elastic bands so that the jaws are held together in correct alignment. The method of reduction and fixation used is determined by the type of fracture and adequacy of the client's teeth. Clients who have a comminuted, compound, or unstable fracture or are edentulous usually require open reduction and internal fixation using interosseous wiring or plates and screws. Those clients with a nondisplaced fracture or a minor degree of displacement and an adequate complement of teeth are more likely to have a closed reduction and intermaxillary fixation.

This care plan focuses on the adult client with a fracture of the mandible hospitalized for closed reduction and intermaxillary fixation. Preoperatively, the goals of care are to reduce fear and anxiety, reduce pain, and educate the client regarding postoperative expectations and management. Postoperatively, the goals of care are to maintain a patent airway, jaw immobilization, an adequate nutritional status, and comfort; prevent complications; and educate the client regarding follow-up care.

DIAGNOSTIC TESTS

X-rays of the mandible
Computed tomography (CT)

DISCHARGE CRITERIA

Prior to discharge, the client will:

- have an adequate respiratory status
- have an adequate oral intake

- have pain controlled
- have no signs and symptoms of infection or postoperative complications
- identify ways to maintain a patent airway
- demonstrate the ability to perform oral hygiene
- verbalize an understanding of dietary modifications and ways to maintain an adequate nutritional status
- identify ways to prevent constipation that may result from temporary dietary modifications
- state signs and symptoms to report to the health care provider
- share thoughts and feelings regarding temporary alterations in diet, speech, and appearance
- verbalize an understanding of and a plan for adhering to recommended follow-up care including future appointments with health care provider and medications prescribed.

NURSING/ COLLABORATIVE DIAGNOSES	**Preoperative**
	1. Anxiety △ 633
	2. Pain: jaw △ 634
	3. Knowledge deficit △ 634
	Postoperative
	1. Risk for aspiration △ 635
	2. Altered nutrition: less than body requirements △ 636
	3. Pain: mouth and jaw △ 637
	4. Altered comfort: nausea and vomiting △ 637
	5. Impaired verbal communication △ 638
	6. Altered oral mucous membrane:
	    a. dry lips
	    b. irritation and breakdown of oral mucosa △ 638
	7. Risk for infection: oral cavity △ 639
	8. Potential complication: respiratory distress △ 640
	9. Body image disturbance △ 640

DISCHARGE TEACHING	10. Knowledge deficit, Ineffective management of therapeutic regimen, or Altered health maintenance △ 641

See Standardized Preoperative and Postoperative Care Plans for additional diagnoses.

PREOPERATIVE

Use in conjunction with the Standardized Preoperative Care Plan.

1. NURSING DIAGNOSIS:

Anxiety

related to:
a. lack of understanding of planned surgery;
b. anticipated effects of general anesthesia or possibility of discomfort during surgery if local anesthesia is planned;
c. unfamiliar environment and separation from significant others;
d. financial concerns associated with hospitalization;
e. anticipated discomfort and effects of surgery and intermaxillary fixation on appearance;
f. anticipated difficulty breathing, swallowing, and talking with jaws wired or banded.

Desired Outcome	Nursing Actions and *Selected Purposes/Rationales*
1. The client will experience a reduction in anxiety (see Standardized Preoperative Care Plan, Nursing Diagnosis 1 [pp. 96–97], for outcome criteria).	1.a. Refer to Standardized Preoperative Care Plan, Nursing Diagnosis 1 (pp. 96–97), for measures related to assessment and reduction of fear and anxiety. b. Implement additional measures *to reduce fear and anxiety:* 1. inform client that the facial swelling and bruising that are present following surgery usually diminish after 2–3 days 2. plan alternative methods of communicating after surgery (e.g. magic slate, pad and pencil); stress that client's difficulty communicating verbally will be temporary and that it will improve as facial swelling subsides and will resolve when intermaxillary fixation device is removed (usually in 4–6 weeks) 3. reassure client that he/she will still be able to breathe and swallow when jaws are wired or banded.

2. NURSING DIAGNOSIS:

Pain: jaw

related to inflammation and tissue and nerve trauma in the area of the fracture.

Desired Outcome	Nursing Actions and *Selected Purposes/Rationales*
2. The client will experience diminished jaw pain as evidenced by: a. verbalization of a reduction in pain b. relaxed facial expression and body positioning c. stable vital signs.	2.a. Assess for signs and symptoms of pain (e.g. verbalization of pain, grimacing, rubbing jaw, reluctance to move, restlessness, diaphoresis, facial pallor, increased B/P, tachycardia). b. Assess client's perception of the severity of pain using a pain intensity rating scale. c. Assess the client's pain pattern (e.g. location, quality, onset, duration, precipitating factors, aggravating factors, alleviating factors). d. Implement measures *to reduce pain:* 1. perform actions *to reduce fear and anxiety about the pain experience* (e.g. assure client that his/her need for pain relief is understood, plan methods for achieving pain control with client) 2. perform actions to reduce fear and anxiety (see Preoperative Nursing Diagnosis 1) *in order to promote relaxation and subsequently increase the client's threshold and tolerance for pain* 3. administer analgesics before activities and procedures that can cause pain and before pain becomes severe 4. apply ice packs to jaw if ordered 5. provide or assist with nonpharmacologic methods for pain relief (e.g. progressive relaxation exercises; restful environment; diversional activities such as watching television, reading, or listening to music) 6. administer analgesics and anti-inflammatory agents if ordered. e. Consult physician if above measures fail to provide adequate pain relief.

Client Teaching

3. NURSING DIAGNOSIS:

Knowledge deficit

regarding the surgical procedure, hospital routines associated with surgery, physical preparation for oral surgery, sensations that normally occur following surgery and anesthesia, and postoperative care.

Desired Outcomes	Nursing Actions and *Selected Purposes/Rationales*

3.a. The client will verbalize an understanding of the surgical procedure, preoperative care, and postoperative sensations and care.	3.a.1. Refer to Standardized Preoperative Care Plan, Nursing Diagnosis 4, actions a.1–4 (pp. 99–100), for information to include in preoperative teaching.
	2. Provide additional information about specific postoperative care following intermaxillary fixation:
	  a. instruct client to avoid trying to open mouth if jaws are wired or banded shut (some surgeons wait until client is fully awake to apply diagonal or vertical wires or bands in order to reduce the risk for aspiration if vomiting occurs)
	  b. inform client that a nasogastric tube may be in place for a short time after surgery to reduce the risk for vomiting
	  c. explain the reason for a liquid or blenderized diet until wires or bands are removed
	  d. instruct client in ways to drink and eat with jaws wired or banded shut:
	    1. sip from a cup or from a spoon
	    2. suck through a straw that has been placed between a gap in teeth
	    3. pour liquid or blenderized food into a bulb syringe attached to a rubber catheter that is placed between a gap in teeth or behind last molar between teeth and cheek
	  e. explain the need for frequent oral hygiene after surgery and instruct client in correct way to rinse mouth and use a low-pressure oral irrigation device (e.g. Water-Pik).
	3. Allow time for questions, clarification, and return demonstration.

3.b The client will demonstrate the ability to perform activities designed to prevent postoperative complications.	3.b.1. Refer to Standardized Preoperative Care Plan, Nursing Diagnosis 4, action b.1 (p. 100), for instructions on ways to prevent postoperative complications.
	2. Provide additional instructions on ways to prevent postoperative complications following intermaxillary fixation:
	  a. demonstrate use of suction equipment; if possible, have client practice suctioning with teeth clenched (suctioning should be done while leaning forward and suction catheter should be inserted through a gap in the teeth or behind last molar between teeth and cheek)
	  b. instruct client to inform staff if nauseated (treatment of nausea helps prevent vomiting, which decreases the risk for aspiration)
	  c. instruct client regarding appropriate actions if vomiting does occur:
	    1. use call signal to summon help
	    2. turn on side if unable to sit up and lean forward
	    3. use fingers to pull cheeks away from teeth and use tongue to push vomitus through spaces between teeth
	    4. suction mouth as instructed.
	3. Allow time for questions, clarification, and return demonstration.

POSTOPERATIVE

Use in conjunction with the Standardized Postoperative Care Plan.

1. NURSING DIAGNOSIS: **Risk for aspiration**

related to:
a. decreased level of consciousness and absent or diminished gag reflex associated with the depressant effect of anesthesia (if a general anesthetic was used) and narcotic (opioid) analgesics;
b. difficulty expelling secretions and/or vomitus associated with intermaxillary fixation;
c. difficulty chewing and swallowing associated with restricted jaw movement.

Desired Outcome	Nursing Actions and *Selected Purposes/Rationales*

1. The client will not aspirate secretions, vomitus, or foods/fluids (see Standardized Postoperative Care Plan, Nursing Diagnosis 18 [p. 119], for outcome criteria).	1.a. Refer to Standardized Postoperative Care Plan, Nursing Diagnosis 18 (p. 119), for measures related to assessment and prevention of aspiration.
	b. Implement additional measures *to prevent aspiration:*
	  1. position client on side with head of bed slightly elevated until he/she is fully awake and able to swallow; then keep head of bed elevated at least 45° *to facilitate swallowing and ability to clear airway*
	  2. perform actions to prevent nausea and vomiting (see Postoperative Nursing Diagnosis 4)
	  3. if vomiting does occur:
	    a. position client on side or assist him/her to sit up and lean forward
	    b. instruct and/or assist client to retract cheeks by holding them out and back with fingers *so vomitus does not pool between cheeks and gingivae*
	    c. instruct client to use tongue to push vomitus through spaces between teeth
	    d. perform and/or assist client with oral and nasopharyngeal suctioning if necessary
	    e. perform good oral hygiene following vomiting episode *to remove vomitus from mouth*
	  4. administer narcotic (opioid) analgesics judiciously *to prevent depression of the gag reflex*
	  5. instruct client to avoid intake of carbonated beverages (*the fizzing in the back of the throat can cause choking*)
	  6. stress to client the importance of adhering to a liquid or blenderized diet (*restricted jaw movement makes it difficult to effectively chew and safely swallow solid food*).

---

2. NURSING DIAGNOSIS: **Altered nutrition: less than body requirements**

related to:
a. decreased oral intake associated with prescribed dietary modifications, nausea, mouth and jaw pain, fear of choking, and dislike of the prescribed diet;
b. inadequate nutritional replacement therapy;
c. loss of nutrients associated with vomiting;
d. increased nutritional needs associated with the increased metabolic rate that occurs during wound healing.

Desired Outcome	Nursing Actions and *Selected Purposes/Rationales*

2. The client will maintain an adequate nutritional status (see Standardized Postoperative Care Plan, Nursing Diagnosis 5 [pp. 105–106], for outcome criteria).	2.a. Refer to Standardized Postoperative Care Plan, Nursing Diagnosis 5 (pp. 105–106), for measures related to assessment and maintenance of an adequate nutritional status.
	b. Implement additional measures *to maintain an adequate nutritional status:*
	  1. perform actions *to increase oral intake:*
	    a. implement measures to reduce mouth and jaw pain (see Postoperative Nursing Diagnosis 3)
	    b. implement measures to prevent nausea and vomiting (see Postoperative Nursing Diagnosis 4)
	    c. allow client to use the technique he/she is most comfortable with when feeding self (e.g. syringe, spoon, straw, cup) *in order to decrease fear of choking*

2. advance diet from clear liquids to blenderized foods with high-protein dietary supplements when allowed and tolerated.

---

3. NURSING DIAGNOSIS: **Pain: mouth and jaw**

related to:
a. tissue trauma associated with the fracture, closed reduction, application of the intermaxillary fixation device, and presence of protruding wire ends in the mouth postoperatively;
b. stretching or compression of nerves associated with operative area edema.

Desired Outcome	Nursing Actions and *Selected Purposes/Rationales*
3. The client will experience diminished mouth and jaw pain (see Standardized Postoperative Care Plan, Nursing Diagnosis 6 [pp. 106–107], for outcome criteria).	3.a. Refer to Standardized Postoperative Care Plan, Nursing Diagnosis 6 (pp. 106–107), for measures related to assessment and reduction of pain. b. Implement additional measures *to reduce mouth and jaw pain:* 1. apply ice packs to jaw for 24–48 hours after surgery if ordered 2. instruct client to avoid intake of hot or cold foods/fluids (*the mouth and teeth are very sensitive for a few days after surgery*) 3. apply topical anesthetics to painful areas in mouth if ordered 4. apply dental or paraffin wax to ends of protruding wires 5. administer corticosteroids (e.g. dexamethasone) if ordered *to reduce edema in the operative area.*

---

4. NURSING DIAGNOSIS: **Altered comfort: nausea and vomiting**

related to stimulation of the vomiting center associated with:
a. stimulation of visceral afferent pathways resulting from the irritating effect of swallowed blood and/or some medications (e.g. corticosteroids) on the gastric mucosa;
b. stimulation of the cerebral cortex resulting from pain, stress, the taste of blood, and/or noxious environmental stimuli (e.g. viewing contents of suction container).

Desired Outcome	Nursing Actions and *Selected Purposes/Rationales*
4. The client will experience relief of nausea and vomiting as evidenced by: a. verbalization of relief of nausea b. absence of vomiting.	4.a. Refer to Standardized Postoperative Care Plan, Nursing Diagnosis 7.B (pp. 108–109), for measures related to assessment and prevention of nausea and vomiting. b. Implement additional measures *to prevent nausea and vomiting:* 1. keep container of suctioned secretions out of client's sight by covering it or placing it at head of the bed (*noxious stimuli can cause stimulation of the vomiting center*) 2. instruct client to remove blood from mouth by suctioning and/or using tongue to push it out through spaces between teeth rather than swallowing it 3. maintain patency of nasogastric tube if present 4. remind client to report nausea so that antiemetics can be given as soon as needed.

5. NURSING DIAGNOSIS: **Impaired verbal communication**

related to restricted jaw movement associated with pain, edema, and presence of intermaxillary fixation device.

Desired Outcome	Nursing Actions and *Selected Purposes/Rationales*

5. The client will successfully communicate needs and desires.	5.a. Assess client for impaired verbal communication (e.g. inability to speak, difficulty forming words or sentences).
	 b. Implement measures *to facilitate communication:*
	   1. answer call signal in person rather than using the intercommunication system
	   2. ask questions that require short answers, eye blinks, or nod of head if client is having difficulty speaking and/or is frustrated or fatigued
	   3. perform actions to reduce mouth and jaw pain (see Postoperative Nursing Diagnosis 3)
	   4. maintain a patient, calm approach; listen attentively and allow ample time for communication
	   5. maintain a quiet environment *so that client does not have to raise voice to be heard*
	   6. provide materials such as magic slate, pad and pencil, or chalk and chalkboard if appropriate; try to ensure that placement of intravenous line does not interfere with client's use of these aids.
	 c. Inform significant others and health care personnel of techniques being used to facilitate client's ability to communicate.

6. NURSING DIAGNOSIS: **Altered oral mucous membrane:**

a. **dry lips** related to inability to moisten lips with tongue associated with jaws being banded or wired shut;
b. **irritation and breakdown of oral mucosa** related to application of intermaxillary fixation device and presence of protruding wires.

Desired Outcome	Nursing Actions and *Selected Purposes/Rationales*

6. The client will experience improved health of the oral mucous membrane as evidenced by:
 a. moist lips
 b. decreased mucosal inflammation
 c. absence of ulcerations
 d. decreasing reports of oral pain.
	6.a. Assess oral mucous membranes frequently (use flashlight and tongue depressor to retract cheeks) being aware that inflammation will be present because of surgical trauma.
	 b. Report any increase in mucosal inflammation, presence of ulcerations, or increased oral pain.
	 c. Implement measures *to maintain or regain integrity of the oral mucous membrane:*
	   1. instruct and assist client with prescribed oral hygiene (e.g. rinsing mouth with saline, diluted hydrogen peroxide, or alkaline mouthwash; brushing teeth with a small, soft-bristle toothbrush; using low-pressure oral irrigation device); avoid use of products that contain lemon and glycerin and use of mouthwashes containing alcohol (*these products have a drying and irritating effect on the oral mucous membrane*)
	   2. avoid using sponge-tipped applicators and cotton swabs to clean teeth (*the sponge or cotton may catch in the intermaxillary fixation device*)

3. stress the importance of performing oral hygiene gently and thoroughly
4. lubricate client's lips frequently
5. encourage client to breathe through nose rather than mouth *in order to reduce dryness of lips*
6. encourage a fluid intake of 2500 ml/day unless contraindicated
7. perform actions to maintain an adequate nutritional status (see Postoperative Nursing Diagnosis 2)
8. instruct client to avoid substances that might further irritate the oral mucosa (e.g. extremely hot, spicy, or acidic foods/fluids)
9. encourage client not to smoke (*smoking dries and irritates the mucosa*)
10. if protruding wires are irritating the oral mucosa, apply or assist client to apply paraffin or dental wax to the ends of the wires (wax should be removed before eating and brushing teeth).
  d. Consult physician about readjustment of wires and/or alternative methods of oral hygiene if irritation and inflammation of oral mucous membrane persist or worsen.

---

7. NURSING DIAGNOSIS: **Risk for infection: oral cavity**

related to:
a. invasion of pathogens associated with breaks in the oral mucous membrane resulting from intermaxillary fixation;
b. colonization of microorganisms in mouth associated with:
  1. difficulty expelling oral secretions and blood resulting from jaws being wired or banded shut
  2. trapping of food particles in intermaxillary fixation device
  3. difficulty performing good oral hygiene;
c. decreased resistance to infection associated with inadequate nutritional status.

Desired Outcome	Nursing Actions and *Selected Purposes/Rationales*
7. The client will remain free of infection in the oral cavity as evidenced by: a. absence of chills and fever b. decreased inflammation and pain in mouth c. absence of ulcerations and white patches in mouth d. absence of foul odor from mouth e. WBC and differential counts returning toward or within normal range f. negative cultures of oral lesions.	7.a. Assess for and report signs and symptoms of oral cavity infection (e.g. chills, fever, increased inflammation of oral mucous membrane, reports of increased mouth pain, presence of ulcerations or white patches in mouth, halitosis). b. Monitor for and report persistent elevation of WBC count and significant change in differential. c. Culture oral lesions as ordered. Report positive results. d. Implement measures *to prevent infection in the oral cavity:* 　1. perform actions to maintain or regain integrity of the oral mucous membrane (see Postoperative Nursing Diagnosis 6, action c) 　2. instruct client to avoid unnecessary handling of wires or bands 　3. suction oral cavity as needed *to remove secretions, blood, and food particles* 　4. perform oral hygiene frequently (usual order is every 2 hours and following meals and snacks) 　5. wash hands thoroughly before performing oral hygiene or suctioning client and instruct client to do the same 　6. administer the following if ordered: 　　a. antimicrobial oral rinse solutions (e.g. Peridex) 　　b. systemic antimicrobial agents.

8. COLLABORATIVE DIAGNOSIS:

Potential complication of jaw surgery: respiratory distress

related to airway obstruction associated with inability to clear airway effectively resulting from:
a. decreased level of consciousness and absent or diminished gag reflex in the early postoperative period;
b. difficulty expelling secretions, blood, and/or vomitus because of jaws being wired or banded shut.

Desired Outcome	Nursing Actions and *Selected Purposes/Rationales*

8. The client will not experience respiratory distress as evidenced by:
a. unlabored respirations at 14–20/minute
b. absence of stridor and sternocleidomastoid muscle retraction
c. usual mental status
d. usual skin color
e. blood gases within normal range.
	8.a. Assess for and immediately report:
	  1. signs and symptoms of respiratory distress (e.g. rapid and/or labored respirations, stridor, sternocleidomastoid muscle retraction, restlessness, agitation, cyanosis)
	  2. abnormal blood gases
	  3. significant decrease in oximetry results.
	b. Obtain an order from physician regarding the circumstances that warrant cutting the wires or bands and specific instructions as to which wires or bands can be cut. Document these orders on the client's nursing care plan.
	c. Have wire cutters or scissors and suction equipment at bedside and tracheostomy tray and oxygen equipment readily available.
	d. Implement measures to prevent aspiration (see Postoperative Nursing Diagnosis 1) *in order to reduce the risk for airway obstruction and subsequent respiratory distress.*
	e. If signs and symptoms of respiratory distress occur:
	  1. place client in a high Fowler's position
	  2. administer oxygen as ordered
	  3. perform oral and nasopharyngeal suctioning as indicated
	  4. use wire cutters or scissors to cut wires or bands if absolutely necessary (specific orders regarding the circumstances in which the wires/bands should be cut and which ones to cut should be strictly adhered to)
	  5. assist with emergency tracheotomy if performed
	  6. provide emotional support to client and significant others.

9. NURSING DIAGNOSIS:

Body image disturbance

related to impaired verbal communication, difficulty eating, and change in appearance associated with facial edema and presence of intermaxillary fixation device.

Desired Outcome	Nursing Actions and *Selected Purposes/Rationales*
9. The client will demonstrate beginning adaptation to the temporary changes in appearance and ability to eat and communicate verbally as evidenced by: a. communication of feelings of self-worth	9.a. Assess for signs and symptoms of a body image disturbance (e.g. verbalization of negative feelings about self, withdrawal from significant others, lack of participation in activities of daily living, refusal to look in mirror). b. Determine the meaning of change in appearance and difficulty eating and communicating verbally to the client by encouraging the communication of feelings and by noting nonverbal responses to these changes. c. Inform client that facial swelling and bruising should start to decrease in

b. maintenance of relationships with significant others
c. active participation in activities of daily living.

2–3 days and that he/she will be able to speak more clearly once the swelling resolves. Stress the temporary nature of jaw immobilization (usually 4–6 weeks).
d. Implement measures *to assist client to increase self-esteem* (e.g. limit negative self-assessment, encourage positive comments about self).
e. Assist the client to identify and utilize coping techniques that have been helpful in the past.
f. Provide privacy during oral hygiene and suctioning. Encourage client to suction self or expectorate frequently *to decrease drooling.*
g. Provide privacy at mealtime if client is embarrassed (client may need to use syringe to feed self and/or may drool while eating).
h. Assist client with usual grooming and makeup habits if necessary.
i. Support behaviors suggesting positive adaptation to changes experienced (e.g. willingness to suction and feed self, attempts at verbal communication).
j. Encourage visits and support from significant others.

Discharge Teaching

━━

10. NURSING DIAGNOSIS: **Knowledge deficit, Ineffective management of therapeutic regimen, or Altered health maintenance***

*The nurse should select the diagnostic label that is most appropriate for the client's discharge teaching needs.

Desired Outcomes	Nursing Actions and *Selected Purposes/Rationales*
10.a. The client will identify ways to maintain a patent airway.	10.a.1. Instruct client regarding ways to maintain a patent airway during period of jaw immobilization:

a. avoid any situation that might lead to nausea and vomiting (e.g. ingestion of foods/fluids that client has not been able to tolerate in the past, noxious sights and odors)
b. reduce the risk of choking by:
  1. sitting up in a chair and leaning forward slightly when eating and drinking
  2. preparing food as recommended (e.g. blenderized)
  3. taking all oral medications in liquid form
  4. avoiding intake of carbonated beverages (the fizzing at the back of the throat can cause choking)
  5. avoiding alcohol intake (alcohol may cause vomiting and/or depress the gag reflex)
c. if vomiting does occur:
  1. sit up, lean forward, and use tongue to push vomitus through spaces between teeth
  2. use fingers to hold cheeks away from teeth to facilitate removal of vomitus
  3. use suction equipment if indicated (a soft, small bulb syringe is usually all that is needed after discharge)
d. perform good oral hygiene after any episode of emesis and after meals to decrease possibility of aspiration
e. avoid swimming and other water activities (increases the risk for aspiration)
f. have wire cutters (if wires present) or scissors (if bands present) readily available at all times and cut the wires or bands per physician's instructions.
2. Provide instructions to significant others regarding circumstances that require cutting the wires or bands and which wires or bands to cut.

Desired Outcomes	Nursing Actions and *Selected Purposes/Rationales*
10.b. The client will demonstrate the ability to perform oral hygiene.	10.b.1. Stress the importance of performing oral hygiene as prescribed. 2. Instruct client in proper oral hygiene techniques (e.g. rinsing mouth with saline, diluted hydrogen peroxide, or alkaline mouthwash; gentle brushing with a small, soft-bristle toothbrush; using a low-pressure oral irrigation device such as Water-Pik). 3. Reinforce the proper method of applying paraffin or dental wax to the protruding wires and removing the wax before meals and oral care. 4. Instruct client to use a lip moisturizer if lips are dry. 5. Allow time for questions, clarification, and return demonstration.
10.c. The client will verbalize an understanding of dietary modifications and ways to maintain an adequate nutritional status.	10.c.1. Reinforce prescribed dietary modifications (client usually progresses rapidly from clear liquids to blenderized foods). 2. Instruct client in ways to maintain an adequate nutritional status: a. plan well-balanced meals that meet caloric needs b. stimulate appetite by looking at and smelling food before it is blenderized c. drink protein supplements between meals d. experiment with spices that may make diet more appetizing and enhance taste sensation e. take vitamin supplements as ordered. 3. Consult dietitian regarding menu planning and food preparation if indicated.
10.d. The client will identify ways to prevent constipation that may result from temporary dietary modifications.	10.d.1. Inform client of the effect that a decrease in dietary fiber will have on bowel habits. 2. Instruct client in ways to prevent constipation: a. drink at least 10 glasses of liquid/day unless contraindicated b. continue with measures previously used to stimulate bowel activity (e.g. drink prune juice) c. take laxatives as prescribed d. use suppositories or enemas if needed.
10.e. The client will state signs and symptoms to report to the health care provider.	10.e.1. Refer to Standardized Postoperative Care Plan, Nursing Diagnosis 21, action c (p. 123), for signs and symptoms to report to the health care provider. 2. Instruct client also to report: a. difficulty breathing b. jaw pain or oral pain unrelieved by prescribed medications c. constipation not controlled by usual methods, laxatives, suppositories, or enemas d. persistent irritation or breakdown of oral mucosa e. facial swelling that persists or increases f. weight loss of 10 pounds or more during the first 6 weeks after surgery g. inability to adhere to prescribed diet h. unusual mouth odor, drainage, or taste i. discoloration of elastic bands (could indicate bands have stretched) and/or loosening of wires or bands.
10.f. The client will verbalize an understanding of and a plan for adhering to recommended follow-up care including future appointments with health care provider and medications prescribed.	10.f.1. Refer to Standardized Postoperative Care Plan, Nursing Diagnosis 21 (pp. 123–124), for routine postoperative instructions and measures to improve client compliance. 2. Explain the rationale for, side effects of, and importance of taking medications prescribed (e.g. laxatives, analgesics, antimicrobials, vitamins, corticosteroids). Inform client of pertinent food and drug interactions. 3. Instruct client to keep teeth clenched and contact physician immediately if wires or bands become loose or disconnected or if it was necessary to cut them.

Bibliography

See pages 897–898 and 907.

PEPTIC ULCER

A peptic ulcer is a break in the continuity of gastrointestinal mucosa that is exposed to acidic digestive secretions. The areas most often involved are the stomach and duodenum. Erosion of these areas can result from direct damage to the mucosa or from an increase in mucosal permeability, which allows gastric acids to diffuse through the mucosal barrier into the underlying tissue. Factors believed to have a role in ulcer development, exacerbation, and/or recurrence include ingestion of alcohol, coffee, certain foods and spices, caffeine, and some medications (e.g. aspirin, nonsteroidal anti-inflammatory agents [NSAIDs], certain chemotherapeutic agents, corticosteroids); presence of the *Helicobacter pylori* (*H. pylori*) bacterium in the stomach; smoking; stress; hypovolemia (can result in ischemia of the gastrointestinal mucosa and subsequent alteration in mucosal permeability); certain disease conditions (e.g. Zollinger-Ellison syndrome, chronic obstructive pulmonary disease, pancreatitis, chronic renal failure); and genetic predisposition.

Peptic ulcers are usually classified by location (e.g. gastric, duodenal) and by the extensiveness of erosion (e.g. acute [superficial erosion with minimal inflammation], chronic [erosion of mucosa and submucosa with scar tissue formation]). Causative factors and the relationship between eating and occurrence of pain vary depending on the location and extensiveness of the ulcer. The characteristic symptom of a peptic ulcer is chronic, intermittent epigastric pain that is described as burning, aching, gnawing, or cramping. Remissions and exacerbations are typical of peptic ulcer disease.

Medical treatment of a peptic ulcer focuses on removing ulcerogenic factors and increasing the gastroduodenal pH. Surgical intervention (e.g. vagotomy, pyloroplasty, partial gastrectomy) may be indicated if symptoms cannot be medically controlled; if ulcers recur frequently; or if complications such as hemorrhage, perforation, or obstruction occur in the ulcerated area(s).

This care plan focuses on the adult client hospitalized for evaluation and medical treatment of a peptic ulcer that has become increasingly symptomatic. The goals of care are to relieve pain, maintain an adequate nutritional status, prevent complications, and educate the client regarding follow-up care.

DIAGNOSTIC TESTS

Endoscopy of the upper gastrointestinal tract
Barium swallow
Cytologic studies
Serum gastrin level
Gastric analysis
Complete blood count (CBC)
Stool analysis for occult blood

DISCHARGE CRITERIA

Prior to discharge, the client will:

- have pain controlled
- have no signs and symptoms of complications
- have an adequate nutritional intake
- identify ways to promote healing of the existing ulcer and prevent recurrence of peptic ulcer
- verbalize an understanding of medications ordered including rationale, food and drug interactions, side effects, schedule for taking, and importance of taking as prescribed
- state signs and symptoms to report to the health care provider
- identify community resources that can assist with making life-style changes necessary to promote healing and prevent recurrence of peptic ulcer
- verbalize an understanding of and a plan for adhering to recommended follow-up care including future appointments with health care provider.

1. NURSING DIAGNOSIS:

Altered nutrition: less than body requirements

related to:
a. decreased oral intake associated with pain (especially with a gastric ulcer because pain often increases after eating);
b. failure to eat a well-balanced diet associated with prescribed or self-imposed dietary modifications.

Desired Outcome	Nursing Actions and *Selected Purposes/Rationales*

Desired Outcome

1. The client will maintain an adequate nutritional status as evidenced by:
   a. weight within normal range for client's age, height, and body frame
   b. normal BUN and serum albumin, Hct, Hb, transferrin, and lymphocyte levels
   c. usual strength and activity tolerance
   d. healthy oral mucous membrane.

Nursing Actions and *Selected Purposes/Rationales*

1.a. Assess for and report signs and symptoms of malnutrition:
   1. weight below normal for client's age, height, and body frame
   2. abnormal BUN and low serum albumin, Hct, Hb, transferrin, and lymphocyte levels (Hct and Hb may also be decreased because of bleeding of the ulcerated area)
   3. weakness and fatigue
   4. sore, inflamed oral mucous membrane
   5. pale conjunctiva.
   b. Monitor percentage of meals and snacks client consumes. Report a pattern of inadequate intake.
   c. Implement measures *to maintain an adequate nutritional status:*
      1. when food or oral fluids are allowed, perform actions *to improve oral intake:*
         a. implement measures to reduce epigastric pain (see Nursing Diagnosis 2, actions e.1.c–g, 2, and 3)
         b. obtain a dietary consult if necessary to assist client in selecting foods/fluids that meet nutritional needs, are appealing, and adhere to personal and cultural preferences as well as dietary modifications
         c. maintain a clean environment and a relaxed, pleasant atmosphere
         d. provide oral hygiene before meals
         e. allow adequate time for meals; reheat foods/fluids if necessary
      2. ensure that meals are well balanced and high in essential nutrients; offer dietary supplements if indicated
      3. administer vitamins and minerals if ordered.
   d. Perform a calorie count if ordered. Report information to dietitian and physician.
   e. Consult physician regarding the need for parenteral nutrition if client does not consume enough food or fluids to meet nutritional needs.

2. NURSING DIAGNOSIS: **Pain: epigastric**

related to:
a. inflammation of the ulcerated area;
b. stimulation of exposed nerve endings and reflex muscle spasm (occurs when gastric or duodenal secretions or other irritants come in contact with the ulcer).

Desired Outcome	Nursing Actions and *Selected Purposes/Rationales*

2. The client will experience diminished pain as evidenced by:
  a. verbalization of a decrease in or absence of pain
  b. relaxed facial expression and body positioning
  c. increased participation in activities.
	2.a. Assess for signs and symptoms of pain (e.g. verbalization of pain, guarding of abdomen, rubbing epigastric area, grimacing, reluctance to move, restlessness).
	b. Assess client's perception of the severity of pain using a pain intensity rating scale.
	c. Assess the client's pain pattern (e.g. location, quality, onset, duration, precipitating factors, aggravating factors, alleviating factors).
	d. Ask the client to describe previous pain experiences and methods used to manage pain effectively.
	e. Implement measures *to reduce epigastric pain:*
	  1. perform actions *to prevent further tissue irritation and/or promote healing of the ulcer:*
	    a. withhold oral intake as ordered *to reduce stimulation of gastric acid secretion*
	    b. insert a nasogastric tube and maintain suction as ordered *to remove gastric secretions*
	    c. administer the following medications if ordered:
	      1. histamine$_2$ receptor antagonists (e.g. cimetidine, famotidine, ranitidine, nizatidine), and/or proton-pump inhibitors (e.g. omeprazole, lansoprazole) *to inhibit gastric acid secretion*
	      2. antacids *to neutralize gastric secretions*
	      3. cytoprotective agents (e.g. sucralfate) *to protect the ulcerated area*
	      4. synthetic prostaglandins (e.g. misoprostol) *to inhibit gastric acid secretion and protect the ulcerated area*
	      5. antimicrobials (e.g. amoxicillin, clarithromycin, tetracycline, metronidazole) *to treat H. pylori if present*
	    d. implement measures to reduce fear and anxiety (see Nursing Diagnosis 4, action b) *in order to reduce stimulation of the vagus nerve and subsequent increase in gastric acid output*
	    e. when foods/fluids are allowed:
	      1. instruct client to:
	        a. avoid intake of coffee, caffeine-containing tea and colas, spices such as black pepper and chili powder, and extremely hot foods/fluids (*these substances typically cause irritation of the gastric mucosa*)
	        b. chew food thoroughly and eat slowly (*a large bolus of food causes an increased output of hydrochloric acid and pepsin*)
	        c. limit intake of milk and milk products and drink milk with rather than between meals (*protein and calcium are potent stimulators of gastrin secretion, which causes increased output of gastric acid*)
	        d. avoid intake of foods/fluids that cause epigastric pain
	      2. provide regularly scheduled meals and snacks as ordered *to neutralize gastric acid* (moderate-sized meals are usually recommended rather than large ones *to help prevent the stimulation of excessive amounts of gastric acid*)
	    f. encourage client to stop smoking

Desired Outcome	Nursing Actions and *Selected Purposes/Rationales*

g. if client is taking medications that are known to be ulcerogenic (e.g. aspirin, NSAIDs, corticosteroids), administer them with meals or snacks *to decrease gastric irritation*

h. prepare client for a vagotomy if planned (*may be done to reduce gastric acid production*)

2. provide or assist with nonpharmacologic measures for pain relief (e.g. massage; position change; progressive relaxation exercises; restful environment; diversional activities such as watching television, reading, or conversing)

3. administer analgesics if ordered.

f. Consult physician if above measures fail to provide adequate pain relief.

■————————————————————————

3. COLLABORATIVE DIAGNOSES:

Potential complications of peptic ulcer:

a. **hypovolemic shock** related to upper gastrointestinal (GI) bleeding associated with:
   1. erosion of numerous small blood vessels (the gastric and duodenal mucosa have a rich blood supply)
   2. erosion of a major blood vessel (can occur if the ulcer is deep);

b. **peritonitis** related to leakage of gastrointestinal contents into the peritoneal cavity associated with perforation of the wall of the stomach or duodenum (can occur if the ulcer is deep);

c. **gastric outlet obstruction** related to narrowing of the pylorus associated with inflammation, spasm, and/or scar tissue formation (can occur if the ulcer is at or near the gastric outlet).

Desired Outcomes	Nursing Actions and *Selected Purposes/Rationales*

3.a. The client will not develop hypovolemic shock as evidenced by:
1. usual mental status
2. stable vital signs
3. skin warm, dry, and usual color
4. palpable peripheral pulses
5. urine output at least 30 ml/hour.

3.a.1. Assess for and report signs and symptoms of upper GI bleeding (e.g. hematemesis, bright red or coffee-ground drainage from nasogastric tube, increased epigastric pain, melena, decreased B/P, increased pulse rate).

2. Monitor RBC, Hct, and Hb levels. Report decreasing values.

3. Assess for and report signs and symptoms of hypovolemic shock:
   a. restlessness, agitation, confusion, or other change in mental status
   b. significant decrease in B/P
   c. postural hypotension
   d. rapid, weak pulse
   e. rapid respirations
   f. cool, moist skin
   g. pallor, cyanosis
   h. diminished or absent peripheral pulses
   i. urine output less than 30 ml/hour.

4. Implement measures to prevent further tissue irritation and/or promote healing of the ulcer (see Nursing Diagnosis 2, action e.1) *in order to prevent upper GI bleeding.*

5. If signs and symptoms of upper GI bleeding occur:
   a. insert nasogastric tube if not already present and maintain suction as ordered
   b. prepare client for diagnostic tests (e.g. endoscopy, angiography) if planned
   c. assist with measures to control bleeding (e.g. gastric lavage, endoscopic electrocoagulation, selective arterial embolization, intravenous or intra-arterial administration of vasopressin) if ordered
   d. prepare client for surgical intervention (e.g. ligation of bleeding vessels, partial gastrectomy) if planned.

6. If signs and symptoms of hypovolemic shock occur:
   a. continue with above measures to control bleeding

b. place client flat in bed with legs elevated unless contraindicated
c. monitor vital signs frequently
d. administer oxygen as ordered
e. administer blood products and/or volume expanders if ordered
f. prepare client for insertion of hemodynamic monitoring devices (e.g. central venous catheter, intra-arterial catheter) if planned
g. provide emotional support to client and significant others.

3.b. The client will not develop peritonitis as evidenced by:
1. no reports of new or increased abdominal pain and tenderness
2. soft, nondistended abdomen
3. afebrile status
4. stable vital signs
5. absence of nausea and vomiting
6. normal bowel sounds
7. WBC count within normal range.

3.b.1. Assess for and report:
a. signs and symptoms of perforation of the gastric or duodenal wall (e.g. sudden, sharp, severe upper abdominal pain; extreme abdominal tenderness; abdominal x-ray showing free air in peritoneal cavity)
b. signs and symptoms of peritonitis (e.g. reports of new or increased abdominal pain; rebound tenderness; distended, rigid abdomen; elevated temperature; tachycardia; tachypnea; hypotension; nausea; vomiting; diminished or absent bowel sounds)
c. increase in WBC count.
2. Implement measures to prevent further tissue irritation and/or promote healing of the ulcer (see Nursing Diagnosis 2, action e.1) *in order to reduce the risk for perforation.*
3. If signs and symptoms of peritonitis occur:
a. withhold oral intake as ordered
b. place client on bed rest in a semi-Fowler's position *to assist in pooling or localizing gastrointestinal contents in the pelvis rather than under the diaphragm*
c. prepare client for diagnostic tests (e.g. abdominal x-ray, computed tomography, ultrasonography) if planned
d. insert a nasogastric tube and maintain suction as ordered
e. administer antimicrobials as ordered
f. administer intravenous fluids and/or blood volume expanders if ordered *to prevent or treat shock (can result from the increased capillary permeability that occurs with inflammation and the subsequent escape of protein, fluid, and electrolytes from the vascular space into the peritoneal cavity)*
g. prepare client for surgical repair of the perforation if indicated
h. provide emotional support to client and significant others.

3.c. The client will not experience gastric outlet obstruction as evidenced by:
1. soft, nondistended epigastric area
2. no reports of epigastric fullness or bloating
3. absence of anorexia, nausea, and vomiting.

3.c.1. Assess for and report signs and symptoms of gastric outlet obstruction (e.g. epigastric distention, reports of epigastric fullness or bloating, anorexia, nausea, vomiting, foul-smelling vomitus containing particles of food ingested many hours earlier).
2. Implement measures to prevent further tissue irritation and/or promote healing of the ulcer (see Nursing Diagnosis 2, action e.1) *in order to reduce the risk of narrowing the lumen of the gastric outlet if the ulcer is at or near the pylorus.*
3. If signs and symptoms of gastric outlet obstruction occur:
a. withhold oral intake as ordered
b. prepare client for diagnostic tests (e.g. endoscopy, barium swallow) if planned
c. insert a nasogastric tube and maintain suction as ordered
d. administer intravenous fluid and electrolyte replacements as ordered
e. prepare client for surgical intervention (e.g. partial gastrectomy, pyloroplasty) if planned
f. provide emotional support to client and significant others.

■

4. NURSING DIAGNOSIS: **Anxiety**

related to pain; lack of understanding of the diagnosis, diagnostic tests, treatment plan, and prognosis; unfamiliar environment; financial concerns; and probable need to change life style in order to control symptoms and prevent ulcer recurrence.

Desired Outcome	Nursing Actions and *Selected Purposes/Rationales*

4. The client will experience a reduction in anxiety as evidenced by:
   a. verbalization of feeling less anxious
   b. usual sleep pattern
   c. relaxed facial expression and body movements
   d. stable vital signs
   e. usual perceptual ability and interactions with others.
	4.a. Assess client for signs and symptoms of anxiety (e.g. verbalization of feeling anxious, insomnia, tenseness, shakiness, restlessness, tachycardia, elevated blood pressure, self-focused behaviors).
	   b. Implement measures *to reduce fear and anxiety:*
	      1. orient client to hospital environment, equipment, and routines
	      2. introduce client to staff who will be participating in care; if possible, maintain consistency in staff assigned to his/her care *to provide feelings of stability and comfort with the environment*
	      3. assure client that staff members are nearby; respond to call signal as soon as possible
	      4. maintain a calm, supportive, confident manner when interacting with client
	      5. encourage verbalization of fear and anxiety; provide feedback
	      6. reinforce physician's explanations and clarify misconceptions client has about the peptic ulcer, the treatment plan, and the prognosis
	      7. explain all diagnostic tests
	      8. perform actions to reduce epigastric pain (see Nursing Diagnosis 2, action e)
	      9. provide a calm, restful environment
	     10. instruct client in relaxation techniques and encourage participation in diversional activities
	     11. assist client to identify specific stressors and ways to cope with them
	     12. provide information based on current needs of client at a level he/she can understand; encourage questions and clarification of information provided
	     13. encourage significant others to project a caring, concerned attitude without obvious anxiousness
	     14. include significant others in orientation and teaching sessions and encourage their continued support of the client
	     15. initiate financial and/or social service referrals if indicated
	     16. administer prescribed antianxiety agents if indicated.
	   c. Consult physician if above actions fail to control fear and anxiety.

---

5. NURSING DIAGNOSIS:

Ineffective management of therapeutic regimen

related to:
a. lack of understanding of the implications of not following the prescribed treatment plan;
b. difficulty modifying personal habits.

Desired Outcome	Nursing Actions and *Selected Purposes/Rationales*

5. The client will demonstrate the probability of effective management of the therapeutic regimen as evidenced by:
   a. willingness to learn about and participate in the treatment plan
   b. statements reflecting ways to modify personal habits
	5.a. Assess for indications that the client may be unable to effectively manage the therapeutic regimen:
	      1. statements reflecting inability to adhere to treatment plan at home
	      2. failure to adhere to treatment plan while in hospital (e.g. refusing medications, not adhering to dietary modifications)
	      3. statements reflecting a lack of understanding of factors that aggravate or cause peptic ulcers
	      4. statements reflecting an unwillingness or inability to modify personal habits and integrate necessary treatments into life style
	      5. statements reflecting view that the peptic ulcer will resolve without

and integrate treatments into life style

c. statements reflecting an understanding of the implications of not following the prescribed treatment plan.

any treatment, that an absence of epigastric pain indicates that the ulcer is cured, or that recurrence and complications are inevitable and efforts to comply with treatments are useless.

b. Implement measures *to promote effective management of the therapeutic regimen:*

1. explain peptic ulcer disease in terms the client can understand; stress the fact that complications can occur and/or ulcer will recur if treatment plan is not followed

2. inform client that prescribed dietary modifications and medication therapy will not be as extensive after the existing ulcer has healed (usually 6–8 weeks)

3. initiate and reinforce the discharge teaching outlined in Nursing Diagnosis 6 *in order to promote a sense of control over disease progression*

4. encourage questions and clarify misconceptions the client has about the peptic ulcer and its effects

5. discuss the importance of developing and utilizing stress reduction techniques (stress can increase gastric acid output and is often a factor contributing to some behaviors such as cigarette smoking, aspirin ingestion, alcohol and/or caffeinated beverage intake, and irregular eating habits that increase the risk for peptic ulcer recurrence or exacerbation)

6. assist client to identify ways treatments can be incorporated into life style; focus on modifications of life style rather than complete change (e.g. drinking decaffeinated rather than caffeine-containing tea and colas)

7. provide a dietary consult to assist client in planning a dietary program that incorporates the prescribed modifications and client's daily routines and personal and cultural preferences

8. provide information about various antacids available if appropriate; instruct client to alternate types of antacids in order to minimize side effects such as diarrhea and constipation

9. assist client in setting up a medication schedule that can be incorporated into daily activities

10. encourage questions and allow time for reinforcement and clarification of information provided

11. provide written instructions about future appointments with health care provider, dietary modifications, medications, and signs and symptoms to report

12. if client has concerns regarding the cost of medications, obtain a social service consult to assist with financial planning and to obtain financial aid if indicated

13. provide information about and encourage utilization of community resources that can assist client to make necessary life-style changes (e.g. smoking cessation programs, stress management classes, counseling services)

14. reinforce behaviors suggesting future compliance with the therapeutic regimen (e.g. participation in the treatment plan, statements reflecting ways to modify personal habits)

15. include significant others in explanations and teaching sessions and encourage their support.

Discharge Teaching

6. NURSING DIAGNOSIS: **Knowledge deficit or Altered health maintenance***

*The nurse should select the diagnostic label that is most appropriate for the client's discharge teaching needs.

Desired Outcomes	Nursing Actions and **Selected Purposes/Rationales**

6.a. The client will identify ways to promote healing of the existing ulcer and prevent recurrence of peptic ulcer.

6.a.1. Instruct client in ways to promote healing of the existing ulcer and prevent recurrence of peptic ulcer:
   a. drink decaffeinated or caffeine-free tea and colas rather than those containing caffeine
   b. avoid drinking coffee and alcohol or drink these beverages only in small amounts during or immediately following a meal
   c. avoid ingestion of foods that are known to irritate gastric mucosa directly or increase gastric acid production (e.g. whole grains, chocolate, rich pastries, spicy foods, meat extracts, extremely hot foods)
   d. avoid intake of any foods and fluids that cause gastric distress
   e. eat regularly scheduled, moderate-sized meals (the number of meals recommended by physicians varies from 3 to 6 meals per day); do not skip meals
   f. eat slowly and chew food thoroughly
   g. maintain a calm, pleasant atmosphere at mealtime and whenever possible
   h. stop smoking
   i. maintain a balance of physical activity and rest
   j. avoid stressful situations
   k. avoid ingestion of over-the-counter medications such as aspirin and ibuprofen; if it is necessary to take these or other ulcerogenic medications (e.g. corticosteroids), take them with antacids or food unless contraindicated and/or take enteric coated or highly buffered preparations of the drugs if available
   l. take medications for ulcer treatment as prescribed.
   2. Obtain a dietary consult if client needs assistance in planning meals that incorporate dietary modifications and his/her daily routines and personal and cultural preferences.
   3. Assist client to identify ways to make necessary life-style changes.

6.b. The client will verbalize an understanding of medications ordered including rationale, food and drug interactions, side effects, schedule for taking, and importance of taking as prescribed.

6.b.1. Explain the rationale for, side effects of, schedule for taking, and importance of taking medications prescribed. Inform client of pertinent food and drug interactions.
   2. If client is discharged on antacid therapy, instruct to:
   a. take as prescribed (usually 7 times/day [1 hour and 3 hours after each meal and at bedtime] or 4 times/day [1 hour after each meal and at bedtime] for 4–6 weeks)
   b. take antacid suspensions rather than tablets whenever possible (suspensions neutralize gastric acid more effectively)
   c. thoroughly chew tablets that are labelled as "chewable"
   d. shake antacid suspensions vigorously before taking dose
   e. check the sodium content of antacids and avoid intake of those high in sodium (e.g. Amphojel, Basaljel, Di-Gel, Delcid) if hypertensive or on a sodium-restricted diet
   f. alternate aluminum-containing antacids (e.g. Amphojel, ALternaGEL) and magnesium-containing antacids (e.g. Milk of Magnesia, Mag-Ox) periodically or take aluminum and magnesium hydroxide combination antacids (e.g. Maalox, Di-Gel, Gaviscon, Mylanta) if constipation or diarrhea develops
   g. avoid excessive intake of antacids high in calcium (e.g. Titralac, Tums) and sodium bicarbonate (e.g. baking soda, Alka-Seltzer, Soda Mint)
   h. expect that stool may be speckled or whitish
   i. observe for and report:
      1. thirst, dry mouth, weakness, lethargy (may indicate hypernatremia resulting from excessive amounts of antacids containing sodium) and/or swelling of extremities and weight gain (can occur with the subsequent water retention)
      2. constipation not resolved by increased fluid intake, laxatives, and switching to an antacid containing magnesium

3. diarrhea not controlled by antidiarrheal medication and switching to an antacid containing aluminum.
3. If client is discharged on sucralfate (Carafate), instruct to:
    a. take it an hour before meals and at bedtime
    b. avoid taking antacids for at least 30 minutes before and after taking the medication
    c. monitor for and report persistent constipation, nausea, or indigestion.
4. If client is discharged on a histamine$_2$ receptor antagonist (e.g. cimetidine, nizatidine, famotidine, ranitidine) or proton-pump inhibitor (e.g. omeprazole, lansoprazole), instruct to:
    a. consult physician or pharmacist about appropriate scheduling if taking antacids or cytoprotective agents (e.g. sucralfate) concurrently
    b. monitor for and report persistent sleepiness, headache, dizziness, diarrhea, or constipation.
5. If client is discharged on misoprostol (e.g. Cytotec), instruct to:
    a. avoid taking it with food or antacids
    b. monitor for and report persistent diarrhea, abdominal pain, or menstrual irregularities (e.g. spotting, cramps, excessive bleeding)
    c. notify physician if pregnancy is suspected (misoprostol may induce miscarriage).
6. Caution client to consult physician before stopping any medication prescribed for peptic ulcer treatment.
7. Instruct client to inform health care providers of medications being taken for the treatment of peptic ulcer (many of these drugs can alter the absorption of other medications).

6.c. The client will state signs and symptoms to report to the health care provider.

6.c. Instruct client to report:
1. black or tarry stools
2. bloody or coffee-ground vomitus
3. abdominal distention
4. persistent epigastric fullness or bloating, nausea, and/or vomiting
5. persistent weight loss
6. persistent or increased epigastric or abdominal pain
7. weakness and fatigue
8. undesirable side effects of medications prescribed (see actions b.2.i, 3.c, 4.b, and 5.b in this diagnosis)
9. persistent high stress levels
10. difficulty taking medications as prescribed.

6.d. The client will identify community resources that can assist with making life-style changes necessary to promote healing and prevent recurrence of peptic ulcer.

6.d.1. Provide information about community resources that can assist client to make life-style changes necessary to promote healing and prevent recurrence of peptic ulcer (e.g. smoking cessation programs, stress management classes, counseling services).
2. Initiate a referral if indicated.

6.e. The client will verbalize an understanding of and a plan for adhering to recommended follow-up care including future appointments with health care provider.

6.e.1. Reinforce the importance of follow-up appointments with health care provider.
2. Refer to Nursing Diagnosis 5, action b, for measures to promote the client's ability to effectively manage the therapeutic regimen.

Bibliography

See pages 897–898 and 907–908.

UNIT FIFTEEN

NURSING CARE OF THE CLIENT WITH DISTURBANCES OF THE LIVER, BILIARY TRACT, AND PANCREAS

ACUTE PANCREATITIS

Acute pancreatitis is an inflammation of the pancreas that occurs when the enzymes it produces become activated in the pancreas rather than in the duodenum. The subsequent autodigestion causes pathologic changes that range from a mild local inflammatory response to a life-threatening situation resulting from severe local and adjacent tissue destruction, hemorrhage, and multi-organ failure. Following an episode of mild to moderate acute pancreatitis, the structure and function of the pancreas often return to normal. However, with more severe episodes of acute pancreatitis, irreversible changes can occur and chronic pancreatitis can develop.

It is theorized that pancreatic duct obstruction, pancreatic ischemia, direct injury to the acinar cells, and reflux of bile into the pancreatic duct are among the mechanisms that trigger the activation of enzymes in the pancreas. The most common causes of acute pancreatitis are biliary tract disease and heavy alcohol intake. Some less frequent causes include external trauma to the abdomen, trauma to the pancreas during pancreatic endoscopy or abdominal surgery, infections, drugs (e.g. azathioprine, valproic acid, estrogen, hydrochlorothiazide, furosemide), and metabolic disorders such as hyperparathyroidism and hyperlipidemia.

The focus of medical treatment is to prevent further autodigestion of the pancreas and prevent systemic complications by decreasing stimulation of the pancreatic enzymes until normal outflow resumes. If the cause of the pancreatitis is biliary tract disease, surgery (e.g. removal of gallstones that may be blocking the pancreatic duct) is usually performed after pancreatic inflammation has subsided and the client is in stable condition.

This care plan focuses on the adult client hospitalized with probable acute pancreatitis. The goals of care are to control pain, maintain an adequate nutritional status and fluid and electrolyte balance, prevent complications, and educate the client regarding follow-up care.

DIAGNOSTIC TESTS

Serum and urine amylase
Pancreatic isoamylase
Serum lipase
White blood cell (WBC) count and differential
Renal amylase/creatinine clearance ratio
Ultrasonography
Computed tomography (CT)
Magnetic resonance imaging (MRI)

DISCHARGE CRITERIA

Prior to discharge, the client will:

- have no signs and symptoms of complications
- have relief of severe pain
- have an adequate nutritional intake
- identify ways to prevent overstimulation of and further trauma to the pancreas
- verbalize an understanding of recommended dietary modifications
- state signs and symptoms to report to the health care provider
- verbalize an understanding of and a plan for adhering to recommended follow-up care including future appointments with health care provider and medications prescribed.

NURSING/ COLLABORATIVE DIAGNOSES	
1. Ineffective breathing pattern △ 655	
2. Altered fluid and electrolyte balance:	
a. fluid volume deficit, hypokalemia, and hypochloremia	
b. hypocalcemia	
c. metabolic alkalosis	
d. third-spacing △ 656	
3. Altered nutrition: less than body requirements △ 657	
4. Pain: abdominal with radiation to the back △ 658	
5A. Altered comfort: nausea and vomiting △ 660	
5B. Altered comfort: abdominal distention and gas pain △ 660	
6. Altered oral mucous membrane: dryness △ 661	

7. Potential complications:
   a. hypovolemic shock
   b. pancreatic necrosis, pseudocyst, or abscess
   c. peritonitis
   d. hyperglycemia
   e. pleural effusion
   f. adult respiratory distress syndrome (ARDS) △ 662
8. Anxiety △ 664

DISCHARGE TEACHING

9. Knowledge deficit, Ineffective management of therapeutic regimen, or Altered health maintenance △ 665

1. NURSING DIAGNOSIS: **Ineffective breathing pattern**

related to:
a. increased rate and decreased depth of respirations associated with fear and anxiety;
b. decreased rate and depth of respirations associated with the depressant effect of some medications (e.g. narcotic [opioid] analgesics);
c. diminished lung/chest wall expansion associated with:
   1. reluctance to breathe deeply because of pain
   2. decreased activity
   3. positioning (client often positions self on side with knees and trunk flexed to reduce pain)
   4. pleural effusion if it occurs
   5. pressure on the diaphragm resulting from accumulation of gastrointestinal gas and fluid and ascites if present.

Desired Outcome	Nursing Actions and *Selected Purposes/Rationales*

1. The client will maintain an effective breathing pattern as evidenced by:
  a. normal rate and depth of respirations
  b. absence of dyspnea
  c. blood gases within normal range.
	1.a. Assess for signs and symptoms of an ineffective breathing pattern (e.g. shallow respirations, dyspnea).
	  b. Monitor for and report the following:
	    1. abnormal blood gases
	    2. significant decrease in oximetry results.
	  c. Implement measures *to improve breathing pattern:*
	    1. perform actions to reduce pain (see Nursing Diagnosis 4, action e)
	    2. perform actions *to reduce pressure on the diaphragm:*
	      a. implement measures to reduce the accumulation of gastrointestinal gas and fluid (see Nursing Diagnosis 5.B, action 3)
	      b. administer albumin infusions if ordered *to reduce ascites*
	    3. perform actions to prevent and treat pleural effusion (see Collaborative Diagnosis 7, actions e.3 and 4)
	    4. when severe pain has subsided, place client in a semi- to high Fowler's position unless contraindicated
	    5. assist client to turn from side to side at least every 2 hours while in bed
	    6. instruct client to deep breathe or use incentive spirometer every 1–2 hours
	    7. increase activity as allowed and tolerated
	    8. administer central nervous system depressants judiciously; hold medication and consult physician if respiratory rate is less than 12/minute.
	  d. Consult physician if:
	    1. ineffective breathing pattern continues

Desired Outcome   Nursing Actions and **Selected Purposes/Rationales**

2. signs and symptoms of atelectasis (e.g. diminished or absent breath sounds, dull percussion note over affected area, increased respiratory rate, dyspnea, tachycardia, elevated temperature) develop
3. signs and symptoms of impaired gas exchange (e.g. restlessness, irritability, confusion, decreased PaO_2 and increased $PaCO_2$ levels) are present.

---

2. NURSING/COLLABORATIVE DIAGNOSIS:

Altered fluid and electrolyte balance:

a. **fluid volume deficit, hypokalemia, and hypochloremia** related to decreased oral intake and excessive loss of fluid and electrolytes associated with vomiting and nasogastric tube drainage;
b. **hypocalcemia** related to:
   1. binding of calcium to the undigested fats in the intestine (enzymes such as lipase and phospholipase A are not released into the intestinal tract to digest fats so calcium binds with the free fats and is excreted in the stool)
   2. hypoalbuminemia associated with increased vascular permeability (albumin is needed to transport nonionized calcium in the blood)
   3. binding of calcium to free fatty acids in areas of tissue necrosis;
c. **metabolic alkalosis** related to hypokalemia, hypochloremia, and excessive loss of hydrochloric acid associated with vomiting and nasogastric tube drainage;
d. **third-spacing** related to increased vascular permeability associated with the inflammatory response and activation of bradykinin and kallidin by kallikrein (the plasma peptide kallikrein is activated by the pancreatic enzyme trypsin, which enters the systemic circulation during acute pancreatitis).

Desired Outcomes   Nursing Actions and **Selected Purposes/Rationales**

2.a. The client will not experience fluid volume deficit, hypokalemia, hypochloremia, hypocalcemia, or metabolic alkalosis as evidenced by:
   1. normal skin turgor
   2. moist mucous membranes
   3. stable weight
   4. B/P and pulse within normal range for client and stable with position change
   5. hand vein filling time less than 3–5 seconds
   6. usual mental status
   7. balanced intake and output
   8. urine specific gravity within normal range
   9. soft, nondistended abdomen with normal bowel sounds
   10. absence of cardiac dysrhythmias, muscle weakness, paresthesias,

2.a.1. Assess for and report signs and symptoms of:
   a. fluid volume deficit:
      1. decreased skin turgor, dry mucous membranes, thirst
      2. sudden weight loss of 2% or greater
      3. postural hypotension and/or low B/P
      4. weak, rapid pulse
      5. delayed hand vein filling time (longer than 3–5 seconds)
      6. change in mental status
      7. decreased urine output with increased specific gravity (reflects an actual rather than potential fluid volume deficit)
      8. increased BUN and Hct
   b. hypokalemia (e.g. cardiac dysrhythmias, postural hypotension, muscle weakness, nausea and vomiting, abdominal distention, hypoactive or absent bowel sounds)
   c. hypochloremia and metabolic alkalosis (e.g. dizziness, irritability, paresthesias, muscle twitching or spasms, hypoventilation)
   d. hypocalcemia (e.g. anxiousness; irritability; numbness or tingling of fingers, toes, or circumoral area; positive Chvostek's and Trousseau's signs; hyperactive reflexes; tetany; seizures).
   2. Monitor serum electrolyte and blood gas results. Report abnormal values.
   3. Implement measures *to prevent or treat fluid volume deficit, hypokalemia, hypochloremia, hypocalcemia, and metabolic alkalosis:*
      a. perform actions to reduce nausea and vomiting (see Nursing Diagnosis 5.A, action 2)
      b. if irrigation of nasogastric tube is indicated, use normal saline rather than water
      c. administer fluid and electrolyte replacements if ordered

muscle twitching or spasms, dizziness, tetany, and seizure activity

11. negative Chvostek's and Trousseau's signs

12. BUN, Hct, serum electrolyte, and blood gases within normal range.

d. maintain a fluid intake of at least 2500 ml/day unless contraindicated

e. when oral intake is allowed:

    1. assist client to select the following foods/fluids:

        a. those high in potassium (e.g. bananas, potatoes, cantaloupe, raisins, apricots)

        b. those high in calcium such as milk and milk products (if client is on a low-fat diet, items such as ice cream, whole milk, butter, and cream should be omitted)

    2. administer pancreatic enzymes (e.g. pancreatin, pancrelipase) if ordered *to promote fat digestion so that there is less fat available for calcium to bind to.*

4. Consult physician if signs and symptoms of fluid volume deficit and electrolyte imbalances persist or worsen.

2.b. The client will experience resolution of third-spacing as evidenced by:

1. resolution of ascites

2. absence of dyspnea

3. audible breath sounds

4. B/P and pulse within normal range for client and stable with position change

5. balanced intake and output.

2.b.1. Assess for and report signs and symptoms of third-spacing:

a. ascites

b. dyspnea and diminished or absent breath sounds

c. evidence of vascular depletion (e.g. postural hypotension; weak, rapid pulse; decreased urine output).

2. Monitor chest x-ray results. Report findings of pleural effusion.

3. Monitor serum albumin levels. Report below-normal levels (*low serum albumin levels result in fluid shifting out of vascular space because albumin normally maintains plasma colloid osmotic pressure*).

4. Implement measures *to prevent further third-spacing and/or promote mobilization of fluid back into vascular space:*

a. encourage client to rest periodically in a recumbent position if tolerated (*lying flat promotes venous return and results in lower venous hydrostatic pressure with subsequent reshifting of fluid back into vascular space*)

b. administer albumin infusions if ordered *to increase colloid osmotic pressure*

c. perform actions to decrease pancreatic stimulation (see Nursing Diagnosis 4, action e.5) *in order to decrease inflammation and activation of kallikrein and subsequently decrease vascular permeability.*

5. Consult physician if signs and symptoms of third-spacing persist or worsen.

---

3. NURSING DIAGNOSIS:

Altered nutrition: less than body requirements

related to:

a. decreased oral intake associated with nausea, pain, prescribed dietary restrictions, and feeling of fullness resulting from abdominal distention;

b. loss of nutrients associated with vomiting;

c. decreased utilization of nutrients associated with impaired digestion of fats, proteins, and carbohydrates resulting from loss of normal outflow of pancreatic enzymes;

d. increased nutritional needs associated with the increased metabolic rate that occurs with pancreatitis.

Desired Outcome	Nursing Actions and *Selected Purposes/Rationales*

3. The client will maintain an adequate nutritional status as evidenced by:
  a. weight within normal range for client's age, height, and body frame
	3.a. Assess for and report signs and symptoms of malnutrition:
	  1. weight below normal for client's age, height, and body frame
	  2. abnormal BUN and low serum albumin, Hct, Hb, transferrin, and lymphocyte levels (albumin levels can also be low because of increased vascular permeability)

Desired Outcome	Nursing Actions and *Selected Purposes/Rationales*

b. normal BUN and serum albumin, Hct, Hb, transferrin, and lymphocyte levels
 	
c. usual strength and activity tolerance
 	
d. healthy oral mucous membrane.
	3. weakness and fatigue
	4. sore, inflamed oral mucous membrane
	5. pale conjunctiva.
	b. When oral intake is allowed, monitor percentage of meals and snacks client consumes. Report a pattern of inadequate intake.
	c. Implement measures *to maintain an adequate nutritional status:*
	  1. administer total parenteral nutrition if ordered
	  2. when food or oral fluids are allowed:
	    a. perform actions *to improve oral intake:*
	      1. implement measures to reduce pain and abdominal distention (see Nursing Diagnoses 4, action e and 5.B, action 3)
	      2. implement measures to reduce nausea and vomiting (see Nursing Diagnosis 5.A, action 2)
	      3. increase activity as allowed and tolerated (*activity usually promotes a sense of well-being and improves appetite*)
	      4. obtain a dietary consult if necessary to assist client in selecting foods/fluids that meet nutritional needs, are appealing, and adhere to personal and cultural preferences as well as the prescribed dietary modifications
	      5. maintain a clean environment and a relaxed, pleasant atmosphere
	      6. provide oral hygiene before meals
	      7. allow adequate time for meals; reheat foods/fluids if necessary
	      8. limit fluid intake with meals (unless the fluids have high nutritional value) *to reduce early satiety and subsequent decreased food intake*
	    b. ensure that meals are well balanced and high in essential nutrients; offer dietary supplements if indicated
	    c. administer the following if ordered:
	      1. vitamins and minerals
	      2. pancreatic enzymes (e.g. pancreatin, pancrelipase) *to facilitate the digestion of proteins, fats, and carbohydrates.*
	d. Perform a calorie count if ordered. Report information to dietitian and physician.
	e. Reassess nutritional status on a regular basis and report decline.

---

4. NURSING DIAGNOSIS: **Pain: abdominal with radiation to the back**

related to:
a. distention of the pancreas associated with inflammation and obstruction of pancreatic ducts;
b. peritoneal irritation associated with escape of activated pancreatic enzymes into the peritoneum.

Desired Outcome	Nursing Actions and *Selected Purposes/Rationales*
4. The client will experience diminished pain as evidenced by: a. verbalization of a decrease in or absence of pain b. relaxed facial expression and body positioning	4.a. Assess for signs and symptoms of pain (e.g. verbalization of pain, guarding of abdomen, rubbing epigastric or flank area, grimacing, reluctance to move, restlessness, diaphoresis, facial pallor, increased B/P, tachycardia). b. Assess client's perception of the severity of pain using a pain intensity rating scale. c. Assess the client's pain pattern (e.g. location, quality, onset, duration, precipitating factors, aggravating factors, alleviating factors).

c. increased participation in
   activities
d. stable vital signs.

d. Ask the client to describe previous pain experiences and methods used to
   manage pain effectively.
e. Implement measures *to reduce pain:*
   1. perform actions *to reduce fear and anxiety about the pain experience*
      (e.g. assure client that his/her need for pain relief is understood, plan
      methods for achieving pain control with client)
   2. perform actions to reduce fear and anxiety (see Nursing Diagnosis 8,
      action b) *in order to promote relaxation and subsequently increase the
      client's threshold and tolerance for pain*
   3. administer analgesics before activities and procedures that can cause
      pain and before pain becomes severe
   4. perform actions to promote rest (e.g. minimize environmental activity
      and noise) *in order to reduce fatigue and subsequently increase the
      client's threshold and tolerance for pain*
   5. perform actions *to reduce pancreatic stimulation:*
      a. withhold all food and oral fluid as ordered (*food and fluid
         [especially those that are acidic or have a high protein or fat
         content] entering the duodenum cause the release of secretin and/
         or cholecystokinin, which stimulates the output of pancreatic
         secretions*)
      b. insert nasogastric tube and maintain suction as ordered *to reduce
         the amount of acid that enters the duodenum* (*hydrochloric acid
         stimulates secretin, which then stimulates the output of pancreatic
         secretions*)
      c. administer the following medications if ordered *to reduce the
         amount of acid-induced secretin release:*
         1. antacids *to neutralize gastric acid*
         2. histamine$_2$ receptor antagonists (e.g. cimetidine, famotidine,
            ranitidine) *to reduce gastric output of hydrochloric acid*
      d. minimize client's exposure to odor and sight of food until
         oral intake is allowed *in order to prevent stimulation of
         gastric secretions and the subsequent output of pancreatic
         secretions*
   6. allow client to sit or lie with knees and trunk flexed (*this position
      relieves pressure on the inflamed pancreas*)
   7. provide or assist with additional nonpharmacologic measures for pain
      relief (e.g. massage; position change; progressive relaxation exercises;
      restful environment; diversional activities such watching television,
      reading, or conversing)
   8. administer analgesics as ordered or encourage client to use patient-
      controlled analgesia (PCA) device as instructed (meperidine is usually
      the analgesic prescribed *because morphine sulfate often intensifies
      pain by increasing spasms of the sphincter of Oddi*)
   9. assist with peritoneal lavage if performed (*may be done to remove
      some of the activated pancreatic enzymes and debris that cause
      peritoneal irritation and subsequent pain*)
   10. when oral intake is allowed, perform actions *to maintain reduced
       pancreatic activity:*
       a. continue to administer antacids and histamine$_2$ receptor antagonists
          as ordered
       b. advance diet slowly
       c. provide small, frequent meals rather than 3 large ones
       d. maintain dietary restrictions of fat intake and caffeinated beverages
          if ordered.
f. Consult physician if above measures fail to provide adequate pain
   relief.

5.A. NURSING DIAGNOSIS: **Altered comfort: nausea and vomiting**

related to stimulation of the vomiting center associated with:
1. stimulation of the visceral afferent pathways resulting from abdominal distention and inflammation of the pancreas;
2. stimulation of the cerebral cortex resulting from pain and stress.

Desired Outcome	Nursing Actions and *Selected Purposes/Rationales*

5.A. The client will experience relief of nausea and vomiting as evidenced by:
1. verbalization of relief of nausea
2. absence of vomiting.
	5.A.1. Assess client for nausea and vomiting.
	  2. Implement measures *to reduce nausea and vomiting:*
	    a. perform actions to reduce fear and anxiety (see Nursing Diagnosis 8, action b)
	    b. perform actions to reduce pain (see Nursing Diagnosis 4, action e)
	    c. perform actions to reduce the accumulation of gastrointestinal gas and fluid (see Nursing Diagnosis 5.B, action 3) *in order to prevent abdominal distention and subsequent visceral irritation*
	    d. maintain food and oral fluid restrictions as ordered
	    e. maintain patency of nasogastric tube (e.g. keep tubing free of kinks, irrigate and maintain suction as ordered) if present
	    f. eliminate noxious sights and odors from the environment (*noxious stimuli can cause stimulation of the vomiting center*)
	    g. encourage client to take deep, slow breaths when nauseated
	    h. instruct client to change positions slowly (*rapid movement can result in chemoreceptor trigger zone stimulation and subsequent excitation of the vomiting center*)
	    i. provide oral hygiene after each emesis
	    j. when oral intake is allowed:
	      1. avoid serving foods with an overpowering aroma; remove lids from hot foods before entering room
	      2. provide small, frequent meals rather than 3 large ones; instruct client to ingest foods and fluids slowly
	      3. instruct client to eat dry foods (e.g. toast, crackers) and avoid drinking liquids with meals if nauseated
	      4. instruct client to avoid foods/fluids that irritate the gastric mucosa (e.g. spicy foods; caffeine-containing beverages such as tea, coffee, and colas)
	      5. instruct client to avoid foods/fluids high in fat (e.g. butter, cream, whole milk, ice cream, fried foods, gravies, nuts) *in order to prevent a delay in gastric emptying and reduce nausea associated with impaired fat digestion*
	      6. instruct the client to rest after eating with head of bed elevated
	    k. administer antiemetics if ordered.
	  3. Consult physician if above measures fail to control nausea and vomiting.

5.B. NURSING DIAGNOSIS: **Altered comfort: abdominal distention and gas pain**

related to accumulation of gastrointestinal gas or fluid associated with:
1. an inability to digest fats properly resulting from obstruction of the flow of lipase;
2. decreased gastrointestinal motility resulting from the depressant effect of some medications (e.g. narcotic [opioid] analgesics) and decreased activity.

Desired Outcome	Nursing Actions and *Selected Purposes/Rationales*

5.B. The client will experience diminished abdominal distention and gas pain as evidenced by:
1. verbalization of same
2. relaxed facial expression and body positioning
3. decrease in abdominal girth.

5.B.1. Assess for verbal reports of abdominal fullness or gas pain.
    2. Assess for nonverbal signs of abdominal distention or gas pain (e.g. grimacing, clutching or guarding of abdomen, restlessness, reluctance to move, increasing abdominal girth).
    3. Implement measures *to reduce the accumulation of gastrointestinal gas and fluid in order to decrease abdominal distention and gas pain:*
      a. encourage and assist client with frequent position changes and ambulation as allowed and tolerated (*activity stimulates peristalsis and expulsion of flatus*)
      b. instruct the client to avoid activities such as gum chewing and smoking *in order to reduce air swallowing*
      c. maintain food and fluid restrictions as ordered
      d. maintain patency of nasogastric tube if present
      e. when oral intake is allowed, instruct client to avoid the following:
        1. carbonated beverages and gas-producing foods (e.g. cabbage, onions, baked beans)
        2. foods/fluids high in fat (e.g. butter, cream, whole milk, ice cream, fried foods, gravies, nuts)
      f. encourage client to eructate and expel flatus whenever the urge is felt
      g. administer the following medications if ordered:
        1. antiflatulents (e.g. simethicone) *to reduce gas accumulation*
        2. pancreatic enzymes (e.g. pancreatin, pancrelipase) *to improve fat digestion*
      h. encourage the use of nonnarcotic analgesics once the period of severe pain has subsided (*narcotic [opioid] analgesics depress gastrointestinal motility*).
    4. Consult physician if signs and symptoms of abdominal distention and gas pain persist or worsen.

---

6. NURSING DIAGNOSIS: **Altered oral mucous membrane: dryness**

related to:
a. fluid volume deficit associated with restricted oral intake and fluid loss resulting from vomiting and nasogastric tube drainage;
b. decreased salivation associated with fluid volume deficit, restricted oral intake, and the side effect of some medications (e.g. narcotic [opioid] analgesics);
c. mouth breathing if nasogastric tube is in place.

Desired Outcome	Nursing Actions and *Selected Purposes/Rationales*

6. The client will maintain a moist, intact oral mucous membrane.

6.a. Assess client for dryness of the oral mucosa.
   b. Implement measures *to decrease dryness of the oral mucous membrane:*
    1. instruct and assist client to perform oral hygiene as often as needed
    2. encourage client to rinse mouth frequently with water
    3. instruct client to avoid use of products that contain lemon and glycerin and use of mouthwashes containing alcohol (*these products have a drying and irritating effect on the oral mucous membrane*)
    4. lubricate client's lips frequently
    5. encourage client to breathe through nose rather than mouth
    6. encourage client not to smoke (*smoking irritates and dries the mucosa*)
    7. maintain intravenous fluid therapy as ordered; when oral intake is allowed, encourage a fluid intake of at least 2500 ml/day unless contraindicated
    8. advance diet as allowed and tolerated *to stimulate salivation.*
   c. Consult physician if dryness persists.

7. COLLABORATIVE DIAGNOSES:

Potential complications of acute pancreatitis:

a. **hypovolemic shock** related to:
   1. fluid volume deficit associated with fluid loss and fluid restrictions
   2. peripheral vasodilation and increased vascular permeability with subsequent third-spacing associated with activation of bradykinin and kallidin (trypsin activates the peptide kallikrein, which then activates these vasoactive substances)
   3. hemorrhage associated with destruction of elastic fibers of the blood vessels by the proteolytic enzyme elastase (elastase is activated in the pancreas by trypsin and causes localized vessel damage in addition to the vessel wall destruction that occurs when it enters the systemic circulation);

b. **pancreatic necrosis, pseudocyst, or abscess** related to destruction of the pancreatic and surrounding tissue by the activated proteolytic enzymes;

c. **peritonitis** related to:
   1. escape of activated pancreatic enzymes from the pancreas into the peritoneum
   2. leakage of necrotic substances into the peritoneum associated with rupture of an abscess or infected pancreatic pseudocyst
   3. suppuration in areas of pancreatic and peripancreatic necrosis;

d. **hyperglycemia** related to:
   1. increased glucagon and decreased insulin output associated with damage to the pancreatic islet cells resulting from activation of pancreatic enzymes in the pancreas
   2. the increased glucagon, cortisol, and catecholamine output that occurs with stress;

e. **pleural effusion** related to:
   1. increased capillary permeability associated with damage to pleural vessels resulting from the escape of activated pancreatic enzymes into the systemic circulation
   2. passage of exudate from the peritoneal cavity to the pleural cavity through the diaphragmatic lymph channels;

f. **adult respiratory distress syndrome (ARDS)** related to increased alveolar-capillary membrane permeability associated with the release of activated pancreatic enzymes into the systemic circulation.

Desired Outcomes	Nursing Actions and *Selected Purposes/Rationales*

7.a. The client will not develop hypovolemic shock as evidenced by:
   1. usual mental status
   2. stable vital signs
   3. skin warm, dry, and usual color
   4. palpable peripheral pulses
   5. urine output at least 30 ml/hour.

7.a.1. Assess for and report signs and symptoms of:
   a. fluid volume deficit and third-spacing (see Nursing Diagnosis 2, actions a.1.a and b.1 for signs and symptoms)
   b. bleeding (e.g. gray-blue discoloration around umbilicus [Cullen's sign], green-blue or purple-blue discoloration of flanks [Grey Turner's sign], increased abdominal or back pain, increased abdominal girth, decreasing B/P and increased pulse rate, decreased Hct and Hb levels)
   c. hypovolemic shock:
      1. restlessness, agitation, confusion, or other change in mental status
      2. significant decrease in B/P
      3. postural hypotension
      4. rapid, weak pulse
      5. rapid respirations
      6. cool, moist skin
      7. pallor, cyanosis
      8. diminished or absent peripheral pulses
      9. urine output less than 30 ml/hour.
   2. Implement measures *to prevent hypovolemic shock:*
      a. perform actions to prevent or treat fluid and electrolyte imbalances (see Nursing Diagnosis 2, actions a.3 and b.4)
      b. perform actions to reduce pancreatic stimulation (see Nursing Diagnosis 4, action e.5) *in order to decrease the amount of elastase*

that is activated and released into the tissue and systemic circulation and thereby reduce the risk for bleeding.

3. If signs and symptoms of hypovolemic shock occur:
   a. continue with above actions
   b. place client flat in bed with legs elevated unless contraindicated
   c. monitor vital signs frequently
   d. administer oxygen as ordered
   e. administer whole blood, blood products, and/or volume expanders if ordered
   f. prepare client for insertion of hemodynamic monitoring devices (e.g. central venous catheter, intra-arterial catheter) if indicated
   g. provide emotional support to client and significant others.

7.b. The client will have resolution of pancreatic necrosis, pseudocyst, or abscess if it develops as evidenced by:
1. decrease in abdominal pain
2. temperature declining toward normal
3. WBC count declining toward normal.

7.b.1. Assess for and report signs and symptoms of pancreatic necrosis, pseudocyst, or abscess (e.g. increased or more constant abdominal pain, persistent or recurrent increase in temperature, further increase in WBC count).

2. If signs and symptoms of pancreatic necrosis, pseudocyst, or abscess occur:
   a. prepare client for diagnostic studies (e.g. computed tomography, ultrasonography, magnetic resonance imaging)
   b. administer antimicrobials if ordered
   c. prepare client for drainage of the necrotic area, pseudocyst, or abscess if planned
   d. assess for and report signs and symptoms of infection (e.g. further increase in temperature; chills; tachycardia; further increase in WBC count; positive results of cultures from necrotic area, pseudocyst, or abscess).

7.c. The client will not develop peritonitis as evidenced by:
1. gradual resolution of abdominal pain
2. soft, nondistended abdomen
3. temperature declining toward normal
4. stable vital signs
5. decreased nausea and vomiting
6. gradual return of normal bowel sounds
7. WBC count declining toward normal.

7.c.1. Assess for and report signs and symptoms of peritonitis (e.g. increase in severity of abdominal pain; generalized abdominal pain; rebound tenderness; distended, rigid abdomen; further increase in temperature; tachycardia; tachypnea; hypotension; increased nausea and vomiting; diminished or absent bowel sounds).

2. Monitor WBC counts. Report levels that increase or fail to return toward normal.

3. Implement measures *to prevent peritonitis:*
   a. perform actions to reduce pancreatic stimulation (see Nursing Diagnosis 4, action e.5) *in order to decrease the activation of pancreatic enzymes within the pancreas and reduce the risk for their escape into the peritoneum*
   b. administer antimicrobials if ordered (*may be ordered prophylactically to prevent peritonitis, especially if culture of drainage from a necrotic area, pseudocyst, or abscess is positive*).

4. If signs and symptoms of peritonitis occur:
   a. withhold oral intake as ordered
   b. place client on bed rest in a semi-Fowler's position *to assist in pooling or localizing gastrointestinal contents in the pelvis rather than under the diaphragm*
   c. prepare client for diagnostic tests (e.g. abdominal x-ray, computed tomography, ultrasonography) if planned
   d. insert a nasogastric tube and maintain suction as ordered
   e. administer antimicrobials as ordered
   f. administer intravenous fluids and/or blood volume expanders if ordered *to prevent or treat shock (can result from the increased capillary permeability that occurs with inflammation and the subsequent escape of protein, fluid, and electrolytes from the vascular space into the peritoneal cavity)*
   g. prepare client for and assist with peritoneal lavage if performed *to remove toxins from the peritoneal cavity*
   h. provide emotional support to client and significant others.

Desired Outcomes	Nursing Actions and *Selected Purposes/Rationales*

7.d. The client will maintain a safe blood glucose level as evidenced by:
  1. absence of polydipsia, polyuria, and polyphagia
  2. usual mental status
  3. serum glucose between 70–200 mg/dl.

7.d.1. Assess for and report signs and symptoms of hyperglycemia (e.g. polydipsia; polyuria; polyphagia; change in mental status).
  2. Monitor blood glucose levels. Report values above 200 mg/dl or greater than the parameter specified by physician.
  3. Implement measures *to prevent hyperglycemia:*
      a. perform actions to reduce pancreatic stimulation (see Nursing Diagnosis 4, action e.5) *in order to prevent further damage to the pancreatic islet cells*
      b. perform actions to reduce fear and anxiety and pain (see Nursing Diagnoses 8, action b and 4, action e) *in order to reduce emotional and physiological stress (stress causes an increased output of epinephrine, norepinephrine, glucagon, and cortisol, which results in a further increase in blood glucose).*
  4. If signs and symptoms of hyperglycemia occur:
      a. administer insulin or oral hypoglycemic agents if ordered
      b. assess for and report signs and symptoms of ketoacidosis (e.g. warm, flushed skin; thirst; weakness; lethargy; hypotension; increased abdominal pain; fruity odor on breath; Kussmaul respirations; blood glucose above 300 mg/dl; ketones in blood and urine; low serum pH and CO_2 content)
      c. if client does not have a history of diabetes or chronic pancreatitis, assure him/her that the hyperglycemia is expected to resolve as the pancreatitis does.

7.e. The client will not experience pleural effusion as evidenced by:
  1. unlabored respirations at 14–20/minute
  2. symmetrical chest movement
  3. resonant percussion note throughout lung fields
  4. normal breath sounds.

7.e.1. Assess for and report signs and symptoms of pleural effusion (e.g. dyspnea, chest pain, decreased chest excursion on affected side, dull percussion note and diminished or absent breath sounds over the affected area).
  2. Monitor chest x-ray results. Report findings of pleural effusion.
  3. Implement measures to reduce pancreatic stimulation (see Nursing Diagnosis 4, action e.5) *in order to reduce the release of activated pancreatic enzymes into the systemic circulation and diaphragmatic lymph channels.*
  4. If signs and symptoms of pleural effusion occur, prepare client for thoracentesis if planned.

7.f. The client will not experience ARDS as evidenced by:
  1. unlabored respirations at 14–20/minute
  2. usual skin color
  3. usual mental status
  4. blood gases within normal range.

7.f.1. Assess for and report signs and symptoms of ARDS (e.g. rapid, shallow respirations; sternocleidomastoid muscle retraction; dusky or cyanotic skin color; drowsiness; confusion).
  2. Monitor for and report:
      a. abnormal blood gas values (progressive arterial hypoxemia even when receiving increasing amounts of oxygen is indicative of ARDS)
      b. significant decrease in oximetry results
      c. findings of atelectasis or pulmonary edema on chest x-ray.
  3. Implement measures to reduce pancreatic stimulation (see Nursing Diagnosis 4, action e.5) *in order to reduce the amount of pancreatic enzymes in the systemic circulation and the subsequent increased risk for damage to the alveolar-capillary membranes.*
  4. If signs and symptoms of ARDS occur:
      a. administer diuretics if ordered *to reduce pulmonary edema*
      b. maintain oxygen therapy as ordered
      c. assist with intubation, mechanical ventilation, and transfer to critical care unit if indicated
      d. provide emotional support to client and significant others.

■

8. NURSING DIAGNOSIS: **Anxiety**

related to severe pain; unknown diagnosis; unfamiliar environment; and lack of understanding of diagnostic tests, treatment plan, and prognosis.

Desired Outcome	Nursing Actions and *Selected Purposes/Rationales*
8. The client will experience a reduction in anxiety as evidenced by: a. verbalization of feeling less anxious b. usual sleep pattern c. relaxed facial expression and body movements d. stable vital signs e. usual perceptual ability and interactions with others.	8.a. Assess client for signs and symptoms of anxiety (e.g. verbalization of feeling anxious, insomnia, tenseness, shakiness, restlessness, diaphoresis, tachycardia, elevated blood pressure, facial pallor, self-focused behaviors). Validate perceptions carefully, remembering that some behavior may be a physiological response to pain. b. Implement measures *to reduce fear and anxiety:* 1. perform actions to reduce pain (see Nursing Diagnosis 4, action e) 2. orient client to hospital environment, equipment, and routines 3. introduce client to staff who will be participating in care; if possible, maintain consistency in staff assigned to his/her care *to provide feelings of stability and comfort with the environment* 4. assure client that staff members are nearby; respond to call signal as soon as possible 5. maintain a calm, supportive, confident manner when interacting with client 6. encourage verbalization of fear and anxiety; provide feedback 7. explain all diagnostic tests 8. reinforce physician's explanations and clarify misconceptions the client has about pancreatitis, the treatment plan, and prognosis 9. provide a calm, restful environment 10. instruct client in relaxation techniques and encourage participation in diversional activities once severe pain has subsided 11. assist client to identify specific stressors and ways to cope with them 12. provide information based on current needs of client at a level he/she can understand; encourage questions and clarification of information provided 13. encourage significant others to project a caring, concerned attitude without obvious anxiousness 14. include significant others in orientation and teaching sessions and encourage their continued support of the client 15. administer prescribed antianxiety agents if indicated. c. Consult physician if above measures fail to control fear and anxiety.

Discharge Teaching

9. NURSING DIAGNOSIS: **Knowledge deficit, Ineffective management of therapeutic regimen, or Altered health maintenance***

*The nurse should select the diagnostic label that is most appropriate for the client's discharge teaching needs.

Desired Outcomes	Nursing Actions and *Selected Purposes/Rationales*
9.a. The client will identify ways to prevent overstimulation of and further trauma to the pancreas.	9.a.1. Instruct client in importance of avoiding overstimulation of the pancreas for the length of time specified by the physician (may be for a few months or for his/her lifetime depending on the cause of the pancreatitis and if permanent pancreatic damage has occurred). 2. Instruct client in ways to prevent overstimulation of and further trauma to the pancreas: a. maintain a balanced program of rest and exercise b. avoid stressful situations c. avoid drinking alcohol d. adhere to recommended dietary modifications (see action b.1 in this diagnosis) e. maintain a relaxed atmosphere during and after meals.

Desired Outcomes	Nursing Actions and *Selected Purposes/Rationales*
	3. Assist client to identify ways he/she can make necessary changes in personal habits and life style.

9.b. The client will verbalize an understanding of recommended dietary modifications.	9.b.1. Instruct client regarding dietary modifications necessary to prevent overstimulation of the pancreas during the recovery period:
	   a. eat small, frequent meals rather than 3 large ones
	   b. avoid foods/fluids high in fat (e.g. butter, cream, whole milk, ice cream, fried foods, gravies, nuts)
	   c. avoid caffeine-containing beverages (e.g. coffee, tea, colas).
	2. Obtain a dietary consult if client needs assistance in planning meals that incorporate dietary modifications.

9.c. The client will state signs and symptoms to report to the health care provider.	9.c. Instruct client to report:
	  1. stools that float and are grayish, greasy, and foul-smelling (indicates a very high fat content resulting from impaired flow of the pancreatic enzyme lipase into the intestinal tract)
	  2. severe abdominal or back pain
	  3. persistent nausea or vomiting
	  4. abdominal distention or increasing feeling of fullness
	  5. excessive thirst or excessive urination
	  6. irritability or confusion
	  7. continued or unexplained weight loss
	  8. bluish areas on the back or abdomen
	  9. elevated temperature that lasts more than 2 days
	 10. tremors or seizures
	 11. difficulty breathing
	 12. reddened, tender nodules on skin (could be indicative of destruction of superficial fatty tissue by activated pancreatic enzymes such as lipase and phospholipase A that have entered the systemic circulation and tissue; if this relatively rare condition occurs, it is usually weeks to months after the episode of acute pancreatitis).

9.d. The client will verbalize an understanding of and a plan for adhering to recommended follow-up care including future appointments with health care provider and medications prescribed.	9.d.1. Reinforce the importance of keeping follow-up appointments with health care provider.
	2. Explain the rationale for, side effects of, and importance of taking medications prescribed (e.g. vitamins, antacids, histamine$_2$ receptor antagonists, pancreatic enzymes). Inform client of pertinent food and drug interactions.
	3. Implement measures to improve client compliance:
	   a. include significant others in teaching sessions if possible
	   b. encourage questions and allow time for reinforcement and clarification of information provided
	   c. provide written instructions on scheduled appointments with health care provider, medications prescribed, and signs and symptoms to report.

Bibliography

See pages 897–898 and 908.

CHOLECYSTECTOMY

A cholecystectomy is the surgical removal of the gall-bladder. It is commonly performed to treat symptomatic cholecystitis and/or cholelithiasis. A cholecystectomy can be done via laparoscopy or through a right subcostal incision (open cholecystectomy). A laparoscopic chole-cystectomy is usually the procedure of choice because of the short hospitalization (less than 2 days), minimal residual scarring, reduced pain, and a more rapid return to usual activities. An open cholecystectomy is war-ranted when the client has a gangrenous gallbladder, a serious bleeding disorder, severe inflammation that obscures the structures of the hepatobiliary triangle, or large stones in the biliary ducts, and when problems are encountered during a laparoscopic cholecystectomy. If stones are found in the common bile duct during an open cholecystectomy, a choledocholithotomy is per-formed and a T tube is usually placed in the common bile duct to maintain adequate flow or drainage of bile until ductal edema subsides.

This care plan focuses on the adult client hospitalized for an open cholecystectomy with common bile duct exploration. Preoperatively, the goals of care are to maintain comfort, reduce fear and anxiety, and prepare the client for the postoperative period. Postoperative goals of care are to maintain comfort, maintain skin integrity, prevent complications, and educate the client regarding follow-up care.

DIAGNOSTIC TESTS

Refer to Care Plan on Cholelithiasis/Cholecystitis.

DISCHARGE CRITERIA

Prior to discharge, the client will:

- have pain controlled
- tolerate prescribed diet
- have evidence of normal healing of surgical wound(s) and normal skin integrity around T tube site
- have clear, audible breath sounds throughout lungs
- have no signs and symptoms of postoperative complications
- demonstrate the ability to appropriately care for T tube and surrounding skin if T tube is present
- verbalize an understanding of the rationale for and components of a low- to moderate-fat diet if prescribed
- state signs and symptoms to report to the health care provider
- verbalize an understanding of and a plan for adhering to recommended follow-up care including future appointments with health care provider, wound care, medications prescribed, and activity level.

NURSING/ COLLABORATIVE DIAGNOSES	**Postoperative**
	1. Ineffective breathing pattern △ 668
	2. Altered nutrition: less than body requirements △ 668
	3. Actual/Risk for impaired tissue integrity △ 669
	4. Potential complications:
	a. abscess formation
	b. peritonitis
	c. continued obstruction of bile flow △ 669
DISCHARGE TEACHING	5. Knowledge deficit, Ineffective management of therapeutic regimen, or Altered health maintenance △ 671

See Care Plan on Cholelithiasis/Cholecystitis and the Standardized Preoperative and Postoperative Care Plans for additional diagnoses.

PREOPERATIVE

Refer to the Care Plan on Cholelithiasis/Cholecystitis and the Standardized Preoperative Care Plan.

POSTOPERATIVE

Use in conjunction with the Standardized Postoperative Care Plan.

---

1. NURSING DIAGNOSIS:

Ineffective breathing pattern

related to:
a. increased rate and decreased depth of respirations associated with fear and anxiety;
b. decreased rate and depth of respirations associated with the depressant effect of anesthesia and some medications (e.g. narcotic [opioid] analgesics);
c. diminished lung/chest wall expansion associated with positioning, weakness, fatigue, abdominal distention, and reluctance to breathe deeply because of a high abdominal incision.

Desired Outcome	Nursing Actions and *Selected Purposes/Rationales*

1. The client will maintain an effective breathing pattern (see Standardized Postoperative Care Plan, Nursing Diagnosis 2 [p. 102], for outcome criteria).	1.a. Refer to Standardized Postoperative Care Plan, Nursing Diagnosis 2 (pp. 102–103), for measures related to assessment and management of an ineffective breathing pattern.
	   b. Implement additional measures *to improve breathing pattern:*
	      1. instruct client to bend knees while coughing and deep breathing *in order to relieve tension on abdominal muscles and incision*
	      2. instruct and assist client to splint incision with hands or pillow when coughing and deep breathing.

---

2. NURSING DIAGNOSIS:

Altered nutrition: less than body requirements

related to:
a. loss of nutrients associated with vomiting and nasogastric tube drainage;
b. decreased oral intake associated with prescribed dietary modifications, pain, fatigue, nausea, dislike of prescribed diet, and feeling of fullness (can occur as a result of abdominal distention);
c. inadequate nutritional replacement therapy;
d. increased nutritional needs associated with the increased metabolic rate that occurs during healing;
e. decreased absorption of fats and fat-soluble vitamins associated with excessive loss or obstructed flow of bile.

Desired Outcome	Nursing Actions and *Selected Purposes/Rationales*
2. The client will maintain an adequate nutritional status (see Standardized Postoperative Care Plan, Nursing Diagnosis 5 [pp. 105–106], for outcome criteria).	2.a. Refer to Standardized Postoperative Care Plan, Nursing Diagnosis 5 (pp. 105–106), for measures related to assessment and maintenance of an adequate nutritional status. b. Clamp T tube before, during, and after meals if ordered and as tolerated (several days following surgery, the T tube is often clamped 1–2 hours before meals and not unclamped until 1–2 hours after meals if tolerated) *to allow bile to drain into the duodenum and aid digestion and the absorption of fat-soluble vitamins.*

3. NURSING DIAGNOSIS:

Actual/Risk for impaired tissue integrity

related to:
a. disruption of tissue associated with the surgical procedure;
b. delayed wound healing associated with factors such as decreased nutritional status and inadequate blood supply to wound area;
c. irritation of skin associated with pressure from tubes, use of tape, and contact with wound and/or T tube drainage (bile is extremely irritating to the skin).

Desired Outcomes	Nursing Actions and *Selected Purposes/Rationales*
3.a. The client will experience normal healing of surgical wounds (see Standardized Postoperative Care Plan, Nursing Diagnosis 9, outcome a [pp. 109–110], for outcome criteria).	3.a. Refer to Standardized Postoperative Care Plan, Nursing Diagnosis 9, action a (pp. 109–110), for measures related to assessment and promotion of wound healing.
3.b. The client will maintain tissue integrity in areas in contact with drainage, tape, and tubings (see Standardized Postoperative Care Plan, Nursing Diagnosis 9, outcome b [p. 110], for outcome criteria).	3.b. Refer to Standardized Postoperative Care Plan, Nursing Diagnosis 9, action b (pp. 110–111), for measures related to assessment and prevention of tissue irritation and breakdown.

4. COLLABORATIVE DIAGNOSES:

Potential complications of cholecystectomy:

a. **abscess formation** related to accumulation of drainage in the surgical area and subsequent invasion of the area by microorganisms and neutrophils;
b. **peritonitis** related to escape of bile into the peritoneal cavity associated with surgical trauma to the gallbladder and biliary duct;
c. **continued obstruction of bile flow** related to residual stones in the biliary duct system or persistent inflammation and/or strictures of the common bile duct associated with surgical trauma.

Desired Outcomes	Nursing Actions and *Selected Purposes/Rationales*

4.a. The client will not develop an abscess as evidenced by:
1. gradual resolution of abdominal pain
2. temperature declining toward normal
3. WBC count declining toward normal.
	4.a.1. Assess for and report signs and symptoms of an abscess (e.g. increased or more constant abdominal pain, increase in temperature and pulse rate, further increase in WBC count).
	2. Implement measures *to prevent accumulation of drainage in the surgical area in order to reduce risk of abscess formation:*
	  a. perform actions *to maintain patency of wound drain and/or T tube if present:*
	    1. implement measures *to prevent stasis and reflux of drainage:*
	      a. keep drainage tubing free of dependent loops and kinks (prevent kinking by placing a gauze roll under the drain tube and anchoring it to the skin with tape)
	      b. keep collection device(s) below drain insertion site(s) unless ordered otherwise (physician may order T tube collection

Desired Outcomes	Nursing Actions and *Selected Purposes/Rationales*
	device to be positioned just slightly below, level with, or above drain insertion site *in order to reduce loss of bile*)
	c. empty collection device(s) as often as necessary and at least every shift
	2. implement measures *to prevent inadvertent removal of wound drain and/or T tube:*
	a. instruct client not to pull on drain(s) and drainage tubing
	b. use caution when changing dressings surrounding drain(s)
	c. attach collection device(s) securely to abdominal dressing
	b. maintain client in a semi- to high-Fowler's position as much as possible when in bed.
	3. If signs and symptoms of an abscess occur:
	a. prepare client for diagnostic tests (e.g. ultrasonography, computed tomography)
	b. administer antimicrobials if ordered
	c. prepare client for surgical intervention (e.g. incision and drainage of abscess) if planned
	d. provide emotional support to client and significant others.

Desired Outcomes	Nursing Actions and *Selected Purposes/Rationales*
4.b. The client will not develop peritonitis as evidenced by: 1. gradual resolution of abdominal pain 2. soft, nondistended abdomen 3. temperature declining toward normal 4. stable vital signs 5. absence of nausea and vomiting 6. gradual return of normal bowel sounds 7. WBC count declining toward normal.	4.b.1. Assess for and report signs and symptoms of peritonitis (e.g. increase in severity of abdominal pain; generalized abdominal pain; rebound tenderness; distended, rigid abdomen; increase in temperature; tachycardia; tachypnea; hypotension; nausea; vomiting; continued diminished or absent bowel sounds). 2. Monitor WBC counts. Report levels that increase or fail to decline toward normal. 3. Implement measures *to prevent peritonitis:* a. perform actions to maintain patency and prevent inadvertent removal of wound drain and/or T tube if present (see actions a.2.a in this diagnosis) *in order to reduce the risk for wound drainage and bile accumulating and leaking into the peritoneum* b. administer antimicrobials if ordered. 4. If signs and symptoms of peritonitis occur: a. withhold oral intake as ordered b. place client on bed rest in a semi-Fowler's position *to assist in pooling or localizing gastrointestinal contents in the pelvis rather than under the diaphragm* c. prepare client for diagnostic tests (e.g. abdominal x-ray, peritoneal aspiration, computed tomography, ultrasonography) d. insert a nasogastric tube or intestinal tube and maintain suction as ordered e. administer antimicrobials as ordered f. administer intravenous fluids and/or blood volume expanders if ordered *to prevent or treat shock (can result from the increased capillary permeability that occurs with inflammation and the subsequent escape of protein, fluid, and electrolytes from the vascular space into the peritoneal cavity)* g. prepare client for surgical intervention (e.g. drainage and irrigation of peritoneum, repair of leakage site) if planned h. provide emotional support to client and significant others.
4.c. The client will have resolution of bile flow obstruction within 7–10 days after surgery as evidenced by: 1. decline in output of bile in T tube to less than 400 ml/day 2. absence of pain, nausea, and feeling of fullness when T tube is clamped	4.c.1. Assess for and report signs and symptoms of continued bile flow obstruction (e.g. T tube draining more than 1000 ml in 24 hours; a marked increase in T tube drainage after it has started to decline; persistent pain, nausea, or feeling of fullness when T tube is clamped; jaundice; clay-colored stools; dark amber urine). 2. If signs and symptoms of bile flow obstruction occur: a. leave T tube unclamped b. perform actions to maintain patency of T tube (see action a.2.a in this diagnosis) c. prepare client for diagnostic tests (e.g. ultrasound, cholangiogram) if planned

3. absence of jaundice, clay-colored stools, and dark amber urine.

d. prepare client for removal of residual stones (e.g. extraction via T tube, endoscopic sphincterotomy with basket removal of stones) or treatment of bile duct stricture (e.g. endoscopic or percutaneous balloon dilatation with or without stent placement, surgical resection of stricture site) if planned

e. provide emotional support to client and significant others.

Discharge Teaching

5. NURSING DIAGNOSIS: **Knowledge deficit, Ineffective management of therapeutic regimen, or Altered health maintenance***

---

*The nurse should select the diagnostic label that is most appropriate for the client's discharge teaching needs.

Desired Outcomes	Nursing Actions and *Selected Purposes/Rationales*
5.a. The client will demonstrate the ability to appropriately care for T tube and surrounding skin if T tube is present.	5.a.1. If the client is to be discharged with a T tube in place, instruct regarding care of the T tube and surrounding skin: a. cleanse the skin around the T tube insertion site daily and cover the site with a dry sterile dressing b. keep the T tube drainage collection device in the position prescribed (usually slightly below the insertion site) c. keep the tubing pinned to the dressing and avoid any kinks or strain on the tubing d. empty the drainage collection device at least twice daily or more often if needed; keep a record of the amount of drainage e. when emptying the drainage collection device, check to see that the tube has not become dislodged (this can be easily monitored if the tube is marked at the skin line before discharge) f. clamp T tube only as instructed. 2. Allow time for questions, clarification, and return demonstration of care of T tube and surrounding skin.
5.b. The client will verbalize an understanding of the rationale for and components of a low- to moderate-fat diet if prescribed.	5.b.1. Explain the rationale for avoiding excessive fat intake for the first 4–6 weeks after surgery (some physicians instruct client to avoid only those foods that cause epigastric discomfort). 2. Instruct client to increase fat intake gradually and introduce foods/fluids high in fat (e.g. butter, cream, whole milk, ice cream, fried foods, gravies, nuts) one at a time.
5.c. The client will state signs and symptoms to report to the health care provider.	5.c.1. Refer to Standardized Postoperative Care Plan, Nursing Diagnosis 21, action c (p. 123), for signs and symptoms to report to health care provider. 2. Instruct client to report these additional signs and symptoms: a. development of increased itchiness or yellowing of skin b. clay-colored stools or dark amber urine c. purulent drainage from the T tube or green-brown drainage around T tube or from wound site d. a significant increase in or more than 500 ml/day of drainage from T tube e. a sudden marked decrease in T tube drainage or increase in length of the T tube (may indicate that the T tube has become dislodged) f. recurrent or persistent abdominal pain g. abdominal distention or rigidity h. recurrent or persistent temperature elevation i. persistent heartburn, feeling of bloating, or nausea j. loose stools that continue for longer than 2–3 months.

Desired Outcomes	Nursing Actions and *Selected Purposes/Rationales*
5.d. The client will verbalize an understanding of and a plan for adhering to recommended follow-up care including future appointments with health care provider, wound care, medications prescribed, and activity level.	5.d.1. Refer to Standardized Postoperative Care Plan, Nursing Diagnosis 21 (pp. 123–124), for routine postoperative instructions and measures to improve client compliance. 2. Instruct client to avoid lifting objects weighing over 10 pounds for 4–6 weeks after surgery.

Bibliography

See pages 897–898 and 908.

 # CHOLELITHIASIS/CHOLECYSTITIS

Cholelithiasis refers to the presence of gallstones in the gallbladder. The two major types of gallstones are cholesterol stones and pigment stones. Cholesterol stones, the most prevalent type, form when bile becomes supersaturated with cholesterol, which then precipitates and starts to form stones. Stones either remain in the gallbladder or migrate into the duct system where they may cause partial or complete obstruction. The severity of the client's symptoms depends on the degree of bile flow obstruction.

Cholecystitis is inflammation of the gallbladder wall. The majority of cases of cholecystitis result from bile stasis, which is most commonly due to obstruction of the cystic duct by a gallstone. The bile trapped in the gallbladder acts as a chemical irritant causing inflammation and edema of the gallbladder wall. The stasis of bile can also lead to bacterial proliferation in the gallbladder. Following the period of acute inflammation, scarring often develops, resulting in loss of normal gallbladder function.

In most cases, the treatment of choice for symptomatic cholelithiasis and cholecystitis is cholecystectomy and choledocholithotomy if stones have migrated into the biliary duct system. A percutaneous cholecystostomy may be done to relieve symptoms if the client has severe symptoms and is a poor surgical risk. Nonsurgical treatment modalities such as endoscopic sphincterotomy with basket removal of stones, dissolution of stones using oral bile acids (e.g. ursodeoxycholic acid [ursodiol, Actigall]), percutaneous or endoscopic instillation of a dissolution agent such as methyl tertiary butyl ether (MTBE) into the gallbladder, and extracorporeal shock-wave lithotripsy or intracorporeal lithotripsy are also options for the treatment of gallstones.

This care plan focuses on the adult client hospitalized with probable cholelithiasis and/or cholecystitis. The goals of treatment are to relieve discomfort, restore or maintain fluid and electrolyte balance, prevent complications, and educate the client regarding follow-up care.

DIAGNOSTIC TESTS

Abdominal x-ray
Ultrasonography
Cholecystography
Percutaneous transhepatic or intravenous cholangiography
Endoscopic retrograde cholangiopancreatography (ERCP)
Radionuclide imaging (e.g. HIDA or DISIDA scan)
Computed tomography (CT)
White blood cell (WBC) count and differential
Serum bilirubin and amylase
Serum transaminases and alkaline phosphatase

DISCHARGE CRITERIA

Prior to discharge, the client will:

- have relief of severe pain
- tolerate prescribed diet
- be free of signs and symptoms of complications
- verbalize an understanding of ways to reduce the risk for recurrent gallbladder attacks
- state signs and symptoms to report to the health care provider
- verbalize an understanding of and a plan for adhering to recommended follow-up care including future appointments with health care provider and medications prescribed.

NURSING/ COLLABORATIVE DIAGNOSES	1. Altered fluid and electrolyte balance: fluid volume deficit, hypokalemia, hypochloremia, and metabolic alkalosis △ 673
	2. Altered nutrition: less than body requirements △ 674
	3. Pain: epigastric area or right upper quadrant of abdomen with radiation to interscapular area or right scapula or shoulder △ 675
	4A. Altered comfort: pruritus △ 676
	4B. Altered comfort: nausea and vomiting △ 676
	4C. Altered comfort: dyspepsia △ 677
	5. Altered oral mucous membrane: dryness △ 678
	6. Potential complications:
	a. abscess or fistula formation
	b. peritonitis
	c. pancreatitis
	d. cholangitis △ 678
	7. Anxiety △ 680
DISCHARGE TEACHING	8. Knowledge deficit, Ineffective management of therapeutic regimen, or Altered health maintenance △ 681

---

1. NURSING/COLLABORATIVE DIAGNOSIS:	**Altered fluid and electrolyte balance: fluid volume deficit, hypokalemia, hypochloremia, and metabolic alkalosis**
	related to decreased oral intake and excessive loss of fluid and electrolytes associated with vomiting and nasogastric tube drainage.

Desired Outcome	Nursing Actions and *Selected Purposes/Rationales*

1. The client will maintain fluid and electrolyte balance as evidenced by:
a. normal skin turgor
b. moist mucous membranes
c. stable weight
d. B/P and pulse within normal range for client and stable with position change
e. hand vein filling time less than 3–5 seconds
	1.a. Assess for and report signs and symptoms of:
	  1. fluid volume deficit:
	    a. decreased skin turgor, dry mucous membranes, thirst
	    b. sudden weight loss of 2% or greater
	    c. postural hypotension and/or low B/P
	    d. weak, rapid pulse
	    e. delayed hand vein filling time (longer than 3–5 seconds)
	    f. change in mental status
	    g. decreased urine output with increased specific gravity (reflects an actual rather than potential fluid volume deficit)
	    h. increased BUN and Hct
	  2. hypokalemia (e.g. cardiac dysrhythmias, postural hypotension, muscle

Desired Outcome	Nursing Actions and *Selected Purposes/Rationales*

f. usual mental status
g. balanced intake and output
h. urine specific gravity within normal range
i. soft, nondistended abdomen with normal bowel sounds
j. absence of cardiac dysrhythmias, muscle weakness, paresthesias, twitching, spasms, and dizziness
k. BUN, Hct, serum electrolytes, and blood gases within normal range.
	weakness, nausea and vomiting, abdominal distention, hypoactive or absent bowel sounds)
	3. hypochloremia and metabolic alkalosis (e.g. dizziness, irritability, paresthesias, muscle twitching or spasms, hypoventilation).
	b. Monitor serum electrolyte and blood gas results. Report abnormal values.
	c. Implement measures *to prevent or treat fluid and electrolyte imbalances:*
	  1. perform actions to reduce nausea and vomiting (see Nursing Diagnosis 4.B, action 2)
	  2. if irrigation of nasogastric tube is indicated, use normal saline rather than water
	  3. maintain a fluid intake of at least 2500 ml/day unless contraindicated; if oral intake is inadequate or contraindicated, maintain intravenous therapy as ordered
	  4. administer electrolyte replacements if ordered
	  5. when oral intake is allowed, assist client to select foods/fluids high in potassium (e.g. bananas, potatoes, raisins, apricots, orange juice, cantaloupe).
	d. Consult physician if signs and symptoms of fluid and electrolyte imbalances persist or worsen.

■————————————————————————————————————

2. NURSING DIAGNOSIS:

Altered nutrition: less than body requirements

related to:
a. decreased oral intake associated with nausea, dyspepsia, pain, and self-imposed or prescribed dietary restrictions;
b. loss of nutrients associated with vomiting;
c. decreased absorption of fats and fat-soluble vitamins associated with bile flow obstruction.

Desired Outcome	Nursing Actions and *Selected Purposes/Rationales*

2. The client will maintain an adequate nutritional status as evidenced by:
a. weight within normal range for client's age, height, and body frame
b. normal BUN and serum albumin, Hct, Hb, transferrin, and lymphocyte levels
c. usual strength and activity tolerance
d. healthy oral mucous membrane.
	2.a. Assess for and report signs and symptoms of malnutrition:
	  1. weight below normal for client's age, height, and body frame
	  2. abnormal BUN and low serum albumin, Hct, Hb, transferrin, and lymphocyte levels
	  3. weakness and fatigue
	  4. sore, inflamed oral mucous membrane
	  5. pale conjunctiva.
	b. Monitor percentage of meals and snacks client consumes. Report a pattern of inadequate intake.
	c. Implement measures *to maintain an adequate nutritional status:*
	  1. when food or oral fluids are allowed, perform actions *to improve oral intake:*
	    a. implement measures to reduce nausea, vomiting, and dyspepsia (see Nursing Diagnoses 4.B, action 2 and 4.C, action 3)
	    b. implement measures to reduce pain (see Nursing Diagnosis 3, action e)
	    c. obtain a dietary consult if necessary to assist client in selecting foods/fluids that meet nutritional needs, are appealing, and adhere to personal and cultural preferences as well as the prescribed dietary modifications
	    d. provide oral hygiene before meals
	    e. maintain a clean environment and a relaxed, pleasant atmosphere
	    f. allow adequate time for meals; reheat foods/fluids if necessary
	  2. ensure that meals are well balanced and high in essential nutrients (diet

may be advanced from powdered protein and carbohydrate supplements in skim milk to a low- to moderate-fat diet); offer dietary supplements if indicated

    3. administer vitamins and minerals (e.g. fat-soluble vitamins) if ordered.

d. Perform a calorie count if ordered. Report information to dietitian and physician.

e. Consult physician regarding an alternative method of providing nutrition (e.g. parenteral nutrition) if client does not consume enough food or fluids to meet nutritional needs.

---

3. NURSING DIAGNOSIS: **Pain: epigastric area or right upper quadrant of abdomen with radiation to interscapular area or right scapula or shoulder**

related to:

a. inflammation and distention of the gallbladder;

b. ductal spasms associated with blockage of bile flow if gallstones are present in the duct system.

Desired Outcome	Nursing Actions and *Selected Purposes/Rationales*

3. The client will experience diminished pain as evidenced by:
   a. verbalization of same
   b. relaxed facial expression and body positioning
   c. increased participation in activities
   d. stable vital signs.

3.a. Assess for signs and symptoms of pain (e.g. verbalization of pain, grimacing, reluctance to move, guarding of abdomen, rubbing right shoulder, restlessness, diaphoresis, facial pallor, increased B/P, tachycardia).

b. Assess client's perception of the severity of pain using a pain intensity rating scale.

c. Assess the client's pain pattern (e.g. location, quality, onset, duration, precipitating factors, aggravating factors, alleviating factors); note that a finding of increased pain with transient inspiratory arrest upon deep palpation of the right upper quadrant (Murphy's sign) is indicative of cholecystitis.

d. Ask the client to describe previous pain experiences and methods used to manage pain effectively.

e. Implement measures *to reduce pain*:
   1. perform actions *to reduce fear and anxiety about the pain experience* (e.g. assure client that his/her need for pain relief is understood, plan methods for achieving pain control with client)
   2. perform actions to reduce fear and anxiety (see Nursing Diagnosis 7, action b) *in order to promote relaxation and subsequently increase the client's threshold and tolerance for pain*
   3. administer analgesics before activities and procedures that can cause pain and before pain becomes severe
   4. perform actions to promote rest (e.g. minimize environmental activity and noise, limit number of visitors and their length of stay) *in order to reduce fatigue and subsequently increase the client's threshold and tolerance for pain*
   5. perform actions *to reduce stimulation of gallbladder contractions*:
      a. maintain NPO status as ordered
      b. insert nasogastric tube and maintain suction if ordered
      c. when oral intake is allowed, maintain dietary restrictions of fat as ordered (avoid foods/fluids high in fat such as butter, cream, whole milk, ice cream, fried foods, gravies, and nuts)
   6. provide or assist with nonpharmacologic measures for pain relief (e.g. position change; restful environment; diversional activities such as watching television, reading, or conversing; progressive relaxation exercises)

Desired Outcome	Nursing Actions and *Selected Purposes/Rationales*

    7. administer the following if ordered:
      a. analgesics (meperidine is often the medication of choice *because morphine sulfate increases spasms of the sphincter of Oddi*)
      b. antimicrobials *to prevent or treat infection and subsequently reduce inflammation of the gallbladder wall*
    8. if client has a patient-controlled analgesia device, encourage him/her to use it as instructed
    9. prepare client for surgery, endoscopic ductal stone removal, endoscopic or percutaneous infusion of cholesterol stone solvent into gallbladder, or lithotripsy if planned.
  f. Consult physician if above measures fail to provide adequate pain relief.

4.A. NURSING DIAGNOSIS: **Altered comfort: pruritus**

related to an accumulation of substances in the blood that act as pruritogens (e.g. bile acid metabolites, endogenous opioid peptides) associated with bile flow obstruction.

Desired Outcome	Nursing Actions and *Selected Purposes/Rationales*

4.A. The client will experience relief of pruritus as evidenced by:
1. verbalization of same
2. no scratching or rubbing of skin.

4.A.1. Assess for the following:
    a. reports of itchiness
    b. persistent scratching or rubbing of skin.
  2. Instruct client in and/or implement measures *to relieve pruritus:*
    a. perform actions *to promote capillary constriction:*
      1. apply cool, moist compresses to pruritic areas
      2. maintain a cool environment
    b. apply emollient creams or ointments frequently *to prevent dryness*
    c. add emollients, cornstarch, or baking soda to bath water
    d. use tepid water and mild soaps for bathing
    e. pat skin dry after bathing, making sure to dry thoroughly
    f. encourage participation in diversional activity
    g. utilize cutaneous stimulation techniques (e.g. massage, pressure, vibration, stroking with soft brush) at the sites of itching or acupressure points
    h. encourage client to wear loose cotton garments
    i. utilize relaxation techniques
    j. administer the following medications if ordered:
      1. antihistamines
      2. bile acid sequestering agents (e.g. cholestyramine, colestipol).
  3. Consult physician if above measures fail to alleviate pruritus or if the skin becomes excoriated.

4.B. NURSING DIAGNOSIS: **Altered comfort: nausea and vomiting**

related to stimulation of the vomiting center associated with:
1. stimulation of the visceral afferent pathways as a result of the visceral irritation that occurs with gallbladder and bile duct inflammation;
2. stimulation of the cerebral cortex resulting from pain and stress.

Desired Outcome	Nursing Actions and *Selected Purposes/Rationales*

4.B. The client will experience relief of nausea and vomiting as evidenced by:
1. verbalization of relief of nausea
2. absence of vomiting.
	4.B.1. Assess client for nausea and vomiting.
	2. Implement measures *to reduce nausea and vomiting:*
	a. maintain patency of nasogastric tube (e.g. keep tubing free of kinks, irrigate and maintain suction as ordered) if present
	b. eliminate noxious sights and odors from the environment (*noxious stimuli can cause stimulation of the vomiting center*)
	c. instruct client to change positions slowly (*rapid movement can result in stimulation of the chemoreceptor trigger zone and subsequent excitation of the vomiting center*)
	d. provide oral hygiene after each emesis
	e. perform actions to reduce fear and anxiety (see Nursing Diagnosis 7, action b)
	f. perform actions to reduce pain (see Nursing Diagnosis 3, action e)
	g. encourage client to take deep, slow breaths when nauseated
	h. withhold oral intake as ordered
	i. when oral intake is allowed:
	 1. advance diet as tolerated
	 2. avoid serving foods with an overpowering aroma; remove lids from hot foods before entering room
	 3. provide small, frequent meals; instruct client to ingest foods and fluids slowly
	 4. instruct client to eat dry foods (e.g. toast, crackers) and avoid drinking liquids with meals if nauseated
	 5. instruct client to avoid the following:
	  a. foods/fluids high in fat (e.g. butter, cream, whole milk, ice cream, fried foods, gravies, nuts)
	  b. foods/fluids that irritate the gastric mucosa (e.g. spicy foods; caffeine-containing beverages such as tea, coffee, and colas)
	 6. instruct client to rest after eating with head of bed elevated
	j. administer antiemetics if ordered (phenothiazines should be used cautiously *because of their potential cholestatic effect*).
	3. Consult physician if above measures fail to control nausea and vomiting.

4.C. NURSING DIAGNOSIS:

Altered comfort: dyspepsia

related to impaired fat digestion associated with bile flow obstruction.

Desired Outcome	Nursing Actions and *Selected Purposes/Rationales*
4.C. The client will verbalize relief of dyspepsia.	4.C.1. Assess client for verbal reports of dyspepsia (e.g. epigastric discomfort, feeling of fullness or bloating, nausea). 2. Determine if particular foods/fluids contribute to dyspepsia (client usually reports an intolerance of fatty foods). 3. Implement measures *to reduce dyspepsia:* a. perform actions to reduce nausea once oral intake is allowed (see Nursing Diagnosis 4.B, action 2.i) b. perform actions *to reduce the accumulation of gas in the gastrointestinal tract:* 1. encourage and assist client with frequent position changes and ambulation as allowed and tolerated (*activity stimulates peristalsis and expulsion of flatus*)

Desired Outcome	Nursing Actions and *Selected Purposes/Rationales*

       2. instruct client to avoid activities such as chewing gum and smoking *in order to reduce air swallowing*
       3. encourage client to avoid the following foods/fluids:
         a. those high in fat (e.g. fried foods, gravies, butter, cream, whole milk, ice cream, nuts)
         b. carbonated beverages
         c. gas-producing foods (e.g. cabbage, onions, beans)
       4. encourage client to eructate and expel flatus whenever the urge is felt
       5. administer antiflatulents (e.g. simethicone) if ordered
    c. administer antacids if ordered.
  4. Consult physician if above measures fail to control dyspepsia.

---

5. NURSING DIAGNOSIS:

Altered oral mucous membrane: dryness

related to:
a. fluid volume deficit associated with restricted oral intake and fluid loss resulting from vomiting and nasogastric tube drainage;
b. decreased salivation associated with fluid volume deficit, restricted oral intake, and treatment with some medications (e.g. narcotic [opioid] analgesics);
c. mouth breathing when nasogastric tube is in place.

Desired Outcome	Nursing Actions and *Selected Purposes/Rationales*

5. The client will maintain a moist, intact oral mucous membrane.

5.a. Assess client for dryness of the oral mucosa.
  b. Implement measures *to relieve dryness of the oral mucous membrane:*
    1. instruct and assist client to perform oral hygiene as often as needed; avoid use of products that contain lemon and glycerin and mouthwashes containing alcohol (*these products have a drying and irritating effect on the oral mucous membrane*)
    2. encourage client to rinse mouth frequently with water
    3. lubricate client's lips frequently
    4. encourage client to breathe through nose rather than mouth
    5. encourage client not to smoke (*smoking irritates and dries the mucosa*)
    6. maintain intravenous fluid administration as ordered *to improve hydration*
    7. provide sips of water frequently if allowed
    8. advance diet as allowed and tolerated *to stimulate salivation.*
  c. Consult physician if dryness, irritation, and/or discomfort persist.

---

6. COLLABORATIVE DIAGNOSES:

Potential complications of cholelithiasis/cholecystitis:

a. **abscess or fistula formation** related to presence of increased cholecystic and ductal pressure (can cause perforation of the gallbladder into localized, contained area [abscess] or wall of an adjacent organ [fistula]);
b. **peritonitis** related to escape of bile into the peritoneal cavity associated with perforation of the gallbladder;
c. **pancreatitis** related to obstruction of the flow of pancreatic secretions as a result of a stone or inflammation in the common bile duct;
d. **cholangitis** related to proliferation of bacteria in the biliary ducts associated with stasis of bile.

Desired Outcomes	Nursing Actions and *Selected Purposes/Rationales*
6.a. The client will experience resolution of any abscess or fistula that develops as evidenced by: 1. decrease in abdominal pain 2. temperature and pulse declining toward normal 3. WBC count declining toward normal.	6.a.1. Assess for and report signs and symptoms of abscess and/or fistula formation (e.g. increased abdominal pain, further increase in temperature and pulse rate, further increase in WBC count). 2. If signs and symptoms of an abscess or fistula occur: a. prepare client for diagnostic studies (e.g. ultrasonography, computed tomography) b. administer antimicrobials as ordered c. prepare client for surgical intervention (e.g. cholecystectomy or cholecystostomy with incision and drainage of abscess or closure of fistula) if planned d. provide emotional support to client and significant others.
6.b. The client will have resolution of peritonitis if it occurs as evidenced by: 1. gradual resolution of abdominal pain 2. soft, nondistended abdomen 3. temperature declining toward normal 4. stable vital signs 5. decreased nausea and vomiting 6. gradual return of normal bowel sounds 7. WBC count declining toward normal.	6.b.1. Assess for and report signs and symptoms of peritonitis (e.g. transient pain relief; diffuse abdominal pain; rebound tenderness; distended, rigid abdomen; further increase in temperature; tachycardia; tachypnea; hypotension; increased nausea and vomiting; diminished or absent bowel sounds). 2. Monitor WBC counts. Report levels that increase or fail to decline toward normal. 3. If signs and symptoms of peritonitis occur: a. withhold oral intake as ordered b. place client on bed rest in a semi-Fowler's position *to assist in pooling or localizing gastrointestinal contents in the pelvis rather than under the diaphragm* c. prepare client for diagnostic tests (e.g. abdominal x-ray, computed tomography, ultrasonography) if planned d. insert a nasogastric tube and maintain suction as ordered e. administer antimicrobials as ordered f. administer intravenous fluids and/or blood volume expanders if ordered *to prevent or treat shock (can result from the increased capillary permeability that occurs with inflammation and the subsequent escape of protein, fluid, and electrolytes from the vascular space into the peritoneal cavity)* g. prepare client for surgery (e.g. cholecystectomy or cholecystostomy with peritoneal lavage) if planned h. provide emotional support to client and significant others.
6.c. The client will experience resolution of pancreatitis if it occurs as evidenced by: 1. gradual resolution of abdominal pain 2. temperature declining toward normal 3. stable B/P and pulse 4. serum amylase and lipase levels declining toward normal 5. renal amylase/creatinine clearance ratio returning toward normal 6. WBC count declining toward normal.	6.c.1. Assess for and report signs and symptoms of pancreatitis (e.g. extension of pain to left upper quadrant or back, further increase in temperature, tachycardia, hypotension, elevated serum amylase and lipase levels). 2. Collect a timed (usually 2-hour) urine specimen if ordered. Report an elevated renal amylase/creatinine clearance ratio. 3. Monitor WBC counts. Report levels that increase or fail to decline toward normal. 4. If signs and symptoms of pancreatitis occur: a. assist client to assume position of greatest comfort (e.g. side-lying or sitting with trunk and knees flexed) b. maintain food and fluid restrictions as ordered c. insert nasogastric tube if not already present and maintain suction as ordered (*removal of gastric secretions reduces pancreatic stimulation*) d. administer the following if ordered: 1. analgesics 2. antacids and histamine$_2$ receptor antagonists (e.g. cimetidine, ranitidine, famotidine) *to decrease the acidity of gastric contents and thereby reduce stimulation of the pancreas (when acidic gastric contents enter the duodenum and jejunum, secretin is released; secretin stimulates pancreatic secretion)* e. prepare client for endoscopic sphincterotomy and stone extraction or surgery to relieve ductal obstruction if planned f. refer to Care Plan on Pancreatitis for additional care measures.

Desired Outcomes	Nursing Actions and *Selected Purposes/Rationales*

6.d. The client will experience resolution of cholangitis if it occurs as evidenced by:
1. gradual resolution of abdominal pain
2. absence of jaundice and chills
3. temperature declining toward normal
4. WBC count declining toward normal.
	6.d.1. Assess for signs and symptoms of cholangitis (e.g. increased abdominal pain, jaundice, chills, increase in temperature). Be aware that lethargy, confusion, and hypotension may indicate septic shock, which can develop with suppurative cholangitis.
	2. Monitor WBC count and serum bilirubin and alkaline phosphatase. Report increased levels.
	3. Obtain blood cultures as ordered. Report positive results.
	4. If signs and symptoms of cholangitis occur:
	  a. prepare client for diagnostic studies (e.g. computed tomography, ultrasonography, endoscopic retrograde cholangiopancreatography [ERCP])
	  b. administer antimicrobials as ordered
	  c. prepare client for endoscopic decompression of biliary system, insertion of a percutaneous transhepatic catheter (to decompress duct), or surgical removal of ductal stone if planned
	  d. provide emotional support to client and significant others.

---

7. NURSING DIAGNOSIS:

Anxiety

related to discomfort, unknown diagnosis, unfamiliar environment, lack of understanding of diagnostic tests and treatments, and possibility of surgery.

Desired Outcome	Nursing Actions and *Selected Purposes/Rationales*

7. The client will experience a reduction in anxiety as evidenced by:
a. verbalization of feeling less anxious
b. usual sleep pattern
c. relaxed facial expression and body movements
d. stable vital signs
e. usual perceptual ability and interactions with others.
	7.a. Assess client for signs and symptoms of anxiety (e.g. verbalization of feeling anxious, insomnia, tenseness, shakiness, restlessness, diaphoresis, tachycardia, elevated blood pressure, facial pallor, self-focused behaviors). Validate perceptions carefully, remembering that some behavior may result from pain.
	b. Implement measures *to reduce fear and anxiety:*
	  1. orient client to hospital environment, equipment, and routines
	  2. introduce client to staff who will be participating in care; if possible, maintain consistency in staff assigned to his/her care *to provide feelings of stability and comfort with the environment*
	  3. assure client that staff members are nearby; respond to call signal as soon as possible
	  4. maintain a calm, supportive, confident manner when interacting with client
	  5. encourage verbalization of fear and anxiety; provide feedback
	  6. explain all diagnostic tests
	  7. reinforce physician's explanations and clarify misconceptions client has about cholelithiasis and/or cholecystitis and the treatment plan
	  8. perform actions to reduce discomfort (see Nursing Diagnoses 3, action e; 4.A, action 2; 4.B, action 2; and 4.C, action 3)
	  9. provide a calm, restful environment
	  10. instruct client in relaxation techniques and encourage participation in diversional activities once severe pain has subsided
	  11. provide information based on current needs of the client at a level he/she can understand; encourage questions and clarification of information provided
	  12. assist client to identify specific stressors and ways to cope with them
	  13. encourage significant others to project a caring, concerned attitude without obvious anxiousness
	  14. include significant others in orientation and teaching sessions and encourage their continued support of the client

15. if surgical intervention is indicated, begin preoperative teaching
16. administer prescribed antianxiety agents if indicated.
   c. Consult physician if above actions fail to control fear and anxiety.

Discharge Teaching

■————————————————————

8. NURSING DIAGNOSIS: **Knowledge deficit, Ineffective management of therapeutic regimen, or Altered health maintenance***

————————

*The nurse should select the diagnostic label that is most appropriate for the client's discharge teaching needs.

Desired Outcomes	Nursing Actions and *Selected Purposes/Rationales*
8.a. The client will verbalize an understanding of ways to reduce the risk for recurrent gallbladder attacks.	8.a. Instruct client regarding ways to reduce the risk for recurrent gallbladder attacks: 1. adhere to a low- to moderate-fat diet (avoid foods/fluids high in fat such as butter, cream, whole milk, ice cream, fried foods, gravies, and nuts) 2. lose weight if obese but avoid rapid weight loss (rapid weight loss has been shown to increase biliary cholesterol saturation) 3. exercise regularly 4. consult physician before starting or resuming use of lipid-lowering agents or estrogen preparations/oral contraceptives (some estrogen preparations and lipid-lowering agents [e.g. clofibrate] increase the risk for gallstones).
8.b. The client will state signs and symptoms to report to the health care provider.	8.b. Instruct client to report the following signs and symptoms: 1. persistent indigestion, flatulence, and loose stools 2. nausea and vomiting 3. recurrent episodes of abdominal pain 4. development of or persistent itching, yellow coloring of skin or eyes, dark color of urine, or clay-colored stools (indicative of bile flow obstruction) 5. persistent or recurrent temperature elevation.

8.c. The client will verbalize an understanding of and a plan for adhering to recommended follow-up care including future appointments with health care provider and medications prescribed.	8.c.1. Reinforce importance of keeping follow-up appointments with health care provider.
	2. Explain the rationale for, side effects of, and importance of taking prescribed medications (e.g. fat-soluble vitamins, cholestyramine, hydrocholeretic agents [e.g. dehydrocholic acid], ursodiol, antimicrobials). Inform client of pertinent food and drug interactions.
	3. Implement measures to improve client compliance:
	  a. include significant others in teaching sessions if possible
	  b. encourage questions and allow time for reinforcement and clarification of information provided
	  c. provide written instructions on future appointments with health care provider, medications prescribed, and signs and symptoms to report.

Bibliography

See pages 897–898 and 908.

CIRRHOSIS

Cirrhosis is a chronic disease of the liver that occurs as a result of extensive destruction of the parenchymal cells in the liver. These cells are eventually replaced by fibrous scar tissue with subsequent change in the structure and functioning of the liver. The structural changes impair portal blood flow which results in venous congestion in other organs and systems such as the spleen and gastrointestinal tract. The four major types of cirrhosis are alcoholic (e.g. Laennec's, portal, nutritional), postnecrotic, biliary, and cardiac. Alcoholic cirrhosis is the most common type seen in North America. Postnecrotic cirrhosis, which can result from viral hepatitis or exposure to toxic chemicals or drugs, is the most common type worldwide. Malnutrition is not a substantiated cause of any type of cirrhosis but is thought to possibly potentiate the harmful effects of alcohol on the liver and augment the development of cirrhosis.

All types of cirrhosis have similar signs and symptoms which are manifestations of impaired liver function and the venous congestion that occurs with portal hypertension. Alcohol-related cirrhosis may have additional manifestations such as cerebral degeneration and demyelinating neuropathies that are thought to be a direct result of the toxic effects of alcohol. Treatment of cirrhosis includes removing the causative factor if possible, providing a diet that prevents further malnutrition and liver damage, and encouraging rest to reduce the metabolic demands on the liver. Colchicine is sometimes used to treat cirrhosis because it has been shown to reduce the amount of fibrosis in the liver and produce clinical improvement in some persons. Liver transplantation is often indicated for treatment of end-stage liver disease. A major criterion used when considering a transplant for a person with alcohol-related cirrhosis is abstinence from alcohol, usually for a minimum of 6 months.

This care plan focuses on the adult client with alcoholic (Laennec's) cirrhosis hospitalized for management of increasing ascites and peripheral edema. The goals of care are to maintain comfort, improve nutritional status and fluid balance, prevent complications, and educate the client regarding follow-up care.

DIAGNOSTIC TESTS

Serum enzymes (e.g. AST [SGOT], ALT [SGPT], GGT [GGTP], LDH, alkaline phosphatase)
Serum proteins and protein electrophoresis
Serum bilirubin
Serum ammonia
Serum cholesterol and electrolytes
Complete blood count (CBC)
Urine bilirubin and urobilinogen
Prothrombin time (PT) or International Normalized Ratio (INR)
Ultrasonography
Computed tomography (CT)
Magnetic resonance imaging (MRI)
Radioisotope scan
Liver biopsy
Angiography or percutaneous transhepatic portography
Esophagoscopy and/or barium contrast esophagography (may be performed to determine the presence of esophageal varices)

DISCHARGE CRITERIA

Prior to discharge, the client will:

- have an adequate nutritional intake
- perform activities of daily living without extreme fatigue or dyspnea
- have a reduction in or resolution of ascites and edema
- have no evidence of life-threatening complications
- identify ways to prevent further liver damage
- verbalize an understanding of the rationale for and components of the recommended diet

- identify ways to reduce stress on esophageal and gastric blood vessels
- identify ways to prevent bleeding
- identify ways to reduce the risk of infection
- identify ways to relieve pruritus
- state signs and symptoms to report to the health care provider
- identify community resources that can assist with home management and adjustment to life-style changes necessary for effective management of cirrhosis
- share concerns and feelings about the diagnosis of cirrhosis; prognosis; and effects of the disease process and its treatment on self-concept, life style, and roles
- verbalize an understanding of and a plan for adhering to recommended follow-up care including future appointments with health care provider, medications prescribed, and activity level.

Use in conjunction with the Care Plan on Immobility.

See Care Plan on Immobility for additional diagnoses.

1. NURSING DIAGNOSIS:

Ineffective breathing pattern

related to diminished lung/chest wall expansion associated with:
a. weakness and decreased mobility;
b. pressure on the diaphragm as a result of peritoneal fluid accumulation;
c. pleural effusion (hepatic hydrothorax) resulting from fluid volume excess and passage of ascitic fluid into the pleural space through a probable pressure-related defect in the diaphragm.

Desired Outcome	Nursing Actions and *Selected Purposes/Rationales*

1. The client will have an improved breathing pattern as evidenced by:
a. normal rate and depth of respirations
b. decreased dyspnea
c. blood gases within normal range.
	1.a. Assess for signs and symptoms of an ineffective breathing pattern (e.g. shallow respirations, dyspnea, tachypnea, use of accessory muscles when breathing).
	b. Monitor for and report the following:
	  1. abnormal blood gases
	  2. significant decrease in oximetry results.
	c. Implement measures *to improve breathing pattern:*
	  1. perform actions to increase strength and activity tolerance (see Nursing Diagnosis 7, action b) *in order to increase client's willingness and ability to move, deep breathe, and use incentive spirometer*
	  2. perform actions to restore fluid balance (see Nursing Diagnosis 2, action a.4) *in order to reduce fluid accumulation in the peritoneal cavity and pleural space*
	  3. assist client to turn from side to side at least every 2 hours while in bed
	  4. place. client in a semi-Fowler's position (a high Fowler's position is uncomfortable if ascites is severe); position with pillows *to prevent slumping*
	  5. instruct client to deep breathe or use incentive spirometer every 1–2 hours
	  6. instruct client to avoid intake of gas-forming foods (e.g. beans, cauliflower, cabbage, onions), carbonated beverages, and large meals *in order to prevent gastric distention and additional pressure on the diaphragm*
	  7. assist with positive airway pressure techniques (e.g. IPPB, continuous positive airway pressure [CPAP], biphasic positive airway pressure [BiPAP], expiratory positive airway pressure [EPAP]) if ordered
	  8. increase activity as allowed and tolerated
	  9. administer central nervous system depressants judiciously; hold medication and consult physician if respiratory rate is less then 12/ minute
	  10. assist with thoracentesis and/or paracentesis if performed *to remove pleural and/or peritoneal fluid in order to allow increased lung expansion.*
	d. Consult physician if:
	  1. ineffective breathing pattern continues
	  2. signs and symptoms of impaired gas exchange (e.g. restlessness, irritability, confusion, decreased PaO_2 and increased $PaCO_2$ levels) are present.

2. NURSING/COLLABORATIVE DIAGNOSIS:

Altered fluid and electrolyte balance:

a. **fluid volume excess** related to:
  1. sodium and water retention associated with an increased aldosterone

level resulting from:
   a. inability of the liver to metabolize aldosterone
   b. activation of the renin-angiotensin-aldosterone mechanism as a result of decreased renal blood flow (occurs because of a decrease in the effective intravascular volume that results from vasodilation and from third-spacing and sequestration of fluid in the splanchnic system)
   2. decreased water excretion associated with increased antidiuretic hormone (ADH) output (a compensatory response to a decrease in the effective intravascular volume that results from vasodilation and from third-spacing and sequestration of fluid in the splanchnic system);
   b. **third-spacing** related to:
      1. low plasma colloid osmotic pressure associated with hypoalbuminemia (a result of decreased hepatic synthesis of albumin and prolonged inadequate nutrition)
      2. increased pressure in the portal system and hepatic lymph system associated with blood flow backup resulting from structural changes in the liver
      3. generalized increase in hydrostatic pressure associated with fluid volume excess;
   c. **hypokalemia** related to excessive potassium loss associated with an increased aldosterone level (aldosterone causes potassium excretion) and diuretic therapy;
   d. **hyponatremia** related to dietary restriction of sodium, hemodilution associated with fluid volume excess, and sodium loss associated with diuretic therapy.

Desired Outcomes	Nursing Actions and *Selected Purposes/Rationales*

2.a. The client will experience resolution of fluid imbalance as evidenced by:
  1. decline in weight toward client's normal
  2. B/P and pulse within normal range for client and stable with position change
  3. absence or resolution of S₃ heart sound
  4. balanced intake and output
  5. usual mental status
  6. serum sodium returning toward normal range
  7. hand vein emptying time less than 3–5 seconds
  8. decreased dyspnea, peripheral edema, and neck vein distention
  9. improved breath sounds
  10. resolution of ascites.
	2.a.1. Assess for signs and symptoms of the following:
	  a. fluid volume excess:
	    1. weight gain of 2% or greater in a short period
	    2. elevated B/P (B/P may not be elevated if fluid has shifted out of the vascular space)
	    3. development or worsening of S₃ heart sound
	    4. intake greater than output
	    5. change in mental status (may also reflect impending hepatic encephalopathy)
	    6. low serum sodium (may also result from diuretic therapy and a low sodium diet)
	    7. delayed hand vein emptying time (longer than 3–5 seconds)
	    8. dyspnea, orthopnea
	    9. peripheral edema
	    10. distended neck veins
	    11. crackles (rales), diminished or absent breath sounds
	  b. third-spacing:
	    1. ascites as evidenced by:
	      a. increase in abdominal girth (abdominal girth should be measured daily at the same time and in the same location on the abdomen with client in same position)
	      b. dull percussion note over abdomen with finding of shifting dullness
	      c. presence of abdominal fluid wave
	      d. protruding umbilicus and bulging flanks
	    2. dyspnea and diminished or absent breath sounds
	    3. evidence of vascular depletion (e.g. postural hypotension; weak, rapid pulse; decreased urine output).
	  2. Monitor chest x-ray results. Report findings of pulmonary vascular congestion, pleural effusion, or pulmonary edema.
	  3. Monitor serum albumin levels. Report below-normal levels (*low serum albumin levels result in fluid shifting out of the vascular space because albumin normally maintains plasma colloid osmotic pressure*).

Desired Outcomes	Nursing Actions and *Selected Purposes/Rationales*

	4. Implement measures *to restore fluid balance:*
	  a. perform actions *to reduce fluid volume excess:*
	    1. restrict sodium intake as ordered
	    2. maintain fluid restrictions if ordered
	    3. implement measures to promote mobilization of fluid back into the vascular space (see action a.4.b. in this diagnosis) *in order to improve renal blood flow and reduce ADH output*
	    4. administer diuretics if ordered (potassium-sparing diuretics [e.g. spironolactone, amiloride, triamterene] are often used initially)
	  b. perform actions *to prevent further third-spacing and promote mobilization of fluid back into the vascular space:*
	    1. implement measures to reduce fluid volume excess (see action a.4.a in this diagnosis)
	    2. encourage client to rest periodically in a recumbent position if tolerated (*lying flat promotes venous return and results in lower venous hydrostatic pressure with subsequent reshifting of fluid into vascular space*)
	    3. administer albumin infusions if ordered *to increase colloid osmotic pressure*
	    4. prepare client for surgical insertion of a peritoneovenous shunt (e.g. Denver shunt, LeVeen shunt) if planned
	  c. assist with paracentesis and follow-up administration of colloid replacement infusions (e.g. albumin, dextran) if performed *to treat ascites*
	  d. prepare client for a portal systemic shunt procedure (e.g. transjugular intrahepatic portosystemic shunt [TIPS]) if planned *to treat portal hypertension and reduce the development of ascites.*
	5. Consult physician if signs and symptoms of fluid imbalance persist or worsen.

2.b. The client will maintain a safe serum potassium level as evidenced by:
  1. regular pulse at 60–100 beats/minute
  2. B/P within normal range for client and stable with position change
  3. usual muscle tone and strength
  4. absence of nausea and vomiting
  5. soft, nondistended abdomen with normal bowel sounds
  6. normal ECG reading
  7. serum potassium within normal range.
	2.b.1. Assess for and report signs and symptoms of hypokalemia (e.g. cardiac dysrhythmias; postural hypotension; muscle weakness; nausea and vomiting; abdominal distention; hypoactive or absent bowel sounds; ECG reading showing ST segment depression, T wave inversion or flattening, and presence of U waves; low serum potassium level).
	  2. Implement measures *to prevent or treat hypokalemia:*
	    a. administer intravenous and oral potassium replacements as ordered (monitor serum potassium and urine output closely when giving supplemental potassium; consult physician if potassium level increases above normal and/or urine output is less than 30 ml/hour)
	    b. if client is taking a potassium-depleting diuretic or if signs and symptoms of hypokalemia are present, encourage intake of foods/fluids high in potassium (e.g. bananas, potatoes, raisins, apricots, cantaloupe).
	  3. Consult physician if signs and symptoms of hypokalemia persist or worsen.

2.c. The client will maintain a safe serum sodium level as evidenced by:
  1. absence of nausea, vomiting, and abdominal cramps
  2. usual mental status
  3. usual muscle strength
  4. absence of seizure activity
  5. serum sodium within normal range.
	2.c.1. Assess for and report signs and symptoms of hyponatremia (e.g. nausea, vomiting, abdominal cramps, lethargy, confusion, weakness, seizures, low serum sodium level).
	  2. Implement measures *to treat hyponatremia:*
	    a. maintain fluid restrictions if ordered
	    b. administer hypertonic saline solutions if ordered (not commonly given until hyponatremia is severe *because of the risk of hypernatremia and intravascular volume overload*); furosemide may be given concurrently *to promote water excretion and reduce the risk for intravascular volume overload.*
	  3. Consult physician if signs and symptoms of hyponatremia persist or worsen.

3. NURSING DIAGNOSIS: **Altered nutrition: less than body requirements**

related to:
a. poor eating habits prior to admission;
b. decreased oral intake associated with abdominal pain, dyspepsia, fatigue, dyspnea, dislike of the prescribed diet, and feeling of fullness (a result of increased intra-abdominal pressure that occurs with ascites);
c. reduced metabolism and storage of nutrients by the liver associated with a reduction of functional liver tissue;
d. malabsorption of fats and fat-soluble vitamins associated with impaired bile production and flow.

Desired Outcome	Nursing Actions and *Selected Purposes/Rationales*

3. The client will have an improved nutritional status as evidenced by:
   a. dry weight approaching normal range for client's age, height, and body frame (dry weight is achieved after fluid volume excess has been resolved)
   b. improved serum albumin, Hct, Hb, transferrin, and lymphocyte levels
   c. improved strength and activity tolerance
   d. healthy oral mucous membrane.

3.a. Assess for and report signs and symptoms of malnutrition:
   1. dry weight below normal for client's age, height, and body frame
   2. decreased serum albumin, Hct, Hb, transferrin, and lymphocyte levels
   3. weakness and fatigue
   4. sore, inflamed oral mucous membrane
   5. pale conjunctiva.
b. Monitor percentage of meals and snacks client consumes. Report a pattern of inadequate intake.
c. Implement measures *to improve nutritional status:*
   1. perform actions *to improve oral intake:*
      a. implement measures to relieve abdominal pain and dyspepsia (see Nursing Diagnoses 4, action e and 5.B, action 3)
      b. obtain a dietary consult if necessary to assist the client in selecting foods/fluids that are appealing and adhere to personal and cultural preferences as well as the prescribed dietary modifications
      c. encourage a rest period before meals *to minimize fatigue*
      d. maintain a clean environment and a relaxed, pleasant atmosphere
      e. provide oral hygiene before meals
      f. serve frequent, small meals rather than large ones if client is weak, fatigues easily, and/or has a poor appetite
      g. elevate head of bed as tolerated for meals *to help relieve dyspnea and feeling of fullness* (a high Fowler's position may be too uncomfortable if ascites is severe)
      h. instruct client to use herbs, spices, and salt substitutes (if approved by physician) *in order to make low-sodium diet more palatable*
      i. allow adequate time for meals; reheat foods/fluids if necessary
      j. increase activity as allowed and tolerated (*activity usually promotes a sense of well-being and improves appetite*)
      k. limit fluid intake with meals (unless the fluid has high nutritional value) *to reduce early satiety and subsequent decreased food intake*
   2. assist and instruct client to adhere to the following dietary recommendations:
      a. avoid skipping meals
      b. consume a diet high in calories (2000–3000 calories/day) and carbohydrates
      c. maintain a moderate to high protein intake (generally at least 1 gm of protein/kg of body weight is recommended unless the serum ammonia level is high or clinical evidence of encephalopathy is present)
      d. consume meals that are well balanced and high in essential nutrients; offer dietary supplements if client's caloric intake is inadequate
   3. administer vitamins and minerals (e.g. fat-soluble vitamins, B-complex vitamins, folic acid, iron) if ordered.

Desired Outcome	Nursing Actions and *Selected Purposes/Rationales*
	d. Perform a calorie count if ordered. Report information to dietitian and physician.
	e. Consult physician about an alternative method of providing nutrition (e.g. parenteral nutrition, tube feedings) if client does not consume enough food or fluids to meet nutritional needs.

---

4. NURSING DIAGNOSIS: **Pain: abdominal**

related to swelling and distention of the liver capsule and distention of the peritoneum associated with excessive fluid accumulation.

Desired Outcome	Nursing Actions and *Selected Purposes/Rationales*

4. The client will experience diminished abdominal pain as evidenced by:
a. verbalization of a decrease in or absence of pain
b. relaxed facial expression and body positioning
c. increased participation in activities.
	4.a. Assess for signs and symptoms of pain (e.g. verbalization of pain, grimacing, guarding of abdomen, reluctance to move, restlessness).
	b. Assess client's perception of the severity of pain using a pain intensity rating scale.
	c. Assess the client's pain pattern (e.g. location, quality, onset, duration, precipitating factors, aggravating factors, alleviating factors).
	d. Ask the client to describe previous pain experiences and methods used to manage pain effectively.
	e. Implement measures *to reduce pain:*
	  1. perform actions *to reduce fear and anxiety about the pain experience* (e.g. assure client that his/her need for pain relief is understood, plan methods for achieving pain control with client)
	  2. perform actions to reduce fear and anxiety (see Nursing Diagnosis 15) *in order to promote relaxation and subsequently increase the client's threshold and tolerance for pain*
	  3. perform actions to promote rest (see Nursing Diagnosis 7, action b.1) *in order to reduce fatigue and subsequently increase the client's threshold and tolerance for pain*
	  4. perform actions to restore fluid balance (see Nursing Diagnosis 2, action a.4) *in order to reduce peritoneal fluid accumulation*
	  5. provide or assist with nonpharmacologic measures for pain relief (e.g. position change; relaxation exercises; restful environment; diversional activities such as watching television, reading, or conversing)
	  6. administer analgesics if ordered; be aware of the following:
	    a. lower doses of opioids (narcotics) are usually ordered *because the liver cannot detoxify them at a normal rate*
	    b. opioid (narcotic) analgesics may cause biliary spasm (particularly morphine sulfate) and the physician should be notified if they fail to relieve or actually intensify pain
	    c. acetaminophen may be ordered (despite its potential hepatotoxic effect) rather than acetylsalicylic acid *because of the increased risk for gastric irritation and bleeding with acetylsalicylic acid.*
	f. Consult physician if above measures fail to provide adequate pain relief.

5.A. NURSING DIAGNOSIS: **Altered comfort: pruritus**

related to an accumulation of substances in the blood that act as pruritogens (e.g. bile acid metabolites, endogenous opioid peptides) associated with bile flow obstruction.

Desired Outcome	Nursing Actions and *Selected Purposes/Rationales*

5.A. The client will experience relief of pruritus as evidenced by:
1. verbalization of same
2. no scratching or rubbing of skin.
	5.A.1. Assess for the following:
	  a. reports of itchiness
	  b. persistent scratching or rubbing of skin.
	  2. Instruct client in and/or implement measures *to relieve pruritus:*
	    a. apply cool, moist compresses to pruritic areas
	    b. apply emollient creams or ointments frequently *to prevent dryness*
	    c. add emollients, cornstarch, or baking soda to bath water
	    d. use tepid water and mild soaps for bathing
	    e. pat skin dry after bathing, making sure to dry thoroughly
	    f. maintain a cool environment
	    g. utilize a room humidifier *to maintain moisture in the air*
	    h. encourage participation in diversional activity
	    i. utilize relaxation techniques
	    j. utilize cutaneous stimulation techniques (e.g. massage, pressure, vibration, stroking with soft brush) at sites of itching or acupressure points
	    k. encourage client to wear loose cotton garments
	    l. administer the following medications if ordered:
	      1. antihistamines
	      2. bile acid sequestering agents (e.g. cholestyramine, colestipol).
	  3. Consult physician if above measures fail to alleviate pruritus or if the skin becomes excoriated.

5.B. NURSING DIAGNOSIS: **Altered comfort: dyspepsia**

related to:
1. impaired fat digestion associated with bile flow obstruction;
2. reflux of gastric contents associated with increased intra-abdominal pressure resulting from ascites;
3. impaired gastrointestinal functioning associated with venous congestion in the gastrointestinal tract (portal hypertensive gastropathy) resulting from portal hypertension;
4. esophagitis/gastritis associated with the irritant effect of alcohol on the esophageal and gastric mucosa.

Desired Outcome	Nursing Actions and *Selected Purposes/Rationales*

5.B. The client will verbalize relief of dyspepsia.	5.B.1. Assess client for verbal reports of dyspepsia (e.g. epigastric discomfort, feeling of fullness or bloating, nausea).
	  2. Determine if particular foods/fluids contribute to dyspepsia.
	  3. Implement measures *to reduce dyspepsia:*
	    a. perform actions *to reduce gastroesophageal reflux:*
	      1. keep head of bed elevated for 2–3 hours after meals
	      2. provide small, frequent meals rather than large ones
	      3. implement measures to restore fluid balance (see Nursing Diagnosis 2, action a.4) *in order to reduce ascites*
	      4. administer gastrointestinal stimulants (e.g. cisapride) if ordered *to promote gastric emptying*
	    b. instruct client to ingest foods and fluids slowly
	    c. instruct client to avoid foods/fluids that may cause gastric irritation (e.g. spicy foods; caffeine-containing beverages such as coffee, tea, and colas; decaffeinated coffee; alcohol)
	    d. instruct client to eat dry foods (e.g. toast, crackers) and avoid drinking liquids with meals if nauseated

Desired Outcome	Nursing Actions and **Selected Purposes/Rationales**
	e. encourage client not to smoke
	f. instruct client to avoid foods high in fat *in order to prevent a delay in gastric emptying and reduce nausea associated with impaired fat digestion*
	g. administer the following medications if ordered:
	1. antacids and histamine$_2$ receptor antagonists (e.g. famotidine, ranitidine) *to reduce acidity of gastric contents and subsequently also reduce esophageal irritation if reflux occurs*
	2. cytoprotective agents (e.g. sucralfate) *to protect the gastric mucosa*
	3. nonselective beta-adrenergic blockers (e.g. propranolol, nadolol) *to reduce venous congestion in the gastrointestinal tract.*
	4. Consult physician if above measures fail to control dyspepsia.

---

6. NURSING DIAGNOSIS: **Risk for impaired tissue integrity**

related to:
a. damage to the skin and/or subcutaneous tissue associated with prolonged pressure on the tissues, friction, and/or shearing if mobility is decreased;
b. increased fragility of the skin associated with edema and malnutrition;
c. excessive scratching associated with pruritus.

Desired Outcome	Nursing Actions and **Selected Purposes/Rationales**

6. The client will maintain tissue integrity as evidenced by:
 a. absence of redness and irritation
 b. no skin breakdown.
	6.a. Inspect the skin (especially bony prominences and dependent, edematous, and pruritic areas) for pallor, redness, and breakdown.
	 b. Refer to Care Plan on Immobility, Nursing Diagnosis 4, action b (pp. 129–130), for measures to prevent tissue breakdown.
	 c. Implement additional measures *to prevent tissue breakdown:*
	   1. perform actions *to prevent skin irritation resulting from scratching:*
	     a. implement measures to relieve pruritus (see Nursing Diagnosis 5.A, action 2)
	     b. keep nails trimmed and/or apply mittens if necessary
	     c. instruct client to apply firm pressure to pruritic areas rather than scratching
	   2. perform actions to improve nutritional status (see Nursing Diagnosis 3, action c)
	   3. perform actions to reduce fluid volume excess (see Nursing Diagnosis 2, action a.4.a.) *in order to reduce edema.*

---

7. NURSING DIAGNOSIS: **Activity intolerance**

related to:
a. tissue hypoxia associated with anemia resulting from:
  1. decreased production of RBCs resulting from a decreased oral intake of vitamins and minerals, an inability of the liver to store vitamins and minerals, and the toxic effect of alcohol on the bone marrow
  2. excessive RBC destruction resulting from hypersplenism (if venous congestion has resulted in splenomegaly, the spleen will destroy RBCs faster than usual)
  3. blood loss if bleeding has occurred;
b. loss of muscle mass, tone, and strength associated with malnutrition and disuse if mobility has been limited for an extended period;

   c. decrease in available energy associated with inability of the liver to
      metabolize glucose, fats, and proteins properly;
   d. difficulty resting and sleeping associated with dyspnea, discomfort, frequent
      assessments and treatments, fear, anxiety, and unfamiliar environment.

Desired Outcome	Nursing Actions and *Selected Purposes/Rationales*

7. The client will demonstrate an increased tolerance for activity as evidenced by:
a. verbalization of feeling less fatigued and weak
b. ability to perform activities of daily living without exertional dyspnea, chest pain, diaphoresis, dizziness, and a significant change in vital signs.
	7.a. Assess for signs and symptoms of activity intolerance:
	  1. statements of fatigue or weakness
	  2. exertional dyspnea, chest pain, diaphoresis, or dizziness
	  3. abnormal heart rate response to activity (e.g. increase in rate of 20 beats/minute above resting rate, rate not returning to preactivity level within 3 minutes after stopping activity, change from regular to irregular rate)
	  4. decreased systolic B/P or a significant increase (10–15 mm Hg) in diastolic pressure with activity.
	  b. Implement measures *to improve activity tolerance:*
	    1. perform actions *to promote rest and/or conserve energy:*
	      a. maintain activity restrictions as ordered
	      b. minimize environmental activity and noise
	      c. organize nursing care to allow for periods of uninterrupted rest
	      d. limit the number of visitors and their length of stay
	      e. assist client with self-care activities as needed
	      f. keep supplies and personal articles within easy reach
	      g. instruct client in energy-saving techniques (e.g. using shower chair when showering, sitting to brush teeth or comb hair)
	      h. implement measures to reduce fear and anxiety (see Nursing Diagnosis 15)
	      i. implement measures to promote sleep (see Nursing Diagnosis 10)
	      j. implement measures to reduce discomfort (see Nursing Diagnoses 4, action e; 5.A, action 2; and 5.B, action 3)
	    2. discourage smoking and excessive intake of beverages high in caffeine such as coffee, tea, and colas (*nicotine and caffeine increase cardiac workload and myocardial oxygen utilization, thereby decreasing oxygen availability*)
	    3. perform actions to improve breathing pattern (see Nursing Diagnosis 1, action c) *in order to decrease dyspnea and improve tissue oxygenation*
	    4. maintain oxygen therapy as ordered
	    5. perform actions to improve nutritional status (see Nursing Diagnosis 3, action c)
	    6. administer packed red blood cells if ordered
	    7. increase client's activity gradually as allowed and tolerated.
	  c. Instruct client to:
	    1. report a decreased tolerance for activity
	    2. stop any activity that causes chest pain, a marked increase in shortness of breath, dizziness, or extreme fatigue or weakness.
	  d. Consult physician if signs and symptoms of activity intolerance persist or worsen.

---

8. NURSING DIAGNOSIS: **Self-care deficit**

related to:
a. weakness, fatigue, and dyspnea;
b. altered thought processes.

Desired Outcome	Nursing Actions and **Selected Purposes/Rationales**

8. The client will demonstrate increased participation in self-care activities within physical and cognitive limitations and prescribed activity restrictions.	8.a. Refer to Care Plan on Immobility, Nursing Diagnosis 7 (p. 132), for measures related to planning for and meeting the client's self-care needs.
	b. Implement measures *to further facilitate the client's ability to perform self-care activities:*
	  1. perform actions to increase strength and activity tolerance (see Nursing Diagnosis 7, action b)
	  2. perform actions to maintain optimal thought processes (see Nursing Diagnosis 9, action c)
	  3. perform actions to improve breathing pattern (see Nursing Diagnosis 1, action c) *in order to decrease dyspnea.*

---

9. NURSING DIAGNOSIS: **Altered thought processes***

related to disturbances in central nervous system functioning associated with accumulation of toxic substances (e.g. ammonia) in the brain, toxic effects of long-term alcohol use, deficiencies of certain vitamins (e.g. thiamine), and hypoxia if anemia is moderate to severe.

---

*The diagnostic label of acute or chronic confusion might be more appropriate depending on the client's symptoms.

Desired Outcome	Nursing Actions and **Selected Purposes/Rationales**

9. The client will demonstrate improvement in thought processes as evidenced by:
a. improved ability to grasp ideas
b. improved memory
c. longer attention span
d. absence or resolution of inappropriate behavior
e. oriented to person, place, and time.
	9.a. Assess client for altered thought processes (e.g. impaired ability to grasp ideas, impaired memory, shortened attention span, inappropriate affect or behavior, disorientation).
	b. Ascertain from significant others client's usual level of cognitive and emotional functioning and whether personality changes have occurred.
	c. Implement measures *to maintain optimal thought processes:*
	  1. perform actions to improve nutritional status (see Nursing Diagnosis 3, action c) *in order to provide vitamins and minerals that are essential for normal neurological functioning and treatment of anemia*
	  2. perform actions to prevent or manage hepatic coma (see Collaborative Diagnosis 13, actions d.3 and 4) *and subsequently reduce levels of cerebral toxins*
	  3. administer central nervous system depressants such as opioids (narcotics), sedative-hypnotics, and antianxiety agents with extreme caution (*many of these agents are metabolized in the liver*); question any order for a normal adult dose of these medications
	  4. administer thiamine if ordered *to prevent progression of neurological manifestations.*
	d. If client shows evidence of altered thought processes:
	  1. reorient client to person, place, and time as necessary
	  2. address client by name
	  3. place familiar objects, clock, and calendar within client's view
	  4. approach client in a slow, calm manner; allow adequate time for communication
	  5. repeat instructions as necessary using clear, simple language and short sentences
	  6. maintain a consistent and fairly structured routine and write out a schedule of activities for client to refer to if desired

7. have client perform only one activity at a time and allow adequate time for performance of activities
8. encourage client to make lists of planned activities, questions, and concerns
9. assist client to problem solve if necessary
10. maintain realistic expectations of client's ability to learn, comprehend, and remember information provided; provide client with a written copy of instructions
11. encourage significant others to be supportive of client; instruct them in methods of dealing with client's altered thought processes
12. inform client and significant others that cognitive and emotional functioning are likely to improve with treatment
13. consult physician if altered thought processes worsen.

---

10. NURSING DIAGNOSIS:

Sleep pattern disturbance

related to unfamiliar environment, frequent assessments and treatments, decreased physical activity, discomfort, fear, anxiety, and inability to assume usual sleep position as a result of orthopnea.

Desired Outcome	Nursing Actions and *Selected Purposes/Rationales*
10. The client will attain optimal amounts of sleep (see Care Plan on Immobility, Nursing Diagnosis 10 [p. 134], for outcome criteria).	10.a. Refer to Care Plan on Immobility, Nursing Diagnosis 10 (pp. 134–135), for measures related to assessment and promotion of sleep. b. Implement additional measures *to promote sleep:* 1. if client has orthopnea, assist him/her to assume a position *that facilitates breathing* (e.g. head of bed elevated with arms supported on pillows, sitting in a chair) 2. maintain oxygen therapy during sleep if indicated 3. perform actions to reduce discomfort (see Nursing Diagnoses 4, action e; 5.A, action 2; and 5.B, action 3) 4. administer prescribed sedative-hypnotics only as necessary remembering that these agents must be used cautiously *because many are metabolized by the liver.*

---

11. NURSING DIAGNOSIS:

Risk for infection

related to:
a. lowered resistance to infection associated with:
   1. diminished function of the Kupffer cells in the liver (these cells normally phagocytize bacteria)
   2. malnutrition
   3. leukopenia resulting from the toxic effect of alcohol on the bone marrow and hypersplenism (if venous congestion has resulted in splenomegaly, the spleen will destroy leukocytes faster than usual)
   4. serum complement deficiency resulting from decreased production of complement proteins by the liver;
b. colonization of bacteria in the ascitic fluid (spontaneous bacterial peritonitis);
c. stasis of secretions in the lungs and urinary stasis if mobility is decreased.

Desired Outcome	Nursing Actions and *Selected Purposes/Rationales*

11. The client will remain free of infection as evidenced by:
    a. absence of fever and chills
    b. pulse within normal limits
    c. normal breath sounds
    d. usual mental status
    e. cough productive of clear mucus only
    f. voiding clear urine without reports of frequency, urgency, and burning
    g. absence of heat, pain, redness, swelling, and unusual drainage in any area
    h. no reports of increased weakness and fatigue
    i. WBC and differential counts within normal range
    j. negative results of cultured specimens
    k. ascitic fluid polymorphonuclear (PMN) leukocyte count within normal limits.

11.a. Assess for signs and symptoms of infection (be aware that some signs and symptoms vary depending on the site of infection, the causative organism, and the age and immune status of the client):
    1. elevated temperature
    2. chills
    3. increased pulse
    4. abnormal breath sounds
    5. change in mental status
    6. loss of appetite
    7. cough productive of purulent, green, or rust-colored sputum
    8. cloudy, foul-smelling urine
    9. reports of frequency, urgency, or burning when urinating
    10. presence of WBCs, bacteria, and/or nitrites in urine
    11. heat, pain, redness, swelling, or unusual drainage in any area
    12. reports of increased weakness or fatigue
    13. abdominal pain and tenderness
    14. elevated WBC count and/or significant change in differential.
  b. Obtain specimens (e.g. urine, vaginal drainage, sputum, blood) for culture as ordered. Report positive results.
  c. Assist with paracentesis if performed to obtain ascitic fluid for examination (e.g. culture, PMN count, appearance).
  d. Implement measures *to prevent infection:*
    1. perform actions to prevent tissue breakdown (see Nursing Diagnosis 6, actions b and c)
    2. maintain the maximum fluid intake allowed
    3. use good handwashing technique and encourage client to do the same
    4. use sterile technique during all invasive procedures (e.g. urinary catheterization, venous and arterial punctures, injections)
    5. rotate intravenous insertion sites according to hospital policy
    6. change equipment, tubings, and solutions used for treatments such as intravenous infusions and respiratory care according to hospital policy
    7. anchor catheters/tubings (e.g. urinary, intravenous) securely *in order to reduce trauma to the tissues and the risk for introduction of pathogens associated with the in-and-out movement of the tubing*
    8. maintain a closed system for drains (e.g. urinary catheter) and intravenous infusions whenever possible
    9. protect client from others with infection
    10. perform actions to improve nutritional status (see Nursing Diagnosis 3, action c)
    11. provide or assist with good oral hygiene
    12. perform actions to reduce stress (e.g. relieve discomfort; explain procedures and treatments; provide a quiet, restful environment) *in order to prevent excessive secretion of cortisol (cortisol inhibits the immune response)*
    13. perform actions *to prevent stasis of respiratory secretions* (e.g. assist client to turn, cough, and deep breathe; increase activity as allowed and tolerated)
    14. perform actions to prevent urinary retention (e.g. instruct client to urinate when the urge is first felt, promote relaxation during voiding attempts) *in order to prevent urinary stasis*
    15. instruct and assist client to perform good perineal care routinely and after each bowel movement
    16. administer prophylactic antimicrobials if ordered (norfloxacin is sometimes ordered for clients with ascites *to help prevent spontaneous bacterial peritonitis*).

e. If signs and symptoms of infection occur:
  1. notify physician
  2. administer antimicrobials as ordered; question any order for aminoglycosides *because they can precipitate the hepatorenal syndrome.*

---

12. NURSING DIAGNOSIS:　　**Risk for trauma:**

a. **falls** related to:
  1. weakness
  2. dizziness (can result from anemia and the postural hypotension that occurs with third-spacing)
  3. balance and gait disturbances that can occur with deficiencies of thiamine and/or vitamin B_{12}
  4. altered thought processes (e.g. agitation, confusion);
b. **burns and lacerations** related to:
  1. paresthesias that can occur with deficiencies of thiamine and vitamin B_{12}
  2. tremors and jerky, restless movements associated with delirium tremens ("DTs") if present.

Desired Outcome	Nursing Actions and *Selected Purposes/Rationales*

12. The client will not experience falls, burns, or lacerations.

12.a. Implement measures *to reduce the risk for trauma*:
  1. perform actions *to prevent falls*:
    a. keep bed in low position with side rails up when client is in bed
    b. keep needed items within easy reach
    c. encourage client to request assistance whenever needed; have call signal within easy reach
    d. instruct and assist client to get out of bed slowly *in order to reduce dizziness associated with postural hypotension*
    e. use lap belt when client is in chair if indicated
    f. instruct client to wear well-fitting slippers/shoes with nonslip soles and low heels when ambulating
    g. keep floor free of clutter and wipe up spills promptly
    h. accompany client during ambulation using a transfer safety belt if he/she is weak or dizzy
    i. provide ambulatory aids (e.g. walker, cane) if the client is weak or unsteady on feet
    j. instruct client to ambulate in well-lit areas and to use handrails if needed
    k. do not rush client; allow adequate time for ambulation to the bathroom and in hallway
    l. perform actions to increase strength and activity tolerance (see Nursing Diagnosis 7, action b)
    m. reinforce instructions from physical therapist on correct transfer and ambulation techniques if client has gait disturbances
    n. make sure that shower has a nonslip bottom surface and that shower chair, secure bath mat, call signal, grab bars, and adequate lighting are present
  2. perform actions *to prevent burns*:
    a. let hot foods and fluids cool slightly before serving
    b. supervise client while smoking if indicated
    c. assess temperature of bath water before and during use
  3. assist client with tasks that require fine motor skills (e.g. shaving) *in order to prevent lacerations*

Desired Outcome	Nursing Actions and *Selected Purposes/Rationales*

4. if client is confused or irrational:
    a. reorient frequently to surroundings and necessity of adhering to safety precautions
    b. provide appropriate level of supervision
    c. consult physician about the temporary use of a bed alarm or jacket or wrist restraints if necessary
    d. administer prescribed antianxiety and antipsychotic medications if indicated
5. administer central nervous system depressants with extreme caution (*many of these agents are metabolized in the liver*); question any order for a normal adult dose of these medications.
b. Include client and significant others in planning and implementing measures to prevent trauma.
c. If injury does occur, initiate appropriate first aid and notify physician.

---

13. COLLABORATIVE DIAGNOSES:

Potential complications of cirrhosis:

a. **bleeding** related to:
    1. decreased production of clotting factors associated with impaired liver function and decreased available vitamin K (can occur from malnutrition, antimicrobial therapy, and impaired absorption of vitamin K as a result of bile flow obstruction)
    2. thrombocytopenia associated with toxic effects of alcohol on the bone marrow and hypersplenism (if venous congestion has resulted in splenomegaly, the spleen will destroy platelets faster than usual);
b. **hepatorenal syndrome** related to decreased renal blood flow possibly associated with:
    1. a decrease in the effective intravascular volume resulting from:
        a. third-spacing and sequestration of fluid in the splanchnic system
        b. treatment-induced fluid loss (e.g. paracentesis, diuretic therapy)
    2. intrarenal vasoconstriction resulting from altered prostaglandin levels and an increase in renin output and sympathetic nervous system activity that occur in response to the decreased effective intravascular volume;
c. **bleeding esophagogastric varices** (varices are a result of the development of collateral circulation in the low-pressure vessels of the esophagus and stomach as a result of portal hypertension) related to:
    1. a further increase in portal pressure associated with factors such as volume overload and a sudden increase in intra-abdominal pressure
    2. increased bleeding tendency;
d. **hepatic (portal-systemic) encephalopathy (hepatic coma)** related to altered brain function associated with:
    1. the effect of toxic substances (e.g. ammonia, mercaptans) on the brain
    2. replacement of true neurotransmitters by false neurotransmitters
    3. increased brain sensitivity to certain substances (e.g. benzodiazepines, gamma-aminobutyric acid [GABA]) and conditions (e.g. hypoxia, metabolic alkalosis).

Desired Outcomes	Nursing Actions and *Selected Purposes/Rationales*

13.a. The client will not experience unusual bleeding as evidenced by:
    1. skin and mucous membranes free of petechiae, purpura, ecchymoses, and active bleeding

13.a.1. Assess client for and report signs and symptoms of unusual bleeding:
    a. petechiae, purpura, ecchymoses
    b. gingival bleeding
    c. prolonged bleeding from puncture sites
    d. epistaxis, hemoptysis
    e. unusual joint pain
    f. further increase in abdominal girth
    g. frank or occult blood in the stool, urine, or vomitus

2. absence of unusual joint pain
3. no further increase in abdominal girth
4. absence of frank and occult blood in stool, urine, and vomitus
5. usual menstrual flow
6. vital signs within normal range for client
7. stable or improved Hct and Hb.

    h. menorrhagia
    i. restlessness, confusion
    j. decreasing B/P and increased pulse rate
    k. decrease in Hct and Hb levels.

2. Monitor platelet count and coagulation test results (e.g. prothrombin time or International Normalized Ratio [INR], activated partial thromboplastin time, bleeding time). Report abnormal values.
3. If platelet count is low, coagulation test results are abnormal, or Hct and Hb levels decrease, test all stools, urine, and vomitus for occult blood. Report positive results.
4. Implement measures *to prevent bleeding:*
   a. perform actions to reduce risk of bleeding from esophagogastric varices (see action c.3 in this diagnosis)
   b. avoid giving injections whenever possible; consult physician about prescribing an alternative route for medications ordered to be given intramuscularly or subcutaneously
   c. when giving injections or performing venous or arterial punctures, use the smallest gauge needle possible and apply gentle, prolonged pressure to the site after the needle is removed
   d. caution client to avoid activities that increase the risk for trauma (e.g. shaving with a straight-edge razor, using stiff-bristle toothbrush or dental floss)
   e. whenever possible, avoid intubations (e.g. nasogastric) and procedures that can cause injury to the rectal mucosa (e.g. taking temperature rectally, inserting a rectal suppository, administering an enema)
   f. pad side rails if client is confused or restless
   g. perform actions to prevent falls (see Nursing Diagnosis 12, action a.1)
   h. instruct client to avoid blowing nose forcefully or straining to have a bowel movement; consult physician about an order for a decongestant and/or laxative if indicated
   i. administer the following if ordered *to improve clotting ability:*
      1. vitamin K (e.g. phytonadione) injections
      2. platelets
      3. fresh frozen plasma (FFP).
5. If bleeding occurs and does not subside spontaneously:
   a. apply firm, prolonged pressure to bleeding area(s) if possible
   b. if epistaxis occurs, place client in a high Fowler's position and apply pressure and ice pack to nasal area
   c. maintain oxygen therapy as ordered
   d. implement measures identified in action c.4 in this diagnosis if gastric or esophageal bleeding occurs
   e. administer vitamin K (e.g. phytonadione) injections, whole blood, or blood products (e.g. fresh frozen plasma, platelets) as ordered
   f. assess for and report signs and symptoms of hypovolemic shock (e.g. restlessness; confusion; significant decrease in B/P; rapid, weak pulse; rapid respirations; cool, pale skin; urine output less than 30 ml/hour)
   g. provide emotional support to client and significant others.

13.b. The client will maintain adequate renal function as evidenced by:
1. BUN and serum creatinine levels within normal range
2. normal urine sodium
3. urine output at least 30 ml/hour.

13.b.1. Assess for and report signs and symptoms of the hepatorenal syndrome (e.g. increased BUN and serum creatinine, low urine sodium, urine output less than 30 ml/hour).
2. Implement measures *to reduce the risk for hepatorenal syndrome:*
   a. perform actions *to maintain adequate renal blood flow:*
      1. maintain an adequate fluid intake; if client is on a fluid restriction, maintain the maximum fluid intake allowed
      2. administer albumin infusions if ordered *to increase the effective intravascular volume*

Desired Outcomes	Nursing Actions and *Selected Purposes/Rationales*

 3. consult physician about reducing the dosage of diuretic ordered if client loses more than 1 kg of weight/day (*vigorous diuresis can reduce the intravascular volume enough to decrease renal blood flow and precipitate the hepatorenal syndrome*)
  b. consult with physician regarding discontinuation of prescribed medications that can precipitate the hepatorenal syndrome (e.g. nonsteroidal anti-inflammatory agents, aminoglycosides).
 3. If signs and symptoms of the hepatorenal syndrome occur:
  a. continue with above actions
  b. consult physician regarding discontinuation of nephrotoxic agents (e.g. neomycin) if any have been ordered
  c. prepare client for dialysis if indicated
  d. refer to Care Plan on Renal Failure for additional care measures.

13.c. The client will not experience bleeding of esophagogastric varices as evidenced by:
 1. absence of hematemesis and melena
 2. B/P and pulse within normal range for client
 3. stable or improved RBC, Hct, and Hb levels.

13.c.1. Assess for and report signs and symptoms of bleeding esophagogastric varices (e.g. hematemesis, melena, decreased B/P, increased pulse).
 2. Monitor RBC, Hct, and Hb levels. Report decreasing values.
 3. Implement measures *to reduce risk of bleeding from esophagogastric varices*:
  a. perform actions to reduce fluid volume excess (see Nursing Diagnosis 2, action a.4.a) *in order to reduce portal hypertension and pressure in esophageal and gastric vessels*
  b. instruct client to avoid activities such as straining to have a bowel movement, coughing, sneezing, and bending at the waist *in order to prevent an increase in intra-abdominal pressure*; consult physician about an order for a laxative, antitussive, and/or decongestant if indicated
  c. administer nonselective beta-adrenergic blockers (e.g. propranolol, nadolol) *to reduce portal pressure*
  d. administer vitamin K and blood products if ordered *to improve clotting ability.*
 4. If signs and symptoms of bleeding esophagogastric varices occur:
  a. turn client on side and suction as necessary *to reduce risk of aspiration*
  b. maintain oxygen therapy as ordered
  c. assist with administration of vasopressin or octreotide acetate (Sandostatin) if ordered *to constrict splanchnic vessels and reduce blood flow to the portal vein* (nitroglycerin or isosorbide may be given concurrently *to lower portal pressure and also reduce the side effects of the vasoconstrictor given*)
  d. prepare client for endoscopic sclerotherapy or ligation of varices if planned
  e. assist with insertion of a gastroesophageal balloon tube (e.g. Sengstaken-Blakemore tube, Minnesota tube); maintain balloon pressure and suction and perform saline lavage as ordered
  f. administer vitamin K (e.g. phytonadione) injections, whole blood, or blood products (e.g. fresh frozen plasma, platelets) as ordered
  g. assess for and immediately report signs and symptoms of hypovolemic shock (e.g. restlessness; confusion; further decrease in B/P and increase in pulse; rapid respirations; cool, pale skin; urine output less than 30 ml/hour)
  h. prepare client for a transjugular intrahepatic portosystemic shunt (TIPS) or surgery (e.g. esophageal transection with reanastomosis, distal splenorenal shunt) if planned
  i. provide emotional support to client and significant others.

13.d. The client will not develop hepatic encephalopathy as evidenced by:
 1. usual speech and handwriting
 2. usual mental status

13.d.1. Assess for and report signs and symptoms of hepatic encephalopathy (e.g. change in handwriting, inability to draw simple figures or numbers, slow or slurred speech, inability to concentrate, emotional lability, disordered sleep, agitation, belligerence, disorientation, lethargy, asterixis, fetor hepaticus [musty or fruity odor on breath], unresponsiveness).
 2. Monitor serum ammonia results. Report elevated values.

3. absence of asterixis and fetor hepaticus
4. serum ammonia level within normal range.

3. Implement measures *to reduce the risk of hepatic coma:*
   a. perform actions *to eliminate or control the following factors that increase levels of ammonia and other nitrogenous substances:*
      1. constipation (*results in increased formation and absorption of ammonia and mercaptans from the gut*)
      2. gastrointestinal hemorrhage (*intestinal bacteria convert the protein in blood to ammonia and other nitrogenous substances*)
      3. hypokalemia and/or metabolic alkalosis (*hypokalemia contributes to alkalosis and increased renal production of ammonia; alkalosis increases the dissociation of NH_4 to NH_3, which more readily crosses the blood brain barrier*)
      4. renal failure (*results in decreased excretion of ammonia*)
      5. excessive protein intake (*intestinal bacteria convert protein to ammonia and other nitrogenous substances*)
      6. infection (*bacteria that produce urease break urea into ammonia*)
      7. dehydration/hypovolemia (*reduced blood flow to the liver results in decreased detoxification of ammonia and other toxins*)
   b. consult physician about discontinuation of prescribed medications that are potential hepatotoxins (e.g. isoniazid, amiodarone, methyldopa, phenytoin) *in order to prevent further liver damage*
   c. administer central nervous system depressants such as narcotics, sedative-hypnotics, and antianxiety agents with extreme caution (*many of these agents are metabolized in the liver and may precipitate nonnitrogenous coma*).
4. If signs and symptoms of hepatic encephalopathy occur:
   a. maintain client on strict bed rest *to reduce metabolic demands on the liver*
   b. maintain dietary protein restrictions as ordered; increase protein intake slowly as encephalopathy resolves and encourage intake of vegetable proteins rather than animal proteins (*vegetable proteins are less ammoniagenic*)
   c. ensure a high carbohydrate intake or administer intravenous glucose or tube feedings as ordered *to provide a rapid energy source and decrease metabolism of endogenous proteins*
   d. administer enemas and/or cathartics as ordered *to hasten expulsion of intestinal contents so that bacteria have less time to convert proteins to ammonia and other nitrogenous substances*
   e. administer the following medications if ordered:
      1. antimicrobials that suppress activity of the intestinal flora (e.g. neomycin, metronidazole) *to decrease dietary protein breakdown and subsequently reduce the formation of nitrogenous substances*
      2. lactulose or lactilol *to stimulate catharsis and create an acidic medium in the intestine (the acidity reduces bacterial growth and the resultant formation of nitrogenous substances and also traps ammonia in the colon by promoting the conversion of NH_3 to the poorly absorbed NH_4*)
      3. benzodiazepine receptor antagonists (e.g. flumazenil) *to block benzodiazepine uptake in the brain*
   f. institute general safety precautions
   g. provide emotional support to client and significant others.

---

14. **NURSING DIAGNOSIS:**   **Sexual dysfunction**

related to:
a. impotence associated with testicular atrophy that can result from:
   1. high levels of circulating estrogen (a result of increased peripheral formation of estrogen associated with decreased hepatic clearance of an estrogen precursor)

2. a possible toxic effect of alcohol on the testes;
b. decreased libido associated with:
  1. hormone deficiencies resulting from hypogonadism (thought to be a direct effect of prolonged alcohol intake)
  2. weakness, fatigue, and an altered self-concept.

Desired Outcome	Nursing Actions and *Selected Purposes/Rationales*

14. The client will demonstrate beginning acceptance of changes in sexual functioning as evidenced by:
 a. verbalization of a perception of self as sexually acceptable and adequate
 b. statements reflecting beginning adjustment to effects of cirrhosis on sexual functioning
 c. maintenance of relationship with significant other.
	14.a. Assess for signs and symptoms of sexual dysfunction (e.g. verbalization of sexual concerns or inability to achieve sexual satisfaction, alteration in relationship with significant other).
	 b. Provide accurate information about the possible effects of cirrhosis and alcohol intake on sexual functioning. Encourage questions and clarify misconceptions.
	 c. Implement measures *to promote optimal sexual functioning:*
	   1. facilitate communication between client and partner; focus on feelings the couple share and assist them to identify changes which may affect their sexual relationship
	   2. discuss ways to be creative in expressing sexuality (e.g. massage, fantasies, cuddling)
	   3. arrange for uninterrupted privacy during hospital stay if desired by the couple
	   4. perform actions to improve client's self-concept (see Nursing Diagnosis 16)
	   5. if impotence is a problem:
	     a. encourage client to discuss impotence and various treatment options (e.g. testosterone, vacuum erection aids, penile prosthesis) with physician
	     b. suggest alternative methods of sexual gratification if appropriate
	   6. encourage client to rest before sexual activity
	   7. include partner in above discussions and encourage continued support of the client.
	 d. Consult physician if counseling appears indicated.

■

15. NURSING DIAGNOSIS:

Anxiety

related to difficulty breathing; discomfort; lack of understanding of diagnosis, diagnostic tests, and treatments; uncertainty of prognosis; financial concerns; unfamiliar environment; and possibility of changes in life style and roles.

Desired Outcome	Nursing Actions and *Selected Purposes/Rationales*

15. The client will experience a reduction in anxiety (see Care Plan on Immobility, Nursing Diagnosis 13 [p. 140], for outcome criteria).	15.a. Refer to Care Plan on Immobility, Nursing Diagnosis 13 (p. 140), for measures related to assessment and reduction of fear and anxiety.
	 b. Implement additional measures *to reduce fear and anxiety:*
	   1. perform actions to improve breathing pattern (see Nursing Diagnosis 1, action c) *in order to decrease dyspnea*
	   2. perform actions to reduce pain and dyspepsia (see Nursing Diagnoses 4, action e and 5.B, action 3).

16. NURSING DIAGNOSIS: **Self-concept disturbance***

related to:
a. changes in appearance (e.g. edema, ascites, jaundice, spider angiomas, palmar erythema, gynecomastia);
b. alterations in sexual functioning;
c. infertility associated with hypogonadism if present;
d. dependence on others to meet self-care needs;
e. altered thought processes;
f. stigma of having a chronic illness;
g. possible changes in life style and roles.

---

*This diagnostic label includes the nursing diagnoses of body image disturbance, self-esteem disturbance, and altered role performance.

Desired Outcome	Nursing Actions and *Selected Purposes/Rationales*
16. The client will demonstrate beginning adaptation to changes in appearance, level of independence, body functioning, life style, and roles (see Care Plan on Immobility, Nursing Diagnosis 14 [p. 141], for outcome criteria).	16.a. Refer to Care Plan on Immobility, Nursing Diagnosis 14 (p. 141), for measures related to assessment and promotion of a positive self-concept. b. Implement additional measures *to assist client to adapt to changes in appearance, level of independence, body functioning, life style, and roles:* 1. encourage client to discuss concerns about fertility with physician; discuss alternative methods of becoming a parent (e.g. adoption, artificial insemination) 2. inform client that many of changes in appearance may be lessened by adherence to treatment regimen 3. perform actions to promote optimal sexual functioning (see Nursing Diagnosis 14, action c) 4. discuss techniques the client can use *to adapt to altered thought processes:* a. encourage client to make lists and jot down messages and refer to these notes rather than relying on memory b. instruct client to place self in a calm environment when making decisions c. encourage client to validate decisions, clarify information, and seek assistance to problem solve 5. assist client *to attain and maintain optimal independence:* a. perform actions to increase client's strength and activity tolerance (see Nursing Diagnosis 7, action b) b. consult social services and occupational therapist about a home evaluation before discharge to identify ways that client's home environment can be modified so that he/she can function more independently c. reinforce benefits of using portable oxygen if it has been prescribed 6. encourage maximum participation in self-care within the prescribed activity restrictions and encourage significant others to allow client to do what he/she is able *so that independence can be re-established and self-esteem redeveloped.*

---

17. NURSING DIAGNOSIS: **Ineffective management of therapeutic regimen**

related to:
a. lack of understanding of the implications of not following the prescribed treatment plan;
b. difficulty modifying personal habits (e.g. dietary habits, alcohol intake);
c. insufficient financial resources.

Desired Outcome	Nursing Actions and **Selected Purposes/Rationales**
17. The client will demonstrate the probability of effective management of the therapeutic regimen as evidenced by: a. willingness to learn about and participate in treatment plan and care b. statements reflecting ways to modify personal habits and integrate treatments into life style c. statements reflecting an understanding of the implications of not following the prescribed treatment plan.	17.a. Assess for indications that the client may be unable to effectively manage the therapeutic regimen: 1. statements reflecting inability to manage care at home 2. failure to adhere to treatment plan while in hospital (e.g. not adhering to dietary modifications and fluid restrictions, refusing medications) 3. statements reflecting a lack of understanding of the factors that will cause further progression of liver failure 4. statements reflecting an unwillingness or inability to modify personal habits and integrate necessary treatments into life style 5. statements reflecting the view that cirrhosis has resolved once he/she is feeling better or that there is no way to control the disease and efforts to comply with treatments are useless. b. Implement measures *to promote effective management of the therapeutic regimen:* 1. explain cirrhosis in terms the client can understand; stress the fact that cirrhosis is a chronic disease and adherence to the treatment plan is necessary in order to delay and/or prevent complications 2. encourage questions and clarify misconceptions client has about cirrhosis and its effects 3. encourage client to participate in the treatment plan 4. initiate and reinforce the discharge teaching outlined in Nursing Diagnosis 18 *in order to promote a sense of control and self-reliance* 5. provide instructions on weighing self and calculating dietary sodium and protein content; allow time for return demonstration; determine areas of difficulty and misunderstanding and reinforce teaching as necessary 6. provide client with written instructions about scheduled appointments with health care provider, medications, signs and symptoms to report, weighing self, and dietary modifications 7. assist client to identify ways treatments can be incorporated into life style; focus on modifications of life style rather than complete change 8. encourage client to discuss concerns about the cost of hospitalization, medications, and lifelong follow-up care; obtain a social service consult to assist with financial planning and to obtain financial aid if indicated 9. provide information about and encourage utilization of community resources that can assist client to make necessary life-style changes (e.g. drug and alcohol rehabilitation programs) 10. reinforce behaviors suggesting future compliance with the therapeutic regimen (e.g. statements reflecting plans for integrating treatments into life style, participation in diet planning, statements reflecting an understanding of the importance of eliminating alcohol intake) 11. include significant others in explanations and teaching sessions and encourage their support; reinforce the need for client to assume responsibility for managing as much of care as possible. c. Consult physician about referrals to community health agencies if continued instruction, support, or supervision is needed.

Discharge Teaching

███

18. NURSING DIAGNOSIS: **Knowledge deficit or Altered health maintenance***

---

*The nurse should select the diagnostic label that is most appropriate for the client's discharge teaching needs.

Desired Outcomes	Nursing Actions and *Selected Purposes/Rationales*

18.a. The client will identify ways to prevent further liver damage.	18.a. Provide the following instructions regarding ways to prevent further liver damage:
	 1. avoid the following hepatotoxic agents:
	   a. alcohol
	   b. cleaning agents containing carbon tetrachloride (these are toxic even when inhaled)
	 2. take acetaminophen (e.g. Tylenol) only when necessary and do not exceed the recommended dose because of its potential toxic effect on the liver
	 3. adhere to the following precautions to prevent hepatitis:
	   a. wash hands thoroughly after having a bowel movement
	   b. eat only in restaurants that have been inspected and approved by health authorities
	   c. if blood transfusions are necessary, receive autologous blood or blood from volunteer donors rather than commercially obtained blood
	   d. avoid sharing food or eating utensils and handling toiletry items of others
	   e. avoid intimate contact with known carrier of hepatitis
	   f. avoid oral-anal sex since it is one of the ways that hepatitis A can be transmitted
	   g. avoid sharing/contact with contaminated needles
	   h. get vaccinations for hepatitis A and B if recommended by health care provider
	   i. if traveling to a developing country:
	     1. receive immune globulin and vaccines for hepatitis (e.g. hepatitis B vaccine, hepatitis A vaccine) as recommended by health care provider
	     2. drink only bottled water and avoid eating raw fruits and vegetables washed or prepared with water when in the country.

18.b. The client will verbalize an understanding of the rationale for and components of the recommended diet.	18.b.1. Explain to client that adherence to the recommended diet will reduce the risk of further liver damage.
	 2. Reinforce the dietary instructions outlined in Nursing Diagnosis 3, action c.2.
	 3. Explain the rationale for a diet low in sodium and provide information about decreasing sodium intake:
	   a. be aware that the terms salt and sodium are often used interchangeably but are not synonymous; there is 40% sodium in table salt
	   b. read food labels and calculate sodium content of items; avoid those products that tend to have a high sodium content (e.g. canned soups and vegetables, tomato juice, commercial baked goods, commercially prepared frozen or canned entrees and sauces)
	   c. do not add salt when cooking foods or to prepared foods; use low-sodium herbs and spices if desired
	   d. avoid cured and smoked foods
	   e. avoid salty snack foods
	   f. avoid commercially prepared fast foods
	   g. avoid routine use of over-the-counter medications with a high sodium content (e.g. some antacids [e.g. Gaviscon], Alka-Seltzer).
	 4. Obtain a dietary consult to assist client in planning meals that will meet prescribed dietary modifications.

18.c. The client will identify ways to reduce stress on esophageal and gastric blood vessels.	18.c. Provide the following instructions about ways to reduce stress on esophageal and gastric blood vessels: 1. adhere to prescribed measures to reduce fluid retention (e.g. fluid restriction, low-sodium diet, diuretics) 2. avoid activities that increase intra-abdominal pressure (e.g. straining to have a bowel movement, coughing, sneezing, lifting heavy objects).
18.d. The client will identify ways to prevent bleeding.	18.d.1. Instruct client about ways to minimize risk of bleeding: a. avoid taking aspirin and other nonsteroidal anti-inflammatory agents (e.g. ibuprofen) on a regular basis

Desired Outcomes	Nursing Actions and *Selected Purposes/Rationales*
	b. use an electric rather than a straight-edge razor
	c. floss and brush teeth gently
	d. cut nails carefully
	e. avoid situations that could result in injury (e.g. contact sports)
	f. avoid blowing nose forcefully
	g. avoid straining to have a bowel movement
	h. avoid putting sharp objects (e.g. toothpicks) in mouth
	i. do not walk barefoot.
	2. Instruct client to control any bleeding by applying firm, prolonged pressure to the area if possible.
18.e. The client will identify ways to reduce the risk of infection.	18.e. Instruct client in ways to reduce risk of infection:
	1. continue with coughing and deep breathing or use of incentive spirometer every 2 hours while awake as long as activity is limited
	2. increase activity as tolerated
	3. avoid contact with persons who have an infection
	4. avoid crowds, especially during flu and cold seasons
	5. decrease or stop smoking
	6. drink at least 10 glasses of liquid/day unless on a fluid restriction
	7. adhere to recommended diet
	8. take supplemental vitamins and minerals as prescribed
	9. maintain good personal hygiene
	10. receive immunizations (e.g. influenza vaccine, pneumococcal vaccine, hepatitis vaccines) if approved by health care provider.
18.f. The client will identify ways to relieve pruritus.	18.f.1. Reinforce instructions in Nursing Diagnosis 5.A, action 2, regarding ways to relieve itching.
	2. Instruct client to take bile acid sequestering agents (e.g. colestipol, cholestyramine) or an antihistamine as prescribed.
18.g. The client will state signs and symptoms to report to the health care provider.	18.g. Stress the importance of reporting the following signs and symptoms:
	1. rapid weight gain or loss
	2. increasing size of abdomen
	3. increased swelling of lower extremities
	4. increasing shortness of breath
	5. increased itchiness or yellowing of skin
	6. temperature elevation that lasts more than 2 days
	7. blood in stools, urine, or vomitus; persistent bleeding from nose, mouth, or skin; prolonged or excessive menses; excessive bruising; severe headache; or sudden abdominal or back pain
	8. persistent impotence or decrease in libido
	9. tremors or changes in behavior, speech, or handwriting.
18.h. The client will identify community resources that can assist with home management and adjustment to life-style changes necessary for effective management of cirrhosis.	18.h.1. Provide information regarding community resources that can assist client and significant others with home management and adjustment to changes necessary for effective management of cirrhosis (e.g. Meals on Wheels, home health agencies, transportation services, drug and alcohol rehabilitation programs, counseling services).
	2. Initiate a referral if indicated.
18.i. The client will verbalize an understanding of and a plan for adhering to recommended follow-up care including future appointments with health care provider, medications prescribed, and activity level.	18.i.1. Reinforce the importance of keeping follow-up appointments with health care provider.
	2. Explain the rationale for, side effects of, and importance of taking medications prescribed. Inform client of pertinent food and drug interactions.
	3. Reinforce physician's instructions regarding activity level. Stress the importance of rest.
	4. Implement measures outlined in Nursing Diagnosis 17, action b, to promote the client's ability to effectively manage the therapeutic regimen.

Bibliography

See pages 897–898 and 908.

▤ HEPATITIS

Hepatitis is widespread inflammation of the liver that results in focal degeneration and necrosis of liver cells with subsequent organized regeneration of the cells in the majority of cases. It can be caused by inhalation, ingestion, or parenteral administration of a hepatotoxic agent (e.g. some drugs, alcohol, industrial chemicals), but the majority of cases are due to a virus.

The five major viruses that cause hepatitis are the hepatitis A virus (HAV), hepatitis B virus (HBV), hepatitis C virus (HCV), hepatitis E virus (HEV), and the delta virus or hepatitis D virus (HDV). Hepatitis A is often referred to as infectious hepatitis and is transmitted almost exclusively by the fecal-oral route. Hepatitis B is transmitted parenterally, sexually, and perinatally. Parenteral transmission occurs primarily in intravenous drug users but can also occur in health care workers who have accidental exposure to infected blood. Percutaneous transmission appears to be the predominant route of transmission of hepatitis C with the majority of cases being associated with intravenous drug abuse and transfusions or occupational exposure to infected blood. Hepatitis D appears to require the presence of the hepatitis B virus for its replication and is seen only in HBV-infected persons. Hepatitis E is similar in many respects to hepatitis A. It is transmitted by the fecal-oral route (usually by sewage-contaminated water) and is seen predominantly in persons who live in or have traveled to developing countries.

The clinical manifestations and course of the disease are similar in all types of viral hepatitis. The majority of signs and symptoms are associated with alterations in the structure and function of the liver. The extrahepatic manifestations (e.g. urticarial rash, arthralgias) that occur in some persons with hepatitis B during the prodromal phase result from activation of the complement system by circulating immune complexes. There are 3 stages or phases of viral hepatitis. The earliest is the preicteric or prodromal phase in which the client experiences a variety of flu-like symptoms. The disease is communicable during this phase and, in many cases, does not progress further. The next phase is the icteric phase. It is characterized by jaundice, dark-colored urine, and light-colored stools, which are manifestations of the cholestasis that is often present during this period. The third phase (posticteric or convalescent phase) lasts several weeks to months. During this time, symptoms subside and liver function tests return to normal.

Acute viral hepatitis is a major public health problem because it is highly communicable, is transmissible prior to the onset of symptoms, and, as yet, has no effective drug treatment. The majority of cases are self-limited and resolve completely without complications but a certain percentage of cases of hepatitis B (up to 10%) and hepatitis C (approximately 50%) do progress to a chronic state. The treatment of acute hepatitis is primarily supportive and directed toward reducing metabolic demands on the liver and promoting cell regeneration. Hospitalization is usually not required but it is indicated for certain high-risk persons (e.g. the elderly, immunocompromised persons, persons with other disease conditions that may be difficult to manage with hepatitis) or for persons with severe disease (indicated by a prothrombin time that is prolonged more than 5 seconds, symptoms of encephalopathy, the presence of edema and/or ascites, an inability to maintain adequate hydration, or laboratory results showing hypoglycemia and/or hypoalbuminemia).

This care plan focuses on the adult client with acute viral hepatitis hospitalized because of persistent nausea and anorexia, worsening of liver function test results, and a prolonged prothrombin time. The goals of care are to ensure adequate rest, maintain an optimal nutritional status, reduce discomfort, prevent complications, and educate the client regarding follow-up care. It is the responsibility of each health care provider to maintain appropriate precautions for the type of hepatitis diagnosed in order to prevent the spread of infection to others.

DIAGNOSTIC TESTS

Serum enzymes (e.g. ALT [SGPT], AST [SGOT], alkaline phosphatase)
Serum and urine bilirubin
Protein electrophoresis and immunoelectrophoresis
Antigen and antibody tests (e.g. HB_sAg, HB_eAg, IgM anti-HB_c, HBV DNA, IgM anti-HAV, anti-HDV, anti-HCV)
White blood count (WBC) and differential
Prothrombin time (PT) or International Normalized Ratio (INR)
Liver biopsy

DISCHARGE CRITERIA

Prior to discharge, the client will:

- have resolution of nausea
- have no evidence of bleeding or progressive liver degeneration
- have an adequate nutritional intake
- perform activities of daily living without fatigue
- identify ways to prevent the spread of hepatitis to others
- identify ways to prevent further liver damage

■ verbalize an understanding of the rationale for and components of the recommended diet

■ state signs and symptoms to report to the health care provider

■ verbalize an understanding of and a plan for adhering to recommended follow-up care including activity level and future appointments with health care provider and for laboratory studies.

NURSING/ COLLABORATIVE DIAGNOSES	**1.** Risk for fluid volume deficit △ 706
	 2. Altered nutrition: less than body requirements △ 707
	 3. Pain: right upper quadrant △ 708
	 4A. Altered comfort: pruritus △ 708
	 4B. Altered comfort: nausea △ 709
	 5. Activity intolerance △ 710
	 6. Potential complications:
	   a. bleeding
	   b. progressive liver degeneration (e.g. fulminant hepatitis, confluent hepatic necrosis, chronic active hepatitis) △ 710
	 7. Anxiety △ 712
	 8. Social isolation △ 713

DISCHARGE TEACHING	**9.** Knowledge deficit, Altered health maintenance, or Ineffective management of therapeutic regimen △ 714

---

1. NURSING DIAGNOSIS:

Risk for fluid volume deficit

related to:
a. decreased oral intake associated with anorexia and nausea;
b. excessive loss of fluid if diaphoresis and/or persistent vomiting is present.

Desired Outcome	Nursing Actions and *Selected Purposes/Rationales*

1. The client will not experience a fluid volume deficit as evidenced by:
 a. normal skin turgor
 b. moist mucous membranes
 c. stable weight
 d. B/P and pulse within normal range for client and stable with position change
 e. hand vein filling time less than 3–5 seconds
 f. balanced intake and output
 g. urine specific gravity within normal range
 h. usual mental status
 i. BUN and Hct within normal range.
	1.a. Assess for and report signs and symptoms of fluid volume deficit:
	   1. decreased skin turgor, dry mucous membranes, thirst
	   2. sudden weight loss of 2% or greater
	   3. postural hypotension and/or low B/P
	   4. weak, rapid pulse
	   5. delayed hand vein filling time (longer than 3–5 seconds)
	   6. decreased urine output with increased specific gravity (reflects an actual rather than potential fluid volume deficit)
	   7. change in mental status
	   8. increased BUN and Hct.
	 b. Implement measures *to prevent fluid volume deficit:*
	   1. perform actions to reduce nausea and prevent vomiting (see Nursing Diagnosis 4.B, action 2)
	   2. perform actions to improve oral intake (see Nursing Diagnosis 2, action c.1)
	   3. perform actions to reduce fever if present (e.g. administer tepid sponge bath, administer antipyretics if ordered) *in order to reduce fluid loss from diaphoresis*
	   4. maintain a fluid intake of at least 2500 ml/day unless contraindicated; if oral intake is inadequate or contraindicated, maintain intravenous therapy as ordered.

2. NURSING DIAGNOSIS: **Altered nutrition: less than body requirements**

related to:
a. decreased oral intake associated with anorexia and nausea;
b. loss of nutrients associated with persistent vomiting if present;
c. reduced metabolism and storage of nutrients by the liver associated with an alteration in normal liver function as a result of inflammation;
d. malabsorption of fats and fat-soluble vitamins associated with impaired bile flow resulting from inflammation of the liver;
e. increased utilization of nutrients associated with the increased metabolic rate that is present with infection.

Desired Outcome	Nursing Actions and *Selected Purposes/Rationales*

2. The client will maintain an adequate nutritional status as evidenced by:
a. weight within normal range for client's age, height, and body frame
b. normal BUN and serum albumin, Hct, Hb, and transferrin levels
c. improved strength and activity tolerance
d. healthy oral mucous membrane.
	2.a. Assess for and report signs and symptoms of malnutrition:
	1. weight below normal for client's age, height, and body frame
	2. abnormal BUN and low serum albumin, Hct, Hb, and transferrin levels (some of these values also reflect impaired liver function)
	3. weakness and fatigue
	4. sore, inflamed oral mucous membrane
	5. pale conjunctiva.
	b. Monitor percentage of meals and snacks client consumes. Report a pattern of inadequate intake.
	c. Implement measures *to maintain an adequate nutritional status:*
	1. perform actions *to improve oral intake:*
	  a. implement measures to reduce nausea and prevent vomiting (see Nursing Diagnosis 4.B, action 2)
	  b. obtain a dietary consult if necessary to assist client in selecting foods/fluids that are appealing and adhere to personal and cultural preferences as well as prescribed dietary modifications
	  c. encourage a rest period before meals *to minimize fatigue*
	  d. maintain a clean environment and a relaxed, pleasant atmosphere
	  e. provide oral hygiene before meals
	  f. serve frequent, small meals rather than large ones if client is weak, fatigues easily, or has a poor appetite
	  g. offer larger meals in the morning *since nausea and anorexia are often not as severe early in the day*
	  h. allow adequate time for meals; reheat foods/fluids if necessary
	  i. limit fluid intake with meals (unless the fluid has high nutritional value) *to reduce early satiety and subsequent decreased food intake*
	  j. increase activity as allowed and tolerated (*activity usually promotes a sense of well-being and improves appetite*)
	2. encourage client to consume meals that are well balanced and high in essential nutrients; offer dietary supplements if client's caloric intake is inadequate
	3. assist and instruct client to adhere to the following dietary recommendations:
	  a. avoid skipping meals
	  b. consume a diet high in calories (2000–3000 calories/day) and carbohydrates; if unable to tolerate food, suck on hard candy and drink fruit juices and regular soft drinks
	  c. maintain a moderate to high protein intake (unless the serum ammonia level is high or clinical evidence of encephalopathy is present) *in order to promote healing of the liver*
	4. administer vitamin preparations (e.g. vitamin K, B-complex vitamins, vitamin C) if ordered.
	d. Perform a calorie count if ordered. Report information to dietitian and physician.

Desired Outcome	Nursing Actions and *Selected Purposes/Rationales*
	e. Consult physician about an alternative method of providing nutrition (e.g. parenteral nutrition, tube feeding) if client does not consume enough food or fluids to meet nutritional needs.

---

3. NURSING DIAGNOSIS: **Pain: right upper quadrant**

related to inflammation of the liver.

Desired Outcome	Nursing Actions and *Selected Purposes/Rationales*

3. The client will experience diminished pain as evidenced by:
  a. verbalization of a decrease in or absence of pain
  b. relaxed facial expression and body positioning
  c. increased participation in activities.
	3.a. Assess for signs and symptoms of pain (e.g. verbalization of pain, reluctance to move, grimacing).
	  b. Assess client's perception of the severity of pain using a pain intensity rating scale.
	  c. Assess the client's pain pattern (the pain is often in the right upper quadrant or epigastric area and aggravated by motions that jar the liver).
	  d. Implement measures *to reduce pain:*
	    1. perform actions to promote rest (see Nursing Diagnosis 5, action b.1) *in order to reduce fatigue and subsequently increase the client's threshold and tolerance for pain*
	    2. provide or assist with nonpharmacologic measures for pain relief (e.g. position change; relaxation exercises; restful environment; diversional activities such as watching television, reading, or conversing)
	    3. administer analgesics if ordered; be aware of the following:
	      a. lower doses of narcotics are usually ordered *because the liver cannot detoxify narcotics at a normal rate*
	      b. acetaminophen may be ordered (despite its potential hepatotoxic effect) rather than acetylsalicylic acid *because of the increased risk of bleeding with acetylsalicylic acid.*
	  e. Consult physician if above measures fail to provide adequate pain relief.

4.A. NURSING DIAGNOSIS: **Altered comfort: pruritus**

related to:
1. an accumulation of substances in the blood that act as pruritogens (e.g. bile acid metabolites, endogenous opioid peptides) associated with bile flow obstruction;
2. rash (sometimes occurs as a result of activation of the complement system by circulating immune complexes that are formed in response to a viral infection).

Desired Outcome	Nursing Actions and *Selected Purposes/Rationales*

4.A. The client will experience relief of pruritus as evidenced by:
  1. verbalization of same
  2. no scratching or rubbing of skin.
	4.A.1. Assess for the following:
	    a. reports of itchiness
	    b. persistent scratching or rubbing of skin.
	  2. Instruct client in and/or implement measures *to relieve pruritus:*
	    a. apply cool, moist compresses to pruritic areas
	    b. apply emollient cream or ointment frequently *to prevent dryness*

    c. add emollients, cornstarch, or baking soda to bath water

    d. use tepid water and mild soaps for bathing

    e. pat skin dry after bathing, making sure to dry thoroughly

    f. maintain a cool environment

    g. encourage participation in diversional activity

    h. utilize relaxation techniques

    i. utilize cutaneous stimulation techniques (e.g. massage, pressure, vibration, stroking with a soft brush) at the sites of itching or acupressure points

    j. encourage client to wear loose cotton garments

    k. administer the following medications if ordered:

        1. antihistamines

        2. bile acid sequestering agents (e.g. cholestyramine, colestipol).

  3. Consult physician if above measures fail to alleviate pruritus or if the skin becomes excoriated.

4.B. NURSING DIAGNOSIS: **Altered comfort: nausea**

related to stimulation of the vomiting center associated with stimulation of the visceral afferent pathways as a result of:

1. inflammation of the gastrointestinal tract resulting from immune complex-mediated tissue responses to the viral infection;
2. gaseous distention resulting from impaired fat digestion if bile flow is obstructed;
3. venous congestion in the gastrointestinal tract if portal hypertension has developed.

Desired Outcome	Nursing Actions and *Selected Purposes/Rationales*

4.B. The client will experience relief of nausea as evidenced by verbalization of same.

4.B.1. Assess client for nausea.

  2. Implement measures *to reduce nausea and prevent vomiting:*

    a. eliminate noxious sights and odors from the environment (*noxious stimuli can cause stimulation of the vomiting center*)

    b. instruct client to change positions slowly (*rapid movement can result in stimulation of the chemoreceptor trigger zone and subsequent excitation of the vomiting center*)

    c. encourage client to take deep, slow breaths when nauseated

    d. encourage client to avoid intake of foods/fluids high in fat (e.g. butter, cream, whole milk, ice cream, fried foods, gravies, nuts) *to prevent a delay in gastric emptying and reduce nausea associated with impaired fat digestion*

    e. avoid serving foods with an overpowering aroma; remove lids from hot foods before entering room

    f. instruct client to eat dry foods (e.g. toast, crackers) and avoid drinking liquids with meals if nauseated

    g. provide small, frequent meals; instruct client to ingest foods and fluids slowly

    h. instruct client to avoid foods/fluids that irritate the gastric mucosa (e.g. spicy foods; caffeine-containing beverages such as tea, coffee, and colas)

    i. instruct client to rest after eating with head of bed elevated

    j. administer antiemetics if ordered (phenothiazines are contraindicated *because of their potential cholestatic effects*).

  3. Consult physician if above measures fail to control nausea.

5. NURSING DIAGNOSIS: **Activity intolerance**

related to:
a. inadequate nutritional status;
b. increased energy utilization associated with the increased metabolic rate present in an infectious process;
c. difficulty resting and sleeping associated with frequent assessments and treatments, discomfort, anxiety, and unfamiliar environment.

Desired Outcome	Nursing Actions and *Selected Purposes/Rationales*

5. The client will demonstrate an increased tolerance for activity as evidenced by:
a. verbalization of feeling less fatigued and weak
b. ability to perform activities of daily living without exertional dyspnea, chest pain, diaphoresis, dizziness, and a significant change in vital signs.
	5.a. Assess for signs and symptoms of activity intolerance:
	  1. statements of fatigue or weakness
	  2. exertional dyspnea, chest pain, diaphoresis, or dizziness
	  3. abnormal heart rate response to activity (e.g. increase in rate of 20 beats/minute above resting rate, rate not returning to preactivity level within 3 minutes after stopping activity, change from regular to irregular rate)
	  4. decreased systolic B/P or a significant increase (10–15 mm Hg) in diastolic pressure with activity.
	b. Implement measures *to improve activity tolerance*:
	  1. perform actions *to promote rest and/or conserve energy*:
	    a. maintain activity restrictions as ordered
	    b. minimize environmental activity and noise
	    c. organize nursing care to allow for periods of uninterrupted rest
	    d. limit the number of visitors and their length of stay
	    e. assist client with self-care activities as needed
	    f. keep supplies and personal articles within easy reach
	    g. instruct client in energy-saving techniques (e.g. using shower chair when showering, sitting to brush teeth or comb hair)
	    h. implement measures to reduce discomfort (see Nursing Diagnoses 3, action d; 4.A, action 2; and 4.B, action 2)
	  2. perform actions to maintain an adequate nutritional status (see Nursing Diagnosis 2, action c)
	  3. increase client's activity gradually as allowed and tolerated.
	c. Instruct client to:
	  1. report a decreased tolerance for activity
	  2. stop any activity that causes chest pain, shortness of breath, dizziness, or extreme fatigue or weakness.
	d. Consult physician if signs and symptoms of activity intolerance persist or worsen.

6. COLLABORATIVE DIAGNOSES: **Potential complications of hepatitis:**

a. **bleeding** related to:
  1. decreased production of clotting factors associated with impaired liver function and impaired vitamin K absorption if bile flow is obstructed (normal bile flow is necessary for absorption of vitamin K)
  2. thrombocytopenia associated with hypersplenism (if venous congestion has resulted in splenomegaly, the spleen will destroy platelets faster than usual);
b. **progressive liver degeneration (e.g. fulminant hepatitis, confluent hepatic necrosis, chronic active hepatitis)** related to continued necrosis of liver cells.

Desired Outcomes	Nursing Actions and *Selected Purposes/Rationales*

6.a. The client will not experience unusual bleeding as evidenced by:

1. skin and mucous membranes free of petechiae, purpura, ecchymoses, and active bleeding
2. absence of unusual joint pain
3. no increase in abdominal girth
4. absence of frank and occult blood in stool, urine, and vomitus
5. usual menstrual flow
6. vital signs within normal range for client
7. stable or improved Hct and Hb.

6.a.1. Assess client for and report signs and symptoms of unusual bleeding:
    a. petechiae, purpura, ecchymoses
    b. gingival bleeding
    c. prolonged bleeding from puncture sites
    d. epistaxis, hemoptysis
    e. unusual joint pain
    f. increase in abdominal girth
    g. frank or occult blood in stool, urine, or vomitus
    h. menorrhagia
    i. restlessness, confusion
    j. decreasing B/P and an increased pulse rate
    k. decrease in Hct and Hb levels.

2. Monitor platelet count and coagulation test results (e.g. prothrombin time or International Normalized Ratio [INR], activated partial thromboplastin time, bleeding time). Report abnormal values.

3. If platelet count is low, coagulation test results are abnormal, or Hct and Hb levels decrease, test all stools, urine, and vomitus for occult blood. Report positive results.

4. Implement measures *to prevent bleeding:*
    a. avoid giving injections whenever possible; consult physician about prescribing an alternative route for medications ordered to be given intramuscularly or subcutaneously
    b. when giving injections or performing venous or arterial punctures, use the smallest gauge needle possible and apply gentle prolonged pressure to the site after the needle is removed
    c. caution client to avoid activities that increase the risk for trauma (e.g. shaving with a straight-edge razor, using stiff-bristle toothbrush or dental floss)
    d. pad side rails if client is confused or restless
    e. whenever possible, avoid intubations (e.g. nasogastric) and procedures that can cause injury to the rectal mucosa (e.g. inserting a rectal suppository or tube, administering an enema)
    f. perform actions *to reduce the risk for falls* (e.g. avoid unnecessary clutter in room, instruct client to wear shoes/slippers with nonslip soles when ambulating)
    g. instruct client to avoid blowing nose forcefully or straining to have a bowel movement; consult physician about an order for a decongestant and/or laxative if indicated
    h. administer the following if ordered *to improve clotting ability:*
        1. vitamin K (e.g. phytonadione) injections
        2. platelets
        3. fresh frozen plasma (FFP).

5. If bleeding occurs and does not subside spontaneously:
    a. apply firm, prolonged pressure to bleeding area(s) if possible
    b. if epistaxis occurs, place client in a high Fowler's position and apply pressure and ice pack to nasal area
    c. maintain oxygen therapy as ordered
    d. if gastric or esophageal bleeding occurs:
        1. turn client on side and suction as necessary *to reduce the risk for aspiration*
        2. assist with administration of vasopressin or octreotide acetate (Sandostatin) if ordered *to constrict splanchnic vessels and reduce blood flow to the portal vein*
        3. prepare client for endoscopic sclerotherapy or ligation of varices if planned
        4. assist with insertion of a gastroesophageal balloon tube (e.g. Sengstaken-Blakemore tube, Minnesota tube); maintain balloon pressure, suction client, and perform saline lavage if ordered
    e. administer vitamin K (e.g. phytonadione) injections, whole blood, or blood products (e.g. fresh frozen plasma [FFP], platelets) as ordered

Desired Outcomes	Nursing Actions and *Selected Purposes/Rationales*

| | f. assess for and report signs and symptoms of hypovolemic shock (e.g. restlessness; confusion; significant decrease in B/P; rapid, weak pulse; rapid respirations; cool, pale skin; urine output less than 30 ml/hour). |
| 6.b. The client will not experience progressive liver degeneration as evidenced by:
 1. resolution of signs and symptoms of hepatitis
 2. absence of edema, ascites, and bleeding
 3. usual mental status
 4. coagulation test results and serum AST (SGOT), ALT (SGPT), alkaline phosphatase, bilirubin, albumin, and glucose levels within or returning toward normal limits. | 6.b.1. Assess for signs and symptoms of progressive liver degeneration:
 a. worsening of signs and symptoms (e.g. increased jaundice, weakness, and pruritus)
 b. edema, ascites
 c. bleeding (see action a.1 in this diagnosis)
 d. encephalopathy (e.g. change in handwriting, slow or slurred speech, emotional lability, agitation, asterixis, disorientation, lethargy)
 e. further increase in prothrombin time
 f. further elevation of serum AST (SGOT), ALT (SGPT), alkaline phosphatase, and bilirubin
 g. low serum albumin and glucose.
 2. Implement measures identified in this care plan to promote healing of the liver.
 3. If signs and symptoms of progressive liver degeneration occur:
 a. implement measures to prevent bleeding (see action a.4 in this diagnosis)
 b. implement measures to prevent and treat nitrogen intoxication (e.g. administer neomycin if ordered, administer lactulose if ordered, maintain prescribed dietary protein restrictions) *in order to prevent or treat hepatic encephalopathy* (*hepatic coma*)
 c. administer osmotic diuretics (e.g. mannitol) if ordered *to treat cerebral edema*
 d. monitor capillary blood glucose (CBG) at least every shift and report glucose levels less than 70 mg/dl or values outside parameters specified by physician
 e. implement measures to reduce the risk for injury (e.g. keep side rails up, maintain seizure precautions)
 f. maintain intravenous therapy if ordered
 g. prepare client for liver transplant if planned. |

---

7. NURSING DIAGNOSIS:

Anxiety

related to:
a. unfamiliar environment and lack of understanding of diagnosis and diagnostic tests;
b. lack of definitive treatment for hepatitis and the possibility of serious complications;
c. discomfort associated with nausea, pain, and pruritus;
d. possible transmission of disease to others and rejection by others because of their fear of contracting hepatitis;
e. temporary restrictions of some of usual activities (e.g. vigorous exercise, contact sports, sexual activity, alcohol consumption).

Desired Outcome	Nursing Actions and *Selected Purposes/Rationales*

| 7. The client will experience a reduction in anxiety as evidenced by:
 a. verbalization of feeling less anxious
 b. usual sleep pattern
 c. relaxed facial expression and body movements | 7.a. Assess client for signs and symptoms of anxiety (e.g. verbalization of feeling anxious, insomnia, tenseness, shakiness, restlessness, diaphoresis, tachycardia, elevated blood pressure, facial pallor, self-focused behaviors).
 b. Implement measures *to reduce fear and anxiety:*
 1. orient client to hospital environment, equipment, and routines
 2. introduce client to staff who will be participating in care; if possible, maintain consistency in staff assigned to his/her care *to provide feelings of stability and comfort with the environment* |

d. stable vital signs
e. usual perceptual ability and interactions with others.

3. assure client that staff members are nearby; respond to call signal as soon as possible
4. maintain a calm, supportive, confident manner when interacting with client
5. encourage verbalization of fear and anxiety; provide feedback
6. reinforce physician's explanations and clarify misconceptions the client has about hepatitis, the treatment plan, and prognosis
7. explain all diagnostic tests
8. perform actions to reduce discomfort (see Nursing Diagnoses 3, action d; 4.A, action 2; and 4.B, action 2)
9. provide a calm, restful environment
10. instruct client in relaxation techniques and encourage participation in diversional activities
11. convey acceptance of client
12. provide information based on current needs of client at a level he/she can understand; encourage questions and clarification of information provided
13. perform actions to decrease social isolation (see Nursing Diagnosis 8, action c)
14. assist client to identify specific stressors and ways to cope with them
15. encourage significant others to visit and to convey a caring, concerned attitude without obvious anxiousness
16. include significant others in orientation and teaching sessions and encourage their continued support of the client
17. administer prescribed antianxiety agents if indicated (use caution when administering these agents *because many are metabolized by the liver*).
   c. Consult physician if above actions fail to control fear and anxiety.

---

8. NURSING DIAGNOSIS: **Social isolation**

related to:
a. temporary restrictions of some usual activities (e.g. vigorous exercise, contact sports, sexual activity, alcohol consumption);
b. limited contact with others associated with fear of transmitting hepatitis and others' fear of contracting hepatitis.

Desired Outcome	Nursing Actions and *Selected Purposes/Rationales*

8. The client will experience a decreased sense of isolation as evidenced by:
a. maintenance of relationships with significant others
b. verbalization of decreasing feelings of aloneness and rejection.
	8.a. Ascertain client's usual degree of social interaction.
	b. Assess for indications of social isolation (e.g. absence of supportive significant others; uncommunicative and withdrawn; expression of feelings of rejection, being different from others, or aloneness imposed by others; hostility; sad, dull affect).
	c. Implement measures *to decrease social isolation:*
	  1. assist client to identify reasons for feeling isolated and alone; aid him/her in developing a plan of action to reduce these feelings
	  2. convey acceptance of client
	  3. encourage significant others to visit
	  4. encourage client to maintain telephone contact with others
	  5. educate client and significant others about mode of disease transmission and ways to prevent spread of infection (see Nursing Diagnosis 9, action a.1) *in order to reduce fear of disease transmission.*

Discharge Teaching

■────────────────────────────────────

| 9. NURSING DIAGNOSIS: | **Knowledge deficit, Ineffective management of therapeutic regimen, or Altered health maintenance*** |

---

*The nurse should select the diagnostic label that is most appropriate for the client's discharge teaching needs.

Desired Outcomes	Nursing Actions and *Selected Purposes/Rationales*

9.a. The client will identify ways to prevent the spread of hepatitis to others.

9.a.1. Provide the following instructions on ways to prevent the spread of hepatitis to others:
  a. if client has hepatitis A, instruct him/her to adhere to the following precautions for 1–2 weeks after the onset of jaundice:
    1. wash hands thoroughly after having a bowel movement
    2. use separate toilet facilities if possible; if separate toilet facilities are not available, clean toilet seat with a chlorine solution after use
    3. wash bedding, towels, and underwear separately from other articles in hot, soapy water
    4. do not donate blood or work in food services until approved by physician
  b. if client has hepatitis B, C, or D, instruct him/her to adhere to the following precautions until certain antigen/antibody tests (e.g. HB_sAg, anti-HB_c, anti-HCV) are negative:
    1. wash hands thoroughly after urinating and having a bowel movement
    2. do not share personal articles (e.g. toothbrush, straight-edge razor, thermometer, washcloth)
    3. use disposable eating utensils or wash utensils separately in hot, soapy water
    4. do not share food, cigarettes, or eating utensils
    5. if any injections (e.g. insulin, vitamin B_{12}) are given at home, use disposable equipment and dispose of it properly to reduce the risk of others coming in contact with contaminated needles
    6. avoid intimate sexual contact; once sexual activity is resumed, avoid intercourse during menstruation and intermenstrual bleeding and make sure that a condom is used during intercourse
    7. do not donate blood.
  2. Instruct client to inform household and sexual contacts to see health care provider for appropriate immunization and testing for early detection of hepatitis.

9.b. The client will identify ways to prevent further liver damage.

9.b. Provide the following instructions regarding ways to prevent further liver damage:
  1. avoid alcohol intake for a minimum of 6 months (many sources recommend a year)
  2. avoid contact with industrial toxins (e.g. paint solvents, cleaning agents containing carbon tetrachloride)
  3. take acetaminophen (e.g. Tylenol) only when necessary and do not exceed the recommended dose because of its potential toxic effect on the liver
  4. take precautions to prevent recurrent hepatitis (client is immune only to the viral type he/she has had):
    a. avoid unnecessary transfusions; if transfusions are necessary, receive autologous blood or blood from volunteer donors rather than commercially obtained blood
    b. avoid intimate sexual contact with known carriers of hepatitis; if sexual partner is a carrier, consult health care provider about receiving a hepatitis B vaccination

c. avoid sharing food and eating utensils and handling toiletry items of others

d. avoid sharing/contact with contaminated needles

e. eat only in restaurants that have been inspected and approved by health authorities

f. get vaccinations for hepatitis A and B if recommended by health care provider

g. avoid oral-anal sex

h. if traveling to a developing country:

    1. receive immune globulin and vaccines for hepatitis (e.g. hepatitis B vaccine, hepatitis A vaccine) as recommended by health care provider

    2. drink only bottled water and avoid eating raw fruits and vegetables washed or prepared with water when in the country.

9.c. The client will verbalize an understanding of the rationale for and components of the recommended diet.	9.c.1. Explain to client that adherence to the recommended diet will promote healing of the liver and reduce the risk of further liver damage. 2. Reinforce the dietary instructions outlined in Nursing Diagnosis 2, action c.3. 3. Instruct client to avoid intake of foods high in fat (e.g. butter, cream, ice cream, pork, fried foods, gravy) until gastrointestinal symptoms such as nausea and indigestion subside.
9.d. The client will state signs and symptoms to report to the health care provider.	9.d. Stress the importance of reporting the following signs and symptoms: 1. persistent or recurrent loss of appetite, nausea, fatigue, or weight loss 2. vomiting 3. increased itchiness or yellowing of skin 4. swelling of lower extremities, rapid weight gain, or increased size of abdomen 5. blood in stools, urine, or vomitus; prolonged or excessive bleeding from nose, mouth, or skin; prolonged or excessive menses; excessive bruising; severe headache; or sudden abdominal or back pain 6. changes in behavior, speech, or handwriting.

9.e. The client will verbalize an understanding of and a plan for adhering to recommended follow-up care including activity level and future appointments with health care provider and for laboratory studies.	9.e.1. Reinforce physician's instructions regarding activity level. Stress the importance of rest during convalescent phase (from 6 weeks to 6 months).
	
	2. Reinforce the importance of keeping follow-up appointments with health care provider and for laboratory studies (liver enzyme levels and serological markers provide information about immunity, presence of a carrier state, and chronicity, which helps determine the need for additional treatment [e.g. interferon alfa-2B] and teaching).
	
	3. Provide client with information about and encourage participation in drug and alcohol rehabilitation programs if indicated.
	
	4. Implement measures to improve client compliance:
	  a. include significant others in teaching sessions if possible
	  b. encourage questions and allow time for reinforcement and clarification of information provided
	  c. provide written instructions regarding scheduled appointments with health care provider and for laboratory studies, activity restrictions, and signs and symptoms to report.

Bibliography

See pages 897–898 and 908.

NURSING CARE OF
THE CLIENT WITH
DISTURBANCES OF
METABOLIC
FUNCTION

⬛ DIABETES MELLITUS

Diabetes mellitus is a chronic systemic syndrome characterized by alterations in carbohydrate, fat, and protein metabolism resulting from an inadequate supply of insulin and/or a defective cellular response to insulin. The hallmark of this metabolic disorder is hyperglycemia. Diabetes* is often complicated by structural and functional abnormalities in the blood vessels and nerves. The atherosclerotic changes that frequently occur in the large vessels (macroangiopathy) affect the cardiac, cerebral, and peripheral circulation. Thickening of the basement membrane of the capillaries (microangiopathy) can also occur and is especially significant when it involves the vessels in the eyes and kidneys. The neurological involvement can be manifested in a wide variety of ways. Some neurological manifestations (particularly the mononeuropathies) are thought to be due to an insufficient blood supply to the nerves. However, much of the neurological involvement is thought to be related to a metabolic defect that activates the polyol pathway. This results in an accumulation of sorbitol and a decrease in myoinositol content in the nerves with subsequent axonal dysfunction and degeneration.

The two major classifications of diabetes are insulin-dependent diabetes mellitus (IDDM), also referred to as type I, and noninsulin-dependent diabetes mellitus (NIDDM), often called type II. Insulin-dependent diabetics have an absolute insulin deficiency and are dependent on insulin therapy to prevent ketosis. The insulin deficiency is a result of pancreatic beta cell destruction that is thought to be related to an environmental injury (e.g. viral infection) that occurs in a person with a genetic predisposition to diabetes and subsequently causes an immune attack on the beta cells. Noninsulin-dependent diabetics have a relative deficiency of insulin due to impaired insulin secretion, decreased tissue responsiveness to insulin, and accelerated hepatic glucose production. The major factors in the development of type II

diabetes are genetics and obesity (there is decreased tissue responsiveness to insulin in obese persons).

A sequence of pathophysiological events occur in diabetes. When an insulin deficiency exists, glucose cannot be transported into the cells for energy metabolism. As a result, glucose accumulates in the blood and starts to spill into the urine once the level exceeds the renal threshold (180 mg/dl or greater). The high blood glucose acts as an osmotic diuretic, which leads to excessive diuresis and subsequent fluid volume deficit. Because the glucose cannot be utilized as an energy source by many cells, protein and fat stores are broken down to provide a source of energy for the starving cells. The free fatty acids that are mobilized from adipose tissue are converted by the liver to ketones (acetoacetate, acetone, β-hydroxybutyrate) to be used as an energy source. The ketones are strong acids and eventually deplete the body's buffer system and respiratory compensatory ability, leading to a state of metabolic acidosis. The simultaneous increase in glucagon release that is present with an insulin deficiency exacerbates the hyperglycemia and ketogenesis. Continuation of these metabolic derangements leads to life-threatening imbalances.

This care plan focuses on the adult client who has had diabetes for many years and is being hospitalized because of difficulty stabilizing blood glucose levels. Many of the long-term vascular and neurological complications have been included in this care plan and should be individualized based on the client's current status. The goals of care are to maintain glucose levels within an optimal range, prevent further complications, and educate the client regarding follow-up care. This care plan should be used in conjunction with the care plans on Heart Failure, Myocardial Infarction, Cerebrovascular Accident, Hypertension, and/or Chronic Renal Failure if the client is also being treated for one of these vascular complications of diabetes.

---

*Diabetes mellitus will be referred to as diabetes throughout this care plan.

DIAGNOSTIC TESTS

Fasting plasma glucose (fasting blood sugar [FBS])
Postprandial blood sugar (PPBS)
Capillary blood glucose (CBG)
Glycosylated hemoglobin (Hb A_{1c})
Serum and urine ketones

DISCHARGE CRITERIA

Prior to discharge, the client will:

- have blood glucose stabilized within a desired range
- have signs and symptoms of vascular and neurological complications at a manageable level
- verbalize a basic understanding of diabetes mellitus
- verbalize an understanding of medications ordered including rationale, food and drug interactions, side effects, schedule for taking, and importance of taking as prescribed
- demonstrate the ability to correctly draw up and administer insulin if prescribed

- verbalize an understanding of the principles of dietary management and be able to calculate and plan meals within the prescribed caloric distribution
- demonstrate the ability to perform blood glucose and urine tests correctly and interpret results accurately
- verbalize an understanding of the role of exercise in the management of diabetes
- identify health care and hygiene practices that should be integrated into life style
- identify appropriate safety measures to follow because of the diagnosis of diabetes
- state signs and symptoms of hypoglycemia and ketoacidosis and appropriate actions for prevention and treatment
- state signs and symptoms to report to the health care provider
- share feelings and concerns about diabetes and its effect on life style
- identify resources that can assist in the adjustment to and management of diabetes
- verbalize an understanding of and a plan for adhering to recommended follow-up care including future appointments with health care provider and for laboratory studies.

NURSING/ COLLABORATIVE DIAGNOSES	1. Altered tissue perfusion △ 719
	2. Risk for fluid volume deficit △ 720
	3. Altered nutrition △ 721
	4A. Altered comfort: burning, aching, cramping, hyperesthesia, numbness, and/or tingling (particularly in lower extremities) △ 722
	4B. Altered comfort: retrosternal discomfort, pyrosis, gastric fullness, and/or nausea △ 723
	5. Sensory/perceptual alteration: visual △ 724
	6. Risk for impaired tissue integrity △ 725
	7. Urinary retention △ 726
	8. Constipation △ 727
	9. Diarrhea △ 727
	10. Risk for infection △ 728
	11. Risk for trauma:
	a. falls
	b. burns
	c. lacerations △ 729
	12. Potential acute metabolic complications:
	a. diabetic ketoacidosis (DKA)
	b. hypoglycemia
	c. hyperosmolar nonketotic coma △ 730
	13. Sexual dysfunction △ 732
	14. Powerlessness △ 733
	15. Ineffective individual coping △ 734
	16. Ineffective management of therapeutic regimen △ 735
DISCHARGE TEACHING	17. Knowledge deficit or Altered health maintenance △ 736

---

1. NURSING DIAGNOSIS:

Altered tissue perfusion

related to:
a. vascular abnormalities (atherosclerosis, microangiopathies) that commonly develop with diabetes;
b. postural hypotension associated with autonomic neuropathy involving the cardiovascular system.

Desired Outcome	Nursing Actions and ***Selected Purposes/Rationales***

1. The client will maintain adequate tissue perfusion as evidenced by:
   a. B/P within normal range for client
   b. usual mental status
   c. extremities warm with absence of pallor and cyanosis
   d. palpable peripheral pulses
   e. capillary refill time less than 3 seconds
   f. absence of edema
   g. absence of exercise-induced pain
   h. urine output at least 30 ml/hour.

1.a. Assess for signs and symptoms of autonomic neuropathy involving the cardiovascular system:
   1. lightheadedness, dizziness, or syncope upon standing
   2. decline in systolic B/P of 30 mm Hg or more when client changes from a lying to sitting or standing position.
  b. Assess for and report signs and symptoms of diminished tissue perfusion (e.g. significant decrease in B/P, restlessness, confusion, cool extremities, pallor or cyanosis of extremities, diminished or absent peripheral pulses, slow capillary refill, edema, claudication, angina, oliguria).
  c. Monitor serum cholesterol, triglycerides, and lipoprotein profile. Report abnormalities. (*Elevated lipid levels may contribute to atherosclerosis.*)
  d. Implement measures *to maintain adequate tissue perfusion:*
   1. perform actions *to promote adequate circulation in lower extremities:*
    a. increase activity as allowed; instruct client with intermittent claudication to walk slowly and alternate activity with periods of rest
    b. discourage positions that compromise blood flow in lower extremities (e.g. crossing legs, pillows under knees, use of knee gatch, prolonged sitting or standing)
    c. instruct client in and assist with active foot and leg exercises every 1–2 hours
   2. perform actions *to reduce postural hypotension:*
    a. instruct client to change from a supine to an upright position slowly *in order to allow time for autoregulatory mechanisms to adjust to upright position*
    b. keep head of bed elevated at least 30°
    c. administer fludrocortisone acetate (Florinef) if ordered *to increase intravascular volume*
   3. instruct client to avoid foods high in saturated fat and cholesterol (e.g. butter, cheese, ice cream, eggs, red meat) *in order to reduce progression of atherogenesis*
   4. perform actions to maintain blood glucose at a near-normal level (see Nursing Diagnosis 3, action d); *maintaining blood glucose at a near-normal level may prevent or delay development of some of the vascular complications*
   5. perform actions to prevent fluid volume deficit (see Nursing Diagnosis 2, action b)
   6. perform actions *to prevent vasoconstriction:*
    a. implement measures *to reduce stress* (e.g. explain procedures, maintain a calm environment, reduce discomfort)
    b. discourage smoking
    c. implement measures *to keep client from getting cold* (e.g. maintain a comfortable room temperature, provide adequate clothing and blankets)
   7. administer the following medications if ordered:
    a. lipid-lowering agents (e.g. lovastatin, gemfibrozil) *to prevent further atherogenesis*
    b. pentoxifylline (Trental) *to improve blood flow* (*increases erythrocyte flexibility and reduces blood viscosity*).
  e. Consult physician if signs and symptoms of diminished tissue perfusion persist or worsen.

---

2. NURSING DIAGNOSIS: **Risk for fluid volume deficit**

related to excessive loss of fluid associated with the osmotic diuresis that can result from hyperglycemia.

Desired Outcome	Nursing Actions and *Selected Purposes/Rationales*
2. The client will not experience a fluid volume deficit as evidenced by: a. normal skin temperature and turgor b. moist mucous membranes c. stable weight d. B/P within normal range for client and stable with position change e. hand vein filling time less than 3–5 seconds f. usual mental status g. balanced intake and output h. urine specific gravity within normal range i. Hct within normal range.	2.a. Assess for and report signs and symptoms of fluid volume deficit: 1. warm, flushed skin 2. decreased skin turgor 3. dry mucous membranes, thirst 4. sudden weight loss of 2% or greater (many clients with diabetes are on weight reduction diets, so some weight loss is expected) 5. postural hypotension and/or low B/P 6. delayed hand vein filling time (longer than 3–5 seconds) 7. change in mental status 8. decreased urine output with increased specific gravity (reflects an actual rather than potential fluid deficit; if client has diabetic nephropathy, specific gravity may not be a useful indicator of hydration status) 9. elevated Hct. b. Implement measures *to prevent fluid volume deficit:* 1. perform actions *to prevent or treat hyperglycemia* (see Collaborative Diagnosis 12, action a.2) *in order to prevent osmotic diuresis* 2. maintain a fluid intake of at least 2500 ml/day unless contraindicated; if oral intake is inadequate or contraindicated, maintain intravenous therapy as ordered.

3. NURSING DIAGNOSIS:

Altered nutrition*

related to:
a. inability to metabolize carbohydrates, fats, and proteins properly associated with insulin deficiency;
b. noncompliance with prescribed dietary regimen.

*This diagnostic label includes altered nutrition: less than and more than body requirements.

Desired Outcome	Nursing Actions and *Selected Purposes/Rationales*
3. The client will maintain an adequate nutritional status as evidenced by: a. maintenance of or return toward normal weight b. serum albumin, Hct, Hb, transferrin, and lymphocyte levels within normal range c. usual strength and activity tolerance.	3.a. Assess for signs and symptoms of an altered nutritional status: 1. abnormal weight for client's age, height, and body frame (many clients with type II diabetes are overweight) 2. low serum albumin, Hct, Hb, transferrin, and lymphocyte levels 3. weakness and fatigue. b. Monitor blood glucose levels regularly. Report values below 70 mg/dl, above 200 mg/dl, or outside of the parameters specified by physician. c. Monitor percentage of meals and snacks client consumes. Report a pattern of inadequate or excessive intake. d. Implement measures *to maintain blood glucose at a near-normal level, achieve ideal weight, and provide necessary nutrients in order to maintain an adequate nutritional status:* 1. obtain a dietary consult to reinforce teaching about the diet prescribed and ways to adapt it to personal and cultural preferences and specific needs (dietary restrictions will vary but are most often prescribed as specific percentages of carbohydrate, fat, and protein within an optimal calorie level; it is recommended that 45–60% of calories be derived from carbohydrate [the majority of which should be complex carbohydrates], 20–30% from fat [saturated fats should be restricted to 10%], and 10–25% from protein; increasing soluble fiber [e.g. fruits, legumes, whole-grain cereals, green leafy vegetables] intake is also often recommended *because of its lipid-lowering effect*)

Desired Outcome	Nursing Actions and *Selected Purposes/Rationales*

2. encourage client to adhere to the diabetic diet prescribed and assist him/her with the selection of appropriate foods
3. provide meals and snacks on time and at evenly spaced intervals *to maintain desired balance between insulin and glucose*
4. administer insulin and/or oral antidiabetic agent(s) as ordered *to enhance cellular utilization of glucose and promote normal metabolism of fats and proteins*
5. perform actions to prevent or treat hypoglycemia (see Collaborative Diagnosis 12, actions b.3 and 4)
6. perform actions to treat gastroparesis and relieve gastroesophageal discomfort if present (see Nursing Diagnosis 4.B, action 3) *in order to promote even absorption of nutrients and an adequate oral intake*
7. reinforce importance of weight loss if client is obese (*studies have shown that obesity is a cause of insulin resistance*).

  e. Perform a calorie count if ordered. Report information to dietitian and physician.

4.A. NURSING DIAGNOSIS:	**Altered comfort: burning, aching, cramping, hyperesthesia, numbness, and/ or tingling (particularly in lower extremities)** related to peripheral polyneuropathy and/or peripheral vascular insufficiency.

Desired Outcome	Nursing Actions and *Selected Purposes/Rationales*

4.A. The client will experience diminished discomfort in extremities as evidenced by:
1. verbalization of same
2. relaxed facial expression and body positioning
3. increased participation in activities
4. stable vital signs.

4.A.1. Assess for signs and symptoms of peripheral polyneuropathy and peripheral vascular insufficiency (most often involves the lower extremities):
  a. persistent burning; sharp, shooting pain; or aching sensation that often becomes worse at night
  b. numbness or tingling
  c. hyperesthesia
  d. intermittent claudication (cramping in calves) precipitated by ambulation (*indicative of insufficient blood flow to legs*).
2. Assess for nonverbal signs of discomfort (e.g. grimacing, guarding of affected area, reluctance to move, restlessness, diaphoresis, facial pallor, increased B/P, tachycardia).
3. Assess client's perception of the severity of the discomfort using an intensity rating scale.
4. Assess the client's pattern of discomfort (e.g. location, quality, onset, duration, precipitating factors, aggravating factors, alleviating factors).
5. Ask the client to describe methods he/she has used to manage the discomfort effectively.
6. Implement measures *to reduce discomfort*:
  a. perform actions *to reduce fear and anxiety about discomfort* (e.g. assure client that his/her need for relief of discomfort is understood; plan methods for control of discomfort with client)
  b. perform actions to reduce stress (e.g. explain procedures, maintain a calm environment) *in order to promote relaxation and subsequently increase the client's threshold and tolerance for discomfort*
  c. administer analgesics before pain becomes severe and before bedtime if discomfort is typically worse at night
  d. if client has hyperesthesia, provide a bed cradle *to keep bedding off affected extremities*
  e. assist client with ambulation if walking relieves discomfort (walking usually relieves lower extremity discomfort associated with

neuropathies of the lower extremities); if client is experiencing intermittent claudication, encourage short, more frequent walks *since longer walks exacerbate pain associated with vascular insufficiency*

f. provide or assist with additional nonpharmacologic measures for relief of discomfort (e.g. position change, relaxation exercises, guided imagery, quiet conversation, restful environment)

g. administer the following medications if ordered *to control discomfort:*

1. analgesics (narcotic [opioid] analgesics are avoided as long as possible *because the pain may be chronic*)
2. tricyclic antidepressants (e.g. amitriptyline) alone or in combination with a phenothiazine (e.g. fluphenazine)
3. carbamazepine or phenytoin (have been useful in treatment of some sharp or stabbing neuralgia pain)
4. capsaicin cream (useful in treatment of superficial burning pain)
5. mexiletine (has been approved for use in treating painful diabetic neuropathy)
6. pentoxifylline (Trental) *to improve blood flow and reduce discomfort associated with intermittent claudication.*

7. Consult physician if above measures fail to provide adequate relief of discomfort.

4.B. NURSING DIAGNOSIS: **Altered comfort: retrosternal discomfort, pyrosis, gastric fullness, and/or nausea**

related to delayed emptying of the esophagus and stomach associated with autonomic neuropathy involving the upper gastrointestinal tract.

Desired Outcome	Nursing Actions and *Selected Purposes/Rationales*

4.B. The client will experience a reduction in esophageal and gastric discomfort as evidenced by:
1. verbalization of same
2. relaxed facial expression and body positioning.

4.B.1. Assess client for verbal reports of discomfort in the retrosternal area, heartburn, gastric fullness or bloating, or nausea.

2. Assess for nonverbal signs of discomfort (e.g. grimacing, rubbing midchest or upper abdomen, restlessness, reluctance to move).

3. Implement measures *to reduce gastroesophageal discomfort:*

a. perform actions *to reduce the accumulation of gas and fluid in the upper gastrointestinal tract:*

1. encourage and assist client with frequent position changes and ambulation as tolerated (*activity stimulates gastrointestinal motility*)
2. have client sit up during meals and for 1–2 hours after meals (*gravity promotes passage of food and fluid through the gastrointestinal tract*)
3. provide small, frequent meals rather than 3 large ones; instruct client to ingest foods and fluids slowly
4. instruct client to avoid foods high in fat (*fat further delays gastric emptying*)
5. instruct client to avoid activities such as gum chewing and smoking *in order to reduce air swallowing*
6. instruct client to avoid intake of carbonated beverages and gas-producing foods (e.g. cabbage, onions, beans)
7. encourage client to eructate whenever the urge is felt
8. administer medications that enhance gastric motility (e.g. metoclopramide, cisapride) if ordered

b. perform actions *to reduce nausea if present:*

1. encourage client to take deep, slow breaths when nauseated

Desired Outcome	Nursing Actions and **Selected Purposes/Rationales**
	2. instruct client to avoid foods/fluids that irritate the gastric mucosa (e.g. spicy foods; caffeine-containing beverages such as coffee, tea, and colas)
	3. eliminate noxious sights and odors from the environment (*noxious stimuli can cause stimulation of the vomiting center*)
	4. instruct client to change positions slowly (*rapid movement can result in stimulation of the chemoreceptor trigger zone and subsequent excitation of the vomiting center*)
	5. avoid serving foods with an overpowering aroma; remove lids from hot foods before entering room
	6. instruct client to eat dry foods (e.g. toast, crackers) and avoid drinking liquids with meals when feeling nauseated
	7. administer antiemetics if ordered
	c. administer antacids and histamine$_2$ receptor antagonists (e.g. cimetidine, ranitidine, famotidine) if ordered *to reduce gastric acidity.*
	4. Consult physician if esophageal or gastric discomfort persists or worsens.

---

5. NURSING DIAGNOSIS:

Sensory/perceptual alteration: visual

related to:
a. osmotic swelling of the lens associated with hyperglycemia;
b. changes in the retinal vessels (retinopathy);
c. presence of cataracts (sorbitol accumulation in the lens appears to be a factor contributing to the increased incidence of cataract formation in persons with diabetes).

Desired Outcome	Nursing Actions and **Selected Purposes/Rationales**
5. The client will not experience further progression of visual disturbances and will demonstrate adaptation to existing ones.	5.a. Assess for visual disturbances (e.g. reports of blurred vision [usually associated with a high blood sugar, which results in accumulation of sugar and fluid in the lens], statements of partial or total loss of vision or the presence of "floaters" or flashing lights).
	b. Implement measures identified in Collaborative Diagnosis 12, action a.2, to prevent or treat hyperglycemia *in order to reduce further progression of visual disturbances* (*studies show that the incidence and progression of changes in the eye can be reduced by optimal glycemic control*).
	c. If vision is impaired:
	1. implement measures to reduce the risk for trauma (see Nursing Diagnosis 11, action a)
	2. avoid startling client (e.g. speak client's name and identify yourself when entering room and before any physical contact, describe activities and reasons for various noises in the room)
	3. assist client with personal hygiene he/she is unable to perform independently
	4. if client has glasses, make sure they are within reach
	5. identify where items are placed on plate and tray, cut food, open packages, and feed client if necessary
	6. assist with activities such as filling out menus and reading mail and legal documents as needed
	7. instruct client in use of appropriate self-help devices (e.g. magnifier for insulin syringe, insulin pen that delivers fixed amount of insulin, needle guide for insulin vial, glucometer that displays blood glucose values in bold numbers); monitor client's accuracy in testing blood glucose and administering insulin
	8. provide auditory rather than visual diversionary activities
	9. inform client of resources available if he/she desires additional information about visual aids (e.g. American Federation for the Blind)

    10. encourage client to discuss options available for treatment of
retinopathy (e.g. laser photocoagulation) and cataracts with physician.
  d. Reassess visual status regularly and consult physician if visual status
worsens.

---

6. NURSING DIAGNOSIS: **Risk for impaired tissue integrity**

related to:
a. increased fragility of the skin associated with inadequate tissue perfusion (a
result of the vascular changes that frequently develop in persons with
diabetes);
b. damage to the skin and/or subcutaneous tissue associated with prolonged
pressure on the tissues, friction, or shearing if mobility is decreased;
c. abnormal pressure distribution on plantar aspect of feet associated with
muscle weakness and/or joint deformity in the feet that may occur as a
result of peripheral neuropathy;
d. undetected foot injuries associated with the diminished sensation that may
be present with peripheral polyneuropathy.

Desired Outcome	Nursing Actions and *Selected Purposes/Rationales*

6. The client will maintain tissue integrity as evidenced by:
a. absence of redness and irritation
b. no skin breakdown.
	6.a. Inspect skin for areas of pallor, redness, and breakdown with particular attention to:
	  1. spaces between toes
	  2. feet and lower legs
	  3. dependent areas
	  4. bony prominences
	  5. areas where sensation is diminished (*client may be unaware of development of blisters and ulcerations*).
	  b. Implement measures *to prevent tissue breakdown:*
	    1. assist client to turn every 2 hours if activity is limited
	    2. gently massage around reddened areas at least every 2 hours
	    3. apply a thin layer of powder or cornstarch to bottom sheet or skin and opposing skin surfaces (e.g. axillae, beneath breasts) if indicated *to absorb moisture and reduce friction*
	    4. limit length of time client is in semi-Fowler's position to 30 minutes (*in this position, client tends to slide down in bed, which can cause skin surface abrasion and shearing*)
	    5. instruct or assist client to shift weight at least every 30 minutes
	    6. use pressure-reducing devices (e.g. pillows, gel or foam cushions) if indicated
	    7. keep skin lubricated, clean, and dry
	    8. keep bed linens dry and wrinkle-free
	    9. increase activity as allowed and tolerated
	    10. perform actions to maintain adequate tissue perfusion (see Nursing Diagnosis 1, action d)
	    11. perform meticulous foot care:
	      a. wash feet daily with warm water and a mild soap
	      b. dry feet thoroughly using a soft towel or cloth, paying particular attention to interdigital spaces
	      c. apply lanolin or other lubricating lotion to feet (except between toes) daily
	    12. perform actions *to prevent trauma to feet:*
	      a. caution client to always wear socks and shoes or sturdy slippers when ambulating
	      b. do not place heating pad on feet
	      c. check the temperature of bath water before client immerses feet.

Desired Outcome	Nursing Actions and *Selected Purposes/Rationales*

	c. If tissue breakdown occurs:
	  1. notify physician
	  2. continue with above measures to prevent further irritation and breakdown
	  3. perform care of involved area(s) as ordered or per hospital procedure
	  4. implement additional measures *to promote wound healing:*
	    a. perform actions *to maintain adequate circulation to the wound area:*
	      1. implement measures to maintain adequate tissue perfusion (see Nursing Diagnosis 1, action d)
	      2. do not apply dressings tightly (*excessive pressure impairs circulation to the area*)
	    b. perform actions to prevent infection in wound (see Nursing Diagnosis 10, action c.12)
	    c. perform actions to maintain an adequate nutritional status (see Nursing Diagnosis 3, action d)
	  5. assess for and report signs and symptoms of impaired wound healing (e.g. increasing redness and swelling at wound site, pale or necrotic tissue in wound, separation of wound edges).

---

7. NURSING DIAGNOSIS: **Urinary retention**

related to loss of bladder sensation and diminished contractility of the detrusor muscle associated with autonomic neuropathy involving the pelvic nerves.

Desired Outcome	Nursing Actions and *Selected Purposes/Rationales*

7. The client will not experience urinary retention as evidenced by:
a. voiding at normal intervals
b. no reports of bladder fullness and suprapubic discomfort
c. absence of bladder distention and dribbling of urine
d. balanced intake and output.
	7.a. Determine client's usual urinary elimination pattern.
	b. Assess for signs and symptoms of urinary retention:
	  1. frequent voiding of small amounts (25–60 ml) of urine
	  2. reports of bladder fullness or suprapubic discomfort
	  3. bladder distention
	  4. dribbling of urine
	  5. output less than intake.
	c. Assist with urodynamic studies (e.g. cystometrogram) if ordered.
	d. Implement measures *to prevent urinary retention:*
	  1. offer bedpan or urinal or assist client to bedside commode or bathroom every 2–3 hours if indicated
	  2. instruct client to urinate when the urge is first felt
	  3. perform actions *that may help trigger the micturition reflex* (e.g. run water, place client's hands in warm water, pour warm water over perineum)
	  4. allow client to assume a normal position for voiding unless contraindicated
	  5. instruct client to lean his/her upper body forward and/or gently press downward on lower abdomen during voiding attempts unless contraindicated *in order to put pressure on the bladder area (pressure helps create a sensation of bladder fullness, which stimulates the micturition reflex)*
	  6. administer cholinergic drugs (e.g. bethanechol) if ordered *to stimulate bladder contraction.*
	e. Consult physician about intermittent catheterization or insertion of an indwelling catheter if above actions fail to alleviate urinary retention.

8. NURSING DIAGNOSIS:

Constipation

related to colonic atony or dilatation associated with autonomic neuropathy involving the large bowel.

Desired Outcome	Nursing Actions and *Selected Purposes/Rationales*

8. The client will not experience or will have resolution of constipation as evidenced by:
a. passage of soft, formed stool every 1–3 days
b. absence of abdominal distention and pain, rectal fullness or pressure, and straining during defecation.
	8.a. Ascertain client's usual bowel elimination habits.
	  b. Assess for signs and symptoms of constipation (e.g. decrease in frequency of bowel movements; passage of hard, formed stools; anorexia; abdominal distention and pain; feeling of fullness or pressure in rectum; straining during defecation).
	  c. Assess bowel sounds. Report a pattern of decreasing bowel sounds.
	  d. Implement measures *to prevent or treat constipation:*
	    1. encourage client to defecate whenever the urge is felt
	    2. assist client to toilet or bedside commode or place in a high Fowler's position on bedpan for bowel movements unless contraindicated
	    3. encourage client to relax, provide privacy, and have call signal within reach during attempts to defecate (*measures to promote relaxation enable client to relax the levator ani muscle and external anal sphincter, which facilitates evacuation of stool*)
	    4. encourage client to establish a regular time for defecation, preferably an hour after a meal
	    5. instruct client to increase intake of foods high in fiber (e.g. bran, whole-grain breads and cereals, fresh fruits and vegetables) unless contraindicated; obtain a dietary consult if indicated to assist client with ways to incorporate high-fiber foods into prescribed diabetic diet
	    6. instruct client to maintain a minimum fluid intake of 2500 ml/day unless contraindicated
	    7. increase activity as allowed and tolerated
	    8. administer laxatives or cathartics and/or enemas if ordered.
	  e. Consult physician if signs and symptoms of constipation persist.

9. NURSING DIAGNOSIS:

Diarrhea

related to autonomic neuropathy involving the small intestine.

Desired Outcome	Nursing Actions and *Selected Purposes/Rationales*

9. The client will have fewer bowel movements and more formed stool if diarrhea occurs.	9.a. Ascertain client's usual bowel elimination habits.
	  b. Assess for and report signs and symptoms of diabetic diarrhea (e.g. frequent, loose stools; episodes of explosive diarrhea; abdominal pain and cramping). Be aware that the diarrhea associated with diabetic neuropathy often occurs at night.
	  c. Administer the following medications if ordered *to control diarrhea* (the diarrhea associated with diabetic neuropathy is typically controlled by medications rather than dietary modifications):
	    1. opiate derivatives (e.g. loperamide, diphenoxylate hydrochloride) *to decrease gastrointestinal motility*
	    2. bulk-forming agents (e.g. methylcellulose, psyllium hydrophilic mucilloid, calcium polycarbophil) *to absorb water in the bowel, which results in a more formed stool*

Desired Outcome	Nursing Actions and *Selected Purposes/Rationales*

        3. antimicrobial agents (*it is thought by some practitioners that diarrhea may be partly due to bacterial overgrowth in the small intestine*)

        4. clonidine (has been used with some success to control diabetic diarrhea).

    d. Consult physician if diarrhea persists.

---

10. NURSING DIAGNOSIS: **Risk for infection**

related to:
a. impaired leukocyte function (appears to be directly related to control of blood glucose levels);
b. delayed healing of any break in skin integrity associated with decreased tissue perfusion and altered nutritional status (there is diminished protein synthesis and tissue repair when insulin is deficient);
c. increased growth and colonization of microorganisms in urinary tract associated with glucosuria (creates a good medium for growth of pathogens) and urinary stasis (can result from retention and decreased mobility if present);
d. stasis of respiratory secretions if mobility is decreased.

Desired Outcome	Nursing Actions and *Selected Purposes/Rationales*

10. The client will remain free of infection as evidenced by:
    a. absence of fever and chills
    b. pulse within normal limits
    c. normal breath sounds
    d. usual mental status
    e. cough productive of clear mucus only
    f. absence of any unusual vaginal discharge
    g. voiding clear urine without reports of frequency, urgency, and burning
    h. absence of heat, pain, redness, swelling, and unusual drainage in any area
    i. WBC and differential counts within normal range
    j. negative results of cultured specimens.

10.a. Assess for and report signs and symptoms of infection (be aware that some signs and symptoms vary depending on the site of infection, the causative organism, and the age and immune status of the client):
    1. elevated temperature
    2. chills
    3. increased pulse
    4. abnormal breath sounds
    5. malaise, lethargy, acute confusion
    6. loss of appetite
    7. cough productive of purulent, green, or rust-colored sputum
    8. unusual vaginal discharge and pruritus in vulvovaginal area
    9. cloudy, foul-smelling urine
    10. reports of frequency, urgency, or burning when urinating
    11. presence of WBCs, bacteria, and/or nitrites in urine
    12. heat, pain, redness, swelling, or unusual drainage in any area
    13. elevated WBC count and/or significant change in differential.

b. Obtain specimens (e.g. urine, vaginal drainage, sputum, blood) for culture as ordered. Report positive results.

c. Implement measures *to prevent infection:*
    1. maintain a fluid intake of at least 2500 ml/day unless contraindicated
    2. perform actions to maintain an adequate nutritional status and a near-normal blood glucose level (see Nursing Diagnosis 3, action d)
    3. instruct and assist client with good oral hygiene
    4. use good handwashing technique and encourage client to do the same
    5. use sterile technique during all invasive procedures (e.g. urinary catheterizations, venous and arterial punctures, injections)
    6. change equipment, tubings, and solutions used for treatments such as intravenous infusions, irrigations, and wound care according to hospital policy
    7. rotate intravenous insertion sites according to hospital policy
    8. anchor catheters/tubings (e.g. urinary, intravenous) securely *in order to reduce trauma to the tissues and the risk for introduction of pathogens associated with the in-and-out movement of the tubing*

9. maintain a closed system for drains (e.g. urinary catheters) and intravenous infusions whenever possible
10. protect client from others with infection
11. perform actions to prevent tissue breakdown (see Nursing Diagnosis 6, action b)
12. perform actions *to prevent infection in any existing wound:*
    a. instruct client to avoid touching dressings or open wounds
    b. maintain sterile technique during all dressing changes and wound care
    c. administer antimicrobials if ordered prophylactically
13. perform actions *to prevent stasis of respiratory secretions* (e.g. assist client to turn, cough, and deep breathe; increase activity as allowed and tolerated)
14. perform actions to prevent urinary retention (see Nursing Diagnosis 7, action d) *in order to prevent urinary stasis*
15. assist female client to perform good perineal care routinely *in order to reduce the risk of vaginal infection.*

---

11. NURSING DIAGNOSIS: **Risk for trauma:**

a. **falls** related to:
   1. gait abnormalities (may result from impaired proprioception, muscle weakness, and/or loss of normal structure of the foot associated with motor and sensory neuropathies)
   2. muscle weakness and diminished or absent reflexes in lower extremity(ies) that may be present with peripheral neuropathy
   3. dizziness and syncope associated with postural hypotension that may be present as a result of autonomic neuropathy
   4. diminished visual acuity;
b. **burns** related to decreased sensation in extremities (may be present as a result of peripheral polyneuropathy);
c. **lacerations** related to visual disturbances and decreased ability to perceive position or movement of a body part (results from neuropathy of proprioceptive fibers).

Desired Outcome	Nursing Actions and *Selected Purposes/Rationales*

11. The client will not experience falls, burns, or lacerations.	11.a. Implement measures *to reduce the risk for trauma:*
	1. perform actions *to prevent falls:*
	  a. keep bed in low position with side rails up when client is in bed
	  b. keep needed items within easy reach
	  c. encourage client to request assistance whenever needed; have call signal within easy reach
	  d. instruct and assist client to get out of bed slowly *in order to reduce dizziness and syncope associated with postural hypotension*
	  e. use lap belt when client is in chair if indicated
	  f. instruct client to wear well-fitting slippers/shoes with nonslip soles and low heels when ambulating
	  g. if vision is impaired, orient client to surroundings and identify obstacles during ambulation
	  h. keep floor free of clutter and wipe up spills promptly
	  i. accompany client during ambulation using a transfer safety belt if he/she is weak or dizzy
	  j. provide ambulatory aids (e.g. walker, cane) if client is weak or unsteady on feet

Desired Outcome	Nursing Actions and *Selected Purposes/Rationales*
	k. instruct client to ambulate in well-lit areas and to use handrails if needed
	l. do not rush client; allow adequate time for ambulation to the bathroom and in hallway
	m. make sure that shower has a nonslip bottom surface and that shower chair, secure bath mat, call signal, grab bars, and adequate lighting are present
	2. perform actions *to prevent burns:*
	a. let hot foods and fluids cool slightly before serving
	b. supervise client while smoking if indicated
	c. assess temperature of bath water and heating pad before and during use
	3. assist client with tasks that require fine motor skills (e.g. shaving) *in order to prevent lacerations*
	4. administer central nervous system depressants judiciously.
	b. Include client and significant others in planning and implementing measures to prevent trauma.
	c. If injury does occur, initiate appropriate first aid measures and notify physician.

---

12. COLLABORATIVE DIAGNOSES:	**Potential acute metabolic complications of diabetes mellitus:**
	a. **diabetic ketoacidosis (DKA)** related to hyperglycemia and accelerated ketogenesis associated with insulin deficiency and glucagon excess (DKA may be precipitated by administration of inadequate amounts of insulin and/or the presence of stressors such as illness, trauma, or infection);
	b. **hypoglycemia** related to administration of too much insulin or oral hypoglycemic agent, inadequate food intake, erratic insulin absorption, and/or decreased excretion of insulin and some oral hypoglycemic agents if renal function is impaired;
	c. **hyperosmolar nonketotic coma** related to severe dehydration associated with sustained osmotic diuresis resulting from uncontrolled hyperglycemia.

Desired Outcomes	Nursing Actions and *Selected Purposes/Rationales*

12.a. The client will not experience ketoacidosis as evidenced by:
 1. stable vital signs
 2. usual skin temperature and color
 3. absence of unusual weakness, lethargy, nausea, vomiting, abdominal pain, and fruity odor on breath
 4. unlabored respirations at 14–20/minute
 5. blood glucose less than 300 mg/dl
 6. absence of ketones in blood and urine
 7. anion gap, blood pH, and bicarbonate level within normal range.
	12.a.1. Assess for and report signs and symptoms of ketoacidosis (clients at greatest risk are insulin-dependent diabetics):
	   a. evidence of fluid volume deficit (e.g. hypotension; weak, rapid pulse; warm, flushed skin; thirst)
	   b. weakness, lethargy
	   c. nausea, vomiting, abdominal pain
	   d. acetone (fruity) odor on breath
	   e. Kussmaul respirations
	   f. blood glucose above 300 mg/dl
	   g. ketones in blood and urine
	   h. increase in the anion gap
	   i. low blood pH and bicarbonate (CO_2 content) level.
	 2. Implement measures to prevent or treat hyperglycemia *in order to prevent ketoacidosis:*
	   a. encourage client to adhere to the diabetic diet prescribed (e.g. American Diabetic Association [ADA] diet, consistent carbohydrate diet)
	   b. administer insulin as ordered and in an area where maximum absorption will occur (*the absorption of insulin can be erratic if it is administered in an area where tissue is hypertrophied*); if client has

an insulin pump, maintain prescribed infusion rate and ensure that client receives preprandial boluses as ordered

  c. administer prescribed oral antidiabetic agent(s) 30–60 minutes before meals

  d. minimize client's exposure to emotional and physiological stress (*stress causes an increased output of epinephrine, glucagon, and cortisol, all of which increase blood sugar*).

3. If signs and symptoms of ketoacidosis occur:
  a. maintain client on bed rest
  b. administer the following if ordered:
    1. insulin (regular insulin is administered intravenously in the initial phase of treatment)
    2. intravenous fluid and electrolyte replacements:
      a. isotonic or half-strength normal saline (usually rapidly infused until B/P is stabilized and urine output is adequate)
      b. combination saline and glucose solutions once blood sugar falls to 250–300 mg/dl (*prevents hypoglycemia that can result with a rapid drop in blood sugar*)
      c. potassium chloride or potassium phosphate (*hypokalemia and hypophosphatemia result from osmotic diuresis and a shift of potassium and phosphorus into the cells during insulin therapy*)
      d. sodium bicarbonate if the serum pH drops below 7.0–7.1; if bicarbonate is administered, it should be discontinued when the pH reaches 7.2–7.3 *because reversing acidosis too quickly has harmful physiological effects.*

12.b. The client will not experience hypoglycemia as evidenced by:
1. pulse rate between 60–100 beats/minute
2. absence of palpitations
3. warm, dry skin
4. usual mental status
5. absence of slurred speech, gait abnormalities, mood swings, and seizures
6. blood glucose above 70 mg/dl.

12.b.1. Assess for and report signs and symptoms of hypoglycemia (at greatest risk are clients taking insulin or long-acting sulfonureas, those having adjustments in insulin dosages or having difficulty maintaining an adequate oral intake, and clients with liver disease or end-stage renal failure):
  a. adrenergic-mediated signs and symptoms—tachycardia; palpitations; cool, pale skin; diaphoresis; weakness; nervousness; tremors (*these signs and symptoms reflect the sympathetic nervous system response to hypoglycemia*); be aware that early sympathetic warning symptoms may not be present in some type I diabetics *because of a decrease in epinephrine output* and that early warning symptoms may also be diminished if client is taking a beta-adrenergic blocking agent
  b. signs and symptoms reflecting central nervous system fuel deprivation—headache, inability to concentrate, somnolence, slurred speech, staggering gait, mood swings, irrational behavior, double or blurred vision, confusion, seizures, coma
  c. blood glucose below 70 mg/dl.

2. Determine from client whether he/she has nightsweats, nightmares, or an early-morning headache (*these symptoms are indicative of hypoglycemia occurring during sleep*).

3. Implement measures *to prevent hypoglycemia:*
  a. administer insulin as ordered being careful to inject it into an area that has adequate subcutaneous tissue
  b. perform actions *to ensure that client has an adequate caloric intake:*
    1. provide a meal within 1 hour after administering insulin (especially routine morning dose) or oral hypoglycemic agent
    2. provide protein snacks in midafternoon and at bedtime if client is receiving an intermediate or long-acting insulin
    3. consult dietitian about appropriate supplements if client does not eat all the meals and snacks provided
  c. consult physician about altering prescribed insulin dose and/or providing alternative forms of intake (e.g. intravenous therapy) if client is to receive nothing by mouth in preparation for a diagnostic test or surgery or is unable to maintain an adequate oral intake.

Desired Outcomes	Nursing Actions and ***Selected Purposes/Rationales***

4. If signs and symptoms of hypoglycemia occur, administer the following depending on the severity of hypoglycemia and hospital protocol:
   a. for a mild (blood glucose less than 70 mg/dl) to moderate reaction, give 4 glucose tablets **OR** 4 oz of a regular soft drink **OR** instant glucose; double these amounts if the blood glucose is less than 45 mg/dl; repeat in 10–15 minutes if symptoms persist; once blood glucose is above 70 mg/dl, give client a complex carbohydrate and protein snack (e.g. glass of milk and 2–3 graham cracker squares) if it will be longer than 30 minutes until the next scheduled meal
   b. for a severe reaction (client unresponsive or having difficulty swallowing), give glucagon **OR** 25 ml of 50% glucose intravenously and repeat in 2–5 minutes if no response; contact physician immediately; when blood glucose is above 70 mg/dl and client can swallow without difficulty, give client a snack (e.g. glass of milk and 2–3 graham cracker squares) or a meal.

12.c. The client will not experience hyperosmolar nonketotic coma as evidenced by:
1. stable vital signs
2. usual skin temperature and color
3. absence of motor and sensory deficits and seizure activity
4. blood glucose less than 600 mg/dl.

12.c.1. Assess for and report signs and symptoms of hyperosmolar nonketotic coma (clients at greatest risk are persons over 60 years of age; noninsulin-dependent diabetics; clients with inadequate fluid intake or excessive fluid loss; those who are experiencing unusual emotional or physical stress [e.g. acute illness, infection, surgery]; and clients receiving corticosteroids, diuretics, phenytoin, hyperalimentation, or dialysis treatments):
   a. evidence of fluid volume deficit (e.g. hypotension; weak, rapid pulse; warm, flushed skin; decreased skin turgor; thirst)
   b. extremely high serum osmolality (above 325 mOsm/liter)
   c. neurological signs such as hemiparesis, aphasia, lethargy, disorientation, and seizures
   d. blood glucose above 600 mg/dl with absent or only slight elevation of ketones in urine and serum.
2. Implement measures *to prevent hyperosmolar nonketotic coma:*
   a. perform actions *to prevent or treat hyperglycemia* (see action a.2 in this diagnosis) *in order to prevent hyperosmolarity and the subsequent osmotic diuresis*
   b. notify physician if client is unable to take in an adequate amount of oral fluids, develops signs and symptoms of infection, has persistent diarrhea or vomiting, or is experiencing unusual emotional stress.
3. If signs and symptoms of hyperosmolar nonketotic coma occur, administer the following if ordered:
   a. fluid replacement (isotonic or half-strength saline is infused rapidly until B/P is stabilized and urine output is adequate; once blood sugar falls to 250–300 mg/dl, 5% glucose is added *to prevent hypoglycemia that can result from the rapid drop in blood sugar*)
   b. insulin (regular insulin is administered intravenously in the initial phase of treatment)
   c. intravenous potassium chloride or potassium phosphate (*hypokalemia and hypophosphatemia result from osmotic diuresis and a shift of potassium and phosphorus into the cells during insulin therapy*).

---

13. NURSING DIAGNOSIS: **Sexual dysfunction**

related to impotence associated with autonomic neuropathy involving nerves that control erection and/or decreased penile blood flow resulting from angiopathy.

Desired Outcome	Nursing Actions and *Selected Purposes/Rationales*

13. The client will perceive self as sexually adequate and acceptable as evidenced by:
a. verbalization of same
b. maintenance of relationship with significant other.
	13.a. Assess for signs and symptoms of sexual dysfunction (e.g. verbalization of sexual concerns or inability to achieve sexual satisfaction, alteration in relationship with significant other).
	b. Provide accurate information about the effects of diabetes on sexual functioning. Encourage questions and clarify misconceptions.
	c. Implement measures *to promote optimal sexual functioning:*
	  1. facilitate communication between client and his/her partner; focus on the feelings the couple share and assist them to identify changes that may affect their sexual relationship
	  2. discuss ways to be creative in expressing sexuality (e.g. massage, fantasies, cuddling)
	  3. arrange for uninterrupted privacy during hospital stay if desired by couple
	  4. if impotence is a problem:
	    a. encourage client to discuss impotence and various treatment options (e.g. discontinuance of sympatholytic agents, penile prosthesis, intracavernosal injections of papaverine and phentolamine) with physician
	    b. suggest alternative methods of sexual gratification if appropriate
	    c. discuss alternative methods of becoming a parent (e.g. adoption, artificial insemination) if of concern to client
	  5. include partner in above discussions and encourage continued support of the client.
	d. Consult physician if counseling appears indicated.

14. NURSING DIAGNOSIS: **Powerlessness**

related to:
a. disease progression despite efforts to comply with treatment regimen;
b. dependence on others for assistance with care;
c. need to modify life style as a result of having diabetes.

Desired Outcome	Nursing Actions and *Selected Purposes/Rationales*
14. The client will demonstrate increased feelings of control over his/her situation as evidenced by: a. verbalization of same b. active participation in planning of care c. participation in self-care and treatment plan.	14.a. Assess for behaviors that may indicate feelings of powerlessness (e.g. verbalization of lack of control over self-care or current situation, anger, irritability, passivity, lack of participation in care planning or self-care). b. Obtain information from client and significant others regarding client's usual response to situations in which he/she has had limited control (e.g. loss of job, financial stress). c. Evaluate client's perception of current situation, strengths, weaknesses, expectations, and parts of current situation which are under his/her control. Correct misinformation and inaccurate perceptions and encourage discussion of feelings about areas in which he/she perceives a lack of control. d. Assist client to establish realistic short- and long-term goals. e. Reinforce physician's explanations about diabetes and the importance of adhering to the treatment plan as a way to prevent and/or delay the development of complications. Clarify misconceptions. f. Implement measures to promote effective coping (see Nursing Diagnosis 15, action c) *in order to promote an increased sense of control over his/her situation.* g. Support realistic hope about ability to control the disease process and prevent or delay the development of complications.

Desired Outcome	Nursing Actions and *Selected Purposes/Rationales*
	h. Remind client of the right to ask questions about diabetes and the prescribed treatment plan.
	i. Support client's efforts to increase knowledge of and control over condition. Provide relevant pamphlets and audiovisual materials.
	j. Include client in the planning of care, encourage maximum participation in the treatment plan, and allow choices whenever possible *to promote a sense of control.*
	k. Inform client of scheduled procedures and tests *so that he/she knows what to expect, which promotes a sense of control.*
	l. Encourage significant others to allow client to do as much as he/she is able *so that a feeling of independence can be maintained.*
	m. Encourage client's participation in self-help groups if indicated.

---

15. NURSING DIAGNOSIS: **Ineffective individual coping**

related to fear of complications and inability to manage them; discomfort; need to alter life style; feeling of powerlessness; and knowledge that condition is chronic and will require lifelong medical supervision, dietary regulation, and medication therapy.

Desired Outcome	Nursing Actions and *Selected Purposes/Rationales*

15. The client will demonstrate effective coping as evidenced by:
  a. verbalization of ability to cope with diabetes and its management
  b. utilization of appropriate problem-solving techniques
  c. willingness to participate in treatment plan and meet basic needs
  d. appropriate use of defense mechanisms
  e. utilization of available support systems.
	15.a. Assess for and report signs and symptoms of ineffective individual coping (e.g. verbalization of inability to cope; inability to problem solve, ask for help, or meet basic needs; insomnia; withdrawal; reluctance to participate in treatment plan; inappropriate use of defense mechanisms; inability to meet role expectations).
	  b. Assess client's perception of current situation.
	  c. Implement measures *to promote effective coping:*
	    1. assist client to recognize and manage inappropriate denial if it is present
	    2. encourage verbalization about current situation and ways comparable situations have been handled in the past
	    3. perform actions to reduce feelings of powerlessness (see Nursing Diagnosis 14, actions c–m)
	    4. assist client to identify personal strengths and resources that can be utilized to facilitate coping with the current situation
	    5. create an atmosphere of trust and support
	    6. assist client to maintain usual daily routines whenever possible
	    7. perform actions to reduce discomfort (see Nursing Diagnoses 4.A, action 6 and 4.B, action 3)
	    8. instruct client in effective problem-solving techniques (e.g. identification of stressors, determination of various options to solve problems)
	    9. provide diversional activities according to client's interests and abilities
	    10. assist client to identify priorities and attainable goals as he/she starts to plan for necessary changes in life style
	    11. assist client to identify and utilize available support systems; provide information regarding available community resources that can assist client and significant others in coping with effects of diabetes (e.g. counseling services, diabetic education classes, diabetes support groups)
	    12. assist client to meet spiritual needs (e.g. arrange for a visit from clergy if desired by client)

13. encourage client to share with significant others the kind of support that would be most beneficial (e.g. listening, inspiring hope, providing reassurance and accurate information)
14. support behaviors indicative of effective coping (e.g. active participation in the treatment plan, verbalization of plans for altering life style, verbalization of ability to cope).

d. Consult physician about psychological counseling if appropriate. Initiate a referral if necessary.

---

16. NURSING DIAGNOSIS:

Ineffective management of therapeutic regimen

related to:
a. lack of understanding of the implications of not following the prescribed treatment plan;
b. feeling of lack of control over disease progression despite efforts to follow prescribed treatment plan;
c. difficulty modifying personal habits and integrating necessary treatments and dietary regimen into life style;
d. insufficient financial resources.

Desired Outcome	Nursing Actions and *Selected Purposes/Rationales*
16. The client will demonstrate the probability of effective management of the therapeutic regimen as evidenced by: a. willingness to learn about and participate in treatments and care b. statements reflecting ways to modify personal habits and integrate treatments into life style c. statements reflecting an understanding of the implications of not following the prescribed treatment plan.	16.a. Assess for indications that client may be unable to effectively manage the therapeutic regimen: 1. statements reflecting inability to manage care at home 2. failure to adhere to treatment plan while in hospital (e.g. refusing medications, not adhering to dietary restrictions) 3. statements reflecting a lack of understanding of factors that contribute to acute and chronic complications 4. statements reflecting an unwillingness or inability to modify personal habits and integrate necessary treatments into life style 5. statements reflecting the view that diabetes is curable or that the situation is hopeless and that efforts to comply with treatments are useless. b. Implement measures *to promote effective management of the therapeutic regimen:* 1. determine client's understanding of diabetes; clarify misconceptions and stress the fact that diabetes is a chronic condition and adherence to the treatment plan may delay and/or prevent complications; caution client that some complications may occur despite strict adherence to treatment plan 2. encourage client to participate in assessments and treatments (e.g. blood glucose monitoring, selection of diet, insulin administration) 3. review prescribed diet with client and his/her technique for drawing up and administering insulin and testing blood glucose; determine areas of difficulty and misunderstanding and reinforce teaching as necessary 4. provide client with written instructions about future appointments with health care provider, diet, medications, exercise, signs and symptoms to report, foot care, and sick day management 5. discuss with client difficulties he/she has had incorporating treatments into life style; assist client to identify ways to modify life style rather than completely change it 6. encourage client to discuss concerns about the cost of medications, food, and supplies; obtain a social service consult to assist with financial planning and obtain financial aid if indicated

Desired Outcome	Nursing Actions and *Selected Purposes/Rationales*
	7. perform actions to reduce feeling of powerlessness and promote effective coping (see Nursing Diagnoses 14, actions c–m and 15, action c)
	8. initiate and reinforce the discharge teaching outlined in Nursing Diagnosis 17 *in order to promote a sense of control and self-reliance*
	9. encourage client to attend follow-up diabetic education classes
	10. provide information about and encourage utilization of resources that can assist client to make necessary life-style changes (e.g. diabetes support groups, counseling services, American Diabetes Association, diabetic cookbooks, publications such as Diabetes Forecast)
	11. reinforce behaviors suggesting future compliance with the therapeutic regimen (e.g. participation in the treatment plan, statements reflecting plans for integrating treatments into life style)
	12. include significant others in explanations and teaching sessions and encourage their support; reinforce the need for client to assume responsibility for managing as much of care as possible.
	c. Consult physician about referrals to community health agencies if continued instruction or supervision is needed.

Discharge Teaching

■

17. NURSING DIAGNOSIS: **Knowledge deficit or Altered health maintenance***

*The nurse should select the diagnostic label that is most appropriate for the client's discharge teaching needs.

Desired Outcomes	Nursing Actions and *Selected Purposes/Rationales*
17.a. The client will verbalize a basic understanding of diabetes mellitus.	17.a.1. Determine client's understanding of diabetes mellitus.
	2. Clarify misconceptions and reinforce teaching as necessary. Utilize available teaching aids (e.g. pamphlets, videotapes).
17.b. The client will verbalize an understanding of medications ordered including rationale, food and drug interactions, side effects, schedule for taking, and importance of taking as prescribed.	17.b.1. Explain the rationale for, side effects of, and importance of taking medications prescribed.
	2. Provide the following instructions if client is to administer own insulin injections after discharge:
	a. keep the bottle(s) of insulin currently being used and cartridges of insulin already placed in an insulin delivery device at room temperature unless the room temperature is above 86° F (insulin is stable for up to 1 month at room temperature)
	b. store unopened bottle(s) of insulin and cartridges containing insulin but not yet placed in delivery device in refrigerator
	c. periodically check expiration date and discard bottle(s) and cartridges of insulin that are outdated
	d. do not use insulin that has changed color or contains granules or clumped particles
	e. let refrigerated insulin return to room temperature before use if possible
	f. do not change type or strength of insulin unless directed by physician
	g. rotate injection sites using the following guidelines:
	1. no site should be used more than once a month
	2. there should be at least 2.5 cm (1 inch) between sites
	3. avoid giving injections right at the waistline or within 2.5 cm (1 inch) of the umbilicus
	4. avoid using an area that will be heavily exercised that day (insulin will be more rapidly absorbed from that area)

     5. do not give injections into areas where the skin appears raised, thickened, or "wasted"

   h. clean insulin delivery devices per manufacturer's instructions

   i. plan meals and snacks keeping the onset, peak action, and length of action of the insulin(s) prescribed in mind

   j. adjust insulin dosage based on blood sugar results and parameters established by physician

   k. consult health care provider immediately if vomiting, severe diarrhea, or inability to tolerate food or fluid persists for more than 4 hours

   l. if local reaction such as itching, redness, or tenderness occurs after injections, consult health care provider

   m. always have a rapid-acting carbohydrate readily available and know actions to take if signs and symptoms of hypoglycemia occur (see action i.1.c in this diagnosis)

   n. consult health care provider if repeated episodes of sweating, nervousness, weakness, hunger, shakiness, slurred speech, blurred or double vision, nightmares, and difficulty concentrating occur (may indicate need to reduce insulin dose)

   o. consult health care provider if experiencing unusual emotional or physical stress (e.g. acute illness, physical trauma, pregnancy) so that insulin dose can be increased to provide adequate coverage.

3. If client is discharged with an insulin pump device, provide instructions regarding its management (e.g. changing the needle and tubing, filling syringes, changing batteries in pump). Allow time for practice and return demonstration.

4. If client is discharged on an oral antidiabetic agent, instruct to:

   a. take medication exactly as prescribed

   b. notify health care provider if unable to tolerate food and fluid

   c. limit alcohol intake to small amounts and be aware that a hypersensitivity to alcohol as evidenced by nausea, shortness of breath, sweating, weakness, flushing of face, or pounding heartbeat sometimes develops when taking a sulfonylurea (most frequently occurs with chlorpropamide)

   d. adhere strictly to the prescribed diet (oral antidiabetic agents are not a substitute for good dietary management)

   e. consult health care provider if experiencing unusual emotional or physical stress (e.g. acute illness, physical injury, pregnancy) so that dosage may be adjusted to provide adequate coverage.

5. Instruct client to consult pharmacist or health care provider before taking other prescription and nonprescription medications (e.g. over-the-counter cold preparations).

6. Instruct client to inform all health care providers of medications being taken.

17.c. The client will demonstrate the ability to correctly draw up and administer insulin if prescribed.	17.c. If client is to be discharged on insulin, reinforce the following instructions regarding preparation and administration:

1. mix insulin before use by gently rotating or rolling bottle between palms or palm and thigh; do not vigorously shake the bottle

2. read the label carefully, making sure the syringe and insulin concentrations match and that it is the correct type of insulin (e.g. regular, NPH)

3. clean the top of the bottle(s) with alcohol

4. withdraw the correct amount of insulin making sure to remove air bubbles

5. if mixing two insulins, withdraw in the same order every time (usually recommended that the rapid-acting insulin be drawn up first in order to reduce the risk of contaminating the vial of rapid-acting insulin with a longer-acting insulin)

6. do not mix lente insulins with regular or NPH insulin

7. insert needle into subcutaneous tissue and inject insulin

8. following insulin injection, apply gentle pressure to site rather than rubbing it.

Desired Outcomes	Nursing Actions and *Selected Purposes/Rationales*
17.d. The client will verbalize an understanding of the principles of dietary management and be able to calculate and plan meals within the prescribed caloric distribution.	17.d.1. Reinforce dietary instructions regarding the prescribed diabetic diet and methods of calculating the foods/fluids allowed (e.g. ADA exchange list, consistent carbohydrate diet). 2. Have client plan sample menus before discharge to ensure that he/she is able to calculate the diet correctly. 3. Explain the purpose of weight reduction if client has been placed on a caloric restriction to reduce weight. Reinforce need to avoid fasting and fad diets. 4. Instruct client on appropriate dietary adjustments that should be made if meal schedule or activity level has been significantly altered. 5. Reinforce the following principles of good dietary management: a. eat 3 or more regularly spaced meals each day and do not skip meals b. weigh or measure foods rather than estimating serving sizes c. avoid intake of concentrated sweets (e.g. sugar, candy, syrups, jams, jellies, cakes, pies, pastries, fruits packed in heavy syrup) and foods high in saturated fat and cholesterol (e.g. butter, cheese, eggs, ice cream, red meat) d. read processed food/fluid labels and avoid those foods/fluids that contain significant amounts of sugar, honey, and nutritive sweeteners such as xylitol, sorbitol, and fructose; use artificial (nonnutritive) sweeteners such as saccharin and aspartame when possible e. if alcoholic beverages are consumed, do not omit anything or substitute alcohol for anything in prescribed diet.
17.e. The client will demonstrate the ability to perform blood glucose and urine tests correctly and interpret results accurately.	17.e.1. Review with client how to perform a capillary blood glucose (CBG) measurement, test urine for ketones, and calibrate and maintain a glucose monitoring device. 2. Have client demonstrate blood and urine tests. Reinforce teaching as necessary. 3. Instruct client to keep a record of test results. 4. Provide instructions on actions client should take when test results are abnormal (some clients are instructed to adjust insulin dose and dietary intake; others are instructed to notify appropriate health care provider).
17.f. The client will verbalize an understanding of the role of exercise in the management of diabetes.	17.f.1. Explain how exercise affects blood sugar levels. 2. Provide the following instructions about exercise and diabetes management: a. maintain a regular exercise program making sure to start exercise slowly and build up gradually b. avoid exercising during insulin peak action time c. try to exercise about 1 hour after a meal and about the same time of the day d. avoid giving insulin in a site that will be heavily exercised e. adjust insulin dosage before exercise according to physician's instructions f. consume extra carbohydrates before vigorous exercise and supplement carbohydrate intake (15–30 gm) at 30–60 minute intervals during vigorous prolonged exercise g. consume an extra bedtime snack on days that exercise has been prolonged or unusually vigorous h. do not exercise at times when blood sugar is greater than 250 and/or ketones are present in urine (vigorous exercise may further increase blood sugar and ketones) i. perform blood glucose tests more frequently during periods of significant variation in activity level j. carry a rapid-acting carbohydrate source (e.g. hard candy, glucose tablets) during exercise (especially if insulin dependent and if exercise is expected to be prolonged or vigorous) k. stop any activity that causes extreme weakness, trembling, incoordination, or nausea.
17.g. The client will identify health care and hygiene	17.g.1. Reinforce the importance of adhering to the following health care practices:

practices that should be integrated into life style.

    a. daily oral hygiene including brushing and flossing teeth
    b. regular dental appointments
    c. regular eye examinations with an ophthalmologist
    d. not smoking (smoking contributes to the risk of cardiovascular complications)
    e. limiting alcohol intake
    f. meticulous care of cuts, burns, and scratches.

2. Provide instructions about foot care:
    a. inspect feet daily for cuts, redness, cracks, blisters, corns, and calluses; use a mirror to check bottoms of feet if necessary
    b. wash feet daily with a mild soap and warm water and dry gently but thoroughly
    c. apply lanolin or other lubricating lotion to feet (except between toes) daily
    d. keep feet dry by wearing cotton socks and avoiding shoes with rubber or plastic soles (cause feet to sweat)
    e. cut nails after a bath or shower; cut them straight across and smooth them with an emery board after cutting
    f. see a podiatrist rather than using home remedies to treat corns, calluses, and ingrown nails or if help is needed with routine nail care
    g. avoid wearing socks, stockings, or garters that are tight (may further compromise peripheral blood flow)
    h. buy shoes that fit well and break them in gradually
    i. do not walk barefoot; wear shoes or slippers when walking to protect feet from injury
    j. do not use a heating pad or hot water bottle on feet (if paresthesias are present, burns may occur); test bath water with bath thermometer, wrist, or elbow before immersing feet (temperature should be between 30–32° C [84–90° F])
    k. protect feet from extreme cold to prevent vasoconstriction and possible frostbite.

17.h. The client will identify appropriate safety measures to follow because of the diagnosis of diabetes.

17.h. Teach client the following safety precautions:
1. always carry an identification card or wear a medical alert bracelet or tag
2. always carry a rapid-acting carbohydrate such as glucose tablets or instant glucose gel
3. if insulin-dependent, always have insulin readily available (carry in purse or briefcase)
4. consult physician about plans for pregnancy and maintain close prenatal supervision
5. keep a glucagon kit readily available and know how and when to use it; make sure significant other is also trained in how to use it
6. if ill but able to tolerate some foods/fluids:
    a. take usual dose of insulin or oral antidiabetic agent unless blood glucose is low
    b. consume soft foods or liquids from bread/starch, milk, fruit, and vegetable exchange list if unable to tolerate usual diet or drink at least 4 ounces of a sugar-containing liquid every hour
    c. test blood glucose and urine ketones every 4 hours and report values outside specified parameters (usually instructed to report ketones in urine; instructions vary regarding blood glucose values to report)
    d. do not exercise
7. notify physician if oral intake is inadequate for longer than 24 hours, vomiting or severe diarrhea persists for more than 4 hours, and/or blood glucose is significantly higher than usual and ketones are present in urine
8. inform all health care providers of diabetic condition.

17.i. The client will state signs and symptoms of hypoglycemia and ketoacidosis and

17.i.1. Reinforce the following information about hypoglycemia:
    a. factors that precipitate hypoglycemia (e.g. too much insulin or oral hypoglycemic agent, insufficient oral intake, excessive exercise, excessive alcohol intake)

Desired Outcomes	Nursing Actions and *Selected Purposes/Rationales*

appropriate actions for prevention and treatment.	b. signs and symptoms of hypoglycemia (e.g. shakiness, nervousness, weakness, hunger, sweating, nightmares, early-morning headache, incoordination, blood sugar less than 70)
	c. actions to take if signs and symptoms of hypoglycemia occur:
	  1. test blood glucose if possible and if less than 80 (or if symptoms are present but glucose testing is not possible), take 15 grams of rapid-acting carbohydrate (e.g. half a glass of regular [sugar-containing] soft drink, 4 glucose tablets, half a tube of instant glucose)
	  2. retest glucose level in 15 minutes, and if still less than 80, take another 15 grams of rapid-acting carbohydrate; if blood glucose level remains below 80 and/or symptoms persist for more than 30 minutes, consult health care provider
	  3. after the hypoglycemic episode, consume a snack (e.g. graham crackers and a glass of milk, half a sandwich and half a glass of milk) if it will be longer than 30 minutes until the next meal.
	2. Teach significant others how to prepare and administer glucagon in case client loses consciousness.
	3. Reinforce the following information about ketoacidosis:
	  a. factors that precipitate ketoacidosis (e.g. emotional stress, infection, failure to take insulin or oral antidiabetic agent)
	  b. signs and symptoms of impending or actual ketoacidosis (e.g. unusual thirst; excessive urination; weakness; warm, flushed skin; blood sugar higher than 300; ketones in urine; abdominal pain; nausea and vomiting)
	  c. immediate actions to take if signs and symptoms of ketoacidosis occur:
	    1. drink a cup or more of broth or tea if able to tolerate it
	    2. administer insulin (if previously instructed in insulin coverage based on blood glucose results)
	    3. consult health care provider.

17.j. The client will state signs and symptoms to report to the health care provider.	17.j. Instruct client to report the following:
	  1. unexplained episodes of hypoglycemia and ketoacidosis (see actions i.1.b and 3.b in this diagnosis for signs and symptoms)
	  2. unusual variations in blood glucose results
	  3. a cut, scratch, or burn that becomes red, swollen, tender, or does not start to heal within 24 hours
	  4. nausea and vomiting or severe diarrhea that lasts more than 4 hours
	  5. temperature elevation that lasts more than 2 days
	  6. change in vision
	  7. development or worsening of symptoms that are indicative of long-term complications (e.g. burning or aching pain in extremity, decreased sensation in extremity, persistent gastric discomfort, frequent urination of small amounts, impotence, gait disturbances, chest pain, extreme fatigue, persistent dizziness or lightheadedness).

17.k. The client will identify resources that can assist in the adjustment to and management of diabetes.	17.k.1. Provide information about resources that can assist client and significant others in adjustment to and management of diabetes (e.g. American Diabetes Association, diabetic education classes, weight loss programs, diabetes support groups, counseling services, publications such as Diabetes Forecast). 2. Initiate a referral if indicated.
17.l. The client will verbalize an understanding of and a plan for adhering to recommended follow-up care including future appointments with health care provider and for laboratory studies.	17.l.1. Reinforce the importance of keeping follow-up appointments with health care provider and for laboratory studies. 2. Refer to Nursing Diagnosis 16, action b, for measures to promote the client's ability to effectively manage the therapeutic regimen.

Bibliography

See pages 897–898 and 908–909.

THYROIDECTOMY

Thyroidectomy is the surgical removal of the thyroid gland. It may be performed to treat thyroid carcinoma, unusually large goiters, or hyperthyroidism that has been refractory to medical treatment. A subtotal thyroidectomy (removal of up to 90% of the thyroid gland) is the preferred procedure unless the surgery is being done to treat a malignancy, in which case a total thyroidectomy will usually be performed. Following a subtotal thyroidectomy, the remaining gland tissue usually hypertrophies enough to supply adequate amounts of thyroid hormone.

The client is often given antithyroid agents for 6–8 weeks prior to hospitalization for a thyroidectomy in order to achieve a euthyroid state and minimize the risk of thyroid crisis. Iodine preparations may also be administered for 7–10 days prior to surgery to reduce vascularity of the thyroid gland and the risk for hemorrhage in the intraoperative and postoperative period. During this prehospitalization period, it is also important that an optimal nutritional state and cardiovascular status be attained.

This care plan focuses on the adult client with hyperthyroidism whose condition has been medically stabilized and who is being hospitalized for a subtotal thyroidectomy. Preoperative goals of care are to reduce fear and anxiety and educate the client regarding postoperative care. Postoperatively, the goals of care are to prevent complications, maintain comfort, and educate the client regarding follow-up care.

DISCHARGE CRITERIA

Prior to discharge, the client will:

- have surgical pain controlled
- have evidence of normal healing of surgical wound
- have no signs and symptoms of complications
- verbalize an understanding of range of motion exercises of the neck
- state signs and symptoms to report to the health care provider
- verbalize an understanding of and a plan for adhering to recommended follow-up care including future appointments with health care provider, medications prescribed, activity level, and wound care.

NURSING/ COLLABORATIVE DIAGNOSES	**Preoperative**
	1. Knowledge deficit △ 742
	Postoperative
	1. Ineffective airway clearance △ 742
	2. Impaired tissue integrity △ 743
	3. Potential complications:
	    a. hemorrhage
	    b. respiratory distress
	    c. hypoparathyroidism
	    d. thyroid storm (thyrotoxic crisis)
	    e. laryngeal nerve damage △ 743

DISCHARGE TEACHING	4. Knowledge deficit, Ineffective management of therapeutic regimen, or Altered health maintenance △ 746

See Standardized Preoperative and Postoperative Care Plans for additional diagnoses.

PREOPERATIVE

Use in conjunction with the Standardized Preoperative Care Plan.

Client Teaching

▄▄

1. NURSING DIAGNOSIS: **Knowledge deficit**

regarding the surgical procedure, hospital routines associated with surgery, physical preparation for a thyroidectomy, sensations that normally occur following surgery and anesthesia, and postoperative care.

Desired Outcomes	Nursing Actions and *Selected Purposes/Rationales*
1.a. The client will verbalize an understanding of the surgical procedure, preoperative care, and postoperative sensations and care.	1.a.1. Refer to Standardized Preoperative Care Plan, Nursing Diagnosis 4, actions a.1–4 (pp. 99–100), for information to include in preoperative teaching. 2. Inform client that he/she will be assessed for voice changes routinely after surgery. Explain that hoarseness is expected for a few days and unnecessary talking should be avoided during that time. 3. Allow time for questions and clarification of information provided.

1.b. The client will demonstrate the ability to perform activities designed to prevent postoperative complications.	1.b.1. Refer to Standardized Preoperative Care Plan, Nursing Diagnosis 4, action b.1 (p. 100), for instructions on ways to prevent postoperative complications.
	2. Provide additional instructions on ways to prevent complications after a thyroidectomy:
	  a. instruct client on ways to minimize stress on the suture line:
	    1. support head and neck with hands when turning head, coughing, and moving in bed for first few days after surgery
	    2. avoid turning head abruptly and hyperextending neck
	  b. inform client that he/she will need to do neck range of motion exercises beginning 2–4 days after surgery; demonstrate flexion, extension, rotation, and lateral movement of head and neck.
	3. Allow time for questions, clarification, and return demonstration.

POSTOPERATIVE

Use in conjunction with the Standardized Postoperative Care Plan.

▄▄

1. NURSING DIAGNOSIS: **Ineffective airway clearance**

related to:
a. occlusion of the pharynx associated with relaxation of the tongue resulting from effects of anesthesia and some medications (e.g. narcotic [opioid] analgesics);
b. stasis of secretions associated with:
  1. decreased activity
  2. poor cough effort resulting from the effect of anesthesia and some medications (e.g. narcotic [opioid] analgesics), pain, weakness, and fear of disrupting incision;
c. increased secretions associated with irritation of the respiratory tract (can result from inhalation anesthetics and endotracheal intubation);
d. tracheal compression associated with swelling and/or bleeding in the surgical area.

Desired Outcome	Nursing Actions and *Selected Purposes/Rationales*

1. The client will maintain clear, open airways (see Standardized Postoperative Care Plan, Nursing Diagnosis 3 [p. 103], for outcome criteria).	1.a. Refer to Standardized Postoperative Care Plan, Nursing Diagnosis 3 (pp. 103–104) for measures related to assessment and promotion of effective airway clearance.
	b. Implement additional measures *to promote effective airway clearance:*
	  1. perform actions *to minimize swelling in the surgical area and subsequently reduce pressure on the trachea:*
	    a. keep head of bed elevated at least 30°
	    b. apply ice packs to neck if ordered *to reduce inflammation*
	  2. perform actions to reduce stress on the incision (see Postoperative Nursing Diagnosis 2, action b) *in order to reduce the risk of bleeding and a subsequent increase in pressure on the trachea.*

---

2. NURSING DIAGNOSIS: **Impaired tissue integrity**

related to:
a. disruption of tissue associated with the surgical procedure;
b. delayed wound healing associated with factors such as decreased nutritional status and unusual stress on incision (can result from excessive movement of head and neck, persistent or vigorous coughing, vomiting, and swelling or hematoma formation at the surgical site).

Desired Outcome	Nursing Actions and *Selected Purposes/Rationales*

2. The client will experience normal healing of surgical wound (see Standardized Postoperative Care Plan, Nursing Diagnosis 9, outcome a [pp. 109–110], for outcome criteria).	2.a. Refer to Standardized Postoperative Care Plan, Nursing Diagnosis 9, action a (pp. 109–110), for measures related to assessment and promotion of wound healing.
	b. Implement additional measures *to reduce stress on the incision and promote wound healing:*
	  1. place client in a semi-Fowler's position with small pillow under head
	  2. maintain client's head and neck in proper alignment using pillows or sandbags if necessary
	  3. support client's head and neck during position change until client is able to do so independently
	  4. reinforce preoperative instructions about supporting head and neck and remind client to avoid turning head abruptly and hyperextending neck
	  5. perform actions to prevent nausea and vomiting (see Standardized Postoperative Care Plan, Nursing Diagnosis 7.B, action 2 [pp. 108–109])
	  6. place personal articles and call signal within easy reach *so client does not have to turn head and neck or strain to reach them*
	  7. focus on deep breathing, use of incentive spirometer, and "huff" coughing rather than vigorous coughing to promote an effective breathing pattern and airway clearance (*vigorous coughing increases stress on suture line*)
	  8. stress importance of doing neck range of motion exercises gently (exercises are usually started 2–4 days postoperatively).

3. COLLABORATIVE DIAGNOSES:

Potential complications of thyroidectomy:

a. **hemorrhage** related to surgery in a highly vascular area;

b. **respiratory distress** related to airway obstruction associated with:
1. tracheal compression resulting from swelling and/or bleeding in the surgical area
2. closure of the glottis resulting from paralysis of the vocal cords (can occur with injury to the bilateral recurrent laryngeal nerves) or laryngeal spasm that can occur with calcium deficiency;

c. **hypoparathyroidism** related to disruption of blood supply to parathyroid gland(s) or damage to or inadvertent removal of the parathyroid gland(s) during surgery;

d. **thyroid storm (thyrotoxic crisis)**—a rare complication that can occur if client was hyperthyroid before surgery and did not receive adequate preoperative preparation with an antithyroid agent;

e. **laryngeal nerve damage** related to trauma to the nerve(s) during surgery and/or pressure on the nerve(s) associated with swelling and/or bleeding in the surgical area.

Desired Outcomes	Nursing Actions and *Selected Purposes/Rationales*

3.a. The client will not have excessive bleeding in the surgical area as evidenced by:
1. absence of feeling of tightness of neck dressing and sensation of pressure or fullness at incision site
2. expected amount of drainage on dressing
3. increasing ease of swallowing
4. absence of choking sensation and respiratory distress
5. stable vital signs.

3.a.1. Assess for and report signs and symptoms of hemorrhage (e.g. increased tightness of neck dressing; complaints of fullness or pressure in neck; excessive bloody drainage on dressing, pillow, or back of neck; statements of persistent or increased difficulty swallowing or a choking sensation; difficulty breathing; tachycardia; decrease in B/P).
2. Implement measures *to reduce the risk of hemorrhage:*
   a. maintain pressure dressing over incision site as ordered
   b. perform actions to reduce stress on the incision (see Postoperative Nursing Diagnosis 2, action b)
   c. perform actions *to decrease venous pressure in the surgical area:*
      1. keep head of bed elevated at least 30°
      2. discourage vigorous coughing
   d. apply ice packs to neck if ordered.
3. If signs and symptoms of bleeding occur:
   a. loosen dressing *to promote drainage of blood and reduce the risk of respiratory distress*
   b. notify physician
   c. assist with suture/clip removal and drainage of hematoma if indicated
   d. assist with emergency tracheostomy if respiratory distress develops
   e. prepare client for surgical intervention (e.g. ligation of bleeding vessels) if planned
   f. provide emotional support to client and significant others.

3.b. The client will not experience respiratory distress as evidenced by:
1. unlabored respirations at 14–20/minute
2. absence of stridor and sternocleidomastoid muscle retraction
3. usual mental status
4. usual skin color
5. blood gases within normal range.

3.b.1. Assess for and immediately report:
   a. increased swelling of the neck or bulging of the wound
   b. persistent or increased difficulty swallowing or choking sensation
   c. signs and symptoms of respiratory distress (e.g. rapid and/or labored respirations, stridor, sternocleidomastoid muscle retraction, restlessness, agitation, cyanosis)
   d. abnormal blood gases
   e. significant decrease in oximetry results.
2. Have oxygen and skin clip or suture removal, tracheostomy, and suction equipment readily available.
3. Implement measures *to prevent respiratory distress:*
   a. perform actions to minimize swelling in the surgical area (see Postoperative Nursing Diagnosis 1, action b.1)

b. perform actions to reduce the risk of hemorrhage or treat bleeding if it occurs (see actions a.2 and 3 in this diagnosis)

c. assess for and immediately report signs and symptoms of hypoparathyroidism (see action c.1 in this diagnosis) *so that treatment of hypocalcemia can be initiated and risk of laryngeal spasm reduced.*

4. If signs and symptoms of respiratory distress occur:
   a. place client in a high Fowler's position unless he/she is hypotensive
   b. loosen dressing on neck *to prevent further compression of trachea*
   c. maintain oxygen therapy as ordered
   d. suction client if indicated
   e. assist with emergency tracheostomy if performed
   f. provide emotional support to client and significant others.

3.c. The client will experience resolution of signs and symptoms of hypoparathyroidism if it occurs as evidenced by:
1. usual mental status
2. absence of numbness and tingling in fingers, toes, and circumoral area
3. negative Chvostek's and Trousseau's signs
4. absence of muscle twitching and spasms and seizure activity
5. serum calcium level within normal range.

3.c.1. Assess for and report signs and symptoms of hypoparathyroidism (e.g. anxiousness; irritability; numbness or tingling of fingers, toes, or circumoral area; positive Chvostek's and Trousseau's signs; muscle twitching or spasms; seizures; low serum calcium).

2. If signs and symptoms of hypoparathyroidism occur:
   a. institute seizure precautions
   b. perform actions to treat respiratory distress if it occurs (see action b.4 in this diagnosis)
   c. administer calcium preparations (e.g. intravenous calcium gluconate, calcium carbonate) as ordered.

3.d. The client will not develop thyroid storm as evidenced by:
1. stable vital signs
2. usual mental status
3. absence of tremors, nausea, and vomiting.

3.d.1. Assess for and report signs and symptoms of thyroid storm:
   a. significant temperature elevation (usually above 39° C)
   b. marked increase in client's usual pulse rate
   c. increasing restlessness
   d. agitation, irritability, tremors
   e. nausea, vomiting
   f. delirium, coma.

2. If signs and symptoms of thyroid storm occur:
   a. utilize hypothermia techniques (e.g. cooling blanket, tepid sponge bath) *to reduce fever*
   b. maintain intravenous fluid and electrolyte therapy as ordered
   c. maintain oxygen therapy as ordered
   d. institute appropriate safety measures if client is irrational, delirious, or comatose
   e. administer the following medications if ordered:
      1. antipyretics *to reduce fever* (avoid aspirin *because it increases free thyroid hormone levels*)
      2. antithyroid agents (e.g. propylthiouracil, methimazole) and iodine preparations (e.g. sodium iodide) *to suppress production and release of thyroid hormone from the remaining thyroid tissue; propylthiouracil also blocks the peripheral conversion of T_4 to the more potent T_3*
      3. glucocorticoids (e.g. dexamethasone, hydrocortisone) *to aid the body in handling stress, replenish endogenous glucocorticoids that have probably been depleted by the increased metabolism, and block the peripheral conversion of T_4 to T_3*
      4. adrenergic inhibiting agents (e.g. propranolol) *to reduce the severity of many of the clinical manifestations*
      5. vitamin supplements *to replace vitamins used during increased metabolism*
   f. provide emotional support to client and significant others.

Desired Outcomes	Nursing Actions and *Selected Purposes/Rationales*

3.e. The client will experience resolution of laryngeal nerve damage if it occurs as evidenced by:
1. improved voice tone and quality
2. gradual resolution of hoarseness
3. absence of respiratory distress.
	3.e.1. Assess for the following indications of laryngeal nerve damage:
	  a. voice changes (e.g. hoarseness; weak, whispery voice; inability to speak)
	  b. respiratory distress (see action b.1.c in this diagnosis for signs and symptoms).
	  2. Implement measures *to reduce the risk of laryngeal nerve damage:*
	    a. perform actions to reduce swelling in the surgical area (see Postoperative Nursing Diagnosis 1, action b.1)
	    b. perform actions to reduce the risk of hemorrhage or treat bleeding if it occurs (see actions a.2 and 3 in this diagnosis).
	  3. If signs and symptoms of laryngeal nerve damage occur:
	    a. encourage client to avoid unnecessary talking in order to rest the vocal cords
	    b. implement measures *to facilitate communication* (e.g. ask questions that require a short answer or nod of head, provide materials such as magic slate or pad and pencil, answer call signal in person rather than using intercommunication system)
	    c. notify physician immediately if signs and symptoms of respiratory distress occur, client is unable to speak, or hoarseness or voice changes worsen.

Discharge Teaching

■━━━

4. NURSING DIAGNOSIS: **Knowledge deficit, Ineffective management of therapeutic regimen, or Altered health maintenance***

---

*The nurse should select the diagnostic label that is most appropriate for the client's discharge teaching needs.

Desired Outcomes	Nursing Actions and *Selected Purposes/Rationales*
4.a. The client will verbalize an understanding of range of motion exercises of the neck.	4.a.1. Reinforce preoperative teaching about range of motion exercises of the neck. Instruct client to do the exercises as prescribed by physician (exercises are usually begun 2–4 days after surgery and are done 3–4 times/day for a few weeks). 2. Allow time for questions and clarification.

4.b. The client will state signs and symptoms to report to the health care provider.	4.b.1. Refer to Standardized Postoperative Care Plan, Nursing Diagnosis 21, action c (p. 123), for signs and symptoms to report to the health care provider.
	  2. Instruct client to also report signs and symptoms of:
	    a. recurrent hyperthyroidism (e.g. insomnia, heat intolerance, diarrhea, restlessness, unexplained weight loss)
	    b. hypothyroidism (e.g. unexplained weight gain, persistent fatigue and weakness, drowsiness, cold intolerance, constipation)
	    c. hypoparathyroidism (e.g. numbness or tingling of toes or fingers or around mouth, muscle twitching or spasms).

4.c. The client will verbalize an understanding of and a plan for adhering to recommended follow-up care including future appointments with health care provider, medications prescribed, activity level, and wound care.	4.c.1. Refer to Standardized Postoperative Care Plan, Nursing Diagnosis 21 (pp. 123–124), for routine postoperative instructions and measures to improve client compliance. 2. Teach client the rationale for, side effects of, schedule for taking, and importance of taking medications prescribed (e.g. thyroid hormone, calcium supplements, vitamin D). Inform client of pertinent food and drug interactions.

Bibliography

See pages 897–898 and 909.

UNIT SEVENTEEN

NURSING CARE OF THE CLIENT WITH DISTURBANCES OF MUSCULOSKELETAL FUNCTION

AMPUTATION

An amputation is the removal of all or part of a limb. Amputation of an upper or lower extremity may be performed to treat conditions such as tumors, uncontrollable infection, gangrene, or congenital anomalies and may be indicated in situations involving tissue destruction as a result of mechanical, thermal, or chemical trauma. The majority of amputations, however, are performed on the lower extremities of persons with severe peripheral vascular disease. In these instances, the ischemic limb is removed to prevent life-threatening infection and/or relieve severe, persistent discomfort. The point of amputation (e.g. above the knee, below the knee) is determined by the adequacy of circulation in the involved extremity and by prosthetic requirements.

The two types of surgical amputations are open and closed. The open type is performed if the client has an infected limb. The wound is left open, treated until infection resolves, and then closed during a second surgical procedure. An open amputation may also be indicated if the client has a very high risk for developing a wound or bone infection postoperatively. A closed amputation, which consists of soft tissue flaps sutured over the bone, is the type of amputation that is more frequently performed. The basic techniques for postoperative management of the residual limb following a closed amputation include use of a soft compression dressing or use of a rigid dressing. The technique selected depends on the client's underlying pathological condition and physiological status and whether prosthetic fitting will be immediate, early (usually within 10–30 days), or delayed or is not expected to occur (unplanned).

This care plan focuses on the adult client hospitalized for a planned below the knee, closed amputation.* Preoperatively, goals of care are to reduce fear and anxiety and educate the client regarding postoperative care and expectations. Goals of postoperative care are to maintain comfort, prevent complications, assist the client to adjust to the change in body image and effects of the amputation on mobility, assist with rehabilitative efforts, and educate the client regarding follow-up care.

---

*If an above the knee amputation is planned, refer to medical-surgical nursing texts for additional nursing diagnoses and related actions that might be appropriate.

DIAGNOSTIC TESTS

Arteriography
Doppler ultrasound
Segmental limb pressure measurements
Plethysmography
Transcutaneous oximetry
Thermography

DISCHARGE CRITERIA

Prior to discharge, the client will:

- have pain controlled
- have evidence of normal healing of the surgical wound
- achieve expected level of mobility
- have no signs and symptoms of postoperative complications
- demonstrate appropriate ways to prevent contractures, increase strength, and improve mobility
- demonstrate correct transfer and ambulation techniques and proper use of ambulatory aids
- identify ways to maintain health of the remaining lower extremity
- demonstrate the ability to care for the residual limb
- verbalize how to care for the prosthesis and residual limb if a permanent prosthesis is planned
- identify ways to manage phantom limb pain if it occurs
- state signs and symptoms to report to the health care provider
- share feelings and thoughts about the change in body image and effects of the amputation on life style and roles
- identify community resources that can assist with home management and adjustment to changes resulting from the amputation
- verbalize an understanding of and a plan for adhering to recommended follow-up care including future appointments with health care provider, prosthetist, and physical therapist; medications prescribed; and activity level.

**NURSING/
COLLABORATIVE
DIAGNOSES**
	Preoperative
	1. Anxiety △ 749
	2. Knowledge deficit △ 750
	Postoperative
	1. Pain:
	   a. incisional pain
	   b. phantom limb pain △ 751
	2. Actual/Risk for impaired tissue integrity △ 752
	3. Impaired physical mobility △ 753
	4. Risk for trauma: falls △ 754
	5. Potential complications:
	   a. hematoma formation
	   b. necrosis of skin flap
	   c. knee and hip contractures on the operative side △ 755
	6. Self-concept disturbance △ 756
	7. Grieving △ 757

DISCHARGE TEACHING	**8.** Knowledge deficit, Ineffective management of therapeutic regimen, or Altered health maintenance △ 758

See Standardized Preoperative and Postoperative Care Plans for additional diagnoses.

PREOPERATIVE

Use in conjunction with the Standardized Preoperative Care Plan.

---

1. NURSING DIAGNOSIS: **Anxiety**

related to:
a. impending disfiguring surgery;
b. lack of understanding of diagnostic tests, reason for amputation, and
   planned surgical procedure;
c. anticipated loss of control associated with effects of anesthesia;
d. unfamiliar environment and separation from significant others;
e. financial concerns associated with hospitalization;
f. anticipated discomfort, surgical findings, change in appearance, and effects
   of amputation on usual life style and roles.

Desired Outcome	Nursing Actions and *Selected Purposes/Rationales*

1. The client will experience a reduction in anxiety (see Standardized Preoperative Care Plan, Nursing Diagnosis 1 [pp. 96–97], for outcome criteria).	1.a. Refer to Standardized Preoperative Care Plan, Nursing Diagnosis 1 (pp. 96–97), for measures related to assessment and reduction of fear and anxiety.
	   b. Implement additional measures *to reduce fear and anxiety:*
	      1. reinforce physician's explanation about the level of amputation planned including that final determination of the level will be made during the surgical procedure once adequacy of circulation in the operative limb is confirmed
	      2. if acceptable to client, arrange for a visit with an individual who has successfully adjusted to the loss of a lower limb.

Client Teaching

∎━━

2. NURSING DIAGNOSIS: **Knowledge deficit**

regarding:
a. the surgical procedure;
b. hospital routines associated with surgery;
c. physical preparation for the amputation;
d. sensations that may occur following surgery and anesthesia;
e. postoperative care and management of the residual limb;
f. postoperative activity and exercises.

Desired Outcomes	Nursing Actions and *Selected Purposes/Rationales*

2.a. The client will verbalize an understanding of the surgical procedure, preoperative care, and postoperative sensations and care.	2.a.1. Refer to Standardized Preoperative Care Plan, Nursing Diagnosis 4, actions a.1–4 (pp. 99–100), for information to include in preoperative teaching.
	2. Explain that following surgery, the client may continue to feel that all or part of the amputated limb is still present. Emphasize that the sensation is typically strongest in the immediate postoperative period and tends to diminish over time.
	3. Provide the following information about postoperative phantom limb pain, including:
	  a. it does not occur in all clients
	  b. it may begin immediately after surgery (especially if the client has been experiencing substantial limb pain preoperatively) but usually starts several weeks postoperatively and disappears gradually over several months to years
	  c. the type of pain experienced varies from client to client and can be similar to pain experienced before the amputation (e.g. burning, squeezing, cramping, electric shock-like or tingling sensations)
	  d. it may be triggered by pressure on other body areas
	  e. measures will be implemented to provide effective control of the pain if it occurs.
	4. Allow time for questions and clarification of information provided.

2.b. The client will demonstrate the ability to perform recommended activities to prevent postoperative complications.	2.b.1. Refer to Standardized Preoperative Care Plan, Nursing Diagnosis 4, action b.1 (p. 100), for instructions on ways to prevent postoperative complications.
	2. Provide additional instructions on ways to prevent residual limb contractures resulting from prolonged flexion of the knee or prolonged flexion, hyperextension, abduction, adduction, or external rotation of the hip:
	  a. avoid sitting for long periods
	  b. avoid placing pillows under residual limb
	  c. maintain residual limb in proper alignment
	  d. lie prone several times during the day unless contraindicated (promotes hip extension)
	  e. perform range of motion exercises as instructed.
	3. Allow time for questions and clarification of information provided and practice and return demonstration of recommended exercises.

2.c. The client will demonstrate ways to improve strength and facilitate mobility postoperatively.	2.c.1. Instruct client in the following exercises performed to improve strength and facilitate mobility postoperatively:
	  a. range of motion exercises
	  b. strengthening exercises for the upper extremities, chest, residual limb, unaffected lower extremity, and abdominal muscles.

2. Provide instructions regarding:
   a. use of overhead trapeze
   b. transfer techniques
   c. use of mobility aids (e.g. crutches, cane, walker).
3. Allow time for practice and return demonstration of exercises, transfer techniques, and use of mobility aids.

2.d. The client will verbalize an understanding of the prosthesis and dressings planned.

2.d.1. Reinforce the physician's explanation about the type of prosthesis and dressings planned.
2. If an immediate prosthetic fitting (immediate postoperative prosthesis [IPOP]) is planned, inform client that:
   a. a rigid plaster dressing will be placed on the residual stump during surgery and the pylon (temporary artificial limb) will attach to the socket that is on the end of this dressing
   b. in addition to providing a means of securing the pylon, the rigid dressing will help shape the residual limb, reduce edema and support tissue in the surgical area, minimize pain during activity, and promote maturation of the residual limb
   c. ambulation using the temporary prosthesis usually begins 24–48 hours after surgery and progresses from walking between parallel bars to using ambulatory aids such as a walker, cane, or crutches if needed (ambulatory aids may be needed if client's gait is not steady or only partial weight bearing is allowed as the surgical area heals)
   d. the rigid dressing will be changed periodically as the residual limb shrinks (the first dressing change usually is done about 7–14 days after surgery)
   e. fitting for a permanent prosthesis will be done when the residual limb size and shape are stable (usually about 3–6 months after surgery).
3. If there are no plans for an immediate prosthetic fitting, inform client that:
   a. a soft compression dressing (soft dressing covered by an elastic bandage or sock) will be placed on the residual limb during surgery (some physicians prefer to apply a rigid dressing to the limb even though there are no plans for an immediate prosthetic fitting) and that the dressing will help reduce edema and support tissue in the surgical area and promote maturation of the residual limb
   b. the elastic bandage or sock will be reapplied if it slips, wrinkles, or loosens
   c. mobility will be accomplished using a wheelchair, walker, and/or crutches
   d. fitting for a temporary prosthesis (if planned) will not occur until after the surgical site has healed (usually 3–6 weeks after surgery).
4. Allow time for questions and clarification of information provided.

POSTOPERATIVE

Use in conjunction with the Standardized Postoperative Care Plan.

1. NURSING DIAGNOSIS:

Pain:

a. **incisional pain** related to tissue trauma and reflex muscle spasms associated with the amputation, irritation from drainage tube, and stress on surgical area associated with movement;
b. **phantom limb pain** related to altered neural transmission associated with interruption in usual nervous system pathways resulting from the amputation.

Desired Outcome	Nursing Actions and *Selected Purposes/Rationales*

1. The client will experience diminished pain (see Standardized Postoperative Care Plan, Nursing Diagnosis 6 [pp. 106–107], for outcome criteria).	1.a. Refer to Standardized Postoperative Care Plan, Nursing Diagnosis 6 (pp. 106–107), for measures related to assessment and management of incisional pain.
	b. Encourage client to report signs and symptoms of phantom limb pain (e.g. burning, squeezing, cramping, electric shock-like or tingling sensations).
	c. Implement measures *to reduce phantom limb pain if it occurs:*
	  1. instruct client to apply pressure on residual limb by walking on pylon or pressing limb against a firm surface unless contraindicated
	  2. consult physician about use of transcutaneous electrical nerve stimulation (TENS)
	  3. instruct client to mentally put absent limb through range of motion exercises
	  4. encourage participation in diversional activities
	  5. perform actions to prevent excessive pressure on any area of the body (e.g. position client properly, assist client to turn or reposition self as often as needed) *in order to reduce the risk of triggering or intensifying phantom limb pain*
	  6. administer the following medications if ordered:
	    a. tricyclic antidepressants (e.g. amitriptyline) *to alter the transmission of pain impulses and/or the client's perception of pain*
	    b. anticonvulsants (e.g. carbamazepine) *to inhibit neurotransmission of pain sensation.*

---

2. NURSING DIAGNOSIS:

Actual/Risk for impaired tissue integrity

related to:
a. disruption of tissue associated with the amputation;
b. delayed wound healing associated with factors such as:
  1. decreased nutritional status
  2. decreased blood supply to wound area resulting from the underlying disease process, edema of the residual limb, and/or excessive or prolonged pressure on operative site (may occur as a result of noncompliance with weight-bearing limitations, improper residual limb wrapping, and/or slippage of the residual limb dressing);
c. irritation of skin associated with contact with wound drainage, pressure from tubings, and use of tape;
d. damage to the skin and/or subcutaneous tissue associated with prolonged pressure on tissues, friction, and/or shearing while mobility is decreased.

Desired Outcomes	Nursing Actions and *Selected Purposes/Rationales*

2.a. The client will experience normal healing of surgical wound (see Standardized Postoperative Care Plan, Nursing Diagnosis 9, outcome a [pp. 109–110], for outcome criteria).	2.a.1. Refer to Standardized Postoperative Care Plan, Nursing Diagnosis 9, action a (pp. 109–110), for measures related to assessment and promotion of wound healing.
	  2. Implement additional measures *to promote wound healing:*
	    a. perform actions *to prevent excessive edema of residual limb:*
	      1. maintain adequate, even pressure on the residual limb (e.g. assist with application of a new rigid dressing if existing one slips or is loose, reapply the elastic bandage or sock of a soft compression dressing if it is wrinkled or slips)
	      2. elevate the residual limb if ordered (usually ordered for the first 24 hours after surgery and then the limb is placed flat to decrease the risk for hip and knee contractures)
	      3. instruct client to keep residual limb in an extended rather than dependent position whenever possible (e.g. when in sitting

position, use an additional chair to support the limb; keep leg support in a raised position when in wheelchair or recliner; do not hang residual limb over side of bed)

b. assess for and report slippage of the residual limb dressing (*can act as a tourniquet and impede circulation*); assist with reapplication if indicated

c. caution client to comply with weight-bearing limitations if prescribed *in order to prevent excessive pressure on wound site.*

2.b. The client will maintain tissue integrity as evidenced by:
1. absence of redness and irritation
2. no skin breakdown.

2.b.1. Inspect the following for pallor, redness, irritation, and breakdown:
a. skin areas in contact with wound drainage, tape, and tubings
b. back, coccyx, and buttocks
c. elbows and remaining heel.

2. Refer to Standardized Postoperative Care Plan, Nursing Diagnosis 9, action b (pp. 110–111), for measures related to prevention of tissue irritation or breakdown resulting from contact with wound drainage, tubings, and/or tape.

3. Implement measures *to prevent tissue irritation and breakdown resulting from decreased mobility:*
a. assist client to turn at least every 2 hours unless contraindicated
b. position client properly; use pressure-reducing or pressure-relieving devices (e.g. pillows, gel or foam cushions, alternating pressure mattress, air-fluidized bed) if indicated
c. instruct client to use overhead trapeze to lift self and shift weight at least every 30 minutes
d. gently massage around reddened areas at least every 2 hours
e. apply a thin layer of powder or cornstarch to bottom sheet or skin and to opposing skin surfaces (e.g. axillae) if indicated *to absorb moisture and/or reduce friction*
f. lift and move client carefully using a turn sheet and adequate assistance
g. limit length of time client is in semi-Fowler's position to 30 minutes (*in this position, client tends to slide down in bed, which can cause skin surface abrasion and shearing*)
h. keep skin lubricated, clean, and dry
i. keep bed linens dry and wrinkle-free
j. increase activity as allowed and tolerated.

4. Implement measures *to prevent irritation and breakdown of elbows and heel:*
a. massage elbows and heel with lotion frequently
b. encourage client to use overhead trapeze to move self rather than pushing up with heel and elbows
c. provide elbow and heel protectors if indicated.

5. If tissue breakdown occurs:
a. notify physician
b. continue with above measures to prevent further irritation and breakdown
c. perform care of involved area(s) as ordered or per standard hospital procedure
d. assess client closely and report signs and symptoms of infection (e.g. elevated temperature; redness, heat, pain, and swelling around area of breakdown; unusual drainage from site).

---

3. **NURSING DIAGNOSIS:**   **Impaired physical mobility**

related to:
a. pain, weakness, and fatigue;
b. depressant effect of anesthesia and some medications (e.g. narcotic [opioid] analgesics);

    c. balance difficulties associated with change in the body's center of gravity as a result of loss of a lower limb;
    d. inability to control prosthesis;
    e. prescribed activity and/or weight-bearing restrictions;
    f. fear of falling and compromising surgical wound.

Desired Outcome	Nursing Actions and *Selected Purposes/Rationales*

3. The client will achieve maximum physical mobility within limitations imposed by the amputation and prescribed activity restrictions.	3.a. Refer to Standardized Postoperative Care Plan, Nursing Diagnosis 11 (p. 112), for measures to increase client's mobility.
	  b. Implement additional measures *to increase mobility:*
	    1. perform actions to reduce pain (see Postoperative Nursing Diagnosis 1, actions a and c)
	    2. reinforce physical therapist's instructions on ways to adapt to the body's new center of gravity (e.g. change position slowly)
	    3. reinforce preoperative instructions about muscle strengthening exercises, transfer and ambulation techniques, and use of ambulatory aids
	    4. assure client that pylon will provide adequate support during ambulation
	    5. reinforce prosthetist's instructions about control and use of prosthesis and correct gait technique
	    6. if only partial weight bearing is allowed or application of a prosthesis is delayed or not planned, assist client with activities to:
	      a. develop standing balance and strength of remaining lower extremity (e.g. knee bends, standing on toes, hopping on the remaining foot while holding on to a chair, balancing on the unoperative leg without support, quadriceps- and gluteal-setting exercises)
	      b. strengthen the residual limb (e.g. quadriceps- and gluteal-setting exercises)
	      c. increase strength of arm and shoulder muscles (e.g. pushups, use of overhead trapeze to move self, flexion and extension of arms holding traction weights or weighted wands, arm pulley exercises) *in order to facilitate use of ambulatory aids*
	    7. perform actions to prevent falls (see Postoperative Nursing Diagnosis 4, actions a and b) *in order to decrease client's fear of injury*
	    8. assist client with ambulation as soon as allowed (usually 24–48 hours after surgery if client had an immediate prosthetic fitting).

■——

4. NURSING DIAGNOSIS: **Risk for trauma: falls**

related to:
a. weakness and fatigue;
b. dizziness or syncope associated with postural hypotension resulting from peripheral pooling of blood and blood loss during surgery;
c. central nervous system depressant effect of some medications (e.g. narcotic [opioid] analgesics);
d. difficulty with balance, prosthesis control, and transfer and ambulation techniques.

Desired Outcome	Nursing Actions and *Selected Purposes/Rationales*
4. The client will not experience falls.	4.a. Refer to Standardized Postoperative Care Plan, Nursing Diagnosis 17 (p. 118), for measures to prevent falls.

    b. Implement additional measures *to reduce the risk for falls:*
1. instruct client in and assist with activities to improve standing balance and strength of remaining lower extremity, residual limb, arms, and shoulders (see Postoperative Nursing Diagnosis 3, action b.6)
2. reinforce physical therapist's instructions regarding correct transfer and ambulation techniques and proper use of prosthesis and ambulatory aids (e.g. walker, crutches, cane)
3. encourage client to ask for assistance until control of the prosthesis, use of ambulatory aids, and transfer and ambulation techniques are mastered.
    c. Include client and significant others in planning and implementing measures to prevent falls.
    d. If client falls, initiate first aid measures if appropriate and notify physician.

5. COLLABORATIVE DIAGNOSES:

Potential complications of amputation:

a. **hematoma formation** related to inadequate hemostasis during or following surgical procedure and/or bleeding associated with trauma to the residual limb following surgery;

b. **necrosis of skin flap** related to impaired wound healing and infection if present;

c. **knee and hip contractures on the operative side** related to:
1. difficulty putting joints through full range of motion associated with decreased mobility, residual limb pain, weakness, and fatigue
2. prolonged periods of hip flexion associated with increased time in sitting position (especially if prosthesis fitting is delayed or not planned)
3. improper positioning of residual limb.

Desired Outcomes	Nursing Actions and *Selected Purposes/Rationales*

5.a. The client will not develop a hematoma at the operative site as evidenced by:
1. expected amount of wound drainage
2. no significant increase in swelling and pain in operative area
3. no increase in skin discoloration at surgical site.
	5.a.1. Assess for and report signs and symptoms of hematoma formation (e.g. less than expected amount of drainage from wound drain; increased swelling, pain, and/or discoloration in surgical area).
	  2. Implement measures *to reduce the risk for hematoma formation:*
	    a. maintain patency of drain if present (e.g. keep tubing free of kinks, empty collection device as often as necessary, maintain suction if ordered)
	    b. ensure that residual limb dressing is applied securely *so that adequate pressure is maintained on the vessels in the surgical area in order to control bleeding*
	    c. perform actions *to protect the residual limb from trauma* (e.g. remove pylon from rigid dressing when in bed [*if pylon remains attached, bedding can catch on it and twist the residual limb*], pad side rails if indicated, assist client with transfer and ambulation as necessary *to reduce the risk for falls*).
	  3. If signs and symptoms of hematoma formation occur, prepare client for surgical ligation of the bleeding vessels and/or drainage of the hematoma if planned.

5.b. The client will not experience necrosis of the skin flap as evidenced by:
1. skin warm and expected color
2. approximated wound edges
	5.b.1. Assess for and report signs and symptoms of:
	    a. impaired blood flow in skin flap (e.g. decreased warmth of skin flap, pallor or cyanosis of skin flap, residual limb capillary refill time greater than 3 seconds)
	    b. skin flap necrosis (e.g. pale, cool, darkened skin flap; separation of wound edges; foul odor from flap area).
	  2. Implement measures *to prevent necrosis of the skin flap:*

Desired Outcomes	Nursing Actions and *Selected Purposes/Rationales*

3. absence of a foul odor from flap area.	a. perform actions to promote wound healing (see Postoperative Nursing Diagnosis 2, action a)
	b. perform actions to prevent and treat wound infection (see Standardized Postoperative Care Plan, Nursing Diagnosis 16, actions b.4 and 5 [pp. 116–117]).
	3. If necrosis occurs:
	  a. prepare client for surgical revision of the skin flap if planned
	  b. provide emotional support to client and significant others.

5.c. The client will not develop knee and hip contractures on the operative side as evidenced by the ability to move joints through their full range of motion.	5.c.1. Assess client for and report development of knee and hip contractures on the operative side (e.g. inability to fully extend knee; inability to extend, adduct, or internally rotate residual limb).
	2. Implement measures *to prevent knee and/or hip contractures on the operative side:*
	  a. if residual limb elevation is ordered postoperatively, place bed in Trendelenburg position unless contraindicated rather than placing limb on pillows
	  b. turn client to prone position several times daily unless contraindicated *in order to promote hip extension*; place a pillow under abdomen and residual limb *to maintain hip extension and stretch flexor muscles*
	  c. place trochanter roll or sandbag along outer aspect of thigh on operative side when client is in a supine or Fowler's position *to prevent external rotation of hip*
	  d. encourage client to keep knee straight when lying or sitting; avoid use of knee gatch and pillows under knee
	  e. limit time that client is in high Fowler's or sitting position (usually no longer than 1 hour at a time)
	  f. perform actions to increase client's mobility (see Postoperative Nursing Diagnosis 3)
	  g. perform actions to reduce pain (see Postoperative Nursing Diagnosis 1) *in order to reduce the risk of client flexing residual limb in response to pain.*
	3. If contractures develop, assist with rehabilitative efforts to improve range of motion of knee and hip.

---

6. NURSING DIAGNOSIS:

Self-concept disturbance*

related to change in appearance, mobility, usual life style and roles, and level of independence associated with the amputation.

---

*This diagnostic label includes the nursing diagnoses of body image disturbance, self-esteem disturbance, and altered role performance.

Desired Outcome	Nursing Actions and *Selected Purposes/Rationales*
6. The client will demonstrate beginning adaptation to changes in appearance, mobility, level of independence, body functioning, life style, and roles as evidenced by: a. verbalization of feelings of self-worth	6.a. Assess for signs and symptoms of a self-concept disturbance (e.g. verbalization of negative feelings about self, withdrawal from significant others, lack of participation in activities of daily living, refusal to look at or touch the residual limb, lack of plan for adapting to necessary changes in life style). b. Determine the meaning of changes in body image and functioning, mobility, level of independence, life style, and roles to the client by encouraging verbalization of feelings and by noting nonverbal responses to changes experienced.

b. maintenance of relationships with significant others

c. active participation in activities of daily living

d. verbalization of a beginning plan for adapting life style to changes resulting from the amputation.

c. Implement measures to facilitate the grieving process (see Postoperative Nursing Diagnosis 7, action b).

d. Stay with client during the first dressing change *to provide support as he/she views the residual limb for the first time.*

e. Discuss with client the availability of a natural-looking prosthesis.

f. Implement measures *to assist client to increase self-esteem* (e.g. limit negative self-assessment, encourage positive comments about self, assist to identify strengths, give positive feedback about accomplishments and behaviors that are indicative of high self-esteem).

g. Assist client to identify and utilize coping techniques that have been helpful in the past.

h. Clarify misconceptions about future limitations on physical activity. Emphasize that a high level of mobility can be achieved with a prosthesis in place and/or use of crutches, walker, or cane.

i. Assist client with usual grooming and makeup habits if necessary.

j. Promote activities which require client to confront the body changes that have occurred (e.g. exercise, bathing, wrapping residual limb). Be aware that integration of the change in body image does not usually occur until 2–6 months after the actual physical change has occurred.

k. Demonstrate acceptance of client using techniques such as touch and frequent visits. Encourage significant others to do the same.

l. Support behaviors suggesting positive adaptation to the amputation (e.g. willingness to care for residual limb, compliance with treatment plan, verbalization of feelings of self-worth, maintenance of relationships with significant others).

m. Encourage significant others to allow client to do what he/she is able *so that independence can be re-established and/or self-esteem redeveloped.*

n. Encourage client contact with others *so that he/she can test and establish a new self-image.*

o. Assist client's and significant others' adjustment by listening, facilitating communication, and providing information.

p. Assist client and significant others to have similar expectations and understanding of future life style and to identify ways that personal and family goals can be adjusted rather than abandoned.

q. Teach client the rationale for treatments and encourage maximum participation in treatment regimen *to enable him/her to maintain a sense of control over life.*

r. Encourage visits and support from significant others.

s. Encourage client to continue involvement in social activities and to pursue usual roles and interests. If previous roles, interests, and hobbies cannot be pursued, encourage development of new ones.

t. If acceptable to client, arrange for a visit with an individual who has successfully adjusted to the loss of a limb.

u. Provide information about and encourage utilization of community agencies and support groups (e.g. National Amputation Foundation; vocational rehabilitation; family, individual, and/or financial counseling).

v. Consult physician about psychological counseling if client desires or seems unwilling or unable to adapt to changes resulting from the amputation.

---

7. NURSING DIAGNOSIS:　　**Grieving***

related to the loss of a limb and changes in body image and usual life style and roles.

---

*This diagnostic label includes anticipatory grieving and grieving following the actual losses.

Desired Outcome	Nursing Actions and *Selected Purposes/Rationales*

7. The client will demonstrate beginning progression through the grieving process as evidenced by:
   a. verbalization of feelings about the amputation
   b. usual sleep pattern
   c. participation in treatment plan and self-care activities
   d. utilization of available support systems
   e. verbalization of a plan for integrating follow-up care into life style.

7.a. Assess for signs and symptoms of grieving (e.g. change in eating habits, inability to concentrate, insomnia, anger, sadness, withdrawal from significant others, denial of loss).
   b. Implement measures *to facilitate the grieving process:*
      1. assist client to acknowledge the losses *so grief work can begin;* assess for factors that may hinder and facilitate acknowledgment
      2. discuss the grieving process and assist client to accept the phases of grieving as an expected response to the loss of a limb and anticipated life-style changes
      3. allow time for client to progress through the phases of grieving (phases vary among theorists but progress from shock and alarm to acceptance); be aware that not every phase is expressed by all individuals, that recurrence of phases is common, and that the grieving process may take months to years
      4. provide an atmosphere of care and concern (e.g. provide privacy, be available and nonjudgmental, display empathy and respect) *so client will feel free to express feelings*
      5. perform actions *to promote trust* (e.g. answer questions honestly, provide requested information)
      6. encourage the verbal expression of anger and sadness about the losses experienced; recognize displacement of anger and assist client to see the actual cause of angry feelings and resentment
      7. encourage client to express feelings in whatever ways are comfortable (e.g. writing, drawing, conversation)
      8. assist client to identify and utilize techniques that have helped him/her cope in previous situations of loss
      9. support realistic hope about successful rehabilitation and the effects of the amputation on his/her life (e.g. increased comfort, prevention of life-threatening infection)
      10. support behaviors suggesting successful grief work (e.g. verbalizing feelings about the amputation, focusing on ways to adapt to the loss of a limb, participating in exercise program and limb care, developing or renewing relationships)
      11. explain the phases of the grieving process to significant others; encourage their support and understanding
      12. facilitate communication between the client and significant others; be aware that they may be in different phases of the grieving process
      13. provide information regarding counseling services and support groups that might assist client in working through grief
      14. when appropriate, assist client to meet spiritual needs (e.g. arrange for a visit from clergy).
   c. Consult physician regarding referral for counseling if signs of dysfunctional grieving (e.g. persistent denial of loss, excessive anger or sadness, emotional lability) occur.

Discharge Teaching

8. NURSING DIAGNOSIS: **Knowledge deficit, Ineffective management of therapeutic regimen, or Altered health maintenance***

*The nurse should select the diagnostic label that is most appropriate for the client's discharge teaching needs.

Desired Outcomes	Nursing Actions and *Selected Purposes/Rationales*

8.a. The client will demonstrate appropriate ways to prevent contractures, increase strength, and improve mobility.	8.a.1. Instruct client in the following ways to prevent contractures, increase strength, and/or improve mobility:
	  a. performing range of motion exercises of residual limb and other extremities
	  b. lying prone several times a day with pillow under abdomen and residual limb (maintains hip extension and stretches flexor muscles)
	  c. performing knee bends, standing on toes, balancing on the unoperative leg without support, and performing quadriceps- and gluteal-setting exercises
	  d. performing pushups, flexion and extension of arms holding weights, and arm pulley exercises (facilitates use of ambulatory aids).
	    2. Allow time for questions, clarification, and return demonstration.

8.b. The client will demonstrate correct transfer and ambulation techniques and proper use of ambulatory aids.	8.b.1. Reinforce instructions about correct transfer and ambulation techniques, amount of weight bearing allowed, and proper use of ambulatory aids (e.g. crutches, walker, cane). 2. Allow time for questions, clarification, practice, and return demonstration.

8.c. The client will identify ways to maintain health of the remaining lower extremity.	8.c.1. Instruct client in ways to maintain health of the remaining lower extremity:
	  a. wear a well-fitting shoe to protect foot from pressure and trauma
	  b. perform foot and nail care using appropriate technique
	  c. avoid breaks in the skin to reduce risk of infection
	  d. stop smoking
	  e. avoid sitting with legs crossed and wearing socks, stockings, or garters that are tight in order to reduce the risk of compromising peripheral blood flow
	  f. adhere to regular follow-up care if diabetes or peripheral vascular disease was a factor leading to the need for amputation.
	    2. Allow time for questions and clarification of information provided.

8.d. The client will demonstrate the ability to care for the residual limb.	8.d.1. Reinforce preoperative teaching about the purpose of the residual limb dressing.
	    2. Instruct client in ways to care for the residual limb while dressing is in place:
	  a. if client has a soft compression dressing over the residual limb:
	    1. demonstrate the technique for rewrapping or changing the elastic bandage or sock; explain that physician may want this to be done routinely during the day and that it should also be done if the dressing slips or the elastic bandage or sock becomes soiled or wrinkled
	    2. demonstrate the technique for changing the soft dressing if client is expected to do this following discharge
	  b. if client has a rigid dressing over the residual limb:
	    1. stress the importance of removing the pylon when in bed to reduce the risk of twisting the residual limb
	    2. explain that the dressing should be positioned securely before applying the pylon (a belt may be needed to maintain the proper position of the rigid dressing during ambulation)
	    3. caution client to adhere to weight-bearing restrictions until the surgical area heals completely.
	    3. Inform client about expected care of the residual limb once the dressings are no longer needed:
	  a. the residual limb will need to be inspected daily using a hand mirror if necessary to check for skin irritation and breakdown
	  b. the residual limb will need to be washed and patted dry daily
	  c. emollients and powders should not be applied to the residual limb.
	    4. Allow time for questions, clarification, and return demonstration.

Desired Outcomes	Nursing Actions and *Selected Purposes/Rationales*

8.e. The client will verbalize how to care for the prosthesis and residual limb if a permanent prosthesis is planned.	8.e.1. Provide the client with information about anticipated care of the prosthesis and residual limb if a permanent prosthesis is planned:
	   a. the residual limb should be toughened by massaging it, pushing it against a firm surface, and/or pulling on it with a hand-held towel (a toughened limb is more resistant to irritation and breakdown from the constant pressure exerted on it by the prosthesis)
	   b. a residual limb sock should be worn next to the skin to reduce friction between residual limb and the socket
	   c. only residual limb socks recommended by the prosthetist should be used; socks should be changed daily, laundered gently in cool water with a mild soap, and laid flat to dry
	   d. worn or damaged residual limb socks should be replaced rather than mended
	   e. a prosthetist should examine the prosthesis on a regular basis and monitor the fit of the socket so that repairs and adjustments can be made when necessary (e.g. as the residual limb continues to shrink, if a weight loss or gain of 5 to 10 pounds occurs)
	   f. the socket should be cleansed daily with a damp cloth and dried thoroughly
	   g. care should be taken to keep the leather or metal components of the prosthesis dry
	   h. shoes worn with the prosthesis should be in good repair to maintain a steady, even gait and avoid damage to the prosthesis
	   i. if skin breakdown occurs, the prosthesis should not be worn until the area has been checked by physician and/or prosthetist
	   j. the prosthesis should be applied on arising and worn for the prescribed length of time to prevent residual limb edema
	   k. a shrinker device may need to be worn whenever the prosthesis is removed (the device will help prevent edema of the residual limb and subsequent difficulty in reapplication of the prosthesis).
	  2. Allow time for questions and clarification of information provided.

8.f. The client will identify ways to manage phantom limb pain if it occurs.	8.f.1. Instruct client in ways to manage phantom limb pain if it occurs:
	   a. apply intermittent pressure to residual limb by walking on pylon or pressing the limb against a firm surface
	   b. mentally put absent limb through range of motion exercises
	   c. participate in diversional activities
	   d. take medications (e.g. amitriptyline, carbamazepine) as prescribed.
	  2. Reassure client that phantom limb pain should gradually disappear.

8.g. The client will state signs and symptoms to report to the health care provider.	8.g.1. Refer to Standardized Postoperative Care Plan, Nursing Diagnosis 21, action c (p. 123), for signs and symptoms to report to the health care provider.
	  2. Instruct client to report these additional signs and symptoms:
	   a. occurrence of and/or persistent phantom limb pain
	   b. persistent or increased residual limb swelling
	   c. difficulty with full extension of residual limb
	   d. inability to maintain balance
	   e. difficulty controlling prosthesis
	   f. numbness, tingling, color changes, or swelling of residual limb and/or remaining extremities
	   g. absent peripheral pulses (teach client how to check peripheral pulses if he/she is to monitor them)
	   h. loosening of rigid dressing.

8.h. The client will identify community resources that can assist with home management and adjustment to changes resulting from the amputation.	8.h.1. Provide information about community resources that can assist the client and significant others with home management and adjustment to changes resulting from the amputation (e.g. home health agency; social services; individual, family, and occupational counseling; amputee support groups; National Amputation Foundation). 2. Initiate a referral if indicated.

8.i. The client will verbalize an understanding of and a plan for adhering to recommended follow-up care including future appointments with health care provider, prosthetist, and physical therapist; medications prescribed; and activity level.

8.i.1. Refer to Standardized Postoperative Care Plan, Nursing Diagnosis 21 (pp. 123–129), for routine postoperative instructions and measures to improve client compliance.
2. Emphasize the importance of adhering to prescribed weight-bearing restrictions and exercise program.

Bibliography

See pages 897–898 and 909.

 # FRACTURED HIP WITH INTERNAL FIXATION OR PROSTHESIS INSERTION

A fractured hip is the term used to describe a fracture of the proximal end of the femur. Hip fractures are classified according to the specific location of the fracture. A common classification system divides hip fractures into three types: femoral neck fractures (also referred to as intracapsular fractures), intertrochanteric fractures, and subtrochanteric fractures (the latter two types are sometimes referred to as extracapsular fractures).

A fractured hip is one of the most common orthopedic injuries in the elderly because of the increased incidence of osteoporosis and falls in the elderly population. Although a fractured hip can be treated by traction for 8–12 weeks, the preferred treatment is surgery because it allows earlier mobility. Surgery involves internal fixation of the fracture or insertion of a femoral head prosthesis. Internal fixation with preservation of the femoral head is the preferred method of treating femoral neck fractures but the femoral head and neck can be replaced with a prosthetic device (e.g. Austin Moore prosthesis)

if factors are present that increase the risk for avascular necrosis and/or nonunion (e.g. a severe comminuted fracture of the femoral head or neck, a pathological fracture, inadequate closed reduction of the fracture in an elderly client). If the fracture occurred in the trochanteric region, internal fixation of the fracture with pins, nails, cannulated screws, or a nail or screw attached to a plate will be performed. Ideally, surgery is performed within 12–24 hours after the injury, especially if the client has a displaced femoral neck. During the preoperative period, traction is usually applied to stabilize and reduce the fracture and reduce muscle spasms and pain.

This care plan focuses on the elderly adult client who is hospitalized for surgical repair of a hip fracture. The goals of preoperative care are to reduce fear and anxiety, maintain comfort, and prevent neurovascular dysfunction. Postoperatively, the goals of care are to maintain comfort, prevent complications, assist the client to regain maximum mobility and independence, and educate the client regarding follow-up care.

DIAGNOSTIC TESTS

X-rays of the hip

DISCHARGE CRITERIA

Prior to discharge, the client will:

- have evidence of normal healing of the surgical wound
- have clear, audible breath sounds throughout lungs
- have expected level of mobility
- have adequate fracture reduction and healing
- have hip pain controlled
- have no signs and symptoms of infection or postoperative complications
- demonstrate correct transfer and ambulation techniques and proper use of ambulatory aids

- demonstrate the ability to correctly perform the prescribed exercises
- verbalize an understanding of activity and position restrictions necessary to prevent dislocation of the prosthesis or internal fixation device
- identify ways to reduce the risk of falls in the home environment
- share thoughts and feelings about the need to transfer to an extended care facility if planned
- state signs and symptoms to report to the health care provider
- identify community resources that can assist with home management and provide transportation
- verbalize an understanding of and a plan for adhering to recommended follow-up care including future appointments with health care provider and physical therapist, medications prescribed, activity level, and wound care.

NURSING/ COLLABORATIVE DIAGNOSES	**Preoperative**
	1. Anxiety △ 762
	2. Pain: hip △ 763
	3. Risk for peripheral neurovascular dysfunction: fractured extremity △ 764
	Postoperative
	1. Risk for peripheral neurovascular dysfunction: operative extremity △ 765
	2. Pain: hip △ 765
	3. Impaired physical mobility △ 766
	4. Risk for infection △ 766
	5. Risk for trauma: falls △ 767
	6. Potential complications:
	   a. dislocation of prosthesis or internal fixation device
	   b. thromboembolism
	   c. avascular necrosis
	   d. delayed healing of the fractured bone △ 768
	7. Powerlessness △ 770

DISCHARGE TEACHING	8. Knowledge deficit, Ineffective management of therapeutic regimen, or Altered health maintenance △ 770

See Standardized Preoperative and Postoperative Care Plans for additional diagnoses.

PREOPERATIVE

Use in conjunction with the Standardized Preoperative Care Plan.

1. NURSING DIAGNOSIS: **Anxiety**

related to:
a. severe pain;
b. lack of understanding of traction device and planned surgical procedure;
c. unfamiliar environment and separation from significant others;
d. anticipated postoperative discomfort and loss of control associated with the effects of anesthesia;
e. financial concerns associated with hospitalization;
f. potential embarrassment or loss of dignity associated with body exposure;
g. possibility of changes in usual life style, permanent disability, or death.

Desired Outcome	Nursing Actions and *Selected Purposes/Rationales*

1. The client will experience a reduction in anxiety (see Standardized Preoperative Care Plan, Nursing Diagnosis 1 [pp. 96–97], for outcome criteria).	1.a. Refer to Standardized Preoperative Care Plan, Nursing Diagnosis 1 (pp. 96–97), for measures related to assessment and reduction of fear and anxiety.
	b. Implement additional measures *to reduce fear and anxiety:*
	   1. perform actions to reduce pain (see Preoperative Nursing Diagnosis 2, action e)
	   2. explain the purpose of traction and how it works
	   3. reassure client that modern treatment methods for a fractured hip have significantly reduced permanent disability and death rates; inform client that he/she will probably begin ambulation by the 2nd postoperative day.

---

2. NURSING DIAGNOSIS: **Pain: hip**

related to fracture of the bone, tissue trauma, and muscle spasms.

Desired Outcome	Nursing Actions and *Selected Purposes/Rationales*

2. The client will experience diminished hip pain as evidenced by:
  a. verbalization of a reduction in pain
  b. relaxed facial expression and body positioning
  c. stable vital signs.
	2.a. Assess for signs and symptoms of pain (e.g. verbalization of pain, grimacing, reluctance to move, clutching hip or thigh, restlessness, diaphoresis, facial pallor, increased B/P, tachycardia).
	b. Assess client's perception of the severity of pain using a pain intensity rating scale.
	c. Assess the client's pain pattern (e.g. location, quality, onset, duration, precipitating factors, aggravating factors, alleviating factors).
	d. Ask the client to describe previous pain experiences and methods used to manage pain effectively.
	e. Implement measures *to reduce pain:*
	   1. perform actions *to reduce fear and anxiety about the pain experience* (e.g. assure client that his/her need for pain relief is understood, plan methods for achieving pain control with client)
	   2. perform actions to reduce fear and anxiety (see Preoperative Nursing Diagnosis 1) *in order to promote relaxation and subsequently increase the client's threshold and tolerance for pain*
	   3. administer analgesics before activities and procedures that can cause pain and before pain becomes severe
	   4. perform actions to promote rest (e.g. minimize environmental activity and noise, limit the number of visitors and their length of stay) *in order to reduce fatigue and subsequently increase the client's threshold and tolerance for pain*
	   5. perform actions *to maintain effective traction on the injured extremity* (client is usually placed in Buck's or Russell's traction preoperatively *to stabilize and reduce the fracture and reduce muscle spasms and pain*):
	     a. ensure that weights are hanging freely
	     b. do not allow footplate or ropes to rest on end of bed
	     c. keep affected heel off bed
	     d. keep knots away from pulley device
	     e. do not remove traction unless specifically ordered
	     f. do not lift the weights in order to facilitate lifting and other care (*this reduces traction pull and can cause severe muscle spasm*)
	     g. limit head of bed elevation to 20–25° except for meals and toileting *in order to maintain the prescribed traction force*
	   6. avoid bumping the traction device

Desired Outcome	Nursing Actions and *Selected Purposes/Rationales*

7. place a trochanter roll or sandbag firmly against the lateral aspect of injured hip and upper thigh (should extend from iliac crest to midthigh) *in order to maintain leg in proper alignment*
8. consult physician if extremity appears out of alignment; do not attempt to realign extremity (*an attempt to realign the extremity may cause further tissue trauma*)
9. move client carefully, keeping injured extremity well supported
10. if turning is allowed, place pillow between legs before turning *in order to prevent adduction and further strain on the fracture site*
11. provide or assist with additional nonpharmacologic measures for pain relief (e.g. relaxation exercises; diversional activities such as watching television, reading, or conversing)
12. administer analgesics and muscle relaxants if ordered.

   f. Consult physician if above measures fail to provide adequate pain relief.

---

3. NURSING DIAGNOSIS: **Risk for peripheral neurovascular dysfunction: fractured extremity**

related to trauma to or excessive pressure on the nerves or blood vessels as a result of the injury; displaced bone fragments; edema; and improper alignment, application of skin traction device, or traction on the injured extremity.

Desired Outcome	Nursing Actions and *Selected Purposes/Rationales*

3. The client will maintain normal neurovascular function in the injured extremity as evidenced by:
  a. palpable pedal pulses
  b. capillary refill time in toes less than 3 seconds
  c. extremity warm and usual color
  d. ability to flex and extend foot and toes
  e. absence of numbness and tingling in leg and foot
  f. absence of foot pain during passive movement of toes and foot
  g. no increase in pain in extremity.

3.a. Assess for and report signs and symptoms of neurovascular dysfunction in the injured extremity:
  1. diminished or absent pedal pulses
  2. capillary refill time in toes greater than 3 seconds
  3. pallor, cyanosis, or coolness of the extremity
  4. inability to flex or extend foot or toes
  5. numbness or tingling in leg or foot
  6. pain in foot during passive motion of toes or foot
  7. increased pain in extremity.

b. Implement measures *to prevent neurovascular dysfunction in injured extremity:*
  1. maintain traction as ordered
  2. place a trochanter roll or sandbag firmly against lateral aspect of injured hip and upper thigh (should extend from the iliac crest to midthigh) *in order to help maintain proper alignment*
  3. do not attempt to realign injured leg unless specifically ordered (*an attempt to align extremity may cause further trauma to the nerves and blood vessels*)
  4. make sure skin traction device (e.g. elastic wraps, foam boot with Velcro strap) is applied properly (if necessary to reapply, obtain assistance *so that one person can maintain traction on the leg during the reapplication process*)
  5. make sure that excessive or prolonged pressure is not exerted on Achilles tendon and medial and lateral aspects of knee and ankle
  6. do not turn client on injured side unless specifically ordered (*may cause further displacement of fracture and decrease blood flow to area*).

c. If signs and symptoms of neurovascular dysfunction occur:
  1. assess for and correct improper positioning of the injured extremity and traction device and external cause of excessive pressure
  2. notify physician if the signs and symptoms persist or worsen

3. prepare client for surgical intervention (e.g. internal fixation, insertion of hip prosthesis).

POSTOPERATIVE

Use in conjunction with the Standardized Postoperative Care Plan.

1. NURSING DIAGNOSIS:

Risk for peripheral neurovascular dysfunction: operative extremity

related to trauma to or excessive pressure on the nerves or blood vessels as a result of surgery and the initial injury, blood accumulation and edema in the surgical area, improper alignment of operative extremity, tight or improperly positioned abductor device straps, or dislocation of prosthesis or internal fixation device.

Desired Outcome	Nursing Actions and *Selected Purposes/Rationales*

1. The client will maintain normal neurovascular function in the operative extremity (see Preoperative Nursing Diagnosis 3, for outcome criteria).	1.a. Assess for signs and symptoms of neurovascular dysfunction in the operative extremity (see Preoperative Nursing Diagnosis 3, action a, for signs and symptoms).
	 b. Implement measures *to prevent neurovascular dysfunction in the operative extremity:*
	   1. maintain extremity in proper alignment
	   2. perform actions to prevent dislocation of prosthesis or internal fixation device (see Postoperative Collaborative Diagnosis 6, action a.2)
	   3. make sure that straps on abductor device are not too tight and are not exerting pressure on the popliteal space, lateral calf immediately below the knee, and lateral malleolus
	   4. apply ice to surgical site if ordered *to reduce edema.*
	 c. If signs and symptoms of neurovascular dysfunction occur:
	   1. assess for and correct improperly applied or tight straps on abductor device and improper positioning of operative extremity; do not attempt to realign extremity if extreme rotation has occurred
	   2. notify physician if the signs and symptoms persist or worsen
	   3. prepare client for closed reduction or return to surgery if planned.

2. NURSING DIAGNOSIS:

Pain: hip

related to tissue trauma and reflex muscle spasms associated with the initial injury, surgery, and strain on the area postoperatively.

Desired Outcome	Nursing Actions and *Selected Purposes/Rationales*

2. The client will experience diminished hip pain (see Standardized Postoperative Care Plan, Nursing Diagnosis 6 [pp. 106–107], for outcome criteria).	2.a. Refer to Standardized Postoperative Care Plan, Nursing Diagnosis 6 (pp. 106–107), for measures related to assessment and reduction of pain.
	 b. Implement additional measures *to reduce pain in operative extremity:*
	   1. adhere to position, activity, and weight-bearing restrictions identified in Postoperative Collaborative Diagnosis 6, actions a.2.b–g *in order to reduce pain associated with strain on the surgical site*
	   2. move the operative extremity gently.

3. NURSING DIAGNOSIS: **Impaired physical mobility**

related to:
a. pain and weakness in weight-bearing extremity associated with the fracture and subsequent surgical repair;
b. prescribed activity and weight-bearing restrictions following internal fixation or prosthesis insertion;
c. generalized weakness associated with surgery;
d. depressant effect of anesthesia and some medications (e.g. narcotic [opioid] analgesics, central-acting muscle relaxants);
e. fear of falling, moving operative hip improperly, and compromising surgical wound.

Desired Outcome	Nursing Actions and *Selected Purposes/Rationales*

3. The client will achieve maximum physical mobility within prescribed activity and weight-bearing restrictions.	3.a. Refer to Standardized Postoperative Care Plan, Nursing Diagnosis 11 (p. 112), for measures to increase client's mobility.
	  b. Implement additional measures *to increase client's mobility:*
	   1. perform actions to reduce pain (see Postoperative Nursing Diagnosis 2)
	   2. instruct client in and assist with isometric quadriceps- and gluteal-setting exercises *to strengthen muscles needed for ambulation*
	   3. encourage client to use overhead trapeze to move self *in order to strengthen arm and shoulder muscles needed for proper use of ambulatory aids*
	   4. reinforce physical therapist's instructions regarding muscle strengthening exercises, transfer and ambulation techniques, and use of ambulatory aids
	   5. perform actions to prevent falls (see Postoperative Nursing Diagnosis 5, actions a and b) *in order to decrease client's fear of injury*
	   6. assist client with ambulation as soon as allowed (usually by the 2nd postoperative day).
	  c. Consult physician if client is unable to achieve expected level of mobility.

4. NURSING DIAGNOSIS: **Risk for infection**

related to:
a. stasis of pulmonary secretions and aspiration (if it occurs);
b. wound contamination associated with introduction of pathogens during or following surgery (risk is increased because of close proximity of wound to perineal area);
c. decreased resistance to infection associated with factors such as an inadequate nutritional status and decreased effectiveness of immune system if client is elderly;
d. increased growth and colonization of microorganisms in the urine associated with urinary stasis if mobility is decreased and introduction of pathogens if indwelling catheter is present.

Desired Outcome	Nursing Actions and *Selected Purposes/Rationales*

4. The client will remain free of infection as evidenced by:
  a. absence of fever and chills
  b. pulse within normal limits
	4.a. Refer to Standardized Postoperative Care Plan, Nursing Diagnosis 16 (pp. 116–117), for measures related to assessment and prevention of infection.
	  b. Assess for and report additional signs and symptoms that may be indicative of wound infection or osteomyelitis:

c. normal breath sounds
d. usual mental status
e. cough productive of clear mucus only
f. voiding clear urine without reports of frequency, urgency, and burning
g. absence of redness, heat, and swelling around wound
h. usual drainage from wound
i. no new or increased discomfort in hip
j. sedimentation rate and WBC and differential counts returning toward normal range
k. negative results of cultured specimens.

1. elevated sedimentation rate
2. reports of increased hip discomfort.

c. Maintain patency of wound drainage system if present (e.g. prevent kinking of tubing, keep collection device below surgical wound, keep suction device compressed) *to prevent the accumulation of drainage and subsequent colonization of pathogens in the surgical area.*

d. If signs and symptoms of wound infection or osteomyelitis occur:
   1. prepare client for surgical debridement of wound and/or irrigation of infected area if planned
   2. administer antimicrobials as ordered.

---

5. NURSING DIAGNOSIS:

Risk for trauma: falls

related to:

a. weakness, fatigue, and postural hypotension associated with the effects of major surgery and physiological changes that may have occurred if client is elderly;
b. central nervous system depressant effect of some medications (e.g. narcotic [opioid] analgesics, central-acting muscle relaxants);
c. weakness and pain in weight-bearing extremity associated with the initial injury and surgery on the hip;
d. difficulty with transfer and ambulation techniques.

Desired Outcome	Nursing Actions and *Selected Purposes/Rationales*

5. The client will not experience falls.

5.a. Refer to Standardized Postoperative Care Plan, Nursing Diagnosis 17, action a (p. 118), for measures to prevent falls.

b. Implement additional measures *to reduce the risk for falls:*
   1. perform actions *to assist client to increase muscle strength:*
      a. instruct and encourage client to perform isometric quadriceps- and gluteal-setting exercises
      b. encourage client to use the overhead trapeze to lift self (*strengthens arm and shoulder muscles which will facilitate use of ambulatory aids*)
   2. reinforce physical therapist's instructions regarding correct transfer and ambulation techniques and proper use of ambulatory aids (e.g. walker)
   3. administer prescribed analgesics before exercise and ambulation sessions *in order to reduce hip pain and subsequently maximize client's ability to utilize proper transfer and ambulation techniques.*

c. Include client and significant others in planning and implementing measures to prevent falls.

d. If client falls, initiate first aid measures if appropriate and notify physician.

6. COLLABORATIVE DIAGNOSES:

Potential complications of prosthesis insertion or internal fixation of hip:

a. **dislocation of prosthesis or internal fixation device** related to improper positioning of operative extremity, early weight-bearing, delayed healing of the fracture, or infection of the bone or surrounding tissue;

b. **thromboembolism** related to:
   1. venous stasis associated with increased blood viscosity (can result from fluid volume deficit), decreased mobility, and pressure exerted on blood vessels by abductor device
   2. hypercoagulability associated with increased release of tissue thromboplastin into the blood (occurs as a result of surgical trauma) and hemoconcentration and increased blood viscosity (can occur as a result of fluid volume deficit)
   3. trauma to vein walls during surgery;

c. **avascular necrosis** related to an inadequate blood supply to the bone (occurs primarily following intracapsular fractures);

d. **delayed healing of the fractured bone** (with eventual nonunion) related to inadequate reduction and internal fixation of fracture, diminished blood supply to fracture site, thin or absent periosteum in neck of femur (decreases the healing potential), inadequate nutritional status, preexisting osteoporosis if present, or development of infection in the fractured bone and/or surrounding tissue.

Desired Outcomes	Nursing Actions and *Selected Purposes/Rationales*

6.a. The client will not experience dislocation of the prosthesis or internal fixation device as evidenced by:
1. continued resolution of hip pain
2. ability to maintain operative leg in proper alignment
3. length of operative leg equal to unoperative leg
4. ability to adhere to exercise and ambulation regimen
5. normal neurovascular status in operative leg.
	6.a.1. Assess for and report signs and symptoms of dislocation of the hip prosthesis or internal fixation device:
	a. sudden, severe pain in operative hip
	b. significant (greater than 10°) external rotation of the operative leg
	c. operative leg more than 2.5 cm (1 inch) shorter than unoperative leg
	d. sudden inability to participate in usual exercise and ambulation regimen
	e. decline in neurovascular status in operative leg.
	2. Implement measures *to reduce the risk for dislocation of the prosthesis or internal fixation device:*
	a. perform actions to promote healing of the fracture (see action c.2 in this diagnosis)
	b. perform actions *to prevent adduction of the operative extremity:*
	  1. keep 2–3 pillows or abductor device between legs at all times
	  2. remind client not to cross legs
	  3. do not move operative extremity past midline
	c. maintain the operative extremity in proper alignment
	d. maintain restrictions on head of bed elevation if ordered (some physicians order a 45–60° maximum elevation for the first few days after surgery) *to reduce hip flexion*
	e. perform actions *to prevent extreme (beyond 90°) hip flexion:*
	  1. instruct client not to lean forward to reach objects on end of bed or on floor or to put on slippers, socks, or shoes
	  2. raise the entire bed to client's midthigh level before he/she gets in or out of bed *in order to reduce the degree of hip flexion that occurs when client sits on edge of bed*
	  3. provide a high, firm chair (or elevate sitting surface with pillows) and an elevated toilet seat for client's use *in order to reduce degree of hip flexion when client sits down*
	  4. do not elevate operative leg when sitting in chair
	f. maintain restrictions on turning (usually allowed to turn on unoperative side only) and always turn client with pillows between legs

g. reinforce weight-bearing limitations ordered (partial weight-bearing is usually allowed as soon as ambulation is started following prosthesis insertion; weight-bearing restrictions vary following internal fixation depending on the stability of the fracture reduction and fixation)

h. perform actions to prevent and treat wound infection and osteomyelitis (see Standardized Postoperative Care Plan, Nursing Diagnosis 16, actions b.4 and 5 [pp. 116–117] and Postoperative Nursing Diagnosis 4, actions c and d).

3. If signs and symptoms of dislocation of prosthesis or internal fixation device occur:

a. maintain client on bed rest

b. prepare client for x-rays of surgical area

c. prepare client for closed reduction or surgical repair of the dislocation if planned

d. provide emotional support to client and significant others.

6.b. The client will not develop a deep vein thrombus or pulmonary embolism (see Standardized Postoperative Care Plan, Collaborative Diagnosis 19, outcomes c.1 and 2 [pp. 120–121], for outcome criteria).	6.b.1. Refer to Standardized Postoperative Care Plan, Collaborative Diagnosis 19, actions c.1 and 2 (pp. 120–121), for measures related to assessment, prevention, and treatment of a deep vein thrombus and pulmonary embolism. 2. Implement additional measures *to prevent thrombus formation:* a. make sure that straps on abductor device do not exert excessive pressure on any area b. encourage client to perform active foot exercises every 1–2 hours while awake; provide adequate analgesia *to promote client compliance* c. administer anticoagulants (e.g. low-dose warfarin, low-molecular-weight or low-dose heparin) or antiplatelet agents (e.g. low-dose aspirin) if ordered d. assist client with ambulation as soon as allowed.

6.c. The client will not experience avascular necrosis or delayed healing of the fracture as evidenced by:
1. resolution of hip pain
2. proper alignment of operative extremity
3. expected progression in prescribed physical therapy program
4. x-rays showing evidence of normal stages of bone healing.
	6.c.1. Assess for and report signs and symptoms of avascular necrosis and/or delayed healing of the fracture:
	a. persistent hip pain
	b. inability to maintain operative leg in proper alignment
	c. inability to make expected progress in physical therapy program
	d. x-rays showing delayed healing of fracture.
	
	2. Implement measures *to promote healing of the fracture:*
	a. maintain operative leg in proper alignment
	b. maintain restrictions on weight-bearing as ordered
	c. maintain an adequate nutritional status (see Standardized Postoperative Care Plan, Nursing Diagnosis 5, action d [p. 106])
	d. encourage client to consume foods/fluids high in calcium and vitamin D (e.g. fortified dairy products)
	e. perform actions to prevent and treat wound infection and osteomyelitis (see Standardized Postoperative Care Plan, Nursing Diagnosis 16, actions b.4 and 5 [pp. 116–117] and Postoperative Nursing Diagnosis 4, actions c and d)
	f. discourage smoking (*evidence strongly suggests that smoking decreases tissue perfusion and may delay bone union*)
	g. administer the following medications if ordered:
	  1. calcium preparations (e.g. calcium carbonate)
	  2. vitamin D (e.g. calcitriol, calcifediol)
	  3. estrogen preparations *to inhibit further bone resorption.*
	
	3. If signs and symptoms of avascular necrosis or delayed healing of the fracture occur:
	a. continue with above measures to promote healing
	b. prepare client for diagnostic tests (e.g. x-ray, magnetic resonance imaging) if planned
	c. prepare client for surgical intervention (e.g. bone grafting, repeat fixation, prosthesis insertion) if planned
	d. provide emotional support to client and significant others.

7. NURSING DIAGNOSIS: **Powerlessness**

related to temporary physical limitations, dependence on others to meet basic needs, and possible change in roles and future living situation.

Desired Outcome	Nursing Actions and *Selected Purposes/Rationales*
7. The client will demonstrate increased feelings of control over his/her situation as evidenced by: a. verbalization of same b. active participation in planning of care and decision-making regarding future living situation c. participation in self-care activities within physical limitations.	7.a. Assess for behaviors that may indicate feelings of powerlessness (e.g. verbalization of lack of control over self-care or current situation, anger, irritability, passivity, lack of participation in self-care or discharge planning). b. Obtain information from client and significant others regarding client's usual response to situations in which he/she has had limited control (e.g. loss of job, financial stress). c. Encourage client to verbalize feelings about current situation and possible changes in roles and living situation (e.g. transfer to an extended care facility, need for a live-in attendant, move to another person's home). Focus on the positive aspects of the planned living arrangement changes. d. Reinforce physician's explanations about the hip surgery and rehabilitation plan. Clarify misconceptions. e. Support realistic hope about effects of rehabilitation and probability of future independence. f. Assist client to establish realistic short- and long-term goals. g. Remind client of the right to ask questions about condition and plan of care. h. Include client in planning of care, encourage maximum participation in the treatment plan, and allow choices whenever possible *to promote a sense of control.* i. Encourage significant others to allow client to do as much as he/she is able *so that a feeling of independence can be maintained.* j. Inform client of schedule (e.g. planned care, physical therapy schedule) *so that he/she knows what to expect, which promotes a sense of control.* k. Assist client to meet spiritual needs (e.g. arrange for a visit from clergy if desired by client). l. Consult occupational therapist if indicated about assistive devices and environmental modifications that would allow client more independence in performing activities of daily living. m. Encourage client to be as active as possible in making decisions about his/her living situation.

Discharge Teaching

8. NURSING DIAGNOSIS: **Knowledge deficit, Ineffective management of therapeutic regimen, or Altered health maintenance***

---

*The nurse should select the diagnostic label that is most appropriate for the client's discharge teaching needs.

Desired Outcomes	Nursing Actions and *Selected Purposes/Rationales*
8.a. The client will demonstrate correct transfer and ambulation techniques and proper use of ambulatory aids.	8.a.1. Reinforce instructions about correct transfer and ambulation techniques, amount of weight-bearing allowed, and proper use of ambulatory aids (a walker is preferable for most elderly clients because it provides the greatest stability).

2. Allow time for questions, clarification, and practice of transfer and ambulation techniques.

8.b. The client will demonstrate the ability to correctly perform the prescribed exercises.

8.b.1. Reinforce instructions on muscle strengthening and range of motion exercises.

2. Explain importance of performing muscle strengthening and range of motion exercises 3–4 times/day.

3. Allow time for questions, clarification, and return demonstration of prescribed exercises.

8.c. The client will verbalize an understanding of activity and position restrictions necessary to prevent dislocation of the prosthesis or internal fixation device.

8.c. Instruct client to adhere to the following activity and position restrictions for at least 2 months (time may vary depending on physician preference) in order to prevent dislocation of prosthesis or internal fixation device:

1. turn only as directed by physician (many physicians allow turning to unoperative side only)
2. keep pillows between legs when lying on back or side and when turning
3. never cross legs
4. do not sit on low chairs, stools, or toilets; place a cushion on low chairs, rent or purchase an elevated toilet seat for home use, and use the high toilets designed for the handicapped when in public facilities
5. do not elevate operative leg higher than hip when sitting
6. sit in chairs with arms and use the arms to raise self off chair
7. support weight on unoperative leg when raising self from a sitting position
8. use assistive devices (e.g. long-handled shoe horn, long-handled grabber) to assist with activities that require flexing hip beyond 90° (e.g. putting on shoes and socks, reaching objects on the floor or in low cupboards or drawers, pulling bed covers up from end of bed)
9. keep operative leg in proper alignment and avoid extreme internal and external rotation of leg
10. when riding in a car:
    a. sit on a firm pillow or cushion to prevent hip flexion of more than 90°
    b. keep operative leg extended (a sudden impact of the knee against the dashboard can dislodge the prosthesis)
11. do not resume sexual activity until approved by physician
12. when sexual activity is resumed, avoid positions that involve extreme rotation of the operative leg, flexing hip beyond 90°, and moving operative leg past the midline
13. avoid lifting heavy objects, excessive twisting and turning of body, walking on uneven surfaces, and activities that place excessive strain on hip (e.g. jogging).

8.d. The client will identify ways to reduce the risk of falls in the home environment.

8.d. If client is to return home, provide the following instructions on how to reduce the risk for falls at home:

1. keep electrical cords out of pathways
2. remove unnecessary furniture and provide wide pathways for ambulation
3. remove scatter rugs
4. provide adequate lighting at all times
5. do not climb stairs until permission is given by physician.

8.e. The client will state signs and symptoms to report to the health care provider.

8.e.1. Refer to Standardized Postoperative Care Plan, Nursing Diagnosis 21, action c (p. 123), for signs and symptoms to report to the health care provider.

2. Instruct client to report these additional signs and symptoms:
    a. persistent or increased pain or spasms in operative extremity
    b. loss of sensation or movement in operative extremity
    c. inability to maintain operative extremity in a neutral position
    d. inability to bear weight on operative extremity once weight-bearing is allowed
    e. shortening of operative extremity (will probably be noticed as a limp once full weight-bearing is resumed).

Desired Outcomes	Nursing Actions and *Selected Purposes/Rationales*
8.f. The client will identify community resources that can assist with home management and provide transportation.	8.f.1. Provide information about community resources that can assist the client and significant others with home management and provide transportation (e.g. home health agencies, Meals on Wheels, church groups, transportation services). 2. Initiate a referral if indicated.
8.g. The client will verbalize an understanding of and a plan for adhering to recommended follow-up care including future appointments with health care provider and physical therapist, medications prescribed, activity level, and wound care.	8.g.1. Refer to Standardized Postoperative Care Plan, Nursing Diagnosis 21 (pp. 123–124), for routine postoperative instructions and measures to improve client compliance. 2. Reinforce the importance of keeping appointments with physical therapist. 3. If client had a hip prosthesis inserted, instruct him/her to inform other health care providers about the hip prosthesis so that prophylactic antimicrobials can be started before any dental work, invasive diagnostic procedures, or surgery is performed.

Bibliography

See pages 897–898 and 909.

 # LAMINECTOMY/DISKECTOMY WITH OR WITHOUT FUSION

A laminectomy is the surgical removal of the lamina of a vertebra. It may be performed to allow for the removal of a neoplasm or bone fragments that are putting pressure on nerve roots or the spinal cord or to enable a rhizotomy or cordotomy to be performed to treat intractable pain. Most commonly, a laminectomy is performed to gain access to a herniated nucleus pulposus (HNP, "ruptured disk") so that a diskectomy (removal of the herniated portion of the disk) can be accomplished.

Disk herniation is usually the result of trauma (e.g. falls, vehicular accidents) or strain caused by factors such as improper or repeated lifting of heavy objects, awkward movement, sneezing, or coughing. Degenerative changes in the disks, supporting ligaments, and vertebrae are known to begin about age 30 and make the disks more prone to rupture. The most common sites of disk herniation are C5–6, C6–7, L4–5, and L5–S1. These areas of the spine are the most flexible and therefore are subjected to a greater amount of movement and strain. Signs and symptoms of lumbar disk herniation can include low back pain which radiates down the buttock, thigh, calf, and ankle on affected side; muscle spasms in lower back; muscle weakness, diminished knee and ankle reflexes, numbness, or tingling in affected lower extremity; constipation; and/or urinary retention. Clinical manifestations of cervical disk herniation can include neck pain which radiates to the shoulder, arm, and fingers on affected side; stiff neck; muscle spasms in neck; and/or muscle weakness, diminished biceps and triceps reflexes, numbness, or tingling in affected upper extremity.

A diskectomy is usually indicated if conservative measures such as bed rest, anti-inflammatory medications, analgesics, and muscle relaxants fail to control pain or if neurological deficits persist or worsen. Disk removal is usually accomplished by a microdiskectomy or laminectomy and can be performed using an anterior or posterior approach. The surgical procedure performed depends on the location and size of the herniated disk and physician preference. If the vertebral column in the surgical area is unstable, a spinal fusion may be performed along with a laminectomy. The surgical immobilization of the unstable area is accomplished using bone from the client's iliac crest or from a bone bank and/or using internal fixation devices such as rods, plates, screws, and wire.

This care plan focuses on the adult client hospitalized for a laminectomy* that is being performed to remove a herniated nucleus pulposus. Preoperatively, goals of care are to reduce fear and anxiety and educate the client regarding postoperative management. Postoperative goals of care are to promote optimal neurological function, maintain comfort, prevent complications, and educate the client regarding follow-up care.

---

*The care of a client hospitalized for a laminectomy with spinal fusion is also discussed. If a fusion is performed and activity is limited for longer than 72 hours, refer to the Care Plan on Immobility.

DIAGNOSTIC TESTS

Spinal x-rays
Computed tomography (CT)
Magnetic resonance imaging (MRI)
Myelography
Electromyography (EMG)

DISCHARGE CRITERIA

Prior to discharge, the client will:

- have improved neurological function
- have evidence of normal healing of the surgical wound
- have intact skin under stabilization device if one is present
- have pain controlled
- have no signs and symptoms of postoperative complications
- identify ways to prevent recurrent disk herniation
- demonstrate the ability to correctly apply and remove stabilization device if one is required
- verbalize an understanding of ways to maintain skin integrity when wearing a stabilization device
- state signs and symptoms to report to the health care provider
- verbalize an understanding of and a plan for adhering to recommended follow-up care including future appointments with health care provider, medications prescribed, activity level, and wound care.

**NURSING/
COLLABORATIVE
DIAGNOSES**

Preoperative
1. Knowledge deficit △   773
Postoperative
1. Risk for peripheral neurovascular dysfunction △   775
2. Pain △   775
3. Actual/Risk for impaired tissue integrity △   776
4. Urinary retention △   777
5. Potential complications:
   a. respiratory distress
   b. cerebrospinal fluid leak
   c. laryngeal nerve damage
   d. paralytic ileus △   778

DISCHARGE TEACHING
6. Knowledge deficit, Ineffective management of therapeutic regimen, or Altered health maintenance △   779

See Standardized Preoperative and Postoperative Care Plans for additional diagnoses.

PREOPERATIVE

Use in conjunction with the Standardized Preoperative Care Plan.

Client Teaching

---

1. NURSING DIAGNOSIS:

Knowledge deficit

regarding the surgical procedure, hospital routines associated with surgery, physical preparation for laminectomy and spinal fusion (if planned), sensations that normally occur following surgery and anesthesia, and postoperative care.

Desired Outcomes | Nursing Actions and **Selected Purposes/Rationales**

1.a. The client will verbalize an
       understanding of the
       surgical procedure,
       preoperative care, and
       postoperative sensations
       and care.

1.a.1. Refer to Standardized Preoperative Care Plan, Nursing Diagnosis 4,
        actions a.1–4 (pp. 99–100), for information to include in preoperative
        teaching.
     2. Provide additional information regarding postoperative care:
         a. if a laminectomy without spinal fusion is planned:
             1. explain that progressive activity will probably begin the evening of
                 or morning after surgery
             2. reinforce physician's explanation about wearing a soft cervical
                 collar (following a cervical laminectomy) or a back brace or corset
                 (following a lumbar laminectomy) if client is expected to need one
                 while the surgical area heals (some physicians order this
                 stabilization device to provide additional support to the operative
                 area for a few weeks postoperatively if the surgery is fairly
                 extensive and/or the client has a tendency to be too active)
         b. if a laminectomy with spinal fusion is planned:
             1. explain that progressive activity usually begins 1–3 days after
                 surgery depending on physician preference and extensiveness of
                 the surgery
             2. reinforce physician's explanation about the type of stabilization
                 device that will need to be worn while the surgical area heals
                 (usually a rigid cervical collar following a cervical fusion and a
                 back brace following a lumbar fusion)
         c. if client has muscle weakness or numbness or tingling in the affected
             extremity, explain that it may take weeks to months to resolve after
             surgery due to surgical trauma and the time it takes the peripheral
             nerves to heal.
     3. Allow time for questions and clarification of information provided.
     4. Allow time for client to practice putting on and removing stabilization
         device if available preoperatively.

1.b. The client will demonstrate
       the ability to perform
       activities designed to
       prevent postoperative
       complications.

1.b.1. Refer to Standardized Preoperative Care Plan, Nursing Diagnosis 4,
        action b.1 (p. 100), for instructions on ways to prevent postoperative
        complications.
     2. Provide additional instructions about ways to prevent postoperative
         complications:
         a. instruct client how to logroll and stress the importance of turning in
             this manner after surgery (the length of time logrolling is necessary
             increases if a fusion was performed)
         b. instruct client to avoid extreme flexion, hyperextension, and twisting
             of the cervical or lumbar spine postoperatively
         c. demonstrate the correct way to change from a lying to standing
             position (e.g. keeping spine in proper alignment, utilizing arm and leg
             muscles)
         d. reinforce physician's or physical therapist's instructions about
             exercises to strengthen arm, shoulder, neck, back, leg, and abdominal
             muscles (increased strength of these muscles decreases strain on the
             spine)
         e. demonstrate proper body alignment and good body mechanics
             and stress the importance of lifelong adherence to these
             principles.
     3. Allow time for questions, clarification, and return demonstration.

POSTOPERATIVE   **Use in conjunction with the Standardized Postoperative Care Plan.**

1. NURSING DIAGNOSIS: **Risk for peripheral neurovascular dysfunction**

related to:
a. trauma to the nerves or blood vessels associated with surgery;
b. blood accumulation and inflammation in the surgical area;
c. dislocation of the bone graft and/or internal fixation devices (if a fusion was performed);
d. excessive external pressure on the nerves or blood vessels associated with improper fit or application of stabilization device (e.g. cervical collar, back brace, corset).

Desired Outcome	Nursing Actions and *Selected Purposes/Rationales*
1. The client will have usual or improved peripheral neurovascular function as evidenced by: a. palpable peripheral pulses b. capillary refill time less than 3 seconds c. extremities warm and usual color d. ability to flex and extend feet and toes and hands and fingers e. usual or improved reflexes, muscle tone, and sensation in extremities f. no new or increased pain in extremities.	1.a. Assess for and report signs and symptoms of peripheral neurovascular dysfunction (check upper extremities after surgery on the cervical area and lower extremities after surgery on the lumbar area): 1. diminished or absent peripheral pulses 2. capillary refill time greater than 3 seconds 3. pallor, cyanosis, or coolness of extremities 4. inability to flex or extend foot or toes or hands or fingers 5. diminished or absent reflexes in extremities 6. development of or increase in muscle weakness, numbness, or tingling in extremities 7. development of or increase in pain in extremities. b. Implement measures *to reduce the risk for peripheral neurovascular dysfunction:* 1. perform actions to reduce strain on the surgical area (see Postoperative Nursing Diagnosis 2, action b.1) *in order to prevent bleeding and subsequent hematoma formation in the surgical area and to reduce the risk for dislocation of the bone graft and/or internal fixation devices (if fusion was performed)* 2. maintain wound suction and patency of wound drain *to reduce the accumulation of blood in the surgical area and subsequently prevent increased pressure on nerves and blood vessels* 3. apply stabilization device properly; notify orthotist if it appears to create excessive pressure on any area 4. administer corticosteroids (e.g. dexamethasone) if ordered *to reduce inflammation in the surgical area.* c. If signs and symptoms of peripheral neurovascular dysfunction occur: 1. assess for and correct improper body alignment and external cause of excessive pressure (e.g. tight or improperly applied stabilization device) 2. notify physician if signs and symptoms persist or worsen 3. prepare client for surgical intervention (e.g. evacuation of hematoma, repositioning of dislocated bone graft and/or internal fixation devices) if planned.

2. NURSING DIAGNOSIS: **Pain**

related to:
a. tissue trauma and reflex muscle spasms associated with the surgery;
b. removal of bone (bone may have been taken from the client's iliac crest to achieve spinal fusion);
c. stretching and compression of sensory nerves associated with blood accumulation and inflammation in the surgical area;
d. irritation from drainage tube (wound drain may be present, especially following a spinal fusion);

  e. stress on surgical area associated with movement;
  f. release of pressure on compressed spinal nerve root following removal of the herniated nucleus pulposus (improved sensory nerve function can cause a temporary increase in pain in area[s] of previously diminished sensation).

Desired Outcome	Nursing Actions and *Selected Purposes/Rationales*

2. The client will experience diminished pain (see Standardized Postoperative Care Plan, Nursing Diagnosis 6 [pp. 106–107], for outcome criteria).	2.a. Refer to Standardized Postoperative Care Plan, Nursing Diagnosis 6 (pp. 106–107), for measures related to assessment and management of pain.
	  b. Implement additional measures *to reduce pain:*
	    1. perform actions *to reduce strain on the surgical area:*
	      a. ensure that client is always positioned with spine in proper alignment
	      b. apply stabilization device if ordered *to provide additional support to surgical area*
	      c. implement measures *to prevent hyperextension, extreme flexion, and/or twisting of spine* (e.g. instruct and assist client to logroll when turning; put needed items within easy reach; if a cervical laminectomy was performed, place a small pillow or folded pad under client's head rather than a full-size pillow; assist with bathing and dressing as needed)
	      d. if lumbar laminectomy was performed, assist client to maintain a position that results in flattening of the lumbosacral spine (e.g. slight knee flexion when supine, knees flexed while in side-lying position, feet elevated on footstool when sitting in chair) *in order to reduce stretching of the nerves and muscles in the lower back*
	      e. instruct client to avoid sitting or standing for longer than 20–30 minute intervals (some physicians instruct clients to sit only during meals and ambulate only short distances when progressive activity begins)
	      f. instruct client to avoid straining to have a bowel movement (especially after lumbar laminectomy) and vigorous coughing; consult physician about an order for a laxative and antitussive if indicated
	    2. if appropriate, perform actions *to reduce pressure on bone graft donor site* (e.g. position client so he/she is not lying on site, protect the site with padding if stabilization device is worn over it)
	    3. administer corticosteroids (e.g. dexamethasone) if ordered *to reduce inflammation in the surgical area.*

---

3. NURSING DIAGNOSIS: **Actual/Risk for impaired tissue integrity**

related to:
a. disruption of tissue associated with the surgical procedure;
b. irritation of skin associated with contact with wound drainage, use of tape, and pressure from tubes and/or stabilization device if present.

Desired Outcomes	Nursing Actions and *Selected Purposes/Rationales*
3.a. The client will experience normal healing of the surgical wound (see Standardized Postoperative Care Plan, Nursing Diagnosis 9, outcome a [pp. 109–110], for outcome criteria).	3.a. Refer to Standardized Postoperative Care Plan, Nursing Diagnosis 9, action a (pp. 109–110), for measures related to assessment and promotion of wound healing.

3.b. The client will maintain tissue integrity in areas in contact with wound drainage, tape, tubings, and stabilization device as evidenced by:
1. absence of redness and irritation
2. no skin breakdown.

3.b.1. Inspect the following for signs and symptoms of skin irritation and breakdown:
  a. areas in contact with wound drainage, tape, and tubings
  b. area under stabilization device.
2. Refer to Standardized Postoperative Care Plan, Nursing Diagnosis 9, action b.2 (pp. 110–111), for measures related to prevention of tissue irritation and breakdown resulting from contact with wound drainage, tape, and tubings.
3. Implement measures *to prevent skin irritation and breakdown under stabilization device:*
  a. apply stabilization device securely enough to keep it from rubbing and irritating the skin but not too tightly
  b. position client so that stabilization device is not causing excessive pressure on any area
  c. assist client to put a cotton T-shirt on under back brace or corset and ensure that the shirt is dry and wrinkle-free
  d. apply a thin layer of powder or cornstarch to skin under stabilization device *in order to absorb moisture and/or reduce friction*
  e. pad areas over bony prominences before applying stabilization device
  f. instruct client to refrain from inserting anything under the stabilization device
  g. consult physician, physical therapist, or orthotist if stabilization device is putting excessive pressure on the skin.
4. If tissue breakdown occurs:
  a. notify physician
  b. continue with above measures to prevent further irritation and breakdown
  c. perform care of involved area(s) as ordered or per standard hospital procedure
  d. assess client closely and report signs and symptoms of infection (e.g. elevated temperature; redness, heat, new or increased pain, and swelling around area of breakdown; unusual drainage from site).

---

4. NURSING DIAGNOSIS:　　**Urinary retention**

related to:
a. incomplete bladder emptying associated with horizontal positioning (client may be on bed rest for a few days following a spinal fusion);
b. increased tone of the urinary sphincters and relaxation of the bladder muscle associated with:
  1. indirect sympathetic nervous system stimulation resulting from pain, fear, and anxiety
  2. direct stimulation of the sympathetic nerves that innervate the bladder (can occur as a result of nerve trauma during a lumbar laminectomy and/or pressure on the nerves as a result of inflammation or accumulation of blood in the surgical area following a lumbar laminectomy);
c. relaxation of the bladder muscle and decreased perception of bladder fullness associated with the depressant effect of anesthesia and some medications (e.g. narcotic [opioid] analgesics, central-acting muscle relaxants).

Desired Outcome	Nursing Actions and *Selected Purposes/Rationales*
4. The client will not experience urinary retention (see Standardized Postoperative Care Plan, Nursing Diagnosis 13 [p. 113], for outcome criteria).	4. Refer to Standardized Postoperative Care Plan, Nursing Diagnosis 13 (pp. 113–114), for measures related to assessment and management of urinary retention.

5. COLLABORATIVE DIAGNOSES:

Potential complications of laminectomy:

a. **respiratory distress** related to:
   1. trauma to the phrenic nerve during surgery and/or compression of the phrenic nerve following surgery associated with inflammation or accumulation of blood in the surgical area (can occur with a cervical laminectomy because the phrenic nerve arises at the C3–5 level)
   2. tracheal compression associated with inflammation or accumulation of blood in the surgical area following a cervical laminectomy (particularly if the anterior approach was used)
   3. closure of the glottis associated with paralysis of the vocal cords (can occur as a result of injury to the bilateral recurrent laryngeal nerves during an anterior cervical laminectomy);

b. **cerebrospinal fluid leak** related to inadvertent damage to and/or incomplete closure of the dura (care is taken during surgery to keep the dura intact; however, it is sometimes necessary to incise dura that extends along the involved nerve);

c. **laryngeal nerve damage** related to surgical trauma or pressure on the nerve(s) associated with inflammation or accumulation of blood in the surgical area (can occur with an anterior cervical laminectomy);

d. **paralytic ileus** related to:
   1. impaired innervation of the intestinal tract following a lumbar laminectomy associated with stimulation of sympathetic nerves and/or loss of parasympathetic nerve function in the operative area
   2. the depressant effect of anesthesia and some medications (e.g. central-acting muscle relaxants, narcotic [opioid] analgesics).

Desired Outcomes	Nursing Actions and *Selected Purposes/Rationales*

5.a. The client will not experience respiratory distress as evidenced by:
1. unlabored respirations at 14–20/minute
2. absence of stridor and sternocleidomastoid muscle retraction
3. usual mental status
4. usual skin color
5. blood gases within normal range.

5.a.1. Following a cervical laminectomy, assess for and immediately report:
   a. increased swelling of the neck or bulging of the wound
   b. statements of difficulty swallowing or choking sensation
   c. signs and symptoms of respiratory distress (e.g. rapid and/or labored respirations, stridor, sternocleidomastoid muscle retraction, restlessness, agitation, cyanosis)
   d. abnormal blood gases
   e. significant decrease in oximetry results.
   2. Have tracheostomy and suction equipment readily available following a cervical laminectomy.
   3. Implement measures *to prevent respiratory distress following a cervical laminectomy:*
      a. perform actions *to reduce inflammation and/or prevent bleeding and subsequent hematoma formation in the surgical area:*
         1. implement measures to reduce strain on the surgical area (see Postoperative Nursing Diagnosis 2, action b.1)
         2. elevate head of bed 30–45° unless contraindicated
         3. apply ice pack to incisional area as ordered
         4. administer corticosteroids (e.g. dexamethasone) if ordered
      b. maintain wound suction and patency of wound drain *to prevent the accumulation of blood in the surgical area.*
   4. If signs and symptoms of respiratory distress occur:
      a. place client in a high Fowler's position unless contraindicated
      b. loosen neck dressing or cervical collar if it appears tight
      c. administer oxygen as ordered
      d. suction client if indicated
      e. assist with intubation or emergency tracheostomy if performed
      f. prepare client for surgical evacuation of hematoma or repair of the bleeding vessel(s) if indicated
      g. provide emotional support to client and significant others.

5.b. The client will have resolution of cerebrospinal fluid leak if it occurs as evidenced by:
   1. absence of cerebrospinal fluid drainage from lower back or neck incision
   2. no reports of headache.

5.b.1. Assess for and report signs and symptoms of a cerebrospinal fluid leak:
   a. presence of glucose in wound drainage as shown by positive results on a glucose reagent strip; be aware that any drainage containing blood will also test positive for glucose
   b. yellowish ring ("halo") around clear, bloody, or serosanguineous drainage on lower back or neck dressing, sheet, or pillowcase
   c. reports of headache.
   2. Implement measures to reduce strain on the surgical area (see Postoperative Nursing Diagnosis 2, action b.1) *in order to promote healing of the dura and subsequent resolution of cerebrospinal fluid leak.*
   3. If signs and symptoms of cerebrospinal fluid leak occur:
   a. maintain activity restrictions as ordered *to reduce stress on the dural tear*
   b. maintain meticulous sterile technique when changing dressing
   c. change dressing as soon as it becomes damp
   d. administer antimicrobials if ordered
   e. assess for and report signs and symptoms of meningitis (e.g. fever; chills; new, increasing, or persistent headache; nuchal rigidity; photophobia; positive Kernig's and Brudzinski's signs)
   f. prepare client for surgical repair of the torn dura if planned (usually the torn dura heals spontaneously within a few days)
   g. provide emotional support to the client and significant others.

5.c. The client will experience resolution of laryngeal nerve damage if it occurs as evidenced by:
   1. improved voice tone and quality
   2. gradual resolution of hoarseness
   3. absence of respiratory distress.

5.c.1. Assess for the following indications of laryngeal nerve damage:
   a. voice changes (e.g. hoarseness; weak, whispery voice; inability to speak)
   b. respiratory distress (see action a.1.c in this diagnosis).
   2. Implement measures to reduce pressure on the laryngeal nerves (see actions a.3.a and b in this diagnosis).
   3. If signs and symptoms of laryngeal nerve damage occur:
   a. encourage client to avoid unnecessary talking *in order to rest the vocal cords*
   b. implement measures *to facilitate communication* (e.g. provide pad and pencil, flash cards, or magic slate; ask questions that require a short answer or nod of head)
   c. reinforce physician's explanation regarding the permanence of voice changes (voice tone and quality usually return to normal as inflammation subsides)
   d. notify physician immediately if signs and symptoms of respiratory distress occur, client is unable to speak, or hoarseness or voice changes worsen.

5.d. The client will not develop a paralytic ileus (see Standardized Postoperative Care Plan, Collaborative Diagnosis 19, outcome d [p. 121], for outcome criteria).

5.d. Refer to Standardized Postoperative Care Plan, Collaborative Diagnosis 19, action d (p. 121), for measures related to assessment and management of a paralytic ileus.

Discharge Teaching

■

6. **NURSING DIAGNOSIS:**   **Knowledge deficit, Ineffective management of therapeutic regimen, or Altered health maintenance***

*The nurse should select the diagnostic label that is most appropriate for the client's discharge teaching needs.

Desired Outcomes	Nursing Actions and *Selected Purposes/Rationales*

6.a. The client will identify ways to prevent recurrent disk herniation.	6.a.1. Inform client about ways to reduce back and/or neck strain and subsequently reduce the risk of recurrent disk herniation:
	  a. lose weight if overweight
	  b. support the spine adequately (e.g. sleep on a firm mattress; sit on firm, straight-backed or contoured chairs; wear stabilization device as prescribed)
	  c. always use proper body mechanics (e.g. bend at the knees rather than waist, push rather than pull heavy objects, carry items close to body)
	  d. always keep spine in good alignment
	  e. adhere to prescribed, progressive exercise program to strengthen back, neck, shoulders, arms, legs, and abdominal muscles when allowed.
	  2. Provide a dietary consult regarding a weight reduction program if indicated.
	  3. Allow time for client to practice proper body alignment when sitting, standing, and walking; proper positioning when resting; and any exercises allowed in immediate postoperative period. Encourage client to think about and plan movements before doing them.
	  4. Allow time for questions, clarification, and return demonstration of proper body mechanics, positioning, and exercises allowed.

6.b. The client will demonstrate the ability to correctly apply and remove stabilization device if one is required.	6.b.1. Reinforce instructions on the correct way to apply and remove stabilization device (e.g. soft or hard cervical collar, back brace, corset) if client needs to wear one after discharge. 2. Allow time for questions, clarification, and return demonstration.

6.c. The client will verbalize an understanding of ways to maintain skin integrity when wearing a stabilization device.	6.c.1. If client is to be discharged with a stabilization device, instruct him/her to examine skin daily when device is off (if device should not be removed, demonstrate how to examine underneath it using a mirror and flashlight).
	  2. Instruct client in ways to maintain skin integrity if a stabilization device needs to be worn:
	    a. apply device properly and maintain spine in good alignment to avoid undue pressure in any area
	    b. wear a cotton T-shirt under back brace or corset and keep shirt dry and wrinkle-free
	    c. apply a thin layer of powder or cornstarch to skin under stabilization device to absorb moisture and reduce irritation caused by friction
	    d. avoid inserting anything under the device
	    e. place padding between stabilization device and bony prominences.

6.d. The client will state signs and symptoms to report to the health care provider.	6.d.1. Refer to Standardized Postoperative Care Plan, Nursing Diagnosis 21, action c (p. 123), for signs and symptoms to report to the health care provider.
	  2. Instruct client to report these additional signs and symptoms:
	    a. decreased movement or sensation in extremities
	    b. coolness or bluish color of extremities
	    c. increasing or recurrent numbness, tingling, or pain in surgical area or extremities
	    d. difficulty standing up straight (after lumbar surgery) or keeping neck straight (after cervical surgery)
	    e. persistent and/or severe headache
	    f. drainage of clear or bloody fluid from incision
	    g. persistent hoarseness or difficulty swallowing (following cervical laminectomy)
	    h. reddened or irritated area on skin underneath stabilization device.

6.e. The client will verbalize an understanding of and a plan for adhering to recommended follow-up care including future appointments with health care provider, medications	6.e.1. Refer to Standardized Postoperative Care Plan, Nursing Diagnosis 21 (pp. 123–124), for routine postoperative instructions and measures to improve client compliance.
	  2. Reinforce physician's instructions regarding activity (the restrictions will vary depending on extensiveness of surgery, client condition, and physician preference):
	    a. avoid lifting objects weighing more than 5–10 pounds

prescribed, activity level, and wound care.

b. progress through exercise program as prescribed
c. avoid sitting or standing for longer than 30 minutes at a time (especially after surgery on lumbar area)
d. schedule adequate rest periods
e. avoid driving a car (causes increased flexion of the spine) and taking long car rides (the vibrations can jar the spine and long periods without significant changes in position can increase stiffness and discomfort) until allowed.

Bibliography

See pages 897–898 and 909.

 # TOTAL HIP REPLACEMENT

A total hip replacement (arthroplasty) is a surgical procedure in which the ball and socket components of the hip joint are replaced with prosthetic devices. There are a variety of prosthetic devices available. The prostheses are either cemented in place using an agent called polymethylmethacrylate or are uncemented (cementless). Uncemented prostheses have porous surfaces that permit bone ingrowth to occur and provide biological fixation. A total hip replacement is performed to relieve joint pain that has been resistant to conservative management and/or improve joint mobility in persons with severe arthritis. It may also be performed to treat avascular necrosis of the femoral head, congenital hip deformity, and failure of previous reconstructive hip surgery.

This care plan focuses on the adult client hospitalized for a total hip replacement. Preoperative goals of care are to reduce fear and anxiety and educate the client regarding ways to prevent postoperative complications and facilitate rehabilitation. Postoperatively, the goals of care are to maintain comfort, prevent complications, assist the client to regain maximum mobility, and educate the client regarding follow-up care. Prevention of infection is of major importance in caring for the client who has had a total hip replacement since infection of the operative hip usually necessitates surgical debridement and/or removal of the prosthesis.

DIAGNOSTIC TESTS

X-rays of the hip, pelvis, and femoral shaft

DISCHARGE CRITERIA

Prior to discharge, the client will:

- have evidence of normal healing of the surgical wound
- have clear, audible breath sounds throughout lungs
- have reduced hip pain
- have expected degree of mobility of hip joint
- have no signs and symptoms of infection or postoperative complications
- demonstrate correct transfer and ambulation techniques and proper use of ambulatory aids
- demonstrate the ability to correctly perform the prescribed exercises
- verbalize an understanding of activity and position restrictions necessary to prevent dislocation of the hip prosthesis
- identify ways to reduce the risk of falls in the home environment
- state signs and symptoms to report to the health care provider
- identify community resources that can assist with home management and provide transportation
- verbalize an understanding of and a plan for adhering to recommended follow-up care including future appointments with health care provider and physical therapist, medications prescribed, activity level, and wound care.

NURSING/	**Preoperative**
COLLABORATIVE	**1.** Knowledge deficit △ 782
DIAGNOSES	**Postoperative**
	1. Risk for peripheral neurovascular dysfunction: operative extremity
	△ 783
	2. Pain: hip △ 784
	3. Actual/Risk for impaired tissue integrity △ 785
	4. Activity intolerance △ 786
	5. Impaired physical mobility △ 787
	6. Risk for infection: operative hip △ 787
	7. Risk for trauma: falls △ 788
	8. Potential complications:
	a. hemorrhage and/or hematoma formation
	b. dislocation of hip prosthesis(es)
	c. thromboembolism △ 789
DISCHARGE TEACHING	**9.** Knowledge deficit, Ineffective management of therapeutic regimen, or
	Altered health maintenance △ 790

See Standardized Preoperative and Postoperative Care Plans for additional diagnoses.

PREOPERATIVE

Use in conjunction with the Standardized Preoperative Care Plan.

Client Teaching

---

1. NURSING DIAGNOSIS: **Knowledge deficit**

regarding the surgical procedure, hospital routines associated with surgery, physical preparation for the total hip replacement, sensations that normally occur following surgery and anesthesia, and postoperative care.

Desired Outcomes	Nursing Actions and *Selected Purposes/Rationales*
1.a. The client will verbalize an understanding of the surgical procedure, preoperative care, and postoperative sensations and care.	1.a.1. Refer to Standardized Preoperative Care Plan, Nursing Diagnosis 4, actions a.1–4 (pp. 99–100), for information to include in preoperative teaching.
	2. Provide additional information on specific preoperative care for clients having a total hip replacement:
	a. explain that the following measures will be performed to reduce the risk of a postoperative hip infection:
	1. the operative hip and thigh will be scrubbed with an antiseptic solution (e.g. povidone-iodine) before surgery
	2. injections will not be given in the operative extremity
	3. existing infections will be treated before surgery; instruct client to report any symptoms of infection (e.g. cough, runny nose, burning on urination)
	4. antimicrobials will probably be administered prophylactically before and after surgery
	b. explain that anticoagulants (e.g. heparin, warfarin) and/or antiplatelet agents (e.g. low-molecular-weight dextran, low-dose aspirin) may be administered before surgery to reduce the risk of postoperative thrombus formation; inform client that coagulation studies are usually done before starting these medications, especially if he/she has been taking aspirin or other nonsteroidal anti-inflammatory agents (e.g. ibuprofen).

3. Inform client that an operative site drain and suction device may be present temporarily after surgery and that this may be an autotransfusion drainage system that can be used for blood replacement if needed.

4. Allow time for questions and clarification of information provided.

1.b. The client will demonstrate the ability to perform activities designed to prevent postoperative complications.

1.b.1. Refer to Standardized Preoperative Care Plan, Nursing Diagnosis 4, action b.1 (p. 100), for instructions on ways to prevent postoperative complications.

2. Provide additional instructions about ways to prevent complications following total hip replacement:

a. reinforce physician's or physical therapist's instructions on:
   1. transfer techniques that can be performed without flexing hip beyond the prescribed limit
   2. exercises (e.g. quadriceps- and gluteal-setting, upper extremity strengthening, active heel slides, straight leg raising)
   3. ambulation techniques and proper use of ambulatory aids (weight-bearing limitations are determined by the physician and vary depending on the type of prostheses used)

b. instruct client in the correct way to use overhead trapeze and unoperative leg to move self

c. explain the following activity and positioning limitations that need to be adhered to postoperatively to prevent dislocation of the prosthesis(es):
   1. operative extremity will be maintained in an abducted position by a balanced suspension device, abduction wedge, or 2–3 pillows for first few days after surgery
   2. operative leg should be kept in proper alignment and should not be brought toward the midline
   3. if turning is allowed, it should be done only with assistance of trained personnel
   4. hip flexion of 45–60° will be permitted initially and then should not exceed 90° during the rehabilitation phase.

3. Allow time for questions, clarification, and return demonstration.

POSTOPERATIVE

Use in conjunction with the Standardized Postoperative Care Plan.

---

1. NURSING DIAGNOSIS:

Risk for peripheral neurovascular dysfunction: operative extremity

related to trauma to or excessive pressure on the nerves or blood vessels associated with surgery, blood accumulation and edema in the surgical area, improper alignment of operative extremity, pressure exerted by balanced suspension device or straps on abductor wedge, and dislocation of the prosthesis(es).

Desired Outcome	Nursing Actions and *Selected Purposes/Rationales*

1. The client will maintain normal neurovascular function in the operative extremity as evidenced by:
   a. palpable pedal pulses
   b. capillary refill time in toes less than 3 seconds

1.a. Assess for and report signs and symptoms of neurovascular dysfunction in the operative extremity:
   1. diminished or absent pedal pulses
   2. capillary refill time in toes greater than 3 seconds
   3. pallor, cyanosis, or coolness of the extremity
   4. inability to flex or extend foot or toes
   5. numbness or tingling in foot or toes

Desired Outcome	Nursing Actions and *Selected Purposes/Rationales*

c. extremity warm and usual color
d. ability to flex and extend foot and toes
e. absence of numbness and tingling in foot and toes
f. absence of foot pain during passive movement of foot and toes
g. no increase in pain in extremity.
	6. pain in foot during passive motion of the toes or foot
	7. increased pain in the extremity.
	b. Implement measures *to prevent neurovascular dysfunction in the operative extremity:*
	  1. perform actions to prevent hematoma formation (see Postoperative Collaborative Diagnosis 8, action a.2)
	  2. make sure that balanced suspension device and straps on abductor wedge are not exerting pressure on the popliteal space, Achilles tendon, and lateral and medial aspects of the knee and ankle
	  3. maintain extremity in proper alignment
	  4. perform actions to prevent dislocation of the prostheses (see Postoperative Collaborative Diagnosis 8, action b.2).
	c. If signs and symptoms of neurovascular dysfunction occur:
	  1. assess for and correct causes of excessive pressure on operative leg (e.g. tight straps on abductor wedge, improper positioning of balanced suspension device)
	  2. notify physician if the signs and symptoms persist
	  3. prepare client for closed reduction (e.g. traction) or surgical intervention (e.g. relocation of prosthesis, hematoma evacuation) if planned.

---

2. NURSING DIAGNOSIS:

Pain: hip

related to tissue trauma and reflex muscle spasms associated with the surgery, blood accumulation and edema in surgical area, and improper positioning of the operative extremity.

Desired Outcome	Nursing Actions and *Selected Purposes/Rationales*

2. The client will experience diminished hip pain (see Standardized Postoperative Care Plan, Nursing Diagnosis 6 [pp. 106–107], for outcome criteria).	2.a. Refer to Standardized Postoperative Care Plan, Nursing Diagnosis 6 (pp. 106–107), for measures related to assessment and reduction of pain.
	b. Implement additional measures *to reduce pain:*
	  1. keep operative extremity in an abducted position (some physicians ensure this position by placing the extremity in balanced suspension for 24 hours after surgery; others order placement of an abduction wedge or 2–3 pillows between legs at all times)
	  2. maintain restrictions on the degree of hip flexion as ordered (usually a 45–60° maximum is allowed for first 2–3 days with a maximum of 90° during rehabilitation period)
	  3. place trochanter roll or sandbag against the operative site for first 24–48 hours after surgery (*pressure on the operative area helps maintain alignment and prevent hematoma formation*)
	  4. maintain patency of wound drainage system (e.g. prevent kinking of tubing, empty collection device as needed, keep collection device below surgical wound, maintain suction as ordered) *to reduce accumulation of fluid in surgical area*
	  5. move operative extremity gently
	  6. if turning is allowed, keep pillows between legs when turning and while in side-lying position *to prevent adduction and resultant strain on surgical site*
	  7. administer prescribed analgesics before exercise and ambulation sessions.

3. NURSING DIAGNOSIS: **Actual/Risk for impaired tissue integrity**

related to:
a. disruption of tissue associated with the surgical procedure;
b. delayed wound healing associated with factors such as decreased nutritional status and inadequate blood supply to wound area;
c. irritation of skin associated with contact with wound drainage, pressure from tubes, and use of tape;
d. excessive or prolonged pressure on tissues from balanced suspension device, straps on abductor wedge, and elastic wraps or stockings;
e. damage to the skin and/or subcutaneous tissue associated with prolonged pressure on tissues, friction, and shearing while mobility is decreased.

Desired Outcomes	Nursing Actions and *Selected Purposes/Rationales*
3.a. The client will experience normal healing of the surgical wound (see Standardized Postoperative Care Plan, Nursing Diagnosis 9, outcome a [pp. 109–110], for outcome criteria).	3.a. Refer to Standardized Postoperative Care Plan, Nursing Diagnosis 9, action a (pp. 109–110), for measures related to assessment and promotion of wound healing.

3.b. The client will maintain tissue integrity as evidenced by:
1. absence of redness and irritation
2. no skin breakdown.
	3.b.1. Inspect the following sites for pallor, redness, and breakdown:
	  a. skin in contact with wound drainage, tape, and tubing
	  b. back, coccyx, and buttocks
	  c. elbows and heels
	  d. pressure points on operative extremity in contact with balanced suspension device
	  e. areas in contact with abductor wedge straps
	  f. areas under elastic wraps or stockings.
	  2. Refer to Standardized Postoperative Care Plan, Nursing Diagnosis 9, action b.2 (pp. 110–111), for measures related to prevention of tissue irritation and breakdown in areas in contact with wound drainage, tubings, and tape.
	  3. Implement measures *to prevent tissue breakdown associated with decreased mobility:*
	    a. position client properly; use pressure-reducing or pressure-relieving devices (e.g. pillows, alternating pressure mattress) if indicated
	    b. instruct client to use overhead trapeze to lift self and shift weight at least every 30 minutes
	    c. gently massage around reddened areas at least every 2 hours
	    d. apply a thin layer of powder or cornstarch to bottom sheet or skin and to opposing skin surfaces (e.g. axillae) if indicated *to absorb moisture and reduce friction*
	    e. lift and move client carefully using a turn sheet and adequate assistance
	    f. limit length of time client is in semi-Fowler's position to 30 minutes (*in this position, client tends to slide down in bed, which can cause skin surface abrasion and shearing*)
	    g. if turning is allowed, turn client every 2 hours (physician may allow client to turn on unoperative side)
	    h. keep skin lubricated, clean, and dry
	    i. keep bed linens dry and wrinkle-free
	    j. increase activity as allowed and tolerated.

Desired Outcomes	Nursing Actions and *Selected Purposes/Rationales*

	4. Implement measures *to prevent tissue breakdown associated with excessive pressure caused by balanced suspension device or abductor wedge:*
	   a. make sure metal parts on suspension device are not resting on any area of extremity
	   b. maintain proper alignment of extremity in suspension device
	   c. make sure that straps holding abductor wedge in place are not too tight.
	 5. Implement measures *to prevent irritation and breakdown on elbows and heels:*
	   a. massage elbows and heels with lotion frequently
	   b. encourage client to use overhead trapeze to move self rather than pushing up with heel and elbows
	   c. provide elbow and heel protectors if indicated.
	 6. Implement measures *to prevent tissue breakdown under elastic wraps or stockings:*
	   a. remove elastic wraps or stockings at least twice daily, bathe and thoroughly dry skin, and reapply smoothly
	   b. check wraps or stockings frequently and reapply if they have slipped or become wrinkled
	   c. if areas of redness develop under wraps or stockings, consult physician before reapplying.
	 7. If tissue breakdown occurs:
	   a. notify physician
	   b. continue with above measures to prevent further irritation and breakdown
	   c. perform care of involved areas as ordered or per standard hospital procedure
	   d. assess client closely and report signs and symptoms of infection (e.g. elevated temperature; redness, heat, pain, and swelling around area of breakdown; unusual drainage from site).

■──

4. NURSING DIAGNOSIS: **Activity intolerance**

related to:
a. tissue hypoxia associated with diminished tissue perfusion and anemia (there is usually significant blood loss because the hip is a very vascular area);
b. difficulty resting and sleeping associated with discomfort, position restrictions, fear, and anxiety.

Desired Outcome	Nursing Actions and *Selected Purposes/Rationales*

4. The client will demonstrate an increased tolerance for activity (see Standardized Postoperative Care Plan, Nursing Diagnosis 10 [p. 111], for outcome criteria).	4.a. Refer to Standardized Postoperative Care Plan, Nursing Diagnosis 10 (pp. 111–112), for measures related to assessment and improvement of activity tolerance.
	  b. Implement additional measures *to help resolve anemia and subsequently improve activity tolerance:*
	   1. encourage client to increase intake of foods high in iron (e.g. organ meats, dried fruits, dark green leafy vegetables, whole-grain or iron-enriched breads and cereals) and vitamin C (*enhances the absorption of iron from plant products*)
	   2. autotransfuse hip drainage and/or administer packed red blood cells if ordered
	   3. administer iron supplements if ordered.

5. NURSING DIAGNOSIS: **Impaired physical mobility**

related to:
a. pain and weakness in weight-bearing extremity associated with surgery on the hip;
b. prescribed activity and weight-bearing restrictions following total hip replacement;
c. generalized weakness associated with surgery;
d. depressant effect of anesthesia and some medications (e.g. narcotic [opioid] analgesics, central-acting muscle relaxants);
e. fear of falling, dislodging drainage tube, dislocating prostheses, and compromising surgical wound.

Desired Outcome	Nursing Actions and *Selected Purposes/Rationales*

5. The client will maintain maximum physical mobility within prescribed activity and weight-bearing restrictions.	5.a. Refer to Standardized Postoperative Care Plan, Nursing Diagnosis 11 (p. 112), for measures to increase client's mobility.
	  b. Implement additional measures *to increase client's mobility:*
	   1. perform actions to reduce pain (see Postoperative Nursing Diagnosis 2)
	   2. instruct client in and assist with quadriceps- and gluteal-setting exercises *to strengthen muscles needed for ambulation*
	   3. encourage client to use overhead trapeze to move self *in order to strengthen arm and shoulder muscles needed for proper use of ambulatory aids*
	   4. reinforce physical therapist's instructions regarding additional muscle strengthening exercises, transfer and ambulation techniques, and use of ambulatory aids
	   5. perform actions to prevent falls (see Postoperative Nursing Diagnosis 7, actions a and b) *to decrease client's fear of injury*
	   6. assist client with ambulation as soon as allowed (usually by the 2nd postoperative day).
	  c. Consult physician if client is unable to achieve expected level of mobility.

6. NURSING DIAGNOSIS: **Risk for infection: operative hip**

related to:
a. introduction of pathogens into the wound during or after surgery;
b. hematoma formation (increases the likelihood of infection by providing a good medium for growth of pathogens and compromising blood flow to the area);
c. increased susceptibility to infection associated with decreased effectiveness of immune system if client is elderly and immunosuppression if client has been taking corticosteroids to treat the joint disorder necessitating the surgery (e.g. rheumatoid arthritis).

Desired Outcome	Nursing Actions and *Selected Purposes/Rationales*

6. The client will remain free of infection in the operative hip (see Standardized Postoperative Care Plan, Nursing Diagnosis 16, outcome b [pp. 116–117], for outcome criteria).	6.a. Assess for and report the following:
	   1. continuous drainage of fluid from incision (*may be indicative of a sinus tract*)
	   2. sloughing or necrosis of skin in the operative area
	   3. signs and symptoms of wound infection (e.g. chills; fever; redness, heat, and swelling of wound area; unusual wound drainage; foul odor from wound area; persistent or increased pain in operative hip; elevated sedimentation rate).

Desired Outcome	Nursing Actions and *Selected Purposes/Rationales*

b. Refer to Standardized Postoperative Care Plan, Nursing Diagnosis 16, actions b.4 and 5 (pp. 116–117), for measures related to prevention and treatment of wound infection.

c. Implement additional measures *to reduce risk for infection in the operative hip:*
   1. use strict sterile technique when performing wound care and emptying wound drainage device
   2. maintain patency of wound drainage system *in order to reduce risk of hematoma formation*
   3. do not administer injections in operative extremity
   4. avoid urinary catheterization but if it becomes necessary, take precautions to prevent urinary tract infection (e.g. use strict sterile technique during catheter insertion, remove catheter as soon as possible); *the presence of a urinary catheter increases the risk for a urinary tract infection, which can lead to lymphatic or hematogenous seeding of the hip wound*
   5. administer prophylactic antimicrobials if ordered (they are usually started before surgery and continued for at least 24 hours after surgery)
   6. prepare client for drainage of hematoma or grafting of any area of tissue sloughing or necrosis if planned.

d. If signs and symptoms of wound infection occur, prepare client for wound irrigation, surgical debridement, and/or removal of prostheses if planned.

---

7. NURSING DIAGNOSIS: **Risk for trauma: falls**

related to:
a. weakness, fatigue, and postural hypotension associated with the effects of major surgery and physiological changes that may have occurred if client is elderly;
b. central nervous system depressant effect of some medications (e.g. narcotic [opioid] analgesics, central-acting muscle relaxants);
c. weakness and pain in weight-bearing extremity associated with surgery on the hip;
d. difficulty with transfer and ambulation techniques.

Desired Outcome	Nursing Actions and *Selected Purposes/Rationales*
7. The client will not experience falls.	7.a. Refer to Standardized Postoperative Care Plan, Nursing Diagnosis 17, action a (p. 118), for measures to prevent falls.

   b. Implement additional measures *to reduce risk of falls:*
   1. reinforce preoperative instructions about and assist client with exercises to improve muscle strength, transfer and ambulation techniques, and use of ambulatory aids
   2. administer prescribed analgesics before exercise and ambulation sessions *in order to reduce hip pain and subsequently maximize client's ability to utilize proper transfer and ambulation techniques*
   3. perform actions to improve activity tolerance (see Nursing Diagnosis 4) *in order to reduce fatigue and weakness.*

   c. Include client and significant others in planning and implementing measures to prevent falls.

   d. If falls occur, initiate first aid measures if appropriate and notify physician.

8. COLLABORATIVE DIAGNOSES:

Potential complications of total hip replacement:

a. **hemorrhage and/or hematoma formation** related to surgical trauma to blood vessels (the hip is a very vascular area) and use of anticoagulants or antiplatelet agents before and after surgery;

b. **dislocation of hip prosthesis(es)** related to weakness of the hip muscles, improper positioning of the operative extremity, and/or noncompliance with weight-bearing limitations;

c. **thromboembolism** related to:
   1. trauma to vein walls during surgery
   2. venous stasis associated with decreased mobility, increased blood viscosity (can result from fluid volume deficit), and pressure exerted on veins by balanced suspension device or abductor wedge
   3. hypercoagulability associated with increased release of tissue thromboplastin into the blood (occurs as a result of surgical trauma) and hemoconcentration and increased blood viscosity (can occur as a result of fluid volume deficit).

Desired Outcomes

Nursing Actions and *Selected Purposes/Rationales*

8.a. The client will not experience hemorrhage or hematoma formation as evidenced by:
1. expected amount of wound drainage
2. no further decrease in RBC, Hct, and Hb
3. no significant increase in hip pain
4. absence of tense swelling in surgical area.

8.a.1. Assess for and report the following:
   a. excessive wound drainage (expected loss is 200–500 ml in the first 24 hours, diminishing to 30 ml/shift by 48 hours after surgery)
   b. significant decrease in RBC, Hct, and Hb levels
   c. signs and symptoms of hematoma formation (e.g. increased pain and tense swelling in buttock and/or thigh).
2. Implement measures *to reduce operative site bleeding and/or prevent hematoma formation:*
   a. maintain pressure dressing over operative site as ordered
   b. keep trochanter roll or sandbag placed firmly against operative site for the first 24–48 hours after surgery *to provide additional pressure on surgical site*
   c. apply ice pack to operative hip if ordered
   d. maintain patency of wound drainage system if present.
3. If signs and symptoms of excessive bleeding or hematoma formation occur, prepare client for return to surgery to ligate bleeding vessels and/or drain hematoma if planned.

8.b. The client will not experience dislocation of the hip prosthesis(es) as evidenced by:
1. continued resolution of hip pain
2. ability to maintain operative leg in proper alignment
3. ability to adhere to expected exercise and ambulation regimen
4. usual length of operative extremity
5. normal neurovascular status in operative leg.

8.b.1. Assess for and report signs and symptoms of dislocation of the hip prosthesis(es):
   a. sudden, severe hip pain followed by continued pain and muscle spasms during hip movement
   b. abnormal rotation of operative leg
   c. inability to move or bear weight on operative leg
   d. shortening of operative leg
   e. decline in neurovascular status in operative leg.
2. Implement measures *to prevent dislocation of the prosthesis(es):*
   a. maintain bed rest as ordered (may be on bed rest for first 24 hours after surgery)
   b. perform actions *to prevent adduction of the operative extremity:*
      1. maintain extremity in abducted position using balanced suspension device, an abduction wedge, or 2–3 pillows between legs
      2. remind client to avoid crossing legs
      3. do not move operative extremity past midline
      4. turn client only as ordered and always with pillows between legs
   c. maintain operative extremity in proper alignment
   d. instruct client to avoid extreme internal and external rotation of operative leg
   e. maintain restrictions on head of bed elevation if ordered (some physicians order a 45–60° maximum for first 2–3 days after surgery) *to reduce hip flexion*

Desired Outcomes	Nursing Actions and *Selected Purposes/Rationales*

      f. perform actions *to prevent extreme (beyond 90°) hip flexion:*

          1. instruct client not to lean forward to reach objects on end of bed or on floor or to put on slippers, socks, or shoes

          2. raise the entire bed to client's midthigh level before he/she gets in or out of bed *in order to reduce the degree of hip flexion that occurs when client sits on edge of bed*

          3. provide a high, firm chair (or elevate sitting surface with pillows) and an elevated toilet seat for client's use *in order to reduce degree of hip flexion when client sits down*

          4. do not elevate operative leg when client is sitting in chair

      g. reinforce importance of adhering to recommended weight-bearing restrictions (the amount of weight-bearing allowed is based on the type of prostheses inserted; with cemented prostheses, partial weight-bearing is usually allowed as soon as ambulation is started)

      h. instruct and assist client to pivot and bear weight on the unoperative leg when transferring from bed to chair and raising self out of chair.

    3. If signs and symptoms of dislocation of the prosthesis(es) occur:

      a. maintain client on bed rest

      b. prepare client for x-rays of the surgical area

      c. prepare client for closed reduction (e.g. traction) or surgical relocation of the prosthesis(es) if planned

      d. provide emotional support to client and significant others.

Desired Outcomes	Nursing Actions and *Selected Purposes/Rationales*

8.c. The client will not develop a deep vein thrombus or pulmonary embolism (see Standardized Postoperative Care Plan, Collaborative Diagnosis 19, outcomes c.1 and 2 [pp. 120–121], for outcome criteria).	8.c.1. Refer to Standardized Postoperative Care Plan, Collaborative Diagnosis 19, actions c.1 and 2 (pp. 120–121), for measures related to assessment, prevention, and treatment of a deep vein thrombus and pulmonary embolism.
	2. Implement additional measures *to prevent thrombus formation:*
	  a. assist client with exercises and ambulation as allowed
	  b. promote active foot and leg exercises by having client rock in a rocking chair once activity is progressed
	  c. perform actions *to reduce risk of compromising venous return:*
	    1. make sure elastic wraps or stockings are not too tight
	    2. make sure that balanced suspension device and elastic wraps or stockings are not exerting pressure on popliteal space
	    3. avoid use of knee gatch or pillows under knees
	    4. discourage prolonged sitting or standing
	    5. make sure that straps on abductor wedge do not exert excessive pressure on any area
	  d. administer anticoagulants (e.g. low-dose warfarin, low-molecular-weight heparin) or antiplatelet agents (e.g. low-dose aspirin) as ordered.

Discharge Teaching

9. NURSING DIAGNOSIS:	**Knowledge deficit, Ineffective management of therapeutic regimen, or Altered health maintenance***

    *The nurse should select the diagnostic label that is most appropriate for the client's discharge teaching needs.

Desired Outcomes	Nursing Actions and *Selected Purposes/Rationales*
9.a. The client will demonstrate correct transfer and ambulation techniques and proper use of ambulatory aids.	9.a.1. Reinforce instructions about correct transfer and ambulation techniques and proper use of walker, quad cane, or crutches. 2. Reinforce physician's instructions about amount of weight-bearing on operative extremity. 3. Allow time for questions, clarification, and practice of transfer and ambulation techniques.

9.b. The client will demonstrate the ability to correctly perform the prescribed exercises.

9.b.1. Reinforce the physical therapist's instructions on prescribed exercises and the importance of continuing the exercises for the prescribed length of time.
2. Inform client that walking and swimming are good aerobic exercises.
3. Allow time for questions, clarification, and return demonstration of prescribed exercises.

9.c. The client will verbalize an understanding of activity and position restrictions necessary to prevent dislocation of the hip prostheses.

9.c. Instruct client to adhere to the following activity and position restrictions in order to prevent dislocation of the hip prostheses (length of time the restrictions are necessary varies but ranges from 2–6 months):
1. turn only as directed by physician (many physicians allow client to turn to unoperative side only)
2. instruct client to keep pillow between legs when lying on back or side and when turning
3. never cross legs
4. do not sit on low chairs, stools, or toilets; place a cushion on low chairs, rent or purchase an elevated toilet seat for home use, and use the high toilets designated for the handicapped when in public facilities
5. do not elevate operative leg higher than hip when sitting
6. sit in chairs with arms and use the arms to raise self off chair
7. support weight on unoperative leg when raising self from a sitting position
8. use assistive devices (e.g. long-handled shoe horn, long-handled grabber) to assist with activities that require flexing hip beyond 90° (e.g. putting on shoes and socks, reaching objects on the floor or in low cupboards or drawers, pulling bed covers up from end of bed)
9. keep operative leg in proper alignment and avoid extreme internal and external rotation of leg
10. when riding in a car:
    a. sit on a firm pillow or cushion to prevent hip flexion of more than 90°
    b. keep operative leg extended (a sudden impact of the knee against the dashboard can dislodge the prostheses)
11. do not resume sexual activity until approved by physician (usually about 6 weeks postoperatively)
12. when sexual activity is resumed, avoid positions that involve extreme rotation of the operative leg, flexing hip beyond 90°, and moving operative leg past the midline
13. avoid lifting heavy objects, excessive twisting and turning of body, and activities that place excessive strain on hip (e.g. jogging, jumping).

9.d. The client will identify ways to reduce the risk of falls in the home environment.

9.d. Provide the following instructions on ways to reduce the risk of falls at home:
1. keep electrical cords out of pathways
2. remove unnecessary furniture and provide wide pathways for ambulation
3. remove scatter rugs
4. provide adequate lighting at all times
5. avoid unnecessary stair climbing.

9.e. The client will state signs and symptoms to report to the health care provider.

9.e.1. Refer to Standardized Postoperative Care Plan, Nursing Diagnosis 21, action c (p. 123), for signs and symptoms to report to the health care provider.
2. Instruct client to report these additional signs and symptoms:
   a. persistent or increased pain or spasms in operative extremity
   b. loss of sensation or movement in operative extremity
   c. inability to bear weight on operative extremity
   d. inability to maintain operative extremity in a neutral position
   e. shortening of operative extremity (will probably be noticed as a limp).

9.f. The client will identify community resources that can assist with home management and provide transportation.

9.f.1. Provide information about community resources that can assist the client and significant others with home management and provide transportation (e.g. home health agencies, Meals on Wheels, church groups, transportation services).
2. Initiate a referral if indicated.

Desired Outcomes	Nursing Actions and *Selected Purposes/Rationales*
9.g. The client will verbalize an understanding of and a plan for adhering to recommended follow-up care including future appointments with health care provider and physical therapist, medications prescribed, activity level, and wound care.	9.g.1. Refer to Standardized Postoperative Care Plan, Nursing Diagnosis 21 (pp. 123–124), for routine postoperative instructions and measures to improve client compliance. 2. Reinforce importance of keeping appointments with physical therapist. 3. Teach client the rationale for, side effects of, schedule for taking, and importance of taking medications prescribed (e.g. iron supplements). Inform client of pertinent food and drug interactions. 4. Instruct client to inform other health care providers of history of total hip replacement so prophylactic antimicrobials can be started before any dental work, invasive diagnostic procedures, or surgery is performed.

Bibliography

See pages 897–898 and 909–910.

 # TOTAL KNEE REPLACEMENT

A total knee replacement (arthroplasty) is a surgical procedure in which the articular surfaces of the tibia and femur and sometimes the patella are replaced with prosthetic devices. It is performed to relieve joint pain that has not been controlled by conservative management and/or improve joint mobility in persons with severe arthritis, congenital knee deformity, hemophilic arthropathy, or severe intra-articular injury.

There are a variety of prostheses available. Most prostheses have a metal femoral component, a metal-backed polyethylene tibial component, and a polyethylene patellar component (the patella is not always replaced). Prostheses may be fully constrained (hinge prosthesis), semi-constrained, or unconstrained (unlinked). Unconstrained prostheses are the type most frequently used. They have separate femoral, tibial, and patellar components, which causes the greatest portion of the load (weight supported) to be absorbed by the surrounding capsule and ligaments as occurs in a normal knee. Fixation of the prostheses is accomplished by using a cement-like agent called polymethylmethacrylate or, if left uncemented, by bone ingrowth into the porous outer surface on the prostheses.

This care plan focuses on the adult client hospitalized for a total knee replacement. Preoperative goals of care are to reduce fear and anxiety and educate the client regarding ways to prevent postoperative complications and facilitate rehabilitation. Postoperatively, the goals of care are to maintain comfort, prevent complications, assist the client to regain maximum mobility, and educate the client regarding follow-up care. Prevention of infection is of major importance in caring for the client who has had a total knee replacement since infection of the operative knee usually necessitates surgical debridement and/or removal of the prosthesis(es).

DIAGNOSTIC TESTS

X-rays of the knee
Magnetic resonance imaging (MRI)

DISCHARGE CRITERIA

Prior to discharge, the client will:

- have evidence of normal healing of the surgical wound
- have clear, audible breath sounds throughout lungs
- have reduced knee pain
- have expected degree of mobility of knee joint
- have no signs and symptoms of infection or postoperative complications
- demonstrate correct transfer and ambulation techniques and proper use of ambulatory aids
- demonstrate the ability to correctly perform the prescribed exercises
- identify ways to reduce the risk of loosening of the prosthesis(es)

- identify ways to reduce the risk of falls in the home environment
- state signs and symptoms to report to the health care provider
- identify community resources that can assist with home management and provide transportation
- verbalize an understanding of and a plan for adhering to recommended follow-up care including future appointments with health care provider and physical therapist, medications prescribed, activity level, and wound care.

NURSING/ COLLABORATIVE DIAGNOSES	**Preoperative**
	1. Knowledge deficit △ 793
	Postoperative
	1. Risk for peripheral neurovascular dysfunction: operative extremity △ 794
	2. Pain: knee △ 795
	3. Actual/Risk for impaired tissue integrity △ 796
	4. Impaired physical mobility △ 797
	5. Risk for infection: operative knee △ 798
	6. Risk for trauma: falls △ 798
	7. Potential complications:
	a. dislocation of knee prosthesis(es) or stress fracture of tibia or femur
	b. thromboembolism △ 799
DISCHARGE TEACHING	**8.** Knowledge deficit, Ineffective management of therapeutic regimen, or Altered health maintenance △ 800

See Standardized Preoperative and Postoperative Care Plans for additional diagnoses.

PREOPERATIVE

Use in conjunction with the Standardized Preoperative Care Plan.

Client Teaching

1. NURSING DIAGNOSIS:

Knowledge deficit

regarding the surgical procedure, hospital routines associated with surgery, physical preparation for total knee replacement, sensations that normally occur following surgery and anesthesia, and postoperative care.

Desired Outcomes	Nursing Actions and *Selected Purposes/Rationales*
1.a. The client will verbalize an understanding of the surgical procedure, preoperative care, and postoperative sensations and care.	1.a.1. Refer to Standardized Preoperative Care Plan, Nursing Diagnosis 4, actions a.1–4 (pp. 99–100), for information to include in preoperative teaching. 2. Provide additional information about specific preoperative care for clients having a total knee replacement: a. explain that the following measures will be performed to reduce the risk of a postoperative knee infection: 1. the operative leg will be scrubbed with an antiseptic solution (e.g. povidone-iodine) before surgery 2. existing infections will be treated before surgery; instruct client to report any symptoms of infection (e.g. cough, runny nose, burning on urination) 3. antimicrobials will probably be administered prophylactically before and after surgery

Desired Outcomes	Nursing Actions and *Selected Purposes/Rationales*
	b. explain that anticoagulants (e.g. heparin, warfarin) and/or antiplatelet agents (e.g. low-molecular-weight dextran, low-dose aspirin) may be administered before surgery to reduce the risk of postoperative thrombus formation; inform client that coagulation studies are usually done before starting these medications, especially if he/she has been taking aspirin or other nonsteroidal anti-inflammatory agents (e.g. ibuprofen) c. explain that a physical therapist will fit crutches or walker and provide instructions on postoperative physical therapy regimen. 3. Allow time for questions and clarification of information provided.

1.b. The client will demonstrate the ability to perform activities designed to prevent postoperative complications.	1.b.1. Refer to Standardized Preoperative Care Plan, Nursing Diagnosis 4, action b.1 (p. 100), for instructions on ways to prevent postoperative complications.
	2. Provide additional instructions about ways to prevent complications following total knee replacement:
	  a. reinforce physician's or physical therapist's instructions on:
	    1. exercises to improve strength and facilitate mobility:
	      a. quadriceps- and gluteal-setting
	      b. upper extremity strengthening
	      c. knee flexion
	      d. sling-assisted and independent straight leg raising
	    2. transfer and ambulation techniques and proper use of ambulatory aids; weight-bearing limitations are determined by the physician and vary depending on the type of prostheses inserted (usually partial weight-bearing is allowed initially with progressive weight-bearing as tolerated)
	  b. instruct client in the correct way to use overhead trapeze and unoperative leg to move self
	  c. inform client that he/she will need to avoid extreme flexion of the knee for first few weeks after surgery in order to prevent dislocation of the prosthesis(es)
	  d. explain the purpose for the continuous passive motion (CPM) machine and the need to leave the extremity in the machine as ordered
	  e. describe or show client knee immobilizer and explain purpose for wearing immobilizer.
	3. Allow time for questions, clarification, and return demonstration.

POSTOPERATIVE

Use in conjunction with the Standardized Postoperative Care Plan.

■————————————————————————————————

1. NURSING DIAGNOSIS:

Risk for peripheral neurovascular dysfunction: operative extremity

related to trauma to or excessive pressure on the nerves or blood vessels associated with surgery; blood accumulation and edema in the surgical area; improper alignment of operative extremity; pressure exerted by the dressing, knee immobilizer, or CPM machine; or dislocation of the prosthesis(es).

Desired Outcome	Nursing Actions and *Selected Purposes/Rationales*

1. The client will maintain normal neurovascular function in the operative extremity as evidenced by:	1.a. Assess for and report signs and symptoms of neurovascular dysfunction in the operative extremity:
	  1. diminished or absent pedal pulses
	  2. capillary refill time in toes greater than 3 seconds

a. palpable pedal pulses
b. capillary refill time in toes less than 3 seconds
c. extremity warm and usual color
d. ability to flex and extend foot and toes
e. absence of numbness and tingling in foot and toes
f. absence of foot pain during passive movement of toes and foot
g. no increase in pain in extremity.

3. pallor, cyanosis, or coolness of the extremity
4. inability to flex or extend foot or toes
5. numbness or tingling in foot or toes
6. pain in foot during passive motion of toes or foot
7. increased pain in extremity.

b. Implement measures *to prevent neurovascular dysfunction in the operative extremity:*
   1. apply ice packs to operative knee for the first 24–48 hours after surgery if ordered *to reduce bleeding and edema in surgical area*
   2. maintain patency of wound drainage system (e.g. prevent kinking of tubing, empty collection device as needed, keep collection device below wound level, maintain suction as ordered) *to reduce accumulation of fluid in the surgical area*
   3. maintain extremity in proper alignment
   4. position leg so that knee immobilizer and CPM machine are not causing excessive pressure on any area
   5. loosen straps of knee immobilizer if it appears to be too tight
   6. notify physician if dressing appears to be too tight
   7. perform actions to prevent dislocation of the prosthesis(es) and stress fracture of the tibia and femur (see Postoperative Collaborative Diagnosis 7, action a.2).

c. If signs and symptoms of neurovascular dysfunction occur:
   1. assess for and correct causes of excessive pressure
   2. notify physician if the signs and symptoms persist
   3. prepare client for closed reduction or surgical intervention (e.g. realignment of the prosthesis) if planned.

---

2. NURSING DIAGNOSIS: **Pain: knee**

related to tissue trauma and reflex muscle spasms associated with the surgery, blood accumulation and edema in the surgical area, and improper positioning of the operative extremity.

Desired Outcome	Nursing Actions and *Selected Purposes/Rationales*

2. The client will experience diminished knee pain (see Standardized Postoperative Care Plan, Nursing Diagnosis 6 [pp. 106–107], for outcome criteria).	2.a. Refer to Standardized Postoperative Care Plan, Nursing Diagnosis 6 (pp. 106–107), for measures related to assessment and reduction of pain.
	b. Implement additional measures *to reduce pain:*
	  1. maintain operative extremity in proper alignment
	  2. move the operative extremity carefully
	  3. apply ice packs to the operative knee for first 24–48 hours after surgery if ordered *to reduce bleeding and edema in the surgical area*
	  4. maintain patency of the wound drainage system if present *to prevent accumulation of fluid in the surgical area*
	  5. remind client to avoid flexing operative knee beyond prescribed limits
	  6. ensure that knee immobilizer is worn as prescribed *in order to prevent strain on the operative area*
	  7. maintain proper placement and function of transcutaneous electrical nerve stimulator (TENS) if ordered
	  8. administer prescribed analgesics before exercise and ambulation sessions
	  9. apply ice packs to operative knee for 20–30 minutes before and after exercise and ambulation sessions as ordered.

3. NURSING DIAGNOSIS: **Actual/Risk for impaired tissue integrity**

related to:
a. disruption of tissue associated with the surgical procedure;
b. delayed wound healing associated with factors such as decreased nutritional status and inadequate blood supply to wound area;
c. irritation of skin associated with contact with wound drainage, pressure from tubes, and use of tape;
d. excessive or prolonged pressure on tissues from compression dressing, knee immobilizer, or CPM machine;
e. damage to the skin and/or subcutaneous tissue associated with prolonged pressure on tissues, friction, and shearing while mobility is decreased.

Desired Outcomes	Nursing Actions and *Selected Purposes/Rationales*

3.a. The client will experience normal healing of the surgical wound (see Standardized Postoperative Care Plan, Nursing Diagnosis 9, outcome a [pp. 109–110], for outcome criteria).

3.b. The client will maintain tissue integrity as evidenced by:
1. absence of redness and irritation
2. no skin breakdown.

3.a. Refer to Standardized Postoperative Care Plan, Nursing Diagnosis 9, action a (pp. 109–110), for measures related to assessment and promotion of wound healing.

3.b.1. Inspect the following areas for pallor, redness, and breakdown:
a. skin in contact with wound drainage, tape, and tubings
b. back, coccyx, and buttocks
c. elbows and heels
d. areas at edges of compression dressing or knee immobilizer
e. areas in contact with CPM machine.
2. Refer to Standardized Postoperative Care Plan, Nursing Diagnosis 9, action b.2 (p. 110–111), for measures related to prevention of tissue irritation and breakdown in areas in contact with wound drainage, tubings, and tape.
3. Implement measures *to prevent tissue breakdown associated with decreased mobility:*
a. position client properly; use pressure-reducing or pressure-relieving devices (e.g. pillows, alternating pressure mattress) if indicated
b. instruct client to use overhead trapeze to lift self and shift weight at least every 30 minutes
c. gently massage around reddened areas at least every 2 hours
d. apply a thin layer of powder or cornstarch to bottom sheet or skin and to opposing skin surfaces (e.g. axillae) if indicated *to absorb moisture and reduce friction*
e. lift and move client carefully using a turn sheet and adequate assistance
f. limit length of time client is in semi-Fowler's position to 30 minutes (*in this position, client tends to slide down in bed, which can cause skin surface abrasion and shearing*)
g. if turning is allowed (some physicians may not allow turning for first 48 hours), turn client every 2 hours keeping pillows between legs and operative knee extended
h. keep skin lubricated, clean, and dry
i. keep bed linens dry and wrinkle-free
j. increase activity as allowed and tolerated.
4. Implement measures *to prevent irritation and breakdown on elbows and heels:*
a. massage elbows and heels with lotion frequently
b. encourage client to use overhead trapeze to move self rather than pushing up with heel and elbows
c. provide elbow and heel protectors if indicated.

5. Implement measures *to prevent tissue breakdown in areas in contact with the compression dressing, knee immobilizer, and CPM machine:*
   a. assess for and report tightness of the dressing or reports of a burning sensation under the dressing or knee immobilizer
   b. loosen straps on knee immobilizer if it appears to be too tight
   c. apply cornstarch to skin under immobilizer *in order to keep skin dry and reduce friction and subsequent skin irritation*
   d. keep dressing dry
   e. position the operative extremity so that the knee immobilizer and CPM machine are not causing excessive pressure on any area
   f. make sure CPM machine is padded adequately
   g. instruct client to refrain from inserting anything inside the dressing or knee immobilizer.
6. If tissue breakdown occurs:
   a. notify physician
   b. continue with above measures to prevent further irritation and breakdown
   c. perform care of involved areas as ordered or per standard hospital procedure
   d. assess client closely and report signs and symptoms of infection (e.g. elevated temperature; redness, heat, pain, and swelling around area of breakdown; unusual drainage from site; foul odor from dressing).

---

4. NURSING DIAGNOSIS: **Impaired physical mobility**

related to:
a. pain and weakness in weight-bearing extremity associated with surgery on the knee;
b. prescribed activity and weight-bearing restrictions following total knee replacement;
c. generalized weakness associated with surgery;
d. depressant effect of anesthesia and some medications (e.g. narcotic [opioid] analgesics, central-acting muscle relaxants);
e. fear of falling, dislocating prostheses, and compromising surgical wound.

Desired Outcome	Nursing Actions and *Selected Purposes/Rationales*
4. The client will maintain maximum physical mobility within prescribed activity and weight-bearing restrictions.	4.a. Refer to Standardized Postoperative Care Plan, Nursing Diagnosis 11 (p. 112), for measures to increase client's mobility. b. Implement additional measures *to increase client's mobility:* 1. perform actions to reduce pain (see Postoperative Nursing Diagnosis 2) 2. maintain prescribed degree of flexion and extension on CPM machine and encourage client to keep operative leg in CPM machine for the prescribed length of time *in order to improve range of motion and prevent stiffening of the knee* 3. encourage client to perform quadriceps- and gluteal-setting, straight leg raising, and knee flexion-extension exercises as soon as allowed (usually started by the 2nd postoperative day) 4. encourage client to use overhead trapeze to move self *in order to strengthen arm and shoulder muscles needed for proper use of ambulatory aids* 5. reinforce physical therapist's instructions regarding transfer and ambulation techniques and use of ambulatory aids (e.g. crutches, walker) 6. perform actions to prevent falls (see Postoperative Nursing Diagnosis 6, actions a and b) *in order to decrease client's fear of injury*

Desired Outcome	Nursing Actions and **Selected Purposes/Rationales**

7. assist client with ambulation as soon as allowed (usually by the 2nd postoperative day).
   c. Consult physician if client is unable to make expected progress with knee flexion or if any other joint motion becomes restricted.

---

5. NURSING DIAGNOSIS:

Risk for infection: operative knee

related to:
a. introduction of pathogens into the wound during or following surgery;
b. increased susceptibility to infection associated with decreased effectiveness of immune system if client is elderly and immunosuppression if client has been taking corticosteroids to treat the joint disorder necessitating the surgery (e.g. rheumatoid arthritis).

Desired Outcome	Nursing Actions and **Selected Purposes/Rationales**

5. The client will remain free of infection in the operative knee (see Standardized Postoperative Care Plan, Nursing Diagnosis 16, outcome b [pp. 116–117], for outcome criteria).

5.a. Assess for and report the following:
   1. continuous drainage of fluid from incision (*may indicate a sinus tract*)
   2. sloughing or necrosis of skin in operative area
   3. signs and symptoms of wound infection (e.g. chills; fever; redness, heat, and swelling of wound area; unusual wound drainage; foul odor from wound area; persistent or increased pain in knee; elevated sedimentation rate).
   b. Refer to Standardized Postoperative Care Plan, Nursing Diagnosis 16, actions b.4 and 5 (pp. 116–117), for measures related to prevention and treatment of wound infection.
   c. Implement additional measures *to reduce risk for infection in the operative knee:*
      1. use strict sterile technique when performing wound care and emptying wound drainage device
      2. maintain patency of the wound drainage device *in order to prevent accumulation of drainage in surgical area*
      3. keep CPM machine off the floor when not in use
      4. avoid urinary catheterization but if it becomes necessary, take precautions to prevent urinary tract infection (e.g. use strict sterile technique during catheter insertion, remove catheter as soon as possible); *the presence of a urinary catheter increases the risk for a urinary tract infection, which can lead to lymphatic or hematogenous seeding of the knee wound*
      5. administer prophylactic antimicrobials if ordered (they are usually started before surgery and continued for 2–5 days after surgery).
   d. If signs and symptoms of wound infection occur, prepare client for wound irrigation, surgical debridement, and/or removal of prostheses if planned.

---

6. NURSING DIAGNOSIS:

Risk for trauma: falls

related to:
a. weakness, fatigue, and postural hypotension associated with the effects of major surgery and physiological changes that may have occurred if client is elderly;
b. central nervous system depressant effect of some medications (e.g. narcotic [opioid] analgesics, central-acting muscle relaxants);

c. weakness and pain in weight-bearing extremity associated with surgery on the knee;
d. improper transfer and ambulation techniques.

Desired Outcome	Nursing Actions and *Selected Purposes/Rationales*

6. The client will not experience falls.	6.a. Refer to Standardized Postoperative Care Plan, Nursing Diagnosis 17, action a (p. 118), for measures to prevent falls.
	b. Implement additional measures *to reduce the risk for falls:*
	    1. reinforce preoperative instructions about and assist client with transfer and ambulation techniques, use of ambulatory aids, and exercises to improve muscle strength
	    2. administer prescribed analgesics and/or apply ice packs to operative knee before exercise and ambulation sessions *in order to reduce knee pain and subsequently maximize the client's ability to use proper transfer and ambulation techniques*
	    3. ensure that client has knee immobilizer on for ambulation sessions *to provide additional support of operative leg.*
	c. Include client and significant others in planning and implementing measures to prevent falls.
	d. If falls occur, initiate first aid measures if appropriate and notify physician.

---

7. **COLLABORATIVE DIAGNOSES:**

Potential complications of total knee replacement:

a. **dislocation of knee prosthesis(es) or stress fracture of tibia or femur** related to rotation of or excessive pressure on the knee;
b. **thromboembolism** related to:
    1. trauma to vein walls during surgery
    2. venous stasis associated with use of a tourniquet on operative leg during surgery; pressure exerted on the veins by the dressing, knee immobilizer, or CPM machine; decreased mobility; and increased blood viscosity (can result from fluid volume deficit)
    3. hypercoagulability associated with increased release of tissue thromboplastin into the blood (occurs as a result of surgical trauma) and hemoconcentration and increased blood viscosity (can occur as a result of fluid volume deficit).

Desired Outcomes	Nursing Actions and *Selected Purposes/Rationales*

7.a. The client will not experience dislocation of the knee prosthesis(es) or stress fracture of tibia or femur as evidenced by:
1. continued resolution of knee pain
2. ability to maintain operative leg in proper alignment
3. ability to adhere to planned exercise and ambulation regimen
4. normal neurovascular status in operative leg.
	7.a.1. Assess for and report signs and symptoms of dislocation of the knee prosthesis(es) and/or stress fracture of tibia or femur:
	    a. sudden, severe knee pain followed by continued pain and muscle spasms during knee movement
	    b. abnormal rotation of the lower portion of operative leg
	    c. inability to move or bear weight on operative leg
	    d. decline in neurovascular status in operative leg.
	  2. Implement measures *to prevent dislocation of the prosthesis(es) and stress fracture of the tibia and femur:*
	    a. instruct client to avoid hyperextension, rotation, and acute flexion of knee
	    b. reinforce physician's instructions regarding the amount of weight-bearing allowed (usual order is partial weight-bearing initially with progressive weight-bearing as tolerated)
	    c. reinforce instructions and assist client with gait training and proper use of ambulatory aids

Desired Outcomes	Nursing Actions and *Selected Purposes/Rationales*
	d. reinforce the importance of wearing knee immobilizer when ambulating.
	3. If signs and symptoms of prosthesis(es) dislocation or stress fracture occur:
	a. maintain client on bed rest
	b. prepare client for x-rays of operative leg
	c. prepare client for closed reduction or surgical intervention (e.g. realignment of prosthesis, internal fixation of fracture) if planned
	d. provide emotional support to client and significant others.
7.b. The client will not develop a deep vein thrombus or pulmonary embolism (see Standardized Postoperative Care Plan, Collaborative Diagnosis 19, outcomes c.1 and 2 [pp. 120–121], for outcome criteria).	7.b.1. Refer to Standardized Postoperative Care Plan, Collaborative Diagnosis 19, actions c.1 and 2 (pp. 120–121), for measures related to assessment, prevention, and treatment of a deep vein thrombus and pulmonary embolism.
	2. Implement additional measures *to prevent thrombus formation:*
	a. perform actions *to improve venous return:*
	1. maintain continuous passive motion of extremity if ordered
	2. assist client to perform leg exercises and ambulate as soon as allowed
	3. implement measures *to reduce risk of compromising venous return:*
	a. consult physician if dressing appears to be too tight
	b. loosen knee immobilizer if it appears to be too tight
	c. make sure exercise sling is not exerting pressure on the popliteal space
	d. avoid use of the knee gatch or pillows under knees
	e. discourage prolonged sitting or standing
	b. administer anticoagulants (e.g. low-dose warfarin, low-molecular-weight heparin) or antiplatelet agents (e.g. low-dose aspirin) as ordered.

Discharge Teaching

---

8. NURSING DIAGNOSIS: **Knowledge deficit, Ineffective management of therapeutic regimen, or Altered health maintenance***

---

*The nurse should select the diagnostic label that is most appropriate for the client's discharge teaching needs.

Desired Outcomes	Nursing Actions and *Selected Purposes/Rationales*
8.a. The client will demonstrate correct transfer and ambulation techniques and proper use of ambulatory aids.	8.a.1. Reinforce instructions about correct transfer and ambulation techniques and proper use of crutches, cane, or walker.
	2. Reinforce the importance of adhering to weight-bearing restrictions if prescribed.
	3. Allow time for questions, clarification, and practice of transfer and ambulation techniques.
8.b. The client will demonstrate the ability to correctly perform the prescribed exercises.	8.b.1. Reinforce the physical therapist's instructions about prescribed exercises.
	2. Reinforce the importance of continuing exercises for the prescribed length of time.
	3. Allow time for questions, clarification, and return demonstration of prescribed exercises.
8.c. The client will identify ways to reduce the risk of loosening of the prosthesis(es).	8.c.1. Inform client of the possibility of loosening of the prosthesis (usually does not occur until 2–3 years after surgery).
	2. Instruct client to report increasing pain or instability of operative knee (may indicate loosening of the prosthesis).
	3. Instruct client regarding ways to minimize risk of loosening of the prosthesis(es):

a. adhere to weight-bearing restrictions if prescribed
b. avoid unusual twisting of knee
c. avoid contact sports
d. do not force knee beyond comfortable degree of flexion and avoid kneeling
e. avoid placing undue stress on knees (e.g. do not lift and carry heavy objects, maintain ideal body weight, avoid activities such as jogging).

8.d. The client will identify ways to reduce the risk of falls in the home environment.

8.d. Provide the following instructions on ways to reduce risk of falls at home:
1. keep electrical cords out of pathways
2. remove unnecessary furniture and provide wide pathways for ambulation
3. remove scatter rugs
4. provide adequate lighting at all times
5. avoid unnecessary stair climbing.

8.e. The client will state signs and symptoms to report to the health care provider.

8.e.1. Refer to Standardized Postoperative Care Plan, Nursing Diagnosis 21, action c (p. 123), for signs and symptoms to report to the health care provider.
2. Instruct client to report these additional signs and symptoms:
a. persistent or increased pain or spasms in operative extremity
b. loss of sensation or movement in operative extremity
c. inability to bear expected amount of weight on operative extremity
d. inability to maintain operative extremity in a neutral position
e. instability of operative extremity (feeling of knee "giving out").

8.f. The client will identify community resources that can assist with home management and provide transportation.

8.f.1. Provide information about community resources that can assist client and significant others with home management and provide transportation (e.g. home health agencies, Meals on Wheels, church groups, transportation services).
2. Initiate a referral if indicated.

8.g. The client will verbalize an understanding of and a plan for adhering to recommended follow-up care including future appointments with health care provider and physical therapist, medications prescribed, activity level, and wound care.

8.g.1. Refer to Standardized Postoperative Care Plan, Nursing Diagnosis 21 (pp. 123–124), for routine postoperative instructions and measures to improve client compliance.
2. Reinforce the importance of keeping appointments with physical therapist.
3. Instruct client to inform other health care providers of history of total knee replacement so prophylactic antimicrobials can be started before any dental work, invasive diagnostic procedures, or surgery is performed.

Bibliography

See pages 897–898 and 910.

UNIT EIGHTEEN

NURSING CARE OF THE CLIENT WITH DISTURBANCES OF THE BREAST AND REPRODUCTIVE SYSTEM

COLPORRHAPHY (ANTERIOR AND POSTERIOR REPAIR)

Colporrhaphy is the surgical tightening of the vagina and repair of incompetent muscles and ligaments of the pelvic floor via an incision in the vaginal wall. An anterior colporrhaphy is performed to correct a cystocele, which is a protrusion or displacement of the bladder through the pubocervical fascia into the vagina and occasionally beyond the introitus. A posterior colporrhaphy is performed to repair a rectocele, which is a protrusion of part of the anterior rectal wall upward into the vagina.

Cystoceles and rectoceles are caused by relaxation of the pelvic musculature and ligaments usually associated with aging and tissue damage during childbirth. Signs and symptoms of a cystocele may include back pain, stress incontinence, urinary urgency and frequency, and a feeling of pelvic pressure. A rectocele is manifested by difficult or incomplete emptying of the rectum, constipation, backache, and a feeling of pelvic pressure. Colporrhaphy is indicated when conservative management (e.g. perineal exercises, insertion of a pessary) no longer controls signs and symptoms.

This care plan focuses on the adult female client hospitalized for an anterior and posterior colporrhaphy. Preoperatively, the goals of care are to reduce fear and anxiety and prepare the client for the surgical experience. The goals of postoperative care are to maintain comfort, prevent complications, and educate the client regarding follow-up care.

DIAGNOSTIC TESTS

Videourodynamic studies
Vaginal examination
Rectal examination
Anorectal physiological studies (if client is experiencing fecal incontinence)

DISCHARGE CRITERIA

Prior to discharge, the client will:

- have evidence of normal healing of surgical wound
- have clear, audible breath sounds throughout lungs
- have adequate urine output
- have surgical pain controlled
- have no signs and symptoms of infection or postoperative complications
- identify ways to decrease the risk of reherniation of the bladder and rectum into the vagina
- identify ways to relieve surgical site discomfort
- state signs and symptoms to report to the health care provider
- verbalize an understanding of and a plan for adhering to recommended follow-up care including future appointments with health care provider, medications prescribed, and limitations on sexual activity.

NURSING/ COLLABORATIVE DIAGNOSES	**Postoperative**
	1. Pain △ 805
	2. Urinary retention △ 805
	3. Constipation △ 806
	4. Risk for infection:
	  a. wound infection
	  b. urinary tract infection △ 806
	5. Potential complications:
	  a. reherniation of the bladder or rectum
	  b. bladder, urethral, or ureteral injury △ 807

DISCHARGE TEACHING	**6.** Knowledge deficit, Ineffective management of therapeutic regimen, or Altered health maintenance △ 808

See Standardized Preoperative and Postoperative Care Plans for additional diagnoses.

PREOPERATIVE   Refer to the Standardized Preoperative Care Plan.

POSTOPERATIVE   Use in conjunction with the Standardized Postoperative Care Plan.

---

1. NURSING DIAGNOSIS: **Pain**

related to tissue trauma and reflex muscle spasms associated with the surgical procedure.

Desired Outcome	Nursing Actions and *Selected Purposes/Rationales*

1. The client will experience diminished pain as evidenced by:
  a. verbalization of a decrease in or absence of pain
  b. relaxed facial expression and body positioning
  c. ability to sit and walk more comfortably
  d. increased participation in activities
  e. stable vital signs.
	1.a. Refer to Standardized Postoperative Care Plan, Nursing Diagnosis 6 (pp. 106–107), for measures related to assessment and management of postoperative pain.
	  b. Implement additional measures *to reduce pain:*
	    1. apply ice packs to the perineal area for the first 24 hours postoperatively if ordered
	    2. instruct client in and assist with sitz baths as ordered
	    3. encourage client to lie flat or in semi-Fowler's position when in bed *in order to minimize pressure on surgical site.*

---

2. NURSING DIAGNOSIS: **Urinary retention**

related to:
a. obstruction of the urethral and/or suprapubic catheter(s);
b. impaired urination following removal of catheter(s) associated with:
    1. edema of the bladder neck and urethra resulting from surgical trauma
    2. increased tone of the urinary sphincters resulting from sympathetic nervous system stimulation (can result from pain, fear, and anxiety)
    3. decreased perception of bladder fullness resulting from the depressant effect of some medications (e.g. narcotic [opioid] analgesics)
    4. relaxation of the bladder muscle resulting from the depressant effect of some medications (e.g. narcotic [opioid] analgesics) and stimulation of the sympathetic nervous system (can result from pain, fear, and anxiety).

Desired Outcome	Nursing Actions and *Selected Purposes/Rationales*

2. The client will not experience urinary retention as evidenced by:
  a. no reports of bladder fullness and suprapubic discomfort
  b. absence of bladder distention
  c. balanced intake and output within 48 hours after surgery
	2.a. Assess for and report the following:
	    1. urinary retention when suprapubic and/or urethral catheter(s) are present (e.g. reports of bladder fullness or suprapubic discomfort, bladder distention, absence of fluid in urinary drainage tubing, output that continues to be less than intake 48 hours after surgery)
	    2. urinary retention following catheter removal (e.g. reports of bladder fullness or suprapubic discomfort, bladder distention, output that continues to be less than intake 48 hours after surgery, frequent voiding of small amounts [25–60 ml] of urine).
	  b. Implement measures *to prevent urinary retention:*
	    1. perform actions *to maintain patency of urinary catheter(s):*

Desired Outcome	Nursing Actions and *Selected Purposes/Rationales*
d. voiding adequate amounts at expected intervals after removal of the catheter(s).	a. keep drainage tubing free of kinks b. keep collection container below level of bladder c. tape catheter tubing securely (suprapubic catheter tubing to abdomen, urethral catheter tubing to thigh) *in order to prevent inadvertent removal* d. irrigate catheter(s) if ordered 2. after urethral catheter is removed, open suprapubic catheter (if one is present) as scheduled and if client is unable to void voluntarily 3. when both urethral and suprapubic catheters have been removed, refer to Standardized Postoperative Care Plan, Nursing Diagnosis 13, actions d and e (pp. 113–114), for measures related to prevention and treatment of urinary retention.

---

3. NURSING DIAGNOSIS: **Constipation**

related to:
a. decreased gastrointestinal motility associated with decreased activity and the depressant effect of the anesthetic and narcotic (opioid) analgesics;
b. reluctance to defecate associated with fear of pain and reherniation of the bladder and rectum;
c. decreased intake of fluids and foods high in fiber.

Desired Outcome	Nursing Actions and *Selected Purposes/Rationales*
3. The client will not experience constipation (see Standardized Postoperative Care Plan, Nursing Diagnosis 14 [p. 114], for outcome criteria).	3.a. Refer to Standardized Postoperative Care Plan, Nursing Diagnosis 14 (pp. 114–115), for measures related to assessment and prevention of constipation. b. Implement additional measures *to prevent constipation:* 1. instruct client to request an analgesic prior to attempting to defecate *in order to ease the surgical site pain associated with the increased intra-abdominal and perineal pressure that occur with defecation* 2. consult physician about an order for a laxative if one has not been prescribed.

---

4. NURSING DIAGNOSIS: **Risk for infection:**

a. **wound infection** related to:
1. wound contamination associated with introduction of pathogens during or following surgery (a high risk with this surgery because of the close proximity of the incisions to the perianal area)
2. decreased resistance to infection (can result if blood flow to wound area is diminished or client has an inadequate nutritional status);
b. **urinary tract infection** related to:
1. increased growth and colonization of microorganisms associated with urinary stasis
2. introduction of pathogens associated with the presence of an indwelling catheter.

Desired Outcomes	Nursing Actions and *Selected Purposes/Rationales*

4.a. The client will remain free of wound infection (see Standardized Postoperative Care Plan, Nursing Diagnosis 16, outcome b [pp. 116–117], for outcome criteria).	4.a.1. Refer to Standardized Postoperative Care Plan, Nursing Diagnosis 16, action b (pp. 116–117), for measures related to assessment, prevention, and management of wound infection.
	2. Implement additional measures *to reduce risk of wound infection:*
	  a. instruct client to wipe from front to back following urination and defecation
	  b. assist client with perineal care every shift and after each bowel movement
	  c. if urethral catheter is present, perform catheter care at least twice a day
	  d. if douches are ordered, use sterile equipment and solution.

4.b. The client will remain free of urinary tract infection (see Standardized Postoperative Care Plan, Nursing Diagnosis 16, outcome c [p. 117], for outcome criteria).	4.b.1. Refer to Standardized Postoperative Care Plan, Nursing Diagnosis 16, action c (p. 117), for measures related to the assessment, prevention, and management of urinary tract infection. 2. Implement measures to prevent urinary retention when urinary catheter is present (see Postoperative Nursing Diagnosis 2, actions b.1 and 2) *in order to further reduce urinary stasis and the subsequent risk for urinary tract infection.*

■───

5. COLLABORATIVE DIAGNOSES:

Potential complications of colporrhaphy:

a. **reherniation of the bladder or rectum** related to stress on suture lines in vagina associated with increased intra-abdominal, bladder, rectal, or vaginal pressure;

b. **bladder, urethral, or ureteral injury** related to accidental tear or ligation during the surgical procedure.

Desired Outcomes	Nursing Actions and *Selected Purposes/Rationales*

5.a. The client will not experience reherniation of the bladder and rectum into the vagina as evidenced by:
1. absence of stress incontinence
2. no difficulty with evacuation of stool
3. absence of urinary frequency and urgency
4. gradual resolution of back pain and pelvic pressure.
	5.a.1. Assess for signs and symptoms of reherniation of the bladder or rectum into the vagina (e.g. stress incontinence, difficulty evacuating stool, urinary frequency and urgency, voiding small amounts, persistent or increasing back pain or pelvic pressure).
	2. Implement measures *to prevent stress on the vaginal suture lines and subsequent reherniation of the bladder and rectum into the vagina:*
	  a. perform actions to prevent urinary retention (see Postoperative Nursing Diagnosis 2, action b) *in order to prevent accumulation of urine in the bladder*
	  b. perform actions to prevent constipation (see Postoperative Nursing Diagnosis 3) *in order to prevent distention of the rectum*
	  c. perform actions *to prevent increased intra-abdominal pressure:*
	    1. instruct client to lie flat or in a semi-Fowler's position while in bed
	    2. instruct client to avoid any activities that may create a Valsalva response (e.g. straining to have a bowel movement, lifting or carrying a heavy object, holding breath while moving up in bed, coughing)
	    3. administer a laxative, antiemetic, and antitussive if ordered *to prevent straining to have a bowel movement and control nausea, vomiting, and persistent cough*
	  d. caution client to avoid prolonged standing and sitting
	  e. if douches are ordered, insert nozzle carefully, slowly instill small amounts of solution, and rotate nozzle gently.

Desired Outcomes	Nursing Actions and *Selected Purposes/Rationales*

	3. If reherniation occurs:
	   a. maintain client on bed rest
	   b. prepare client for surgical repair of the vaginal wall
	   c. provide emotional support to client and significant others.

5.b. The client will experience healing of bladder, urethral, or ureteral injury if it occurs as evidenced by:
   1. gradual resolution of hematuria and backache
   2. urine output greater than 200 ml within 6–8 hours after surgery.
	5.b.1. Assess for and report signs and symptoms of bladder, urethral, or ureteral injury (e.g. persistent or increasing hematuria or backache, urine output less than 200 ml in first 6–8 hours after surgery).
	   2. If signs and symptoms of bladder, urethral, or ureteral injury are present:
	   a. continue to monitor output carefully
	   b. prepare client for surgical repair if indicated
	   c. provide emotional support to client and significant others.

Discharge Teaching

■────────────────────────────────

6. NURSING DIAGNOSIS: **Knowledge deficit, Ineffective management of therapeutic regimen, or Altered health maintenance***

──────────────

*The nurse should select the diagnostic label that is most appropriate for the client's discharge teaching needs.

Desired Outcomes	Nursing Actions and *Selected Purposes/Rationales*

6.a. The client will identify ways to decrease the risk of reherniation of the bladder and rectum into the vagina.	6.a.1. Provide the following instructions on ways to minimize pressure on the suture lines and decrease the risk of reherniation of the bladder and/or rectum:
	   a. reinforce instructions about avoiding prolonged sitting and standing and any activity that may create a Valsalva response (e.g. straining to have a bowel movement, lifting or carrying heavy objects, holding breath while moving, coughing) for at least 6 weeks
	   b. instruct client to urinate whenever she feels the urge or at least every 4 hours
	   c. if douches are ordered, instruct client to carefully insert nozzle, slowly instill small amounts of solution, and rotate nozzle gently
	   d. reinforce instructions about how to prevent constipation (e.g. drink at least 8 glasses of water daily, increase intake of foods high in fiber, take stool softeners as prescribed).
	   2. Instruct client in additional ways to reduce the risk of reherniation of the bladder and rectum:
	   a. do perineal exercises (e.g. stopping and starting urinary stream, alternately contracting and relaxing the gluteal muscles) when healing is complete (usually in 6 weeks) in order to improve vaginal tone
	   b. adhere to a weight reduction diet and exercise program if overweight.

6.b. The client will identify ways to relieve surgical site discomfort.	6.b. Provide the following instructions regarding ways to relieve discomfort in the surgical area:
	   1. take a sitz bath 2–3 times/day
	   2. avoid prolonged sitting and standing
	   3. sit on a foam pad or pillow
	   4. take analgesics as prescribed.

6.c. The client will state signs and symptoms to report to the health care provider.	6.c.1. Refer to Standardized Postoperative Care Plan, Nursing Diagnosis 21, action c (p. 123), for signs and symptoms to report to the health care provider.
	   2. Instruct the client to report these additional signs and symptoms:
	   a. foul-smelling vaginal discharge
	   b. heavy, bright red vaginal bleeding or the passage of clots that are thumb-size or larger

c. stress incontinence

d. presence of urine or stool in vaginal drainage

e. excessive perineal edema or pain.

6.d. The client will verbalize an understanding of and a plan for adhering to recommended follow-up care including future appointments with health care provider, medications prescribed, and limitations on sexual activity.

6.d.1. Refer to Standardized Postoperative Care Plan, Nursing Diagnosis 21 (pp. 123–124), for routine postoperative instructions and measures to improve client compliance.

2. Instruct client not to have sexual intercourse until permitted by physician (usually 6 weeks).

3. Inform client that loss of vaginal sensation is usually temporary but may persist for several months.

Bibliography

See pages 897–898 and 910.

HYSTERECTOMY WITH SALPINGECTOMY AND OOPHORECTOMY

A total hysterectomy is the surgical removal of the uterus and cervix. A panhysterectomy is removal of the uterus, cervix, fallopian tubes, and ovaries and is also referred to as total abdominal hysterectomy with bilateral salpingectomy and oophorectomy (TAH-BSO). The most frequent reasons for hysterectomy are to treat cancer of the cervix, uterus, and ovaries; uterine leiomyomas; symptomatic endometriosis; and uterine prolapse. A vaginal or abdominal approach can be used to perform a hysterectomy. The approach used depends on factors such as the woman's pelvic anatomy and size of the uterus, whether repairs to the vaginal wall or pelvic floor are needed, the presence of other medical conditions, previous abdominal surgeries, and whether the surgery is being done to treat cancer.

This care plan focuses on the adult female client hospitalized for a total abdominal hysterectomy with salpingectomy and oophorectomy. Preoperatively, the goals of care are to reduce fear and anxiety and prepare the client for the surgical experience. Postoperative goals are to maintain comfort, prevent complications, assist the client to adjust to changes in body image, and educate her regarding follow-up care.

DIAGNOSTIC TESTS

Pap smear

Colposcopy with cervical biopsy

Cervical conization or loop electrosurgery excision procedure (LEEP)

Endometrial biopsy

Dilatation and curettage (D & C)

Pelvic ultrasonography

Intravenous pyelography (to locate the position of the ureters and detect concomitant urological anomalies)

DISCHARGE CRITERIA

Prior to discharge, the client will:

- have evidence of normal healing of surgical wound
- have clear, audible breath sounds throughout lungs
- be voiding adequate amounts of urine
- have surgical pain controlled
- tolerate expected level of activity
- have no signs and symptoms of postoperative complications

- verbalize an understanding of the effects of surgical menopause
- identify ways to achieve sexual satisfaction
- verbalize an understanding of medications ordered including rationale, food and drug interactions, side effects, schedule for taking, and importance of taking as prescribed
- state signs and symptoms to report to the health care provider
- share feelings about the loss of reproductive ability
- verbalize an understanding of and a plan for adhering to recommended follow-up care including future appointments with health care provider, activity limitations, and wound care.

**NURSING/
COLLABORATIVE
DIAGNOSES**
	Preoperative
	1. Anxiety △ 810
	Postoperative
	1. Urinary retention △ 811
	2. Potential complications:
	   a. bladder or ureteral injury
	   b. thromboembolism △ 811
	3. Altered sexuality patterns △ 812
	4. Body image disturbance △ 813
	5. Grieving △ 813

DISCHARGE TEACHING	6. Knowledge deficit, Ineffective management of therapeutic regimen, or Altered health maintenance △ 814

See Standardized Preoperative and Postoperative Care Plans for additional diagnoses.

PREOPERATIVE

Use in conjunction with the Standardized Preoperative Care Plan.

1. NURSING DIAGNOSIS:

Anxiety

related to:
a. anticipated loss of control associated with the effects of anesthesia;
b. anticipated effects of surgery on femininity and reproductive ability;
c. fear of rejection by partner;
d. unfamiliar environment and separation from significant others;
e. potential embarrassment or loss of dignity associated with body exposure during preoperative care, surgery, and postoperative care;
f. lack of understanding of the surgical procedure;
g. anticipated surgical findings and postoperative discomfort;
h. financial concerns associated with hospitalization;
i. diagnosis of cancer (if present) and prognosis.

Desired Outcome	Nursing Actions and *Selected Purposes/Rationales*

1. The client will experience a reduction in anxiety (see Standardized Preoperative Care Plan, Nursing Diagnosis 1 [pp. 96–97], for outcome criteria).	1.a. Refer to Standardized Preoperative Care Plan, Nursing Diagnosis 1 (pp. 96–97), for measures related to assessment and reduction of fear and anxiety.
	   b. Implement additional measures *to reduce fear and anxiety:*
	     1. encourage client to verbalize concerns and feelings about loss of ovarian function and reproductive ability; provide feedback

2. discuss alternative methods of becoming a parent (e.g. adoption) if of concern to client

3. assure client she will not suffer needless body exposure during preoperative care, surgery, and postoperative care.

POSTOPERATIVE

Use in conjunction with the Standardized Postoperative Care Plan.

---

1. NURSING DIAGNOSIS:

Urinary retention

related to:
a. decreased perception of bladder fullness associated with the depressant effect of some medications (e.g. anesthetic agents, narcotic [opioid] analgesics);
b. increased tone of the urinary sphincters associated with sympathetic nervous system stimulation resulting from pain, fear, and anxiety;
c. relaxation of the bladder muscle associated with:
    1. nerve trauma and/or edema in the bladder area resulting from surgical manipulation
    2. the depressant effect of some medications (e.g. anesthetic agents, narcotic [opioid] analgesics)
    3. stimulation of the sympathetic nervous system (can result from pain, fear, and anxiety).

Desired Outcome	Nursing Actions and *Selected Purposes/Rationales*
1. The client will not experience urinary retention (see Standardized Postoperative Care Plan, Nursing Diagnosis 13 [p. 113], for outcome criteria).	1. Refer to Standardized Postoperative Care Plan, Nursing Diagnosis 13 (pp. 113–114), for measures related to assessment, prevention, and treatment of urinary retention (client will usually have an indwelling urinary catheter for the first 24–48 hours after surgery).

---

2. COLLABORATIVE DIAGNOSES:

Potential complications of total abdominal hysterectomy:

a. **bladder or ureteral injury** related to accidental tear or ligation during the surgical procedure;
b. **thromboembolism** related to:
    1. trauma to the pelvic veins during surgery
    2. venous stasis associated with:
        a. decreased activity
        b. increased blood viscosity (can result from fluid volume deficit)
        c. pelvic congestion resulting from inflammation in the surgical area
        d. abdominal distention (the distended intestine may put pressure on the abdominal vessels)
    3. hypercoagulability associated with increased release of tissue thromboplastin into the blood (occurs as a result of surgical trauma) and hemoconcentration and increased blood viscosity (can result from fluid volume deficit).

Desired Outcomes	Nursing Actions and *Selected Purposes/Rationales*
2.a. The client will experience resolution of bladder or ureteral injury if it occurs as evidenced by: 　　1. gradual resolution of hematuria and backache 　　2. urine output greater than 200 ml within 6–8 hours after surgery.	2.a.1. Assess for and report signs and symptoms of bladder or ureteral injury (e.g. hematuria, backache, urine output less than 200 ml in first 6–8 hours after surgery). 　　2. If signs and symptoms of bladder or ureteral injury are present: 　　　a. continue to monitor output carefully 　　　b. prepare client for surgical repair of the bladder or ureter if planned 　　　c. provide emotional support to client and significant others.
2.b. The client will not develop a deep vein thrombus or pulmonary embolism (see Standardized Postoperative Care Plan, Collaborative Diagnosis 19, outcomes c.1 and 2 [pp. 120–121], for outcome criteria).	2.b.1. Refer to Standardized Postoperative Care Plan, Collaborative Diagnosis 19, actions c.1 and 2 (pp. 120–121), for measures related to assessment, prevention, and treatment of a deep vein thrombus and pulmonary embolism. 　　2. Implement additional measures *to prevent thrombus formation:* 　　　a. avoid having client in a high Fowler's position 　　　b. encourage client to lie flat for short periods at least every 4 hours *to increase blood return from the legs* 　　　c. assist client with ambulation as soon as allowed.

███ ──

3. NURSING DIAGNOSIS:　　**Altered sexuality patterns**

related to:
a. perceived loss of femininity and sexuality;
b. decreased libido associated with postoperative weakness, fatigue, and changes in hormone levels;
c. dyspareunia associated with presence of the cervical stump suture line and vaginal changes that occur with decreased estrogen levels (e.g. dryness, thinning).

Desired Outcome	Nursing Actions and *Selected Purposes/Rationales*
3. The client will verbalize a perception of self as sexually adequate and acceptable.	3.a. Determine the client's perception of desired sexuality and concerns about the impact of a hysterectomy and oophorectomy on sexuality. 　b. Implement measures *to promote an optimal sexuality pattern:* 　　1. facilitate communication between client and partner; focus on feelings shared by the couple and assist them to identify changes that may affect their sexual relationship 　　2. discuss ways to be creative in expressing sexuality (e.g. massage, fantasies, cuddling) 　　3. arrange for uninterrupted privacy during hospital stay if desired by couple 　　4. inform client that removal of the uterus and cervix should not affect the ability to have sexual intercourse and physiological sexual responses but that surgical menopause created by removal of the ovaries may cause some changes such as decreased libido and painful intercourse; encourage client to discuss these changes and estrogen replacement therapy with physician 　　5. instruct client in ways *to reduce dyspareunia:* 　　　a. use a water-soluble lubricant before sexual intercourse *to reduce vaginal dryness* 　　　b. experiment with different positions during intercourse that might reduce the depth of penetration 　　　c. take estrogen as prescribed *to reduce vaginal dryness and thinning of the vaginal epithelium*

6. reinforce the importance of rest before sexual activity
7. include partner in above discussions and encourage continued support of the client.
c. Consult physician if counseling appears indicated.

---

4. **NURSING DIAGNOSIS:**   **Body image disturbance**

related to:
a. loss of reproductive organs with subsequent inability to bear children;
b. feeling of loss of femininity and sexuality.

Desired Outcome	Nursing Actions and *Selected Purposes/Rationales*
4. The client will demonstrate beginning adaptation to changes in body image and functioning as evidenced by: a. verbalization of feelings of self-worth and sexual adequacy b. maintenance of relationships with significant others c. active participation in activities of daily living.	4.a. Assess for signs and symptoms of a body image disturbance (e.g. verbalization of negative feelings about self, withdrawal from significant others, lack of participation in activities of daily living). b. Determine the meaning of the loss of reproductive organs to the client by encouraging verbalization of feelings and by noting nonverbal responses to the changes experienced. c. Implement measures to facilitate the grieving process (see Postoperative Nursing Diagnosis 5, action b). d. Implement measures *to assist client to increase self-esteem* (e.g. limit negative self-assessment, encourage positive comments about self, assist to identify strengths, give positive feedback about accomplishments and behaviors that are indicative of high self-esteem). e. Implement measures to promote an optimal sexuality pattern (see Postoperative Nursing Diagnosis 3, action b). f. Assist client to identify and utilize coping techniques that have been helpful in the past. g. Assist client with usual grooming and makeup habits if necessary. h. Support behaviors suggesting positive adaptation to loss of reproductive organs (e.g. active interest in personal appearance, verbalization of feelings of self-worth, maintenance of relationships with significant others). i. Assist client's and significant others' adjustment by listening, facilitating communication, and providing information. j. Encourage visits and support from significant others. k. If client expresses an interest in the adoption of children, provide names of appropriate community agencies. l. Consult physician about psychological counseling if client desires or seems unwilling or unable to adapt to changes resulting from the surgery.

---

5. **NURSING DIAGNOSIS:**   **Grieving***

related to loss of reproductive organs and its effect on body image and functioning (e.g. surgical menopause, inability to reproduce).

---

*This diagnostic label includes anticipatory grieving and grieving following the actual losses.

Desired Outcome	Nursing Actions and **Selected Purposes/Rationales**

5. The client will demonstrate beginning progression through the grieving process as evidenced by:
   a. verbalization of feelings about the loss of reproductive organs
   b. usual sleep pattern
   c. participation in treatment plan and self-care activities
   d. utilization of available support systems.

5.a. Assess for signs and symptoms of grieving (e.g. change in eating habits, inability to concentrate, insomnia, anger, sadness, withdrawal from significant others, denial of loss).
   b. Implement measures *to facilitate the grieving process:*
   1. assist client to acknowledge the losses *so grief work can begin*; assess for factors that may hinder and facilitate acknowledgment
   2. discuss the grieving process and assist client to accept the phases of grieving as an expected response to loss of her reproductive organs and usual body functioning
   3. allow time for client to progress through the phases of grieving (phases vary among theorists but progress from shock and alarm to acceptance); be aware that not every phase is expressed by all individuals, that recurrence of phases is common, and that the grieving process may take months to years
   4. provide an atmosphere of care and concern (e.g. provide privacy, be available and nonjudgmental, display empathy and respect) *so that client will feel free to express feelings*
   5. perform actions *to promote trust* (e.g. answer questions honestly, provide requested information)
   6. encourage the verbal expression of anger and sadness about the losses experienced; recognize displacement of anger and assist client to see the actual cause of angry feelings and resentment
   7. encourage client to express feelings in whatever ways are comfortable (e.g. writing, drawing, conversation)
   8. assist client to identify and utilize techniques that have helped her cope in previous situations of loss
   9. support behaviors suggesting successful grief work (e.g. verbalizing feelings about changes in physical functioning, expressing sorrow, focusing on ways to adapt to loss of reproductive function)
   10. explain the phases of the grieving process to significant others; encourage their support and understanding
   11. facilitate communication between client and significant others; be aware that they may be in different phases of the grieving process
   12. provide information about counseling services and support groups that might assist client in working through grief
   13. when appropriate, assist client to meet spiritual needs (e.g. arrange for visit from clergy).
   c. Consult physician about referral for counseling if signs of dysfunctional grieving (e.g. persistent denial of losses, excessive anger or sadness, emotional lability) occur.

Discharge Teaching

▆━━━

6. NURSING DIAGNOSIS: **Knowledge deficit, Ineffective management of therapeutic regimen, or Altered health maintenance***

*The nurse should select the diagnostic label that is most appropriate for the client's discharge teaching needs.

Desired Outcomes	Nursing Actions and **Selected Purposes/Rationales**

6.a. The client will verbalize an understanding of the effects of surgical menopause.

6.a.1. Reinforce the physician's explanation of surgical menopause and its possible effects (e.g. hot flashes, facial hair growth, decrease in vaginal lubrication, insomnia, fatigue, nervousness, palpitations, depression).
   2. Allow time for questions and clarification of information provided.

6.b. The client will identify ways to achieve sexual satisfaction.

6.b.1. Explain the effects of the surgery on sexual functioning (e.g. painful intercourse because of vaginal dryness).

2. Instruct client in ways to promote sexual satisfaction:
   a. use a water-soluble lubricant in the vagina to prevent pain during intercourse (the amount of vaginal lubrication decreases as a result of the effects of surgically-induced menopause)
   b. take hormone replacements (e.g. estrogen) as prescribed
   c. try different positions for intercourse to determine whether some positions are more comfortable than others.

3. Reinforce physician's instructions regarding when client can resume sexual intercourse (usually 4–6 weeks).

6.c. The client will verbalize an understanding of medications ordered including rationale, food and drug interactions, side effects, schedule for taking, and importance of taking as prescribed.

6.c.1. Explain the rationale for, side effects of, schedule for taking, and importance of taking medications prescribed.

2. If client is discharged on estrogen replacement therapy, instruct her to:
   a. apply patch as prescribed; take oral medication with food or at bedtime to prevent nausea
   b. be aware that depression, headache, weight gain, acne, increased skin pigmentation, nausea, and tender breasts are potential side effects of estrogen therapy
   c. wear a supportive bra if breasts are tender
   d. stop smoking (smoking may increase the incidence of the thromboembolic side effect of estrogen)
   e. report the following to the health care provider:
      1. side effects that are not controlled or tolerable
      2. visual blurring or acuity changes or contact lens intolerance
      3. numbness, swelling, pain, or redness of an extremity
      4. sudden onset of chest pain or shortness of breath
   f. keep scheduled follow-up appointments with health care provider while on estrogen replacement therapy.

3. Inform client of pertinent interactions between estrogen and other medications she is taking.

4. Instruct client to inform physician of any other prescription and nonprescription medications she is taking and to inform all health care providers of medications being taken.

6.d. The client will state signs and symptoms to report to the health care provider.

6.d.1. Refer to Standardized Postoperative Care Plan, Nursing Diagnosis 21, action c (p. 123), for signs and symptoms to report to the health care provider.

2. Instruct the client to report these additional signs and symptoms:
   a. foul-smelling vaginal discharge (it is normal to have an increased amount of discharge about 2 weeks postoperatively when internal sutures are absorbed)
   b. heavy, bright red vaginal bleeding or the passage of clots that are thumb-size or larger
   c. excessive depression or difficulty dealing with changes in body image
   d. excessive discomfort associated with effects of surgical menopause.

6.e. The client will verbalize an understanding of and a plan for adhering to recommended follow-up care including future appointments with health care provider, activity limitations, and wound care.

6.e.1. Refer to Standardized Postoperative Care Plan, Nursing Diagnosis 21 (pp. 123–124), for routine postoperative instructions and measures to promote client compliance.

2. Reinforce the physician's instructions regarding the need to:
   a. avoid lifting objects over 10 pounds, sitting for long periods, stair climbing, and strenuous physical activity (e.g. vacuuming, aerobics) for 6–8 weeks postoperatively
   b. avoid driving for at least a week after surgery
   c. avoid douching and the use of tampons for 4–6 weeks postoperatively.

Bibliography

See pages 897–898 and 910.

≣ MAMMOPLASTY

A mammoplasty is the surgical reconstruction of the breast(s) that is performed to augment or reduce breast size, lift the breasts or correct asymmetry, or shape and build a new breast mound following a mastectomy. Augmentation mammoplasty is done by placing an implant in a surgically created pocket between the capsule of the breast and the pectoral fascia. Reduction mammoplasty is performed by resecting wedges of tissue from the upper and lower quadrants of the breast and then removing excess skin and relocating the areola and nipple. Breast reconstruction is the rebuilding of a breast mound following a mastectomy and can be done at the time of the mastectomy or several months to years after the mastectomy. The extent of reconstruction done depends on the type of mastectomy that was performed; the amount, condition, and laxness of the skin on the chest wall; the availability of donor tissue; and the presence of other medical conditions and factors that may affect healing and recovery.

Reconstruction of the breast is accomplished using autologous tissue flaps from the transverse rectus abdominis muscle (TRAM flap), latissimus dorsi muscle, buttocks, or lower abdomen or by implanting a prosthesis in the subpectoral plane. Tissue expander prostheses are now the most common type of implant utilized. A tissue expander prosthesis is an inflatable device that is placed beneath the pectoral muscle and gradually filled with saline over a period of weeks to months. Once the tissue expander has adequately stretched the skin, it is usually removed and replaced with a permanent prosthesis (some tissue expanders are available that can serve as a permanent prosthesis). Construction of a nipple-areola complex is usually delayed until satisfactory breast symmetry has been achieved and placement can be more accurately determined. Many women who undergo breast reconstruction following a mastectomy choose to have surgery (e.g. reduction, augmentation, mastopexy) on the contralateral breast in order to achieve symmetry.

This care plan focuses on the adult female client who has previously had a mastectomy and is now hospitalized for breast reconstruction. Preoperatively, the goals of care are to reduce fear and anxiety and educate the client regarding postoperative expectations and management. Postoperative goals of care are to prevent complications and educate the client regarding follow-up care.

DISCHARGE CRITERIA

Prior to discharge, the client will:

- have evidence of normal healing of surgical wound
- have clear, audible breath sounds throughout lungs
- be able to perform activities of daily living
- have no signs and symptoms of postoperative complications
- demonstrate ways to prevent capsule formation around breast implant
- demonstrate the ability to care for wound drain insertion site, empty collection device, measure wound drainage, and re-establish negative pressure in collection device if a wound drainage device is present
- state signs and symptoms to report to the health care provider
- share feelings and thoughts about the change in body image
- verbalize an understanding of and a plan for adhering to recommended follow-up care including future appointments with health care provider, medications prescribed, activity restrictions, and wound care.

NURSING/ COLLABORATIVE DIAGNOSES	**Preoperative**
	1. Knowledge deficit △ 817
	Postoperative
	1. Self-care deficit △ 818
	2. Potential complications:
	  a. hematoma formation
	  b. seroma formation
	  c. necrosis of skin flap
	  d. tissue expander failure △ 818

DISCHARGE TEACHING	3. Knowledge deficit, Ineffective management of therapeutic regimen, or Altered health maintenance △ 819

See Standardized Preoperative and Postoperative Care Plans for additional diagnoses.

PREOPERATIVE

Client Teaching

Use in conjunction with the Standardized Preoperative Care Plan.

■

1. NURSING DIAGNOSIS:

Knowledge deficit

regarding:
a. the surgical procedure and hospital routines associated with surgery;
b. physical preparation for the mammoplasty;
c. sensations that normally occur following surgery and anesthesia;
d. postoperative care;
e. appearance of the breast following reconstruction.

Desired Outcomes	Nursing Actions and *Selected Purposes/Rationales*

1.a. The client will verbalize an understanding of the surgical procedure, preoperative care, and postoperative sensations and care.	1.a.1. Refer to Standardized Preoperative Care Plan, Nursing Diagnosis 4, actions a.1–4 (pp. 99–100), for information to include in preoperative teaching.
	2. Provide information about expected sensations associated with breast reconstruction:
	  a. if the use of a tissue expander is planned, explain that a feeling of tightness and pressure in the chest will be present
	  b. if a latissimus dorsi flap will be used, explain that a feeling of back stiffness or tightness may be present as a result of muscle loss
	  c. explain that a loss of sensitivity in grafted tissue and skin around the suture lines is a common occurrence.
	3. Allow time for questions and clarification. Provide feedback.

1.b. The client will demonstrate the ability to perform activities designed to prevent postoperative complications.	1.b.1. Refer to Standardized Preoperative Care Plan, Nursing Diagnosis 4, action b.1 (p. 100), for instructions on ways to prevent postoperative complications. 2. Inform client that she will need to keep upper arm on operative side close to her body for a week after surgery (length of time may vary according to physician preference) in order to prevent tension on the suture lines and subsequent hematoma and seroma formation. 3. Allow time for questions and clarification of information provided.

1.c. The client will verbalize an awareness of the expected appearance of her breast after reconstruction.	1.c.1. Provide the following information on expected appearance of the breast after reconstruction:
	  a. reinforce physician's explanation that the goal of reconstructive surgery after a mastectomy is to achieve a normal appearance in clothing; emphasize that it is impossible to duplicate the size, shape, and contour of a natural breast
	  b. explain that the operative breast will be swollen and discolored in the immediate postoperative period and may appear unusually high on the chest wall if a subpectoral implant has been done; assure client and significant other that this is temporary.
	2. Allow time for questions and clarification of information provided.
	3. Consult physician if client has unrealistic expectations about the postoperative appearance of her breast.

POSTOPERATIVE

Use in conjunction with the Standardized Postoperative Care Plan.

1. NURSING DIAGNOSIS:

Self-care deficit

related to impaired physical mobility associated with pain, the depressant effect of some medications (e.g. narcotic [opioid] analgesics), fear of injury to surgical site, and prescribed arm movement restrictions on the operative side.

Desired Outcome	Nursing Actions and *Selected Purposes/Rationales*
1. The client will perform self-care activities within physical limitations and postoperative activity restrictions.	1.a. Refer to Standardized Postoperative Care Plan, Nursing Diagnosis 12 (p. 113), for measures related to planning for and meeting client's self-care needs. b. Assist client with personal hygiene tasks that require extension and abduction of the arm on the operative side (e.g. bathing, combing and washing hair).

2. COLLABORATIVE DIAGNOSES:

Potential complications of mammoplasty:

a. **hematoma formation** related to inadequate hemostasis during surgical procedure, stress on vessels in operative area, and impaired drainage from the operative area;

b. **seroma formation** related to delayed or impaired flap adherence associated with irregular shape of chest wall, impaired wound drainage, and movement of operative site with use of arm;

c. **necrosis of skin flap** related to:
   1. inadequate blood supply in skin flap associated with stretching or rotation of blood vessels in grafted tissue during operative procedure and hematoma or seroma formation
   2. presence of infection;

d. **tissue expander failure** related to accidental puncture during operative procedure, defect in device, or excessive pressure on chest wall.

Desired Outcomes	Nursing Actions and *Selected Purposes/Rationales*

2.a. The client will not develop a hematoma at the surgical site as evidenced by:
  1. no unusual increase in pain, swelling, and skin discoloration in operative area
  2. expected amount of wound drainage in collection device.
	2.a.1. Assess for and report signs and symptoms of hematoma formation (e.g. increased pain, swelling, and skin discoloration in operative area; less than expected amount of wound drainage in collection device).
	  2. Implement measures *to prevent hematoma formation:*
	    a. caution client to adhere to prescribed arm movement restrictions after surgery *in order to prevent strain on the surgical site and reduce the risk of subsequent bleeding*
	    b. maintain patency of wound drains (e.g. keep tubing free of kinks)
	    c. maintain wound drain suction as ordered.
	  3. If signs and symptoms of hematoma formation occur, prepare client for evacuation of hematoma and repair of bleeding vessels if planned.

2.b. The client will not develop a seroma at the surgical site as evidenced by:
  1. no unusual swelling around incision
  2. absence of continued drainage from incision
  3. expected amount of wound drainage in collection device.
	2.b.1. Assess for and report signs and symptoms of seroma formation (e.g. unusual swelling around incision site, continued drainage from incision, less than expected amount of wound drainage in collection device).
	  2. Implement measures *to prevent seroma formation:*
	    a. maintain patency of wound drains (e.g. keep tubing free of kinks)
	    b. maintain wound drain suction as ordered
	    c. place needed items within easy reach *to prevent unnecessary arm movement*
	    d. reinforce importance of adhering to prescribed arm movement restrictions.

3. If seroma formation occurs:
   a. prepare client for needle aspiration of excessive fluid if planned
   b. assist with application of compression dressing if planned
   c. administer antimicrobials if ordered.

2.c. The client will not experience necrosis of the skin flap as evidenced by:
1. skin flap warm and expected color
2. approximated wound edges
3. absence of foul odor from flap area.

2.c.1. Assess for and report signs and symptoms of:
   a. impaired blood flow in skin flap (e.g. decreased warmth of skin flap pallor or cyanosis of skin flap, capillary refill time greater than 3 seconds)
   b. skin flap necrosis (e.g. pale, cool, darkened tissue; separation of wound edges; foul odor from flap area).
2. Implement measures *to prevent necrosis of skin flap:*
   a. perform actions *to maintain adequate circulation to wound area:*
      1. implement measures to prevent and treat hematoma and seroma formation (see actions a.2 and 3 and b.2 and 3 in this diagnosis)
      2. ascertain that dressings and clothing are not too tight
      3. keep client warm *to prevent generalized vasoconstriction*
      4. position client on unoperative side or back *to prevent pressure on the surgical area*
      5. encourage client not to smoke (*smoking causes vasoconstriction*)
   b. perform actions to promote healing of surgical incision and prevent and treat wound infection (see Standardized Postoperative Care Plan, Nursing Diagnoses 9, action a.2 [p. 110] and 16, actions b.4 and 5 [pp. 116–117])
   c. use caution when changing dressings, being careful not to disturb graft site.
3. If signs and symptoms of necrosis of the skin flap occur:
   a. prepare client for surgical revision of reconstructed area
   b. provide emotional support to client and significant others.

2.d. The client will maintain a functional and intact tissue expander as evidenced by:
1. maintenance of inflation of breast mound
2. statements of feeling of skin and chest tightness and pressure in reconstructed breast in early postoperative period.

2.d.1. Assess for and report signs and symptoms of tissue expander failure (e.g. deflation of breast mound, sudden reduction in sensations of tightness or pressure in reconstructed breast in early postoperative period).
2. Implement measures *to prevent excessive pressure on reconstructed area in order to reduce the risk for tissue expander failure:*
   a. notify physician if dressings appear to be too tight
   b. make sure that clothing worn over area is loose
   c. instruct client to lie on unoperative side or back.
3. If signs and symptoms of tissue expander failure occur:
   a. prepare client for surgical replacement or removal of expander if planned
   b. provide emotional support to client and significant others.

Discharge Teaching

3. NURSING DIAGNOSIS: **Knowledge deficit, Ineffective management of therapeutic regimen, or Altered health maintenance***

*The nurse should select the diagnostic label that is most appropriate for the client's discharge teaching needs.

Desired Outcomes	Nursing Actions and *Selected Purposes/Rationales*

3.a. The client will demonstrate ways to prevent capsule formation around breast implant.

3.a.1. If client had a subpectoral breast implant, instruct her in the following:
   a. the massage technique that is used to maintain mobility of the implant and prevent capsule formation
   b. the necessity of massaging and moving the implant at least 4 times/ day as soon as permitted by physician and for the length of time prescribed (usually for several months postoperatively).
2. Allow time for questions and clarification.

Desired Outcomes	Nursing Actions and *Selected Purposes/Rationales*

3.b. The client will demonstrate the ability to care for wound drain insertion site, empty collection device, measure wound drainage, and re-establish negative pressure in collection device if a wound drainage device is present.	3.b.1. If client is to be discharged with a wound drain and suction device, provide instructions on:
	  a. cleaning of drain insertion site
	  b. emptying collection device
	  c. measuring and recording the amount of wound drainage
	  d. establishing negative pressure in collection device.
	2. Allow time for questions, clarification, and return demonstration.

3.c. The client will state signs and symptoms to report to the health care provider.	3.c.1. Refer to Standardized Postoperative Care Plan, Nursing Diagnosis 21, action c (p. 123), for signs and symptoms to report to the health care provider.
	2. Instruct client to report these additional signs and symptoms:
	  a. thinning, change of color, or breakdown of skin over implant or flap site
	  b. increasing redness of or drainage from donor site if grafting was done
	  c. sudden change in position of implant.

3.d. The client will verbalize an understanding of and a plan for adhering to recommended follow-up care including future appointments with health care provider, medications prescribed, activity restrictions, and wound care.	3.d.1. Refer to Standardized Postoperative Care Plan, Nursing Diagnosis 21 (pp. 123–124), for routine postoperative instructions and measures to improve client compliance.
	2. Reinforce physician's instructions about when client can resume wearing a bra (physicians usually recommend that a bra not be worn for several months following insertion of an implant in order to reduce discomfort that can occur as a result of pressure on the surgical site and to allow the prosthesis to settle and reduce the risk of capsule formation).
	3. If client had a tissue expander inserted:
	  a. emphasize importance of keeping scheduled appointments to enlarge expander; explain that a sterile solution will be added until a slight feeling of tightness is felt around the expander
	  b. instruct her to report pain, change in color of tissue over expander, redness of area, and/or separation of incision edges.
	4. Caution client to limit arm movement as prescribed.
	5. Caution client to avoid pressure on chest wall during sexual activity and to avoid sleeping on operative side or in prone position until healing is complete.
	6. Instruct client to avoid lifting or pushing heavy objects (over 5–10 pounds) for at least a month in order to prevent strain on pectoral muscles.
	7. Reinforce the importance of doing a breast self-examination (BSE) routinely and having follow-up breast exams and mammography as prescribed.

Bibliography

See pages 897–898 and 910.

MASTECTOMY

A mastectomy is the surgical removal of all or part of the breast and is usually performed to treat breast cancer. The type of mastectomy is based on factors such as the location, type, and size of the tumor; the number of tumors; breast size; whether the client has received prior irradiation of the breast; and client preference. The two major types of mastectomies performed today are a modified radical mastectomy and breast-conserving surgery (e.g. lumpectomy, quadrantectomy, partial [segmental] mastectomy). A modified radical mastectomy includes removal of the breast, some or all of the axillary nodes, and possibly the pectoralis minor muscle. The pectoralis major muscle is preserved with this procedure which allows the client to retain the shape of her chest and facilitates reconstructive surgery. Reconstruction may be performed at the time of the mastectomy or may be delayed for several months depending on physician and client preference and additional treatment planned. Breast-conserving surgery followed by irradiation of the breast is an option today for women with grades I and II breast cancer instead of a more extensive mastectomy. It involves excision of the tumor and a surrounding margin of normal tissue and an axillary node dissection.

A course of radiation therapy is done following breast-conserving surgery to eradicate any residual tumor and reduce the risk for tumor recurrence.

This care plan focuses on the adult female client hospitalized for a modified radical mastectomy. Goals of preoperative care are to reduce fear and anxiety and prepare the client for the postoperative period. Postoperatively, the goals of care are to maintain comfort, prevent complications, assist the client to adjust to the change in body image, and educate her regarding follow-up care. This care plan should be used in conjunction with the Care Plan on Mammoplasty if breast reconstruction is performed with the mastectomy.

DIAGNOSTIC TESTS

Mammography
Ultrasonography
Breast biopsy
Bone scan, chest x-ray, liver function tests (may be done to determine whether metastasis has occurred)
Hormone receptor assays (to help determine the response to antiestrogen therapy)

DISCHARGE CRITERIA

Prior to discharge, the client will:

- have evidence of normal healing of surgical wounds
- have clear, audible breath sounds throughout lungs
- have surgical pain controlled
- be able to perform activities of daily living
- have no signs and symptoms of postoperative complications
- identify ways to reduce the risk of trauma to and infection in the arm on the operative side
- identify ways to prevent and treat lymphedema of the arm on the operative side
- demonstrate the ability to care for wound drainage device if present
- demonstrate the ability to perform the prescribed exercises and verbalize an understanding of additional exercises to be done once the sutures are removed
- verbalize an understanding of the importance of doing a routine breast self-examination (BSE) on the remaining breast and operative site
- demonstrate the ability to perform a BSE correctly
- state the factors to consider in selecting a breast prosthesis
- state signs and symptoms to report to the health care provider
- share thoughts and feelings about the change in body image
- identify community resources that can assist with home management and adjustment to the diagnosis of cancer and the loss of a breast
- verbalize an understanding of and a plan for adhering to recommended follow-up care including future appointments with health care provider, medications prescribed, activity level, and wound care.

NURSING/ COLLABORATIVE DIAGNOSES	**Preoperative**
	1. Anxiety △ 822
	2. Knowledge deficit △ 823
	Postoperative
	1. Self-care deficit △ 824
	2. Potential complications:
	  a. lymphedema of arm on operative side
	  b. motor and sensory impairment of the arm and/or shoulder on the operative side
	  c. seroma formation
	  d. hematoma formation
	  e. necrosis of skin flap △ 824
	3. Self-concept disturbance △ 826
	4. Ineffective individual coping △ 827
	5. Grieving △ 828

DISCHARGE TEACHING	**6.** Knowledge deficit, Ineffective management of therapeutic regimen, or Altered health maintenance △ 829

See Standardized Preoperative and Postoperative Care Plans for additional diagnoses.

PREOPERATIVE

Use in conjunction with the Standardized Preoperative Care Plan.

---

1. NURSING DIAGNOSIS: **Anxiety**

related to:
a. diagnosis of cancer, treatment plan, and prognosis;
b. anticipated loss of control associated with the effects of anesthesia;
c. anticipated loss of femininity and physical attractiveness and possible change in relationship with significant other associated with the disfiguring effect of the mastectomy;
d. unfamiliar environment and separation from significant others;
e. anticipated surgical findings and postoperative discomfort;
f. lack of understanding of the surgical procedure;
g. potential embarrassment or loss of dignity associated with body exposure;
h. financial concerns associated with hospitalization.

Desired Outcome	Nursing Actions and *Selected Purposes/Rationales*

1. The client will experience a reduction in anxiety (see Standardized Preoperative Care Plan, Nursing Diagnosis 1 [pp. 96–97], for outcome criteria).	1.a. Refer to Standardized Preoperative Care Plan, Nursing Diagnosis 1 (pp. 96–97), for measures related to assessment and reduction of preoperative fear and anxiety.
	b. Implement additional measures *to reduce fear and anxiety:*
	  1. arrange for a Reach to Recovery volunteer to visit client if appropriate
	  2. if immediate reconstruction is not planned, reinforce information from physician about the possibility of future breast reconstruction if desired by client
	  3. reinforce physician's explanations and clarify misconceptions the client has about the surgery (e.g. the size and location of the incision, the amount of tissue surrounding the breast that will be removed, probability of removing all of the tumor, expected mobility of arm on operative side)
	  4. reinforce physician's explanation about the positive effects of the mastectomy on her prognosis.

Client Teaching

■ ──

2. NURSING DIAGNOSIS: **Knowledge deficit**

regarding the surgical procedure, hospital routines associated with surgery, physical preparation for a mastectomy, sensations that may occur following surgery and anesthesia, and postoperative care.

Desired Outcomes	Nursing Actions and *Selected Purposes/Rationales*

2.a. The client will verbalize an understanding of the surgical procedure, preoperative care, and postoperative sensations and care.

2.a.1. Refer to Standardized Preoperative Care Plan, Nursing Diagnosis 4, actions a.1–4 (pp. 99–100), for information to include in preoperative teaching.

    2. Provide the following information about sensations that may occur after a mastectomy:

      a. explain to client that it is common to have sensations of coldness, heaviness, pain, numbness, and tingling in the operative area

      b. explain that abnormal sensations usually subside within a year but that numbness may persist in the operative area and upper inner arm

      c. assure client that the sense that both breasts are present (phantom breast sensation) is common

      d. explain to client that she may feel a change in balance at first, particularly if breasts are large.

    3. Allow time for questions and clarification of information provided.

2.b. The client will demonstrate the ability to perform activities designed to prevent postoperative complications.

2.b.1. Refer to Standardized Preoperative Care Plan, Nursing Diagnosis 4, action b.1 (p. 100), for instructions on ways to prevent postoperative complications.

    2. Provide additional instructions regarding ways to prevent complications following a mastectomy:

      a. inform the client that she must keep upper arm on operative side close to her body for about a week after surgery (length of time will vary according to physician preference) in order to prevent tension on the suture lines and subsequent hematoma and seroma formation

      b. explain that exercise of the hand, arm, and shoulder on the operative side is essential in order to facilitate and improve lymphatic and blood circulation, maintain muscle tone, and prevent contractures

      c. demonstrate recommended postmastectomy exercises (e.g. flexion and extension of the fingers and wrist, wall climbing, rope pulley exercises, rope turning); inform client that hand and wrist exercises are usually begun the day after surgery with gradual progression to full range of motion of shoulder on operative side when sutures are removed

      d. explain that a sling may be used initially when ambulating to support the arm on the operative side

      e. instruct client on ways to minimize or prevent lymphedema of the arm on operative side:

        1. keep arm on operative side elevated on pillows with elbow at heart level and hand higher than elbow in the early postoperative period

        2. perform recommended postmastectomy exercises as soon as allowed

        3. avoid having B/P measurements, injections, blood draws, and intravenous infusions in arm on operative side (these procedures increase risk of infection or trauma and subsequent lymphedema).

    3. Allow time for questions, clarification, practice, and return demonstration of exercises.

POSTOPERATIVE

Use in conjunction with the Standardized Postoperative Care Plan.

---

1. NURSING DIAGNOSIS:

Self-care deficit

related to impaired physical mobility associated with pain, the depressant effect of some medications (e.g. narcotic [opioid] analgesics), fear of dislodging tubes and compromising surgical wound, and prescribed arm movement restrictions on the operative side.

Desired Outcome	Nursing Actions and *Selected Purposes/Rationales*
1. The client will perform self-care activities within physical limitations and postoperative activity restrictions.	1.a. Refer to Standardized Postoperative Care Plan, Nursing Diagnosis 12 (p. 113), for measures related to planning for and meeting client's self-care needs. b. Instruct and assist client with postmastectomy exercises as soon as allowed *in order to strengthen extremity on operative side and increase client's ability to perform self-care.* c. Assist client with personal hygiene tasks that require extension and abduction of arm on operative side (e.g. combing and washing hair, bathing).

---

2. COLLABORATIVE DIAGNOSES:

Potential complications of modified radical mastectomy:

a. **lymphedema of arm on operative side** related to interruption in usual lymph flow associated with surgical removal of axillary lymph nodes and channels, edema in the operative area, and infection of or trauma to operative arm;

b. **motor and sensory impairment of the arm and/or shoulder on the operative side** related to:
   1. transection of or trauma to the nerves during surgical procedure
   2. pressure on nerves associated with lymphedema if it occurs
   3. noncompliance with prescribed exercise program;

c. **seroma formation** related to:
   1. presence of dead space beneath flap associated with dissection of breast tissue and lymph nodes
   2. delayed or impaired flap adherence associated with irregular shape of chest wall, impaired wound drainage, and movement of operative area with arm and shoulder use;

d. **hematoma formation** related to inadequate hemostasis during surgical procedure, stress on vessels in operative area, and impaired drainage from the operative area;

e. **necrosis of skin flap** related to inadequate blood supply in flap or infection of surgical wound.

Desired Outcomes	Nursing Actions and *Selected Purposes/Rationales*
2.a. The client will not develop lymphedema of the arm on the operative side as evidenced by:	2.a.1. Assess for and report signs and symptoms of lymphedema of the arm on the operative side: a. sensory or motor deficits b. pain, sensation of heaviness

1. normal motor and sensory function of the arm
2. absence of pain and edema in the arm.

    c. edema (measure arm on operative side at points 5–10 cm above and below elbow).
2. Implement measures *to prevent lymphedema of arm on operative side:*
    a. place client in a semi-Fowler's position during the immediate postoperative period; elevate arm on the operative side on pillows, keeping elbow at heart level and hand higher than elbow
    b. place a sign above bed to remind personnel not to use arm on operative side for intravenous therapy, blood draws, injections, and B/P measurement *in order to decrease risk of infection or trauma and subsequent lymphedema*
    c. perform actions to prevent and treat wound infection (see Standardized Postoperative Care Plan, Nursing Diagnosis 16, actions b.4 and 5 [pp. 116–117])
    d. instruct and assist client to perform postmastectomy exercises as soon as allowed *in order to promote adequate lymphatic drainage.*
3. If signs and symptoms of lymphedema occur:
    a. continue with above measures
    b. apply an elastic bandage or elastic pressure gradient sleeve to the affected arm if ordered *to reduce edema*
    c. assist and instruct client in use of sequential compression device on affected arm if ordered
    d. restrict sodium intake if ordered
    e. administer antimicrobial agents if ordered *to prevent or treat cellulitis.*

2.b. The client will have expected motor and sensory function of the arm and shoulder on the operative side as evidenced by:
1. ability to put hand, arm, and shoulder through expected range of motion
2. no reports of tingling or increased numbness or weakness in arm.

2.b.1. Assess for and report signs and symptoms of motor and/or sensory impairment of the arm and shoulder on operative side (e.g. inability to move joints through expected range of motion, reports of tingling or increased numbness or weakness in arm).
2. Implement measures *to prevent arm and shoulder dysfunction:*
    a. perform actions to prevent lymphedema (see action a.2 in this diagnosis) *in order to reduce pressure on the nerves*
    b. initiate postmastectomy exercises as soon as allowed
    c. encourage use of arm on operative side to perform activities of daily living as soon as allowed.
3. If signs and symptoms of impaired arm or shoulder function occur:
    a. continue with above measures
    b. assist with prescribed physical therapy
    c. provide emotional support to client and significant others.

2.c. The client will not develop a seroma at the surgical site as evidenced by:
1. no unusual swelling around incision
2. expected amount of wound drainage in collection device
3. absence of continued drainage from incision.

2.c.1. Assess for and report signs and symptoms of seroma formation (e.g. unusual swelling around incision site, less than expected amount of drainage in collection device, continued drainage from incision).
2. Implement measures *to prevent seroma formation:*
    a. maintain compression dressing over operative site if one is in place *to promote skin flap adherence and help prevent the accumulation of fluid in any dead space beneath the flap*
    b. maintain patency of wound drainage system (e.g. prevent kinking of tubing, empty collection device as needed, keep collection device below surgical wound, maintain suction as ordered)
    c. place needed items within easy reach *to prevent unnecessary arm and shoulder movement*
    d. if a sling is ordered, apply it to client's arm before she gets out of bed *in order to support the arm and reduce strain on the surgical site*
    e. reinforce importance of adhering to arm and shoulder movement restrictions.
3. If seroma formation occurs:
    a. prepare client for needle aspiration of excessive fluid if planned
    b. assist with application of compression dressing if not already present
    c. administer antimicrobials if ordered.

2.d. The client will not develop a hematoma at the surgical site as evidenced by:
1. no unusual increase in

2.d.1. Assess for and report signs and symptoms of hematoma formation (e.g. increased pain, swelling, and discoloration of operative site; less than expected amount of wound drainage in collection device).
2. Implement measures *to prevent hematoma formation:*

Desired Outcomes	Nursing Actions and *Selected Purposes/Rationales*
pain, swelling, and skin discoloration in operative area 2. expected amount of wound drainage in collection device.	a. caution client to adhere to arm and shoulder movement restrictions *in order to prevent strain on the surgical site and subsequent bleeding* b. maintain compression dressing over operative site if one is in place c. maintain patency of wound drainage system (e.g. prevent kinking of tubing, empty collection device as needed, keep collection device below surgical wound, maintain suction as ordered). 3. If signs and symptoms of hematoma formation occur, prepare client for evacuation of hematoma and repair of bleeding vessels if planned.
2.e. The client will not experience necrosis of the skin flap as evidenced by: 1. skin flap warm and expected color 2. approximated wound edges 3. absence of foul odor from flap area.	2.e.1. Assess for and report signs and symptoms of: a. impaired blood flow in skin flap (e.g. decreased warmth of skin flap, pallor or cyanosis of skin flap, capillary refill time greater than 3 seconds) b. skin flap necrosis (e.g. pale, cool, darkened tissue; separation of wound edges; foul odor from flap area). 2. Implement measures *to prevent skin flap necrosis:* a. perform actions *to maintain adequate circulation to wound area:* 1. implement measures to prevent and treat seroma and hematoma formation (see actions c.2 and 3 and d.2 and 3 in this diagnosis) 2. consult physician regarding loosening the dressing if client reports increased tightness of dressing or if dressing appears too restrictive 3. position client on unoperative side or back 4. encourage client not to smoke (*smoking causes vasoconstriction*) b. perform actions to promote healing of surgical incision and prevent and treat wound infection (see Standardized Postoperative Care Plan, Nursing Diagnoses 9, action a.2 [p. 110] and 16, actions b.4 and 5 [pp. 116–117]). 3. If signs and symptoms of skin flap necrosis occur: a. prepare client for surgical revision of flap b. provide emotional support to client and significant others.

■

3. NURSING DIAGNOSIS:

Self-concept disturbance*

related to:
a. loss of a breast;
b. dependence on others for assistance with self-care associated with restricted arm movement;
c. possible altered sexuality patterns associated with decreased libido, perceived loss of femininity, and fear of rejection by partner.

---

*This diagnostic label includes the nursing diagnoses of body image disturbance, self-esteem disturbance, and altered role performance.

Desired Outcome	Nursing Actions and *Selected Purposes/Rationales*
3. The client will demonstrate beginning adaptation to the loss of her breast and integration of the change in body image as evidenced by: a. verbalization of feelings of self-worth and sexual adequacy b. active participation in activities of daily living	3.a. Assess for signs and symptoms of a self-concept disturbance (e.g. verbalization of negative feelings about self, lack of participation in activities of daily living, refusal to look at mastectomy site, withdrawal from significant others). b. Determine the meaning of the loss of a breast to the client by encouraging verbalization of feelings and by noting nonverbal responses to the loss experienced. c. Implement measures to facilitate the grieving process (see Postoperative Nursing Diagnosis 5, action b). d. Implement measures to assist client to cope with the effects of the mastectomy (see Postoperative Nursing Diagnosis 4, action c).

c. willingness to look at surgical site
d. maintenance of relationships with significant others.

e. Implement measures *to assist client to increase self-esteem* (e.g. limit negative self-assessment, encourage positive comments about self, assist to identify strengths, give positive feedback about accomplishments and behaviors that are indicative of high self-esteem).

f. Implement measures *to facilitate client's adjustment to the effects of the loss of a breast on her sexuality:*
   1. facilitate communication between client and partner; focus on the feelings the couple share and assist them to identify factors which may affect their sexual relationship
   2. arrange for uninterrupted privacy during hospital stay if desired by the couple.

g. If appropriate, involve partner in care of the client's wound *to facilitate partner's adjustment to the change in client's appearance and subsequently decrease the possibility of partner's rejection of client.*

h. Assist client with usual grooming and makeup habits.

i. Demonstrate acceptance of client using techniques such as touch and frequent visits. Encourage significant others to do the same.

j. Stay with client during first dressing change and encourage her to express feelings about appearance of incision and change in body. Be aware that integration of the change in body image does not occur until 2–6 months after the actual physical change has occurred.

k. If the client is reluctant to look at the surgical site, provide support and encouragement to do so before discharge.

l. If breast reconstruction has not been performed:
   1. encourage client to discuss possibilities for future reconstruction of breast with the physician if desired
   2. discuss the variety of prostheses available and ways to obtain one.

m. Assist client's and significant others' adjustment by listening, facilitating communication, and providing information.

n. Support behaviors suggesting positive adaptation to the loss of a breast (e.g. willingness to look at and care for wound, compliance with exercise program, maintenance of relationships with significant others).

o. Encourage significant others to allow client to do what she is able *so that independence can be re-established and/or self-esteem redeveloped.*

p. Encourage client contact with others *so that she can test and establish a new self-image.*

q. Encourage visits and support from significant others.

r. Encourage client to pursue usual roles and interests and to continue involvement in social activities.

s. Provide information about and encourage utilization of community agencies and support groups (e.g. Reach to Recovery; sexual, family, and individual counseling services).

t. Consult physician about psychological counseling if client desires or seems unwilling or unable to adapt to the loss of her breast.

4. **NURSING DIAGNOSIS:** **Ineffective individual coping**

related to:
a. perceived loss of femininity and embarrassment associated with loss of a breast;
b. fear of rejection by significant others;
c. fear, anxiety, and feelings of loss of control associated with the diagnosis of cancer, adjuvant therapy (e.g. chemotherapy, radiation therapy) if planned, and possibility of disease recurrence.

Desired Outcome	Nursing Actions and *Selected Purposes/Rationales*

4. The client will demonstrate effective coping as evidenced by:
  a. verbalization of ability to cope with the loss of a breast
  b. utilization of appropriate problem-solving techniques
  c. willingness to participate in treatment plan and meet basic needs
  d. absence of destructive behavior toward self and others
  e. appropriate use of defense mechanisms
  f. utilization of available support systems.
	4.a. Assess for and report signs and symptoms of ineffective individual coping (e.g. verbalization of inability to cope; inability to ask for help, problem solve, or meet basic needs; insomnia; withdrawal; reluctance to participate in the treatment plan; destructive behavior toward self or others; inappropriate use of defense mechanisms; inability to meet role expectations).
	  b. Assess client's perception of current situation.
	  c. Implement measures *to promote effective coping:*
	    1. allow time for client to begin to adjust to the mastectomy; inform client that a peak period of emotional distress may occur several weeks postoperatively
	    2. assist client to recognize and manage inappropriate denial if it is present
	    3. if acceptable to client, arrange for a visit with a Reach to Recovery volunteer
	    4. perform actions to improve self-concept (see Postoperative Nursing Diagnosis 3, actions e–s)
	    5. reinforce physician's explanations and clarify misconceptions about adjuvant therapy if planned
	    6. perform actions to facilitate the grieving process (see Postoperative Nursing Diagnosis 5, action b)
	    7. encourage verbalization about current situation
	    8. assist client to identify personal strengths and resources that can be utilized to facilitate coping with the current situation
	    9. demonstrate acceptance of client but set limits on inappropriate behavior
	    10. create an atmosphere of trust and support
	    11. include client in planning of care, encourage maximum participation in treatment plan, and allow choices when possible *to enable her to maintain a sense of control*
	    12. instruct client in effective problem-solving techniques (e.g. accurate identification of stressors, determination of various options to solve problem)
	    13. assist client to maintain usual daily routines whenever possible
	    14. assist client through methods such as role playing to prepare for negative reactions from others because of the loss of her breast and the diagnosis of cancer
	    15. administer antianxiety and/or antidepressant agents if ordered
	    16. assist client to identify and utilize available support systems; provide information about available community resources that can assist client and significant others in coping with the mastectomy (e.g. I Can Cope, Reach to Recovery, counselors, mastectomy support groups)
	    17. encourage the client to share with significant others the kind of support that would be most beneficial (e.g. listening, inspiring hope, providing reassurance and accurate information)
	    18. support behaviors indicative of effective coping (e.g. participation in wound care, exercises, and self-care activities; verbalization of the ability to cope; utilization of effective problem-solving strategies).
	  d. Consult physician about psychological counseling if appropriate. Initiate a referral if necessary.

---

5. NURSING DIAGNOSIS: **Grieving***

related to:
a. loss of a breast and subsequent change in body image;
b. potential for premature death associated with the diagnosis of cancer.

---

*This diagnostic label includes anticipatory grieving and grieving following the actual loss.

Desired Outcome	Nursing Actions and *Selected Purposes/Rationales*

5. The client will demonstrate beginning progression through the grieving process as evidenced by:
a. verbalization of feelings about the loss of a breast and diagnosis of cancer
b. usual sleep pattern
c. participation in treatment plan and self-care activities
d. utilization of available support systems.
	5.a. Assess for signs and symptoms of grieving (e.g. change in eating habits, inability to concentrate, insomnia, anger, sadness, withdrawal from significant others, denial of loss and diagnosis).
	b. Implement measures *to facilitate the grieving process:*
	  1. assist client to acknowledge the changes resulting from loss of her breast and the diagnosis of cancer *so grief work can begin*; assess for factors that may hinder and facilitate acknowledgment
	  2. discuss the grieving process and assist client to accept the phases of grieving as an expected response to loss of a breast and the diagnosis of cancer
	  3. allow time for client to progress through the phases of grieving (phases vary among theorists but progress from shock and alarm to acceptance); be aware that not every phase is expressed by all individuals, that recurrence of phases is common, and that the grieving process may take months to years
	  4. provide an atmosphere of care and concern (e.g. provide privacy, be available and nonjudgmental, display empathy and respect) *so client will feel free to express feelings*
	  5. perform actions *to promote trust* (e.g. answer questions honestly, provide requested information)
	  6. encourage the verbal expression of anger and sadness about the diagnosis of cancer and the loss of a breast; recognize displacement of anger and assist client to see the actual cause of angry feelings and resentment
	  7. encourage client to express feelings in whatever ways are comfortable (e.g. writing, drawing, conversation)
	  8. perform actions to promote effective coping (see Postoperative Nursing Diagnosis 4, action c)
	  9. support realistic hope about the effect of surgery on the disease process and the possibility of breast reconstruction if it has not been done
	  10. support behaviors suggesting successful grief work (e.g. verbalizing feelings about loss of a breast, expressing sorrow)
	  11. explain the phases of the grieving process to significant others; encourage their support and understanding
	  12. facilitate communication between the client and significant others; be aware that they may be in different phases of the grieving process
	  13. provide information regarding counseling services and support groups that might assist client in working through grief
	  14. when appropriate, assist client to meet spiritual needs (e.g. arrange for visit from clergy).
	c. Consult physician regarding referral for counseling if signs of dysfunctional grieving (e.g. persistent denial of loss, excessive anger or sadness, emotional lability) occur.

Discharge Teaching

6. NURSING DIAGNOSIS: **Knowledge deficit, Ineffective management of therapeutic regimen, or Altered health maintenance***

*The nurse should select the diagnostic label that is most appropriate for the client's discharge teaching needs.

Desired Outcomes	Nursing Actions and *Selected Purposes/Rationales*
6.a. The client will identify ways to reduce the risk of	6.a.1. Provide the following instructions regarding ways to reduce the risk of trauma to and infection in the arm on operative side:

Desired Outcomes	Nursing Actions and *Selected Purposes/Rationales*
trauma to and infection in the arm on the operative side.	a. avoid cuts by pushing cuticles back instead of cutting them and trimming fingernails carefully b. use heavy work gloves when gardening and rubber gloves when in contact with steel wool, harsh chemicals or abrasive compounds, or water for prolonged periods c. use insulated gloves when reaching into a hot oven d. use a thimble when sewing in order to avoid pinpricks e. avoid wearing tight jewelry or constrictive clothing on the affected arm to prevent unnecessary pressure f. carry heavy objects such as purse or packages with the unaffected arm g. offer only the unaffected arm for blood pressure readings, injections, blood drawing, and intravenous therapy h. wash any break in the skin on the affected arm with soap and water and cover the area with a protective dressing i. use an electric rather than a straight-edge razor when shaving underarm area j. apply a lanolin hand cream several times/day to prevent drying and cracking of the skin k. avoid prolonged exposure to the sun in order to prevent burns. 2. Instruct client to contact physician immediately if any injury to the arm on the operative side occurs. 3. Instruct client to wear a medical alert bracelet or tag warning others not to draw blood, give injections, insert an intravenous access device, or measure blood pressure in arm on operative side.
6.b. The client will identify ways to prevent and treat lymphedema of the arm on the operative side.	6.b.1. Instruct client in ways to prevent lymphedema of the arm on operative side: a. elevate the affected arm for 30 minutes at least 3 times a day for the next 6–8 weeks b. sleep on unaffected side or back with affected arm elevated for the next 6–8 weeks c. adhere to recommended measures for reducing the risk of trauma to and preventing infection in the arm on the operative side (see action a.1 in this diagnosis) d. adhere to the prescribed exercise regimen. 2. Reinforce physician's instructions regarding ways to treat lymphedema if present: a. adhere to a diet low in sodium b. take antimicrobials if prescribed c. use elastic bandage or pressure gradient sleeve as recommended.
6.c. The client will demonstrate the ability to care for wound drainage device if present.	6.c.1. If the client is to be discharged with wound drains and a suction device, demonstrate how to empty and establish negative pressure in the collection device and provide these additional instructions: a. keep the collection device positioned below the insertion site b. keep the tubing pinned to the dressing and avoid any kinks or strain on the tubing c. empty the collection device at least twice daily or more often if needed d. keep a record of drainage (drains will typically be removed once the drainage is less than 20–25 ml in 24 hours). 2. Allow time for questions, clarification, and return demonstration.
6.d. The client will demonstrate the ability to perform the prescribed exercises and verbalize an understanding of additional exercises to be done once the sutures are removed.	6.d.1. Reinforce teaching about postmastectomy exercises. 2. Emphasize the need to perform hand and elbow exercises regularly and begin full range of motion exercises of the arm and shoulder once the sutures are removed. 3. Allow time for questions, clarification, and return demonstration.
6.e. The client will verbalize an understanding of the importance of doing a	6.e.1. Explain the reasons for monthly BSE of the remaining breast and operative site. 2. Explore with client ways to remember to carry out BSE. The examination

routine breast self-examination (BSE) on the remaining breast and operative site.

6.f. The client will demonstrate the ability to perform a BSE correctly.

6.g. The client will state the factors to consider in selecting a breast prosthesis.

should be done a week after conclusion of menses or on a specific date if postmenopausal.

6.f.1. Demonstrate, using a model, film, or chart, how to do a BSE.
2. Allow time for questions, clarification, and return demonstration.

6.g.1. If acceptable to client, invite a Reach to Recovery volunteer or prosthetist to share information about the various prostheses available.
2. Suggest that client wear a soft, temporary prosthesis until complete healing of the incision has occurred.
3. Encourage the client to take significant other or a close friend with her for the initial fitting of the prosthesis in order to provide emotional support.
4. Emphasize that it is important to select or make a prosthesis that will balance the chest in order to avoid difficulties with posture and subsequent back, shoulder, and neck discomfort.

6.h. The client will state signs and symptoms to report to the health care provider.

6.h.1. Refer to Standardized Postoperative Care Plan, Nursing Diagnosis 21, action c (p. 123), for signs and symptoms to report to the health care provider.
2. Instruct client to report these additional signs and symptoms:
   a. tingling or increased numbness in hand, arm, or shoulder on operative side (explain that numbness is expected and may persist in the chest wall and upper inner arm)
   b. increasing weakness of the affected arm
   c. warmth or redness of the affected arm
   d. increase in size of arm on affected side (client may be instructed to measure arm circumference weekly at points about 4 inches above and below elbow and compare with unaffected arm); inform client that transient edema may occur as she increases use of the affected arm and that this should subside as collateral lymphatic circulation develops
   e. decreased ability to move shoulder or arm on operative side through full range of motion (full range of motion should be regained within 3–6 months)
   f. increased swelling around incision(s)
   g. continued drainage from incision site(s) with saturation of dressing more than once a day.

6.i. The client will identify community resources that can assist with home management and adjustment to the diagnosis of cancer and the loss of a breast.

6.j. The client will verbalize an understanding of and a plan for adhering to recommended follow-up care including future appointments with health care provider, medications prescribed, activity level, and wound care.

6.i.1. Provide information about community resources that can assist the client and significant others with home management and adjustment to the diagnosis of cancer and the mastectomy (e.g. American Cancer Society, Reach to Recovery, I Can Cope, mastectomy support groups, social services, home health agencies, individual and family counselors).
2. Initiate a referral if appropriate.

6.j.1. Refer to Standardized Postoperative Care Plan, Nursing Diagnosis 21 (pp. 123–124), for routine postoperative instructions and measures to improve client compliance.
2. Reinforce physician's explanations and instructions regarding future treatment (e.g. chemotherapy, radiation therapy, breast reconstruction) if planned.
3. Explain the importance of having follow-up breast exams and mammography as prescribed.
4. Reinforce the physician's instructions regarding activity limitations. Instruct client to:
   a. avoid lifting heavy objects (over 5–10 pounds) until wound has healed (usually about 4–6 weeks)
   b. avoid driving until approved by physician (usually about 2 weeks).

Bibliography
See pages 897–898 and 910–911.

RADICAL PROSTATECTOMY

A radical prostatectomy involves removal of the prostate gland, prostatic capsule, seminal vesicles, and part of the vas deferens. In addition, a portion of the bladder neck is sometimes removed prior to anastomosis of the remaining urethra to the bladder neck. The surgery is accomplished via a retropubic or perineal approach depending on the size and position of the prostate and physician preference. A pelvic lymphadenectomy may be done concurrently. Radical prostatectomy is a curative treatment for cancer of the prostate if the cancer is basically confined to the prostate gland. Surgery may be followed by a course of external radiation therapy (teletherapy) if there is evidence of metastasis to the lymph nodes.

This care plan focuses on the adult male client with cancer of the prostate who is admitted for a radical prostatectomy. The goals of preoperative care are to reduce fear and anxiety, provide emotional support, and prepare the client for the surgical experience. Postoperatively, goals of care are to maintain comfort, prevent complications, facilitate the client's adjustment to the changes in body functioning and diagnosis, and educate him regarding follow-up care.

DIAGNOSTIC TESTS*

Blood studies (e.g. prostatic acid phosphatase [PAP], prostate-specific antigen [PSA])
Biopsy of the prostate
Transrectal ultrasonography (TRUS)
Computed tomography (CT)
Bone scan
Magnetic resonance imaging (MRI)
Lymphangiography
Intravenous pyelography (IVP)

---

*May be performed to confirm the diagnosis and/or stage the disease.

DISCHARGE CRITERIA

Prior to discharge, the client will:

- have adequate urine output
- have normal healing of the surgical wound
- have clear, audible breath sounds throughout lungs
- have surgical pain controlled
- have no signs and symptoms of infection or postoperative complications
- demonstrate the ability to perform care related to the urinary catheter and drainage system
- identify ways to manage urinary incontinence if it occurs following catheter removal
- identify ways to manage bowel incontinence if present
- share feelings and concerns about the diagnosis of cancer, the prognosis, and changes in body functioning that may occur as a result of a radical prostatectomy
- state signs and symptoms to report to the health care provider
- verbalize an understanding of and a plan for adhering to recommended follow-up care including future appointments with health care provider, medications prescribed, activity level, wound care, and plans for subsequent treatment.

NURSING/ COLLABORATIVE DIAGNOSES

Preoperative
1. Anxiety △   833
Postoperative
1. Pain △   834
2. Urinary retention △   834

3. Bowel incontinence △   835
4. Risk for infection:
   a. wound infection
   b. urinary tract infection △   835
5. Potential complications:
   a. hypovolemic shock
   b. thromboembolism △   836
6. Sexual dysfunction △   837
7. Self-concept disturbance △   838
8. Grieving △   839

DISCHARGE TEACHING   9. Knowledge deficit, Ineffective management of therapeutic regimen, or Altered health maintenance △   840

See Standardized Preoperative and Postoperative Care Plans for additional diagnoses.

PREOPERATIVE

Use in conjunction with the Standardized Preoperative Care Plan.

---

1. NURSING DIAGNOSIS: **Anxiety**

related to:
a. diagnosis of cancer, treatment plan, and prognosis;
b. potential embarrassment or loss of dignity associated with body exposure during preoperative care, surgery, and postoperative assessments and treatments;
c. anticipated loss of control associated with effects of anesthesia;
d. lack of understanding of the surgical procedure and postoperative expectations and care;
e. anticipated surgical findings and postoperative discomfort;
f. changes in body functioning expected to occur as a result of radical prostatectomy;
g. unfamiliar environment and separation from significant others;
h. financial concerns associated with hospitalization.

Desired Outcome	Nursing Actions and *Selected Purposes/Rationales*

1. The client will experience a reduction in anxiety (see Standardized Preoperative Care Plan, Nursing Diagnosis 1, [pp. 96–97], for outcome criteria).	1.a. Refer to Standardized Preoperative Care Plan, Nursing Diagnosis 1 (pp. 96–97), for measures related to assessment and reduction of fear and anxiety.
	b. Implement additional measures *to reduce fear and anxiety:*
	  1. allow time for verbalization of concerns regarding the effects of the radical prostatectomy on body functioning (e.g. sterility, possible impotence, possible urinary and/or bowel incontinence); reinforce physician's explanation that if incontinence occurs, it often resolves over time and that nerve-sparing surgical techniques have greatly reduced the incidence of impotence
	  2. instruct client to expect the following postoperatively *so that he is not overly concerned when they occur:*
	    a. presence of a urinary catheter (the catheter is usually removed about 2–3 weeks after surgery)
	    b. frequent dressing changes and/or presence of wound drainage collection device for the first 2–4 days after surgery
	    c. possible need for bladder irrigations to keep catheter patent
	    d. presence of some blood in urine (can occur occasionally during the first 1–3 days after surgery)

Desired Outcome	Nursing Actions and *Selected Purposes/Rationales*
	3. reinforce physician's explanation about the positive effects of surgery (when diagnosed and treated in early stages, prostatic cancer is a highly curable disease)
	4. assure client that privacy will be maintained during preoperative care and postoperative assessments and treatments
	5. assure client that he will receive thorough instructions about management of the urinary catheter prior to discharge.

POSTOPERATIVE

Use in conjunction with the Standardized Postoperative Care Plan.

---

1. NURSING DIAGNOSIS:

Pain

related to tissue trauma and reflex muscle spasms associated with the surgery; irritation from drainage tubes; and stress on surgical area associated with movement, sitting (especially following a perineal approach), and straining to have a bowel movement.

Desired Outcome	Nursing Actions and *Selected Purposes/Rationales*
1. The client will experience diminished pain (see Standardized Postoperative Care Plan, Nursing Diagnosis 6 [pp. 106–107], for outcome criteria).	1.a. Refer to Standardized Postoperative Care Plan, Nursing Diagnosis 6 (pp. 106–107), for measures related to assessment and management of pain.
	b. Implement additional measures *to reduce pain:*
	1. instruct client to avoid straining to have a bowel movement *in order to prevent increased pressure on operative site*; consult physician about an order for a laxative if indicated
	2. if client has a perineal incision:
	a. provide a pillow or foam pad for him to sit on if desired
	b. assist with sitz baths if ordered following removal of perineal wound drains (some physicians do not order sitz baths until the urinary catheter is also removed).

---

2. NURSING DIAGNOSIS:

Urinary retention

related to obstruction of the urinary catheter.

Desired Outcome	Nursing Actions and *Selected Purposes/Rationales*
2. The client will not experience urinary retention as evidenced by:	2.a. Assess for and report signs and symptoms of urinary retention (e.g. reports of bladder fullness or suprapubic discomfort, bladder distention, absence of urine in urinary catheter drainage tubing, output that continues to be less than intake 48 hours after surgery).
a. no reports of bladder fullness and suprapubic discomfort	b. Implement measures *to maintain patency of urinary catheter in order to prevent urinary retention:*
b. absence of bladder distention	1. keep drainage tubing free of kinks
	2. keep collection container below level of bladder

c. balanced intake and output within 48 hours after surgery.

3. tape catheter securely to abdomen or thigh *in order to prevent inadvertent removal*
4. perform bladder irrigations as ordered *to flush out blood clots if present (the clots could obstruct the catheter).*

c. Consult physician if signs and symptoms of urinary retention persist.

---

3. NURSING DIAGNOSIS:

Bowel incontinence

related to:
a. unavoidable or inadvertent damage to the anal sphincter or to the pudendal nerve during surgery (this nerve controls the anal sphincter);
b. compression of the pudendal nerve associated with edema in the surgical area;
c. loss of perineal muscle tone associated with surgical incision if a perineal approach was used.

Desired Outcome	Nursing Actions and *Selected Purposes/Rationales*

3. The client will maintain optimal bowel control as evidenced by absence of or decrease in episodes of incontinence.

3.a. Monitor for episodes of bowel incontinence.
b. Implement measures *to reduce the risk of bowel incontinence:*
  1. instruct client to perform perineal exercises (e.g. squeezing buttocks together, then relaxing the muscles) regularly when allowed *in order to increase anal sphincter tone and strengthen pelvic floor muscles (helps maintain a normal anorectal angle)*
  2. have bedside commode or bedpan readily available to client and provide easy access to bathroom *in order to reduce delays in toileting.*
c. If bowel incontinence occurs, consult physician about initiating a bowel care program *so that client is able to routinely evacuate contents of lower colon and reduce the risk of incontinence.*

---

4. NURSING DIAGNOSIS:

Risk for infection:

a. **wound infection** related to wound contamination associated with introduction of pathogens during or following surgery (especially with a perineal approach because incision is close to the anus);
b. **urinary tract infection** related to:
  1. introduction of pathogens associated with presence of indwelling catheter
  2. increased growth and colonization of microorganisms associated with urinary stasis.

Desired Outcomes	Nursing Actions and *Selected Purposes/Rationales*

4.a. The client will remain free of wound infection (see Standardized Postoperative Care Plan, Nursing Diagnosis 16, outcome b [pp. 116–117], for outcome criteria).

4.a.1. Refer to Standardized Postoperative Care Plan, Nursing Diagnosis 16, action b (pp. 116–117), for measures related to assessment, prevention, and treatment of wound infection.
  2. If a perineal approach was used, implement additional measures *to prevent wound infection:*
    a. instruct and assist client to perform good perineal care immediately after bowel movements

Desired Outcomes	Nursing Actions and *Selected Purposes/Rationales*
	b. use a double-tailed T-binder, scrotal support, or jockey shorts to secure perineal dressings (*movement of loose dressings can cause skin irritation and subsequent breakdown*)
	c. assist with sitz baths if ordered *to cleanse the wound and promote healing* (sitz baths are often ordered following removal of the perineal wound drains although some physicians wait until the catheter is also removed).
4.b. The client will remain free of urinary tract infection as evidenced by: 1. clear urine 2. no unusual odor to urine 3. absence of chills and fever 4. absence of nitrites, bacteria, and WBCs in urine 5. negative urine culture.	4.b.1. Assess for and report signs and symptoms of urinary tract infection (e.g. cloudy, foul-smelling urine; chills; elevated temperature). 2. Monitor urinalysis and report presence of nitrites, bacteria, and/or WBCs. 3. Obtain a urine specimen for culture and sensitivity if ordered. Report abnormal results. 4. Implement measures *to prevent urinary tract infection:* a. perform actions to prevent urinary retention and subsequent stasis of urine (see Postoperative Nursing Diagnosis 2, action b) b. maintain a fluid intake of at least 2500 ml/day unless contraindicated *to promote urine formation and subsequent flushing of pathogens from the bladder* c. maintain sterile technique during bladder irrigations if performed d. perform catheter care as often as needed *to prevent accumulation of mucus and blood around the meatus* e. keep urine collection container below bladder level at all times *to prevent reflux or stasis of urine* f. anchor tubing securely *to reduce the amount of in-and-out movement of the catheter* (*this movement can result in the introduction of pathogens into the urinary tract and can cause tissue trauma, which can result in colonization of microorganisms*) g. if frequent bladder irrigations are necessary, consult physician about initiation of continuous, closed system irrigation (*frequent intermittent irrigations increase the risk of introduction of pathogens*) h. increase activity as allowed and tolerated *to decrease urinary stasis.* 5. If signs and symptoms of urinary tract infection are present: a. continue with the above actions b. administer antimicrobials if ordered.

---

5. COLLABORATIVE DIAGNOSES:

Potential complications of radical prostatectomy:

a. **hypovolemic shock** related to:
   1. fluid volume deficit associated with excessive fluid loss and inadequate fluid replacement
   2. hemorrhage associated with surgical trauma to the highly vascular prostate gland, opening of wound (can occur as a result of inadequate wound closure, stress on incision line, and/or poor wound healing), slippage of closures on ligated vessels, and/or disruption of clots at incision site;

b. **thromboembolism** related to:
   1. trauma to pelvic veins during surgery
   2. venous stasis associated with:
      a. pressure on the pelvic and calf vessels during surgery if client was in lithotomy position (this position is used during a perineal approach)
      b. decreased activity
      c. increased blood viscosity (can result from fluid volume deficit)
      d. abdominal distention (the distended intestine can put pressure on the abdominal vessels)
   3. hypercoagulability associated with increased release of tissue thromboplastin into the blood (occurs as a result of surgical trauma) and hemoconcentration and increased blood viscosity (can occur as a result of fluid volume deficit).

Desired Outcomes	Nursing Actions and *Selected Purposes/Rationales*

5.a. The client will not develop hypovolemic shock (see Standardized Postoperative Care Plan, Collaborative Diagnosis 19, outcome a [p. 120], for outcome criteria).	5.a.1. Assess for and report the following:
	a. excessive operative site bleeding:
	  1. excessive bloody drainage on dressings or from drains
	  2. increased swelling and/or blue-black discoloration in surgical area
	  3. persistent redness of or blood clots in urine
	  4. significant decrease in RBC, Hct, and Hb levels
	b. persistent vomiting
	c. difficulty maintaining intravenous or oral fluid intake
	d. signs and symptoms of hypovolemic shock (see Standardized Postoperative Care Plan, Collaborative Diagnosis 19, action a.3 [p. 120]).
	2. Refer to Standardized Postoperative Care Plan, Collaborative Diagnosis 19, actions a.4 and 5 (p. 120), for measures to prevent and treat hypovolemic shock.
	3. Implement measures *to minimize pressure on the operative area in order to prevent hemorrhage and subsequently reduce the risk of hypovolemic shock:*
	a. perform actions to prevent urinary retention (see Postoperative Nursing Diagnosis 2, action b) *in order to prevent distention of the bladder and subsequent strain on the suture lines and newly coagulated blood vessels*
	b. instruct client to avoid sitting for long periods
	c. instruct client to avoid straining to have a bowel movement; consult physician regarding an order for a laxative if indicated
	d. instruct client to return to bed and limit activity for a few hours if urine becomes red when ambulating or sitting in chair.

5.b. The client will not develop a deep vein thrombus or pulmonary embolism (see Standardized Postoperative Care Plan, Collaborative Diagnosis 19, outcomes c.1 and 2 [pp. 120–121], for outcome criteria).	5.b. Refer to Standardized Postoperative Care Plan, Collaborative Diagnosis 19, actions c.1 and 2 (pp. 120–121), for measures related to assessment, prevention, and treatment of a deep vein thrombus and pulmonary embolism. Be aware that prophylactic anticoagulant and antiplatelet medications may be contraindicated *because of the high risk of hemorrhage during and following surgery on the prostate gland.*

■━━

6. NURSING DIAGNOSIS:

Sexual dysfunction

related to:
a. decreased libido associated with fear of bowel incontinence, fear of urinary incontinence following catheter removal, surgical site discomfort, anxiety, and depression;
b. impotence (erectile dysfunction) associated with psychological factors and damage to the pudendal nerve and/or neurovascular supply to the corpora cavernosa during surgery if physician was unable to use a nerve-sparing technique (the possibility of impotence is higher with the perineal approach);
c. absence of ejaculation associated with removal of the seminal vesicles, prostate gland, and a portion of the vas deferens.

Desired Outcome	Nursing Actions and *Selected Purposes/Rationales*
6. The client will demonstrate beginning acceptance of changes in sexual functioning as evidenced by:	6.a. Assess for signs and symptoms of sexual dysfunction (e.g. verbalization of sexual concerns, alteration in relationship with significant other, limitations imposed by effects of radical prostatectomy). b. Provide accurate information about the effects of the radical prostatectomy on sexual functioning. Encourage questions and clarify misconceptions.

Desired Outcome	Nursing Actions and **Selected Purposes/Rationales**

a. verbalization of a perception of self as sexually acceptable and adequate
b. statements reflecting beginning adjustment to effects of radical prostatectomy on sexual functioning
c. maintenance of relationship with significant other.
	c. Implement measures *to promote optimal sexual functioning:*
	  1. facilitate communication between client and partner; focus on the feelings the couple share and assist them to identify changes which may affect their sexual relationship
	  2. discuss ways to be creative in expressing sexuality (e.g. massage, fantasies, cuddling)
	  3. arrange for uninterrupted privacy during hospital stay if desired by the couple
	  4. perform actions to facilitate client's psychological adjustment to the diagnosis and effects of the surgery (see Postoperative Nursing Diagnoses 7, actions e–p and 8, action b)
	  5. if impotence is a problem:
	    a. encourage client to discuss it and various treatment options (e.g. penile prosthesis) with physician
	    b. suggest alternative methods of sexual gratification if appropriate
	  6. if bowel incontinence is a problem and/or urinary incontinence is anticipated following catheter removal, encourage client to defecate and/or urinate just before intercourse and other sexual activity
	  7. if client is concerned that operative site discomfort will interfere with usual sexual activity:
	    a. assure him that the discomfort is temporary and will diminish as incision heals
	    b. encourage alternatives to intercourse and, when intercourse is allowed, use of positions that decrease pressure on the surgical site (e.g. side-lying)
	  8. include partner in above discussions and encourage continued support of the client.
	d. Consult physician if counseling appears indicated.

---

7. NURSING DIAGNOSIS: **Self-concept disturbance***

related to:
a. temporary presence of urinary catheter (the catheter is usually not removed until 2–3 weeks after surgery);
b. bowel incontinence if present and possible urinary incontinence following removal of the catheter;
c. sterility associated with removal of the prostate gland, seminal vesicles, and a portion of the vas deferens;
d. alteration in sexual functioning.

---

*This diagnostic label includes the nursing diagnoses of body image disturbance, self-esteem disturbance, and altered role performance.

Desired Outcome	Nursing Actions and **Selected Purposes/Rationales**
7. The client will demonstrate beginning adaptation to changes in body functioning as evidenced by: a. verbalization of feelings of self-worth and sexual adequacy	7.a. Assess for signs and symptoms of a self-concept disturbance (e.g. verbalization of negative feelings about self, withdrawal from significant others, lack of participation in activities of daily living, refusal to look at or touch urinary catheter or perform catheter care). b. Determine the meaning of changes in body functioning to the client by encouraging the verbalization of feelings and by noting nonverbal responses to the changes experienced.

b. maintenance of relationships with significant others

c. active participation in activities of daily living.

c. Implement measures to promote optimal sexual functioning (see Postoperative Nursing Diagnosis 6, action c).

d. Implement measures to facilitate the grieving process (see Postoperative Nursing Diagnosis 8, action b).

e. Discuss with client improvements in bowel, bladder, and sexual function that can realistically be expected.

f. Implement measures *to assist client to increase self-esteem* (e.g. limit negative self-assessment, encourage positive comments about self, assist to identify strengths, give positive feedback about accomplishments and behaviors that are indicative of high self-esteem).

g. Assist client to identify and utilize coping techniques that have been helpful in the past.

h. Assist client with usual grooming if necessary.

i. Inform client that when he is discharged, he will be able to connect his urinary catheter to a leg bag and that this bag will not be visible to others when he is dressed.

j. If client is incontinent of stool and/or if incontinence of urine is an anticipated problem following catheter removal:
   1. reinforce the importance of doing perineal exercises when allowed *in order to improve bowel and bladder control*
   2. assist him to establish a routine bowel care program *to reduce the risk of bowel incontinence*
   3. instruct in ways to minimize incontinence *so that social interaction is possible* (e.g. placing disposable liners in underwear, wearing absorbent undergarments such as Attends).

k. Because sterility is expected and impotence may occur, discuss alternative methods of becoming a parent (e.g. adoption) if of concern to client.

l. Support behaviors suggesting positive adaptation to changes that have occurred (e.g. verbalization of feelings of self-worth, compliance with treatment plan, maintenance of relationships with significant others).

m. Assist client's and significant others' adjustment by listening, facilitating communication, and providing information.

n. Encourage visits and support from significant others.

o. Encourage client to pursue usual roles and interests and to continue involvement in social activities.

p. Provide information about and encourage utilization of community agencies and support groups (e.g. sexual, family, or individual counseling).

q. Consult physician about psychological counseling if client desires or seems unwilling or unable to adapt to changes resulting from the radical prostatectomy.

---

8. NURSING DIAGNOSIS:　　**Grieving***

related to impotence and loss of bowel control (if they occur), possible loss of bladder control following removal of the urinary catheter, loss of reproductive ability, the diagnosis of cancer, and possibility of premature death.

---

*This diagnostic label includes anticipatory grieving and grieving following the actual losses.

Desired Outcome	Nursing Actions and *Selected Purposes/Rationales*
8. The client will demonstrate beginning progression through the grieving process as evidenced by:	8.a. Assess for signs and symptoms of grieving (e.g. change in eating habits, inability to concentrate, insomnia, anger, sadness, withdrawal from significant others, denial of losses). b. Implement measures *to facilitate the grieving process:*

Desired Outcome	Nursing Actions and **Selected Purposes/Rationales**
a. verbalization of feelings about changes in body functioning and diagnosis of cancer b. usual sleep pattern c. participation in treatment plan and self-care activities d. utilization of available support systems.	1. assist client to acknowledge the losses *so grief work can begin*; assess for factors that may hinder and facilitate acknowledgment 2. discuss the grieving process and assist client to accept the phases of grieving as an expected response to actual and/or anticipated losses 3. allow time for client to progress through the phases of grieving (phases vary among theorists but progress from shock and alarm to acceptance); be aware that not every phase is expressed by all individuals, that recurrence of phases is common, and that the grieving process may take months to years 4. provide an atmosphere of care and concern (e.g. provide privacy, be available and nonjudgmental, display empathy and respect) *so client will feel free to express feelings* 5. perform actions *to promote trust* (e.g. answer questions honestly, provide requested information) 6. encourage the verbal expression of anger and sadness about the losses experienced; recognize displacement of anger and assist client to see the actual cause of angry feelings and resentment 7. encourage client to express feelings in whatever ways are comfortable (e.g. writing, drawing, conversation) 8. assist client to identify and utilize techniques that have helped him cope in previous situations of loss 9. if appropriate, support realistic hope that bowel and/or bladder control will improve if he continues to do perineal exercises 10. support behaviors suggesting successful grief work (e.g. verbalizing feelings about losses, focusing on ways to adapt to losses, learning needed skills, developing or renewing relationships) 11. explain the phases of the grieving process to significant others; encourage their support and understanding 12. facilitate communication between the client and significant others; be aware that they may be in different phases of the grieving process 13. provide information about counseling services and support groups that might assist client in working through grief 14. when appropriate, assist client to meet spiritual needs (e.g. arrange for a visit from clergy). c. Consult physician regarding referral for counseling if signs of dysfunctional grieving (e.g. persistent denial of losses, excessive anger or sadness, emotional lability) occur.

Discharge Teaching

■━━

9. NURSING DIAGNOSIS: **Knowledge deficit, Ineffective management of therapeutic regimen, or Altered health maintenance***

---

*The nurse should select the diagnostic label that is most appropriate for the client's discharge teaching needs.

Desired Outcomes	Nursing Actions and **Selected Purposes/Rationales**
9.a. The client will demonstrate the ability to perform care related to the urinary catheter and drainage system.	9.a.1. Instruct client in care related to the urinary catheter and drainage system including: a. washing the urinary meatus with soap and water at least twice a day b. anchoring the catheter tubing securely to abdomen or thigh c. keeping catheter and urine collection bag tubing free of kinks d. keeping urine collection bag below the level of the bladder e. changing from the leg bag to bedside collection bag when lying down for more than a few hours

f. emptying the leg bag and the bedside collection bag

g. measuring and recording the amount of urine output if necessary.

2. Allow time for questions, clarification, practice, and return demonstration.

9.b. The client will identify ways to manage urinary incontinence if it occurs following catheter removal.

9.b.1. Provide information about ways to reduce the risk of urinary incontinence following removal of the urinary catheter (incontinence can occur as a result of trauma to urinary sphincters during surgery and/or irritation from the urinary catheter, damage to pelvic nerves during surgery, and/or a temporary decrease in bladder capacity because of the continued decompression of the bladder while the catheter was in place):

a. try to urinate every 2–3 hours and when the urge is felt

b. urinate in a standing or sitting position to facilitate complete bladder emptying

c. avoid drinking large quantities of liquid (especially alcohol) over a short period

d. avoid drinking caffeine-containing beverages (e.g. coffee, tea, colas)

e. stop drinking liquids a few hours before bedtime (reduces risk of nighttime incontinence)

f. avoid activities that make it difficult to empty bladder as soon as the urge is felt (e.g. long car rides, lengthy meetings).

2. Reinforce the importance of performing perineal exercises (e.g. stopping and starting stream during voiding; squeezing buttocks together, then relaxing the muscles) regularly when allowed in order to improve urinary control. Assist client to set up a schedule that will remind him to do the exercises (e.g. before and after each meal, during television commercials, when talking on telephone).

3. Inform client that if urinary incontinence occurs following catheter removal, he should:

a. wash and dry perineal area after each episode of incontinence

b. wear disposable underwear liners or absorbent undergarments such as Attends if needed.

9.c. The client will identify ways to manage bowel incontinence if present.

9.c. If client is experiencing bowel incontinence, instruct him to:

1. adhere to a routine bowel care program

2. perform perineal exercises (e.g. stopping and starting stream during voiding; squeezing buttocks together, then relaxing the muscles) regularly when allowed in order to improve bowel control

3. wash and dry perineal area after each episode of incontinence

4. wear disposable underwear liners or absorbent undergarments such as Attends if needed.

9.d. The client will state signs and symptoms to report to the health care provider.

9.d.1. Refer to Standardized Postoperative Care Plan, Nursing Diagnosis 21, action c (p. 123), for signs and symptoms to report to the health care provider.

2. Instruct client to also report:

a. unexpected loss of bladder or bowel control

b. urinary incontinence that persists longer than expected, worsens, or interferes with daily life

c. persistent, unexpected impotence

d. difficulty coping with the diagnosis of cancer and/or the effects of the radical prostatectomy on body functioning.

9.e. The client will verbalize an understanding of and a plan for adhering to recommended follow-up care including future appointments with health care provider, medications prescribed, activity level, wound care, and plans for subsequent treatment.

9.e.1. Refer to Standardized Postoperative Care Plan, Nursing Diagnosis 21 (pp. 123–124), for routine postoperative instructions and measures to improve client compliance.

2. Reinforce physician's explanations and instructions regarding adjuvant therapy (e.g. radiation therapy) if planned.

Bibliography

See pages 897–898 and 911.

TRANSURETHRAL RESECTION OF THE PROSTATE (TURP)

Transurethral resection of the prostate (TURP) is the surgical removal of a prostatic adenoma through the urethra, while leaving the true prostate and its fibrous capsule intact. It may be performed to remove a small cancerous prostatic tumor but most frequently is done to remove a benign prostatic neoplasm that has enlarged enough to block the bladder neck or urethra. The most common cause of a benign neoplasm is benign prostatic hyperplasia (BPH).

BPH is common in men over 50 years of age and results from age-associated changes in androgen levels. Hyperplasia usually occurs gradually and involves the medial portion of the prostate gland which surrounds the urethra. Treatment is indicated when signs and symptoms of prostatism (e.g. urgency, frequency, hesitancy, decreased force of urinary stream, nocturia, postvoid dribbling) become problematic or when complications such as recurrent urinary tract infection, urinary retention, hematuria, renal calculi, or hydronephrosis occur. TURP is the most common surgical method for treating BPH. If the prostate gland is quite large, an open prostatectomy using a suprapubic, retropubic, or perineal approach may be necessary. Nonsurgical methods that may be used to treat symptomatic BPH include medication therapy (e.g. terazosin, finasteride), balloon dilatation of the prostatic urethra, laser prostatectomy, and thermal therapy. Factors influencing the treatment method selected include the client's age and health status, size of the enlarged prostate, presence of complications, and physician preference and expertise.

This care plan focuses on the adult male client with BPH who is hospitalized for a transurethral resection of the prostate. Preoperative goals of care are to reduce fear and anxiety, promote adequate urinary elimination, and educate the client regarding postoperative management. Postoperatively, goals of care are to maintain comfort, maintain fluid balance, prevent complications, and educate the client regarding follow-up care.

DIAGNOSTIC TESTS

Measurement of postvoid residual urine
Urodynamic studies (e.g. uroflowmetry)
Urethrocystoscopy
Transrectal ultrasonography (TRUS)

DISCHARGE CRITERIA

Prior to discharge, the client will:

- have adequate urine output
- have bladder spasms controlled
- have no signs and symptoms of infection or postoperative complications
- identify ways to prevent bleeding in the surgical area
- identify ways to regain or maintain control of bladder emptying
- state signs and symptoms to report to the health care provider
- verbalize an understanding of and a plan for adhering to recommended follow-up care including future appointments with health care provider, medications prescribed, and activity level.

NURSING/ COLLABORATIVE DIAGNOSES

Preoperative
1. Urinary retention △ 843
2. Knowledge deficit △ 843

Postoperative
1. Altered fluid balance: fluid volume excess or water intoxication ("TUR syndrome") △ 845
2. Altered comfort: bladder spasms △ 845
3. Altered urinary elimination:
   a. retention
   b. incontinence following catheter removal △ 846
4. Risk for infection: urinary tract △ 848

5. Potential complications:
   a. hypovolemic shock
   b. thromboembolism △   848
DISCHARGE TEACHING   **6.** Knowledge deficit, Ineffective management of therapeutic regimen, or Altered health maintenance △   849

See Standardized Preoperative and Postoperative Care Plans for additional diagnoses.

PREOPERATIVE

Use in conjunction with the Standardized Preoperative Care Plan.

1. NURSING DIAGNOSIS: **Urinary retention**

related to:
a. obstruction of the urethra and/or bladder neck by the enlarged prostate;
b. loss of bladder muscle tone associated with hypertrophy of the bladder wall (as BPH develops, the detrusor muscle hypertrophies in an attempt to increase its ability to push urine past the bladder neck or urethral obstruction; this hypertrophied muscle has poor contractility).

Desired Outcome	Nursing Actions and *Selected Purposes/Rationales*

1. The client will experience resolution of urinary retention if it occurs as evidenced by:
   a. no reports of bladder fullness and suprapubic discomfort
   b. absence of bladder distention
   c. balanced intake and output.
	1.a. Assess for signs and symptoms of urinary retention:
	      1. reports of bladder fullness or suprapubic discomfort
	      2. bladder distention
	      3. output less than intake.
	   b. Implement measures *to treat urinary retention if present:*
	      1. insert or assist with insertion of a urethral catheter as ordered (if insertion is difficult because of obstruction of the prostatic urethra or bladder neck, it may be necessary to use a stylet or a firm, specially angled catheter)
	      2. assist with insertion of a suprapubic catheter if unable to insert a urethral catheter because of obstruction.
	   c. If a urinary catheter is present, implement measures *to maintain patency of the catheter in order to prevent urinary retention:*
	      1. keep drainage tubing free of kinks
	      2. keep collection container below level of bladder
	      3. tape catheter securely to abdomen or thigh *in order to prevent inadvertent removal.*
	   d. Consult physician if signs and symptoms of urinary retention persist despite implementation of above actions.

Client Teaching

2. NURSING DIAGNOSIS: **Knowledge deficit**

regarding surgical procedure, hospital routines associated with surgery, physical preparation for the TURP, sensations that normally occur following surgery and anesthesia, and postoperative care.

Desired Outcomes	Nursing Actions and *Selected Purposes/Rationales*

2.a. The client will verbalize an understanding of the surgical procedure, preoperative care, and postoperative sensations and care.	2.a.1. Refer to Standardized Preoperative Care Plan, Nursing Diagnosis 4, actions a.1–4 (pp. 99–100), for information to include in preoperative teaching.
	2. Provide additional information regarding care following a TURP:
	  a. explain that bed rest is usually ordered for 6–18 hours after surgery; activity is then increased gradually (the level of activity allowed depends on physician preference, extensiveness of the resection, and the amount of postoperative bleeding client experiences)
	  b. explain that a urinary catheter will be in place for 24–72 hours after surgery (a urethral catheter with 3 lumens is usually inserted to allow drainage of bladder and simultaneous infusion of irrigation solution if needed)
	  c. describe the procedure and rationale for intermittent and continuous bladder irrigations
	  d. explain that traction may be applied to the catheter for 4–6 hours postoperatively and again as needed so that the catheter balloon puts pressure on the surgical site in order to control bleeding (traction is accomplished by pulling down on the urethral catheter and anchoring it securely to the client's leg so that tension is maintained)
	  e. explain that the following can be expected:
	    1. red urine that gradually lightens in color (urine color usually goes from bright red to pink within 24–36 hours and to light pink or dark amber within 72 hours) but often temporarily becomes more red when activity increases
	    2. some blood clots in urine
	    3. some bloody drainage from urethra
	  f. describe signs and symptoms that can be indicative of bladder spasms (e.g. leakage of urine around catheter, feeling of an urgent need to urinate or defecate, pressure in bladder); stress that these signs and symptoms should be reported to the nurse so that catheter patency can be checked and medication can be given as needed to reduce discomfort
	  g. explain that after the catheter is removed:
	    1. a mild to moderate burning sensation may be experienced when urinating and that this is expected to decrease with each voiding and resolve within 1–2 days
	    2. urinary symptoms experienced preoperatively (e.g. urgency, frequency, hesitancy, postvoid dribbling) may still be present or may even increase temporarily postoperatively due to poor bladder muscle tone and/or tissue trauma from the surgery and catheter (these symptoms are expected to resolve within 2–3 weeks).
	3. Reinforce physician's explanation regarding effects of TURP on sexual functioning (after surgery, the client usually experiences retrograde ejaculation as a result of direct trauma to the internal urinary sphincter and/or widening of the bladder neck; normal ejaculatory function usually returns within weeks or months).
	4. Allow time for questions and clarification of information provided.

2.b. The client will demonstrate the ability to perform activities designed to prevent postoperative complications.	2.b.1. Refer to Standardized Preoperative Care Plan, Nursing Diagnosis 4, action b.1 (p. 100), for instructions on ways to prevent postoperative complications.
	2. Provide additional instructions about ways to prevent complications following TURP:
	  a. when oral fluid intake is allowed after surgery, drink one glass of fluid each hour while awake to keep urine dilute (helps keep catheter patent and reduces the risk for urinary tract infection)
	  b. avoid activities that can put excessive pressure on the surgical area (e.g. straining to have a bowel movement, attempting to urinate around catheter, pulling on catheter, walking or sitting for too long).
	3. Allow time for questions, clarification, and return demonstration.

POSTOPERATIVE

Use in conjunction with the Standardized Postoperative Care Plan.

---

1. NURSING DIAGNOSIS:

Altered fluid balance: fluid volume excess or water intoxication ("TUR syndrome")

related to:
a. vigorous fluid therapy during and immediately after surgery;
b. increased secretion of antidiuretic hormone (output of ADH is stimulated by trauma, pain, and anesthetic agents);
c. excessive absorption of irrigation solution via the prostatic veins during and following surgery.

Desired Outcome	Nursing Actions and *Selected Purposes/Rationales*

1. The client will not experience fluid volume excess or water intoxication (see Standardized Postoperative Care Plan, Nursing Diagnosis 4, outcome b [p. 105], for outcome criteria).	1.a. Refer to Standardized Postoperative Care Plan, Nursing Diagnosis 4, action b (p. 105), for measures related to assessment, prevention, and treatment of fluid volume excess and water intoxication.
	b. Implement measures *to reduce absorption of fluid via the prostatic veins in order to further reduce the risk for fluid volume excess and/or water intoxication:*
	  1. use normal saline rather than hypotonic solutions for bladder irrigations
	  2. do not increase frequency of bladder irrigations or speed up continuous irrigation unless indicated.

---

2. NURSING DIAGNOSIS:

Altered comfort: bladder spasms

related to:
a. irritation of the bladder wall associated with tissue trauma during surgery, presence of urinary catheter, rapid infusion of irrigation solution, and distention of the bladder (can occur if urine flow becomes obstructed);
b. increased pressure on the bladder neck and prostatic fossa if traction is applied to the urethral catheter (traction may be applied to pull the catheter balloon into the prostatic fossa in order to put pressure on bleeding vessels).

Desired Outcome	Nursing Actions and *Selected Purposes/Rationales*

2. The client will experience relief of bladder spasms as evidenced by:
a. verbalization of relief of suprapubic discomfort
b. no reports of an urgent need to urinate or defecate
c. no leakage of urine around the urinary catheter.
	2.a. Assess for signs and symptoms of bladder spasms:
	  1. reports of suprapubic discomfort
	  2. statements of an urgent need to urinate or defecate
	  3. leakage of urine around the urinary catheter.
	b. Implement measures *to decrease the risk of bladder spasms:*
	  1. maintain patency of catheter (e.g. irrigate as needed, keep tubing free of kinks) *to prevent distention of bladder*
	  2. perform actions *to keep urinary catheter from irritating the bladder mucosa:*
	    a. tape catheter securely to client's abdomen or thigh
	    b. instruct client to avoid pulling on and twisting the catheter
	  3. release traction on the catheter as soon as ordered *to reduce pressure on the bladder neck and prostatic fossa*

Desired Outcome	Nursing Actions and *Selected Purposes/Rationales*

4. do not increase frequency of bladder irrigations or speed up continuous irrigation unless bleeding is noted or blood clots are present (*excessive or rapid bladder irrigation can irritate the bladder mucosa*)

5. instruct client to avoid attempting to urinate around the catheter and straining to urinate after catheter is removed (*attempts to forcefully contract bladder can stimulate bladder spasms*)

6. perform actions to prevent urinary retention following removal of catheter (see Postoperative Nursing Diagnosis 3, action a.3) *in order to prevent distention of the bladder.*

c. If bladder spasms occur:
1. encourage client to take short, frequent walks unless contraindicated (*walking seems to reduce spasms*)
2. decrease the rate of continuous bladder irrigation if urine is not red and blood clots are not present
3. administer belladonna and opium (B&O) rectal suppositories if ordered (this combination of an antimuscarinic and narcotic analgesic *reduces spasm of the bladder muscle and the client's perception of discomfort*; it is usually only prescribed when the urinary catheter is present *because it can cause urinary retention*).

d. Consult physician if above measures fail to control bladder spasms.

---

3. NURSING DIAGNOSIS: **Altered urinary elimination:**

a. **retention** related to:
1. obstruction of the urinary catheter
2. difficulty urinating following removal of the catheter associated with:
   a. loss of bladder muscle tone resulting from hypertrophy of the detrusor muscle as BPH developed, overdistention of the bladder preoperatively, and/or decompression of the bladder when the catheter was present
   b. relaxation of the bladder muscle resulting from stimulation of the sympathetic nervous system (can result from surgical site discomfort, fear, and anxiety) and the depressant effect of some medications (e.g. narcotic [opioid] analgesics)
   c. decreased perception of bladder fullness resulting from the depressant effect of some medications (e.g. narcotic [opioid] analgesics)
   d. obstruction of the urethra and bladder neck by blood clots and/or edema resulting from tissue trauma (can occur as a result of surgical instrumentation, irritation from the urethral catheter, and/or pressure from the catheter balloon if traction was applied postoperatively);

b. **incontinence following catheter removal** related to trauma to the urinary sphincter(s) associated with surgical instrumentation, irritation from the urethral catheter, and/or pressure from the catheter balloon if traction was applied postoperatively.

Desired Outcomes	Nursing Actions and *Selected Purposes/Rationales*

3.a. The client will not experience urinary retention as evidenced by:
1. no reports of bladder fullness and suprapubic discomfort
2. absence of bladder distention
3. balanced intake and output within 48 hours after surgery

3.a.1. Assess for and report signs and symptoms of the following:
a. urinary retention when catheter is present (e.g. reports of bladder fullness or suprapubic discomfort, bladder distention, absence of fluid in urinary drainage tubing, output that continues to be less than intake 48 hours after surgery)
b. progressive narrowing of the urethra or bladder neck after catheter removal (e.g. reports of decreasing size of urinary stream, increasing need to strain to empty bladder, and increasing urgency)
c. urinary retention following removal of catheter (e.g. reports of bladder fullness or suprapubic discomfort, frequent voiding of small amounts [25–60 ml] of urine, bladder distention, output that continues to be less than intake 48 hours after surgery).

4. voiding adequate amounts at expected intervals after removal of catheter.

2. Implement measures *to maintain patency of the urinary catheter in order to prevent urinary retention:*
   a. keep drainage tubing free of kinks
   b. keep collection container below level of bladder
   c. tape catheter securely to abdomen or thigh *in order to prevent inadvertent removal*
   d. perform bladder irrigations as ordered *to flush out blood clots if present* (*the clots could obstruct the catheter*).
3. Following removal of the catheter, implement measures *to prevent urinary retention:*
   a. offer urinal or assist client to bathroom every 2–3 hours if indicated
   b. instruct client to urinate when the urge is first felt (*a hypotonic bladder can easily become distended*)
   c. perform actions *to promote relaxation during voiding attempts* (e.g. provide privacy, hold a warm blanket against abdomen, encourage client to read)
   d. perform actions to relieve discomfort (see Postoperative Nursing Diagnosis 2, actions b and c)
   e. perform actions *that may help trigger the micturition reflex and promote a sense of relaxation during voiding attempts* (e.g. run water, place client's hands in warm water, encourage client to urinate when in shower)
   f. allow client to assume a normal position for voiding unless contraindicated.
4. If signs and symptoms of urinary retention occur after removal of the catheter, consult physician about intermittent catheterization or reinsertion of an indwelling catheter.

3.b. The client will experience urinary continence.

3.b.1. Assess for urinary incontinence after removal of the urinary catheter (catheter is usually removed 1–3 days after surgery).
2. Implement measures *to prevent trauma to the urinary sphincter(s) while the catheter is in place in order to reduce the risk of urinary incontinence following removal of the catheter:*
   a. if urethral catheter traction is ordered to control bleeding, release it as soon as allowed (traction should not be maintained for longer than 4–6 hours without being released) *in order to reduce pressure on and possible damage to the internal urinary sphincter*
   b. tape catheter securely to client's abdomen or thigh *in order to prevent excessive movement of the catheter.*
3. Following removal of the catheter, implement measures *to reduce the risk of urinary incontinence:*
   a. keep urinal within client's reach and provide easy access to bathroom *in order to reduce delays in toileting*
   b. allow client to assume a normal position for voiding unless contraindicated *in order to promote complete bladder emptying*
   c. instruct client to perform perineal exercises (e.g. stopping and starting stream during voiding; squeezing buttocks together, then relaxing the muscles) regularly *in order to strengthen pelvic floor muscles and improve tone of the external urinary sphincter*
   d. limit oral fluid intake in the evening *to decrease the possibility of nighttime incontinence*
   e. instruct client to avoid drinking beverages containing caffeine (*caffeine is a mild diuretic and a bladder irritant; both effects may make urinary control more difficult*)
   f. instruct client to space fluids evenly throughout the day rather than drinking a large quantity at one time (*rapid filling of bladder can result in incontinence if client has decreased urinary sphincter tone*).
4. If urinary incontinence persists, consult physician regarding intermittent catheterization, reinsertion of an indwelling catheter, or use of external catheter.

4. NURSING DIAGNOSIS:

Risk for infection: urinary tract

related to:
a. introduction of pathogens associated with instrumentation of urinary tract during surgery, presence of indwelling catheter, and frequent bladder irrigations;
b. increased growth and colonization of microorganisms associated with urinary stasis resulting from decreased activity and urinary retention if it occurs.

Desired Outcome	Nursing Actions and *Selected Purposes/Rationales*
4. The client will remain free of urinary tract infection (see Standardized Postoperative Care Plan, Nursing Diagnosis 16, outcome c [p. 117], for outcome criteria).	4.a. Refer to Standardized Postoperative Care Plan, Nursing Diagnosis 16, action c (p. 117), for measures related to assessment, prevention, and treatment of urinary tract infection. b. Implement additional measures *to prevent urinary tract infection:* 1. perform actions to prevent urinary retention (see Postoperative Nursing Diagnosis 3, actions a.2 and 3) 2. consult physician about removal of the catheter as soon as the urine is clear and free of blood clots (*risk of urinary tract infection increases the longer the catheter is in place*).

5. COLLABORATIVE DIAGNOSES:

Potential complications of TURP:

a. **hypovolemic shock** related to hemorrhage (the prostate gland is very vascular) and inadequate fluid replacement;
b. **thromboembolism** related to venous stasis associated with pressure on the pelvic and calf vessels during surgery (the client is usually in lithotomy position) and decreased activity.

Desired Outcomes	Nursing Actions and *Selected Purposes/Rationales*
5.a. The client will not develop hypovolemic shock (see Standardized Postoperative Care Plan, Collaborative Diagnosis 19, outcome a [p. 120], for outcome criteria).	5.a.1. Assess for and report the following: a. excessive operative site bleeding: 1. bright red drainage (could indicate arterial bleeding) or persistent darker drainage (venous bleeding) and blood clots in urinary catheter 2. persistent redness of and blood clots in urine after removal of the catheter 3. significant decrease in RBC, Hct, and Hb levels b. signs and symptoms of hypovolemic shock (see Standardized Postoperative Care Plan, Collaborative Diagnosis 19, action a.3 [p. 120]). 2. Refer to Standardized Postoperative Care Plan, Collaborative Diagnosis 19, actions a.4 and 5 (p. 120), for measures to prevent and treat hypovolemic shock. 3. Implement additional measures *to prevent or control hemorrhage in order to prevent hypovolemic shock:* a. maintain traction on the urethral catheter as ordered (*provides direct pressure on the bleeding vessels*) b. perform actions *to prevent trauma to and/or unnecessary pressure on the prostatic area:*

1. tape catheter tubing securely to client's abdomen or thigh *in order to minimize movement of catheter*
2. caution client to avoid pulling on the catheter
3. instruct client to take short rather than long walks and to avoid sitting for long periods
4. instruct client to avoid straining to have a bowel movement; consult physician regarding an order for a laxative if indicated
5. implement measures to prevent urinary retention (see Postoperative Nursing Diagnosis 3, actions a.2 and 3) *in order to prevent distention of the bladder and subsequent stretching of the newly coagulated blood vessels in the operative area*

c. instruct client to return to bed and limit activity for a few hours if urine becomes more red when ambulating or sitting in chair.

Desired Outcomes	Nursing Actions and *Selected Purposes/Rationales*
5.b. The client will not develop a deep vein thrombus or pulmonary embolism (see Standardized Postoperative Care Plan, Collaborative Diagnosis 19, outcomes c.1 and 2 [pp. 120–121], for outcome criteria).	5.b. Refer to Standardized Postoperative Care Plan, Collaborative Diagnosis 19, actions c.1 and 2 (pp. 120–121), for measures related to assessment, prevention, and treatment of a deep vein thrombus and pulmonary embolism. Be aware that prophylactic anticoagulant and antiplatelet medications are usually contraindicated *because of the risk of hemorrhage during and following surgery on the highly vascular prostate gland.*

Discharge Teaching

■━━━━━━━━━━━━━━━━━━━━━━━━━━━━━━━━━━━━━

6. NURSING DIAGNOSIS: **Knowledge deficit, Ineffective management of therapeutic regimen, or Altered health maintenance***

---

*The nurse should select the diagnostic label that is most appropriate for the client's discharge teaching needs.

Desired Outcomes	Nursing Actions and *Selected Purposes/Rationales*
6.a. The client will identify ways to prevent bleeding in the surgical area.	6.a.1. Instruct client in ways to prevent bleeding in the surgical area: a. avoid straining during defecation (provide instructions about increasing fluid intake and intake of foods high in fiber if client tends to be constipated) b. avoid long walks, prolonged sitting, long car rides, running, climbing stairs quickly, strenuous exercise, sexual intercourse, and lifting objects over 5–10 pounds for as long as recommended by physician (usually for 3–6 weeks after discharge). 2. Allow time for questions and clarification of information provided.
6.b. The client will identify ways to regain or maintain control of bladder emptying.	6.b.1. Instruct client in ways to regain or maintain control of bladder emptying: a. try to urinate every 2–3 hours and whenever the urge is felt b. urinate in a standing or sitting position to facilitate bladder emptying c. avoid drinking large quantities of liquids (especially alcohol) over a short period d. avoid drinking caffeine-containing beverages (e.g. coffee, tea, colas) e. stop drinking liquids a few hours before bedtime (reduces risk of urine retention and nighttime incontinence) f. avoid activities that make it difficult to empty bladder as soon as the urge is felt (e.g. long car rides, lengthy meetings) in order to prevent retention and the subsequent risk for incontinence g. perform perineal exercises (e.g. stopping and starting stream during voiding; squeezing buttocks together, then relaxing the muscles) 10–20 times/hour while awake until urinary control is regained; assist client to set up a schedule that will remind him to do the exercises (e.g. before and after each meal, during television commercials, when talking on telephone).

Desired Outcomes	Nursing Actions and *Selected Purposes/Rationales*
	2. If client is experiencing urinary incontinence, instruct him to: a. wear disposable underwear liners or absorbent undergarments such as Attends if necessary b. consult physician if urinary incontinence persists, worsens, or interferes with daily life so that various options (e.g. external urinary catheter, insertion of artificial urinary sphincter) can be discussed.
6.c. The client will state signs and symptoms to report to the health care provider.	6.c.1. Refer to Standardized Postoperative Care Plan, Nursing Diagnosis 21, action c (p. 123), for signs and symptoms to report to the health care provider. 2. Instruct client to report these additional signs and symptoms: a. persistent burgundy colored or bright red urine (inform client that some blood is expected intermittently for 2–3 weeks after surgery but that urine should become pink to amber after he rests and increases fluid intake for a couple of hours) b. presence of large blood clots or continued passage of smaller clots c. development of or increase in frequency, burning, or pain when urinating d. decrease in urine output or force and caliber of urinary stream e. bladder distention f. unexpected loss of bladder control g. cloudy urine unrelated to orgasm (it is expected that urine will be cloudy after orgasm if client is experiencing retrograde ejaculation) h. persistent or increased bladder spasms.
6.d. The client will verbalize an understanding of and a plan for adhering to recommended follow-up care including future appointments with health care provider, medications prescribed, and activity level.	6.d.1. Refer to Standardized Postoperative Care Plan, Nursing Diagnosis 21 (pp. 123–124), for routine postoperative instructions and measures to improve client compliance. 2. Reinforce the physician's instructions regarding the importance of lying down and increasing fluid intake for a few hours if amount of blood or number of blood clots in the urine increases. 3. Explain the importance of having a digital rectal examination and a blood test for prostatic-specific antigen (PSA) done each year (cancer of the prostate and recurrent BPH can develop since the entire prostate gland is not removed during a TURP).

Bibliography

See pages 897–898 and 911.

UNIT NINETEEN

NURSING CARE OF THE CLIENT WITH DISTURBANCES OF THE HEAD AND NECK

TOTAL LARYNGECTOMY WITH RADICAL NECK DISSECTION

A total laryngectomy with radical neck dissection is the usual treatment for cancer of the larynx with metastasis to regional lymph nodes and/or adjacent neck structures. A total laryngectomy includes removal of the larynx, the hyoid bone, cricoid cartilage, epiglottis, and 2 to 3 tracheal rings. The extent of metastasis is a major factor in determining which additional neck structures are removed during the concurrent radical neck dissection. A comprehensive radical neck dissection usually involves only one side of the neck and includes removal of the tumor, regional lymph nodes and lymphatic channels, sternocleidomastoid muscle, spinal accessory nerve, and internal jugular vein. The current trend, however, is to perform a modified (selective) radical neck dissection whenever possible. With this procedure, the spinal accessory nerve, the sternocleidomastoid muscle, and/or the internal jugular vein are spared. Myocutaneous flaps using the pectoralis major, latissimus dorsi, or the lateral trapezius muscle or free flaps are commonly used in reconstruction of the neck and oral cavity if remaining tissue does not adequately cover the surgical area.

A tracheoesophageal puncture (TEP) may also be performed at the time of the surgery to create a fistula for the insertion of a voice prosthesis early in the postoperative period. The prosthesis allows for diversion of exhaled air into the pharynx by occlusion of the stoma. Sound is produced by the vibration of the mucosa above the expired air stream and is converted to speech by the client's tongue, lips, teeth, and palate.

This care plan focuses on the adult client with cancer of the larynx hospitalized for a laryngectomy with radical neck dissection. Preoperatively, the goals of care are to reduce fear and anxiety and prepare the client for the postoperative period. The goals of postoperative care are to maintain an adequate respiratory and nutritional status, facilitate communication, prevent infection and complications, assist the client to cope with the change in body image and functioning, and educate the client regarding follow-up care. The care plan will need to be individualized according to the extensiveness of the dissection, the amount and type of reconstructive surgery performed, and the physiological and psychological status of the client. If the client has received a preoperative course of radiation therapy, refer to the Care Plan on External Radiation Therapy for specific nursing care measures related to side effects the client may still be experiencing.

DIAGNOSTIC TESTS

Laryngoscopy
Biopsies of larynx, lymph nodes, and neck
X-rays of the chest and neck
Computed tomography (CT)
Magnetic resonance imaging (MRI)
Barium swallow

DISCHARGE CRITERIA

Prior to discharge, the client will:

- have an adequate respiratory status
- be able to communicate effectively
- have an adequate nutritional status
- have evidence of normal healing of surgical wounds
- have surgical pain controlled
- have no signs and symptoms of infection or postoperative complications
- demonstrate appropriate stomal care, suctioning, tracheostomy tube care, oral hygiene, and tube feeding techniques
- demonstrate the ability to effectively use and care for an artificial larynx
- demonstrate the ability to care for the tracheoesophageal puncture (TEP) and voice prosthesis if in place
- identify appropriate safety precautions related to the presence of a tracheostomy and nerve damage resulting from surgery
- identify signs and symptoms to report to the health care provider
- share feelings and thoughts about the effects of the laryngectomy and radical neck dissection on body image and usual life style and roles
- identify community resources that can assist with home management and adjustment to the effects of surgery

communicate an understanding of and a plan for adhering to recommended follow-up care including future appointments with health care provider and speech pathologist, medications prescribed, exercises, activity level, and wound care.

NURSING/ COLLABORATIVE DIAGNOSES	**Preoperative**
	1. Anxiety △ 853
	2. Knowledge deficit △ 854
	Postoperative
	1. Ineffective airway clearance △ 855
	2. Altered nutrition: less than body requirements △ 856
	3. Impaired swallowing △ 857
	4. Impaired verbal communication △ 857
	5. Actual/Risk for impaired tissue integrity △ 858
	6. Risk for infection: wound △ 859
	7. Potential complications:
	a. hypovolemic shock
	b. necrosis of the skin flaps
	c. salivary fistula
	d. thoracic duct fistula
	e. shoulder and neck dysfunction △ 860
	8. Self-concept disturbance △ 862
	9. Ineffective individual coping △ 864
	10. Grieving △ 865
DISCHARGE TEACHING	11. Knowledge deficit, Ineffective management of therapeutic regimen, or Altered health maintenance △ 866

See Standardized Preoperative and Postoperative Care Plans for additional diagnoses.

PREOPERATIVE

Use in conjunction with the Standardized Preoperative Care Plan.

---

1. NURSING DIAGNOSIS:

Anxiety

related to:
a. impending surgery that will result in loss of normal speech and a marked change in appearance and body functioning;
b. lack of understanding of diagnostic tests, surgical procedure, and care required for the tracheostomy and voice prosthesis (if planned);
c. anticipated loss of control associated with effects of anesthesia;
d. financial concerns associated with hospitalization;
e. unfamiliar environment and separation from significant others;
f. possible rejection by significant others;
g. anticipated discomfort, surgical findings, and changes in usual life style and roles;
h. diagnosis of cancer with uncertain prognosis.

Desired Outcome	Nursing Actions and *Selected Purposes/Rationales*
1. The client will experience a reduction in anxiety (see Standardized Preoperative	1.a. Refer to Standardized Preoperative Care Plan, Nursing Diagnosis 1 (pp. 96–97), for measures related to assessment and reduction of fear and anxiety.

Desired Outcome	Nursing Actions and *Selected Purposes/Rationales*

Care Plan, Nursing Diagnosis 1 [pp. 96–97], for outcome criteria).	b. Implement additional measures *to reduce fear and anxiety:*
	   1. support client's decision to have a total laryngectomy with radical neck dissection
	   2. discuss and plan with client and speech pathologist a method of communicating during the postoperative period (e.g. artificial larynx, paper and pencil, picture or word board, magic slate, flash cards)
	   3. if acceptable to client, arrange for a visit with an individual who has successfully adjusted to a laryngectomy.

Client Teaching

2. NURSING DIAGNOSIS:	**Knowledge deficit** regarding the surgical procedure, hospital routines associated with surgery, physical preparation for the laryngectomy and radical neck dissection, sensations that normally occur following surgery and anesthesia, and postoperative care and expectations.

Desired Outcomes	Nursing Actions and *Selected Purposes/Rationales*

2.a. The client will verbalize an understanding of the surgical procedure, preoperative care, and postoperative sensations and care.	2.a.1. Refer to Standardized Preoperative Care Plan, Nursing Diagnosis 4, actions a.1–4 (pp. 99–100), for information to include in preoperative teaching.
	   2. Explain purpose of each part of a tracheostomy tube and how it works. Allow client to handle a tube and use pictures or a model to show where the tube will be inserted and what the stoma will look like when the tube is removed.
	   3. Provide additional information regarding specific expectations and care after laryngectomy and radical neck dissection:
	     a. length of time the tracheostomy tube will be in place (usually 3–6 weeks but depends on physician preference and length of healing time)
	     b. purpose, frequency, and procedure for tracheostomy care
	     c. suctioning procedure and purpose and sensations (e.g. pressure) that client may experience during the procedure
	     d. techniques that will be used to provide moisture to inspired air (e.g. nebulizer, humidifier)
	     e. temporary need for nasogastric or gastrostomy tube feedings to minimize contamination of internal suture lines and to prevent fluid from leaking through the suture line into the trachea; assure client that oral feedings will be initiated as soon as suture line has healed and edema has subsided (usually 8–10 days after surgery, but a longer healing time [12–14 days] may be necessary if client has had radiation therapy to the operative area)
	     f. presence and purpose of closed wound drainage system
	     g. involvement in wound care, suctioning, and tube feeding very early in the postoperative period
	     h. appearance of neck if a tracheoesophageal puncture (TEP) is planned during the surgical procedure (will return from surgery with a stent or catheter protruding from stoma and taped to neck; the stent or catheter will be removed and the voice prosthesis will be inserted about 5–7 days after surgery)
	     i. different methods of speech production (e.g. esophageal speech, artificial larynx) that can be learned postoperatively if a TEP is not performed or is planned as a subsequent surgery.
	   4. Allow time for questions and clarification. Provide feedback.

2.b. The client will demonstrate the ability to perform activities designed to	2.b.1. Refer to Standardized Preoperative Care Plan, Nursing Diagnosis 4, action b.1 (p. 100), for teaching related to prevention of postoperative complications.

prevent postoperative complications.

2. Provide additional instructions on ways to prevent complications associated with a laryngectomy and radical neck dissection:
   a. demonstrate oral hygiene techniques that will be used postoperatively (e.g. low-pressure power spray, irrigations with saline or hydrogen peroxide and water)
   b. demonstrate exercises (e.g. shoulder flexion, abduction, and external rotation; wall climbing with fingers; pulley exercises) that may be ordered to prevent or treat shoulder and neck dysfunction on the affected side
   c. emphasize the need to stop smoking in order to promote healing and reduce the risk for respiratory infection after surgery.
3. Allow time for questions, clarification, practice, and return demonstration of exercises and oral hygiene techniques.

POSTOPERATIVE

Use in conjunction with the Standardized Postoperative Care Plan.

---

1. NURSING DIAGNOSIS:

Ineffective airway clearance

related to:
a. obstruction or dislodgment of tracheostomy tube;
b. stasis of secretions associated with:
   1. depressed ciliary function resulting from effects of anesthesia
   2. difficulty coughing up secretions resulting from the depressant effect of anesthesia and some medications (e.g. narcotic [opioid] analgesics), pain, weakness, fatigue, presence of tenacious secretions (can occur as a result of fluid volume deficit and loss of normal humidification since inspired air no longer passes through the nose and mouth), and inability to raise intrathoracic pressure following removal of the larynx;
c. increased secretions associated with irritation of the respiratory tract resulting from inhalation anesthetics, endotracheal intubation, and presence of tube in trachea;
d. tracheal compression associated with edema and/or bleeding in operative area.

Desired Outcome	Nursing Actions and *Selected Purposes/Rationales*

1. The client will maintain clear, open airways (see Standardized Postoperative Care Plan, Nursing Diagnosis 3 [p. 103], for outcome criteria).	1.a. Refer to Standardized Postoperative Care Plan, Nursing Diagnosis 3 (pp. 103–104), for measures related to assessment and promotion of effective airway clearance.
	b. Implement additional measures *to promote effective airway clearance:*
	  1. perform actions *to decrease risk of dislodgment of tracheostomy tube:*
	    a. obtain adequate assistance when changing tracheostomy tube ties (if assistance is not available, do not remove old ties until new ones are securely in place)
	    b. fasten tracheostomy tube ties securely; check them frequently to be sure that they have not become loose
	    c. minimize movement of outer cannula when suctioning or performing tracheostomy care (*movement of the tracheostomy tube can irritate the trachea and stimulate coughing*)
	    d. ensure that dressings placed around the tracheostomy site are made of a nonraveling material *to prevent lint from entering tube and stimulating coughing*
	    e. discourage vigorous coughing
	    f. consult physician about an order for an antitussive if client is coughing excessively

Desired Outcome	Nursing Actions and *Selected Purposes/Rationales*

2. if tracheostomy tube does become dislodged, perform or assist with immediate replacement according to hospital procedure (proper size tracheostomy tube should be kept at the bedside)
3. perform tracheal suctioning and clean tracheostomy tube as necessary *in order to remove excessive secretions*
4. perform additional measures *to thin and facilitate removal of tenacious pulmonary secretions:*
   a. instill small amounts (usually 2–5 ml) of sterile normal saline into tracheostomy tube before suctioning
   b. maintain humidification of inspired air (e.g. place humidifier in room, provide oxygen mist by nebulizer as ordered)
5. perform actions *to prevent tracheal compression:*
   a. keep head of bed elevated at least 30° *to reduce edema in surgical area*
   b. implement measures to reduce stress on the surgical site (see Postoperative Nursing Diagnosis 5, actions a.2.c.2–7) *in order to prevent bleeding and hematoma formation.*

---

2. NURSING DIAGNOSIS: **Altered nutrition: less than body requirements**

related to:
a. decreased oral intake associated with:
   1. prescribed dietary modifications
   2. anorexia resulting from factors such as discomfort, weakness, fatigue, depression, and an impaired sense of taste and smell (olfactory stimulation does not occur because client no longer breathes through nose)
   3. impaired swallowing;
b. inadequate nutritional replacement therapy;
c. increased nutritional needs associated with the increased metabolic rate that occurs during wound healing.

Desired Outcome	Nursing Actions and *Selected Purposes/Rationales*

2. The client will maintain an adequate nutritional status (see Standardized Postoperative Care Plan, Nursing Diagnosis 5 [pp. 105–106], for outcome criteria).

2.a. Refer to Standardized Postoperative Care Plan, Nursing Diagnosis 5 (pp. 105–106), for measures related to assessment and maintenance of nutritional status.
  b. Implement additional measures *to maintain an adequate nutritional status:*
  1. administer nasogastric or gastrostomy tube feedings as ordered
  2. perform actions *to improve oral intake when allowed* (oral feedings are usually initiated 7–10 days after surgery):
     a. implement measures to improve client's ability to swallow (see Postoperative Nursing Diagnosis 3, action b)
     b. implement measures *to compensate for impaired sense of taste and smell* (assure client that both senses usually return to some degree):
        1. provide extra sweeteners for foods/fluids
        2. encourage client to experiment with spices and other seasonings (e.g. lemon, garlic, onion, mint)
     c. implement measures to facilitate client's psychological adjustment to the effects of the surgery (see Postoperative Nursing Diagnoses 8, actions e–w; 9, action c; and 10, action b) *in order to reduce depression and improve appetite*
     d. provide support during mealtime if needed by staying with client and offering encouragement.

3. NURSING DIAGNOSIS: **Impaired swallowing**

related to:
a. edema of surgical area;
b. impaired tongue movement (can occur if the hypoglossal nerve was damaged during surgery);
c. throat and neck discomfort;
d. structural changes in the pharynx (results in difficulty moving food bolus from pharynx into esophagus);
e. dry mouth and viscous oral secretions (can occur as a result of fluid volume deficit and/or destruction of salivary glands if client had radiation therapy preoperatively).

Desired Outcome	Nursing Actions and *Selected Purposes/Rationales*

3. The client will experience an improvement in swallowing as evidenced by:
   a. communication of same
   b. absence of food in oral cavity after swallowing
   c. absence of choking when eating and drinking.

3.a. Assess for signs and symptoms of impaired swallowing (e.g. communication of difficulty swallowing, stasis of food in oral cavity, choking when eating or drinking).
   b. Implement measures *to improve ability to swallow:*
      1. place client in high Fowler's position for meals and snacks
      2. perform actions *to reduce throat and neck discomfort* (e.g. medicate before meals)
      3. when oral intake is first allowed, provide thick rather than thin fluids or add a thickening agent (e.g. "Thick-it," gelatin, baby cereal) to thin fluids
      4. assist client to select foods that have a distinct texture and are easy to swallow (e.g. custard, canned fruit, mashed potatoes)
      5. avoid serving foods that are sticky (e.g. peanut butter, soft bread, honey)
      6. moisten dry foods with gravy or sauces (e.g. catsup, sour cream, salad dressings)
      7. utilize assistive devices (e.g. long-handled spoon) to place food that does not need to be chewed (e.g. gelatin, custard, mashed potatoes) in back of mouth if tongue movement is impaired
      8. if client has a dry mouth and/or viscous oral secretions:
         a. perform actions *to stimulate salivation at mealtime:*
            1. provide oral hygiene before meals
            2. provide a piece of hard candy for client to suck on just before meals unless contraindicated
            3. serve foods that are visually pleasing
            4. place a piece of lemon or sour pickle on client's plate
         b. encourage a fluid intake of 2500 ml/day unless contraindicated
         c. encourage client to use artificial saliva if indicated
      9. encourage client to avoid milk, milk products, and chocolate (*when combined with saliva, these produce very thick secretions*)
      10. instruct client to avoid putting too much food/fluid in mouth at one time
      11. encourage client to concentrate on the act of swallowing
      12. consult speech pathologist about methods for dealing with impaired swallowing; reinforce recommended exercises and techniques.
   c. Consult physician if swallowing difficulties persist or worsen.

4. NURSING DIAGNOSIS: **Impaired verbal communication**

related to surgical removal of the larynx.

Desired Outcome	Nursing Actions and **Selected Purposes/Rationales**

4. The client will successfully communicate needs and desires.	4.a. Implement measures *to facilitate communication:*
	  1. maintain a patient, calm approach; listen attentively and allow ample time for communication
	  2. answer call signal in person rather than using the intercommunication system
	  3. if client is frustrated or fatigued, try to anticipate needs *in order to minimize the necessity of communication attempts*
	  4. ask questions that require short answers, eye blinks, or nod of head if client is having difficulty communicating and/or is frustrated or fatigued
	  5. provide materials such as magic slate, pad and pencil, word cards, and/or picture board; try to ensure that placement of intravenous line does not interfere with client's use of these communication aids
	  6. reinforce communication techniques prescribed by speech pathologist
	  7. if a TEP has been performed and the voice prosthesis is in place (usually inserted 5–7 days after surgery), reinforce instructions from speech pathologist about its use
	  8. assist client to operate artificial larynx if indicated.
	b. Post a sign on the door, intercommunication system, and above bed to remind health care personnel that the client is nonverbal.
	c. Inform significant others and health care personnel of techniques being used to facilitate client's ability to communicate. Stress the importance of consistent use of these techniques.

---

5. NURSING DIAGNOSIS: **Actual/Risk for impaired tissue integrity**

related to:
a. disruption of tissue associated with the surgical procedure and grafting (if performed);
b. delayed wound healing associated with factors such as:
  1. compromised circulation in wound area resulting from preoperative radiation to tumor site and/or excessive pressure or stress on surgical site
  2. fluid accumulation under skin flaps
  3. inadequate nutritional status;
c. irritation of skin associated with contact with wound drainage, pressure from tubes, and use of tape.

Desired Outcomes	Nursing Actions and **Selected Purposes/Rationales**

5.a. The client will experience normal healing of surgical wounds (see Standardized Postoperative Care Plan, Nursing Diagnosis 9, outcome a [pp. 109–110], for outcome criteria).	5.a.1. Refer to Standardized Postoperative Care Plan, Nursing Diagnosis 9, action a (pp. 109–110), for measures related to assessment and promotion of wound healing.
	  2. Implement additional measures *to promote wound healing:*
	    a. clean peristomal area gently with normal saline or a hydrogen peroxide solution
	    b. use a bed cradle if indicated *to protect donor site from pressure of linens*
	    c. perform actions *to reduce stress on and trauma to graft site, suture lines, and/or surrounding tissue:*
	      1. position client as ordered (e.g. support head and neck with pillows, elevate head of bed at least 30°) *to maintain head alignment and promote venous and lymphatic drainage*

2. instruct client to avoid manipulation of nasogastric tube if present
3. support client's head and neck during position change until client is able to do so
4. instruct client to support head and neck with hands when moving in bed and to avoid turning head abruptly, flexing neck, and hyperextending neck
5. place personal articles and call signal within easy reach *so client does not have to turn or strain to reach them*
6. maintain patency of wound drainage system *in order to prevent fluid accumulation under the skin flaps*
7. instruct client to focus on deep breathing rather than vigorous coughing to promote effective airway clearance (some physicians prefer that their clients not cough *because it increases stress on the suture line*)
8. make sure that tracheostomy tube ties are not too tight
9. soak adherent dressings with sterile normal saline before removal

d. perform actions to maintain an adequate nutritional status (see Postoperative Nursing Diagnosis 2)
e. perform actions to prevent and treat wound infection (see Postoperative Nursing Diagnosis 6).

Desired Outcome	Nursing Actions and *Selected Purposes/Rationales*
5.b. The client will maintain tissue integrity in areas in contact with wound drainage, tubings, and tape as evidenced by: 1. absence of redness and irritation 2. no skin breakdown.	5.b.1. Refer to Standardized Postoperative Care Plan, Nursing Diagnosis 9, action b (pp. 110–111), for measures related to assessment, prevention, and treatment of tissue irritation and breakdown resulting from contact with wound drainage, tubings, and tape. 2. Implement additional measures *to prevent tissue irritation and breakdown:* a. make sure that tracheostomy tube ties are not too tight b. soak adherent dressings with sterile normal saline before removal c. change dressings when damp *to prevent maceration of skin.*

---

6. NURSING DIAGNOSIS: **Risk for infection: wound**

related to:
a. wound contamination associated with introduction of pathogens during or following surgery;
b. increased colonization of microorganisms associated with accumulation of drainage around tracheostomy and beneath flaps (can result from a large dead space and/or obstruction of the wound drainage system);
c. decreased resistance to infection associated with factors such as inadequate nutritional status and diminished tissue perfusion of wound area.

Desired Outcome	Nursing Actions and *Selected Purposes/Rationales*
6. The client will remain free of wound infection (see Standardized Postoperative Care Plan, Nursing Diagnosis 16, outcome b [pp. 116–117], for outcome criteria).	6.a. Refer to Standardized Postoperative Care Plan, Nursing Diagnosis 16, action b (pp. 116–117), for measures related to assessment, prevention, and management of wound infection. b. Implement additional actions *to prevent wound infection:* 1. perform actions to promote wound healing (see Postoperative Nursing Diagnosis 5, action a.) 2. apply an antimicrobial ointment to tracheal stoma and suture lines if ordered 3. perform tracheostomy care as needed *to prevent the accumulation of secretions.*

7. COLLABORATIVE DIAGNOSES:

Potential complications of laryngectomy and radical neck dissection:

a. **hypovolemic shock** related to:
1. hemorrhage associated with:
   a. opening of wound (can occur as a result of inadequate wound closure, stress on incision line, and/or poor wound healing), slippage of closures on ligated vessels, and/or disruption of clots at incision site
   b. carotid artery rupture resulting from prolonged exposure of vessel during and/or following surgery (causes drying and subsequent destruction of the vessel wall) and weakening of the vessel wall (can occur if client had radiation therapy to the tumor site prior to surgery)
2. fluid volume deficit associated with excessive fluid loss and inadequate fluid replacement;

b. **necrosis of the skin flaps** related to:
1. inadequate blood supply in flaps associated with excessive tension on wound margins, preoperative radiation to wound area, mechanical obstruction of blood flow within the flap, vascular congestion (can result from pressure differences in blood flow to and from flap), and development of hematoma or seroma under flaps
2. infection of surgical wound;

c. **salivary fistula** related to dehiscence or necrosis of suture line in pharynx associated with wound infection, inadequate nutritional status, excessive tension on suture line resulting from removal of a large amount of tissue, and impaired vascularity of the wound;

d. **thoracic duct fistula** related to injury to the thoracic duct or one of its tributaries during the surgical procedure (can occur if the neck dissection is on the left side);

e. **shoulder and neck dysfunction** related to removal of or damage to the sternocleidomastoid muscle and/or spinal accessory nerve during surgery.

Desired Outcomes	Nursing Actions and *Selected Purposes/Rationales*
7.a. The client will not develop hypovolemic shock (see Standardized Postoperative Care Plan, Collaborative Diagnosis 19, outcome a [p. 120], for outcome criteria).	7.a.1. Assess for and report: a. signs and symptoms of impending carotid artery rupture (e.g. slight amount of bright red bleeding from wound [occurs 24–48 hours before rupture], sternal or high epigastric discomfort [often present a few hours before rupture]) b. profuse bleeding from wound, tracheostomy, or mouth c. decreasing RBC, Hct, and Hb levels d. signs and symptoms of hypovolemic shock (see Standardized Postoperative Care Plan, Collaborative Diagnosis 19, action a.3 [p. 120], for signs and symptoms). 2. Have suction equipment, gloves, cuffed tracheostomy tube (if one is not already in place), and absorbent dressings at bedside in case of carotid artery rupture. 3. Refer to Standardized Postoperative Care Plan, Collaborative Diagnosis 19, actions a.4 and 5 (p. 120), for measures related to prevention and treatment of hypovolemic shock. 4. Implement measures *to prevent carotid artery rupture and further reduce the risk of hypovolemic shock:* a. perform actions to promote healing of the surgical incision (see Postoperative Nursing Diagnosis 5, action a) and prevent and treat wound infection (see Postoperative Nursing Diagnosis 6) *in order to prevent exposure, drying, and erosion of the carotid artery* b. assess for and report pulsation of tracheostomy tube (*indicates tip is in close proximity to carotid artery and may be causing undue pressure on the vessel*) c. maintain tracheostomy tube in midtracheal position at all times d. if the carotid artery is exposed, keep it covered with loosely packed gauze moistened with sterile normal saline solution as ordered.

5. If carotid artery rupture occurs:
   a. apply firm, prolonged, continuous pressure to bleeding area using absorbent dressings
   b. position client in high Fowler's position with head turned to side or in side-lying position and ensure that tracheostomy cuff is inflated *to prevent aspiration*; assist with insertion of a cuffed tracheostomy tube if one is not in place
   c. suction as necessary *to clear oral cavity and airway*
   d. prepare client for ligation of carotid artery if planned
   e. provide emotional support to client and significant others
   f. administer medications such as intravenous morphine sulfate or diazepam if ordered *to allay anxiety* (client is typically alert).

7.b. The client will not experience necrosis of skin flaps as evidenced by:
1. skin flaps warm and expected color
2. approximated wound edges
3. absence of foul odor from flap area.

7.b.1. Assess for and report:
   a. signs and symptoms of impaired blood flow in skin flaps (e.g. paleness or cyanosis of skin flaps; capillary refill time greater than 3 seconds)
   b. signs and symptoms of skin flap necrosis (e.g. pale, cool, darkened tissue; separation of wound edges; foul odor from flap area).
2. Implement measures to promote wound healing (see Postoperative Nursing Diagnosis 5, action a) and prevent and treat wound infection (see Postoperative Nursing Diagnosis 6) *in order to prevent skin flap necrosis.*
3. If signs and symptoms of skin flap necrosis occur:
   a. prepare client for surgical revision of flap(s)
   b. provide emotional support to client and significant others.

7.c. The client will not develop a salivary fistula as evidenced by:
1. absence of redness, edema, and tenderness near incision
2. afebrile status
3. usual drainage from incision
4. intact skin around incision.

7.c.1. Assess for and report signs and symptoms of a salivary fistula (e.g. redness, edema, and tenderness near incision; increased temperature; drainage of saliva or oral foods/fluids through incision or a cutaneous opening near incision).
2. Implement measures *to prevent a salivary fistula:*
   a. perform actions to prevent and treat wound infection (see Postoperative Nursing Diagnosis 6)
   b. perform actions to maintain an adequate nutritional status (see Postoperative Nursing Diagnosis 2)
   c. maintain patency of drain catheter if in place (the catheter may be inserted in the pharynx during surgery and left in place for 7–10 days *to allow for controlled drainage of saliva, which decreases the risk of breakdown of the pharyngeal incision*).
3. If signs and symptoms of a salivary fistula occur:
   a. continue with above actions
   b. withhold oral food and fluid as ordered
   c. maintain intravenous therapy and tube feedings as ordered until fistula closes
   d. perform wound care as ordered
   e. administer antimicrobials if ordered
   f. prepare client for surgical closure of fistula if planned
   g. provide emotional support to client and significant others.

7.d. The client will experience resolution of a thoracic duct fistula if it occurs as evidenced by:
1. usual amount and character of drainage from incision
2. wound drainage negative for chylomicrons.

7.d.1. Assess for and report signs and symptoms of a thoracic duct fistula (e.g. sudden increase in drainage from wound; cloudy, milky-appearing fluid in drain system; wound drainage positive for chylomicrons).
2. If signs and symptoms of a thoracic duct fistula occur:
   a. apply pressure dressing over fistula site if ordered
   b. accurately assess amount of fistula drainage
   c. administer fluid and electrolytes *to replace those lost via the fistula*
   d. prepare client for surgical repair of fistula if planned
   e. provide emotional support to client and significant others.

7.e. The client will regain optimal shoulder and neck function on affected side as evidenced by:

7.e.1. Assess for and report signs and symptoms of sternocleidomastoid muscle and/or spinal accessory nerve damage on the affected side (e.g. inability to abduct arm, drooping shoulder, continued pain in neck and shoulder).
2. If shoulder and neck dysfunction occur:

Desired Outcomes	Nursing Actions and *Selected Purposes/Rationales*
1. improved range of motion of shoulder 2. ability to maintain shoulder in near-normal position 3. gradual resolution of pain in shoulder and neck.	a. instruct client to support affected arm in a sling when ambulating and rest it on a chair arm, table, or pillow when sitting b. assist client with self-care activities as needed c. reinforce the need to begin neck and shoulder exercises (e.g. wall climbing with fingers, shoulder swing, pulley exercises, range of motion of neck) as soon as allowed *in order to improve tone and strength of muscles on the affected side* (exercises are usually started 10 days to 6 weeks postoperatively depending on extensiveness of surgery and stage of healing process) d. assure client that partial neck and shoulder function may be regained if exercise program and physical therapy schedule are adhered to.

---

8. NURSING DIAGNOSIS: **Self-concept disturbance***

related to:
a. changes in appearance (e.g. disfigurement of neck, presence of tracheostomy, drooling and loss of facial expression if facial nerve was damaged during surgery, drooping of shoulder if spinal accessory nerve was removed or damaged during surgery, facial edema resulting from disruption of lymphatic channels in the neck);
b. alteration in usual body functioning:
  1. loss of ability to speak normally, sing, produce crying and laughing sounds, and whistle
  2. loss of sense of taste and smell and ability to blow nose associated with neck breathing
  3. loss of normal shoulder and neck movement and strength (can occur if the spinal accessory nerve and sternocleidomastoid muscle were removed or damaged during surgery)
  4. impaired swallowing and tongue movement (can occur if the hypoglossal nerve was damaged during surgery);
c. possible altered sexuality patterns associated with decreased libido, perceived loss of femininity/masculinity and physical attractiveness, and fear of rejection by partner;
d. temporary dependence on others to meet self-care needs;
e. possible life-style and role changes.

---

*This diagnostic label includes the nursing diagnoses of body image disturbance, self-esteem disturbance, and altered role performance.

Desired Outcome	Nursing Actions and *Selected Purposes/Rationales*
8. The client will demonstrate beginning adaptation to changes in appearance, body functioning, life style, and roles as evidenced by: a. communication of feelings of self-worth and sexual adequacy b. maintenance of relationships with significant others c. active participation in activities of daily living, tracheostomy care, and speech therapy	8.a. Assess for signs and symptoms of a self-concept disturbance (e.g. communication of negative feelings about self; withdrawal from significant others; lack of participation in activities of daily living, tracheostomy care, or speech therapy; refusal to look at or touch neck area; lack of plan for adapting to changes in life style). b. Determine the meaning of the changes in appearance, body functioning, life style, and roles to the client by encouraging communication of feelings and by noting nonverbal responses to the changes experienced. c. Implement measures to assist client to cope with the effects of the laryngectomy and radical neck dissection (see Postoperative Nursing Diagnosis 9, action c). d. Implement measures to facilitate the grieving process (see Postoperative Nursing Diagnosis 10, action b). e. Implement measures *to facilitate client's adjustment to the effects of changes in appearance and body functioning on his/her sexuality:*

d. communication of a beginning plan for adapting life style to changes resulting from the laryngectomy and radical neck dissection.

1. facilitate communication between client and partner; focus on feelings the couple share and assist them to identify factors which may affect their sexual relationship
2. perform actions *to decrease the possibility of rejection by partner:*
   a. if appropriate, involve partner in care of client's wound and suctioning *to facilitate adjustment to the changes in client's appearance and functioning*
   b. instruct client to suction and clean stoma and cover it with a porous shield just before sexual activity
3. if client is concerned that operative site discomfort will interfere with usual sexual activity, assure him/her that discomfort is temporary and will diminish as incision heals
4. arrange for uninterrupted privacy during hospital stay if desired by couple.

f. Implement measures *to assist client to increase self-esteem* (e.g. limit negative self-assessment, encourage positive communication about self, assist to identify strengths, give positive feedback about accomplishments and behaviors that are indicative of high self-esteem).

g. Implement measures *to reduce drooling if it occurs:*
   1. instruct client to wipe mouth or suction oral cavity frequently (if circumoral paresthesias are present, client may be unaware of drooling)
   2. perform actions to improve client's ability to swallow (see Postoperative Nursing Diagnosis 3, action b).

h. Provide privacy for client when eating if indicated *to reduce embarrassment associated with swallowing difficulties.*

i. Remain with client for the first look at the operative area after removal of dressings. Explain that some of the physical changes will not be as severe once edema and redness have subsided and the tracheostomy tube is out. (Facial edema that may occur with a radical neck dissection peaks by the fifth postoperative day and may take 2–6 months to resolve totally).

j. If client is experiencing impaired movement and strength of neck and shoulder on the affected side, inform him/her that improvement usually occurs if the prescribed exercise and physical therapy regimen is followed and that wearing clothing with shoulder padding can help camouflage a drooping shoulder.

k. Suggest clothing styles and accessories that help camouflage the stoma (e.g. stoma bibs, neck scarves, ties, ascots, clothing with high collars) and accessories that help to draw attention away from the neck area (e.g. hats, belts).

l. Encourage client to pursue available options for regaining speech (e.g. voice prosthesis, esophageal speech, artificial larynx).

m. Assist client with usual grooming and makeup habits if necessary.

n. Promote activities that require client to confront the physical changes that have occurred (e.g. suctioning, tracheostomy care, tube feeding). Be aware that integration of the changes in body image do not usually occur until 2–6 months after the actual physical changes have occurred.

o. Demonstrate acceptance of client using techniques such as touch and frequent visits. Encourage significant others to do the same.

p. Support behaviors suggesting positive adaptation to changes that have occurred (e.g. willingness to participate in wound and tracheostomy care, tube feedings, and suctioning; compliance with treatment plan; communication of feelings of self-worth; maintenance of relationships with significant others).

q. Encourage significant others to allow client to do what he/she is able *so that independence can be re-established and/or self-esteem redeveloped.*

r. Encourage client contact with others *so that he/she can test and establish a new self-image.*

s. Assist client's and significant others' adjustment by listening, facilitating communication, and providing information.

t. If client appears to be rejecting significant others, explain to them that this is a common occurrence (client rejects family and/or spouse before they have a chance to reject him/her). Encourage them to visit often and persist in offering understanding and support for the client.

Desired Outcome	Nursing Actions and *Selected Purposes/Rationales*
	u. Assist client and significant others to have similar expectations and understanding of future life style and to identify ways that personal and family goals can be adjusted rather than abandoned.
	v. Encourage client to pursue usual roles and interests and to continue involvement in social activities. If previous roles, interests, and hobbies cannot be pursued, encourage development of new ones.
	w. Provide information about and encourage utilization of community resources and support groups (e.g. Lost Chord Club; New Voice Club; American Cancer Society; vocational rehabilitation; sexual, family, individual, and/or financial counseling).
	x. Consult physician about psychological counseling if client desires or seems unwilling or unable to adapt to changes resulting from the laryngectomy and radical neck dissection.

■

9. NURSING DIAGNOSIS: **Ineffective individual coping**

related to:
a. loss of ability to speak normally and audibly laugh and cry;
b. difficulty mastering new speech techniques;
c. fear of rejection by significant others;
d. fear, anxiety, and/or loss of control associated with changes in appearance and body functioning, the diagnosis of cancer, and possibility of disease recurrence;
e. self-care expectations regarding tube feeding and wound and tracheostomy care.

Desired Outcome	Nursing Actions and *Selected Purposes/Rationales*

9. The client will demonstrate effective coping as evidenced by:
 a. communication of ability to cope with the effects of the laryngectomy and radical neck dissection
 b. utilization of appropriate problem-solving techniques
 c. willingness to participate in treatment plan and meet basic needs
 d. absence of destructive behavior toward self and others
 e. appropriate use of defense mechanisms
 f. utilization of available support systems.
	9.a. Assess for and report signs and symptoms of ineffective individual coping (e.g. communication of inability to cope; inability to ask for help, problem solve, or meet basic needs; insomnia; withdrawal; reluctance to participate in treatment plan; destructive behavior toward self or others; inappropriate use of defense mechanisms; inability to meet role expectations).
	 b. Assess client's perception of current situation.
	 c. Implement measures *to promote effective coping:*
	   1. expect and encourage client to participate in tracheostomy and wound care, tube feeding, and suctioning as soon as possible (*active participation in care in the early postoperative period facilitates adjustment to changes experienced*)
	   2. assist client to recognize and manage inappropriate denial if it is present
	   3. if acceptable to client, arrange for a visit with another individual who has successfully adjusted to the loss of the larynx
	   4. perform actions to assist the client to adapt to changes in appearance, body functioning, life style, and roles (see Postoperative Nursing Diagnosis 8, actions d–w)
	   5. perform actions to facilitate communication (see Postoperative Nursing Diagnosis 4, action a)
	   6. reinforce physician's explanations and clarify misconceptions about the diagnosis and prognosis
	   7. encourage client to communicate feelings about current situation
	   8. assist client to identify personal strengths and resources that can be utilized to facilitate coping with the current situation
	   9. create an atmosphere of trust and support
	   10. include client in planning of care, encourage maximum participation in treatment plan, and allow choices when possible *to enable him/her to maintain a sense of control*

11. instruct client in effective problem-solving techniques (e.g. accurate identification of stressors, determination of various options to solve problem)
12. assist client to maintain usual daily routines whenever possible
13. assist client to identify priorities and attainable goals as he/she starts to plan for necessary life-style and role changes
14. assist client through methods such as role playing to prepare for negative reactions from others because of changes in appearance and inability to speak normally
15. administer antianxiety and/or antidepressant agents if ordered
16. assist client to identify and utilize available support systems; provide information about available community resources that can assist client and significant others in coping with effects of surgery (e.g. New Voice Club, Lost Chord Club, American Cancer Society, vocational rehabilitation, International Association of Laryngectomees)
17. encourage client to share with significant others the kind of support that would be most beneficial (e.g. being there, inspiring hope, providing reassurance and accurate information)
18. support behaviors indicative of effective coping (e.g. participating in treatment plan and self-care activities, communication of ability to cope, recognition and utilization of available support systems and effective problem-solving strategies).

    d. Consult physician about psychological and vocational counseling if appropriate. Initiate a referral if necessary.

---

10. NURSING DIAGNOSIS:	**Grieving***

related to:

a. changes in appearance and body functioning (e.g. neck breathing; loss of ability to speak normally, sing, blow nose, and audibly laugh and cry; impaired sense of smell and taste; impaired shoulder movement);
b. possible changes in life style and roles.

---

*This diagnostic label includes anticipatory grieving and grieving following the actual losses.

Desired Outcome	Nursing Actions and *Selected Purposes/Rationales*

10. The client will demonstrate beginning progression through the grieving process as evidenced by:
   a. communication of feelings about the effects of the laryngectomy and radical neck dissection on appearance, body functioning, life style, and roles
   b. usual sleep pattern
   c. participation in treatment plan and self-care activities
   d. utilization of available support systems.

10.a. Assess for signs and symptoms of grieving (e.g. change in eating habits, inability to concentrate, insomnia, anger, sadness, withdrawal from significant others, denial of loss).
  b. Implement measures *to facilitate the grieving process:*
    1. assist client to acknowledge the losses *so grief work can begin;* assess for factors that may hinder and facilitate acknowledgment
    2. discuss the grieving process and assist client to accept the phases of grieving as an expected response to actual and/or anticipated losses
    3. allow time for client to progress through the phases of grieving (phases vary among theorists but progress from shock and alarm to acceptance); be aware that not every phase is expressed by all individuals, that recurrence of phases is common, and that the grieving process may take months to years
    4. provide an atmosphere of care and concern (e.g. provide privacy, be available and nonjudgmental, display empathy and respect) *so client will feel free to express feelings*
    5. perform actions *to promote trust* (e.g. answer questions honestly, provide requested information)

Desired Outcome	Nursing Actions and *Selected Purposes/Rationales*
	6. encourage the expression of anger and sadness about the losses experienced; recognize displacement of anger and assist client to see the actual cause of angry feelings and resentment
	7. encourage client to express feelings in whatever ways are comfortable (e.g. writing, drawing)
	8. perform actions to promote effective coping (see Postoperative Nursing Diagnosis 9, action c)
	9. support realistic hope regarding ability to resume usual activities and regain speech
	10. support behaviors suggesting successful grief work (e.g. communicating feelings about the loss of speech and changes in body functioning, focusing on ways to adapt to losses, learning needed skills, developing or renewing relationships)
	11. explain the phases of the grieving process to significant others; encourage their support and understanding
	12. provide information regarding counseling services and support groups that might assist client in working through grief
	13. facilitate communication between the client and significant others; be aware that they may be in different phases of the grieving process
	14. when appropriate, assist client to meet spiritual needs (e.g. arrange for a visit from clergy).
	c. Consult physician regarding referral for counseling if signs of dysfunctional grieving (e.g. persistent denial of losses, excessive anger or sadness, emotional lability) occur.

Discharge Teaching

∎━━

11. NURSING DIAGNOSIS: **Knowledge deficit, Ineffective management of therapeutic regimen, or Altered health maintenance***

*The nurse should select the diagnostic label that is most appropriate for the client's discharge teaching needs.

Desired Outcomes	Nursing Actions and *Selected Purposes/Rationales*
11.a. The client will demonstrate appropriate stomal care, suctioning, tracheostomy tube care, oral hygiene, and tube feeding techniques.	11.a.1. Reinforce instructions and demonstrate the following if appropriate: a. procedure for insertion of new tracheostomy tube in an emergency situation b. procedure for cleaning stoma and changing tracheostomy tube ties and dressing c. methods for maintaining skin integrity around stoma (e.g. keep skin clean and dry) d. removal and cleaning of the inner cannula e. oral and tracheal suctioning f. ways to increase moisture content of inspired air (e.g. use humidifier, wear a moist bib, place pans of water throughout the home) g. administration of nasogastric or gastrostomy tube feedings h. oral care (e.g. irrigation with normal saline or a solution of hydrogen peroxide and water). 2. Allow time for questions, clarification, practice, and return demonstration.
11.b. The client will demonstrate the ability to effectively use and care for an artificial larynx.	11.b.1. Reinforce instructions from speech pathologist about use and care of artificial larynx if appropriate. 2. Allow time for questions, clarification, and return demonstration.

11.c. The client will demonstrate the ability to care for the tracheoesophageal puncture (TEP) and voice prosthesis if in place.	11.c.1. Provide the following instructions about care of the TEP and voice prosthesis if in place: a. clean and reinsert voice prosthesis as instructed by physician or speech pathologist (some models are removed daily and cleaned with a hydrogen peroxide solution while others are left in place and cleaned with an applicator) b. maintain the TEP site by inserting a catheter (stent) when the prosthesis is out for cleaning or for any other reason (the puncture site will close in 1–2 hours if stent or prosthesis is not in place); if unable to insert catheter or prosthesis, call physician or go to the closest medical emergency care facility immediately to have it done c. secure prosthesis strap to skin above stoma with nonallergenic tape d. take antifungal medication (e.g. Mycelex troche) as prescribed to prevent or control growth of *Candida albicans* on the prosthesis (a fungal infection can eventually interfere with function of the valve in the prosthesis) e. instruct client to report leakage of food/fluids or saliva around TEP site f. have prosthesis replaced as often as instructed by physician. 2. Emphasize the importance of indicating on his/her medical alert bracelet or tag that a voice prosthesis is in place. 3. Allow time for questions, clarification, and return demonstration.
11.d. The client will identify appropriate safety precautions related to the presence of a tracheostomy and nerve damage resulting from surgery.	11.d. Provide the following instructions regarding appropriate safety precautions related to the presence of a tracheostomy and nerve damage resulting from surgery: 1. always keep an obturator and outer cannula available for an emergency situation 2. always wear a medical alert bracelet or tag indicating neck breather status 3. reduce the risk of injury in surgical area (the area will remain numb for several months after surgery): a. use an electric rather than a straight-edge razor in order to decrease risk of cuts in surgical area b. avoid extremely hot foods/fluids to decrease risk of burning the oral cavity or esophagus 4. have smoke detectors installed in home because of impaired sense of smell 5. prevent blockage of stoma and/or entrance of foreign particles into stoma: a. do not wear constrictive clothing around neck b. wear a protective shield over stoma (e.g. crocheted bib, moistened 4 × 4 gauze pad, scarf, ascot) at all times c. prevent water from entering stoma (e.g. do not swim unless wearing special snorkel device designed for neck breathers, direct shower nozzle well below stoma, use stoma guard or shield while bathing) d. apply shaving cream by hand rather than spraying directly on face and neck e. cover stoma while shaving or getting a hair cut f. avoid close contact with animals that shed 6. if shoulder and neck movement are impaired, use caution when driving.
11.e. The client will identify signs and symptoms to report to the health care provider.	11.e.1. Refer to Standardized Postoperative Care Plan, Nursing Diagnosis 21, action c (p. 123), for signs and symptoms to report to the health care provider. 2. Instruct client to report these additional signs and symptoms: a. persistent choking or difficulty swallowing b. bloody oral secretions c. presence of blood or ingested liquid, food, or tube feeding formula in secretions from stoma d. darkening of skin flaps or separation of wound edges

Desired Outcomes	Nursing Actions and *Selected Purposes/Rationales*
	e. increased weakness of arm on affected side
	f. persistent pain in or drooping of shoulder on affected side
	g. nausea, vomiting, diarrhea, and/or cramping associated with tube feeding.
11.f. The client will identify community resources that can assist with home management and adjustment to the effects of surgery.	11.f.1. Provide information about community resources that can assist the client and significant others with home management and adjustment to the surgery (e.g. American Cancer Society, home health agencies, counselors, social service agencies, New Voice Club, Lost Chord Club, vocational rehabilitation, International Association of Laryngectomees, church groups, American Speech and Hearing Association).
	2. Initiate a referral if indicated.
11.g. The client will communicate an understanding of and a plan for adhering to recommended follow-up care including future appointments with health care provider and speech pathologist, medications prescribed, exercises, activity level, and wound care.	11.g.1. Refer to Standardized Postoperative Care Plan, Nursing Diagnosis 21 (pp. 123–124), for routine postoperative instructions and measures to improve client compliance.
	2. Caution client to avoid lifting more than 2 pounds with the affected arm until healing occurs and strength improves.
	3. Emphasize the importance of adhering to prescribed exercise program to strengthen shoulder and neck muscles on the affected side.
	4. Encourage client to follow up with speech rehabilitation if appropriate.

Bibliography

See pages 897–898 and 911.

▦ Appendix
Nursing Diagnoses Approved by NANDA* Through 1996†

ACTIVITY INTOLERANCE
Definition

A state in which an individual has insufficient physiological or psychological energy to endure or complete required or desired daily activities.

Defining Characteristics

*Verbal report of fatigue or weakness; abnormal heart rate or blood pressure response to activity; exertional discomfort or dyspnea; electrocardiographic changes reflecting arrhythmias or ischemia.

Related Factors

Bedrest/immobility; generalized weakness; sedentary life style; imbalance between oxygen supply/demand.

---

*Critical defining characteristic.

ACTIVITY INTOLERANCE, RISK FOR
Definition

A state in which an individual is at risk of experiencing insufficient physiological or psychological energy to endure or complete required or desired daily activities.

Defining Characteristics
Presence of risk factors such as:

History of previous intolerance; deconditioned status; presence of circulatory/respiratory problems; inexperience with the activity.

Related Factors

See risk factors.

ADJUSTMENT, IMPAIRED
Definition

The state in which the individual is unable to modify his/her life style/behavior in a manner consistent with a change in health status.

Defining Characteristics
Major

Verbalization of nonacceptance of health status change; nonexistent or unsuccessful ability to be involved in problem solving or goal setting.

---

*North American Nursing Diagnosis Association.

†These diagnostic labels with definitions, defining characteristics, and related factors are reprinted from NANDA Nursing Diagnoses: Definitions & Classification 1997–1998 published by North American Nursing Diagnosis Association, 1211 Locust Street, Philadelphia, PA 19107.

Minor

Lack of movement toward independence; extended period of shock, disbelief, or anger regarding health status change; lack of future-oriented thinking.

Related Factors

Disability requiring change in life style; inadequate support systems; impaired cognition; sensory overload; assault to self-esteem; altered locus of control; incomplete grieving.

AIRWAY CLEARANCE, INEFFECTIVE
Definition

A state in which an individual is unable to clear secretions or obstructions from the respiratory tract.

Defining Characteristics

Abnormal breath sounds (crackles, gurgles, wheezes); cough, ineffective or absent; reports difficulty with sputum; reports chest congestion.

Recommend Further Research for the Following Defining Characteristics

Change in rate and depth of respiration, effective cough, tenacious and copious sputum, fatigue.

Related Factors

Decreased energy; tracheobronchial infection, obstruction, secretion; perceptual/cognitive impairment; trauma.

ANXIETY
Definition

A vague uneasy feeling whose source is often nonspecific or unknown to the individual.

Defining Characteristics

Subjective: increased tension; apprehension; painful and persistent increased helplessness; uncertainty; fearful; scared; regretful; overexcited; rattled; distressed; jittery; feelings of inadequacy; shakiness; fear of unspecific consequences; expressed concerns about change in life events; worried; anxious.

Objective: *sympathetic stimulation-cardiovascular excitation, superficial vasoconstriction, pupil dilation; restlessness; insomnia; glancing about; poor eye contact; trembling/hand tremors; extraneous movement (foot shuffling, hand/arm movements); facial tension; voice

---

*Critical defining characteristics.

quivering; focus on self; increased wariness; increased perspiration.

Related Factors

Unconscious conflict about essential values/goals of life; threat to self-concept; threat of death; threat to or change in health status; threat to or change in role functioning; threat to or change in environment; threat to or change in interaction patterns; situational/maturational crises; interpersonal transmission/contagion; unmet needs.

ASPIRATION, RISK FOR
Definition

The state in which an individual is at risk for entry of gastrointestinal secretions, oropharyngeal secretions, or solids or fluids into tracheobronchial passages.

Defining Characteristics
Presence of risk factors such as:

Reduced level of consciousness; depressed cough and gag reflexes; presence of tracheostomy or endotracheal tube; incompetent lower esophageal sphincter; gastrointestinal tubes; tube feedings; medication administration; situations hindering elevation of upper body; increased intragastric pressure; increased gastric residual; decreased gastrointestinal motility; delayed gastric emptying; impaired swallowing; facial/oral/neck surgery or trauma; wired jaws.

Related Factors

See risk factors.

BODY IMAGE DISTURBANCE
Definition

Disruption in the way one perceives one's body image.

Defining Characteristics

A *or* B must be present to justify the diagnosis of body image disturbance. *A = verbal response to actual or perceived change in structure and/or function; *B = nonverbal response to actual or perceived change in structure and/or function. The following clinical manifestations may be used to validate the presence of A *or* B.

Objective: missing body part; actual change in structure and/or function; not looking at body part; not touching body part; hiding or overexposing body part (intentional or unintentional); trauma to nonfunctioning part; change in social involvement; change in ability to estimate spatial relationship of body to environment.

Subjective: verbalization of: change in life style; fear of rejection or of reaction by others; focus on past strength, function, or appearance; negative feelings about body; and feelings of helplessness, hopelessness, or powerlessness; preoccupation with change or loss; emphasis on remaining strengths, heightened achievement; extension of body boundary to incorporate environmental objects; personalization of part or loss by name; depersonalization of part or loss by impersonal pronouns; refusal to verify actual change.

---

*Critical defining characteristics.

Related Factors

Biophysical; cognitive/perceptual; psychosocial; cultural or spiritual.

BODY TEMPERATURE, RISK FOR, ALTERED
Definition

The state in which the individual is at risk for failure to maintain body temperature within normal range.

Defining Characteristics
Presence of risk factors such as:

Extremes of age; extremes of weight; exposure to cold/cool or warm/hot environments; dehydration; inactivity or vigorous activity; medications causing vasoconstriction/vasodilation; altered metabolic rate; sedation; inappropriate clothing for environmental temperature; illness or trauma affecting temperature regulation.

Related Factors

See risk factors.

BOWEL INCONTINENCE
Definition

A state in which an individual experiences a change in normal bowel habits characterized by involuntary passage of stool.

Defining Characteristics

Involuntary passage of stool.

Related Factors

Gastrointestinal disorders; neuromuscular disorders; colostomy; loss of rectal sphincter control; impaired cognition.

BREASTFEEDING, EFFECTIVE
Definition

The state in which a mother-infant dyad/family exhibits adequate proficiency and satisfaction with breastfeeding process.

Defining Characteristics
Major

Mother able to position infant at breast to promote a successful latch-on response; infant is content after feeding; regular and sustained suckling/swallowing at the breast; appropriate infant weight patterns for age; effective mother/infant communication patterns (infant cues, maternal interpretation and response).

Minor

Signs and/or symptoms of oxytocin release (let down or milk ejection reflex); adequate infant elimination patterns for age; eagerness of infant to nurse; maternal verbalization of satisfaction with the breastfeeding process.

Related Factors

Basic breastfeeding knowledge; normal breast structure; normal infant-oral structure; infant gestational age greater than 34 weeks; support sources; maternal confidence.

BREASTFEEDING, INEFFECTIVE

Definition

The state in which a mother, infant, or child experiences dissatisfaction or difficulty with the breastfeeding process.

Defining Characteristics

Major

Unsatisfactory breastfeeding process.

Minor

Actual or perceived inadequate milk supply; infant inability to attach onto maternal breast correctly; no observable signs of oxytocin release; observable signs of inadequate infant intake; nonsustained suckling at the breast; insufficient emptying of each breast per feeding; persistence of sore nipples beyond the first week of breastfeeding; insufficient opportunity for suckling at the breast; infant exhibiting fussiness and crying within the first hour after breastfeeding; unresponsive to other comfort measures; infant arching and crying at the breast; resisting latching on.

Related Factors

Prematurity; infant anomaly; maternal breast anomaly; previous breast surgery; previous history of breastfeeding failure; infant receiving supplemental feedings with artificial nipple; poor infant sucking reflex; nonsupportive partner/family; knowledge deficit; interruption in breastfeeding; maternal anxiety or ambivalence.

BREASTFEEDING, INTERRUPTED

Definition

A break in the continuity of the breastfeeding process as a result of inability or inadvisability to put baby to breast for feeding.

Defining Characteristics

Major

Infant does not receive nourishment at the breast for some or all of feedings.

Minor

Maternal desire to maintain lactation and provide (or eventually provide) her breastmilk for her infant's nutritional needs; separation of mother and infant; lack of knowledge regarding expression and storage of breastmilk.

Related Factors

Maternal or infant illness; prematurity; maternal employment; contraindications to breastfeeding (e.g. drugs, true breastmilk jaundice); need to abruptly wean infant.

BREATHING PATTERN, INEFFECTIVE

Definition

A state in which the rate, depth, timing, rhythm or chest/abdominal wall excursion during inspiration, expiration or both does not maintain optimum ventilation for the individual.

Defining Characteristics

Dyspnea, shortness of breath; respiratory rate (adults [ages 14 or greater] <11 or >24, infants <25 or >60, ages 1–4 <20 or >30, ages 5–14 <15 or >25); depth of breathing (adults VT <200 ml or >500 ml at rest, infants 6–8 ml/kilo); timing ratio of inspiration and expiration (if measured): inspiratory time <1:2 or >2:4), fractional inspiratory time <.36 or >.47, inspiration longer than expiration; irregular breathing rhythm (e.g. apnea, frequent sighs, use of accessory muscles of breathing inappropriate to level of activity, asynchronous thoracoabdominal motion); grunting; nasal flaring (infants); paradoxical breathing patterns; use of accessory muscles; altered chest excursion.

Recommend Further Research for the Following Defining Characteristics

Fremitus, abnormal arterial blood gas, cyanosis, cough, assumption of a 3-point position, pursed lip breathing, prolonged expiratory phases, increased anteroposterior diameter.

Related Factors

Neuromuscular impairment; pain; musculoskeletal impairment; perception/cognitive impairment; anxiety; decreased energy/fatigue.

CARDIAC OUTPUT, DECREASED

Definition

A state in which the blood pumped by the heart is inadequate to meet the metabolic demands of the body.

Defining Characteristics

Variations in BP readings; arrhythmias; fatigue; jugular venous distention (JVD); skin color changes; rales; oliguria; decreased peripheral pulses; cold, clammy skin; dyspnea; orthopnea/paroxysmal nocturnal dyspnea (PND); restlessness; chest pain; weight gain; wheezing; edema; elevated PA pressures; increased respiratory rate; use of accessory muscles; ECG changes; ejection fraction <40%; abnormal chest x-ray (pulmonary vascular congestion); abnormal cardiac enzymes; altered mental status.

Recommend Further Research for the Following Defining Characteristics

Decreased peripheral pulses, decreased CO by thermodilution method, increased heart rate, S_3 or S_4, cough, mixed venous O_2 (SaO_2).

Related Factors

To be developed.

CAREGIVER ROLE STRAIN
Definition

A caregiver's felt difficulty in performing the family caregiver role.

Defining Characteristics

Caregivers report they: do not have enough resources to provide the care needed; find it hard to do specific caregiving activities; worry about such things as the care receiver's health and emotional state, having to put the care receiver in an institution, and who will care for the care receiver if something should happen to the caregiver; feel that caregiving interferes with other important roles in their lives. Feel loss because the care receiver is like a different person compared to before caregiving began or, in the case of a child, that the care receiver was never the child the caregiver expected; feel family conflict around issues of providing care; feel stress or nervousness in their relationship with the care receiver; feel depressed.

Related Factors

Pathophysiological/Physiological: illness severity of the care receiver; addiction or codependency; premature birth/congenital defect; discharge of family member with significant home care needs; caregiver health impairment; unpredictable illness course or instability in the care receiver's health; caregiver is female.
Developmental: caregiver is not developmentally ready for caregiver role, e.g. young adult needing to provide for a middle-aged parent; developmental delay or retardation of the care receiver or caregiver.
Psychosocial: psychological or cognitive problems in care receiver; marginal family adaptation or dysfunction prior to the caregiving situation; marginal caregiver's coping patterns; past history of poor relationship between caregiver and care receiver; caregiver is spouse; care receiver exhibits deviant, bizarre behavior.
Situational: presence of abuse or violence; presence of situational stressors which normally affect families, such as: significant loss, disaster or crisis, poverty or economic vulnerability, major life events, e.g. birth, hospitalization, leaving home, returning home, marriage, divorce, employment, retirement, death; duration of caregiving required; inadequate physical environment for providing care, e.g. housing, transportation, community services, equipment; family/caregiver isolation; lack of respite and recreation for caregiver; inexperience with caregiving; caregiver's competing role commitments; complexity/amount of caregiving tasks.

CAREGIVER ROLE STRAIN, RISK FOR
Definition

A caregiver is vulnerable for felt difficulty in performing the family caregiver role.

Risk Factors

Pathophysiological/Physiological: illness severity of the care receiver; addiction or codependency; premature birth/congenital defect; discharge of family member with significant home care needs; caregiver health impairment; unpredictable illness course or instability in the care receiver's health; caregiver is female; psychological or cognitive problems in care receiver.
Developmental: caregiver is not developmentally ready for caregiver role, e.g. young adult needing to provide for a middle-aged parent; developmental delay or retardation of the care receiver or caregiver.
Psychosocial: marginal family adaptation or dysfunction prior to the caregiving situation; marginal caregiver's coping patterns; past history of poor relationship between caregiver and care receiver; caregiver is spouse; care receiver exhibits deviant, bizarre behavior.
Situational: presence of abuse or violence; presence of situational stressors which normally affect families, such as significant loss, disaster or crisis, poverty or economic vulnerability, major life events, e.g. birth, hospitalization, leaving home, returning home, marriage, divorce, employment, retirement, death; duration of caregiving required; inadequate physical environment for providing care, e.g. housing, transportation, community services, equipment; family/caregiver isolation; lack of respite and recreation for caregiver; inexperience with caregiving; caregiver's competing role commitments; complexity/amount of caregiving tasks.

Related Factors

See risk factors.

COMMUNICATION, IMPAIRED VERBAL
Definition

The state in which an individual experiences a decreased or absent ability to use or understand language in human interaction.

Defining Characteristics

*Unable to speak dominant language; *speaks or verbalizes with difficulty; *does not or cannot speak; stuttering; slurring; difficulty forming words or sentences; difficulty expressing thought verbally; inappropriate verbalization; dyspnea; disorientation.

Related Factors

Decrease in circulation to brain; brain tumor; physical barrier (tracheostomy, intubation); anatomical defect, cleft palate; psychological barriers (psychosis, lack of stimuli); cultural difference; developmental or age-related.

---

*Critical defining characteristics.

CONFUSION, ACUTE
Definition

The abrupt onset of a cluster of global, transient changes and disturbances in attention, cognition, psychomotor activity level of consciousness, and/or sleep/wake cycle.

Defining Characteristics
Major

Fluctuation in cognition; fluctuation in sleep/wake cycle; fluctuation in level of consciousness; fluctuation in psychomotor activity, increased agitation or restlessness; misperceptions; lack of motivation to initiate and/or follow through with goal-directed or purposeful behavior.

Minor

Hallucinations.

Related Factors

Over 60 years of age; dementia; alcohol abuse; drug abuse; delirium.

CONFUSION, CHRONIC
Definition

An irreversible, long-standing and/or progressive deterioration of intellect and personality characterized by decreased ability to interpret environmental stimuli, decreased capacity for intellectual thought processes and manifested by disturbances of memory, orientation, and behavior.

Defining Characteristics

Major

Clinical evidence of organic impairment; altered interpretation/response to stimuli; progressive/long-standing cognitive impairment.

Minor

No change in level of consciousness; impaired socialization; impaired memory (short term, long term); altered personality.

Related Factors

Alzheimer's disease; Korsakoff's psychosis; Multi-infarct Dementia; cerebral vascular accident; head injury.

CONSTIPATION
Definition

A state in which an individual experiences a change in normal bowel habits characterized by a decrease in frequency and/or passage of hard, dry stools.

Defining Characteristics

Decreased activity level; frequency less than usual pattern; hard, formed stools; palpable mass; reported feeling of pressure in rectum; reported feeling of rectal fullness; straining at stool.

Other Possible Characteristics

Abdominal pain; appetite impairment; back pain; headache; interference with daily living; use of laxatives.

Related Factors

To be developed.

CONSTIPATION, COLONIC
Definition

The state in which an individual's pattern of elimination is characterized by hard, dry stool that results from a delay in passage of food residue.

Defining Characteristics

Major

Decreased frequency; hard, dry stool; straining at stool; painful defecation; abdominal distention; palpable mass.

Minor

Rectal pressure; headache; appetite impairment; abdominal pain.

Related Factors

Less than adequate fluid intake; less than adequate dietary intake; less than adequate fiber; less than adequate physical activity; immobility; lack of privacy; emotional disturbances; chronic use of medication and enemas; stress; change in daily routine; metabolic problems, e.g. hypothyroidism, hypocalcemia, hypokalemia.

CONSTIPATION, PERCEIVED
Definition

The state in which an individual makes a self-diagnosis of constipation and ensures a daily bowel movement through abuse of laxatives, enemas, and suppositories.

Defining Characteristics

Major

Expectation of a daily bowel movement with the resulting overuse of laxatives, enemas, and suppositories; expected passage of stool at same time every day.

Related Factors

Cultural/family health beliefs; faulty appraisal; impaired thought processes.

COPING, COMMUNITY, INEFFECTIVE
Definition

A pattern of community activities for adaptation and problem solving that is unsatisfactory for meeting the demands or needs of the community.

Defining Characteristics

Major

None.

Minor

Community does not meet its own expectations; deficits in community participation; deficits in communication methods; excessive community conflicts; expressed difficulty in meeting demands for change; expressed vulnerability; high illness rates; stressors perceived as excessive.

Related Factors

Deficits in social support; inadequate resources for problem solving; powerlessness.

COPING, COMMUNITY, POTENTIAL FOR ENHANCED
Definition

A pattern of community activities for adaptation and problem solving that is satisfactory for meeting the demands or needs of the community but can be improved for management of current and future problems/stressors.

Defining Characteristics

Major

Deficits in one or more characteristics that indicate effective coping.

Minor

Active planning by community for predicted stressors; active problem solving by community when faced with issues; agreement that community is responsible for stress management; positive communication among community members; positive communication between community/aggregates and larger community; programs available for recreation and relaxation; resources sufficient for managing stressors.

Related Factors

Social supports available; resources available for problem solving; community has a sense of power to manage stressors.

COPING, DEFENSIVE

Definition

The state in which an individual repeatedly projects falsely positive self-evaluation based on a self-protective pattern that defends against underlying perceived threats to positive self-regard.

Defining Characteristics

Major

Denial of obvious problems/weaknesses; projection of blame/responsibility; rationalizes failures; hypersensitive to slight criticism; grandiosity.

Minor

Superior attitude toward others; difficulty establishing/maintaining relationships; hostile laughter or ridicule of others; difficulty in reality testing perceptions; lack of follow-through or participation in treatment or therapy.

COPING, FAMILY: POTENTIAL FOR GROWTH

Definition

Effective managing of adaptive tasks by family member involved with the client's health challenge, who now is exhibiting desire and readiness for enhanced health and growth in regard to self and in relation to the client.

Defining Characteristics

Family member attempting to describe growth impact of crisis on his/her own values, priorities, goal, or relationships; family member moving in direction of health-promoting and enriching life style that supports and monitors maturational processes, audits and negotiates treatment programs, and generally chooses experiences that optimize wellness; individual expressing interest in making contact on a one-to-one basis or on a mutual-aid group basis with another person who has experienced a similar situation.

Related Factors

Needs sufficiently gratified and adaptive tasks effectively addressed to enable goals of self-actualization to surface.

COPING, FAMILY: INEFFECTIVE, COMPROMISED

Definition

A usually supportive primary person (family member or close friend) is providing insufficient, ineffective, or compromised support, comfort, assistance, or encouragement which may be needed by the client to manage or master adaptive tasks related to his or her health challenge.

Defining Characteristics

Subjective: client expresses or confirms a concern or complaint about significant other's response to his or her health problem; significant person describes preoccupation with personal reaction (e.g. fear, anticipatory grief, guilt, anxiety to illness, disability, or to other situational or developmental crises); significant person describes or confirms an inadequate understanding or knowledge base which interferes with effective assistive or supportive behaviors.

Objective: significant person attempts assistive or supportive behaviors with less than satisfactory results; significant person withdraws or enters into limited or temporary personal communication with the client at the time of need; significant person displays protective behavior disproportionate (too little or too much) to the abilities or need for autonomy.

Related Factors

Inadequate or incorrect information or understanding by a primary person; temporary preoccupation by a significant person who is trying to manage emotional conflicts and personal suffering and is unable to perceive or act effectively in regard to needs; temporary family disorganization and role changes; other situational or developmental crises or situations the significant person may be facing; little support provided by client, in turn, for primary person; prolonged disease or disability progression that exhausts supportive capacity of significant people.

COPING, FAMILY: INEFFECTIVE, DISABLING

Definition

Behavior of significant person (family member or other primary person) that disables his or her own capacities and the capacity to effectively address tasks essential to either person's adaptation to the health challenge.

Defining Characteristics

Neglectful care of the client in regard to basic human needs and/or illness treatment; distortion of reality regarding the health problem, including extreme denial about its existence or severity; intolerance; rejection; abandonment; desertion; carrying on usual routines, disregarding needs; psychosomaticism; taking on illness signs of client; decisions and actions by family which are detrimental to economic or social well-being; agitation, depression, aggression, hostility; impaired restructuring of a meaningful life for self, impaired individualization, prolonged overconcern for client; neglectful relationships with other family members; client's development of helpless, inactive dependence.

Related Factors

Significant person with chronically unexpressed feelings of guilt, anxiety, hostility, despair, etc.; dissonant discrepancy of coping styles for dealing with adaptive tasks by the significant person and client or among significant people; highly ambivalent family relationships; arbitrary handling of family's resistance to treatment, which tends to solidify defensiveness, as it fails to deal adequately with underlying anxiety.

COPING, INDIVIDUAL: INEFFECTIVE
Definition

Impairment of adaptive behaviors and abilities of a person in meeting life's demands and roles.

Defining Characteristics

*Verbalization of inability to cope or inability to ask for help; inability to meet role expectations; inability to meet basic needs; *inability to problem-solve; alteration in societal participation; destructive behavior toward self or others; inappropriate use of defense mechanisms; change in usual communication patterns; verbal manipulation; high illness rate; high rate of accidents; expression of anxiety, depression, fear, impatience, frustration, irritability, discouragement, and life stress.

Related Factors

Situational crises; maturational crises; vulnerability.

---

*Critical defining characteristics.

DECISIONAL CONFLICT (SPECIFY)
Definition

The state of uncertainty about course of action to be taken when choice among competing actions involves risk, loss, or challenge to personal life values.

Defining Characteristics
Major

Verbalized uncertainty about choices; verbalization of undesired consequences of alternative actions being considered; vacillation between alternative choices; delayed decision making.

Minor

Verbalized feeling of distress while attempting a decision; self-focusing; physical signs of distress or tension (increased heart rate, increased muscle tension, restlessness, etc.); questioning personal values and beliefs while attempting a decision.

Related Factors

Unclear personal values/beliefs; perceived threat to value system; lack of experience or interference with decision making; lack of relevant information; support system deficit; multiple or divergent sources of information.

DENIAL, INEFFECTIVE
Definition

The state of a conscious or unconscious attempt to disavow the knowledge or meaning of an event to reduce anxiety/fear to the detriment of health.

Defining Characteristics
Major

Delays seeking or refuses health care attention to the detriment of health; does not perceive personal relevance of symptoms or danger.

Minor

Uses home remedies (self-treatment) to relieve symptoms; does not admit fear of death or invalidism; minimizes symptoms; displaces source of symptoms to other organs; unable to admit impact of disease on life pattern; makes dismissive gestures or comments when speaking of distressing events; displaces fear of impact of the condition; displays inappropriate affect.

DIARRHEA
Definition

A state in which an individual experiences a change in normal bowel habits characterized by the frequent passage of loose, fluid, unformed stools.

Defining Characteristics

Abdominal pain; cramping; increased frequency; increased frequency of bowel sounds; loose, liquid stools; urgency.

Other Possible Characteristics

Change in color.

Related Factors

Gastrointestinal disorders; metabolic disorders; nutritional disorders; endocrine disorders; infectious processes; tube feedings; fecal impaction; change in dietary intake; adverse effects of medications; high stress levels.

DISUSE SYNDROME, RISK FOR
Definition

A state in which an individual is at risk for deterioration of body systems as the result of prescribed or unavoidable musculoskeletal inactivity.*

Defining Characteristics
Presence of risk factors such as:

Paralysis; mechanical immobilization; prescribed immobilization; severe pain; altered level of consciousness.

Related Factors

See risk factors.

---

*Complications from immobility can include pressure ulcer, constipation, stasis of pulmonary secretions, thrombosis, urinary tract infection/retention, decreased strength/endurance, orthostatic hypotension, decreased range of joint motion, disorientation, body image disturbance, and powerlessness.

DIVERSIONAL ACTIVITY DEFICIT
Definition

The state in which an individual experiences a decreased stimulation from (or interest or engagement in) recreational or leisure activities.

Defining Characteristics

Patient's statements regarding: boredom, wish there was something to do, to read, etc.; usual hobbies cannot be undertaken in hospital.

Related Factors

Environmental lack of diversional activity, as in long-term hospitalization, frequent lengthy treatments.

DYSREFLEXIA
Definition

The state in which an individual with a spinal cord injury at T7 or above experiences a life-threatening uninhibited sympathetic response of the nervous system to a noxious stimulus.

Defining Characteristics
Major

Individual with spinal cord injury (T7 or above) with: paroxysmal hypertension (sudden periodic elevated blood pressure where systolic pressure is over 140 mm Hg and diastolic is above 90 mm Hg); bradycardia or tachycardia (pulse rate of less than 60 or over 100 beats/minute); diaphoresis (above the injury); red splotches on skin (above the injury); pallor (below the injury); headache (a diffuse pain in different portions of the head and not confined to any nerve distribution area).

Minor

Chilling; conjunctival congestion; Horner's syndrome (contraction of the pupil, partial ptosis of the eyelid, enophthalmos and sometimes loss of sweating over the affected side of the face); paresthesia; pilomotor reflex (gooseflesh formation when skin is cooled); blurred vision; chest pain; metallic taste in mouth; nasal congestion.

Related Factors

Bladder distention; bowel distention; skin irritation; lack of patient and caregiver knowledge.

ENERGY FIELD DISTURBANCE
Definition

A disruption of the flow of energy surrounding a person's being which results in a disharmony of the body, mind, and/or spirit.

Defining Characteristics

Temperature change (warmth/coolness); visual changes (image/color); disruption of the field (vacant/hold/spike/bulge); movement (wave/spike/tingling/dense/flowing); sounds (tone/words).

ENVIRONMENTAL INTERPRETATION SYNDROME, IMPAIRED
Definition

Consistent lack of orientation to person, place, time, or circumstances over more than three to six months necessitating a protective environment.

Defining Characteristics
Major

Consistent disorientation in known and unknown environments; chronic confusional states.

Minor

Loss of occupation or social functioning from memory decline; inability to follow simple directions, instructions; inability to reason; inability to concentrate; slow in responding to questions.

Related Factors

Dementia (Alzheimer's disease, Multi-infarct Dementia, Pick's Disease, AIDS Dementia); Parkinson's Disease; Huntington's Disease; depression; alcoholism.

FAMILY PROCESS: ALCOHOLISM, ALTERED
Definition

The state in which the psychosocial, spiritual, and physiological functions of the family unit are chronically disorganized, leading to conflict, denial of problems, resistance to change, ineffective problem-solving, and a series of self-perpetuating crises.

Defining Characteristics
Major

Feelings: decreased self-esteem/worthlessness; anger/suppressed rage; frustration; powerlessness; anxiety/tension/distress; insecurity; repressed emotions; responsibility for alcoholic's behavior; lingering resentment; shame/embarrassment; hurt; unhappiness; guilt; emotional isolation/loneliness; vulnerability; mistrust; hopelessness; rejection.
Roles and Relationships: deterioration in family relationships/disturbed family dynamics; ineffective spouse communication/marital problems; altered role function/disruption of family roles; inconsistent parenting/low perception of parental support; family denial; intimacy dysfunction; chronic family problems; closed communication systems.
Behaviors: expression of anger inappropriately; difficulty with intimate relationships; loss of control of drinking; impaired communication; ineffective problem-solving skills; enabling to maintain drinking; inability to meet emotional needs of its members; manipulation; dependency; criticizing; alcohol abuse; broken promises; rationalization/denial of problems; refusal to get help/inability to accept and receive help appropriately; blaming; inadequate understanding or knowledge of alcoholism.

Minor

Feelings: being different from other people; depression; hostility; fear; emotional control by others; confusion; dissatisfaction; loss; misunderstood; abandonment; confused love and pity; moodiness; failure; being unloved; lack of identity.

Roles and Relationships: triangulating family relationships; reduced ability of family members to relate to each other for mutual growth and maturation; lack of skills necessary for relationships; lack of cohesiveness; disrupted family rituals; family unable to meet security needs of its members; family does not demonstrate respect for individuality and autonomy of its members; pattern of rejection; economic problems; neglected obligations.

Behaviors: inability to meet spiritual needs of its members; inability to express or accept wide range of feelings; orientation toward tension relief rather than achievement of goals; family special occasions are alcohol centered; escalating conflict; lying; contradictory, paradoxical communication; lack of dealing with conflict; harsh self-judgment; isolation; nicotine addiction; difficulty having fun; self-blaming; unresolved grief; controlling communication/power struggles; inability to adapt to change; immaturity; stress-related physical illnesses; inability to deal with traumatic experiences constructively; seeking approval and affirmation; lack of reliability; disturbances in academic performance in children; disturbances in concentration; chaos; substance abuse other than alcohol; failure to accomplish current or past developmental tasks/difficulty with life cycle transitions; verbal abuse of spouse or parent; agitation; diminished physical contact.

Related Factors

Abuse of alcohol; family history of alcoholism, resistance to treatment; inadequate coping skills; genetic predisposition; addictive personality; lack of problem-solving skills; biochemical influences.

FAMILY PROCESSES, ALTERED

Definition

The state in which a family that normally functions effectively experiences a dysfunction.

Defining Characteristics

Family system unable to meet physical needs of its members; family system unable to meet emotional needs of its members; family system unable to meet spiritual needs of its members; parents do not demonstrate respect for each other's views on child-rearing practices; inability to express/accept wide range of feelings; inability to express/accept feelings of members; family unable to meet security needs of its members; inability of the family members to relate to each other for mutual growth and maturation; family uninvolved in community activities; inability to accept/receive help appropriately; rigidity in function and roles; family not demonstrating respect for individuality and autonomy of its members; family unable to adapt to change/deal with traumatic experience constructively; family failing to accomplish current/past developmental task; unhealthy family decision-making process; failure to send and receive clear messages; inappropriate boundary maintenance; inappropriate/poorly communicated family rules, rituals, symbols; unexamined family myths; inappropriate level and direction of energy.

Related Factors

Situation transition and/or crisis; developmental transition and/or crisis.

FATIGUE

Definition

An overwhelming sustained sense of exhaustion and decreased capacity for physical and mental work.

Defining Characteristics

Major

Verbalization of an unremitting and overwhelming lack of energy; inability to maintain usual routines.

Minor

Perceived need for additional energy to accomplish routine tasks; increase in physical complaints; emotionally labile or irritable; impaired ability to concentrate; decreased performance; lethargic or listless; disinterest in surroundings/introspection; decreased libido; accident prone.

Related Factors

Decreased/increased metabolic energy production; overwhelming psychological or emotional demands; increased energy requirements to perform activity of daily living; excessive social and/or role demands; states of discomfort; altered body chemistry (e.g. medications, drug withdrawal, chemotherapy).

FEAR

Definition

Feeling of dread related to an identifiable source that the person validates.

Defining Characteristics

Ability to identify object of fear.

Related Factors

To be developed.

FLUID VOLUME DEFICIT

Definition

The state in which an individual experiences decreased intravascular, interstitial and/or intracellular fluid. This refers to dehydration, water loss alone without change in sodium.

Defining Characteristics

Decreased urine output; increased urine concentration; sudden weight loss; decreased venous filling; increased hematocrit; decreased skin/tongue turgor; decreased BP; dry skin/mucous membranes.

Defining Characteristics That Require Further Study

Thirst; increased pulse rate; decreased pulse volume/pressure; change in mental state; increased body temperature; weakness.

Related Factors

Active fluid volume loss; failure of regulatory mechanisms.

FLUID VOLUME DEFICIT, RISK FOR
Definition

The state in which an individual is at risk of experiencing vascular, cellular, or intracellular dehydration.

Defining Characteristics
Presence of risk factors such as:

Extremes of age; extremes of weight; excessive losses through normal routes, e.g. diarrhea; loss of fluid through abnormal routes, e.g. indwelling tubes; deviations affecting access to or intake or absorption of fluids, e.g. physical immobility; factors influencing fluid needs, e.g. hypermetabolic state; knowledge deficiency related to fluid volume; medications, e.g. diuretics.

Related Factors

See risk factors.

FLUID VOLUME EXCESS
Definition

The state in which an individual experiences increased isotonic fluid retention.

Defining Characteristics

Edema; effusion; anasarca; weight gain; shortness of breath; intake greater than output; abnormal breath sounds, rales (crackles); decreased hemoglobin and hematocrit; increased central venous pressure;* jugular vein distention;* positive hepatojugular reflex.

Defining Characteristics That Require Further Study

Clinical evidence lacking in fluid volume excess studies; orthopnea; S_3 heart sound; pulmonary congestion; change in respiratory pattern; change in mental status; blood pressure changes; pulmonary artery pressure changes; oliguria; specific gravity changes; azotemia; altered electrolytes; restlessness; anxiety.

Related Factors

Compromised regulatory mechanism; excess fluid intake; excess sodium intake.

---

*NOTE: Minimal clinical evidence present and needs further research.

GAS EXCHANGE, IMPAIRED
Definition

A state in which an individual experiences an excess or deficit in oxygenation and/or carbon dioxide elimination at the alveolar-capillary membrane (specify: hypercapnia or hypoxemia).

Defining Characteristics

Dyspnea; confusion; abnormal ABGs; hypoxia; hypercapnia (headache upon awakening, vision disturbances); cyanosis (in neonates only); confusion; somnolence; restlessness; irritability.

Related Factors

Ventilation-perfusion imbalance.

GRIEVING, ANTICIPATORY
Definition

Intellectual and emotional responses and behaviors by which individuals (families, communities) work through the process of modifying self-concept based on the perception of potential loss.

Defining Characteristics

Potential loss of significant object; expression of distress at potential loss; denial of potential loss; denial of the significance of the loss; guilt; anger; sorrow; bargaining; alteration in: eating habits, sleep patterns, dream patterns, activity level, libido; altered communication patterns; difficulty taking on new or different roles; resolution of grief prior to the reality of loss.

Related Factors

To be developed.

GRIEVING, DYSFUNCTIONAL
Definition

Extended, unsuccessful use of intellectual and emotional responses by which individuals (families, communities) attempt to work through the process of modifying self-concept based upon the perception of loss.

Defining Characteristics

Repetitive use of ineffectual behaviors associated with attempts to reinvest in relationships; reliving of past experiences with little or no reduction (diminishment) of intensity of the grief; prolonged interference with life functioning; onset or exacerbation of somatic or psychomatic responses; expression of distress at loss; denial of loss; expression of guilt; expression of unresolved issues; anger; sadness; crying; difficulty in expressing loss; alterations in: eating habits, sleep patterns, dream patterns, activity level, libido, concentration and/or pursuit of tasks; idealization of lost object; reliving of past experiences; interference with life functioning; developmental regression; labile affect.

Related Factors

Actual or perceived object loss (object loss is used in the broadest sense); objects may include: people, possessions, a job, status, home, ideals, parts and processes of the body.

GROWTH AND DEVELOPMENT, ALTERED
Definition

The state in which an individual demonstrates deviations in norms from his/her age group.

Defining Characteristics

Major

Delay or difficulty in performing skills (motor, social, or expressive) typical of age group; altered physical growth; inability to perform self-care or self-control activities appropriate for age.

Minor

Flat affect; listlessness, decreased responses.

Related Factors

Inadequate caretaking: indifference, inconsistent responsiveness, multiple caretakers; separation from significant others; environmental and stimulation deficiencies; effects of physical disability; prescribed dependence.

HEALTH MAINTENANCE, ALTERED

Definition

Inability to identify, manage, and/or seek out help to maintain health.

Defining Characteristics

Demonstrated lack of knowledge regarding basic health practices; demonstrated lack of adaptive behaviors to internal/external environmental changes; reported or observed inability to take responsibility for meeting basic health practices in any or all functional pattern areas; history of lack of health seeking behavior; expressed interest in improving health behaviors; reported or observed lack of equipment, financial, and/or other resources; reported or observed impairment of personal support systems.

Related Factors

Lack of or significant alteration in communication skills (written, verbal, and/or gestural); lack of ability to make deliberate and thoughtful judgments; perceptual/cognitive impairment (complete/partial lack of gross and/or fine motor skills); ineffective individual coping; dysfunctional grieving; unachieved developmental tasks; ineffective family coping; disabling spiritual distress; lack of material resources.

HEALTH SEEKING BEHAVIORS (SPECIFY)

Definition

A state in which an individual in stable health is actively seeking ways to alter personal health habits and/or the environment in order to move toward a higher level of health.*

Defining Characteristics

Major

Expressed or observed desire to seek a higher level of wellness.

Minor

Expressed or observed desire for increased control of health practice; expression of concern about current en-

---

*Stable health status is defined as age-appropriate illness prevention measures are achieved; client reports good or excellent health; and signs and symptoms of disease, if present, are controlled.

vironmental conditions on health status; stated or observed unfamiliarity with wellness community resources; demonstrated or observed lack of knowledge in health promotion behaviors.

HOME MAINTENANCE MANAGEMENT, IMPAIRED

Definition

Inability to independently maintain a safe growth-promoting immediate environment.

Defining Characteristics

Subjective: *household members express difficulty in maintaining their home in a comfortable fashion; *household members request assistance with home maintenance; *household members describe outstanding debts or financial crises.

Objective: disorderly surroundings; *unwashed or unavailable cooking equipment, clothes, or linen; *accumulation of dirt, food wastes, or hygienic wastes; offensive odors; inappropriate household temperature; *overtaxed family members, e.g. exhausted, anxious; lack of necessary equipment or aids; presence of vermin or rodents; *repeated hygienic disorders, infestations, or infections.

Related Factors

Individual/family member disease or injury; insufficient family organization or planning; insufficient finances; unfamiliarity with neighborhood resources; impaired cognitive or emotional functioning; lack of knowledge; lack of role modeling; inadequate support systems.

---

*Critical defining characteristics.

HOPELESSNESS

Definition

A subjective state in which an individual sees limited or no alternatives or personal choices available and is unable to mobilize energy on own behalf.

Defining Characteristics

Major

Passivity, decreased verbalization; decreased affect; verbal cues (despondent content, "I can't," sighing).

Minor

Lack of initiative; decreased response to stimuli; decreased affect; turning away from speaker; closing eyes; shrugging in response to speaker; decreased appetite; increased/decreased sleep; lack of involvement in care/passively allowing care.

Related Factors

Prolonged activity restriction creating isolation; failing or deteriorating physiological condition; long-term stress; abandonment; lost belief in transcendent values/God.

HYPERTHERMIA

Definition

A state in which an individual's body temperature is elevated above his/her normal range.

Defining Characteristics

Major

Increase in body temperature above normal range.

Minor

Flushed skin; warm to touch; increased respiratory rate; tachycardia; seizures/convulsions.

Related Factors

Exposure to hot environment; vigorous activity; medications/anesthesia; inappropriate clothing; increased metabolic rate; illness or trauma; dehydration; inability or decreased ability to perspire.

HYPOTHERMIA
Definition

The state in which an individual's body temperature is reduced below normal range.

Defining Characteristics

Major

Reduction in body temperature below normal range; shivering (mild); cool skin; pallor (moderate).

Minor

Slow capillary refill; tachycardia; cyanotic nail beds; hypertension; piloerection.

Related Factors

Exposure to cool or cold environment; illness or trauma; damage to hypothalamus; inability or decreased ability to shiver; malnutrition; inadequate clothing; consumption of alcohol; medications causing vasodilation; evaporation from skin in cool environment; decreased metabolic rate; inactivity; aging.

INCONTINENCE, FUNCTIONAL
Definition

The state in which an individual experiences an involuntary, unpredictable passage of urine.

Defining Characteristics

Major

Urge to void or bladder contractions sufficiently strong to result in loss of urine before reaching an appropriate receptacle.

Related Factors

Altered environment; sensory, cognitive, or mobility deficits.

INCONTINENCE, REFLEX
Definition

The state in which an individual experiences an involuntary loss of urine, occurring at somewhat predictable intervals when a specific bladder volume is reached.

Defining Characteristics

Major

No awareness of bladder filling; no urge to void or feelings of bladder fullness; uninhibited bladder contraction/spasm at regular intervals.

Related Factors

Neurological impairment (e.g. spinal cord lesion that interferes with conduction of cerebral messages above the level of the reflex arc).

INCONTINENCE, STRESS
Definition

The state in which an individual experiences a loss of urine of less than 50 cc occurring with increased abdominal pressure.

Defining Characteristics

Major

Reported or observed dribbling with increased abdominal pressure.

Minor

Urinary urgency; urinary frequency (more often than every 2 hours).

Related Factors

Degenerative changes in pelvic muscles and structural supports associated with increased age; high intraabdominal pressure (e.g. obesity, gravid uterus); incompetent bladder outlet; overdistention between voidings; weak pelvic muscles and structural supports.

INCONTINENCE, TOTAL
Definition

The state in which an individual experiences a continuous and unpredictable loss of urine.

Defining Characteristics

Major

Constant flow of urine occurs at unpredictable times without distention or uninhibited bladder contractions/spasm; unsuccessful incontinence refractory to treatments; nocturia.

Minor

Lack of perineal or bladder filling awareness; unawareness of incontinence.

Related Factors

Neuropathy preventing transmission of reflex indicating bladder fullness; neurological dysfunction causing triggering of micturition at unpredictable times; independent contraction of detrusor reflex due to surgery; trauma or disease affecting spinal cord nerves; anatomical (fistula).

INCONTINENCE, URGE

Definition

The state in which an individual experiences involuntary passage of urine occurring soon after a strong sense of urgency to void.

Defining Characteristics

Major

Urinary urgency; frequency (voiding more often than every 2 hours); bladder contracture/spasm.

Minor

Nocturia (more than 2 times per night); voiding in small amounts (less than 100 cc) or in large amounts (more than 550 cc); inability to reach toilet in time.

Related Factors

Decreased bladder capacity (e.g. history of PID, abdominal surgeries, indwelling urinary catheter); irritation of bladder stretch receptors causing spasm (e.g. bladder infection); alcohol; caffeine; increased fluids; increased urine concentration; overdistention of bladder.

INFANT BEHAVIOR, DISORGANIZED

Definition

Alteration in integration and modulation of the physiological and behavioral systems of functioning (i.e. autonomic, motor, state, organizational, self-regulatory, and attentional-interactional systems).

Defining Characteristics

Major

Change from baseline physiologic measures; tremors, startles, twitches; hyperextension of arms and legs; diffuse/unclear sleep; deficient self-regulatory behaviors; deficient response to visual/auditory stimuli.

Minor

Yawning; apnea.

Related Factors

Pain; oral/motor problems; feeding intolerance; environmental overstimulation; lack of containment/boundaries; prematurity; invasive/painful procedures.

INFANT BEHAVIOR, DISORGANIZED, RISK FOR

Definition

Risk for alteration in integration and modulation of the physiological and behavioral systems of functioning (i.e. autonomic, motor, state, organizational, self-regulatory, and attentional-interactional systems).

Risk Factors

Pain; oral/motor problems; environmental overstimulation; lack of containment/boundaries; prematurity; invasive/painful procedures.

INFANT BEHAVIOR, ORGANIZED, POTENTIAL FOR ENHANCED

Definition

A pattern of modulation of the physiological and behavioral systems of functioning of an infant (i.e. autonomic, motor, state, organizational, self-regulatory, and attentional-interactional systems) that is satisfactory but that can be improved, resulting in higher levels of integration in response to environmental stimuli.

Defining Characteristics

Stable physiologic measures; definite sleep-wake states; use of some self-regulatory behaviors; response to visual/auditory stimuli.

Related Factors

Prematurity; pain.

INFANT FEEDING PATTERN, INEFFECTIVE

Definition

A state in which an infant demonstrates an impaired ability to suck or coordinate the suck-swallow response.

Defining Characteristics

Major

Inability to initiate or sustain an effective suck; inability to coordinate sucking, swallowing and breathing.

Minor

None.

Related Factors

Prematurity; neurological impairment/delay; oral hypersensitivity; prolonged NPO; anatomic abnormality.

INFECTION, RISK FOR

Definition

The state in which an individual is at increased risk for being invaded by pathogenic organisms.

Defining Characteristics

Presence of risk factors such as:

Inadequate primary defenses (broken skin, traumatized tissue, decrease in ciliary action, stasis of body fluids, change in pH secretions, altered peristalsis); inadequate secondary defenses (e.g. decreased hemoglobin, leukopenia, suppressed inflammatory response) and immunosuppression; inadequate acquired immunity; tissue destruction and increased environmental exposure; chronic disease; invasive procedures; malnutrition; pharmaceutical agents; trauma; rupture of amniotic membranes; insufficient knowledge to avoid exposure to pathogens.

Related Factors

See risk factors.

INJURY, RISK FOR

Definition

A state in which the individual is at risk of injury as a result of environmental conditions interacting with the individual's adaptive and defensive resources.

Defining Characteristics

Presence of risk factors such as:

Internal: biochemical, regulatory function (sensory dysfunction, integrative dysfunction, effector dysfunction); tissue hypoxia; malnutrition; immunoautoimmune; abnormal blood profile (leukocytosis/leukopenia; altered clotting factors; thrombocytopenia; sickle cell, thalassemia; decreased hemoglobin); physical (broken skin, altered mobility); developmental age (physiological, psychosocial); psychological (affective, orientation).

External: biological (immunization level of community, microorganism); chemical (pollutants, poisons, drugs, pharmaceutical agents, alcohol, caffeine, nicotine, preservatives, cosmetics and dyes); nutrients (vitamins, food types); physical (design, structure, and arrangement of community, building, and/or equipment); mode of transport/transportation; people/provider (nosocomial agents; staffing patterns; cognitive, affective, and psychomotor factors).

Related Factors

See risk factors.

INTRACRANIAL, ADAPTIVE CAPACITY, DECREASED

Definition

A clinical state in which intracranial fluid dynamic mechanisms that normally compensate for increases in intracranial volumes are compromised, resulting in repeated disproportionate increases in intracranial pressure (ICP) in response to a variety of noxious and nonnoxious stimuli.

Defining Characteristics

Major

Repeated increases in ICP of greater than 10 mm Hg for more than 5 minutes following any of a variety of external stimuli.

Minor

Disproportionate increase in ICP following single environmental or nursing maneuver stimulus; elevated P2 ICP waveform; volume-pressure response test variation (volume-pressure ratio >2, pressure-volume index <10); baseline ICP equal to or greater than 10 mm Hg; wide amplitude ICP waveform.

Related Factors

Brain injuries; sustained increase in ICP ≥ 10–15 mm Hg; decreased cerebral perfusion pressure ≤ 50–60 mm Hg; systemic hypotension with intracranial hypertension.

KNOWLEDGE DEFICIT (SPECIFY)

Definition

Absence or deficiency of cognitive information related to specific topic.

Defining Characteristics

Verbalization of the problem; inaccurate follow-through of instruction; inaccurate performance of test; inappropriate or exaggerated behaviors, e.g. hysterical, hostile, agitated, apathetic.

Related Factors

Lack of exposure; lack of recall; information misinterpretation; cognitive limitation; lack of interest in learning; unfamiliarity with information resources.

LONELINESS, RISK FOR

Definition

A subjective state in which an individual is at risk of experiencing vague dysphoria.

Risk Factors

Affectional deprivation; physical isolation; cathectic deprivation; social isolation.

MANAGEMENT OF THERAPEUTIC REGIMEN: COMMUNITY, INEFFECTIVE

Definition

A pattern of regulating and integrating into community processes programs for treatment of illness and the sequelae of illness that are unsatisfactory for meeting health-related goals.

Defining Characteristics

Deficits in persons and programs to be accountable for illness care of aggregates; deficits in advocates for aggregates; deficits in community activities for secondary and tertiary prevention; illness symptoms above the norm expected for the number and type of population; number of health care resources are insufficient for the incidence or prevalence of illness(es); unavailable health care resources for illness care; unexpected acceleration of illness(es).

MANAGEMENT OF THERAPEUTIC REGIMEN: FAMILIES, INEFFECTIVE

Definition

A pattern of regulating and integrating into family processes a program for treatment of illness and the sequelae of illness that are unsatisfactory for meeting health goals.

Defining Characteristics

Major

Inappropriate family activities for meeting the goals of a treatment or prevention program.

Minor

Acceleration (expected or unexpected) of illness symptoms of a family member; lack of attention to illness and its sequelae; verbalized desire to manage the treatment of illness and prevention of the sequelae; verbalized difficulty with regulation/integration of one or more effects or prevention of complication; verbalizes that family did not take action to reduce risk factors for progression of illness and sequelae.

Related Factors

Complexity of health care system; complexity of therapeutic regimen; decisional conflicts; economic difficulties; excessive demands made on individual or family; family conflict.

MANAGEMENT OF THERAPEUTIC REGIMEN: INDIVIDUAL, EFFECTIVE

Definition

A pattern of regulating and integrating into daily living a program for treatment of illness and its sequelae that is satisfactory for meeting specific health goals.

Defining Characteristics

Appropriate choices of daily activities for meeting the goals of a treatment or prevention program; illness symptoms are within a normal range of expectation; verbalized desire to manage the treatment of illness and prevention of sequelae; verbalized intent to reduce risk factors for progression of illness and sequelae.

MANAGEMENT OF THERAPEUTIC REGIMEN (INDIVIDUAL), INEFFECTIVE

Definition

A pattern of regulating and integrating into daily living a program for treatment of illness and the sequelae of illness that is unsatisfactory for meeting specific health goals.

Defining Characteristics

Major

Choices of daily living ineffective for meeting the goals of a treatment or prevention program.

Minor

Acceleration (expected or unexpected) of illness symptoms of a family member; verbalized desire to manage the treatment of illness and prevention of sequelae; verbalized difficulty with regulation/integration of one or more prescribed regimens for treatment of illness and its effects or prevention of complications; verbalized that did not take action to include treatment regimens in daily routines; verbalized that did not take action to reduce risk factors for progression of illness and sequelae.

Related Factors

Complexity of health care system; complexity of therapeutic regimen; decisional conflicts; economic difficulties; excessive demands made on individual or family; family conflict; family patterns of health care; inadequate number and types of cues to action; knowledge deficits; mistrust of regimen and/or health care personnel; perceived seriousness; perceived susceptibility; perceived barriers; perceived benefits; powerlessness; social support deficits.

MEMORY, IMPAIRED

Definition

The state in which an individual experiences the inability to remember or recall bits of information or behavioral skills. Impaired memory may be attributed to pathophysiological or situational causes that are either temporary or permanent.

Defining Characteristics

Major

Observed or reported experiences of forgetting; inability to determine if a behavior was performed; inability to learn or retain new skills or information; inability to perform a previously learned skill; inability to recall factual information; inability to recall recent or past events.

Minor

Forgets to perform a behavior at a scheduled time.

Related Factors

Acute or chronic hypoxia; anemia; decreased cardiac output; fluid and electrolyte imbalance; neurological disturbances; excessive environmental disturbances.

NEUROVASCULAR DYSFUNCTION, PERIPHERAL, RISK FOR

Definition

A state in which an individual is at risk of experiencing a disruption in circulation, sensation, or motion of an extremity.

Risk Factors

Fractures; mechanical compression, e.g. tourniquet, cast, brace, dressing, or restraint; orthopedic surgery; trauma; immobilization; burns; vascular obstruction.

NONCOMPLIANCE (SPECIFY)

Definition

A person's informed decision not to adhere to a therapeutic recommendation.

Defining Characteristics

*Behavior indicative of failure to adhere (by direct observation or by statements of patient or significant others); objective tests (physiological measures, detection of markers); evidence of development of complications; evidence of exacerbation of symptoms; failure to keep appointments; failure to progress.

Related Factors

Patient value system: health beliefs, cultural influences, spiritual values; client-provider relationships.

---

*Critical defining characteristic.

NUTRITION: LESS THAN BODY REQUIREMENTS, ALTERED

Definition

The state in which an individual experiences an intake of nutrients insufficient to meet metabolic needs.

Defining Characteristics

Loss of weight with adequate food intake; body weight 20% or more under ideal; reported inadequate food intake less than RDA (recommended daily allowance); weakness of muscles required for swallowing or mastication; reported or evidence of lack of food; aversion to eating; reported altered taste sensation; satiety immediately after ingesting food; abdominal pain with or without pathology; sore, inflamed buccal cavity; capillary fragility; abdominal cramping; diarrhea and/or steatorrhea; hyperactive bowel sounds; lack of interest in food; perceived inability to ingest food; pale conjunctiva and mucous membranes; poor muscle tone; excessive loss of hair; lack of information, misinformation; misconceptions.

Related Factors

Inability to ingest or digest food or absorb nutrients due to biological, psychological, or economic factors.

NUTRITION: MORE THAN BODY REQUIREMENTS, ALTERED
Definition

The state in which an individual is experiencing an intake of nutrients that exceeds metabolic needs.

Defining Characteristics

Weight 10% over ideal for height and frame; *weight 20% over ideal for height and frame; *triceps skinfold greater than 15 mm in men, 25 mm in women; sedentary activity level; reported or observed dysfunctional eating pattern: pairing food with other activities; concentrating food intake at the end of day; eating in response to external cues such as time of day, social situation; eating in response to internal cues other than hunger, e.g. anxiety.

Related Factors

Excessive intake in relation to metabolic need.

---

*Critical defining characteristics.

NUTRITION: POTENTIAL FOR MORE THAN BODY REQUIREMENTS, ALTERED
Definition

The state in which an individual is at risk of experiencing an intake of nutrients that exceeds metabolic needs.

Defining Characteristics

Presence of risk factors such as:

*Reported or observed obesity in one or both parents; *rapid transition across growth percentiles in infants or children; reported use of solid food as major food source before 5 months of age; observed use of food as reward or comfort measure; reported or observed higher baseline weight at beginning of each pregnancy; dysfunctional eating patterns: pairing food with other activities; concentrating food intake at end of day; eating in response to external cues such as time of day, social situa-

---

*Critical defining characteristics.

tion; eating in response to internal cues other than hunger such as anxiety.

Related Factors

See risk factors.

ORAL MUCOUS MEMBRANE, ALTERED
Definition

The state in which an individual experiences disruptions in the tissue layers of the oral cavity.

Defining Characteristics

Oral pain/discomfort; coated tongue; xerostomia (dry mouth); stomatitis; oral lesions or ulcers; lack of or decreased salivation; leukoplakia; edema; hyperemia; oral plaque; desquamation; vesicles; hemorrhagic gingivitis; carious teeth; halitosis.

Related Factors

Pathological conditions—oral cavity (radiation to head or neck); dehydration; trauma (chemical, e.g. acidic foods, drugs, noxious agents, alcohol; mechanical, e.g. ill-fitting dentures, braces, tubes [endotracheal/nasogastric], surgery in oral cavity); NPO for more than 24 hours; ineffective oral hygiene; mouth breathing; malnutrition; infection; lack of or decreased salivation; medication.

PAIN
Definition

An unpleasant sensory and emotional experience arising from actual or potential tissue damage or described in terms of such damage (International Association for the Study of Pain); sudden or slow onset of any intensity from mild to severe with an anticipated or predictable end and a duration of less than 6 months.

Defining Characteristics

Major

Verbal or coded report; observed evidence; antalgic position; protective behavior; guarding behavior; antalgic gestures; facial mask; sleep disturbance (eyes lack luster, fixed or scattered movement, grimace).

Minor

Self focus; narrowed focus (altered time perception, impaired thought process, reduced interaction with people and environment); distraction behavior (pacing, seeking out other people and/or activities, repetitive activities); autonomic alteration in muscle tone (may span from listless to rigid); autonomic responses (diaphoresis, blood pressure, respiration, pulse change, pupillary dilatation); expressive behavior (restlessness, moaning, crying, vigilance, irritability, sighing); changes in appetite and eating.

Related Factors

Injury agents (biological, chemical, physical, psychological).

PAIN, CHRONIC

Definition

An unpleasant sensory and emotional experience arising from actual or potential tissue damage or described in terms of such damage (International Association for the Study of Pain); sudden or slow onset of any intensity from mild to severe, constant or recurring without an anticipated or predictable end and a duration of greater than 6 months.

Defining Characteristics

Major

Verbal or coded report or observed evidence of protective behavior; guarding behavior; facial mask; irritability; self focusing; restlessness; depression.

Minor

Atrophy of involved muscle group; changes in sleep pattern; weight changes; fatigue; fear of reinjury; reduced interaction with people; altered ability to continue previous activities; sympathetic mediated responses (temperature, cold, changes of body position, hypersensitivity); anorexia.

Related Factors

Chronic physical/psychosocial disability.

PARENTAL ROLE CONFLICT

Definition

The state in which a parent experiences role confusion and conflict in response to crisis.

Defining Characteristics

Major

Parent(s) expresses concerns/feelings of inadequacy to provide for child's physical and emotional needs during hospitalization or in the home; demonstrated disruption in caretaking routines; parent(s) expresses concerns about changes in parental role, family functioning, family communication, family health.

Minor

Expresses concern about perceived loss of control over decisions relating to child; reluctant to participate in usual caretaking activities even with encouragement and support; verbalizes/demonstrates feelings of guilt, anger, fear, anxiety, and/or frustrations about effect of child's illness on family process.

Related Factors

Separation from child due to chronic illness; intimidation with invasive or restrictive modalities (e.g. isolation, intubation), specialized care centers, policies; home care of a child with special needs (e.g. apnea monitoring, postural drainage, hyperalimentation); change in marital status; interruptions of family life due to home care regimen (treatments, caregivers, lack of respite).

PARENTING, ALTERED

Definition

The state in which a nurturing figure experiences an inability to create an environment that promotes the optimal growth and development of another human being.†

Defining Characteristics

Abandonment; runaway; verbalization cannot control child; incidence of physical and psychological trauma; lack of parental attachment behaviors; inappropriate visual, tactile, auditory stimulation; negative identification of infant's/child's characteristics; negative attachment of meanings to infant's/child's characteristics; constant verbalization of disappointment in gender or physical characteristics of the infant/child; verbalization of resentment toward the infant/child; verbalization of role inadequacy; *inattentive to infant's/child's needs; verbal disgust at body functions of infant/child; noncompliance with health appointments for self and/or infant/child; *inappropriate caretaking behavior (toilet training, sleep/rest, feeding); inappropriate or inconsistent discipline practices; frequent accidents; frequent illness; growth and development lag in the child; *history of child abuse or abandonment by primary caretaker; verbalizes desire to have child call him/herself by first name versus traditional cultural tendencies; child receives care from multiple caretakers without consideration for the needs of the infant/child; compulsively seeking role approval from others.

---

†It is important to state as a preface to this diagnosis that adjustment to parenting in general is a normal maturational process that elicits nursing behaviors of prevention of potential problems and health promotion.
*Critical defining characteristics.

Related Factors

Lack of available role model; ineffective role model; physical and psychosocial abuse of nurturing figure; lack of support between/from significant other(s); unmet social/emotional maturation needs of parenting figures; interruption in bonding process, i.e. maternal, paternal, other; unrealistic expectation for self, infant, partner; perceives threat to own survival, physical and emotional; mental and/or physical illness; presence of stress (financial, legal, recent crisis, cultural move); lack of knowledge; limited cognitive functioning; lack of role identity; lack or inappropriate response of child to relationship; multiple pregnancies.

PARENTING, RISK FOR ALTERED

Definition

The state in which a nurturing figure is at risk to experience an inability to create an environment that promotes the optimal growth and development of another human being.†

Defining Characteristics

Presence of risk factors such as:

Lack of parental attachment behaviors; inappropriate visual, tactile, auditory stimulation; negative identification of infant's/child's characteristics; negative attachment of meanings to infant's/child's characteristics; constant ver-

---

†It is important to state as a preface to this diagnosis that adjustment to parenting in general is a normal maturational process that elicits nursing behaviors of prevention of potential problems and health promotion.

balization of disappointment in gender or physical characteristics of the infant/child; verbalization of resentment toward the infant/child; verbalization of role inadequacy; *inattentive to infant's/child's needs; verbal disgust at body functions of infant/child; noncompliance with health appointments for self and/or infant/child; *inappropriate caretaking behaviors (toilet training, sleep/rest, feeding); inappropriate or inconsistent discipline practices; frequent accidents; frequent illness; growth and development lag in the child; *history of child abuse or abandonment by primary caretaker; verbalizes desire to have child call him/herself by first name versus traditional cultural tendencies; child receives care from multiple caretakers without consideration for the needs of the infant/child; compulsively seeking role approval from others.

Related Factors

Lack of available role model; ineffective role model; physical and psychosocial abuse of nurturing figure; lack of support between/from significant other(s); unmet social/emotional maturation needs of parenting figures; interruption in bonding process, i.e. maternal, paternal, other; unrealistic expectation for self, infant, partner; perceive threat to own survival, physical and emotional; mental and/or physical illness; presence of stress (financial, legal, recent crisis, cultural move); lack of knowledge; limited cognitive functioning; lack of role identity; lack or inappropriate response of child to relationship; multiple pregnancies.

*Critical defining characteristics.

PARENT/INFANT/CHILD ATTACHMENT, ALTERED, RISK FOR
Definition

Disruption of the interactive process between parent/significant other and infant that fosters the development of a protective and nurturing reciprocal relationship.

Risk Factors

Inability of parents to meet the personal needs; anxiety associated with the parent role; substance abuse; premature infant, ill infant/child who is unable to effectively initiate parental contact due to altered behavioral organization; separation; physical barriers; lack of privacy.

PERIOPERATIVE POSITIONING INJURY, RISK FOR
Definition

A state in which the client is at risk for injury as a result of the environmental conditions found in the perioperative setting.

Risk Factors

Disorientation; immobilization, muscle weakness; sensory/perceptual disturbances due to anesthesia; obesity; emaciation; edema.

PERSONAL IDENTITY DISTURBANCE
Definition

Inability to distinguish between self and nonself.

Defining Characteristics
To be developed.

Related Factors
To be developed.

PHYSICAL MOBILITY, IMPAIRED
Definition

A state in which the individual experiences a limitation of ability for independent physical movement.

Defining Characteristics

Inability to purposefully move within the physical environment, including bed mobility, transfer, and ambulation; reluctance to attempt movement; limited range of motion; decreased muscle strength, control, and/or mass; imposed restrictions of movement, including mechanical, medical protocol; impaired coordination.

Related Factors

Intolerance to activity/decreased strength and endurance; pain/discomfort; perceptual/cognitive impairment; neuromuscular impairment; musculoskeletal impairment; depression/severe anxiety.

Suggested Functional Level Classification†

0 = Completely independent.
1 = Requires use of equipment or device.
2 = Requires help from another person, for assistance, supervision, or teaching.
3 = Requires help from another person and equipment device.
4 = Dependent, does not participate in activity.

†Code adapted from Jones, E., et al. Patient classification for long-term care: users' manual. HEW, Publication No. HRA-74-3107, November, 1974.

POISONING, RISK FOR
Definition

Accentuated risk of accidental exposure to or ingestion of drugs or dangerous products in doses sufficient to cause poisoning.

Defining Characteristics
Presence of risk factors such as:

Internal (individual): reduced vision; verbalization of occupational setting without adequate safeguards; lack of safety or drug education; lack of proper precaution; cognitive or emotional difficulties; insufficient finances.
External (environmental): large supplies of drugs in house; medicines stored in unlocked cabinets accessible to children or confused persons; dangerous products placed or stored within the reach of children or confused persons; availability of illicit drugs potentially contaminated by poisonous additives; flaking, peeling paint or plaster in presence of young children; chemical contamination of food and water; unprotected contact with heavy metals or chemicals; paint, lacquer, etc. in poorly ventilated areas or without effective protection; presence of poisonous vegetation; presence of atmospheric pollutants.

Related Factors

See risk factors.

POST-TRAUMA RESPONSE
Definition

The state of an individual experiencing a sustained painful response to an overwhelming traumatic event.

Defining Characteristics

Major

Re-experience of the traumatic event that may be identified in cognitive, affective, and/or sensory motor activities (flashbacks, intrusive thoughts, repetitive dreams or nightmares, excessive verbalization of the traumatic event, verbalization of survival guilt or guilt about behavior required for survival).

Minor

Psychic/emotional numbness (impaired interpretation of reality, confusion, dissociation or amnesia, vagueness about traumatic event, constricted affect); altered life style (self-destructiveness such as substance abuse, suicide attempt or other acting out behavior; difficulty with interpersonal relationship; development of phobia regarding trauma; poor impulse control/irritability and explosiveness).

Related Factors

Disasters, wars, epidemics, rape, assault, torture, catastrophic illness or accident.

POWERLESSNESS

Definition

Perception that one's own action will not significantly affect an outcome; a perceived lack of control over a current situation or immediate happening.

Defining Characteristics

Severe: verbal expressions of having no control or influence over situation; verbal expressions of having no control or influence over outcome; verbal expressions of having no control over self-care; depression over physical deterioration that occurs despite patient compliance with regimens; apathy.

Moderate: nonparticipation in care or decision making when opportunities are provided; expressions of dissatisfaction and frustration over inability to perform previous tasks and/or activities; does not monitor progress; expression of doubt regarding role performance; reluctance to express true feelings; fearing alienation from caregivers; passivity; inability to seek information regarding care; dependence on others that may result in irritability, resentment, anger, and guilt; does not defend self-care practices when challenged.

Low: expressions of uncertainty about fluctuating energy levels; passivity.

Related Factors

Health care environment; interpersonal interaction; illness-related regimen; life style of helplessness.

PROTECTION, ALTERED

Definition

The state in which an individual experiences a decrease in the ability to guard the self from internal or external threats such as illness or injury.

Defining Characteristics

Major

Deficient immunity; impaired healing; altered clotting; maladaptive stress response; neurosensory alteration.

Minor

Chilling; perspiring; dyspnea; cough; itching; restlessness; insomnia; fatigue; anorexia; weakness; immobility; disorientation; pressure sores.

Related Factors

Extremes of age; inadequate nutrition; alcohol abuse; abnormal blood profiles (leukopenia, thrombocytopenia, anemia, coagulation); drug therapies (antineoplastic, corticosteroid, immune, anticoagulant, thrombolytic); treatments (surgery, radiation) and diseases such as cancer and immune disorders.

RAPE-TRAUMA SYNDROME

Definition

Forced, violent sexual penetration against the victim's will and consent. The trauma syndrome that develops from this attack or attempted attack includes an acute phase of disorganization of the victim's life style and a long-term process of reorganization of life style.*

Defining Characteristics

Acute phase: emotional reactions (anger, embarrassment, fear of physical violence and death, humiliation, revenge, self-blame); multiple physical symptoms (gastrointestinal irritability, genitourinary discomfort, muscle tension, sleep pattern disturbance).

Long-term phase: changes in life style (change in residence; dealing with repetitive nightmares and phobias; seeking family support; seeking social network support).

Related Factors

To be developed.

---

*This syndrome includes the following three subcomponents: rape-trauma, compound reaction, and silent reaction. In the NANDA list, each appears as a separate diagnosis.

RAPE-TRAUMA SYNDROME: COMPOUND REACTION

Definition

Forced, violent sexual penetration against the victim's will and consent. The trauma syndrome that develops from this attack or attempted attack includes an acute phase of disorganization of the victim's life style and a long-term process of reorganization of life style.*

Defining Characteristics

Acute phase: emotional reaction (anger, embarrassment, fear of physical violence and death, humiliation, revenge, self-blame); multiple physical symptoms (gastrointestinal irritability, genitourinary discomfort, muscle tension, sleep pattern disturbance); reactivated symptoms of such previous conditions, i.e. physical illness, psychiatric illness; reliance on alcohol and/or drugs.

Long-term phase: change in life style (changes in residence; dealing with repetitive nightmares and phobias; seeking family support; seeking social network support).

---

*This syndrome includes the following three subcomponents: rape-trauma, compound reaction, and silent reaction. In the NANDA list, each appears as a separate diagnosis.

Related Factors

To be developed.

RAPE-TRAUMA SYNDROME: SILENT REACTION
Definition

Forced, violent sexual penetration against the victim's will and consent. The trauma syndrome that develops from this attack or attempted attack includes an acute phase of disorganization of the victim's life style and a long-term process of reorganization of life style.*

Defining Characteristics

Abrupt changes in relationships with men; increase in nightmares; increased anxiety during interview, i.e. blocking of associations, long periods of silence, minor stuttering, physical distress; pronounced changes in sexual behavior; no verbalization of the occurrence of rape; sudden onset of phobic reactions.

Related Factors

To be developed.

_____

*This syndrome includes the following three subcomponents: rape-trauma, compound reaction, and silent reaction. In the NANDA list, each appears as a separate diagnosis.

ROLE PERFORMANCE, ALTERED
Definition

Disruption in the way one perceives one's role performance.

Defining Characteristics

Change in self-perception of role; denial of role; change in others' perception of role; conflict in roles; change in physical capacity to resume role; lack of knowledge of role; change in usual patterns of responsibility.

Related Factors

To be developed.

RELOCATION STRESS SYNDROME
Definition

Physiological and/or psychosocial disturbances as a result of transfer from one environment to another.

Defining Characteristics
Major

Change in environment/location; anxiety; apprehension; increased confusion (elderly population); depression; loneliness.

Minor

Verbalization of unwillingness to relocate; sleep disturbance; change in eating habits; dependency; gastrointestinal disturbances; increased verbalization of needs; insecurity; lack of trust; restlessness; sad affect; unfavorable comparison of post/pre-transfer staff; verbalization of being concerned/upset about transfer; vigilance; weight change; withdrawal.

Related Factors

Past, current, and recent losses; losses involved with decision to move; feeling of powerlessness; lack of adequate support system; little or no preparation for the impending move; moderate to high degree of environmental change; history and types of previous transfers; impaired psychosocial health status; decreased physical health status.

SELF-CARE DEFICIT: BATHING/HYGIENE†
Definition

A state in which the individual experiences an impaired ability to perform or complete bathing/hygiene activities for oneself.

Defining Characteristics

*Inability to wash body or body parts; inability to obtain or get to water source; inability to regulate temperature or flow.

Related Factors

Intolerance to activity, decreased strength and endurance; pain, discomfort; perceptual or cognitive impairment; neuromuscular impairment; musculoskeletal impairment; depression, severe anxiety.

_____

†See suggested Functional Level Classification under diagnosis of Physical Mobility, Impaired.
*Critical defining characteristic.

SELF-CARE DEFICIT: DRESSING/GROOMING†
Definition

A state in which the individual experiences an impaired ability to perform or complete dressing and grooming activities for oneself.

Defining Characteristics

*Impaired ability to put on or take off necessary items of clothing; impaired ability to obtain or replace articles of clothing; impaired ability to fasten clothing; inability to maintain appearance at a satisfactory level.

Related Factors

Intolerance to activity, decreased strength and endurance; pain, discomfort; perceptual or cognitive impairment; neuromuscular impairment; musculoskeletal impairment; depression, severe anxiety.

_____

†See suggested Functional Level Classification under diagnosis of Physical Mobility, Impaired.
*Critical defining characteristic.

SELF-CARE DEFICIT: FEEDING†
Definition

A state in which the individual experiences an impaired ability to perform or complete feeding activities for oneself.

_____

†See suggested Functional Level Classification under diagnosis of Physical Mobility, Impaired.

Defining Characteristics

Inability to bring food from a receptacle to the mouth.

Related Factors

Intolerance to activity, decreased strength and endurance; pain, discomfort; perceptual or cognitive impairment; neuromuscular impairment; musculoskeletal impairment; depression, severe anxiety.

SELF-CARE DEFICIT: TOILETING†
Definition

A state in which the individual experiences an impaired ability to perform or complete toileting activities for oneself.

Defining Characteristics

*Unable to get to toilet or commode; *unable to sit on or rise from toilet or commode; *unable to manipulate clothing for toileting; *unable to carry out proper toilet hygiene; unable to flush toilet or commode.

Related Factors

Impaired transfer ability; impaired mobility status; intolerance to activity, decreased strength and endurance; pain, discomfort; perceptual or cognitive impairment; neuromuscular impairment; musculoskeletal impairment; depression, severe anxiety.

---

†See suggested Functional Level Classification under diagnosis of Physical Mobility, Impaired.
*Critical defining characteristics.

SELF ESTEEM, CHRONIC LOW
Definition

Long-standing negative self evaluation/feelings about self or self-capabilities.

Defining Characteristics
Major

Long-standing or chronic: self-negating verbalization; expressions of shame/guilt; evaluates self as unable to deal with events; rationalizes away/rejects positive feedback and exaggerates negative feedback about self; hesitant to try new things/situations.

Minor

Frequent lack of success in work or other life events; overly conforming, dependent on others' opinions; lack of eye contact; nonassertive/passive; indecisive; excessively seeks reassurance.

Related Factors

To be developed.

SELF ESTEEM, SITUATIONAL LOW
Definition

Negative self evaluation/feelings about self which develop in response to a loss or change in an individual who previously had a positive self evaluation.

Defining Characteristics
Major

Episodic occurrence of negative self appraisal in response to life events in a person with a previous positive self evaluation; verbalization of negative feelings about self (helplessness, uselessness).

Minor

Self-negating verbalizations; expressions of shame/guilt; evaluates self as unable to handle situations/events; difficulty making decisions.

Related Factors

To be developed.

SELF-ESTEEM DISTURBANCE
Definition

Negative self evaluation/feelings about self or self-capabilities, which may be directly or indirectly expressed.

Defining Characteristics

Self-negating verbalization; expressions of shame/guilt; evaluates self as unable to deal with events; rationalizes away/rejects positive feedback and exaggerates negative feedback about self; hesitant to try new things/situations; denial of problems obvious to others; projection of blame/responsibility for problems; rationalizing personal failures; hypersensitive to slight or criticism; grandiosity.

Related Factors

To be developed.

SELF-MUTILATION, RISK FOR
Definition

A state in which an individual is at risk to perform an act upon the self to injure, not kill, which produces tissue damage and tension relief.

Defining Characteristics

Inability to cope with increased psychological/physiological tension in a healthy manner; feelings of depression, rejection, self-hatred, separation anxiety, guilt, and depersonalization; fluctuating emotions; command hallucinations; need for sensory stimuli; parental emotional deprivation; dysfunctional family.

Risk Factors

Groups at risk: Clients with borderline personality disorder, especially females 16-25 years of age; clients in psychotic state—frequently males in young adulthood; emotionally disturbed and/or battered children; mentally retarded and autistic children; clients with a history of self-injury; history of physical, emotional, or sexual abuse.

Related Factors

See risk factors.

SENSORY/PERCEPTUAL ALTERATIONS (SPECIFY) (VISUAL, AUDITORY, KINESTHETIC, GUSTATORY, TACTILE, OLFACTORY)

Definition

A state in which an individual experiences a change in the amount or patterning of oncoming stimuli accompanied by a diminished, exaggerated, distorted, or impaired response to such stimuli.

Defining Characteristics

Disoriented in time, in place, or with persons; altered abstraction; altered conceptualization; change in problem-solving abilities; reported or measured change in sensory acuity; change in behavior pattern; anxiety; apathy; change in usual response to stimuli; indication of body image alteration; restlessness; irritability; altered communication patterns.

Other Possible Characteristics

Complaints of fatigue; alteration in posture; change in muscular tension; inappropriate responses; hallucinations.

Related Factors

Altered environmental stimuli, excessive or insufficient; altered sensory reception, transmission, and/or integration; chemical alterations, endogenous (electrolyte), exogenous (drugs, etc.); psychological stress.

SEXUAL DYSFUNCTION

Definition

The state in which an individual experiences a change in sexual function that is viewed as unsatisfying, unrewarding, inadequate.

Defining Characteristics

Verbalization of problem; alterations in achieving perceived sex role; actual or perceived limitation imposed by disease and/or therapy; conflicts involving values; alteration in achieving sexual satisfaction; inability to achieve desired satisfaction; seeking confirmation of desirability; alteration in relationship with significant other; change of interest in self and others.

Related Factors

Biopsychosocial alteration of sexuality; ineffectual or absent role models; physical abuse; psychosocial abuse, e.g. harmful relationships; vulnerability; values conflict; lack of privacy; lack of significant other; altered body structure or function (pregnancy, recent childbirth, drugs, surgery, anomalies, disease process, trauma, radiation); misinformation or lack of knowledge.

SEXUALITY PATTERNS, ALTERED

Definition

The state in which an individual expresses concern regarding his/her sexuality.

Defining Characteristics

Major

Reported difficulties, limitations, or changes in sexual behaviors or activities.

Related Factors

Knowledge/skill deficit about alternative responses to health-related transitions, altered body function or structure, illness or medical treatment; lack of privacy; lack of significant other; ineffective or absent role models; conflicts with sexual orientation or variant preferences; fear of pregnancy or of acquiring a sexually transmitted disease; impaired relationship with a significant other.

SKIN INTEGRITY, IMPAIRED

Definition

A state in which the individual's skin is adversely altered.

Defining Characteristics

Disruption of skin surface; destruction of skin layers; invasion of body structures.

Related Factors

External (environmental): hyper- or hypothermia; chemical substance; mechanical factors (shearing forces, pressure, restraint); radiation; physical immobilization; humidity.
Internal (somatic): medication; altered nutritional state (obesity, emaciation); altered metabolic state; altered circulation; altered sensation; altered pigmentation; skeletal prominence; developmental factors; immunological deficit; alterations in turgor (change in elasticity).

SKIN INTEGRITY, RISK FOR IMPAIRED

Definition

A state in which the individual's skin is at risk of being adversely altered.

Defining Characteristics

Presence of risk factors such as:

External (environmental): hypo- or hyperthermia; chemical substance; mechanical factors (shearing forces, pressure, restraint); radiation; physical immobilization; excretions/secretions; humidity.
Internal (somatic): medication; alterations in nutritional state (obesity, emaciation); altered metabolic state; altered circulation; altered sensation; altered pigmentation; skeletal prominence; developmental factors; alter-

ations in skin turgor (change in elasticity); psychogenic; immunological.

Related Factors

See risk factors.

SLEEP PATTERN DISTURBANCE
Definition

Disruption of sleep time causes discomfort or interferes with desired life style.

Defining Characteristics

*Verbal complaints of difficulty falling asleep; *awakening earlier or later than desired; *interrupted sleep; *verbal complaints of not feeling well rested; changes in behavior and performance (increasing irritability, restlessness, disorientation, lethargy, listlessness); physical signs (mild fleeting nystagmus, slight hand tremor, ptosis of eyelid, expressionless face, dark circles under eyes, frequent yawning, changes in posture); thick speech with mispronunciation and incorrect words.

Related Factors

Sensory alterations: internal (illness, psychological stress); external (environmental changes, social cues).

_____

*Critical defining characteristics.

SOCIAL INTERACTION, IMPAIRED
Definition

The state in which an individual participates in an insufficient or excessive quantity or ineffective quality of social exchange.

Defining Characteristics
Major

Verbalized or observed discomfort in social situations; verbalized or observed inability to receive or communicate a satisfying sense of belonging, caring, interest, or shared history; observed use of unsuccessful social interaction behaviors; dysfunctional interaction with peers, family, and/or others.

Minor

Family report of change of style or pattern of interaction.

Related Factors

Knowledge/skill deficit about ways to enhance mutuality; communication barriers; self-concept disturbance; absence of available significant others or peers; limited physical mobility; therapeutic isolation; sociocultural dissonance; environmental barriers; altered thought processes.

SOCIAL ISOLATION
Definition

Aloneness experienced by the individual and perceived as imposed by others and as a negative or threatened state.

Defining Characteristics

Objective: *absence of supportive significant other(s) [family, friends, group]; sad, dull affect; inappropriate or immature interests/activities for development age/stage; uncommunicative, withdrawn, no eye contact; preoccupation with own thoughts, repetitive meaningless actions; projects hostility in voice, behavior; seeks to be alone, or exists in a subculture; evidence of physical/mental handicap or altered state of wellness; shows behavior unaccepted by dominant cultural group.

Subjective: *expresses feelings of aloneness imposed by others; *expresses feelings of rejection; experiences feelings of difference from others; inadequacy in or absence of significant purpose in life; inability to meet expectations of others; insecurity in public; expresses values acceptable to the subculture but unacceptable to the dominant cultural group; expresses interests inappropriate to the developmental age/stage.

Related Factors

Factors contributing to the absence of satisfying personal relationships, such as: delay in accomplishing developmental tasks; immature interests; alterations in physical appearance; alterations in mental status; unaccepted social behavior; unaccepted social values; altered state of wellness; inadequate personal resources; inability to engage in satisfying personal relationships.

_____

*Critical defining characteristics.

SPIRITUAL DISTRESS (DISTRESS OF THE HUMAN SPIRIT)
Definition

Disruption in the life principle that pervades a person's entire being and that integrates and transcends one's biological and psychosocial nature.

Defining Characteristics

*Expresses concern with meaning of life/death and/or belief systems; anger toward God; questions meaning of suffering; verbalizes inner conflict about beliefs; verbalizes concern about relationship with deity; questions meaning of own existence; unable to participate in usual religious practices; seeks spiritual assistance; questions moral/ethical implications of therapeutic regimen; gallows humor; displacement of anger toward religious representatives; description of nightmares/sleep disturbances; alteration in behavior/mood evidenced by anger, crying, withdrawal, preoccupation, anxiety, hostility, apathy, and so forth.

Related Factors

Separation from religious/cultural ties; challenged belief and value system, e.g. due to moral/ethical implications of therapy, due to intense suffering.

_____

*Critical defining characteristic.

SPIRITUAL WELL-BEING, ENHANCED, POTENTIAL FOR
Definition

Spiritual well-being is the process of an individual's developing/unfolding of mystery through harmonious interconnectedness that springs from inner strengths.

Defining Characteristics

Inner strengths: a sense of awareness, self consciousness, sacred source, unifying force, inner core, and transcendence; unfolding mystery: one's experience about life's purpose and meaning, mystery, uncertainty, and struggles; harmonious interconnectedness: relatedness, connectedness, harmony with self, others, higher power/God, and the environment.

SUFFOCATION, RISK FOR

Definition

Accentuated risk of accidental suffocation (inadequate air available for inhalation).

Defining Characteristics

Presence of risk factors such as:

Internal (individual): reduced olfactory sensation; reduced motor abilities; lack of safety education; lack of safety precautions; cognitive or emotional difficulties; disease or injury process.

External (environmental): pillow placed in an infant's crib; propped bottle placed in an infant's crib; vehicle warming in closed garage; children playing with plastic bags or inserting small objects into their mouths or noses; discarded or unused refrigerators or freezers without removed doors; children left unattended in bathtubs or pools; household gas leaks; smoking in bed; use of fuel-burning heaters not vented to outside; low-strung clothesline; pacifier hung around infant's head; person who eats large mouthfuls of food.

Related Factors

See risk factors.

SWALLOWING, IMPAIRED

Definition

The state in which an individual has decreased ability to voluntarily pass fluids and/or solids from the mouth to the stomach.

Defining Characteristics

Major

Observed evidence of difficulty in swallowing, e.g. stasis of food in oral cavity, coughing/choking.

Minor

Evidence of aspiration.

Related Factors

Neuromuscular impairment (e.g. decreased or absent gag reflex, decreased strength or excursion of muscles involved in mastication, perceptual impairment, facial paralysis); mechanical obstruction (e.g. edema, tracheostomy tube, tumor); fatigue; limited awareness; reddened, irritated oropharyngeal cavity.

THERMOREGULATION, INEFFECTIVE

Definition

The state in which the individual's temperature fluctuates between hypothermia and hyperthermia.

Defining Characteristics

Major

Fluctuations in body temperature above or below the normal range. See also major and minor characteristics present in hypothermia and hyperthermia.

Related Factors

Trauma or illness; immaturity; aging; fluctuating environmental temperature.

THOUGHT PROCESSES, ALTERED

Definition

A state in which an individual experiences a disruption in cognitive operations and activities.

Defining Characteristics

Inaccurate interpretation of environment; cognitive dissonance; distractibility; memory deficit/problems; egocentricity; hyper- or hypovigilance.

Other Possible Characteristics

Inappropriate nonreality-based thinking.

Related Factors

To be developed.

TISSUE INTEGRITY, IMPAIRED

Definition

A state in which an individual experiences damage to mucous membrane, corneal, integumentary, or subcutaneous tissue.

Defining Characteristics

Major

Damaged or destroyed tissue (cornea, mucous membrane, integumentary, or subcutaneous).

Related Factors

Altered circulation; nutritional deficit/excess; fluid deficit/excess; knowledge deficit; impaired physical mobility; irritants, chemical (including body excretions, secretions, medications); thermal (temperature extremes); mechanical (pressure, shear, friction); radiation (including therapeutic radiation).

TISSUE PERFUSION, ALTERED (SPECIFY TYPE) (RENAL, CEREBRAL, CARDIOPULMONARY, GASTROINTESTINAL, PERIPHERAL)†

Definition

The state in which an individual experiences a decrease in nutrition and oxygenation at the cellular level due to a deficit in capillary blood supply.

---

†Further work and development are required for the subcomponents, specifically cerebral, renal, and gastrointestinal.

Defining Characteristics

Estimated sensitivities and specificities

	Chances that characteristic will be present in given diagnosis:	Chances that characteristic will not be explained by any other diagnosis:
Skin temperature: cold extremities	High	Low
Skin color:		
Dependent blue or purple	Moderate	Low
*Pale on elevation, color does not return on lowering of leg	High	High
*Diminished arterial pulsations	High	High
Skin quality: shining	High	Low
Lack of lanugo Round scars covered with atrophied skin	High	Moderate
Gangrene	Low	High
Slow-growing, dry brittle nails	High	Moderate
Claudication Blood pressure changes in extremities	Moderate	High
Bruits	Moderate	Moderate
Slow healing of lesions	High	Low

Related Factors

Interruption of flow, arterial; interruption of flow, venous; exchange problems; hypovolemia; hypervolemia.

*Critical defining characteristic.

TRAUMA, RISK FOR

Definition

Accentuated risk of accidental tissue injury, e.g. wound, burn, fracture.

Defining Characteristics

Presence of risk factors such as:

Internal (individual): weakness; poor vision; balancing difficulties; reduced temperature and/or tactile sensation; reduced large or small muscle coordination; reduced hand-eye coordination; lack of safety education; lack of safety precautions; insufficient finances to purchase safety equipment or effect repairs; cognitive or emotional difficulties; history of previous trauma.

External (environmental): slippery floors, e.g. wet or highly waxed; snow or ice collected on stairs, walkways; unanchored rugs; bathtub without hand grip or antislip equipment; use of unsteady ladders or chairs; entering unlighted rooms; unsturdy or absent stair rails; unanchored electric wires; litter or liquid spills on floors or stairways; high beds; children playing without gates at the top of the stairs; obstructed passageways; unsafe window protection in homes with young children; inappropriate call-for-aid mechanisms for bedresting client; pot handles facing toward front of stove; bathing in very hot water, e.g. unsupervised bathing of young children; potential igniting gas leaks; delayed lighting of gas burner or oven; experimenting with chemical or gasoline; unscreened fires or heaters; wearing plastic apron or flowing clothes around open flame; children playing with matches, candles, cigarettes; inadequately stored combustible or corrosives, e.g. matches, oily rags, lye; highly flammable children's toys or clothing; overloaded fuse boxes; contact with rapidly moving machinery, industrial belts, or pulleys; sliding on coarse bed linen or struggling within bed restraints; faulty electric plugs, frayed wires, or defective appliances; contact with acids or alkalies; playing with fireworks or gunpowder; contact with intense cold; overexposure to sun, sun lamps, radiotherapy; use of cracked dishware or glasses; knives stored uncovered; guns or ammunition stored unlocked; large icicles hanging from the roof; exposure to dangerous machinery; children playing with sharp-edged toys; high crime neighborhood and vulnerable clients; driving a mechanically unsafe vehicle; driving after partaking of alcoholic beverages or drugs; driving at excessive speeds; driving without necessary visual aids; children riding in the front seat in car; smoking in bed or near oxygen; overloaded electrical outlets; grease waste collected on stoves; use of thin or worn potholders or misuse of necessary headgear for motorized cyclists or young children carried on adult bicycles; unsafe road or road-crossing conditions; play or work near vehicle pathways, e.g. driveways, laneways, railroad tracks; nonuse or misuse of seat restraints.

Related Factors

See risk factors.

UNILATERAL NEGLECT

Definition

A state in which an individual is perceptually unaware of and inattentive to one side of the body.

Defining Characteristics

Major

Consistent inattention to stimuli on an affected side.

Minor

Inadequate self-care; positioning and/or safety precautions in regard to the affected side; does not look toward affected side; leaves food on plate on the affected side.

Related Factors

Effects of disturbed perceptual abilities, e.g. hemianopsia; one-sided blindness; neurological illness or trauma.

URINARY ELIMINATION, ALTERED

Definition

The state in which the individual experiences a disturbance in urine elimination.

Defining Characteristics

Dysuria; frequency; hesitancy; incontinence; nocturia; retention; urgency.

Related Factors

Multiple causality, including: anatomical obstruction, sensory motor impairment, urinary tract infection.

URINARY RETENTION

Definition

The state in which the individual experiences incomplete emptying of the bladder.

Defining Characteristics

Major

Bladder distention; small, frequent voiding or absence of urine output.

Minor

Sensation of bladder fullness; dribbling; residual urine; dysuria; overflow incontinence.

Related Factors

High urethral pressure caused by weak detrusor; inhibition of reflex arc; strong sphincter; blockage.

VENTILATION, SPONTANEOUS, INABILITY TO SUSTAIN

Definition

A state in which the response pattern of decreased energy reserves results in an individual's inability to maintain breathing adequate to support life.

Defining Characteristics

Major

Dyspnea; increased metabolic rate.

Minor

Increased restlessness; apprehension; increased use of accessory muscles; decreased tidal volume; increased heart rate; decreased pO_2; increased PCO_2; decreased cooperation; decreased SaO_2.

Related Factors

Metabolic factors; respiratory muscle fatigue.

VENTILATORY WEANING RESPONSE, DYSFUNCTIONAL (DVWR)

Definition

A state in which a patient cannot adjust to lowered levels of mechanical ventilator support, which interrupts and prolongs the weaning process.

Defining Characteristics

Mild DVWR

Major

Responds to lowered levels of mechanical ventilator support with: restlessness; slight increased respiratory rate from baseline.

Minor

Responds to lowered levels of mechanical ventilator support with: expressed feelings of increased need for oxygen; breathing discomfort; fatigue; warmth; queries about possible machine malfunction; increased concentration on breathing.

Moderate DVWR

Major

Responds to lowered levels of mechanical ventilator support with: slight increase from baseline blood pressure < 20 mm Hg; slight increase from baseline heart rate < 20 beats/minute; baseline increase in respiratory rate < 5 breaths/minute.

Minor

Hypervigilance to activities; inability to respond to coaching; inability to cooperate; apprehension; diaphoresis; eye widening, wide-eyed look; decreased air entry on auscultation; color changes; pale, slight cyanosis; slight respiratory accessory muscle use.

Severe DVWR

Major

Responds to lowered levels of mechanical ventilator support with: agitation; deterioration in arterial blood gases from current baseline; increase from baseline blood pressure > 20 mm Hg; increase from baseline heart rate > 20 beats/minute; respiratory rate increases significantly from baseline.

Minor

Profuse diaphoresis; full respiratory accessory muscle use; shallow, gasping breaths; paradoxical abdominal breathing; discoordinated breathing with the ventilator; decreased level of consciousness; adventitious breath sounds, audible airway secretions; cyanosis.

Related Factors

Physical: ineffective airway clearance; sleep pattern disturbance; inadequate nutrition; uncontrolled pain or discomfort.
Psychological: knowledge deficit of the weaning process, patient role; patient perceived inefficacy about the ability to wean; decreased motivation; decreased self-esteem; anxiety (moderate, severe); fear; hopelessness; powerlessness; insufficient trust of the nurse.
Situational: uncontrolled episodic energy demands or problems; inappropriate pacing of diminished ventilator support; inadequate social support; adverse environment (noisy, active environment, negative events in the room, low nurse-patient ratio, extended nurse absence from bedside, unfamiliar nursing staff); history of ventilator dependence > 1 week; history of multiple unsuccessful weaning attempts.

VIOLENCE, RISK FOR: DIRECTED AT OTHERS
Definition

Behaviors in which an individual demonstrates that he/she can be physically, emotionally, and/or sexually harmful to others.

Defining Characteristics
Presence of risk factors such as:

History of violence: 1) against others (hitting someone, kicking someone, spitting at someone, scratching someone, throwing objects at someone, biting someone, attempted rape, rape, sexual molestation, urinating/defecating on a person; 2) threats (verbal threats against property, verbal threats against person, social threats, cursing, threatening notes/letters, threatening gestures, sexual threats); 3) against self (suicidal threats or attempts, hitting or injuring self, banging head against wall); 4) social (stealing, insistent borrowing, insistent demands for privileges, insistent interruption of meetings, refusal to eat, refusal to take medication, ignoring instructions); 5) indirect (tearing off clothes, ripping objects off walls, writing on walls, urinating on floor, defecating on floor, stamping feet, temper tantrum, running in corridors, yelling, throwing objects, breaking a window, slamming doors, sexual advances).

Other factors: neurological impairment (positive EEG, CAT, or MRI, head trauma, positive neurological findings, seizure disorders); cognitive impairment (learning disabilities, attention deficit disorder, decreased intellectual functioning); history of childhood abuse; history of witnessing family violence; cruelty to animals; firesetting; prenatal and perinatal complications/abnormalities; history of drug/alcohol abuse; pathological intoxication; psychotic symptomatology (auditory, visual, command hallucinations; paranoid delusions; loose, rambling, or illogical thought processes); motor vehicle offenses (frequent traffic violations, use of motor vehicle to release anger); suicidal behavior; impulsivity; availability and/or possession of weapon(s); body language; rigid posture, clenching of fists and jaw, hyperactivity, pacing, breathlessness, and threatening stances.

Related Factors

Antisocial character; battered women; catatonic excitement; child abuse; manic excitement; organic brain syndrome; panic states; rage reactions; suicidal behavior; temporal lobe epilepsy; toxic reactions to medication.

VIOLENCE, RISK FOR: SELF-DIRECTED
Definition

Behaviors in which an individual demonstrates that he/she can be physically, emotionally, and/or sexually harmful to self.

Defining Characteristics
Presence of risk factors such as:

Age 15–19, over 45; marital status: single, widowed, divorced; employment: unemployed, recent job loss/failure; occupation: executive, administrator/owner of business, professional, semi-skilled worker; interpersonal relationships: conflictual; family background: chaotic or conflictual, history of suicide; sexual orientation: bisexual (active), homosexual (inactive); physical health: hypochondriac, chronic or terminal illness; mental health: severe depression, psychosis, severe personality disorder, alcoholism or drug abuse; emotional status: hopelessness, despair, increased anxiety, panic, anger, hostility; history of multiple attempts; suicidal ideation: frequent, intense prolonged; suicidal plan: clear and specific; lethality: method and availability of destructive means; personal resources: poor achievement, poor insight, affect unavailable and poorly controlled; social resources: poor rapport, socially isolated, unresponsive family; verbal clues: talking about death, better off without me, asking questions about lethal dosages of drugs; behavioral clues: writing forlorn love notes, directing angry messages at a significant other who has rejected the person, giving away personal items, taking out a large life insurance policy; persons who engage in autoerotic sexual acts.

Bibliography

General Bibliography

Abrams, AC, & Goldsmith, TL. Clinical drug therapy (4th ed.). Philadelphia: J.B. Lippincott Company, 1995.

Acute Pain Management Guideline Panel. Acute pain management: operative or medical procedures and trauma. Clinical practice guideline. AHCPR Pub. No. 92-0032. Rockville, MD: Agency for Health Care Policy and Research, Public Health Service, U.S. Department of Health and Human Services, 1992.

Bates, B. A guide to physical examination (6th ed.). Philadelphia: J.B. Lippincott Company, 1995.

Beare, PG, & Meyers, JL. Principles and practice of adult health nursing (2nd ed.). St. Louis: Mosby-Year Book, 1994.

Bennett, JC, & Plum, F (Eds.). Cecil textbook of medicine (20th ed.). Philadelphia: W.B. Saunders Company, 1996.

Black, JM, & Matassarin-Jacobs, E. Luckmann and Sorensen's medical-surgical nursing: clinical management for continuity of care (5th ed.). Philadelphia: W.B. Saunders Company, 1997.

Bolander, VB. Sorensen and Luckmann's basic nursing: a psychophysiological approach (3rd ed.). Philadelphia: W.B. Saunders Company, 1994.

Bullock, BL. Pathophysiology: adaptations and alterations in function (4th ed.). Philadelphia: J.B. Lippincott Company, 1996.

Carpenito, LJ. Nursing care plans and documentation (2nd ed.). Philadelphia: J.B. Lippincott Company, 1995.

Copstead, LC. Perspectives on pathophysiology. Philadelphia: W.B. Saunders Company, 1995.

Damjanov, I, & Linder, J (Eds.). Anderson's pathology (10th ed.). St. Louis: Mosby-Year Book, 1996.

Dantzker, DR. Cardiopulmonary critical care (2nd ed.). Philadelphia: W.B. Saunders Company, 1991.

Deglin, JH, & Vallerand, AH. Davis's drug guide for nurses (5th ed.). Philadelphia: F.A. Davis Company, 1997.

Doenges, ME, Moorhouse, MF, & Geisler, AC. Nursing care plans: guidelines for planning patient care (3rd ed.). Philadelphia: F.A. Davis Company, 1993.

Dudek, SG. Nutrition handbook for nursing practice (2nd ed.). Philadelphia: J.B. Lippincott Company, 1993.

Fishbach, F. A manual of laboratory & diagnostic tests (5th ed.). Philadelphia: J.B. Lippincott Company, 1996.

Guyton, AC, & Hall, JE. Textbook of medical physiology (9th ed.). Philadelphia: W.B. Saunders Company, 1996.

Hardman, JG, & Limbrid, LE (Eds.). Goodman & Gilman's the pharmacological basis of therapeutics (9th ed.). New York: McGraw-Hill, 1996.

Holloway, NM. Medical surgical care planning (2nd ed.). Springhouse, PA: Springhouse Corporation, 1993.

Hudak, CM, & Gallo, BM. Critical care nursing: a holistic approach (6th ed.). Philadelphia: J.B. Lippincott Company, 1994.

Huether, SE, & McHance, KL. Understanding pathophysiology. St. Louis: Mosby-Year Book, 1996.

Ignatavicius, DD, & Bayne, MV. Medical-surgical nursing: a nursing process approach (2nd ed.). Philadelphia: W.B. Saunders Company, 1995.

Isselbacher, KJ, Braunwald, E, Wilson, JD, et al. (Eds.). Harrison's principles of internal medicine (13th ed.). New York: McGraw-Hill, 1994.

Jarvis, C. Physical examination and health assessment (2nd ed.). Philadelphia: W.B. Saunders Company, 1996.

Kim, MJ, McFarland, GK, & McLane, AM. Pocket guide to nursing diagnoses (6th ed.). St. Louis: Mosby-Year Book, 1995.

Kozier, B, Erb, G, Blais, K, & Wilkinson, JM. Fundamentals of nursing: concepts, process, and practice (5th ed.). Redwood City, CA: Addison-Wesley, 1995.

Lee, CAB, Barrett, CA, & Ignatavicius, DD. Fluids and electrolytes: a practical approach (4th ed.). Philadelphia: F.A. Davis Company, 1996.

LeMone, P, & Burke, KM. Medical-surgical nursing: critical thinking in client care. Menlo Park, CA: Addison-Wesley, 1996.

Lewis, SM, Collier, IC, & Heitkemper, MM. Medical-surgical nursing: assessment and management of clinical problems (4th ed.). St. Louis: Mosby-Year Book, 1996.

Mahan, LK, & Escott-Stump, S. Krause's food, nutrition, & diet therapy (9th ed.). Philadelphia: W.B. Saunders Company, 1996.

Maher, AB, Salmond, SW, & Pellino, TA. Orthopaedic nursing. Philadelphia: W.B. Saunders Company, 1994.

Malarkey, LM, & McMorrow, ME. Laboratory tests and diagnostic procedures. Philadelphia: W.B. Saunders Company, 1996.

McCance, KL, & Huether, S. Pathophysiology: the biological basis for disease in adults and children (2nd ed.). St. Louis: Mosby-Year Book, 1994.

McEvoy, GK (Ed.). Drug information '96. Bethesda, MD: American Society of Hospital Pharmacists, 1996.

McKenry, LM, & Salerno, E. Mosby's pharmacology in nursing (19th ed.). St. Louis: Mosby-Year Book, 1995.

Metheny, NM. Fluid and electrolyte balance: nursing considerations (3rd ed.). Philadelphia: J.B. Lippincott Company, 1996.

Morton, PG. Health assessment in nursing (2nd ed.). Philadelphia: F.A. Davis Company, 1993.

Murray, RB, & Zenter, JP. Nursing assessment and health promotion: strategies through the health span (5th ed.). Norwalk, CT: Appleton & Lange, 1993.

NANDA. Nursing diagnoses: definitions and classification: 1997-1998. Philadelphia: North American Nursing Diagnosis Association, 1996.

Panel for Prediction and Prevention of Pressure Ulcers in Adults. Pressure ulcers in adults: prediction and prevention. Clinical practice guideline, number 3. AHCPR Publication No. 92-0047. Rockville, MD: Agency for Health Care Policy and Research, Public Health Service, U.S. Department of Health and Human Services, 1992.

Phipps, WJ, Cassmeyer, VL, Sands, JK, & Lehman, MK. Medical-surgical nursing: concepts and clinical practice (5th ed.). St. Louis: Mosby-Year Book, 1995.

Physicians' desk reference. Montvale, NJ: Medical Economics Data, 1996.

Polaski, AL, & Tatro, SE. Luckmann's core principles and practice of medical-surgical nursing. Philadelphia: W.B. Saunders Company, 1996.

Porth, CM. Pathophysiology: concepts of altered health states (4th ed.). Philadelphia: J.B. Lippincott Company, 1994.

Potter, PA, & Perry, AG. Fundamentals of nursing: concepts, process, and practice (4th ed.). St. Louis: Mosby-Year Book, 1996.

Price, SA, & Wilson, LM. Pathophysiology: clinical concepts of disease processes (5th ed.). St. Louis: Mosby-Year Book, 1996.

Rakel, RE (Ed.). Conn's current therapy. Philadelphia: W.B. Saunders Company, 1996.

Sabiston, DC. Atlas of general surgery. Philadelphia: W.B. Saunders Company, 1994.

Sabiston, DC, & Lyerly, HK. Textbook of surgery: the biological basis of modern surgical practice (15th ed.). Philadelphia: W.B. Saunders Company, 1997.

Sabiston, DC, & Lyerly, HK. Sabiston essentials of surgery (2nd ed.). Philadelphia: W.B. Saunders Company, 1994.

Schlafer, M. The nurse, pharmacology, and drug therapy (2nd ed.). Redwood City, CA: Addison-Wesley, 1993.

Schwartz, SI (Ed.). Principles of surgery (6th ed.). New York: McGraw-Hill, 1994.

Shannon, MT, Wilson, BA, & Stang, CL. Govoni & Hayes' drugs and nursing implications (8th ed.). Norwalk, CT: Appleton & Lange, 1995.

Shils, ME, Olson, JA, & Shike, M (Eds.). Modern nutrition in health and disease (8th ed.). Philadelphia: Lea & Febiger, 1994.

Skidmore-Roth, L. Mosby's drug guide for nurses. St. Louis: Mosby-Year Book, 1996.

Smeltzer, SC, & Bare, BG. Brunner & Suddarth's textbook of medical-surgical nursing (8th ed.). Philadelphia: J.B. Lippincott Company, 1996.

Stein, JH (Ed.). Internal medicine (4th ed.). St. Louis: Mosby-Year Book, 1994.

Stuart, GW, & Sundeen, SJ. Principles & practice of psychiatric nursing (5th ed.). St. Louis: Mosby-Year Book, 1995.

Thompson, JM, McFarland, GK, Hirsch, JE, et al. Mosby's manual of clinical nursing (4th ed.). St. Louis: Mosby-Year Book, 1997.

Thompson, JM, & Wilson, SF. Health assessment for nursing practice. St. Louis: Mosby-Year Book, 1996.

Tierney, LM, McPhee, SJ, & Papadakis, MA (Eds.). Current medical diagnosis and treatment (35th ed.). Stamford, CT: Appleton & Lange, 1996.

Townsend, MC. Nursing diagnoses in psychiatric nursing: a pocket guide for care plan construction (3rd ed.). Philadelphia: F.A. Davis Company, 1994.

Treseler, KM. Clinical laboratory and diagnostic tests: significance and nursing implications (3rd ed.). Norwalk, CT: Appleton & Lange, 1995.

Way, LW (Ed.). Current surgical diagnosis and treatment (10th ed.). Norwalk, CT: Appleton & Lange, 1994.

Wilson, HS, & Kneisl, CR. Psychiatric nursing (5th ed.). Menlo Park, CA: Addison-Wesley, 1996.

UNIT III. Nursing Care of the Elderly Client

Anderson, MA, & Braun, JV. Caring for the elderly client. Philadelphia: F.A. Davis Company, 1995.

Brocklehurst, JC, Tallis, RC, & Fillit, HM (Eds). Textbook of geriatric medicine and gerontology (4th ed.). New York: Churchill Livingstone, 1992.

Carnevali, DL, & Patrick, M (Eds.). Nursing management for the elderly (3rd ed.). Philadelphia: J.B. Lippincott Company, 1993.

Drake, A, & Romano, E. How to protect your older patient from the hazards of polypharmacy. Nursing 95, 25(6):35–42, 1995.

Eliopoulos, C. Gerontological nursing (4th ed.). Philadelphia: J.B. Lippincott Company, 1997.

Freedham, JF. Gerontological nursing. Albany, NY: Delmar Publishers, 1993.

Funk, SG, Tornquist, EM, Champagne, MT, & Weise, RA (Eds.). Key aspects of elder care: managing falls, incontinence, and cognitive impairment. New York: Springer Publishing Company, 1992.

Hogstel, M. Clinical manual of gerontological nursing. St. Louis: Mosby-Year Book, 1992.

Luekenotte, A. Gerontologic nursing. St. Louis: Mosby-Year Book, 1996.

McCormick, KA, Newman, DK, Colling, J, & Pearson, BD. Clinical guidelines: urinary incontinence in adults. American Journal of Nursing, 92(10):75–93, 1992.

Needham, JF. Gerontological nursing. Albany, NY: Delmar Publishers, 1995.

Urinary Incontinence Guideline Panel. Urinary incontinence in adults. Clinical practice guideline. AHCPR Publication No. 92-0038. Rockville, MD: Agency for Health Care Policy and Research, Public Health Service, U.S. Department of Health and Human Services, March, 1992.

Vorhies, D, & Riley, BE. Deconditioning . . . changes in organ system physiology . . . induced by inactivity and reversed by activity. Clinics in Geriatric Medicine, 9(4):745–763, 1993.

Waltman, RE. 5 goals for managing older patients. Nursing 93, 23(1):63–64, 1993.

Wold, G. Basic geriatric nursing. St. Louis: Mosby-Year Book, 1993.

UNIT IV. Nursing Care of the Client Having Surgery

IV. 2. Postoperative Care

Bowell, B. Infection control: protecting the patient at risk. Nursing Times, 88(3):32–35, 1992.

Bowen, KJ, & Vukelja, SJ. Hypercoagulable states: their cause and management. Postgraduate Medicine, 91(3):117–118, 123, 125, 128, 131–132, 1992.

Calianno, C. Nosocomial pneumonia: repelling a deadly invader. Nursing 96, 26(5):32–39, 1996.

George, S, & Bugwadia, N. Nutrition and wound healing. MEDSURG Nursing, 5(4):272–275, 1996.

Good, M. Relaxation techniques for surgical patients. American Journal of Nursing, 95(5):39–43, 1995.

Griffin, K. They should have washed their hands. Health, 10(7):82–91, 1996.

Hall, GR, Karstens, M, Rakel, B, et al. Managing constipation using a research-based protocol. MEDSURG Nursing, 4(1):11–20, 1995.

Hickey, A. Catching deep vein thrombosis in time. Nursing 94, 24(10):34–41, 1994.

Hinojosa, RJ. Nursing interventions to prevent or relieve postoperative nausea and vomiting. Journal of Post Anesthesia Nursing, 7(1):3–14, 1992.

Hiyama, DT, & Zinner, MJ. Surgical complications. In Schwartz, SI (Ed.), Principles of surgery (6th ed.). New York: McGraw-Hill, 1994, pp. 455–484.

Kane, AV, & Kurlowicz, LH. Improving the postoperative care of acutely-confused older adults. MEDSURG Nursing, 3(6):453–458, 1994.

Majoros, KA, & Moccia, JM. Pulmonary embolism. Nursing 96, 26(4):27–31, 1996.

Maklebust, J, & Palleschi, M. Promoting surgical wound healing. Nursing 96, 26(6):24c–24h, 1996.

McCaffery, M. Analgesics: mapping out pain relief. Nursing 96, 26(1):41–46, 1996.

Metzler, DJ, & Fromm, CG. Laying out a care plan for the elderly postoperative patient. Nursing 93, 23(4):67–74, 1993.

Murray, CK. Helping your patient relax. Nursing 96, 26(2):32h–32n, 1996.

O'Donohue, WJ. Postoperative pulmonary complications. Postgraduate Medicine, 91(3):167–170+, 1992.

Pasero, CL, & McCaffery, M. Managing postoperative pain in the elderly. American Journal of Nursing, 96(10):39–45, 1996.

Peden, L. Helping postoperative patients sleep. RN, 55(4):24–26, 1992.

Russell, S. Hypovolemic shock. Nursing 94, 24(4):34–43, 1994.

UNIT V. Nursing Care of the Immobile Client

Corcoran, PJ. Use it or lose it—the hazards of bed rest and inactivity. Western Journal of Medicine, 154(5):536–538, 1991.

Hall, GR, Karstens, M, Rakel, B, et al. Managing constipation using a research-based protocol. MEDSURG Nursing, 4(1):11–20, 1995.

Hickey, A. Catching deep vein thrombosis in time. Nursing 94, 24(10):34–41, 1994.

Hunt, AH, Civitelli, R, & Halstead, L. Evaluation of bone resorption: a common problem during impaired mobility. Sci Nursing, 12(3):90–4, 1995.

Ludwig, LM. Preventing footdrop. Nursing 95, 25(8):32C–32D, 32F, 32J, 1995.

Majoros, KA, & Moccia, JM. Pulmonary embolism. Nursing 96, 26(4):27–31, 1996.

Mobily, PR, & Kelley, LS. Iatrogenesis in the elderly: factors of immobility. Journal of Gerontological Nursing, 17(9):5–10, 1991.

Von Rueden, KT, & Harris, JR. Pulmonary dysfunction related to immobility in the trauma patient. AACN Clinical Issues: Advanced Practice in Acute & Critical Care, 6(2):212–228, 1995.

Vorhies, D, & Riley, BE. Deconditioning . . . changes in organ system physiology . . . induced by inactivity and reversed by activity. Clinics in Geriatric Medicine, 9(4):745–763, 1993.

UNIT VI. Nursing Care of the Client Who Is Dying

Barnum, B. The challenge of providing nursing care for the dying. Nursing Leadership Forum, 2(1):34–37, 1996.

Breitbart, W, & Jacobsen, PB. Psychiatric symptom management in terminal care. Clinics in Geriatric Medicine, 12(2):329–347, 1996.

Davis, BD, Cowley, SA, & Ryland, RK. The effects of terminal illness on patients and their carers. Journal of Advanced Nursing, 23(3):512–520, 1996.

Fisher, R. Dealing with death: tools of the heart. American Journal of Nursing, 96(7):56–57, 1996.

Hall, GR, Karstens, M, Rakel, B, et al. Managing constipation using a research-based protocol. MEDSURG Nursing, 4(1):11–20, 1995.

Herbst, LH, Lynn, J, Mermann, AC, et al. What do dying patients want and need? Patient Care, 29(4):27–35, 39, 1995.

Kemp, C. Terminal illness: a guide to nursing care. Philadelphia: J.B. Lippincott Company, 1995.

Kristjanson, LJ, & Ashcroft, T. The family's cancer journey: a literature review. Cancer Nursing, 17(1):1–17, 1994.

Martinez, J, & Wagner, S. Hospice care. In Groenwald, SL, Frogge, MH, Goodman, M, & Yarbro, CH (Eds.), Cancer nursing: principles and practice (3rd ed.). Boston: Jones and Bartlett Publishers, 1993, pp. 1432–1450.

McCue, JD. The naturalness of dying. Journal of the American Medical Association, 273(13):1039–1043, 1995.

Meyer, C. 'End-of-life' care: patients' choices, nurses' challenges. American Journal of Nursing, 93(2):40–47, 1993.

Pickett, M. Cultural awareness in the context of terminal illness. Cancer Nursing, 16(2):102–106, 1993.

Rhymes, JA. Barriers to effective palliative care of terminal patients. Clinics in Geriatric Medicine, 12(2):407–416, 1996.

Schaefer, MS. Speak up! Letting patients go. RN, 59(6):72, 1996.

Solari-Twadell, PA, et al. The pinwheel model of bereavement. IMAGE: Journal of Nursing Scholarship, 27(4):323–326, 1995.

UNIT VII. Nursing Care of the Client Receiving Treatment for Neoplastic Disorders

VII. 1. Brachytherapy

Brunner, DW, Iwamoto, R, Keane, K, & Strohl, R (Eds.). Manual for radiation oncology nursing practice and education. Pittsburgh: Oncology Nursing Society, 1992.

Bucholtz, JD. Implications of radiation therapy for nursing. In Clark, JC, & McGee, RF (Eds.), Core curriculum for oncology nursing (2nd ed.). Philadelphia: W.B. Saunders Company, 1992, pp. 319–328.

Clarke, SEM. Antitumor therapy: radionuclide therapy in oncology. Cancer Treatment Reviews, 20:51–71, 1994.

Dow, KH, & Hilderly, LJ. Nursing care in radiation oncology. Philadelphia: W.B. Saunders Company, 1992.

Dunne-Daly, CF. Programmed instruction: radiation therapy—brachytherapy. Cancer Nursing, 17(4):355–364, 1994.

Dunne-Daly, CF. Programmed instruction: radiation therapy—education and nursing care of brachytherapy patients. Cancer Nursing, 17(5):435–445, 1994.

Hellman, S. Principles of radiation therapy. In DeVita, VT, Jr, Hellman, S, & Rosenberg, SA (Eds.), Cancer: principles and practice of oncology (4th ed.). Philadelphia: J.B. Lippincott Company, 1993, pp. 249–250, 271.

Hilderly, LJ. Radiotherapy. In Groenwald, SL, Frogge, MH, Goodman, M, & Yarbro, CH (Eds.), Cancer nursing: principles and practice (3rd ed.). Boston: Jones and Bartlett Publishers, 1993, pp. 264–269.

Perez, CA, & Brady, LW (Eds.). Principles and practice of radiation oncology (2nd ed.). Philadelphia: W.B. Saunders Company, 1992.

Porter, AT, Blasko, JC, Grimm, PD, et al. Brachytherapy for prostate cancer. Ca:A Cancer Journal for Clinicians, 45(3):165–178, 1995.

Shank, B. Radiotherapy: implications for general patient care. In McDonald, JS, Haller, DG, & Mayer, RJ, Manual of oncologic therapeutics (3rd ed.). Philadelphia: J.B. Lippincott Company, 1995, pp. 78–79.

Weichselbaum, RR, Hallahan, DE, & Chen, GTY. Biological and physical basis to radiation oncology. In Holland, JF, Frei, E III, Bast, RC, Jr, et al (Eds.), Cancer medicine (4th ed.) (Vol. 1). Philadelphia: Lea and Febiger, 1997, p. 720.

VII. 2. Chemotherapy

Aldag, JC, & Smith, RA. Nausea and retching/vomiting control in ondansetron and no-ondansetron groups receiving highly toxic chemotherapy. Oncology Nursing Forum, 21(2):347, 1994.

Bandyk, EA, & Gilmore, MA. Perceived concerns of pregnant women with breast cancer treated with chemotherapy. Oncology Nursing Forum, 22(6):975–977, 1995.

Basser, RL, & Green, MD. Strategies for prevention of anthracycline cardiotoxicity. Cancer Treatment Reviews, 19(1):55–77, 1993.

Bissett, D, Setanoians, A, Cassidy, J, et al. Phase 1 pharmacokinetic study of Taxotere (RP56976) administered as a 24 hr. infusion. Cancer Research, 53(3):523–527, 1993.

Boyle, DM, & Engelking, C. Vesicant extravasation: myths and realities. Oncology Nursing Forum, 22(1):57–67, 1995.

Brogden, JM, & Nevidjon, B. Vinorelbine (Navelbine): drug profile and nursing implications of a new vinca alkaloid. Oncology Nursing Forum, 22(4):635–646, 1995.

Cain, JW, & Bender, CM. Ifosfamide-induced neurotoxicity: associated symptoms and nursing implications. Oncology Nursing Forum, 22(4):659–668, 1995.

Carter, L. Bacterial translocation: nursing implications in the care of patients with neutropenia. Oncology Nursing Forum, 21(5):857–867, 1994.

Carter, LW. Influences of nutrition and stress on people at risk for neutropenia: nursing implications. Oncology Nursing Forum, 20(8):1241–1250, 1993.

DeVita, VT, Jr, Hellman, S, & Rosenberg, SA (Eds.). Cancer: principles and practice of oncology (5th ed.). Philadelphia: J.B. Lippincott Company, 1997.

Egan, AP, Taggart, JR, & Bender, CM. Management of chemotherapy-related nausea and vomiting using a serotonin antagonist. Oncology Nursing Forum, 19(5):791–795, 1992.

Ezzone, S, Jolly, D, Replogle, D, et al. Survey of oral hygiene regimens among bone marrow transplant centers. Oncology Nursing Forum, 20(9):1375–1381, 1993.

Facione, NC, Dodd, MJ, & Dibble, SL. Multiple methods to describe the prevalence and experience of chemotherapy induced oral mucositis. Oncology Nursing Forum, 20(2):341, 1993.

Fox, SM, & Haney, LG. Taxol: new hope for cancer patients. RN, 57(11):33–36, 1994.

Furlong, TG. Neurologic complications of immunosuppressive cancer therapy. Oncology Nursing Forum, 20(9):1337–1352, 1993.

Groenwald, SL, Frogge, MH, Goodman, M, & Yarbro, CH (Eds.). Cancer nursing: principles and practice (3rd ed.). Boston: Jones and Bartlett Publishers, 1993.

Hagopian, GA. Cognitive strategies used in adapting to a cancer diagnosis. Oncology Nursing Forum, 20(11):759–763, 1993.

Holland, JF, Bast, RC, Morton, DL, et al (Eds.). Cancer medicine (4th ed.). Baltimore: Williams & Wilkins, 1997.

Hooper, PJ, & Santas, EJ. Peripheral blood cell transplantation. Oncology Nursing Forum, 20(8):1215–1221, 1993.

Kintzel, PE, & Dorr, RT. Anticancer drug renal toxicity and elimination: dosing guidelines for altered renal function. Cancer Treatment Reviews, 21(1):33–64, 1995.

Langer, CJ, Leighton, JC, Comis, RL, et al. Paclitaxel and carboplatin in combination in the treatment of advanced non-small-cell lung cancer: a phase II toxicity, response, and survival analysis. Journal of Clinical Oncology, 13(8):1860–1870, 1995.

Lassiter, M, & Meisenbert, B. The prevention of hemorrhagic cystitis with high-dose cyclophosphamide therapy. Oncology Nursing Forum, 21(2):341, 1994.

Lieschke, GJ, Ramenghi, V, O'Connor, MP, et al. Studies of oral neutrophil levels in patients receiving G-CSF after autologous bone marrow transplant. British Journal of Haematology, 82(3):589–595, 1992.

McGuire, D, Altomonte, V, Peterson, DE, et al. Patterns of mucositis and pain in patients receiving preparative chemotherapy and bone marrow transplant. Oncology Nursing Forum, 20(10):1493–1502, 1993.

Mock, V, Burke, MB, Sheehan, P, et al. A nursing rehabilitation program for women with breast cancer receiving adjuvant chemotherapy. Oncology Nursing Forum, *21*(5):899–907, 1994.

Reiger, PT, & Haeuber, D. A new approach to managing chemotherapy-related anemia: nursing implications of epoetin alfa. Oncology Nursing Forum, *22*(1):71–81, 1995.

Rogers, BB. Taxol: a promising new drug of the 90's. Oncology Nursing Forum, *20*(10):1483–1489, 1993.

Skalla, KA, & LaCasse, C. Patient education for fatigue. Oncology Nursing Forum, *19*(10):1537–1541, 1992.

Smith, DB, & Babaian, RJ. The effects of treatment for cancer on male fertility and sexuality. Cancer Nursing, *15*(4):271–275, 1992.

Sonis, ST, Lindquist, L, Vav Vugt, A, et al. Prevention of chemotherapy-induced ulcerative mucositis by transforming growth factor beta 3. Cancer Research, *54*(5):1135–1138, 1994.

Stahel, RA, Jost, LM, Pichert, G, & Widmer, L. High dose chemotherapy and autologous bone marrow transplant for malignant lymphoma. Cancer Treatment Reviews, *21*(1):3–32, 1995.

Stuckey, LA. Acute tumor lysis syndrome: assessment and nursing implications. Oncology Nursing Forum, *20*(1):49–57, 1993.

Troesch, LM, Rodehaver, CB, Delaney, E, & Yanes, B. The influence of guided imagery on chemotherapy-related nausea and vomiting. Oncology Nursing Forum, *20*(8):1179–1185, 1993.

Tuxen, MK, & Hansen, SW. Neurotoxicity secondary to antineoplastic drugs. Cancer Treatment Reviews, *20*(2):191–214, 1994.

Vasterling, J, Jenkins, RA, Tope, DM, & Burich, TG. Cognitive distraction and relaxation training for the control of side effects due to chemotherapy. Journal of Behavioral Medicine, *16*(1):65–80, 1993.

Weaver-McClure, LL, Wexler, LH, & Horowitz, ME. Doxorubicin induced cardiotoxicity: understanding the cause and reducing the risks with ICRF-187. Oncology Nursing Forum, *22*(2):387, 1995.

Winningham, ML, Nail, LM, Burke, MB, et al. Fatigue and the cancer experience: the state of knowledge. Oncology Nursing Forum, *21*(1): 23–34, 1994.

Wood, LS, & Gullo, SM. IV vesicants: how to avoid extravasation. American Journal of Nursing, *93*(4):42–46, 1993.

Workman, M, Ellenhorst-Ryan, J, & Hargrave-Koertge, V. Nursing care of the immunocompromised patient. Philadelphia: W.B. Saunders Company, 1993.

Young-McCaughan, S. Sexual functioning in women treated with chemoendocrine therapy for breast cancer. Oncology Nursing Forum, *22*(2):371, 1995.

VII. 3. External Radiation Therapy

Bruner, DK, Iwamoto, R, Keane, K, & Strohl, R (Eds.). Manual for radiation oncology nursing practice and education. Pittsburgh: Oncology Nursing Society, 1992.

Cartwright-Alcarese, F. Addressing sexual dysfunction following radiation therapy for a gynecologic malignancy. Oncology Nursing Forum, *22*(8):1227–1232, 1995.

DeVita, VT, Jr, Hellman, S, & Rosenberg, SA (Eds.). Cancer: principles and practice of oncology (5th ed.). Philadelphia: J.B. Lippincott Company, 1997.

Dini, D, Macchia, R, Gozza, A, et al. Management of acute radiodermatitis: pharmacological or nonpharmacological remedies? Cancer Nursing, *16*(5):366–370, 1993.

Dow, KH, & Hilderly, LJ. Nursing care in radiation oncology. Philadelphia: W.B. Saunders Company, 1992.

Dunne-Daly, CF. Programmed instruction: radiation therapy—external radiation therapy self-learning module. Cancer Nursing, *17*(2):156–169, 1994.

Dunne-Daly, CF. Programmed instruction: radiation therapy—nursing care and adverse reactions of external radiation therapy: a self-learning module. Cancer Nursing, *17*(3):236–256, 1994.

Dunne-Daly, CF. Programmed instruction: radiation therapy—potential long-term and late effects from radiation therapy. Cancer Nursing, *18*(1):67–79, 1995.

Dunne-Daly, CF. Programmed instruction: radiation ther-

apy—skin and wound care in radiation oncology. Cancer Nursing, *18*(2):144–162, 1995.

Dusenbery, KE, McGuire, WA, Holt, PJ, et al. Erythropoetin increases hemoglobin during radiation therapy for cervical cancer. International Journal of Radiation Oncology Biology and Physics, *29*(5):1079–1084, 1994.

Foote, RL, Loprinzi, CL, Frank, AR, et al. Randomized trial of chlorhexidine mouthwash for alleviation of radiation-induced mucositis. Journal of Clinical Oncology, *12*(12):2630–2633, 1994.

Gallagher, J. Management of cutaneous symptoms. Seminars in Oncology Nursing, *11*(4):239–247, 1995.

Ganley, BJ. Mouth care for the patient undergoing head and neck radiation therapy: survey of radiation oncology nurses. Oncology Nursing Forum, *23*(10):1619–1622, 1996.

Gomez, EG. A teaching booklet for patients receiving mantle field irradiation. Oncology Nursing Forum, *22*(1):121–126, 1995.

Graydon, JE, Bubela, N, Irvine, D, & Vincent, L. Fatigue-reducing strategies used by patients receiving treatment for cancer. Cancer Nursing, *18*(1):23–28, 1994.

Hagopian, GA. Cognitive strategies used in adapting to a cancer diagnosis. Oncology Nursing Forum, *20*(11):759–763, 1993.

Hagopian, GA. The effects of informational audiotapes on knowledge and self-care behaviors of patients undergoing radiation therapy. Oncology Nursing Forum, *23*(4):697–700, 1996.

Hahnfeldt, P, & Hlatky, L. Resensitization due to redistribution of cells in the phases of the cell cycle during arbitrary radiation protocols. Radiation Research, *145*:134–143, 1996.

Hilderly, LJ. Radiotherapy. In Groenwald, SL, Frogge, MH, Goodman, M, & Yarbro, CH (Eds.), Cancer nursing: principles and practice (3rd ed.). Boston: Jones and Bartlett Publishers, 1993, pp. 235–264.

Holland, JF, Bast, RC, Morton, DL, et al (Eds.). Cancer medicine (4th ed.). Baltimore: Williams & Wilkins, 1997.

Irvine, D, Vincent, L, Graydon, JE, et al. The prevalence and correlates of fatigue in patients receiving treatment with chemotherapy and radiotherapy: a comparison with the fatigue experienced by healthy individuals. Cancer Nursing, *17*(5):367–378, 1994.

Lichter, AS, & Lawrence, TS. Recent advances in radiation oncology. The New England Journal of Medicine, *332*(6):371–377, 1995.

Lichter, AS, & Ten Haken, RK. Three-dimensional treatment planning and conformal radiation dose delivery. In DeVita, VT, Hellman, S, & Rosenberg, SA (Eds.), Important advances in oncology. Philadelphia: J.B. Lippincott Company, 1995, pp. 95–109.

Madeya, ML. Oral complications from cancer therapy: part 1—pathophysiology and secondary complications. Oncology Nursing Forum, *23*(5):801–807, 1996.

Madeya, ML. Oral complications from cancer therapy: part 2—nursing implications for assessment and treatment. Oncology Nursing Forum, *23*(5):808–819, 1996.

Moonen, L, & Bartelink, H. Fractionation in radiotherapy. Cancer Treatment Reviews, *20*(4):365–378, 1994.

Parker, RG, & Withers, RJ. Principles of radiation oncology. In Haskell, CM, Cancer treatment. Philadelphia: W.B. Saunders Company, 1995, pp. 23–31.

Perez, CA, & Brady, LW (Eds.). Principles and practice of radiation oncology (2nd ed.). Philadelphia: W.B. Saunders Company, 1992.

Poroch, D. The effect of preparatory patient education on the anxiety and satisfaction of cancer patients receiving radiation therapy. Cancer Nursing, *18*(3):206–214, 1995.

Ransier, A, Epstein, JB, Lunn, R, & Spinelli, J. A combined analysis of a toothbrush, foam brush, and a chlorhexidine-soaked foam brush in maintaining oral hygiene. Cancer Nursing, *18*(5):393–396, 1995.

Rubin, DB, Drab, EA, Kang, HJ, et al. WR-1065 and radioprotection of vascular endothelial cells: 1. cell proliferation, DNA synthesis and damage. Radiation Research, *145*:210–216, 1996.

Shank, B. Radiotherapy: implications for general patient care.

In Macdonald, JS, Haller, DG, & Mayer, RJ, Manual of oncologic therapeutics (3rd ed.). Philadelphia: J.B. Lippincott Company, 1995, pp. 73–78.

Workman, M, Ellenhorst-Ryan, J, & Hargrave-Koertge, V. Nursing care of the immunocompromised patient. Philadelphia: W.B. Saunders Company, 1993.

UNIT VIII. Nursing Care of the Client with Disturbances of Neurological Function

VIII. 1. Cerebrovascular Accident

Adams, HP, Brott, TG, Crowell, RM, et al. American Heart Association: guidelines for the management of patients with acute ischemic stroke. Circulation, 90(3):1588–1601, 1994.

Arbour, R. What you can do to reduce increased i.c.p. Nursing 93, 23(11):41–46, 1993.

Barnett, JF, Eliasziw, M, & Meldrum, HE. Drugs and surgery in the prevention of ischemic stroke. New England Journal of Medicine, 332(4):238–248, 1995.

Benson, C, & Lusardi, P. Neurologic antecedents to patient falls. Journal of Neuroscience Nursing, 27(6):331–337, 1995.

Cammermeyer, M, & Appeldorn, C (Eds.). Core curriculum for neuroscience nursing (3rd ed. update). Chicago: American Association of Neuroscience Nurses, 1996.

Caplan, LR. Cerebrovascular disease (stroke). In Stein, JH (Ed.), Internal medicine (4th ed.). St. Louis: Mosby-Year Book, 1994, pp. 1074–1087.

Cochran, I, et al. Stroke care. Nursing 94, 24(6):34–41, 1994.

Counsell, C, et al. Pharmacology update. Nimodipine: a drug therapy for treatment of vasospasm. Journal of Neuroscience Nursing, 27(1):53–56, 1995.

Dancer, S. Redesigning care for the nonhemorrhagic stroke patient. Journal of Neuroscience Nursing, 28(3):183–189, 1996.

Davis, AE, Arrington, K, Fields-Ryan, S, & Pruitt, JO. Preventing feeding-associated aspiration. MEDSURG Nursing, 4(2):111–119, 1995.

Fowler, SB. Deep vein thrombosis and pulmonary emboli in neuroscience patients. Journal of Neuroscience Nursing, 27(4):224–228, 1995.

Fowler, S, Durkee, CM, & Webb, DJ. Rehabilitating stroke patients in the acute care setting. MEDSURG Nursing, 5(5):327–332, 1996.

Gresham, GE, Duncan, PW, Stason, WB, et al. Post-stroke rehabilitation: assessment, referral, and patient management. Clinical practice guideline, number 16. AHCPR Publication No. 95-0662. Rockville, MD: Agency for Health Care Policy and Research, Public Health Service, U.S. Department of Health and Human Services, May, 1995.

Hickey, JV. The clinical practice of neurological and neurosurgical nursing (4th ed.). Philadelphia: J.B. Lippincott Company, 1996.

Janowski, MJ. A road map for stroke recovery. RN, 59(3):26–30, 1996.

Killen, JM. Understanding dysphagia: interventions for care. MEDSURG Nursing, 5(2):99–101, 104–105, 1996.

Lucke, KT, Kerr, ME, & Chovanes, GI. Continuous bedside cerebral blood flow monitoring. Journal of Neuroscience Nursing, 27(3):164–173, 1995.

Macabasco, AC, & Hickman, JL. Thrombolytic therapy for brain attack. Journal of Neuroscience Nursing, 27(3):138–149, 1995.

Meyer, FB. Sundt's occlusive cerebrovascular disease (2nd ed.). Philadelphia: W.B. Saunders Company, 1994.

Moore, K. Stroke: the long road back. RN, 57(3):50–54, 1994.

Moore, K, & Trifiletti, E. Stroke: the first critical days. RN, 57(2):22–27, 1994.

Murphy, KB. Depression and stroke patients: the keys to successful adaptation. MEDSURG Nursing, 4(3):225–228, 1995.

Robinson-Smith, G, & Mahoney, C. Coping and marital equilibrium after stroke. Journal of Neuroscience Nursing, 27(2):83–89, 1995.

Shantz, D, & Spitz, MC. What you need to know about seizures. Nursing 93, 23(11):34–40, 1993.

Sikes, PJ, & Nolan, S. Pharmacologic management of cerebral vasospasm. Critical Care Nursing Quarterly, 15(4):78–88, 1993.

Specht, DM. Cerebral edema: bringing the brain back down to size. Nursing 95, 25(11):34–38, 1995.

Tickle, EH, & Hull, KV. Family members' roles in long-term care. MEDSURG Nursing, 4(4):300–304, 1995.

Warlow, CP. Cerebrovascular disease. In Weatherall, DJ, Ledingham, JGG, & Warrell, DA (Eds.), Oxford textbook of medicine (3rd ed.) (Vol. 3). New York: Oxford University Press, 1996, pp. 3946–3964.

VIII. 2. Craniocerebral Trauma

Arbour, R. What you can do to reduce increased i.c.p. Nursing 93, 23(11):41–46, 1993.

Benson, C, & Lusardi, P. Neurologic antecedents to patient falls. Journal of Neuroscience Nursing, 27(6):331–337, 1995.

Cammermeyer, M, & Appeldorn, C (Eds.). Core curriculum for neuroscience nursing (3rd ed. update). Chicago: American Association of Neuroscience Nurses, 1996.

Chestnut, R, Marshal, L, et al. The role of secondary brain injury in determining outcomes from severe head injury. Journal of Trauma, 34(2):216–222, 1993.

Counsell, C, et al. Pharmacology update. Nimodipine: a drug therapy for treatment of vasospasm. Journal of Neuroscience Nursing, 27(1):53–56, 1995.

Davis, AE, Arrington, K, Fields-Ryan, S, & Pruitt, JO. Preventing feeding-associated aspiration. MEDSURG Nursing, 4(2):111–119, 1995.

Geary, SM. Nursing management of cranial nerve dysfunction. Journal of Neuroscience Nursing, 27(2):102–108, 1995.

Hickey, JV. The clinical practice of neurological and neurosurgical nursing (4th ed.). Philadelphia: J.B. Lippincott Company, 1996.

Hilton, G. Secondary brain injury and the role of neuroprotective agents. Journal of Neuroscience Nursing, 26(4):251–255, 1994.

Johnson, CC. After brain injury: clearing up the confusion. Nursing 95, 25(11):39–45, 1995.

Lucke, KT, Kerr, ME, & Chovanes, GI. Continuous bedside cerebral blood flow monitoring. Journal of Neuroscience Nursing, 27(3):164–173, 1995.

Maroon, JC, Bailes, JE, Yates, A, & Norwig, J. Assessing closed head injuries. The Physician and Sports Medicine, 20(4):37–44, 1992.

Meissner, JE. Caring for patients with meningitis. Nursing 95, 25(7):50–51, 1995.

Mitchell, DH, & Owens, B. Replacement therapy: arginine vasopressin (AVP), growth hormone (GH), cortisol, thyroxine, testosterone and estrogen. Journal of Neuroscience Nursing, 28(3):140–152, 1996.

Paraobek, V, & Alaimo, I. Fluid and electrolyte management in the neurologically-impaired patient. Journal of Neuroscience Nursing, 28(5):322–328, 1996.

Rosenwasser, RH. Critical care management of head injury. Trauma Quarterly, 8(2):30–57, 1992.

Rowland, LP. Head injury. In Rowland, LP (Ed.), Merritt's textbook of neurology (9th ed.). Baltimore: Williams & Wilkins, 1995, pp. 417–439.

Schinner, KM, Chisholm, AH, Grap, MJ, et al. Effects of auditory stimuli on intracranial pressure and cerebral perfusion pressure in traumatic brain injury. Journal of Neuroscience Nursing, 27(6):348–354, 1995.

Shantz, D, & Spitz, MC. What you need to know about seizures. Nursing 93, 23(11):34–40, 1993.

Specht, DM. Cerebral edema: bringing the brain back down to size. Nursing 95, 25(11):34–38, 1995.

Teasdale, GM. Head injuries. In Weatherall, DJ, Ledingham, JGG, & Warrell, DA (Eds.), Oxford textbook of medicine (3rd ed.) (Vol. 3). New York: Oxford University Press, 1996, pp. 4044–4050.

Tickle, EH, & Hull, KV. Family members' roles in long-term care. MEDSURG Nursing, 4(4):300–304, 1995.

VIII. 3. Craniotomy

Apuzzo, MLJ (Ed.). Brain surgery: complication avoidance and management. New York: Churchill Livingstone, 1993.

Cammermeyer, M, & Appeldorn, C (Eds.). Core curriculum for

neuroscience nursing (3rd ed. update). Chicago: American Association of Neuroscience Nurses, 1996.

Counsell, C, et al. Pharmacology update. Nimodipine: a drug therapy for treatment of vasospasm. Journal of Neuroscience Nursing, *27*(1):53–56, 1995.

Geary, SM. Nursing management of cranial nerve dysfunction. Journal of Neuroscience Nursing, *27*(2):102–108, 1995.

Hickey, JV. The clinical practice of neurological and neurosurgical nursing (4th ed.). Philadelphia: J.B. Lippincott Company, 1996.

Lucke, KT, Kerr, ME, & Chovanes, GI. Continuous bedside cerebral blood flow monitoring. Journal of Neuroscience Nursing, *27*(3):164–173, 1995.

Meissner, JE. Caring for patients with meningitis. Nursing 95, *25*(7):50–51, 1995.

Mitchell, DH, & Owens, B. Replacement therapy: arginine vasopressin (AVP), growth hormone (GH), cortisol, thyroxine, testosterone and estrogen. Journal of Neuroscience Nursing, *28*(3):140–152, 1996.

Paraobek, V, & Alaimo, I. Fluid and electrolyte management in the neurologically-impaired patient. Journal of Neuroscience Nursing, *28*(5):322–328, 1996.

Rengachary, SS, & Wilkins, RH (Eds.). Principles of neurosurgery. London: Mosby-Wolfe, 1994.

Zejdik, CP. Management of spinal cord injury (2nd ed.). Boston: Jones and Bartlett Publishers, 1992.

VIII. 4. Spinal Cord Injury

Cammermeyer, M, & Appeldorn, C (Eds.). Core curriculum for neuroscience nursing (3rd ed. update). Chicago: American Association of Neuroscience Nurses, 1996.

Fowler, SB. Deep vein thrombosis and pulmonary emboli in neuroscience patients. Journal of Neuroscience Nursing, *27*(4):224–228, 1995.

Gundy, DJ. Spinal cord injury and the management of paraplegia. In Weatherall, DJ, Ledingham, JGG, & Warrell, DA (Eds.), Oxford textbook of medicine (3rd ed.) (Vol. 3). New York: Oxford University Press, 1996, pp. 3895–3902.

Gutierrez, PA, Vulpe, M, & Young, RR. Spinal cord injury. In Stein, JH (Ed.), Internal medicine (4th ed.). St. Louis: Mosby-Year Book, 1994, pp. 1134–1144.

Hickey, JV. The clinical practice of neurological and neurosurgical nursing (4th ed.). Philadelphia: J.B. Lippincott Company, 1996.

Marotta, JT. Spinal injury. In Rowland, LP (Ed.), Merritt's textbook of neurology (9th ed.). Baltimore: Williams & Wilkins, 1993, pp. 440–446.

Matthews, WB. Spinal cord. In Weatherall, DJ, Ledingham, JGG, & Warrell, DA (Eds.), Oxford textbook of medicine (3rd ed.) (Vol. 3). New York: Oxford University Press, 1996, pp. 3891–3895.

Pontieri-Lewis, V. Therapeutic beds: an overview. MEDSURG Nursing, *4*(4):323–324, 330, 1995.

Richmond, TS, et al. Requirement for nursing care services and associated costs in acute spinal cord injury. Journal of Neuroscience Nursing, *27*(1):47–52, 1995.

Segatore, M. Understanding chronic pain after spinal cord injury. Journal of Neuroscience Nursing, *26*(4):230–235, 1994.

UNIT IX. Nursing Care of the Client with Disturbances of Cardiovascular Function

IX. 1. Angina Pectoris

Braunwald, E (Ed.). Heart disease: a textbook of cardiovascular medicine (4th ed.). Philadelphia: W.B. Saunders Company, 1992.

Braunwald, E, Mark, DB, Jones, RH, et al. Diagnosing and managing unstable angina. Quick reference guide for clinicians, number 10 (amended). AHCPR Publication No. 94-0603. Rockville, MD: Agency for Health Care Policy and Research and National Heart, Lung, and Blood Institute, Public Health Service, U.S. Department of Health and Human Services, May, 1994.

Cody, RJ, Conti, CR, & Samet, P. Managing angina and concomitant disease. Patient Care, *27*(12):45–46, 49, 52, 1993.

Cooke, DH. To stabilize unstable angina. Emergency Medicine, *24*(9):98–104, 1992.

Fleury, J. Long-term management of the patient with stable angina. Nursing Clinics of North America, *27*(1):205–230, 1992.

Futterman, LG, & Lemberg, L. Cardiology case book. Angina, linked angina, chest pain: an enigma within a dilemma. American Journal of Critical Care, *4*(4):325–331, 1995.

Holcomb, SS. Atherectomy. Nursing 93, *23*(2):44–47, 1993.

Hurst, JW (Ed.). The heart (8th ed.). New York: McGraw-Hill, 1994.

Leibovitch, ER. Chest pain: how to distinguish between cardiac and noncardiac causes. Geriatrics, *50*(9):32–36, 39–40, 1995.

Matrisciano, L. Unstable angina. Critical Care Nurse, *12*(8):30–38, 1992.

Obrych, DD. Interpreting CPK and LDH results. Nursing 93, *23*(1):48–49, 1993.

Waite, LG. Commentary on double-blind trial of aspirin in primary prevention of myocardial infarction in patients with stable chronic angina pectoris. AACN Nursing Scan in Critical Care, *3*(3):4, 1993.

IX. 2. Heart Failure

Ahrens, SG. Managing heart failure: a blueprint for success. Nursing 95, *25*(12):26–32, 1995.

Amsterdam, EA, Cohn, JN, Konstam, MA, & Pitt, B. Treating heart failure: a waiting game no longer. . . .second in a three-part series. Patient Care, *29*(5):74–82, 85–88, 93–94, 1995.

Braunwald, E (Ed.). Heart disease: a textbook of cardiovascular medicine (4th ed.). Philadelphia: W.B. Saunders Company, 1992.

Brown, KK. Boosting the failing heart with inotropic drugs. Nursing 93, *23*(4):34–43, 1993.

Cash, LA. Advanced practice nursing: heart failure from diastolic dysfunction. Dimensions of Critical Care Nursing, *15*(4):170–178, 1996.

Clochesy, JM, Breu, C, Cardin, S, et al. Critical care nursing. Philadelphia: W.B. Saunders Company, 1993.

Dalen, R, & Roberts, SL. Nursing management of congestive heart failure—Part I. Intensive & Critical Care Nursing, *11*(5):272–279, 1995.

Dalen, R, & Roberts, SL. Nursing management of congestive heart failure—Part II. Intensive & Critical Care Nursing, *11*(6):322–328, 1995.

Devereaux, RB, Diodati, JG, & Levy, D. Cardiac hypertrophy: practice implications. Patient Care, *26*(9):88–92, 95–102, 110–112, 121–122, 1992.

Fowler, JP. From chronic to acute: when CHF turns deadly. . . . congestive heart failure. Nursing 95, *25*(1):54–55, 1995.

Kennedy, GT. Acute congestive heart failure: pharmacologic intervention. Critical Care Nursing Clinics of North America, *4*(2):365–375, 1992.

Konstam, M, Dracup, K, Baker, D, et al. Heart failure: evaluation and care of patients with left-ventricular systolic dysfunction. Clinical practice guideline, number 11. AHCPR Publication No. 94-0612. Rockville, MD: Agency for Health Care Policy and Research, Public Health Service, U.S. Department of Health and Human Services, June, 1994.

Letterer, RA, Carew, B, Reid, M, & Woods, P. Learning to live with congestive heart failure. Nursing 92, *22*(5):34–42, 1992.

Moser, DK. Maximizing therapy in the advanced heart failure patient. Journal of Cardiovascular Nursing, *10*(2):29–46, 1996.

Skillings, J. Improving survival in congestive heart failure: the role of ACE inhibitors. Physician Assistant, *19*(7):26–28, 31–38, 45, 1995.

Weeks, SM. Caring for patients with heart failure. Nursing 96, *26*(3):52, 1996.

Wright, JM. Pharmacologic management of congestive heart failure. Critical Care Nursing Quarterly, *18*(1):32–44, 1995.

IX. 3. Heart Surgery: Coronary Artery Bypass Grafting (CABG) or Valve Replacement

Allen, JK. Trends in coronary artery bypass surgery: implications for rehabilitation. Journal of Cardiopulmonary Rehabilitation, *14*(1):30–34, 1994.

Braunwald, E (Ed.). Heart disease: a textbook of cardiovascular medicine (5th ed.). Philadelphia: W.B. Saunders Company, 1996.

Coleman, B, Lavieri, MC, & Gross, S. Patients undergoing cardiac surgery. In Clochesy, JM, Breu, C, Cardin, S, et al, Critical care nursing. Philadelphia: W.B. Saunders Company, 1993, pp. 385–429.

Earp, JK. The gastroepiploic arteries as alternative coronary artery bypass conduits. Critical Care Nurse, *14*(1):24–30, 1994.

Kirklin, JW, & Barratt-Boyes, B. Cardiac surgery (2nd ed.). New York: Churchill Livingstone, 1995.

Lewis-Sims, L. Practical innovations. Minimizing patients' hypothermia and bleeding after cardiac surgery. AORN Journal, *61*(4):731, 733–736, 1995.

Shinn, JA. Management of a patient undergoing myocardial revascularization: coronary artery bypass graft surgery. Nursing Clinics of North America, *27*(1):243–256, 1992.

IX. 4. Hypertension

Amsterdam, EA, Mathews, JJ, Messerli, FH, et al. Urgent, emergent—and safe—BP reduction. Patient Care, *28*(14):80–82, 85, 88, 1994.

Braunwald, E (Ed.). Heart disease: a textbook of cardiovascular medicine (5th ed.). Philadelphia: W.B. Saunders Company, 1996.

Clochesy, JM, Breu, C, Cardin, S, et al. Critical care nursing. Philadelphia: W.B. Saunders Company, 1993.

Cuddy, RP. Hypertension: keeping dangerous blood pressure down. Nursing 95, *25*(8):35–41, 1995.

Eaton, LE, Buck, EA, & Catanzaro, JE. The nurse's role in facilitating compliance in clients with hypertension. MEDSURG Nursing, *5*(5):339–345, 359, 1996.

Fifth report of the Joint National Committee on Detection, Evaluation, and Treatment of High Blood Pressure. Archives of Internal Medicine, *153*(2):154–183, 1993.

Fox, K. Hypertension and heart disease. Nursing Standard, *10*(23):52, 1996.

Futterman, LG, & Lemberg, L. Hypertension, stroke, and noncompliance: an unavoidable triad. American Journal of Critical Care, *5*(3):227–233, 1996.

Hurst, JW (Ed.). The heart (8th ed.). New York: McGraw-Hill, 1994.

Hutchins, LN. Drug therapy for hypertension and hyperlipidemia. Journal of Cardiovascular Nursing, *9*(2):37–53, 1995.

Johansen, JM. Update: guidelines for treating hypertension. American Journal of Nursing, *93*(3):42–49, 1993.

Laragh, JH, & Brenner, BM. Hypertension: pathophysiology, diagnosis, and management. New York: Raven Press, 1995.

Redeker, NS, & Sadowski, AV. Update on cardiovascular drugs and elders. American Journal of Nursing, *95*(9):34–41, 1995.

IX. 5. Myocardial Infarction

Apple, S. New trends in thrombolytic therapy. RN, *59*(1):30–34, 1996.

Braunwald, E (Ed.). Heart disease: a textbook of cardiovascular medicine (5th ed.). Philadelphia: W.B. Saunders Company, 1996.

Cairns, JA. Economics and efficacy in choosing oral anticoagulants or aspirin after myocardial infarction. Journal of American Medical Association, *273*(12):965–967, 1995.

Cerrato, PL. What's new in drugs. This ACE inhibitor may help save acute MI patients. . . .lisinopril (Prinivil). RN, *59*(2):78–79, 1996.

Clochesy, JM, Breu, C, Cardin, S, et al. Critical care nursing. Philadelphia: W.B. Saunders Company, 1993.

Holcomb, SS. Atherectomy. Nursing 93, *23*(2):44–47, 1993.

Huth, MM, O'Brien, KD, & Kennedy, JW. Acute myocardial infarctions: assessment and management. Physical Medicine and Rehabilitation Clinics of North America, *6*(1):69–95, 1995.

Lewis, PS. Clinical implications of non-Q-wave (subendocardial) myocardial infarctions. Focus on Critical Care AACN, *19*(1):29–33, 1992.

Lynn, LA, & Kissinger, JF. Coronary precautions: should caffeine

be restricted in patients with myocardial infarction? Heart and Lung, *21*(4):365–371, 1992.

Nyamathi, A, Alison, J, Constancia, P, et al. Coping and adjustment of spouses of critically ill patients with cardiac disease. Heart and Lung, *21*(2):160–165, 1992.

Obrych, DD. Interpreting CPK and LDH results. Nursing 93, *23*(1):48–49, 1993.

O'Donnell, L. Complications of MI beyond the acute stage. American Journal of Nursing, *96*(9):24–31, 1996.

Paul, S. The pathophysiologic process of ventricular remodeling: from infarct to failure. Critical Care Nursing Quarterly, *18*(1):7–21, 1995.

Pfeffer, MA. ACE inhibition in acute myocardial infarction. New England Journal of Medicine, *332*(2):118–120, 1995.

Roberts, R, Morris, D, Pratt, CM, & Alexander, RW. Pathophysiology, recognition, and treatment of acute myocardial infarction and its complications. In Hurst, JW (Ed.), The heart. New York: McGraw-Hill, 1994, pp. 1107–1166.

Scherck, KA. Coping with acute myocardial infarction. Heart and Lung, *21*(4):327–334, 1992.

Stovsky, B. Nursing intervention for risk factor reduction. Nursing Clinics of North America, *27*(1):257–270, 1992.

Weston, CFM. Current status of thrombolytic therapy, part 1: acute myocardial infarction and unstable angina. Care of the Critically Ill, *12*(3):106–108, 1996.

IX. 6. Pacemaker Insertion

Buckingham, TA, Janosik, DL, & Pearson, AC. Pacemaker hemodynamics: clinical implications. Progress in Cardiovascular Disease, *34*(5):347–366, 1992.

Goldberger, AL, & Goldberger, E. Clinical electrocardiography (5th ed.). St. Louis: Mosby-Year Book, 1994.

Hasemeier, CS. Clinical snapshot. Permanent pacemaker. American Journal of Nursing, *96*(2):30–31, 1996.

Hurst, JW (Ed.). The heart (8th ed.). New York: McGraw-Hill, 1994.

Jones, JV, MacConnell, TJ, & Evans, SJ. Pacemakers. Care of the Critically Ill, *11*(2):53–55, 1995.

Lascelles, K. Permanent pacemakers. Nursing Standard, *9*(20):52–53, 1995.

Levine, PA. Benefits of dual-chambered pacemakers. Western Journal of Medicine, *156*(1):70–71, 1992.

Mercer, ME. Electrical support for the heart: rate-responsive pacers. RN, *55*(5):34–37, 1992.

Porterfield, LM, & Porterfield, JG. Third generation pacemaker-cardioverter-defibrillator. Critical Care Nurse, *15*(2):43–45, 1995.

Pulice, C. Heeding that "inner voice". . .pacemaker failure to capture. Nursing 95, *25*(10):66, 1995.

UNIT X. Nursing Care of the Client with Disturbances of Peripheral Vascular Function

X. 1. Abdominal Aortic Aneurysm Repair

Anderson, LA. An update on the cause of AAA. Journal of Vascular Nursing, *12*(4):95–100, 1994.

Fahey, VA (Ed.). Vascular nursing (2nd ed.). Philadelphia: W.B. Saunders Company, 1994.

Fellows, E. Abdominal aortic aneurysm: warning flags to watch for. American Journal of Nursing, *95*(5):27–33, 1995.

Green, RM, & Ouriel, K. Peripheral arterial disease. In Schwartz, SI (Ed.), Principles of surgery (6th ed.). New York: McGraw-Hill, 1994, pp. 925–940.

Greenfield, LJ, et al (Eds.). Surgery: scientific principles and practice (2nd ed.). Philadelphia: J.B. Lippincott Company, 1997.

Hatswell, EM. Abdominal aortic aneurysm surgery, part I: an overview and discussion of immediate perioperative complications. Heart Lung, *23*(3):228–241, 1994.

Matula, PA. Aortic rupture! RN, *59*(11):38–41, 1996.

Rutherford, RB (Ed.). Vascular surgery (4th ed.). Philadelphia: W.B. Saunders Company, 1995.

Warbinek, E, & Wyness, MA. Caring for patients with complications after elective AAA surgery: a case study. Journal of Vascular Nursing, *12*(3):73–79, 1994.

X. 2. Carotid Endarterectomy

Cammermeyer, M, & Appeldorn, C (Eds.). Core curriculum for neuroscience nursing (3rd ed. update). Chicago: American Association of Neuroscience Nurses, 1996.

Colburn, MD, & Moore, WS. Carotid endarterectomy. In Jamieson, CW, & Yao, JST (Eds.), Rob & Smith's operative surgery (5th ed.). London: Chapman & Hall Medical, 1994, pp. 123–139.

Fahey, VA (Ed.). Vascular nursing (2nd ed.). Philadelphia: W.B. Saunders Company, 1994.

Greenfield, LJ, et al (Eds.). Surgery: scientific principles and practice (2nd ed.). Philadelphia: J.B. Lippincott Company, 1997.

Hertzer, NR. Postoperative management and complications following carotid endarterectomy. In Rutherford, RB (Ed.), Vascular surgery (4th ed.) (Vol. 2). Philadelphia: W.B. Saunders Company, 1995, pp. 1637–1659.

Hickey, JV. The clinical practice of neurological and neurosurgical nursing (4th ed.). Philadelphia: J.B. Lippincott Company, 1996.

Meyer, FB. Sundt's occlusive cerebrovascular disease (2nd ed.). Philadelphia: W.B. Saunders Company, 1994.

Sundt, TM, et al. Prevention and management of postoperative complications. In Meyer, FB, Sundt's occlusive cerebrovascular disease (2nd ed.). Philadelphia: W.B. Saunders Company, 1994, pp. 248–263.

X. 3. Deep Vein Thrombosis

Apple, S. New trends in thrombolytic therapy. RN, 59(1):30–34, 1996.

Berkman, SA. Current concepts in anticoagulation. Hospital Practice, 27(2):187–194, 199–200, 1992.

Bick, RL. Oral anticoagulants in thromboembolic disease. Laboratory Medicine, 26(3):188–193, 1995.

Coffman, JD. Venous thrombosis and the diagnosis of pulmonary emboli. Hospital Practice, 27(4A):99–102, 107–112, 1992.

Grant, BJB, & El-Solh, AA. Thromboembolic disease: optimizing recognition. Hospital Medicine, 31(11):14–17, 21–22, 24, 1995.

Gray, BH, & Graor, RA. Deep vein thrombosis and pulmonary embolism: the importance of heightened awareness. Postgraduate Medicine, 91(1):207–210, 213–214, 217–218, 1992.

Hickey, A. Catching deep vein thrombosis in time. Nursing 94, 24(10):34–41, 1994.

Majoros, KA, & Moccia, JM. Pulmonary embolism. Nursing 96, 26(4):27–31, 1996.

X. 4. Femoropopliteal Bypass

Fahey, VA (Ed.). Vascular nursing (2nd ed.). Philadelphia: W.B. Saunders Company, 1994.

Green, RM, & Ouriel, K. Peripheral arterial disease. In Schwartz, SI (Ed.), Principles of surgery (6th ed.). New York: McGraw-Hill, 1994, pp. 953–956.

Greenfield, LJ, et al (Eds.). Surgery: scientific principles and practice (2nd ed.). Philadelphia: J.B. Lippincott Company, 1997.

Inahara, T, & Mukherjee, D. Femoral and popliteal thromboendarterectomy. In Rutherford, RB (Ed.), Vascular surgery (4th ed.). Philadelphia: W.B. Saunders Company, 1995, pp. 835–848.

Jamieson, CW. Femoral and popliteal embolectomy. In Jamieson, CW, & Yao, JST (Eds.), Rob & Smith's operative surgery (5th ed.). London: Chapman & Hall Medical, 1994, pp. 384–391.

UNIT XI. Nursing Care of the Client with Disturbances of Respiratory Function

XI. 1. Cancer of the Lung

Baum, GL, & Wolinsky, E. Textbook of pulmonary diseases (5th ed). Boston: Little, Brown & Company, 1994.

Boyer, CL. Three cancer complications that can't wait. Nursing 93, 23(10):34–41, 1993.

DesJardins, T, & Burton, GG. Clinical manifestations and assessment of respiratory disease (3rd ed.). St. Louis: Mosby-Year Book, 1995.

DeVita, VT, Jr, Hellman, S, & Rosenberg, SA (Eds.). Cancer: principles and practice of oncology (5th ed.). Philadelphia: J.B. Lippincott Company, 1997.

Fox, JM. Malignant pleural effusion. MEDSURG Nursing, 3(5):353–359, 1994.

Groenwald, SL, Frogge, MH, Goodman, M, & Yarbro, CH (Eds.). Cancer nursing: principles and practice (4th ed.). Boston: Jones and Bartlett Publishers, 1997.

Handerhan, B. Responding to pleural effusion. Nursing 94, 24(7):32C–32D, 32F, 1994.

Haskell, CM. Cancer treatment (4th ed.). Philadelphia: W.B. Saunders Company, 1995.

Held, JL. Caring for a patient with lung cancer. Nursing 95, 25(10):34–43, 1995.

Holland, JF, Bast, RC, Morton, DL, et al (Eds.). Cancer medicine (4th ed.). Baltimore: Williams & Wilkins, 1997.

McCorkle, R, Grant, M, Frank-Stromborg, M, & Baird, SB. Cancer nursing: a comprehensive textbook (2nd ed.). Philadelphia: W.B. Saunders Company, 1996.

Roth, JA, Ruckdeschel, JC, & Weisenburger, TH. Thoracic oncology (2nd ed.). Philadelphia: W.B. Saunders Company, 1995.

Sabiston, DC, Jr, & Spencer, FC. Surgery of the chest (6th ed.). Philadelphia: W.B. Saunders Company, 1995.

Sarna, L. Correlates of symptom distress in women with lung cancer. Cancer Practice, 1(1):21–28, 1993.

Seale, DD, & Beaver, BM. Pathophysiology of lung cancer. Nursing Clinics of North America, 27(3):603–613, 1992.

Turner, JAT. Nursing care of the terminal lung cancer patient. Nursing Clinics of North America, 27(3):691–702, 1992.

XI. 2. Chronic Obstructive Pulmonary Disease

Ahrens, SG. Managing heart failure: a blueprint for success. Nursing 95, 25(12):26–31, 1995.

Barnes, TA. Core textbook of respiratory care practice (2nd ed.). St. Louis: Mosby-Year Book, 1994.

Dantzker, DR. Obstructive lung disease. In Dantzker, DR, MacIntyre, NR, & Bakow, ED, Comprehensive respiratory care. Philadelphia: W.B. Saunders Company, 1995, pp. 692–713.

DesJardins, T, & Burton, GG. Clinical manifestations and assessment of respiratory disease (3rd ed.). St. Louis: Mosby-Year Book, 1995.

Edelman, NH, Kaplan, RM, Buist, AS, et al. Chronic obstructive pulmonary disease. Chest, 102(3):234S–256S, 1992.

Hagedorn, DS. Acute exacerbation of COPD. Postgraduate Medicine, 91(1):105–107, 110–112, 1992.

Ingram, RH, Jr. Chronic bronchitis, emphysema, and airways obstruction. In Isselbacher, KJ, Braunwald, E, Wilson, JD, et al (Eds.), Harrison's principles of internal medicine (13th ed.). New York: McGraw-Hill, 1994, pp. 1197–1206.

Janowski, MJ. Managing heart failure. RN, 59(2):34–38, 1996.

Niewoehner, DE. Clinical aspects of chronic obstructive pulmonary disease. In Baum, GL, & Wolinsky, E (Eds.), Textbook of pulmonary diseases (5th ed.) (Vol. 2). Boston: Little, Brown & Company, 1994, pp. 995–1027.

Scanlan, CL, Spearman, CB, & Sheldon, RL (Eds.). Egan's fundamentals of respiratory care (6th ed.). St. Louis: Mosby-Year Book, 1995.

Weeks, SM. Caring for patients with heart failure. Nursing 96, 26(3):52–53, 1996.

XI. 3. Pneumonia

Baum, GL, & Wolinsky, E (Eds.). Textbook of pulmonary diseases (5th ed.). Boston: Little, Brown and Company, 1994.

Calianno, C. Nosocomial pneumonia: repelling a deadly invader. Nursing 96, 26(5):34–40, 1996.

Fein, AM, & Niederman, MS. Severe pneumonia in the elderly. Clinics in Geriatric Medicine, 10(1):121–143, 1994.

George, RB, Light, RW, Matthay, MA, & Matthay, RA (Eds.). Chest medicine: essentials of pulmonary and critical care medicine (3rd ed.). Baltimore: Williams & Wilkins, 1995.

Mandell, GL, Bennett, JE, & Dolin, R (Eds.). Mandell, Douglas and Bennett's principles and practice of infectious diseases (4th ed.). New York: Churchill Livingstone, 1995.

XI. 4. Pneumothorax

Abolnik, IZ, Lossos, IS, Gillis, D, & Breuer, R. Primary spontaneous pneumothorax in men. American Journal of Medical Science, *305*(5):297–303, 1993.

Connors, AF, & Altose, MD. Hemothorax, chylothorax, pneumothorax, and other pleural disorders. In Baum, GL, & Wolinsky, E (Eds.), Textbook of pulmonary diseases (5th ed.) (Vol. 2). Boston: Little, Brown & Company, 1994, pp. 1869–1873.

DesJardins, T, & Burton, GG. Clinical manifestations and assessment of respiratory disease (3rd ed.). St. Louis: Mosby-Year Book, 1995.

Lazzara, D. Why is the Heimlich chest drain valve making a comeback? Nursing 96, *26*(12):50–53, 1996.

Zane, RE, et al. Video thoracoscopy: routine application for recurrent spontaneous pneumothorax. Journal of National Medical Association, *86*(7):527–529, 1994.

XI. 5. Pulmonary Embolism

Ahrens, SG. Managing heart failure: a blueprint for success. Nursing 95, *25*(12):26–31, 1995.

Apple, S. New trends in thrombolytic therapy. RN, *59*(1):30–34, 1996.

Bone, RC. Pulmonary embolism: new approaches to a complex problem. Emergency Medicine, *24*(14):144–146, 149–152, 1992.

Catania, U. Monitoring coumadin therapy. RN, *57*(2):29–34, 1994.

DesJardins, T, & Burton, GG. Clinical manifestations and assessment of respiratory disease (3rd ed.). St. Louis: Mosby-Year Book, 1995.

Gonzalez-Juanatey, JR, Amaro, A, Iglesias, C, et al. Treatment of massive pulmonary thromboembolism with low intrapulmonary dosages of urokinase. Chest, *102*(2):341–346, 1992.

Gray, BH, & Graor, RA. Deep venous thrombosis and pulmonary embolism. Postgraduate Medicine, *91*(1):207–210, 213–214, 217–218+, 1992.

Janowski, MJ. Managing heart failure. RN, *59*(2):34–38, 1996.

Majoros, KA, & Moccia, JM. Pulmonary embolism. Nursing 96, *26*(4):27–31, 1996.

Moser, KM. Pulmonary embolism. In Baum, GL, & Wolinsky, E (Eds.), Textbook of pulmonary diseases (5th ed.) (Vol. 2). Boston: Little, Brown & Company, 1994, pp. 1305–1325.

Weeks, SM. Caring for patients with heart failure. Nursing 96, *26*(3):52–53, 1996.

Weinberger, SE. Principles of pulmonary medicine. Philadelphia: W.B. Saunders Company, 1992.

XI. 6. Thoracic Surgery

Hazelrigg, SR, Nunchick, SK, & LeCicero, J. Video assisted thoracic surgery study group data. Annals of Thoracic Surgery, *56*(5):1039–1044, 1993.

Pearson, FG. Current status of surgical resection for lung cancer. Chest, *106*(6):337S–339S, 1994.

Sabiston, DC, & Spencer, FC. Surgery of the chest (6th ed.). Philadelphia: W.B. Saunders Company, 1995.

Waller, DA, Gebitekin, C, Saunders, NR, & Walker, DR. Noncardiogenic pulmonary edema complicating lung resection. Annals of Thoracic Surgery, *55*(1):140–143, 1993.

UNIT XII. Nursing Care of the Client with Disturbances of the Kidney and Urinary Tract

XII. 1. Bladder Neck Suspension (Vesicourethral Suspension)

Abrams, P. Bladder neck suspension procedures. In Whitfield, HN (Ed.), Rob & Smith's operative surgery (5th ed.). Oxford: Butterworth-Heinemann, 1993.

Bergman, A, & Elia, G. Three surgical procedures for genuine stress incontinence. American Journal of Obstetrics and Gynecology, *173*(1):66–71, 1995.

Carnevali, DL, & Patrick, M. Nursing management for the elderly (3rd ed.). Philadelphia: J.B. Lippincott Company, 1993.

Gillenwater, JY, Grayhack, JT, Howards, SS, & Duckett, JW. Adult and pediatric urology (3rd ed.). St. Louis: Mosby-Year Book, 1996.

Karlowicz, KA (Ed.). Urologic nursing: principles and practice. Philadelphia: W.B. Saunders Company, 1995.

McCormick, KA, Newman, DK, Colling, J, & Pearson, BD. Clinical guidelines: urinary incontinence in adults. American Journal of Nursing, *92*(10):75–93, 1992.

Raz, S, Little, NA, & Juma, S. Female urology. In Walsh, PC, Retik, AB, Stamey, TA, & Vaughan, ED, Jr (Eds.), Campbell's urology (6th ed.)(Vol. 3). Philadelphia: W.B. Saunders Company, 1992, pp. 2782–2812.

Reilly, NJ. Urinary incontinence: new attitudes and treatment options. Innovations in Urology Nursing, *III*(2):1–15, 1992.

Stamey, TA. Urinary incontinence in the female: the Stamey endoscopic suspension of the vesical neck for stress urinary incontinence. In Walsh, PC, Retik, AB, Stamey, TA, & Vaughan, ED, Jr (Eds.), Campbell's urology (6th ed.) (Vol. 3). Philadelphia: W.B. Saunders Company, 1992, pp. 2829–2849.

Tanagho, EA, & McAninch, JW (Eds.). Smith's general urology (14th ed.). Norwalk, CT: Appleton & Lange, 1995.

Thompson, JD, Wall, LL, Growdon, WA, & Ridley, JH. Urinary stress incontinence. In Thompson, JD, & Rock, JA, TeLinde's operative gynecology (7th ed.). Philadelphia: J.B. Lippincott Company, 1992, pp. 904–914.

XII. 2. Chronic Renal Failure

Alfrey, AC, & Chan, L. Chronic renal failure: manifestations and pathogenesis. In Schrier, RW (Ed.), Renal and electrolyte disorders (4th ed.). Boston: Little, Brown & Company, 1992, pp. 539–579.

Brenner, BM, & Lazarus, JM. Chronic renal failure. In Isselbacher, KJ, Braunwald, E, Wilson, JD, et al (Eds.), Harrison's principles of internal medicine (13th ed.). New York: McGraw-Hill, 1994, pp. 1274–1281.

Gillenwater, JY, Grayhack, JT, Howards, SS, & Duckett, JW (Eds.). Adult and pediatric urology (3rd ed.). St. Louis: Mosby-Year Book, 1996.

Kutner, NG. Rehabilitation, aging, and chronic renal disease. American Journal of Physical Medicine and Rehabilitation, *71*(2):97–101, 1992.

Luke, RG, & Strom, TB. Chronic renal failure. In Stein, JH (Ed.), Internal medicine (4th ed.). St. Louis: Mosby-Year Book, 1994, pp. 2622–2645.

Tanagho, EA, & McAninch, JW (Eds.). Smith's general urology (14th ed.). Norwalk, CT: Appleton & Lange, 1995.

Walsh, PC, Retik, AB, Stamey, TA, & Vaughan, ED, Jr (Eds.). Campbell's urology (6th ed.) (Vol 3). Philadelphia: W.B. Saunders Company, 1992.

XII. 3. Cystectomy with Urinary Diversion

Benson, MC, & Olsson, CA. Urinary diversion. Urologic Clinics of North America, *19*(4):779–795, 1992.

Carroll, PR, & Barbour, S. Urinary diversion and bladder substitution. In Tanagho, EA, & McAninch, JW (Eds.), Smith's general urology (14th ed.). Norwalk, CT: Appleton & Lange, 1995, pp. 448–461.

DeVita, VT, Jr, Hellman, S, & Rosenberg, SA. Important advances in oncology 1995. Philadelphia: J.B. Lippincott Company, 1995.

Gillenwater, JY, Grayhack, JT, Howards, SS, & Duckett, JW (Eds.). Adult and pediatric urology (3rd ed.). St. Louis: Mosby-Year Book, 1996.

Groenwald, SL, Frogge, MH, Goodman, M, & Yarbro, CH (Eds.). Cancer nursing: principles and practice (4th ed.). Boston: Jones and Bartlett Publishers, 1997.

Hampton, BG, & Bryant, RA (Eds.). Ostomies and continent diversions: nursing management. St. Louis: Mosby-Year Book, 1992.

Holland, JF, Bast, RC, Morton, DL, et al (Eds.). Cancer medicine (4th ed.). Baltimore: Williams & Wilkins, 1997.

Walsh, PC, Retik, AB, Stamey, TA, & Vaughan, ED, Jr (Eds.). Campbell's urology (6th ed.) (Vol 3). Philadelphia: W.B. Saunders Company, 1992.

Whitfield, HN (Ed.). Rob & Smith's operative surgery: genitourinary surgery (5th ed.) (Vol. 1). Oxford: Butterworth-Heinemann, 1993.

XII. 4. Nephrectomy

Gillenwater, JY, Grayhack, JT, Howards, SS, & Duckett, JW (Eds.). Adult and pediatric urology (3rd ed.). St. Louis: Mosby-Year Book, 1996.

Groenwald, SL, Frogge, MH, Goodman, M, & Yarbro, CH (Eds.). Cancer nursing: principles and practice (4th ed.). Boston: Jones and Bartlett Publishers, 1997.

Latal, D, & Marberger, M. Operations for renal ablation: simple nephrectomy. In Whitfield, HN (Ed.), Rob & Smith's operative surgery: genitourinary surgery (5th ed.) (Vol. 1). Oxford: Butterworth-Heinemann, 1993, pp. 62–67.

Tanagho, EA, & McAninch, JW (Eds.). Smith's general urology (14th ed.). Norwalk, CT: Appleton & Lange, 1995.

Walsh, PC, Retik, AB, Stamey, TA, & Vaughan, ED, Jr (Eds.). Campbell's urology (6th ed.) (Vol 3). Philadelphia: W.B. Saunders Company, 1992.

UNIT XIII. Nursing Care of the Client with Disturbances of Hematopoietic and Lymphatic Function

XIII. 1. Human Immunodeficiency Virus (HIV) Infection and Acquired Immune Deficiency Syndrome (AIDS)

Anastasi, JK. AIDS update. Nursing 93, 23(8):68–70, 1993.

Anastasi, JK, & Lee, VS. HIV wasting: how to stop the cycle. American Journal of Nursing, 94(6):18–24, 1994.

Anonymous. A new class of anti-HIV drugs debuts. American Journal of Nursing, 96(7):59–63, 1996.

Anonymous. New drugs for HIV infection. Medical Letter on Drugs & Therapeutics, 38(972):35–37, 1996.

Bartlett, JG. Johns Hopkins Hospital guide to medical care of patients with HIV infection (5th ed.). Baltimore: Williams & Wilkins, 1995.

Beal, JE, & Martin, BM. The clinical management of wasting and malnutrition in HIV/AIDS. AIDS Patient Care, 9(2):66–74, 1995.

Beal, JE, Olson, R, Laubenstein, L, et al. Dronabinol as a treatment for anorexia associated with weight loss in patients with AIDS. Journal of Pain and Symptom Management, 10(2):89–97, 1995.

Carpenter, CC, Fischl, MA, Hammer, SM, et al. Antiretroviral therapy for HIV infection in 1996: recommendations of an international panel. JAMA, 276(2):146–154, 1996.

Collier, AC, Coombs, RW, Schoenfeld, DA, et al. Treatment of human immunodeficiency virus infection with saquinavir, zidovudine, and zalcitabine. New England Journal of Medicine, 334(16):1011–1017, 1996.

Cowley, G, & Hager, M. New AIDS optimism. . . .can a blend of three drugs collar the virus? Newsweek, 128(4):68, 1996.

Fields, BN, Knipe, DM, & Howley, PM (Eds.). Fields virology (3rd ed.). Philadelphia: Lippincott-Raven, 1996.

Flaskerud, JH, & Ungvarski, PJ. HIV/AIDS: a guide to nursing care (3rd ed) Philadelphia: W.B. Saunders Company, 1993.

Forstein, M. The neuropsychiatric aspects of HIV infection. Primary Care, 19(1):97–117, 1992.

Grimes, DE, & Grimes, RM. AIDS and HIV infection. St. Louis: Mosby-Year Book, 1994.

Holzemer, WL, Henry, SB, Reilly, CA, & Portillo, CJ. Problems of persons with HIV/AIDS hospitalized for *Pneumocystis carinii* pneumonia. Journal of the Association of Nurses in AIDS Care, 6(3):23–30, 1995.

Karp, JE, Groopman, JE, & Broder, S. Cancer in AIDS. In DeVita, VT, Jr, Hellman, S, & Rosenberg, SA (Eds.), Cancer: principles and practice of oncology (4th ed.). Philadelphia: J.B. Lippincott Company, 1993, pp. 2093–2110.

Kelleher, AD, Carr, A, Zaunders, J, & Cooper, DA. Alterations in the immune response of human immunodeficiency virus (HIV)-infected subjects treated with an HIV-specific protease inhibitor, ritonavir. Journal of Infectious Diseases, 173(2):321–329, 1996.

Kenny, P. Managing HIV infection: how to bolster your patient's fragile health. Nursing 96, 26(8):26–35, 1996.

Law, C. Basic research plays a key role in new patient treatments. Journal of the National Cancer Institute, 88(13):869, 1996.

Libman, H, & Witzburg, RA (Eds.). HIV infection: a clinical manual (2nd ed.). Boston: Little, Brown and Company, 1993.

Markowitz, M, Saag, M, Powderly, WG, et al. A preliminary study of ritonavir, an inhibitor of HIV-1 protease, to treat HIV-1 infection. New England Journal of Medicine, 333(23):1534–1539, 1995.

Moran, TA. AIDS-related malignancies. In Groenwald, SL, Frogge, MH, Goodman, M, & Yarbro, CH (Eds.), Cancer nursing: principles and practice (3rd ed.). Boston: Jones and Bartlett, 1993, pp. 861–876.

Ownby, KK. Management of the hematological manifestations of HIV infection and AIDS. Journal of the Association of Nurses in AIDS Care, 6(4):9–15, 17–18, 1995.

Sande, MA, & Volberding, PA. The medical management of AIDS (4th ed.). Philadelphia: W.B. Saunders Company, 1995.

Schneider, H. What's your diagnosis? AIDS-related cachexia. Consultant, 35(3):379–380, 382, 1995.

Smith, AR, & Chang, BL. Nursing diagnoses for hospitalized patients with AIDS. Nursing Diagnosis, 7(1):9–18, 1996.

Ungvarski, PJ. Waging war on HIV wasting. RN, 59(2):27–32, 1996.

USPHS/IDSA Guidelines for the prevention of opportunistic infections in persons infected with human immunodeficiency virus: a summary. Annals of Internal Medicine, 124(3):349–361, 1996.

Winson, G. Winning a losing battle. . .wasting, physiology, nutrition. . . the most devastating aspects of AIDS. Nursing Times, 91(23):40–43, 1995.

Workman, M, Ellenhorst-Ryan, J, & Koertge, V. Nursing care of the immunocompromised patient. Philadelphia: W.B. Saunders Company, 1993.

XIII. 2. Splenectomy

Athens, JW. The reticuloendothelial (mononuclear phagocyte) system and the spleen. In Lee, GR, Bithell, TC, Foerster, J, et al (Eds.), Wintrobe's clinical hematology (9th ed.) (Vol. 1). Philadelphia: Lea & Febiger, 1993, pp. 311–325.

Bartley, MK, & Laskowski-Jones, L. Understanding postsplenectomy sepsis. American Journal of Nursing, 95(1):56A, 56D, 1995.

Gares, D. Preventing infection after splenectomy. Nursing 94, 24(5):32M, 1994.

Lewis, SM, & Swirsky, D. The spleen and its disorders. In Weatherall, DJ, Ledingham, JGG, & Warrell, DA (Eds.), Oxford textbook of medicine (3rd ed.). New York: Oxford University Press, 1996, pp. 3587–3596.

Russell, S. Septic shock. Nursing 94, 24(4):40–46, 1994.

Schwartz, SI. Spleen. In Schwartz, SI (Ed.), Principles of surgery (6th ed.). New York: McGraw-Hill, 1994, pp. 1433–1447.

UNIT XIV. Nursing Care of the Client with Disturbances of the Gastrointestinal Tract

XIV. 1. Appendectomy

Calder, JD, & Gajraj, H. Recent advances in the diagnosis and treatment of acute appendicitis. British Journal of Hospital Medicine, 54(4):129–133, 1995.

Haubrich, WS, Schaffner, F, & Berk, JE. Bockus gastroenterology (5th ed.). Philadelphia: W.B. Saunders Company, 1995.

Yamada, T (Ed.). Textbook of gastroenterology (2nd ed.). Philadelphia: J.B. Lippincott Company, 1995.

XIV. 2. Bowel Diversion: Ileostomy

Allison, M. Comparing methods of stoma formation. Nursing Standard, 9(24):25–28, 1995.

Black, PK. Common problems following stoma surgery. British Journal of Nursing, 3(8):413–414, 416–417, 1994.

Brennecke, A. Peristomal pyoderma gangrenosum: review and case study. MEDSURG Nursing, 5(3):195–198, 1996.

Epps, CK. The delicate business of ostomy care. RN, 59(11):32–36, 1996.

Fazio, VW. Preventing and managing ileostomy complications. Journal of Enterostomal Nursing, 19(2):48–53, 1992.

Hampton, BG, & Bryant, RA. Ostomies and continent diversions: nursing management. St. Louis: Mosby-Year Book, 1992.

Haubrich, WS, Schaffner, F, & Berk, JE (Eds.). Bockus gastroenterology (5th ed.) (Vol. 2). Philadelphia: W.B. Saunders Company, 1995.

Kelly, KA. Approach to the patient with ileostomy and ileal pouch. In Yamada, T, Alpers, DH, Owyang, C, et al (Eds.), Textbook of gastroenterology (2nd ed.). Philadelphia: J.B. Lippincott Company, 1995, pp. 880–893.

Kirsner, JB, & Shorter, RG (Eds.). Inflammatory bowel disease (4th ed.). Baltimore: Williams & Wilkins, 1995.

Nadler, LH. General considerations and complications of the ileostomy. Ostomy/Wound Management, 38(4):18–20, 1992.

Paulford-Lecher, N. Getting your patient started with an ostomy pouch. Nursing 95, 25(4):32L, 1995.

Salter, M. Advances in ileostomy care. Nursing Standard, 10(49):33–39, 1995.

Todd, D. Ileoanal reservoirs: construction and management. Journal of Enterostomal Nursing, 20(1):26–35, 1993.

Wilson, RE. Patient education sheets: a guide to educating the patient with a urostomy, colostomy, and ileostomy. Ostomy/Wound Management, 38(4):45–46, 48–50, 52, 1992.

XIV. 3. Gastrectomy

Cave, DR. Therapeutic approaches to recurrent peptic ulcer disease. Hospital Practice, 27(9A):33–40, 43, 47–48, 49, 1992.

Gitnick, G (Ed.). Principles and practice of gastroenterology and hepatology (2nd ed.). Norwalk, CT: Appleton & Lange, 1994.

Haubrich, WS, Schaffner, F, & Berk, JE (Eds.). Bockus gastroenterology (5th ed.) (Vol. 1). Philadelphia: W.B. Saunders Company, 1995.

Maier, RV, Mitchell, D, & Gentilello, I. Optimal therapy for stress gastritis. Annals of Surgery, 220(3):353–360, 1994.

Sleisenger, MH, & Fordtran, JS (Eds.). Gastrointestinal disease: pathophysiology/diagnosis/management (5th ed.). Philadelphia: W.B. Saunders Company, 1993.

Spiro, HM. Clinical gastroenterology (4th ed.). New York: McGraw-Hill, 1993.

Yamada, T, Alpers, DH, Owyang, C, et al (Eds.). Textbook of gastroenterology (2nd ed.). Philadelphia: J.B. Lippincott Company, 1995.

XIV. 4. Gastric Reduction

Bo-Linn, GW. Obesity, anorexia nervosa, bulimia, and other eating disorders. In Sleisenger, MH, & Fordtran, JS (Eds.), Gastrointestinal disease: pathophysiology/diagnosis/management (5th ed.) (Vol. 2). Philadelphia: W.B. Saunders Company, 1993, pp. 2109–2136.

Brolin, RL, Robertson, LB, Kenler, HA, et al. Weight loss and dietary intake after vertical banded gastroplasty and Roux-en-Y gastric bypass. Annals of Surgery, 220(6):782–790, 1994.

Capella, JF, & Capella, RF. The weight reduction operation of choice: vertical banded gastroplasty or gastric bypass. American Journal of Surgery, 171(1):74–79, 1996.

Cucchi, SG, Pories, WJ, MacDonald, KG, et al. Gastrogastric fistulas. A complication of divided gastric bypass surgery. Annals of Surgery, 221(4):387–391, 1995.

Kual, JG. Therapy for severe obesity. In Haubrich, WS, Schaffner, F, & Berk, JE (Eds.), Bockus gastroenterology (5th ed.) (Vol. 4). Philadelphia: W.B. Saunders Company, 1995, pp. 3231–3240.

Rhode, BM, Arseneau, P, Cooper, BA, et al. Vitamin B-12 deficiency after gastric surgery for obesity. American Journal of Clinical Nutrition, 63(1):103–109, 1996.

Sarr, MG, Felty, CL, Hilmer, DM, et al. Technical and practical considerations involved in operations on patients weighing more than 270 kg. Archives of Surgery, 130(1):102–105, 1995.

Spiro, HM. Clinical gastroenterology (4th ed.). New York: McGraw-Hill, 1993.

XIV. 5. Inflammatory Bowel Disease: Ulcerative Colitis and Crohn's Disease

Cox, J. Inflammatory bowel disease: implications for the medical-surgical nurse. MEDSURG Nursing, 4(6):427–437, 1995.

Doughty, DB. What you need to know about inflammatory bowel disease. American Journal of Nursing, 94(7):24–31, 1994.

Gitnick, G (Ed.). Principles and practice of gastroenterology and hepatology (2nd ed.). Norwalk, CT: Appleton & Lange, 1994.

Haubrich, WS, Schaffner, F, & Berk, JE. Bockus gastroenterology (5th ed.). Philadelphia: W.B. Saunders Company, 1995.

Kirsner, JB, & Shorter, RG (Eds.). Inflammatory bowel disease (4th ed.). Baltimore: Williams & Wilkins, 1995.

Mahan, LK, & Escott-Stump, S. Krause's food, nutrition, and diet therapy (9th ed.). Philadelphia: W.B. Saunders Company, 1996.

Naccarini, DAL, & Minor, ML. Cyclosporine and 6-mercaptopurine in pediatric inflammatory bowel disease. Gastroenterology Nursing, 16(4):169–175, 1994.

Nelson, JK, Moxness, KE, Jensen, MD, & Gastineau, CF. Mayo clinic diet manual (7th ed.). St. Louis: Mosby-Year Book, 1994.

Phillips, S. Gut reaction. . .bowel disease. Nursing Times, 91(1):44–45, 1995.

Phillips, S, & Warren, J. Supporting the patient with inflammatory bowel disease. Nursing Times, 91(27):38–39, 1995.

Sleisenger, MH, & Fordtran, JS. Gastrointestinal disease: pathophysiology/diagnosis/management (5th ed.). Philadelphia: W.B. Saunders Company, 1993.

Spiro, HM. Clinical gastroenterology (4th ed.). New York: McGraw-Hill, 1993.

Welage, J. Insight into IBD. . .what you need to know about inflammatory bowel disease. American Journal of Nursing, 94(11):20, 22, 1994.

Yamada, T (Ed.). Textbook of gastroenterology (2nd ed.). Philadelphia: J.B. Lippincott Company, 1995.

XIV. 6. Mandibular (Jaw) Fracture with Intermaxillary Fixation

Cohen, M (Ed.). Mastery of plastic and reconstructive surgery. Boston: Little, Brown & Company, 1994.

Finn, RA. Treatment of comminuted mandibular fractures by closed reduction. Journal of Oral and Maxillofacial Surgery, 54(3):320–327, 1996.

Leach, J, & Truelson, J. Traditional methods vs. rigid internal mandible fractures. Archives of Otolaryngology, Head and Neck Surgery, 121(7):750–753, 1995.

Smith, BR, & Teenier, TJ. Treatment of comminuted mandibular fractures by open reduction and rigid internal fixation. Journal of Oral and Maxillofacial Surgery, 54(3):328–331, 1996.

Stanley, RB. Maxillofacial trauma. In Cummings, CW, & Krause, CJ (Eds.), Otolaryngology—head and neck surgery (2nd ed.) (Vol. 1). St. Louis: Mosby-Year Book, 1993, pp. 374–402.

Terris, DJ, Lalakea, ML, Tuffo, KM, et al. Mandible fracture repair: specific indications for newer techniques. Otolaryngology, Head and Neck Surgery, 111(6):751–757, 1994.

XIV. 7. Peptic Ulcer

Cave, DR. Therapeutic approaches to recurrent peptic ulcer disease. Hospital Practice, 27(9A):33–40, 43, 47–48, 49, 1992.

Ching, CK, & Lam, SK. Drug therapy of peptic ulcer disease. British Journal of Hospital Medicine, 54(2–3):101–106, 1995.

Gitnick, G (Ed.). Principles and practice of gastroenterology and hepatology (2nd ed.). Norwalk, CT: Appleton & Lange, 1994.

Hatlebakk, JG, Nesje, LB, Hausken, T, et al. Lansoprazole capsules and amoxicillin oral suspension in the treatment of peptic ulcer disease. Scandinavian Journal of Gastroenterology, 30(11):1053–1057, 1995.

Haubrich, WS, Schaffner, F, & Berk, JE (Eds.). Bockus gastroenterology (5th ed.) (Vol. 1). Philadelphia: W.B. Saunders Company, 1995.

Heslin, JM. Peptic ulcer disease: making a case against the prime suspect. Nursing 97, 27(1):34–39, 1997.

Maier, RV, Mitchell, D, & Gentilello, I. Optimal therapy for stress gastritis. Annals of Surgery, 220(3):353–360, 1994.

Rauws, EA, & van der Hulst, RW. Current guidelines for the eradication of Helicobacter pylori in peptic ulcer disease. Drugs, 50(6):984–990, 1995.

Soll, AH. Medical treatment of peptic ulcer disease. Journal of the American Medical Association, 275(8):622–629, 1996.

Spiro, HM. Clinical gastroenterology (4th ed.). New York: McGraw-Hill, 1993.

Toyoda, H, Nakano, S, Takeda, I, et al. Transcatheter arterial embolization for massive bleeding from duodenal ulcers not controlled by endoscopic hemostasis. Endoscopy, 27(4):304–307, 1995.

Yamada, T, Alpers, DH, Owyang, C, et al (Eds.). Textbook of

gastroenterology (2nd ed.). Philadelphia: J.B. Lippincott Company, 1995.

UNIT XV. Nursing Care of the Client with Disturbances of the Liver, Biliary Tract, and Pancreas

XV. 1. Acute Pancreatitis

Ambrose, MS. Pancreatitis. Nursing 96, *26*(4):33–39, 1996.

Berry, SM, & Fink, AS. Acute pancreatitis. In Rakel, RE (Ed.), Conn's current therapy. Philadelphia: W.B. Saunders Company, 1996, pp. 458–463.

Bradley, EL (Ed.). Acute pancreatitis: diagnosis and therapy. New York: Raven Press, 1994.

Frey, CF. Management of necrotizing pancreatitis. Western Journal of Medicine, *159*(6):675–680, 1993.

Gorelick, FS. Acute pancreatitis. In Yamada, T, Alpers, DH, Owyang, C, et al (Eds.), Textbook of gastroenterology (2nd ed.) (Vol. 2.). Philadelphia: J.B. Lippincott Company, 1995, pp. 2064–2091.

Greenberger, NJ, Toskes, PP, & Isselbacher, KJ. Acute and chronic pancreatitis. In Isselbacher, KJ, Braunwald, KE, Wilson, JD, et al (Eds.), Harrison's principles of internal medicine (13th ed.). New York: McGraw-Hill, 1994, pp. 1520–1532.

Handerhan, B. Responding to pleural effusion. Nursing 94, *24*(7):32C–32D, 32F, 1994.

Jones, MA, Hoffman, LA, & Delgado, E. A.R.D.S. revisited. Nursing 94, *24*(12):34–43, 1994.

Krumberger, JM. Acute pancreatitis. Critical Care Nursing Clinics of North America, *5*(1):185–202, 1993.

Sleisenger, MH, & Fordtran, JS (Eds.). Gastrointestinal disease: pathophysiology/diagnosis/management (5th ed.). Philadelphia: W.B. Saunders Company, 1993.

XV. 2. Cholecystectomy

Royal, K. A case management experience with cholecystectomies. Seminars in Perioperative Nursing, *3*(1):3–12, 1994.

Shade, RR, & Cattano, CJ. Trends in gallbladder disease and its treatment. Hospital Medicine, *28*(11):30, 32, 37–40+, 1992.

Sherlock, S, & Dooley, J. Diseases of the liver and biliary system (9th ed.). Oxford: Blackwell Scientific Publications, 1993.

Sleisenger, MH, & Fordtran, JS. Gastrointestinal disease: pathophysiology/diagnosis/management (5th ed.). Philadelphia: W.B. Saunders Company, 1993.

Stillman, A. Laparoscopic cholecystectomy: an electrosurgical approach to biliary disease. AORN Journal, *57*(2):429–430, 432–436, 1993.

Yamada, T (Ed.). Textbook of gastroenterology (2nd ed.). Philadelphia: J.B. Lippincott Company, 1995.

XV. 3. Cholelithiasis/Cholecystitis

Gitnick, G (Ed.). Principles and practice of gastroenterology and hepatology (2nd ed.). Norwalk, CT: Appleton & Lange, 1994.

Haubrich, WS, Schaffner, F, & Berk, JE. Bockus gastroenterology (5th ed.). Philadelphia: W.B. Saunders Company, 1995.

Sherlock, S, & Dooley, J. Diseases of the liver and biliary system (9th ed.). Oxford: Blackwell Scientific Publications, 1993.

Sleisenger, MH, & Fordtran, JS. Gastrointestinal disease: pathophysiology/diagnosis/management (5th ed.). Philadelphia: W.B. Saunders Company, 1993.

Yamada, T (Ed.). Textbook of gastroenterology (2nd ed.). Philadelphia: J.B. Lippincott Company, 1995.

Yee, JM, & Telegrafi, S. Gallbladder sonography: review and update. Applied Radiology, *24*(11):51–53, 1995.

XV. 4. Cirrhosis

Butler, RW. Managing the complications of cirrhosis. American Journal of Nursing, *94*(3):46–49, 1994.

Caregaro, L, Alberino, F, Amodio, P, et al. Malnutrition in alcoholic and virus-related cirrhosis. American Journal of Clinical Nutrition, *63*(4):602–609, 1996.

Cerrato, PL. When your patient has liver disease. RN, *55*(3):77–78, 80, 1992.

Doherty, MM, & Carver, DK. New relief for esophageal varices. American Journal of Nursing, *93*(4):58–63, 1993.

Gitnick, G (Ed.). Principles and practice of gastroenterology and hepatology (2nd ed.). Norwalk, CT: Appleton & Lange, 1994.

Goddard, CJR, & Warnes, TW. Primary biliary cirrhosis: how should we evaluate new treatments? Lancet, *343*(8909):1305–1306, 1994.

Haubrich, WS, Schaffner, F, & Berk, JE. Bockus gastroenterology (5th ed.). Philadelphia: W.B. Saunders Company, 1995.

Kelso, LA. Fluid and electrolyte disturbances in hepatic failure. AACN Clinical Issues in Critical Care Nursing, *3*(3):681–687, 1992.

Meissner, JE. Caring for patients with cirrhosis. Nursing 94, *24*(9):44–45, 1994.

Miller, F. Using a stent to treat patients with portal hypertension. Nursing Standard, *10*(26):42–45, 1996.

Mudge, C, et al. Hepatorenal syndrome. AACN Clinical Issues in Critical Care Nursing, *3*(3):614–632, 1992.

Schiff, L, & Schiff, ER. Diseases of the liver (7th ed.). Philadelphia: J.B. Lippincott Company, 1993.

Sherlock, S, & Dooley, J. Diseases of the liver and biliary system (9th ed.). Oxford: Blackwell Scientific Publications, 1993.

Sleisenger, MH, & Fordtran, JS. Gastrointestinal disease: pathophysiology/diagnosis/management (5th ed.). Philadelphia: W.B. Saunders Company, 1993.

Smith, SL, & Ciferni, ML. Liver transplantation. Critical Care Nursing Clinics of North America, *4*(1):131–148, 1992.

Zakim, D, & Boyer, TD. Hepatology: a textbook of liver disease (3rd ed.). Philadelphia: W.B. Saunders Company, 1996.

XV. 5. Hepatitis

Aach, RD. The emerging clinical significance of hepatitis C. Hospital Practice, *27*(5A):19–22, 1992.

Aach, R, Hirschman, SZ, & Holland, PV. The ABCs of viral hepatitis. Patient Care, *26*(13):34–38, 40, 44–46, 1992.

Fields, BN, Knipe, DM, & Howley, PM (Eds.). Fields virology (3rd ed.). Philadelphia: Lippincott-Raven Publishers, 1996.

Gitnick, G (Ed.). Principles and practice of gastroenterology and hepatology (2nd ed.). Norwalk, CT: Appleton & Lange, 1994.

Haubrich, WS, Schaffner, F, & Berk, JE. Bockus gastroenterology (5th ed.). Philadelphia: W.B. Saunders Company, 1995.

Herreid, JA. Hepatitis C: past, present, and future. MEDSURG Nursing, *4*(3):179–184, 1995.

Konigsberg, AJ. Interferon: new therapy for chronic viral hepatitis. Physician Assistant, *16*(10):53–55, 59–60, 109–112, 1992.

Konigsberg, AJ. Keeping up with viral hepatitis: recertification series. Physician Assistant, *16*(7):25–30, 32, 35–36, 1992.

Kools, AM. Hepatitis A, B, C, D, and E. Postgraduate Medicine, *91*(3):109–112, 114, 187–189, 1992.

Marx, JF. Viral hepatitis: unscrambling the alphabet. Nursing 93, *23*(1):34–42, 1993.

Petersen, T. Hepatitis C: a new enemy. Nursing Times, *91*(36):31–33, 1995.

Schiff, L, & Schiff, ER. Diseases of the liver (7th ed.). Philadelphia: J.B. Lippincott Company, 1993.

Sherlock, S, & Dooley, J. Diseases of the liver and biliary system (9th ed.). Oxford: Blackwell Scientific Publications, 1993.

Zakim, D, & Boyer, TD. Hepatology: a textbook of liver disease (3rd ed.). Philadelphia: W.B. Saunders Company, 1996.

UNIT XVI. Nursing Care of the Client with Disturbances of Metabolic Function

XVI. 1. Diabetes Mellitus

Abramowicz, M (Ed.). Metformin for non-insulin-dependent diabetes mellitus. The Medical Letter, *37*(948):41–42, 1995.

Bihm, B, & Wilson, BA. Metformin [Glucophage]: new treatment for NIDDM. MEDSURG Nursing, *4*(3):236–238, 254, 1995.

Cirone, N. Diabetes in the elderly: Part I. Nursing 96, *26*(3):34–45, 1996.

Coniff, RF, Shapiro, JA, Robbins, D, et al. Reduction of glycosylated hemoglobin and postprandial hyperglycemia by acarbose in patients with NIDDM: a placebo-controlled dose-comparison study. Diabetes Care, *18*(6):817–824, 1995.

Degroot, LJ (Ed.). Endocrinology (3rd ed.). Philadelphia: W.B. Saunders Company, 1995.

Dillinger, J, & Yass, C. Carbohydrate counting in the management of diabetes. Diabetes Educator, 21(6):547–550, 552, 1995.

Draeger, E. Clinical profile of glimepiride. Diabetes Research and Clinical Practice, 28 Suppl:S139–146, 1995.

Felig, P, Baxter, JD, & Frohman, LA (Eds.). Endocrinology and metabolism (3rd ed.). New York: McGraw-Hill, 1995.

Gleeson, CA. Diabetic peripheral neuropathies. MEDSURG Nursing, 4(2):121–125, 1995.

Josse, RG. Acarbose for the treatment of type II diabetes: the results of a Canadian multi-centre trial. Diabetes Research and Clinical Practice, 28 Suppl:S167–172, 1995.

Kahn, CR, & Weir, GC (Eds.). Joslin's diabetes mellitus (13th ed.). Philadelphia: Lea & Febiger, 1994.

Kestel, F. Using blood glucose meters: what you and your patient need to know. Nursing 93, 23(5):51–54, 1993.

Kestel, F. Feet first. Nursing 96, 26(6):24t, 24v, 1996.

LeMone, P. Differentiating and treating altered glycemic responses. MEDSURG Nursing, 5(4):257–261, 1996.

Levin, ME, O'Neal, LW, & Bowker, JH. The diabetic foot (5th ed.). St. Louis: Mosby-Year Book, 1993.

Macheka, MK. Diabetic hypoglycemia: how to keep the threat at bay. American Journal of Nursing, 93(4):26–30, 1993.

Pfeifer, MA, & Schumer, MP. Clinical trials of diabetic neuropathy: past, present, and future. Diabetes, 44(12):1355–1361, 1995.

Rogell, GD. Keeping an eye on eye disease. Diabetes Forecast, 45(6):48–52, 1992.

Watkins, PJ, Drury, PL, & Howell, SL. Diabetes and its management (5th ed.). Cambridge, MA: Blackwell Science, 1996.

Yamanouchi, K, Shinozaki, T, Chikada, K, et al. Daily walking combined with diet therapy is a useful means for obese NIDDM patients not only to reduce body weight but also to improve insulin sensitivity. Diabetes Care, 18(6):775–778, 1995.

XVI. 2. Thyroidectomy

Degroot, LJ (Ed.). Endocrinology (3rd ed.). Philadelphia: W.B. Saunders Company, 1995.

Felig, P, Baxter, JD, & Frohman, LA (Eds.). Endocrinology and metabolism (3rd ed.). New York: McGraw-Hill, 1995.

Lammon, CA, & Hart, G. Recognizing thyroid crisis. Nursing 93, 23(4):33, 1993.

UNIT XVII. Nursing Care of the Client with Disturbances of Musculoskeletal Function

XVII. 1. Amputation

Bowker, JH, & Michael, JW (Eds.). Atlas of limb prosthetics: surgical, prosthetic, and rehabilitation principles. St. Louis: Mosby-Year Book, 1992.

Folsom, D, King, T, & Rubin, JR. Lower-extremity amputation with immediate postoperative prosthetic placement. American Journal of Surgery, 58(8):474–477, 1992.

Krupski, MD, William, C, Skinner, H, & Effeney, DJ. Amputation. In Way, LW (Ed.), Current surgical diagnosis and treatment (10th ed.). Norwalk, CT: Appleton & Lange, 1994, pp. 772–780.

Maher, A, Salmond, S, & Pellino, T. Orthopaedic nursing. Philadelphia: W.B. Saunders Company, 1994.

Moore, TJ. Amputation of the lower extremities. In Chapman, MW (Ed.), Operative orthopaedics (2nd ed.). Philadelphia: J.B. Lippincott Company, 1993, pp. 2443–2455.

Patterson, JW. Banishing phantom pain. Nursing 94, 24(9):64, 1994.

Pinzur, MS, Goltschalk, F, et al. Functional outcome of below-knee amputation in peripheral vascular insufficiency. Clinical Orthopaedics, 286(2):247–249, 1996.

Schwartz, SI. Amputation. In Schwartz, SI (Ed.), Principles of surgery (6th ed.). New York: McGraw-Hill, 1994, pp. 1967–1977.

Sieggreen, M, & Mauchline, S. Lower extremity amputation: getting your patient back on track. Nursing 96, 26(6):24j, 24m–n, 1996.

Tooms, RE. General principles of amputations. In Crenshaw, AH (Ed.), Campbell's operative orthopedics (8th ed.) (Vol. 2). St. Louis: Mosby-Year Book, 1992, pp. 677–702.

XVII. 2. Fractured Hip with Internal Fixation or Prosthesis Insertion

Chapman, MW, & Madison, M (Eds.). Operative orthopaedics (2nd ed.) (Vol. 3). Philadelphia: J.B. Lippincott Company, 1993.

Cuckler, JM, & Tamarapalli, JR. An algorithm for the management of femoral neck fractures. Orthopedics, 17(9):789–792, 1994.

Dykes, P. Minding the five Ps of neurovascular assessment. American Journal of Nursing, 93(6):38–39, 1993.

Houldin, AD, & Hogan-Quigley, B. Psychological intervention for older hip fracture patients. Journal of Gerontological Nursing, 21(12):20–26, 48–49, 1995.

Johnson, EE, Kay, RM, & Dorey, FJ. Heterotopic ossification prophylaxis following operative treatment of acetabular fracture. Clinical Orthopaedics, 305:88–95, 1994.

Lu-Yao, GL, Baron, JA, Barrett, JA, & Fisher, ES. Treatment and survival among elderly Americans with hip fractures: a population-based study. American Journal of Public Health, 84(8):1287–1291, 1994.

Rockwood, CA, Green, DP, Bucholz, RW, & Heckman, JD (Eds.). Fractures in adults (4th ed.) (Vol. 2). Philadelphia: J.B. Lippincott Company, 1996.

Rogers, FB, Shackford, SR, & Keller, MS. Early fixation reduces morbidity and mortality in elderly patients with hip fractures from low-impact falls. Journal of Trauma, 39(2):261–265, 1995.

Weinstein, SL, & Buckwalter, JA. Turek's orthopaedics (5th ed). Philadelphia: J.B. Lippincott Company, 1994.

XVII. 3. Laminectomy/Diskectomy with or without Fusion

Hardy, RW, Jr (Ed.). Lumbar disc disease (2nd ed.). New York: Raven Press, 1993.

Hickey, JV. The clinical practice of neurological and neurosurgical nursing (4th ed.). Philadelphia: J.B. Lippincott Company, 1996.

Maurice-Williams, RS. Disorders of the spinal nerve roots. In Weatherall, DJ, Ledingham, JGG, & Warrell, DA (Eds.), Oxford textbook of medicine (3rd ed.). New York: Oxford University Press, 1996, pp. 3902–3909.

Netherlin, JS, et al. Body image in preoperative and postoperative lumbar laminectomy patients. Journal of Neuroscience Nursing, 27(1):43–46, 1995.

Rothman, RH, & Simeone, FA (Eds.). The spine (3rd ed.). Philadelphia: W.B. Saunders Company, 1992.

Rowland, LP (Ed.). Merritt's textbook of neurology (9th ed.). Baltimore: Williams & Wilkins, 1995.

Schultz, DL. The role of the neuroscience nurse in lumbar fusion. Journal of Neuroscience Nursing, 27(2):90–95, 1995.

XVII. 4. Total Hip Replacement

Altizer, L. Total hip arthroplasty. Orthopaedic Nursing, 14(4):7–19, 1995.

Brander, VA, Stulberg, SD, & Chang, RW. Rehabilitation following hip and knee arthroplasty. Physical Medicine and Rehabilitation Clinics of North America, 5(4):815–836, 1994.

Chapman, MW, & Madison, M (Eds.). Operative orthopaedics (2nd ed.) (Vol. 3). Philadelphia: J.B. Lippincott Company, 1993.

Dore, DD, & Rubash, E. Primary total hip arthroplasty in the older patient: optimizing the results. In Schafer, M (Ed.), Instructional course lectures (Vol. 43). American Academy of Orthopaedic Surgeons.

Dykes, P. Minding the five Ps of neurovascular assessment. American Journal of Nursing, 93(6):38–39, 1993.

Erikkson, BI, Ekman, S, Kalebo, P, et al. Prevention of deep-vein thrombosis after total hip replacement: direct thrombin inhibition with recombinant hirudin, CGP 39393. Lancet, 347(9002):635–639, 1996.

Harris, WH. The case for cemented fixation of the femur in every patient. In Schafer, M (Ed.), Instructional course lectures (Vol. 43). American Academy of Orthopaedic Surgeons, 1994.

Hickey, A. Catching deep vein thrombosis in time. Nursing 94, 24(10):34–42, 1994.

John, L. Care before and after surgery for total hip replacement. Nursing Times, 90(21):43–45, 1994.

King, L. Safe handling of hip replacement patients. Nursing Standard, 8(47):31–35, 1994.

Lewallen, DG. Heterotopic ossification following total hip arthroplasty. In Jackson, DW (Ed.), Instructional course lectures (Vol. 44). American Academy of Orthopaedic Surgeons, 1995.

Lotke, PA, Palevsky, H, Keenan, AM, et al. Aspirin and warfarin for thromboembolic disease after total joint arthroplasty. Clinical Orthopaedics, 324:251–258, 1996.

Scarcella, JB, & Cohn, BT. The effect of cold therapy on the postoperative course of total hip and knee arthroplasty patients. American Journal of Orthopedics, 24(11):847–852, 1995.

Spica, MM, & Schwab, MD. Sexual expression after total joint replacement. Orthopaedic Nursing, 15(5):41–44, 1996.

Yandrich, TJ. Preventing infection in total joint replacement surgery. Orthopaedic Nursing, 14(2):15–19, 1995.

XVII. 5. Total Knee Replacement

Brander, VA, Stulberg, SD, & Chang, RW. Rehabilitation following hip and knee arthroplasty. Physical Medicine and Rehabilitation Clinics of North America, 5(4):815–836, 1994.

Chapman, MW, & Madison, M (Eds.). Operative orthopaedics (2nd ed.) (Vol. 3). Philadelphia: J.B. Lippincott Company, 1993.

Colwell, CW, Jr, Spiro, TE, Trowbridge, AA, et al. Efficacy and safety of enoxaparin versus unfractionated heparin for prevention of deep venous thrombosis after elective knee arthroplasty. Clinical Orthopaedics, 321:19–27, 1995.

Crutchfield, J, Zimmerman, L, Nieveen, J, et al. Preoperative and postoperative pain in total knee replacement patients. Orthopaedic Nursing, 15(2):65–72, 1996.

Dykes, P. Minding the five Ps of neurovascular assessment. American Journal of Nursing, 93(6):38–39, 1993.

Fitzgerald, RH, Jr. Preventing DVT following total knee replacement: a review of recent clinical trials. Orthopedics, 18 Suppl:10–11, 1995.

Furia, JP, & Pellegrini, VD, Jr. Heterotopic ossification following primary total knee arthroplasty. Journal of Arthroplasty. 10(4):413–419, 1995.

Hickey, A. Catching deep vein thrombosis in time. Nursing 94, 24(10):34–42, 1994.

Idusuyi, OB, & Morrey, BF. Peroneal nerve palsy after total knee arthroplasty: assessment of predisposing and prognostic factors. Journal of Bone and Joint Surgery (American Volume), 78(2):177–184, 1996.

Larson, RL, & Grana, WA (Eds.). The knee. Philadelphia: W.B. Saunders Company, 1993.

Leutz, DW, & Harris, H. Continuous cold therapy in total knee arthroplasty. American Journal of Knee Surgery, 8(4):121–123, 1995.

Lotke, PA, Palevsky, H, Keenan, AM, et al. Aspirin and warfarin for thromboembolic disease after total joint arthroplasty. Clinical Orthopaedics, 324:251–258, 1996.

Marks, RM, Vaccaro, AR, Balderston, RA, et al. Postoperative blood salvage in total knee arthroplasty using the Solcotrans autotransfusion system. Journal of Arthroplasty, 10(4):433–437, 1995.

Moak, E. The perioperative nurse's role in total knee replacement. Today's OR Nurse, 14(5):11–15, 30–31, 1992.

Moran, MC, Brick, GW, Sledge, CB, et al. Supracondylar femoral fracture following total knee arthroplasty. Clinical Orthopaedics, 324:196–209, 1996.

Morris, J. The value of continuous passive motion in rehabilitation following total knee replacement. Physiotherapy, 81(9):557–562, 1995.

Rawes, ML, Patsalis, T, & Gregg, PJ. Subcapital stress fractures of the hip complicating total knee replacement. Injury, 26(6):421–423, 1995.

Scarcella, JB, & Cohn, BT. The effect of cold therapy on the postoperative course of total hip and knee arthroplasty patients. American Journal of Orthopedics, 24(11):847–852, 1995.

Ververeli, PA, Sutton, DC, Hearn, SL, et al. Continuous passive motion after total knee arthroplasty: analysis of cost and benefits. Clinical Orthopaedics, 321:208–215, 1995.

Yandrich, TJ. Preventing infection in total joint replacement surgery. Orthopaedic Nursing, 14(2):15–19, 1995.

UNIT XVIII. Nursing Care of the Client with Disturbances of the Breast and Reproductive System

XVIII. 1. Colporrhaphy (Anterior and Posterior Repair)

Gillenwater, JY, Grayhack, JT, Howards, SS, & Duckett, JW. Adult and pediatric urology (3rd ed.). St. Louis: Mosby-Year Book, 1996.

Harris, RL, Yancey, CA, Wiser, WL, et al. Comparison of anterior colporrhaphy and retropubic urethropexy for patients with genuine stress urinary incontinence. American Journal of Obstetrics and Gynecology, 173(6):1671–1675, 1995.

Karlowicz, KA (Ed.). Urologic nursing: principles and practice. Philadelphia: W.B. Saunders Company, 1995.

Mellgren, A, Anzen, B, Nilsson, BY, et al. Results of rectocele repair: a prospective study. Diseases of the Colon and Rectum, 38(1):7–13, 1995.

Stanton, SL. Anterior and posterior colporrhaphy. In Whitfield, HN (Ed.), Rob & Smith's operative surgery (5th ed.) (Vol. 1). Oxford: Butterworth-Heinemann, 1993.

Thompson, JD, & Rock, JA. TeLinde's operative gynecology (7th ed.). Philadelphia: J.B. Lippincott Company, 1992.

XVIII. 2. Hysterectomy with Salpingectomy and Oophorectomy

DeCherney, AH, & Pernoll, ML (Eds.). Current obstetric and gynecologic diagnosis and treatment (8th ed.). Norwalk, CT: Appleton & Lange, 1994.

Hall, L. And now, a positive word on hysterectomy. RN, 57(9):9, 1994.

McDonald, TW. Hysterectomy—indications, types, and alternatives. In Copeland, LJ, Textbook of gynecology. Philadelphia: W.B. Saunders Company, 1993, pp. 779–797.

Scriven, A, & Chesterton, A. Information needs of hysterectomy patients. Nursing Standard, 9(7):36, 1994.

Segal, S. Nursing rounds: postoperative TAH/BSO. . .total abdominal hysterectomy/bilateral salpingoophorectomy. American Journal of Nursing, 96(1):45, 57, 1996.

Thompson, JD, & Rock, JA. TeLinde's operative gynecology (7th ed.). Philadelphia: J.B. Lippincott Company, 1992.

XVIII. 3. Mammoplasty

Akerlund, E, Odams, E, Larsson, I, & Fridlund, B. Nipple necrosis after reduction mammoplasty: a case report. International Journal of Rehabilitation & Health, 1(4):285–289, 1995.

Ellis, C. Nursing care for the mastectomy patient who has immediate tram flap breast reconstruction. Nursing Interventions in Oncology, 5:10–11, 1993.

Giomuso, CB, & Suster, V. Free flap breast reconstruction. MEDSURG Nursing, 3(1):9–24, 1994.

Goodman, M, & Chapman, DD. Breast cancer. In Groenwald, SL, Frogge, MH, Goodman, M, & Yarbro, CH (Eds.), Cancer nursing: principles and practice (3rd ed.). Boston: Jones and Bartlett Publishers, 1993, pp. 939–943.

Hart, D. Women and saline breast implant surgery. Plastic Surgical Nursing, 15(3):161–165, 176–178, 1995.

Haskel, CM. Cancer treatment (4th ed.). Philadelphia: W.B. Saunders Company, 1995.

Kroll, SS. Mastectomy with immediate autogenous tissue reconstruction. Nursing Interventions in Oncology, 5:8–9, 1993.

Kroll, SS, & Baldwin, B. Comparison of outcomes using three different methods of breast reconstruction. Plastic and Reconstructive Surgery, 90(3):455–462, 1992.

Mangan, MA. Current concepts in breast reconstruction. Nursing Clinics of North America, 29(4):763–776, 1994.

Schuster, RH, Kuske, RR, Young, VL, & Fineberg, B. Breast reconstruction in women treated with radiation therapy for breast cancer: cosmesis, complications, and tumor control. Plastic and Reconstructive Surgery, 90(3):445–451, 1992.

XVIII. 4. Mastectomy

Appling, SE. One in nine: risks and prevention strategies for breast cancer. MEDSURG Nursing, 5(1):62–64, 1996.

Brennan, MJ, DePompolo, RW, & Garden, FH. Focused review:

postmastectomy lymphedema. Archives of Physical Medicine & Rehabilitation, *77*(3S Suppl):S74–80, 1996.

Buyske, J, MacKarem, G, Ulmer, BC, & Hughes, KS. Breast cancer in the nineties. AORN Journal, *64*(1):64–65, 67–72, 1996.

Ellis, C. Nursing care for the mastectomy patient who has immediate tram flap breast reconstruction. Nursing Interventions in Oncology, *5*:10–11, 1993.

Goodman, M, & Chapman, DD. Breast cancer. In Groenwald, SL, Frogge, MH, Goodman, M, & Yarbro, CH (Eds.), Cancer nursing: principles and practice (3rd ed.). Boston: Jones and Bartlett Publishers, 1993, pp. 939–943.

Gross, RE, Burnett, CB, & Borelli, M. Coping responses to the diagnosis of breast cancer in postmastectomy patients. Cancer Practice: A Multidisciplinary Journal of Cancer Care, *4*(4):204–211, 1996.

Harwood, K. Straight talk about breast cancer. Nursing 96, *26*(10):39–44, 1996.

Haskel, CM. Cancer treatment (4th ed.). Philadelphia: W.B. Saunders Company, 1995.

Hopkins, E. Sequential compression to treat lymphoedema. Professional Nurse, *11*(6):397–398, 1996.

Kinney, CK. Transcending breast cancer: reconstructing one's self. Issues in Mental Health Nursing, *17*(3):201–216, 1996.

Kroll, SS. Mastectomy with immediate autogenous tissue reconstruction. Nursing Interventions in Oncology, *5*:8–9, 1993.

Kwekkeboom, K. Postmastectomy pain syndromes. Cancer Nursing, *19*(1):37–43, 1996.

Sternberger, C. Breast self-examination: how nurses can influence performance. MEDSURG Nursing, *3*(5):367–371, 1994.

Wainstock, JM. Breast cancer: psychosocial consequences for the patient. Seminars in Oncology Nursing, *7*(3):207–215, 1991.

Whitman, M. Breast surgery: helping patients choose. Nursing 94, *24*(8):25, 1994.

Wilmoth, MC, & Townsend, J. A comparison of the effects of lumpectomy versus mastectomy on sexual behaviors. Cancer Practice: A Multidisciplinary Journal of Cancer Care, *3*(5):279–285, 1995.

XVIII. 5. Radical Prostatectomy

Cali-Ascani, MA. Caring for patients with prostate cancer. Nursing 94, *24*(6):32C–32D, 1994.

Davison, BJ, Degner, LF, & Morgan, TP. Information and decision-making preferences of men with prostate cancer. Oncology Nursing Forum, *22*(9):1402–1408, 1995.

DeVita, VT, Hellman, S, & Rosenberg, SA (Eds.). Important advances in oncology 1995. Philadelphia: J.B. Lippincott Company, 1995.

Gillenwater, JY, Grayhack, JT, Howards, SS, & Duckett, JW (Eds.). Adult and pediatric urology (3rd ed.) (Vol. 1). St. Louis: Mosby-Year Book, 1996.

Holland, JF, Bast, RC, Morton, DL, et al (Eds.). Cancer medicine (4th ed.) (Vol. 2). Baltimore: Williams & Wilkins, 1997.

Klimaszewski, AD, & Karlowicz, KA. Cancer of the male genitalia. In Karlowicz, KA (Ed.), Urological nursing: principles and practice. Philadelphia: W.B. Saunders Company, 1995, pp. 271–286.

Lerner, SE, Blute, MI, Lieber, MM, et al. Morbidity of contemporary radical retropubic prostatectomy for localized prostate cancer. Oncology, *9*(5):379–382, 1995.

Lind, J, Kravitz, K, & Greig, B. Urologic and male genital malignancies. In Groenwald, SL, Frogge, MH, Goodman, M, & Yarbro, CH (Eds.), Cancer nursing: principles and practice (3rd ed.). Boston: Jones and Bartlett Publishers, 1993, pp. 1258–1279.

Mahon, SM. Using brochures to educate the public about the early detection of prostate and colorectal cancer. Oncology Nursing Forum, *22*(9):1413–1415, 1995.

Narayan, P. Neoplasms of the prostate gland. In Tanagho, EA, & McAninch, JW (Eds.), Smith's general urology (14th ed.). Norwalk, CT: Appleton & Lange, 1995, pp. 410–433.

Seidman, EJ. Negotiating the complications of radical prostatectomy. Contemporary Urology, *6*(3):68–75, 1993.

Whitfield, HN (Ed.). Rob & Smith's operative surgery: genitourinary surgery (5th ed.) (Vol. 2). Oxford: Butterworth-Heinemann, 1993.

XVIII. 6. Transurethral Resection of the Prostate (TURP)

Benign Prostatic Hyperplasia Guideline Panel. Benign prostatic hyperplasia: diagnosis and treatment. AHCPR Publication No. 94-0582. Rockville, MD: Agency for Health Care Policy and Research, Public Health Service, U.S. Department of Health and Human Services, February, 1994.

Grayhack, JT, & Kozlowski, JM. Benign prostatic hypertrophy. In Gillenwater, JY, Grayhack, JT, Howards, SS, & Duckett, JW (Eds.), Adult and pediatric urology (3rd ed.) (Vol. 1). St. Louis: Mosby-Year Book, 1996, pp. 1501–1574.

Karlowicz, KA (Ed.). Urological nursing: principles and practice. Philadelphia: W.B. Saunders Company, 1995.

Narayan, P. Neoplasms of the prostate gland. In Tanagho, EA, & McAninch, JW (Eds.), Smith's general urology (14th ed.). Norwalk, CT: Appleton & Lange, 1995, pp. 392–410.

UNIT XIX. Nursing Care of the Client with Disturbances of the Head and Neck

XIX. 1. Total Laryngectomy with Radical Neck Dissection

Bildstein, CY. Head and neck malignancies. In Groenwald, SL, Frogge, MH, Goodman, M, & Yarbro, CH (Eds.), Cancer nursing: principles and practice (3rd ed.). Boston: Jones and Bartlett Publishers, 1993, pp. 1128–1145.

Calcaterra, TC, & Juillard, GJF. Larynx and hypopharynx. In Haskell, CM, Cancer treatment (4th ed.). Philadelphia: W.B. Saunders Company, 1995, pp. 726–732.

Cummings, CW (Ed.). Otolaryngology—head and neck surgery (3rd ed.). St. Louis: Mosby-Year Book, 1997.

Ganley, BJ. Effective mouth care for head and neck radiation therapy patients. MEDSURG Nursing, *4*(2):133–141, 1995.

Holland, JF, Bast, RC, Morton, DL, et al (Eds.). Cancer medicine (4th ed.). Baltimore: Williams & Wilkins, 1997.

Larson, DL. Principles of composite resection and neck dissection for carcinoma of the oropharynx. In Cohen, M (Ed.), Mastery of plastic and reconstructive surgery. Boston: Little, Brown & Company, 1994, pp. 931–938.

Lockhart, JS, & Bryce, J. Restoring speech with tracheoesophageal puncture. Nursing 93, *23*(1):59–61, 1993.

Roth, JA, Ruckdeschel, JC, & Weisenburger, TH. Thoracic oncology (2nd ed.). Philadelphia: W.B. Saunders Company, 1995.

Index